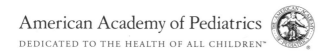

American Academy of Pediatrics
DEDICATED TO THE HEALTH OF ALL CHILDREN™

**American College of
Emergency Physicians**®

# APLS Steering Committee

**February 2006**

**Marianne Gausche-Hill, MD, FAAP, FACEP**
*Chair, APLS Steering Committee*
*Representative, American College of Emergency
 Physicians*
*Editor, APLS Fourth Edition and Revised Fourth
 Edition*
Professor of Medicine
Geffen School of Medicine at UCLA
Director, EMS and Pediatric Emergency Medicine
 Fellowships
Department of Emergency Medicine
Harbor-UCLA Medical Center
Torrance, California

**Francois P. Belanger, MD, FRCP(C)**
*Liaison, Canadian Association of Emergency
 Physicians*
Past President
Canadian Association of Emergency Physicians
Assistant Clinical Professor
University of Calgary
Medical Director and Division Chief
Emergency Department
Alberta Children's Hospital
Calgary, Alberta

**Susan Fuchs, MD, FAAP, FACEP**
*Representative, American Academy of Pediatrics*
*Editor, APLS Fourth Edition and Revised Fourth
 Edition*
Professor of Pediatrics
Feinberg School of Medicine
Northwestern University
Associate Director, Pediatric Emergency Medicine
Children's Memorial Hospital
Chicago, Illinois

**Michael Gerardi, MD, FAAP, FACEP**
*Representative, American College of Emergency
 Physicians*
Assistant Clinical Professor of Medicine
UMDNJ-New Jersey Medical School
Director, Pediatric Emergency Medicine
Goryeb Children's Hospital
Department of Emergency Medicine
Morristown Memorial Hospital
Morristown, New Jersey

**D. Anna Jarvis, MB, BS, FRCPC, FAAP**
*Liaison, Canadian Paediatric Society*
Professor, Department of Paediatrics
Director, Office of Student Affairs
University of Toronto
Division of Emergency Medicine
The Hospital for Sick Children
Toronto, Ontario

**Stephen R. Karl, MD, FAAP, FACS**
*Representative, American Academy of Pediatrics*
Principal Investigator
South Dakota EMS for Children Project
Director, Pediatric Surgery
Avera McKennan Hospital and University Health
 Center
Sioux Falls, South Dakota

**Brent R. King, MD, FAAP, FACEP**
*Representative, American College of Emergency
 Physicians*
Professor of Emergency Medicine and Pediatrics
Chairman, Department of Emergency Medicine
The University of Texas Medical School at
 Houston
Houston, Texas

**Loren Yamamoto, MD, MPH, MBA, FAAP, FACEP**
*Representative, American Academy of Pediatrics*
*Editor, APLS Fourth Edition and Revised Fourth
 Edition*
Professor of Pediatrics
University of Hawaii
John A. Burns School of Medicine
Director, Pediatric Emergency Medicine
Kapiolani Medical Center for Women and
 Children
Honolulu, Hawaii

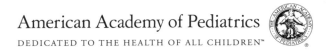
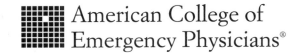

American Academy of Pediatrics
DEDICATED TO THE HEALTH OF ALL CHILDREN™

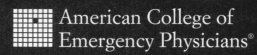
American College of
Emergency Physicians®

# APLS

# The Pediatric Emergency Medicine Resource

## REVISED FOURTH EDITION

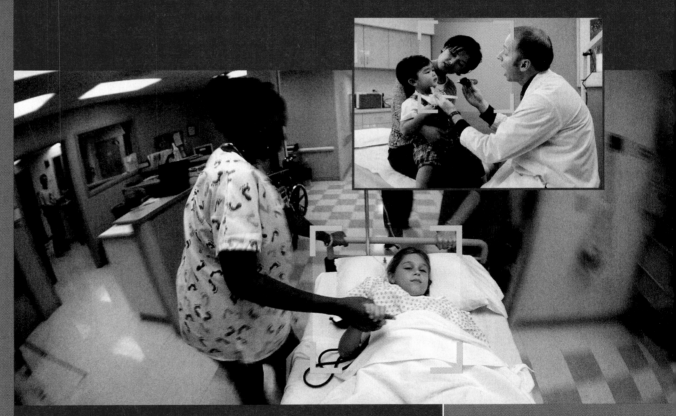

*Marianne Gausche-Hill, MD, FAAP, FACEP*
Editor

*Susan Fuchs, MD, FAAP, FACEP*
Editor

*Loren Yamamoto, MD, MPH, MBA, FAAP, FACEP*
Editor

*Children are one-fourth of our population— and all of our future.*

JONES AND BARTLETT PUBLISHERS
*Sudbury, Massachusetts*
BOSTON   TORONTO   LONDON   SINGAPORE

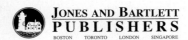
**JONES AND BARTLETT PUBLISHERS**
BOSTON    TORONTO    LONDON    SINGAPORE

**Jones and Bartlett World Headquarters**
40 Tall Pine Drive
Sudbury, MA 01776
978-443-5000
info@jbpub.com
www.APLSonline.com
www.jbpub.com

Jones and Bartlett Publishers Canada
2406 Nikanna Road
Mississauga, Ontario
Canada L5C 2WG

Jones and Bartlett Publishers International
Barb House, Barb Mews
London W6 7PA
United Kingdom

American Academy of Pediatrics
DEDICATED TO THE HEALTH OF ALL CHILDREN™

Eileen Schoen, Manager, Life Support Programs
Wendy Simon, MA, CAE, Director, Life Support Programs
Robert Perelman, MD, Director, Department of Education
Tina Patel, Life Support Assistant

**American Academy of Pediatrics**
141 Northwest Point Boulevard
Post Office Box 927
Elk Grove Village, IL 60009-0927
847-434-4795
www.APLSonline.com
www.aap.org

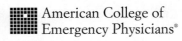
American College of
Emergency Physicians®

Marta Foster, Director, Educational
and Professional Publications
Tom Werlinich, Associate Executive Director, Educational
and Professional Products Division

**American College of Emergency Physicians**
1125 Executive Circle
Post Office Box 619911
Dallas, TX 75261-9911
800-798-1822
www.APLSonline.com
www.acep.org

### Production Credits

Chief Executive Officer: Clayton Jones
Chief Operating Officer: Don W. Jones, Jr.
Executive V.P. & Publisher: Robert W. Holland, Jr.
V.P., Sales and Marketing: William J. Kane
V.P., Design and Production: Anne Spencer
V.P., Manufacturing and Inventory Control: Therese Bräuer
Publisher—Public Safety Group: Kimberly Brophy

Marketing Director: Alisha Weisman
Production Editor: Anne Spencer
Cover and Text Design: Anne Spencer
Composition: Carlisle Communications
Printing and Binding: Courier Companies
Cover Printing: John Pow Printing

Copyright © 2004, 2007 By American Academy of Pediatrics and American College of Emergency Physicians

**Library of Congress Cataloging-in-Publication Data**

Advanced pediatric life support / editors, Susan Fuchs, Marianne
Gausche-Hill, Loren Yamamoto.-- revised 4th ed.
    p. ; cm.
Rev. ed. of: APLS : the pediatric emergency medicine course / editors,
Susan Fuchs, Marianne Gausche-Hill, Loren Yamamoto. 4th ed. c2004.
 ISBN-13: 978-0-7637-4414-4
 ISBN-10: 0-7637-4414-X (Jones & Bartlett : hardcover)
1.  Pediatric emergencies. 2.  CPR (First aid) for children.
 [DNLM: 1.  Cardiopulmonary Resuscitation--Child. 2.  Cardiopulmonary
Resuscitation--Infant. 3.  Emergencies--Child. 4.  Emergencies--Infant.
WS 205 A2444 2007] I. Fuchs, Susan. II. Gausche-Hill, Marianne. III.
Yamamoto, Loren. IV. American Academy of Pediatrics. V. American College
of Emergency Physicians. VI. APLS.
RJ370.A35 2006
 618.92'0025--dc22                        2007016862

Printed in the United States of America
10    09    08    07    06            10   9   8   7   6   5   4   3   2   1

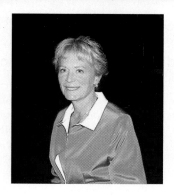

# Dr. Martha Jane Smith Bushore-Fallis

In the late 1970s, Martha Bushore-Fallis, MD, FAAP, FACEP, FCCM, was corresponding with Jerry Foster, MD, at the Children's Hospital in Columbus, Ohio, to find other physicians who were providing emergency care to children, in an effort to establish dialogue, share concerns, and set some goals. From their efforts evolved the American Academy of Pediatrics (AAP) Section on Emergency Medicine. And when Dr. Bushore-Fallis became Chair of the Section, the pursuit of a course for physicians in this "new" field of pediatric emergency medicine became her mission—and her passion.

Armed with a concept, but no endorsement and no funding, not to mention a lack of accepted clinical guidelines for many critical conditions, Dr. Bushore-Fallis and several colleagues began working on a manual based on the courses they had been teaching for several years. When all the chapters were finished, and with a bit of grant money, the books were printed and bound. She then presented them to the American Academy of Pediatrics' Committee on Hospital Care for its endorsement. Eventually, the course was approved by the AAP and the American College of Emergency Physicians (ACEP).

In 1983, pediatric life support education evolved into two groups. One group became the forerunner of the American Heart Association Subcommittee on Pediatric Resuscitation, focusing on pediatric resuscitation and the development of the Pediatric Advanced Life Support Course (PALS). The other—"the rest of us, established as the critical condition recognition and stabilization group," according to Dr. Bushore-Fallis—was the forerunner of the Advanced Pediatric Life Support (APLS) Joint Task Force, now the APLS Steering Committee, responsible for the development of the APLS program.

The first APLS course was implemented in 1984. Five years and thousands of hours of development work later, the first edition of the APLS course student manual was published by the AAP and ACEP. Dr. Martha Bushore-Fallis, along with Gary Fleisher, MD, James Seidel, MD, and David Wagner, MD, were the editorial board for the original edition. The first edition was published in 1989, a second edition in 1993, and a third edition in 1998, all guided by the APLS Joint Task Force, and all built on the foundation laid by Dr. Bushore-Fallis and her colleagues.

Dr. Bushore-Fallis retired in 1999 after a 30-year career of caring for children at the University of Tennessee Hospital and East Tennessee Children's Hospital, both in Knoxville, Good Samaritan Hospital in West Palm Beach, Florida, Emory University School of Medicine (multiple sites) in Atlanta, St. Joseph Hospital, Tampa, and Bayfront Hospital, St. Petersburg. She currently resides in both Clearwater, Florida, and Toronto, Ontario, with her husband Jim Fallis, a pediatric surgeon.

The members of the APLS Steering Committee, the editors, and the authors proudly dedicate this fourth edition to Dr. Martha Jane Smith Bushore-Fallis in recognition of her vision and diligence that made APLS possible. For Dr. Bushore-Fallis, it's always been about "doing it for the children." And for those of us who continue her work, it always will be.

The American Academy of Pediatrics, American College of Emergency Physicians, and Editors acknowledge with appreciation the contributions of the following individuals in the development of this resource.

**Terry A. Adirim, MD, MPH, FAAP**
Assistant Professor of Pediatrics and Emergency
    Medicine
George Washington University School of
    Medicine
Attending Physician
Division of Emergency Medicine
Children's National Medical Center
Washington, DC

**Jeffrey R. Avner, MD, FAAP**
Director, Children's Emergency Service
Children's Hospital at Montefiore
Professor of Clinical Pediatrics
Albert Einstein College of Medicine
Bronx, NY

**Carol D. Berkowitz, MD, FAAP**
Vice-President of American Academy of
    Pediatrics
Acting Director of Medical Education
Executive Vice-Chair, Department of Pediatrics
Professor of Clinical Pediatrics
UCLA, School of Medicine
Los Angeles, CA

**Rodney B. Boychuk, MD, FAAP**
Professor of Pediatrics and Surgery
John A. Burns School of Medicine
University of Hawaii
Honolulu, HI

**David J. Burchfield, MD, FAAP**
Professor and Chief of Neonatology
Department of Pediatrics
University of Florida
Gainesville, FL

**Meta Carroll, MD, FAAP, FACEP**
Assistant Professor of Pediatrics
Division of Pediatric Emergency Medicine
Department of Pediatrics
Northwestern University Feinberg School of
    Medicine
Children's Memorial Hospital
Chicago, IL

**Mary E. Cataletto, MD, FAAP**
Associate Professor of Clinical Pediatrics
State University of New York, Stonybrook
Associate Director, Pediatric Pulmonology
Winthrop University Hospital
Mineola, NY

**Wendy C. Coates, MD, FACEP**
Director, Medical Education
Department of Emergency Medicine
Harbor-UCLA Medical Center
Torrance, CA
Associate Professor of Medicine and Vice-Chair
Acute Care College
David Geffen School of Medicine at UCLA
Los Angeles, CA

**Andrew D. DePiero, MD**
Attending Physician
Division of Pediatric Emergency Medicine
A.I. duPont Hospital for Children
Wilmington, DE

**Ronald A. Dieckmann, MD, MPH, FAAP, FACEP**
Department of Emergency Services
San Francisco General Hospital
University of California
San Francisco, CA

**Gregory M. Enns, MB, ChB**
Assistant Professor of Pediatrics
Director, Biochemical Genetics Program
Stanford University
Stanford, CA

**Timothy B. Erickson, MD, FACEP, FACMT**
Associate Professor
Department of Emergency Medicine
University of Illinois, Chicago
Director, Emergency Medicine Residency Program
Director, Division of Clinical Toxicology
Chicago, IL

**Mary E. Fallat, MD, FAAP, FACS**
Professor of Surgery
University of Louisville
Director of Trauma
Kosair Children's Hospital
Louisville, KY

**Laura Fitzmaurice, MD, FAAP, FACEP**
Professor of Pediatrics
Children's Mercy Hospital
School of Medicine
University of Missouri, Kansas City
Kansas City, MO

**George L. Foltin, MD, FAAP, FACEP**
Director, Center for Pediatric Emergency
  Medicine
Associate Professor of Pediatrics and Emergency
  Medicine
New York University School of Medicine
Bellevue Hospital Center
New York, NY

**Michael J. Gerardi, MD, FAAP, FACEP**
Director, Pediatric Emergency Medicine
Goryeb Children's Hospital and Atlantic Health
  System
Attending Physician
Department of Emergency Medicine
Morristown Memorial Hospital
Clinical Instructor
University of Medicine and Dentistry
New Jersey Medical School
Morristown, NJ

**Nicole Glaser, MD, FAAP**
Assistant Professor of Pediatrics
School of Medicine
University of California, Davis
Davis, CA

**Katherine Gnauck, MD, FAAP**
Department of Pediatrics
St. Louis Children's Hospital at Washington
  University Medical Center
St. Louis, MO

**Fred M. Henretig, MD, FAAP**
Medical Director
Poison Control Center
Children's Hospital of Philadelphia
Philadelphia, PA

**Barry A. Hicks, MD, FAAP**
Associate Professor, Pediatric Surgery
Interim Chair, Pediatric Surgery
Children's Medical Center of Dallas
The University of Texas Southwestern
Medical Center at Dallas
Dallas, TX

**Dee Hodge III, MD, FAAP**
Associate Professor of Pediatrics
Associate Director of Clinical Affairs
School of Medicine
Washington University
St Louis Children's Hospital
St Louis, MO

**Daniel J. Isaacman, MD, FAAP**
Eastern Virginia Medical School
Norfolk, VA

**Brent R. King, MD, FAAP, FACEP, FAAEM**
Professor of Emergency Medicine and Pediatrics
Chairman, Department of Emergency Medicine
Medical School
The University of Texas, Houston
Houston, TX

**Christopher King, MD, FACEP**
Associate Professor of Emergency Medicine and
  Pediatrics
School of Medicine
University of Pittsburgh
Pittsburgh, PA

**Jane F. Knapp, MD, FAAP, FACEP**
Professor of Pediatrics
Children's Mercy Hospital
University of Missouri, Kansas City
School of Medicine
Kansas City, MO

**Nathan Kuppermann, MD, MPH, FAAP**
Associate Professor, Emergency Medicine and
  Pediatrics
Director of Research, Emergency Medicine
University of California, Davis
School of Medicine
Davis, CA

**Brian Lee, MD**
Assistant Clinical Professor of Medicine
UCLA David Geffen School of Medicine
Los Angeles, CA
Clinical Faculty
Harbor-UCLA Medical Center
Torrance, CA
Department of Emergency Medicine
St. Joseph's Hospital/Children's Hospital of
  Orange County
Orange, CA

**Michele R. McKee, MD, FAAP**
Children's National Medical Center
Washington, DC

**Kemedy K. McQuillen, MD**
Advocate Christ Medical Center
Oak Lawn, IL

**Thomas M. Moriarty, MD, PhD**
Chief, Pediatric Neurosurgery
Kosair Children's Hospital
University of Louisville
Louisville, KY

**Pamela J. Okada, MD, FAAP**
Assistant Professor of Pediatrics
Division of Emergency Medicine
Department of Pediatrics
The University of Texas Southwestern
Medical Center at Dallas
Dallas, TX

**Ronald I. Paul, MD, FAAP, FACEP**
School of Medicine
University of Louisville
Louisville, KY

**Lou E. Romig, MD, FAAP, FACEP**
Pediatric Emergency Medicine
Attending Physician and EMS Liaison
Miami Children's Hospital
Miami, FL

**Steven G. Rothrock, MD, FAAP, FACEP**
Associate Professor of Emergency Medicine
University of Florida College of Medicine
Orlando Regional Medical Center
Orlando, FL

**Alfred Sacchetti, MD, FACEP**
Associate Director, Department of Emergency
  Medicine
Our Lady of Lourdes Medical Center
Camden, NJ
Assistant Clinical Professor, Emergency Medicine
Thomas Jefferson University
Philadelphia, PA

**John P. Santamaria, MD, FAAP, FACEP**
Medical Director
After Hours Pediatrics
Clinical Associate Professor of Pediatrics
School of Medicine
University of South Florida
Tampa, FL

**James S. Seidel, MD, PhD, FAAP**
Chief, General and Emergency Pediatrics
Harbor-UCLA Medical Center
Torrance, CA

**Steven M. Selbst, MD, FAAP, FACEP**
Professor of Pediatrics
A.I. duPont Hospital for Children
Wilmington, DE
Jefferson Medical College
Philadelphia, PA

**Ghazala Q. Sharieff, MD, FAAP, FACEP, FAAEM**
Assistant Clinical Professor
Department of Emergency Medicine
University of Florida
Director of Pediatric Emergency Medicine
Palomar-Pomerado Hospitals
San Diego, CA

**Phyllis Hendry Stenklyft, MD, FAAP, FACEP**
Associate Professor of Emergency Medicine and
  Pediatrics
University of Florida Health Science Center
Director of Pediatric Emergency Services
Shands Jacksonville
Jacksonville, FL

**Joseph J. Tepas III, MD, FAAP, FACS**
Professor of Surgery and Pediatrics
College of Medicine
University of Florida
Jacksonville, FL

**Jennifer L. Trainor, MD, FAAP**
Assistant Professor of Pediatrics
Feinberg School of Medicine
Northwestern University
Children's Memorial Hospital
Chicago, IL

**Michael G. Tunik, MD, FAAP**
Department of Pediatrics and Emergency
  Medicine
New York University School of Medicine
Bellevue Hospital Center
New York, NY

The editors acknowledge the work of Benjamin K. Silverman, MD, FAAP, not only for his stewardship as editor of the first and second editions, but also for the countless hours spent on his in-depth review of *APLS: The Pediatric Emergency Medicine Resource,* Fourth Edition.

The editors also acknowledge the work of all former APLS Joint Task Force members. Their efforts served as the basis for prior editions and contributed to the inspiration of the APLS Steering Committee and their development of *APLS: The Pediatric Emergency Medicine Resource,* Fourth Edition.

Martha Bushore-Fallis, MD, FAAP, FACEP, FCCM
Gary Fleisher, MD, FAAP, FACEP
Alex Haller, MD, FAAP, FACS
Carden Johnston, MD, FAAP
Robert Luten, MD, FAAP
Cheri Nijssen-Jordan, MD, FAAP, FRCP(C)
James Seidel, MD, PhD, FAAP
Benjamin K. Silverman, MD, FAAP
Johnathan Singer, MD, FAAP
David Wagner, MD, FACEP

The editors thank William T. Zempsky, MD, FAAP, for his review of pertinent information on behalf of the AAP Committee on Pediatric Emergency Medicine, and Lynne Maxwell, MD, FAAP, for her review of pertinent information on behalf of the AAP Committee on Drugs.

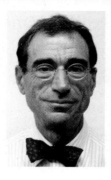

In memory of
James S. Seidel, MD, PhD, FAAP
June 24, 1943 – July 25, 2003

The editors of APLS would like to honor James S. Seidel for a lifetime of achievement and dedication in the field of pediatric emergency medicine. He was a teacher, scientist, a child advocate to the core, and a wonderful friend to many. He is best known for his brilliance, his tenacity, and his determination to fight for what was right and just. It is these qualities that led to a lifetime of contribution in the field of pediatric emergency medicine. He was a member of the original APLS Task Force and to this end was a pioneer in education for health care professionals in pediatric emergency medicine.

Dr. Seidel won many honors including the Outstanding Teacher Award from Harbor-UCLA Medical Center (1994); Section on Pediatric Emergency Medicine, American Academy of Pediatrics Outstanding Service Award (1994); Los Angeles County EMS Agency Award for Contributions to the Development of EMS in LA County (2000); and the EMS-C National Hero Award for Lifetime Achievement in Emergency Medical Services for Children, Maternal and Child Health Bureau HRSA/National Highway Traffic Safety Administration (2000), just to name a few. In addition, several awards have been named in his honor, including the Ambulatory Pediatric Association Ludwig-Seidel Award for outstanding work by research fellows in pediatric emergency medicine, the American Academy of Pediatrics Emergency Medicine Section Award for Outstanding Service, and a classroom in Universidad de Valle, Cali, Colombia that was named in his honor to recognize his efforts in fostering international pediatric resuscitation education.

The field of pediatric emergency medicine has been enriched by your presence and more importantly, your efforts have saved many children's lives. Bravo, Jim Seidel. We salute you and will miss you.

# Brief Contents

# Contents

# Contents

Working in crisis situations is demanding and requires that you be at your best. Prepare yourself with APLS, the definitive resource on pediatric emergency medicine. This resource is the core of the APLS course with features that will reinforce and expand on the essential information. These features include:

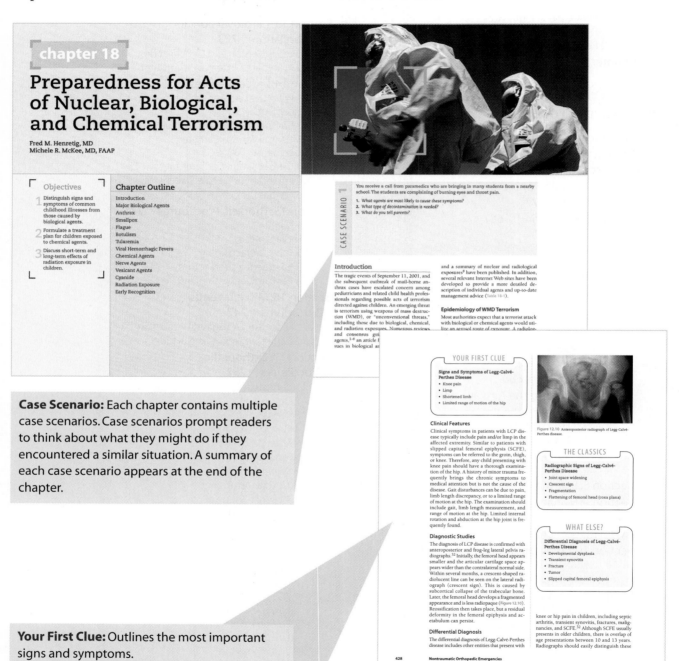

**Case Scenario:** Each chapter contains multiple case scenarios. Case scenarios prompt readers to think about what they might do if they encountered a similar situation. A summary of each case scenario appears at the end of the chapter.

**Your First Clue:** Outlines the most important signs and symptoms.
**The Classics:** Outlines significant diagnostic study findings.
**What Else?:** Outlines important points of differential diagnosis.

and the pain can be reproduced by having the patient extend the knee against resistance or by squatting with the knee in full flexion. History usually reveals that running, going up and down stairs, and jumping cause increased pain.

### Diagnostic Studies

The diagnosis of Osgood-Schlatter disease is usually clinical. Radiographs are frequently obtained to rule out other conditions, including neoplasm, cysts, infections, stress fractures, and other musculoskeletal diseases involving the knee. Although a lateral knee radiograph might reveal a fracture through the tibial tubercle, frequently only soft tissue swelling is seen. Some patients who present with radiographic fragmentation of the tubercle will develop chronic symptoms. Those with no fragmentation are usually asymptomatic at long-term followup.[49]

### Management

Management of patients with Osgood-Schlatter disease is almost always nonsurgical and depends on the extent of the presenting symptoms.[48] Patients with mild symptoms should be given nonsteroidal anti-inflammatory drugs

and be advised to avoid activities that cause repeated quadriceps contraction. For many adolescents, the latter advice is frequently hard to follow. Symptoms usually improve in weeks to months. More advanced cases can be treated with a knee immobilizer (and, rarely, a cylindrical cast). Steroid injections are not indicated. Rarely, patients with unresolved lesions will require surgery directed at excision of all the intratendon ossicles and possible removal of the tibial tubercle.[50] In most patients, the condition is self-limiting and results in no long-term complications.

### Summary

The approach to children with orthopedic complaints should be based on age, history of symptoms, and physical findings. Causes of nontraumatic orthopedic conditions vary significantly with age, and a complete history and physical examination will be necessary to exclude systemic disease.

#### KEY POINTS

**Management of Osgood-Schlatter Disease**

- Mild to moderate symptoms
  - decrease activity; nonsteroidal anti-inflammatory agents
- Moderate to severe symptoms
  - knee immobilizer or cylindrical cast
- Very severe cases
  - surgical intervention (rare)

#### THE BOTTOM LINE

- Causes of nontraumatic orthopedic emergencies vary with patient age.
- Obtain a complete history to include character, location, quality, and time course of symptoms.
- Establish if the condition is associated with an acute traumatic event or repetitive activity.
- Always examine the hips in any patient with knee pain.
- Radiographs might be needed to establish the diagnosis.
- Prompt orthopedic or primary care referral is necessary.

Summary    437

**Key Points:** Outlines critical management steps.
**The Bottom Line:** Brief summary of crucial chapter concepts.

## CHAPTER REVIEW

### Check Your Knowledge

1. A biological weapons attack would most likely resemble which of the following mass casualty emergencies?
   A. Earthquake
   B. Large bomb blast
   C. Release of chlorine from a train wreck
   D. Severe influenza epidemic
   E. Tornado
2. Which of the following syndromes is common to most of the high threat biological agents?
   A. Characteristic rash
   B. Encephalopathy
   C. Febrile prodrome
   D. Pneumonia
   E. Renal failure
3. Distinguishing features of botulism from other causes of paralysis include which of the following?
   A. Hallucinations
   B. High fever
   C. Intact sensation
   D. Normal bulbar function
   E. Severe paresthesias
4. Which of the following patients poses the least potential hazard to health care providers?
   A. An adolescent with untreated pneumonic plague
   B. An asymptomatic adolescent with mustard agent on skin
   C. Children exposed to high doses of ionizing radiation
   D. A child with fever and extensive lesions of smallpox
   E. An infant with nerve agent on clothing

### References

1. Inglesby TV, Henderson DA, Bartlett JG, et al. Anthrax as a biological weapon: medical and public health management [consensus statement]. JAMA. 1999;281:1735–1745.
2. Henderson DA, Inglesby TV, Bartlett JG, et al. Smallpox as a biological weapon: medical and public health management [consensus statement]. JAMA. 1999;281:2127–2137.

3. Inglesby TV, Dennis DT, Henderson DA, et al. Plague as a biological weapon: medical and public health management [consensus statement]. JAMA. 2000;283:2281–2290.
4. Arnon SS, Schechter R, Inglesby TV, et al. Botulinum toxin as a biological weapon: medical and public health management [consensus statement]. JAMA. 2001;285:1059–1070.
5. Dennis DT, Inglesby TV, Henderson DA, et al. Tularemia as a biological weapon: medical and public health management [consensus statement]. JAMA. 2001;285:2763–2773.
6. Inglesby TV, O'Toole T, Henderson DA, et al. Anthrax as a biological weapon, 2002: updated recommendations for management. JAMA. 2002;287:2236–2252.
7. Henretig FM, Cieslak TJ, Eitzen EM Jr. Medical Progress: biological and chemical terrorism. J Pediatr. 2002; 141:311–326. Corrections J Pediatr. 2002; 141:743–746.
8. Mettler FA, Voelz GL. Major radiation exposure: what to expect and how to respond. N Engl J Med. 2002;346:1554–1561.
9. White S, Henretig F, Dukes R. Vulnerable populations in the setting of bioterrorism. Emerg Med Clin North Am. 2002;20:365–392.
10. Torok TJ, Tauxe RE, Wise RP, et al. A large community outbreak of salmonellosis caused by intentional contamination of restaurant salad bars. JAMA. 1997;278:389–395.
11. US Army Medical Research Institute of Infectious Diseases. Medical Management of Biological Casualties Handbook. Ft Detrick, MD: US Army Medical Research Institute of Infectious Diseases; 1998.
12. Okumura T, Takasu N, Ishimatsu S, et al. Report on 640 victims of the Tokyo subway sarin attack. Ann Emerg Med. 1996;28:129–135.
13. US Army Medical Research Institute of Chemical Defense. Medical Management of Chemical Casualties, 3rd ed. Aberdeen Proving Ground, Md: US Army Medical Research Institute of Chemical Defense; 1999.
14. Macintyre AG, Christopher GW, Eitzen E Jr, et al. Weapons of mass destruction events with contaminated casualties: effective planning for health care facilities. JAMA. 2000;283:242–249.
15. Mettler FA, Voelz GL. Major radiation exposure: what to expect and how to respond. N Engl J Med. 2002;346:1554–1561.
16. Helfand I, Forrow L, Tiwari J. Nuclear terrorism. BMJ. 2002;324:356–359.
17. IAEA News. Calculating the new global nuclear terrorism threat. Sci Total Env 2002;284:269–272.
18. Jarrett DG. Medical Management of Radiation Casualties Handbook. Bethesda, Md: Armed Forces Radiobiology Research Institute; 1999.

Chapter Review

**Check Your Knowledge:** End-of-chapter questions for your own self-assessment or Category I CME credit.

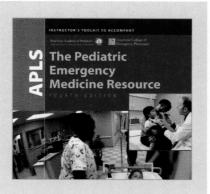

### Instructor's ToolKit CD-ROM

0-7637-4592-8

Preparation is made easy with the resources found on this CD-ROM, including:

*PowerPoint Presentations,* providing a powerful way to make presentations that are educational and engaging to your students. The slides can be modified to meet your needs.

*Lecture Outlines,* providing you with complete ready to use lecture notes. The lecture outlines can be customized to fit your personal style.

*Image Bank,* providing you with a selection of the most important images found in the textbook. You can use these to incorporate more images into the PowerPoint presentations, make handouts, or enlarge a specific image for further discussion.

*Table Bank,* providing access to the many tables found in the Fourth Edition.

*Administrative Information,* and forms, and skill station tips for APLS Course Directors and Instructors.

And much more.

The fourth edition of *APLS: The Pediatric Emergency Medicine Resource* represents quantum leaps both in the content and in the scope of the course. Originally conceived as a course in the basic elements of pediatric emergency medicine for physicians who did not regularly care for ill or injured children, the course now attempts to be the definitive resource in pediatric emergency medicine education for physicians and physician extenders in training and in practice. The expanded horizon of the fourth edition is neatly captured in the mission statement adopted by the APLS Steering Committee:

*The American Academy of Pediatrics and the American College of Emergency Physicians APLS Steering Committee will transform the APLS program into the pre-eminent source of continuing education in pediatric emergency medicine. A flexible, modular information database will be the core of the fourth edition.*

This state-of-the-art multimedia educational program embraces not only the traditional 2-day intensive course format, but also an abbreviated 1-day course format for practicing physicians who wish to focus on key skills. For the first time, wallet-sized, time-limited course completion cards will be issued to participants who successfully complete course segments.

The cornerstone of pediatric resuscitation education continues to be the Pediatric Assessment Triangle that was developed by the *Pediatric Education for Paramedics* (PEP) course, and later refined by the *Pediatric Education for Prehospital Professionals* (PEPP) course. The Pediatric Assessment Triangle provides the pediatric emergency professional with a structured mnemonic for reliable formation of a first impression of severity of illness or injury that serves to guide the initial assessment of the child who presents in an urgent condition.

It is almost cliché to describe a document as living, breathing, and circulating, but *APLS: The Pediatric Emergency Medicine Resource* is becoming just that, not only in terms of its content, but also in terms of its vitality. It is the goal of the APLS Steering Committee henceforth to provide online updates to the resource on a regular basis, aided by the tools available through modern technology. To reach its goal, the APLS Steering Committee needs the help of every member of its family—and you are now part of that family! Your feedback is invaluable to the Steering Committee. Technology now enables us to deliver up-to-date information directly to you via a Web site, reflecting the very latest thoughts and practices in pediatric emergency care. The future is now, and at your fingertips, whether you are reading this book in your lap, or learning on your computer, in your office, or at your patient's bedside—today and tomorrow.

High praise is due to the editors and authors of the fourth edition. The editors, Marianne Gausche-Hill, MD, Susan Fuchs, MD, and Loren Yamamoto, MD, were assisted by Francois Belanger, MD, Arthur Cooper, MD, Michael Gerardi, MD, Daniel Isaacman, MD, Anna Jarvis, MB, BS, and Robert Wiebe, MD. The editorial staff was superbly supported by the staffs of both the AAP, including Robert Perelman, MD, Linda Lipinsky, and Eileen Schoen, and ACEP, including Michael Gallery, Thomas Werlinich, and Marta Foster. Special thanks are also due to the Boards of Directors of both organizations, who supported the vision of the APLS Steering Committee and encouraged their extraordinary partnership with Jones and Bartlett Publishers. We also wish to thank Publisher Kimberly Brophy of Jones and Bartlett, whose exceptional commitment ensured that this quality resource resulted in state-of-the-art educational materials that set a new "gold standard" for continuing education in pediatric emergency medicine.

Children are our most valuable resource, and all of our future. On behalf of the entire APLS family, thank you for caring enough to learn to care for them well.

Arthur Cooper, MD, MS, FAAP, FACS, FCCM
*Chair, APLS Steering Committee*
*October 2003*

A lot has changed since the American Academy of Pediatrics (AAP) and the American College of Emergency Physicians (ACEP) began collaborating on the first edition of *APLS: The Pediatric Emergency Medicine Course*. Through the years, the dedication and expertise of task force and committee members, editors, course directors, and instructors continually enriched the course and all related materials. The pattern continued, and perhaps reached one of many peaks, when the current APLS Steering Committee decided to "reach for the stars" and craft a mission to establish APLS as the foremost body of knowledge in pediatric emergency medicine.

The fourth edition of APLS has become more than a course, and much more than just another acronym. *APLS: The Pediatric Emergency Medicine Resource* has been designed to meet the growing needs of physicians and other health care professionals. It will not be a book that sits on the shelf after it is used as a course study guide. If you want the newest, most comprehensive reference on pediatric emergency medicine, you will want to keep APLS at your fingertips—full color, almost three times larger than previous editions, and a flexible modular format—all in one program! It is the culmination of 2 years of work and the writing of nearly 50 contributors.

The book in your hand is but one component of a unique teaching and learning system. Complimenting the textbook is the *APLS Instructor's ToolKit CD-ROM*. In it, you will find presentations with embedded lecture notes for 20 modules, an image and table bank, and instructions for implementing skill stations and emergency procedures, as well as other teaching adjuncts. All this is in a user-friendly electronic format that can be exported into an instructor's customized presentation.

In the past, the heart of APLS has been the live 2-day course. For the fourth edition, we designed a new 2-day course with more options (including a PALS renewal), as well as a 1-day course with prescribed self-study. Completion of either course entitles the student to receive the new APLS Course Completion Card after the new APLS Course Completion Examination. Speaking of examinations, our evolution continues with an online component (www.APLSonline.com) and self-directed CME.

The APLS Steering Committee has designed the fourth edition to meet your needs, whether you are an instructor or residency director, and whether you use APLS materials as a course guide, a reference book, for a single topic lecture, or to reinforce hands-on skills. The fourth edition of *APLS: The Pediatric Emergency Medicine Resource* has been created with you in mind and with the welfare of children at heart.

Marianne Gausche-Hill, MD, FAAP, FACEP
Susan Fuchs, MD, FAAP, FACEP
Loren Yamamoto, MD, MPH, MBA, FAAP, FACEP
*Editors*
*October 2003*

When *APLS: The Pediatric Emergency Medicine Resource*, Fourth Edition, was published in 2003, the APLS Steering Committee knew that a subsequent edition would be necessary at some point to address new information and recommendations in the field of pediatric emergency medicine. That opportunity arose in November 2005 with the release of the *American Heart Association 2005 Guidelines for Cardiopulmonary Resuscitation and Emergency Cardiovascular Care*. As a result, we decided to update the fourth edition of APLS to reflect the 2005 resuscitation guidelines, including the new algorithms for care of dysrhythmias and cardiopulmonary arrest. This revision also gave us the opportunity to conduct a thoughtful, comprehensive review of all of the APLS content—updating other chapters, correcting errors, and replacing a few images—to bring you the best information for 2006 and beyond.

The textbook in your hands, the Revised Fourth Edition of APLS, is the result of that effort. It is but one component of a unique teaching-and-learning system. The APLS system is an exciting curriculum designed to present the information physicians need to assess and care for critically ill and injured children during the first hours in the emergency department or office-based setting. Complementing this textbook is the *APLS Instructor's ToolKit CD-ROM*, also available from ACEP, AAP, and Jones and Bartlett. In it you will find 29 presentations, with embedded lecture notes for each, an image and table bank, and instructions for implementing skill stations in emergency procedures as well as other teaching adjuncts. All of this is in a user-friendly electronic format that can be exported into an instructor's customized presentation. The textbook is complementary to these materials and provides 22 chapters covering the breadth of pediatric emergency medicine.

In the past, the heart of APLS has been the live 2-day course. For the Fourth Edition, we designed a new 2-day course with more options, including a PALS renewal, as well as a 1-day course with prescribed self-study. Completion of either course format and the APLS Course Completion Examination entitles the student to receive the APLS Course Completion Card.

Also new to the APLS resource materials is APLS Online (www.APLSonline.com). APLS Online has a number of new features, including: APLS Case Presentations, which provide enhanced knowledge to information already printed in the APLS materials; APLS Community, which has a bulletin board that allows you to post your comments and questions about APLS (all clinical questions are answered by APLS Steering Committee members); and APLS "Check Your Knowledge" Online CME, which allows health care providers easy access to online modules and CME credits.

The APLS Steering Committee has designed the APLS teaching-and-learning system to meet your needs whether you are an instructor or residency director and whether you use APLS materials as a course guide, a reference book, or a single topic lecture, or to reinforce hands-on skills. It has been created with you in mind, and with the welfare of children at heart.

Marianne Gausche-Hill, MD, FAAP, FACEP
Susan Fuchs, MD, FAAP, FACEP
Loren Yamamoto, MD, MPH, MBA, FAAP, FACEP
*Editors*
*May 2006*

# chapter 1

# Preparedness for Pediatric Emergencies

James Seidel, MD, PhD, FAAP
Jane F. Knapp, MD, FAAP, FACEP

## Objectives

1 Provide guidelines for the preparation of the general emergency department to care for pediatric patients.

2 List the equipment and supplies necessary to care for pediatric patients in the emergency department.

3 Discuss the staffing and continuing education needs for pediatric emergency care.

4 Outline the importance of having emergency department policies that address patient transfer, child abuse and neglect, and interpersonal violence.

## Chapter Outline

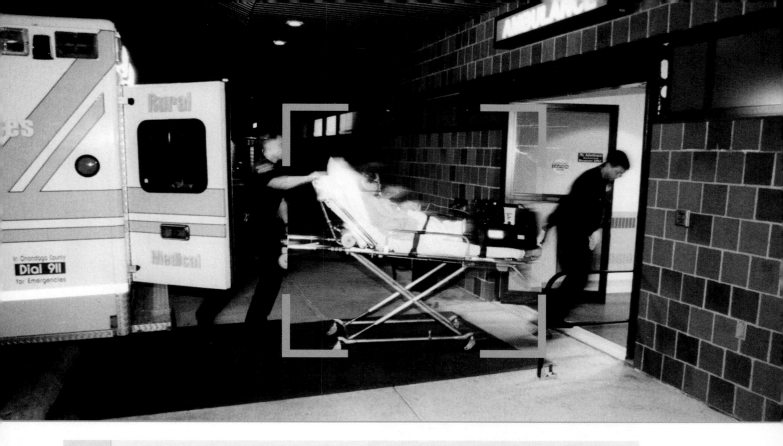

**CASE SCENARIO 1**

A 3-year-old boy is found at the bottom of a Jacuzzi by his grandparents. Paramedics arrive 4 minutes later to find the grandfather performing CPR. Paramedics gently ask the grandfather to step aside and note that the child's appearance is unconscious and unresponsive to surroundings, work of breathing is absent, and color is pale. Further assessment shows the child has a weak brachial pulse. Bag-mask ventilation is begun, and the boy is transported to your emergency department.

1. *How would this child be triaged?*
2. *What will you do to prepare for his arrival?*
3. *How will you determine the size of equipment and dosage of medications to be used for this boy?*

## Introduction

In 1993, the Institute of Medicine reported on the state of emergency medical services (EMS) for children (EMS-C) in the United States. This expert panel made a number of recommendations, including that all agencies with jurisdiction over hospitals "require that hospital emergency departments . . . have available and maintain equipment and supplies appropriate for the emergency care of children" and that they begin to "address the issues of categorization and regionalization and overseeing the development of EMS-C and its integration in the state and regional EMS system."[1]

The public expects any hospital with an emergency department (ED) to be prepared to care for all patients, no matter what their problem or age, 24 hours a day. Not all hospitals have the same capacity to attend to the special needs of children. Most children who present for emergency care are seen in community EDs. These departments can ensure good care by creating child-friendly environments, using pediatric protocols, providing pediatric training for staff, and making sure appropriate pediatric equipment and supplies are available. Hospitals that do not have a pediatric inpatient service or a pediatric intensive care unit should have transfer agreements

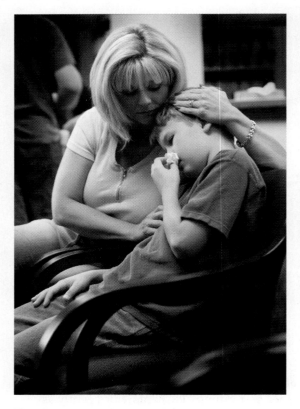

Figure 1.1 Most children are brought to the ED by their caregivers.

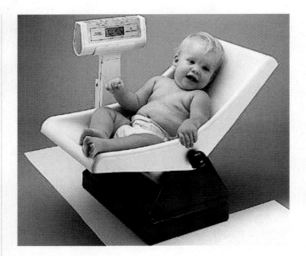

Figure 1.2 Pediatric scale.

and protocols in place to allow for rapid and efficient transfer of seriously ill or injured children from the ED to another facility with a higher level of care.

Systems of care are often based on facility categorization. EMS agencies may have transportation policies that bypass general hospitals to get patients to specialty centers. Only a small percentage of children are transported to the ED by ambulance. Most children are brought to the ED by their caregivers (Figure 1.1). All practitioners should know the EMS clinical care and destination policies in regard to pediatric patients, as well as the pediatric emergency and critical care services available in their areas.

## Emergency Department Preparedness

When a person with an ill child enters an ED, there are several unique features. The first is the triage process, often followed by sitting in a waiting room, which might have a separate area for children. This is followed by placement in an examination room, which might have child-friendly decorations. These and certain other key factors help define an ED prepared to handle children.

## Triage

Triage is the first point of service for all patients in EDs. Under most state laws, a registered nurse or a physician must perform this function. At triage, each patient is assigned a level of acuity. The assignment of this level usually determines in which area and in what time frame the patient will be seen. Pediatric triage criteria are age specific; thus, what is assigned a high level of acuity differs with age and associated signs and symptoms. For example, a temperature of 39°C in a 1-month-old is an emergency and is in the emergent acuity triage level. The same fever in a 7-year-old who appears well, is considered urgent but not as emergent. All triage areas should have pediatric scales, appropriate-sized blood pressure cuffs for infants, children, and adolescents, and pulse oximetry monitors with probes appropriate for infants and children (Figure 1.2). In addition, the patient's temperature (rectal in infants and oral or ear in older children) should be determined. The triage personnel will obtain a brief history of the present illness and past medical

| TABLE 1-1 | Pediatric Emergency Triage Categories |
|---|---|

- Level I—Resuscitation: Child/infant in respiratory failure, shock, coma, or cardiopulmonary arrest; any child or infant who requires continuous assessment and intervention to maintain physiological stability (e.g., coma, seizures, critical asthma, severe respiratory distress, unconsciousness, major burns, severe trauma, significant bleeding, and cardiopulmonary arrest).
- Level II—Emergent: Any physiologically unstable child with moderate respiratory distress, altered level of consciousness, or severe dehydration. Dehydration is difficult to accurately assess. Any suspicion (or evidence) should cause concern. Any infant/child who requires comprehensive assessment and multiple interventions to prevent further deterioration.

  Fever—Age <3 months, >38°C. Temperature is not always a reliable indicator of the severity of illness. Younger patients can have significant infections and serious problems even though the signs and symptoms may be subtle (e.g., sepsis, altered level of consciousness [GCS< 13], toxic ingestion, severe asthma, seizure [postictal], DKA, child abuse with ongoing risk, purpuric rash [a rash that does not blanch with pressure, e.g., petechiae], fever, open fractures, toxic ingestion/overdose, violent patients, severe testicular pain, lacerations or orthopedic injuries with neurovascular compromise, or dental injury with an avulsed permanent tooth).
- Level III—Urgent: Child/infant who is alert, oriented, well hydrated, with minor alterations in vital signs. Interventions include assessment and simple procedures. Febrile child >3 months with a temperature >38.5°C, mild respiratory distress, and minor head injuries. Level III patients need carefully planned reassessment while awaiting care since critical illness in children may present with common symptoms and evolve rapidly (e.g. simple burns, fractures, dental injuries, pneumonia without distress, history of seizure, suicide ideation, ingestion requiring observation only, head trauma GCS 14 or 15, alert/vomiting).
- Level IV—Less Urgent: Child/infant who is alert, oriented, and may have a condition that causes distress and may progress with the development of complications (e.g., vomiting/diarrhea and no dehydration, age >2, simple lacerations/sprains/strains, fever and simple complaints such as ear pain, sore throat or nasal congestion, or head trauma with no symptoms).
- Level V—Nonurgent: Child/infant who is afebrile, alert, oriented, well hydrated, with normal vital signs. Interventions are not usually required other than assessment/discharge instruction. These patients may be referred to other areas of the hospital or healthcare system for management.

Source: Canadian Pediatric Triage and Acuity Scale. *Canadian Journal of Emergency Medicine*. October 2001. Vol 3;No 4 (Suppl):www.CAEP.ca. Reprinted with permission.

history and will assess the patient, including vital signs and the ABCs (airway, breathing, and circulation). Patients considered in the highest level of acuity are immediately taken to a bed and registered at the bedside. Others might be registered at the registration area. An example of pediatric triage criteria can be found in Table 1-1 and Figure 1.3.

## Child-Friendly Area

Infants, children, and adolescents should be examined in a designated pediatric area if possible. Better care might be facilitated by separating the pediatric patients from frightening sights and sounds. Child-proofing the area with plug covers, locks on cabinets, and keeping dangerous equipment out of reach of the child should ensure patient safety. The sharps container should be out of reach, and all trash cans should be tall and covered. The room can easily be made child friendly by simple decorations and soothing colors (Figure 1.4). Infants and young children typically present with a caregiver, and the examination often is best done with the patient sitting on that person's lap. Thus, a comfortable chair for the caregiver, and a stool for the examining physician, are important. Studies have demonstrated that parents perceive their child has received better care when the physician sits during the interview.[2] Entertainment such as a television with a VCR or DVD player can provide distraction for the child who is undergoing treatment.[3] Coloring books and reading materials are also helpful but need replenishing frequently. Local charitable groups are often willing to provide these materials to the ED. Policies and procedures must be in place to ensure that all "distracters"/toys provided are age appropriate, checked frequently for safety, and cleaned between uses if necessary.

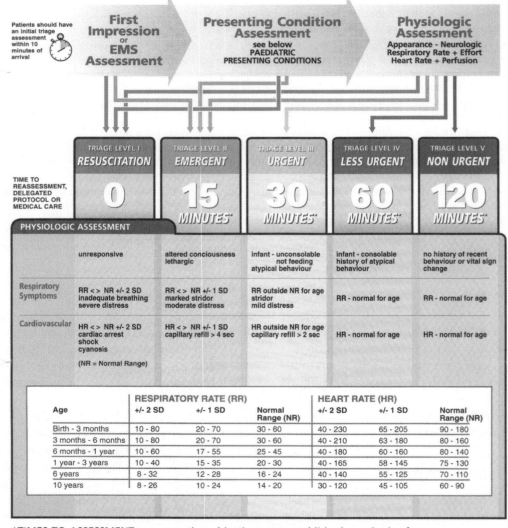

Figure 1.3 A Canadian Pediatric Triage and Acuity Scale. 1.3A. Triage level and rapid pediatric assessment.

| | TRIAGE LEVEL I RESUSCITATION | TRIAGE LEVEL II EMERGENT | TRIAGE LEVEL III URGENT | TRIAGE LEVEL IV LESS URGENT | TRIAGE LEVEL V NON URGENT |
|---|---|---|---|---|---|
| **PAEDIATRIC PRESENTING CONDITIONS** | | | | | |
| Respiratory | airway compromise | marked stridor | stridor | | |
| | severe distress | moderate distress | mild distress | | |
| | critical asthma | severe asthma | moderate asthma | mild asthma | |
| | chest trauma with respiratory distress | FB aspiration with respiratory distress | FB aspiration with no respiratory distress | possible FB aspiration with no distress | |
| | | inhalation of toxic substance | constant cough - distressed | minor chest injury no shortness of breath | |
| Neurological | major head injury GCS < 10 | moderate head injury GCS ≤ 13 | minor head injury GCS ≤ 15 | minor head injury | |
| CNS | unresponsive | altered consciousness | history of altered consciousness | no vomiting or altered consciousness | |
| | actively seizuring | headache severe sudden onset | headache | chronic headache | |
| | | ill - shunt dysfunction | possible shunt dysfunction | | |
| | | new neurologic findings | previous seizure | | |
| Cardiovascular | cardiac arrest | tachycardia ++ | tachycardia | normal heart rate | well hydrated |
| Circulation | shock | bradycardia | | chest pain | |
| | hypotension | severe dehydration | signs of dehydration | | |
| | exsanguinating haemorrhage | uncontrollable major haemorrhage | uncontrollable minor haemorrhage | | |
| Musculo-skeletal | major trauma | traumatic amputation - digit | | | |
| | traumatic amputation -extremity | open fracture fracture with neuro-vascular deficit | fracture no neuro-vascular deficit tight cast | greenstick fracture | |
| | hypothermia | back pain with neurologic symptom | joint pain with fever | extremity swelling sprain/strain | |
| | | avulsed 2° tooth | dental trauma | | |
| Skin | burn, > 25 % BSA or airway involved | burn > 10 % BSA burn- face, hand, foot chemical /electrical purpuric rash | burn < 10 % BSA frostbite cellulitis - ill / fever complex lacerations | minor burn minor cold injury local cellulitis simple laceration | superficial burn abrasion, contusion, local rash minor insect bite |
| Gastrointestinal | penetrating or blunt trauma with shock | acute bleeding - vomitus or rectal | persistent or bilious vomiting acute vomiting/ diarrhea age < 2 | constipation / pain acute vomiting / diarrhea age > 2 | vomiting or diarrhea no pain, no dehydration |
| | difficulty swallowing with airway compromise | abdominal pain with vomiting / diarrhea / abnormal vital signs | ? appendicitis | | |
| Genitourinary | vaginal bleed - unstable | severe testicular pain | moderate testicular pain / swelling | scrotal trauma | |
| Gynecologic | | ? ectopic pregnancy | inguinal mass / pain | possible UTI | |
| | | urine retention >24 hr | urine retention > 8 hrs | | |
| | | severe vaginal bleed paraphimosis | vaginal bleeding | | |
| Ear/Nose/Throat | airway compromise | amputation ear | foreign body nose epistaxis controlled puncture palate | ear drainage earache | sore throat mouth sores nasal congestion laryngitis |
| | | uncontrolled epistaxis | tonsillar pustules with difficulty swallowing | | |
| | | sore throat with drooling, stridor | hearing problem | | |
| | | difficulty swallowing hoarseness after trauma | Post T& A bleed | | |
| Eye | | chemical exposure penetrating injury orbital infection | vision change periorbital infection | tearing, discharge affecting function corneal FB | conjunctivitis |
| Hematologic | anaphylaxis | bleeding disorder sickle cell crisis | | | |
| Immunologic | | fever- neutropenic / immune suppressed | moderate allergic reaction | local allergic reaction | |
| Endocrine | diabetic- altered consciousness | diabetic- ketoacidosis hypoglycemia | hyperglycemia | | |
| Psychiatry | | toxic overdose | ingestion requiring observation | low risk of harm to self/ others | chronic symptoms with no change |
| | | high risk of harm to self / others | moderate risk of harm to self / others | | |
| | | violent behaviour | disruptive/distressed | depression | |
| Behaviour Change | unresponsive | lethargic child infant < 7 days old | unconsolable infant infant not feeding | irritable- consolable atypical behaviour | |
| Infection | septic shock | infant < 3 mon 36< temperature ≥ 38 toxic appearance - any age | infant 3-36 mon with temperature > 38.5 | Infant > 36 mon with temperature > 38.5 non toxic appearance | |
| Child Abuse | unstable situation or conflict | ongoing risk | physical assault sexual abuse <48 hr | signs / history of family violence | |
| Pain | | Severe  8 - 10 / 10 | Moderate   4 - 7 / 10 | Mild  1 - 3 / 10 | |

**Figure 1.3 B** Pediatric Presenting Conditions.

Source: Canadian Pediatric ED Triage and Acuity Scale. *Canadian Journal of Emergency Medicine*. Reprinted with permission.

B

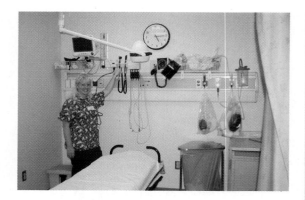

Figure 1.4 A child-friendly examining room.

## Staffing

Clerical and nursing staff should be child friendly. Pediatric nursing is a recognized specialty. The assessment skills necessary for appropriate triage, ongoing assessment, and pediatric care are critical for good outcomes in the ED. Nurses can be educated through years of experience on a pediatric unit, through formal education in professional schools (clinical nurse specialist), or through specific continuing medical education such as the *Emergency Nurse Pediatric Course* (ENPC) given through the Emergency Nurses Association.[4] In addition, several self-learning programs are available.[5,6] *The Pediatric Advanced Life Support Course* (PALS), offered by the American Heart Association prepares physicians and nurses improve their pediatric resuscitation skills.[7]

Physician education is also important. The PALS course or an equivalent is helpful to physicians who do not frequently resuscitate children in the ED. *APLS: The Pediatric Emergency Medicine Resource* is also helpful for reviewing pediatric emergency medicine. Conducting routine mock codes will enable the ED team to practice resuscitation skills.[8] Phlebotomists and respiratory therapists should also be familiar with the special needs of children, and the latter be skilled in the delivery of pediatric emergency care.

## Interface With Out-of-Hospital Care

Hospitals that have either online (direct) or offline (indirect) medical oversight responsibilities for out-of-hospital providers should have pediatric treatment and destination protocols in place. If it is determined in the field that a child will require intensive care, he or she should be primarily transported to a hospital that can offer that level of care, unless the transport time is too long or the child requires immediate stabilization. Emergency physicians working with the pediatric community can develop destination policies based on local needs and resources. It is also crucial that all ambulances and basic and paramedic EMS units be equipped and supplied for pediatric emergencies. The American College of Emergency Physicians (ACEP) and the Committee on Trauma of the American College of Surgeons published guidelines in 2001 for equipping ambulances (Table 1-2). Continuing education in pediatric emergency care designed specifically for EMS providers such as the *Pediatric Education for Prehospital Providers* (PEPP) course can be used to ensure that EMS personnel have the knowledge to care for pediatric emergencies.[9]

## Equipment and Supplies

In 2001, Canadian investigators surveyed 737 EDs for pediatric equipment availability. Table 1-3 lists the equipment items that were not available. EDs with low pediatric volumes were statistically more likely to have less equipment availability than higher volumes EDS. There are no comparative data in the United States; however, the Consumer Product Safety Commission surveyed 101 hospitals with EDs that were enrolled in the National Electronic Injury Surveillance System to identify the state of pediatric preparedness. The results of this survey were then extrapolated to the 5,312 EDs in the United States. The survey showed that, although one third of hospitals had a pediatric ward or pediatrics department, almost 76% of hospitals still

**TABLE 1-2    Equipment for BLS and ALS Ambulances**

**Basic Level Providers**

A. **Ventilation and Airway Equipment**
1. Portable and fixed suction apparatus
   - Wide-bore tubing, rigid pharyngeal curved suction tip; tonsillar and flexible suction catheters, 5F–14F
2. Portable and fixed oxygen equipment
   - Variable flow regulator
3. Oxygen administration equipment
   - Adequate length tubing; mask (adult, child, and infant sizes), transparent, non-rebreathing, Venturi, and valveless; nasal cannulas (adult, child, and infant sizes)
4. Pocket mask with one-way valve
5. Bag-valve mask
   - Hand-operated, self-reexpanding bag (adult and infant sizes), with oxygen reservoir/accumulator; clear mask (adult, child, infant, and neonate sizes); valve (clear, disposable, operable in cold weather)
6. Airways
   - Nasopharyngeal, oropharyngeal (adult, child, and infant sizes)

B. **Monitoring and Defibrillation**
   Automatic external defibrillator is strongly recommended for systems that do not have immediate availability of an advanced life support service.

C. **Immobilization Devices**
1. Cervical collars
   - Rigid for children ages 2 years or older, infant, child, and adult sizes (small, medium, large, and other available sizes)
2. Head immobilization device (not sandbags)
   - Firm padding or commercial device
3. Lower extremity (femur) traction devices
   - Lower extremity, limb-support slings, padded ankle hitch, padded pelvic support, traction strap (adult and child sizes)
4. Upper and lower extremity immobilization devices
   - Joint-above and joint-below fracture (adult and child sizes), rigid-support appropriate material (cardboard, metal, pneumatic, vacuum, wood, or plastic)
5. Radiolucent backboards (long, short) and extrication device
   - Joint-above and joint-below fracture site (chin strap alone should not be used for head immobilization), adult and child sizes, with

padding for children, hand holds for moving patients, short (extrication, head-to-pelvis length), long (transport, head to feet), with at least 3 appropriate restraint straps

D. **Bandages**
1. Burn pack
   - Standard package, clean burn sheets (or towels for children)
2. Triangular bandages
   - Minimum 2 safety pins each
3. Dressings
   - Sterile multitrauma dressings (various large and small sizes)
   - ABDs, 10"×12" or larger
   - 4"×4" gauze sponges
4. Gauze rolls
   - Sterile (various sizes)
5. Elastic bandages
   - Nonsterile (various sizes)
6. Occlusive dressing
   - Sterile, 3"×8" or larger
7. Adhesive tape
   - Various sizes (including 2" or 3") hypoallergenic
   - Various sizes (including 2" or 3") adhesive

E. **Communication**
   - Two-way radio communication (UHS, VHF) between EMT, dispatcher, and medical direction (physician)
   - Two-way disaster communication
   - Cellular phone

F. **Obstetrical**
1. Kit (separate sterile kit)
   - Towels, 4"×4" dressing, umbilical tape, sterile scissors or other cutting utensil, bulb suction, clamps for cord, sterile gloves, blanket
2. Thermal absorbent blanket and head cover, aluminum foil roll, or appropriate heat-reflective material (enough to cover newborn)
3. Appropriate heat source for ambulance compartment

G. **Miscellaneous**
1. Sphygmomanometer (infant, pediatric, and adult regular and large, for example, thigh sizes)
2. Stethoscope (pediatric and adult)
3. Length/weight-based chart for pediatric equipment sizing
4. Thermometer with low temperature capability

*(continues)*

**TABLE 1-2    Equipment for BLS and ALS Ambulances (Continued)**

5. Heavy bandage or paramedic scissors for cutting clothing, belts, and boots
6. Cold packs
7. Sterile saline solution for irrigation (1-liter bottles or bags)
8. Flashlights (2) with extra batteries and bulbs
9. Blankets
10. Sheets, linen, or paper (minimum 4), and pillows
11. Towels
12. Triage tags
13. Disposable emesis bags or basins
14. Disposable bedpan
15. Disposable urinal
16. Wheeled cot (properly secured patient transport system)
17. Folding stretcher
18. Stair chair or carry chair
19. Patient care charts/forms
20. Lubricating jelly (water soluable)

### H. Infection Control*
*Latex-free equipment should be available.
1. Eye protection (full peripheral glasses or goggles, face shield)
2. Masks
3. Gloves, nonsterile
4. Jumpsuits or gowns
5. Shoe covers
6. Disinfectant hand wash, commercial antimicrobial (towelette, spray, liquid)
7. Disinfectant solution for cleaning equipment
8. Standard sharps containers (EMT-Basic, -Intermediate, and -Paramedic)
9. Disposable trash bags (identifiable color, such as red)
10. HEPA mask

### I. Injury Prevention Equipment
1. Appropriate restraints (seat belts, air bags) for patient, crew, and family members
2. Child safety restraints
3. Protective helmet and coat with reflective material (1 each per crew member)
4. Fire extinguisher
5. Hazardous material reference guide
6. Traffic signaling devices (reflective material triangles or other reflective, nonigniting devices)

### J. Optional Basic Equipment
1. Pneumatic antishock garment (PASG)
   - Compartmentalized (legs and abdomen separate), control valves (closed/open), inflation pump, lower leg to lower rib cage (does not include chest)
2. Respirator
   - Volume-cycled valve, on/off operation, 100% oxygen, 40–50 psi pressure (child/infant capabilities)

## Advanced Level Providers

For EMT-Paramedic, include all the equipment listed for the basic level provider plus the following additional equipment and supplies. For EMT-Intermediate (and other nonparamedic advanced levels), include all the equipment for the basic level provider and selected equipment and supplies from the following list, as appropriate.

### A. Vascular Access
1. Intravenous administration equipment (fluid must be in bags, not bottles)
2. Crystalloid solutions, Ringer's lactate or normal saline solution (1,000-mL bags × 4), 5% dextrose in water (optional)
3. Antiseptic solution (alcohol wipes and povidone-iodine wipes preferred)
4. IV pole or roof hook
5. Intravenous catheters 14G–24G, 1" long
6. Intraosseous needles
7. Tourniquet, rubber bands
8. Syringes of various sizes, including tuberculin
9. Needles, sizes 19G–25G
10. Intravenous administration sets (microdrip and macrodrip), Burretrol, and in-line blood pump (as differentiated from intravenous tubing with an in-line blood filter)
11. Intravenous arm boards, adult and pediatric

### B. Airway and Ventilation Equipment
1. Laryngoscope handle with extra batteries and bulbs, adult and pediatric
2. Laryngoscope blades, sizes 0, 1, and 2, straight; sizes 3 and 4, straight and curved
3. Endotracheal tubes, sizes 2.5–6.0 mm uncuffed and 6.5–8.0 mm cuffed (2 each), other sizes optional
4. Meconium aspirator
5. 10-mL non-Luerlock syringes
6. Stylettes for endotracheal tubes, adult and pediatric

*(continues)*

**TABLE 1-2    Equipment for BLS and ALS Ambulances** *(Continued)*

7. Magill forceps, adult and pediatric
8. Lubricating jelly (water soluble)
9. Nasogastric tubes, pediatric sizes 5F and 8F, Salem sump sizes 14F, 16F, and 18F
10. End-tidal $CO_2$ detectors
    - Colorimetric or quantitative

### C. Cardiac

1. Portable, battery-operated monitor/defibrillator
   - With tape write-out/recorder, defibrillator pads, quick-look paddles or hands-free patches, ECG leads, adult and pediatric chest attachment electrodes, adult and pediatric paddles, with capability to provide electrical discharge below 25 watt-seconds.
2. Transcutaneous cardiac pacemaker
   - Either stand-alone unit or integrated into monitor/defibrillator

### D. Other Advanced Equipment

1. Nebulizer
2. Glucometer or blood glucose measuring device
   - With reagent strips
3. Pulse oximetry with pediatric and adult probes

### E. Medications (pre-load when available)

Medications used on advanced level ambulances should be compatible with current standards as indicated by the American Heart Association's Emergency Cardiac Care Committee, as reflected in the Advanced Cardiac Life Support Course, or other such organizations and publications (ACEP, ACS, National Association of EMS Physicians, and so on). In general, medications should include:

- Cardiovascular medication, such as 1:10,000 epinephrine, atropine, lidocaine, bretylium tosylate,* adenosine, diltiazem hydrochloride, propranolol, nitroglycerin tablets, aspirin, dopamine
- Cardiopulmonary/respiratory medications, such as albuterol (or other inhaled beta agonist), 1:1,000 epinephrine, furosemide
- 50% dextrose solution (and sterile dilutent or 25% dextrose solution for pediatrics)
- Analgesics, such as morphine, meperidine hydrochloride, nitrous oxide
- Antiepileptic medications, such as diazepam or midazolam

---

* *Editor's note: Bretylium is no longer available and is not used.*

- Activated charcoal, sodium bicarbonate, magnesium sulfate, glucagon, naloxone hydrochloride, flumazenil
- Bacteriostatic water and sodium chloride for injection

### F. Optional Advanced Equipment

1. Portable automatic ventilators
2. Alternative airway devices (double lumen tube airways)
3. Umbilical vein catheters (sizes 3.5F and 5F)
4. Blood sample tubes, adult and pediatric
5. Automatic blood pressure device

## Extrication Equipment

Adequate extrication equipment must be readily available to the EMS responders, but is more often found on heavy rescue vehicles than on the primary responding ambulance.

In general, the devices or tools used for extrication fall into several broad categories: disassembly, spreading, cutting, pulling, protective, and patient-related.

The following is necessary equipment that should be available either on the primary response vehicle or on a heavy rescue vehicle.

### Disassembly Tools

- Wrenches (adjustable)
- Screwdrivers (flat and Phillips head)
- Pliers
- Bolt cutter
- Tin snips
- Hammer
- Spring-loaded center punch
- Axes (pry, fire)
- Bars (wrecking, crow)
- Ram (4 ton)

### Spreading Tools

- Hydraulic jack/spreader combination
- Boss tool with spreading device

### Cutting Tools

- Saws (hacksaw, fire, windshield, pruning, reciprocating)
- Air-cutting gun kit

### Pulling Tools/Devices

- Ropes/chains
- Come-along
- Hydraulic truck jack
- Air bags

*(continues)*

TABLE 1-2    Equipment for BLS and ALS Ambulances *(Continued)*

**Protective Devices**
- Reflectors/flares
- Hard hats
- Safety goggles
- Fireproof blanket
- Leather gloves
- Jackets/coats/boots

**Patient-Related Devices**
- Swiss seat
- Stokes basket

**Miscellaneous**
- Shovel
- Lubricating oil
- Wood/wedges
- Generator
- Floodlights

Local extrication needs may necessitate additional equipment, that is, water, aerial, or mountain rescue.

Source: American College of Emergency Physicians, American College of Surgeons. *Equipment for ambulances* [Policy Resource and Education Paper]. American College of Emergency Physicians Web site. Reprinted with permission.

| TABLE 1-3 | Percentage of Canadian EDs Lacking Equipment Items | |
| --- | --- | --- |
| • | Intraosseous needles | 15.9% |
| • | Pediatric drug dose guidelines | 6.6% |
| • | Infant BP cuff | 14.8% |
| • | Pediatric defibrillator paddles | 10.5% |
| • | Infant warming device | 59.4% |
| • | Pediatric pulse oximeter | 18.0% |
| • | 3.0 ET tubes | 2.5% |
| • | Infant laryngoscope blade | 3.5% |

Source: McGillivray D, Nijssen-Jordan C, Kramer MS, Yang H, Platt R.: Critical pediatric equipment availability in Canadian hospital emergency departments. *Ann Emerg Med.* 2001;37:371–376. Reprinted with permission.

admitted pediatric patients to adult wards. About 7% of the hospitals had a separate pediatric ED. EDs were more likely to lack pediatric than adult emergency equipment and supplies.[10]

In 2001, the American Academy of Pediatrics (AAP) and ACEP published joint ED preparedness guidelines for children in "Care of Children in the Emergency Department: Guidelines for Preparedness." These guidelines were supported in concept by 17 national organizations. The guidelines outline equipment and supplies for EDs that care for children. Tables 1-4 and 1-5 list recommended medications, equip-

ment, and supplies that should be available. This includes scales to obtain weights in kilograms and appropriate-sized blood pressure cuffs. Both infant and adult pulse oximetry probes should be available. Appropriate supplies for vascular access, including intraosseous needles, should be readily available. Monitors and defibrillators should be equipped with pediatric and adult leads and paddles. Resuscitation drugs and equipment should be placed in an identified area or cart and contain a table and or tape for length-based weight determination (Figure 1.5). Some EDs use a color coding system based on the child's length to store all supplies and equipment (Figure 1.6).[11]

## Other Preparedness Issues

Other aspects of the ED visit cover a broad range of topics. Some of these are issues dealt within the ED, while others require decisions that could affect a patients ultimate outcome.

## Interpersonal Violence

Family violence, which includes child abuse and neglect, intimate partner violence (IPV), and elder abuse, affects as many as 25% of individuals in the United States during their life-

| TABLE 1-4 | Guidelines for Medications for Use in Pediatric Patients in the EDs |
|---|---|

| Resuscitation Medications | Other Drug Groups |
|---|---|
| • Atropine<br>• Adenosine<br>• Bretylium tosylate*<br>• Calcium chloride<br>• Dextrose<br>• Epinephrine (1:1000, 1:10,000)<br>• Lidocaine<br>• Naloxone hydrochloride<br>• Sodium bicarbonate (4.2%)<br><br>*  *Editor's note: Bretylium is no longer available and is not used.* | • Activated charcoal<br>• Analgesics<br>• Antibiotics (parenteral)<br>• Resuscitation medications<br>• Anticonvulsants<br>• Antidotes (common antidotes should be accessible to the ED)[†]<br>• Antipyretics<br>• Bronchodilators<br>• Corticosteroids<br>• Inotropic agents<br>• Neuromuscular blocking agents<br>• Oxygen<br>• Sedatives |

[†]For less frequently used antidotes, a procedure for obtaining them should be in place.

Source: American Academy of Pediatrics, Committee on Pediatric Emergency Medicine; and American College of Emergency Physicians, Pediatric Committee. Care of children in the emergency department: guidelines for preparedness. *Pediatrics.* 2001;107:777–781. American Academy of Pediatrics, Committee on Pediatric Emergency Medicine; and American College of Emergency Physicians, Pediatric Committee. Care of children in the emergency department: guidelines for preparedness. *Ann Emerg Med.* 2001;37:423–427. Reprinted with permission.

times.[12] Child abuse and neglect or child maltreatment generally refers to physical abuse, sexual abuse, emotional abuse, and neglect. Child abuse and neglect are defined by statute in all 50 states, the District of Columbia, Guam, Puerto Rico, and the United States Virgin Islands. The ED is an important area for the identification of child abuse and neglect. ED personnel should have knowledge of child abuse and neglect indicators and their jurisdiction's legal definition and reporting requirements. In addition, they should have intervention and documentation skills. To assist in this process, all EDs should have written protocols for the care of the abused child. It is also important to have an identified source for expert consultation and referral.

In addition to violence perpetrated against them, millions of children are affected by witnessing IPV, especially against their mothers. Professional organizations such as the AAP and ACEP have recommended routine screening for IPV at child health visits and in the ED. The AAP Committee on Child Abuse and Neglect asserts that intervening on behalf of battered women is an active form of child abuse prevention.[13] With this in mind, EDs that care for children should have routine screening protocols in place and ensure that ED health professionals are competent in IPV screening and knowledgeable of state laws for reporting and local resources for intervention and referral.

## Parental Presence

Research has demonstrated that families and patients benefit from having family members present during procedures and cardiopulmonary resuscitation (CPR). Even when there is a fatal outcome, families feel comforted and have an easier time with the grieving process when they have witnessed the resuscitation.[14,15] Children undergoing placement of an intravenous cannula also benefit from having parents present during the procedure.[16] All EDs should have a policy

## TABLE 1-5    Guidelines for Equipment and Supplies for Use in Pediatric Patients in the ED

### Monitoring Equipment
- Cardiorespiratory monitor with strip recorder
- Defibrillator with pediatric and adult paddles (4.5 cm and 8 cm) or corresponding adhesive pads
- Pediatric and adult monitor electrodes
- Pulse oximeter with sensors and probe sizes for children
- Thermometer or rectal probe†
- Sphygmomanometer
- Doppler blood pressure device
- Blood pressure cuffs (neonatal, infant, child, and adult arm and thigh cuffs)
- Method to monitor tracheal tube and placement‡
- Stethoscope

### Airway Management
- Portable oxygen regulators and canisters
- Clear oxygen masks (standard and nonrebreathing – neonatal infant, child, and adult)
- Oropharyngeal airways (sizes 0–5)
- Nasopharyngeal airways (12F–30F)
- Bag-valve-mask resuscitator, self-inflating (450- and 1000-mL sizes)
- Nasal cannulae (child and adult)
- Tracheal tubes: uncuffed (2.5, 3.0, 3.5, 4.0, 4.5, 5.0, 5.5, and 6.0 mm) and cuffed (6.5, 7.0, 7.5, 8.0, and 9.0 mm)
- Stylets (infant, pediatric, and adult)
- Laryngoscope handle (pediatric and adult)
- Laryngoscope blades: straight or Miller (0, 1, 2, and 3) and Macintosh (2 and 3)
- Magill forceps (pediatric and adult)
- Nasogastric/feeding tubes (5F through 18F)
- Suction catheters—flexible (6F, 8F, 10F, 12F, 14F, and 16F)
- Yankauer suction tip
- Bulb syringe
- Chest tubes (8F through 40F)§
- Laryngeal mask airway** (sizes 1, 1.5, 2, 2.5, 3, 4, and 5)

### Vascular Access
- Butterfly needles (19–25 gauge)
- Catheter-over-needle devices (14–24 gauge)
- Rate limiting infusion device and tubing§¶
- Intraosseous needles (may be satisfied by standard bone needle aspiration needles)
- Arm boards**
- Intravenous fluid and blood warmers§
- Umbilical vein catheters§# (size 5F feeding tube may be used)
- Seldinger technique vascular access kit§

### Miscellaneous
- Infant and standard scales
- Infant formula and oral rehydrating solutions§
- Heating source (may be met by infrared lamps or overhead warmer)§
- Towel rolls, blanket rolls, or equivalent
- Pediatric restraining devices
- Resuscitation board
- Sterile linen*
- Length-based resuscitation tape or precalculated drug or equipment list based on weight

### Specialized Pediatric Trays
- Tube thoracostomy with water seal drainage capability§
- Lumbar puncture
- Pediatric urinary catheters
- Obstetric pack
- Newborn kit§
- Umbilical vessel cannulation supplies§
- Venous cutdown§
- Needle cricothyrotomy tray
- Surgical airway kit (may include a tracheostomy tray or a surgical cricothyrotomy tray)§

### Fracture Management
- Cervical immobilization equipment§††
- Extremity splints§
- Femur splints§

### Medical Photography Capability

†Suitable for hypothermic and hyperthermic measurements with temperature capability from 25°C to 44°C

‡May be satisfied by a disposable $CO_2$ detector of appropriate size for infants and children. For children 5 years or older who are >5 yrs 20 kg in body weight, an esophageal detection bulb or syringe also may be used

§Equipment that is essential but may be shared with the nursery, pediatric ward, or other inpatient service and is readily available to the ED

**Equipment or supplies that are desirable but not essential

¶To regulate rate and volume

#Ensure availability of pediatric sizes within the hospital

*Available within hospital for burn care

††Many types of cervical immobilization devices are available, including wedges and collars. The type of device chosen depends on local preferences and policies and procedures. Chosen device should be stocked in sizes to fit infants, children, adolescents, and adults. Use of sandbags to meet this requirement is discouraged, because they may cause injury if the patient has to be turned.

Source: American Academy of Pediatrics, Committee on Pediatric Emergency Medicine and American College of Emergency Physicians, Pediatric Committee. Care of children in the emergency department: guidelines for preparedness. *Pediatrics*. 2001;107:777–781. American Academy of Pediatrics, Committee on Pediatric Emergency Medicine and American College of Emergency Physicians, Pediatric Committee. Care of children in the emergency department: guidelines for preparedness. *Ann Emerg Med*. 2001;37:423–427. Reprinted with permission.

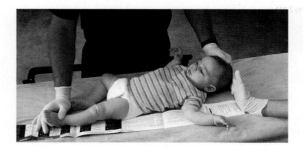

Figure 1.5 Length-Based Resuscitation Tape.

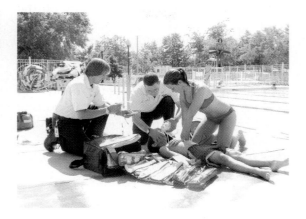

Figure 1.6 Color-coded equipment bag for pediatrics.

AGREEMENT

This AGREEMENT is made between SPECIALIZED REFERRAL CENTER (CENTER)*

LOCATED AT _____

and HOSPITAL located at _____ ,

henceforth referred to as HOSPITAL or referring hospital.


This Agreement serves as documentation of the arrangements, policies, and procedures governing the transfer of critically ill and/or injured pediatric patients (. . . Add other types of patients or services, if desired . . .) between the above named institutions in order to facilitate timely transfer, continuity of care, and appropriate transport for these patients.


THE CENTER AND HOSPITAL DO MUTUALLY AGREE AS FOLLOWS:

Figure 1.7 Sample pediatric interfacility transfer agreement.

that describes the circumstances under which family members are permitted to be present during procedures and CPR. Additional personnel such as social workers, clergy, and volunteers can be helpful resources for families so that they are comforted and have the procedures and resuscitation explained to them. Most protocols make sure that family members are never in the treatment room without a designated support person.

## Transfer to a Higher Level of Care

EDs that do not have pediatric inpatient units or pediatric intensive care units sometimes must transfer patients to other hospitals for a higher level of care. All EDs should have a policy or procedure in place for interfacility transfers (Figure 1.7).[17] Sometimes transfers are between hospitals in different states, and these agreements are particularly important for reimbursement issues. Physician-to-physician and nurse-to-nurse communication should always take place between the referring and receiving hospital staff. Communication should be reinforced with complete written documentation to be transmitted at the time of transfer. The decision on mode of transport (air versus ground) will depend on a variety of factors, including weather, time to definitive care, and availability of resources.

## Disasters

All hospital and ED disaster plans should address the special needs of children. This includes family-centered care and psychological first aid for pediatric patients who have been victims of violence or have witnessed a disaster.[3] See Chapter 17, Disaster Management.

## Check Your Knowledge

1. A 2-month-old presents to the ED with a temperature of 40°C. He is irritable but in no obvious distress. The triage nurse should consider this patient to be which of the following?
   A. A Level IV triage, and place in the waiting room
   B. A Level III triage, and place in the waiting room
   C. A Level II triage, and place in an examination room to see the physician
   D. A Level II triage, and requires immediate medical attention

2. Which of the following statements regarding a child-friendly examination room is correct?
   A. Involves both décor and safety-proofing the room
   B. Is generally not necessary in a busy ED
   C. Requires placing children in a separate part of the ED
   D. Means having toys in the room

3. All EDs in the United States:
   A. Admit children to pediatric wards
   B. Have appropriate equipment and supplies for pediatrics
   C. Transfer all pediatric patients when necessary for higher levels of care
   D. None of the above

4. Which of the following statements is correct?
   A. Most children are brought to hospital EDs by EMS
   B. Most children are brought to hospital EDs by police
   C. Most children are referred to EDs from schools
   D. Most children are transported by caregivers to the ED

## References

1. Institute of Medicine, Committee on Pediatric Emergency Medical Services. Durch JS, Lohr KN, eds. *Institute of Medicine Report: Emergency Medical Services for Children.* Washington, DC: National Academy Press; 1993.
2. Korsch BM, Gotti EK, Francis V. Gaps in doctor-patient communication: doctor-patient interaction and patient satisfaction. *Pediatrics.* 1968;42:855–871.
3. Seidel JS, Knapp JF, eds. *Childhood Emergencies in the Office, Hospital and Community: Organizing Systems of Care.* Elk Grove Village, Il: American Academy of Pediatrics, 2000.
4. Emergency Nurses Association. *The Emergency Nursing Pediatric Course Provider Manual.* Park Ridge, Il: ENA; 1993.
5. Henderson DP, Seidel JS. *The Acutely Ill or Injured Pediatric Patient: An Interactive Educational Program.* Los Angeles, Ca: NERA; 2001.
6. Henderson DP, Brownstein D, eds. *Pediatric Emergency Nursing Manual.* New York, NY: Springer Publishing; 1994.
7. Hazinski MF et al., eds. *Pediatric Advanced Life Support Manual.* Dallas, Tex: American Heart Association; 2002.
8. Roback MG, Teach SJ, eds. *Pediatric Resuscitation: A Practical Approach.* Dallas, Tex: American College of Emergency Physicians; 2005.
9. Dieckmann RA, ed. *Pediatric Education for Prehospital Professionals.* 2nd Ed. Sudbury, Mass: American Academy of Pediatrics, Jones and Bartlett Publishers; 2006.
10. Athey J, Dean JM, Ball J et al. Ability of hospitals to care for pediatric emergency patients. *Pediatr Emerg Care.* 2001;17:170–174.
11. Lanoix R, Golden J. The facilitated pediatric resuscitation room. *J Emerg Med.* 1999;17:363–366.
12. Centers for Disease Control. Prevalence of intimate partner violence and injuries—Washington, 1998. *MMWR.* 2000; 49(26):589–592.
13. American Academy of Pediatrics Committee on Child Abuse and Neglect. The role of the pediatrician in recognizing and intervening on behalf of abused women. *Pediatrics.* 1998;101: 1091–1092.
14. Hanson C, Strawser D. Family presence during cardiopulmonary resuscitation: Foote hospital emergency department's nine-year perspective. *J Emerg Nurs.* 1996;18(2):104–106.
15. Eichhorn DJ, Meyers TA, Mitchell TG, Guzzetta CE. Opening the doors: family presence during resuscitation. *J Cardiovasc Nurs.* 1996;10(4):59–70.
16. Wolfram RW, Turner ED, Phipput C. Effects of parental presence on children's venipuncture. *Pediatr Emerg Care.* 1997;13:325–328.
17. Henderson DP, Seidel JS, et al. *Development and Implementation of Emergency Medical Services for Children: A Step by Step Approach.* Los Angeles, Ca: NERA; 2000.

CASE SUMMARY 1

A 3-year-old boy is found at the bottom of a Jacuzzi by his grandparents. Paramedics arrive 4 minutes later to find the grandfather performing CPR. Paramedics gently ask the grandfather to step aside and note that the child's appearance is unconscious and unresponsive to surroundings, work of breathing is absent, and color is pale. Further assessment shows the child has a weak brachial pulse. Bag-mask ventilation is begun, and the boy is transported to your emergency department.

1. *How would this child be triaged?*
2. *What will you do to prepare for his arrival?*
3. *How will you determine the size of equipment and dosage of medications to be used for this boy?*

This child is critically ill and would be triaged as a Level I or immediate care patient. He must be immediately placed in an appropriate resuscitation area.

An organized approach to resuscitation will provide the child optimal care. This could mean gathering team members and briefing them on their responsibilities, gathering appropriate-sized equipment and needed supplies, and notifying subspecialists, as needed, about the imminent arrival of the patient.

There is no time to weigh the boy, but a length-based resuscitation tape (i.e., Broselow tape) can be used to quickly estimate weight. Equipment sizes and precalculated drug dosages are printed on the tape. Some emergency departments estimate weight based on the age of the patient, then precalculate drug dosages prior to the patient's arrival in the emergency department.

# chapter 2

# Pediatric Assessment

Ronald A. Dieckmann, MD, MPH, FAAP, FACEP

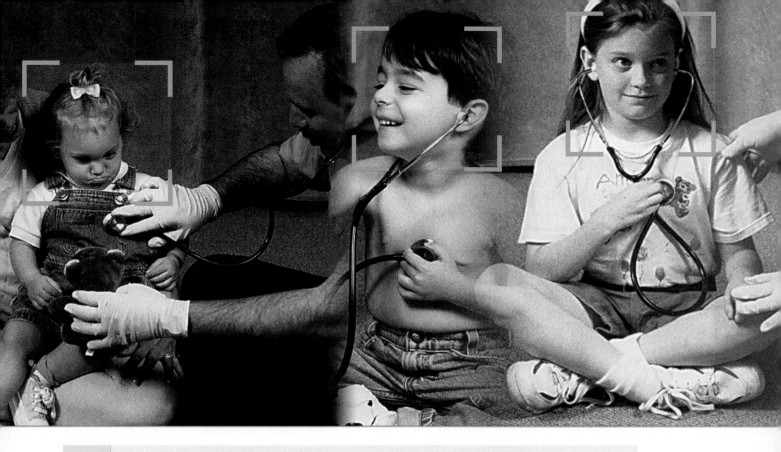

**CASE SCENARIO 1**

A 6-month-old boy who has had persistent vomiting for 24 hours presents to the emergency department. The infant is lying still and has poor muscle tone. He is irritable if touched, and his cry is weak. There are no abnormal airway sounds, retractions, or flaring. He is pale and mottled. The respiratory rate is 45 breaths/min, heart rate is 170 beats per minute (bpm), and blood pressure is 50/palp. Air movement is normal, and breath sounds are clear to auscultation. The skin feels cool, and capillary refill time is 4 seconds. The brachial pulse is weak. His abdomen is distended.

1. *What are the key signs of serious illness in this infant?*
2. *How helpful are heart rate, respiratory rate, and blood pressure in evaluating cardiopulmonary function?*

## Introduction

Accurate physical assessment of a child with an acute illness or injury requires special knowledge of growth and development and pediatric-specific evaluation skills. Time-honored, adult-oriented assessment techniques can have limited value in acutely ill and injured children, especially preschool-aged children, in whom measurements of heart rate, respiratory rate, and blood pressure, or findings on physical assessment such as auscultation and palpation, are sometimes misinterpreted. A developmentally appropriate approach to physical assessment will help adjust assessment approaches to the child's expected behavior and permit more subtle evaluation.

Physical assessment is a different process than diagnosis. Assessment is a clinical evaluation, the primary goals of which are identification of abnormal anatomy and physiology, estimation of severity, and determination of urgency for emergency treatment. It is mainly a clinical process, so diagnostic imaging and laboratory investigations are not essential components. Assessment directs general and specific treatment to restore normal body homeostasis and physiology, and to prevent deterioration to respiratory or circulatory failure, but it might not establish a diagnosis. Exact diagnosis is a secondary goal of initial assessment and is rarely necessary in the first phases of general life support. During the second phase of physical assessment, the comprehensive history and physical examination of the stable child, clinical diagnosis becomes a primary goal.

For patients of all ages, the physical assessment has several steps. First is the initial assessment, which includes the general visual and auditory impression using the pediatric assessment triangle (PAT) and the hands-on ABCDEs (airway, breathing, circulation, disability, and exposure). The initial assessment is designed to assess the presence of life-threatening emergencies. It requires modification to accommodate different developmental stages of childhood. Second is the additional assessment, which includes a focused history and physical examination to detect more subtle abnormal anatomy and physiology, and to identify dangerous signs and symptoms. The additional assessment also integrates traditional, detailed history-taking and physical examination and is done when the patient is stable. Additional assessment is oriented toward anatomic rather than physiologic abnormalities and focuses on clinical diagnosis and the staging of ancillary testing with laboratory investigations and imaging. In life-threatening conditions, additional assessment might not be possible because of overwhelming requirements for basic physiologic support. Ongoing assessment is another component of additional assessment and is appropriate for all patients. Ongoing assessment includes repeated physical assessments and monitoring intended to evaluate trends of physiologic response to therapy.

## Background

Children experience a diverse array of acute illnesses and injuries, many of them unique to the vulnerable anatomy, immature immunology and physiology, and normal exploratory behavior of youth. Fortunately, most pediatric emergencies are minor and can be readily managed with simple first aid measures at home or in school, or by a primary medical provider in a community office, clinic, or hospital pediatric ambulatory practice. Sometimes, pediatric illness or injury is of high acuity or life threatening, or involves serious pain, and the more sophisticated medical capabilities of the emergency department (ED) are necessary.[1]

## Epidemiology

The National Hospital Ambulatory Medical Care Survey (NHAMCS) is a national probability sample survey of visits to hospital emergency and outpatient departments of nonfederal, short-stay, and general hospitals in the United States. In 2000, there were 108 million ED visits, with 21.7% (23,890,000) visits by children younger than 15 years.[2] An additional 16.4% (17,664,000) visits were by adolescents and young adults 15 to 24 years old.[2] This survey indicated that among children less than 15 years of age, the rate of ED visits (the number of visits per 100 persons per year), was higher for males (42.9) than females (34.4), and higher for African-Americans (58.9) in this age group than Caucasians (36).[2]

These recent data are supported by the American College of Emergency Physicians, which reports that, across the country, about one third of ED patients per year are children.[3] The majority of children are seen in the 4,000 general EDs throughout the United States, and the rest in about 70 pediatric EDs in children's hospitals.[2] Most pediatric ED patients arrive by private vehicle or are walk-ins and have either private insurance or Medicaid.[2]

These data pertain only to ED pediatric patients, who can be significantly different in their demographic characteristics from children with emergency conditions cared for in private offices or clinics. Several physician surveys have found an important role for pediatricians in out-of-hospital management of many moderate to severe childhood emergencies, including meningitis, severe asthma, severe dehydration, seizures, altered mental status, anaphylaxis, and cardiopulmonary arrest.[4,5] Illnesses seem to predominate in office and clinic pediatric emergency experiences, while injuries are the most common childhood complaints in EDs. Information based on earlier NHAMCS data shows that, for children, 43% of all ED visits were injury related, with the highest number of visits by those 0 to

2 years and 18 to 20 years old.[6] Moreover, other data suggest that children with many minor acute conditions easily treatable in the office or clinic are often managed in the ED.[7]

**Prehospital and In-Hospital Epidemiology**

In the prehospital setting, about 10% of ambulance runs are for infants, children, and adolescents.[8] This rate is variable, however, depending on the geographic location of the EMS system. Trauma represents a disproportionately high number of pediatric prehospital complaints, comprising approximately 50% to 65% of transported cases.[9] The most frequent mechanisms of injury are motor vehicle crashes, falls, and burns. Among prehospital illness complaints, the most common are seizures, metabolic/toxic exposures, and cardiopulmonary problems (Table 2-1).[8] The epidemiology of prehospital pediatrics is age dependent, with illness complaints more common among younger children and injury more common with increasing age.

In fact, the 2000 NHAMCS data show that among all patients seen in the ED, 14% arrive by ambulance. For children under 15 years, only 5.3% arrive by ambulance, in contrast to 10.3% for those 15 to 24 years, and 43.1% for patients 75 years and older.[2]

Overall, 16.9% (range 10% to 25%) of pediatric ED visits result in hospitalization,[10] while only 5% of injured children appear to require hospitalization.[6] However, these data vary widely in different communities depending on transfer rates, primary physician ED utilization patterns, and the overall socioeconomic status of the population. Another factor in pediatric hospitalization rates might be the hospital site of ED evaluation; one review found a 3.8% pediatric admission rate from the general ED, versus an 11% rate for a pediatric ED.[11] In contrast, a 2002 Canadian report on admission rates for bronchiolitis in Calgary found a 24% admission rate for children seen in pediatric EDs, compared to a 43% admission rate for those seen with similar characteristics in general EDs.[12] Admission experiences can vary widely in geographic locations, and children's hospital EDs might care for children with different levels of illness and acuity than general EDs.

Types of illness complaint can also vary among hospitals. The most common medical admission diagnoses for general and pediatric EDs are outlined in Table 2-2.[11]

**Injuries**

Injuries are the most common reason for pediatric presentations to the ED, and unintentional injuries are the leading cause of death in children older than 1 year. In the ED survey, the highest rate of injury occurred in 15-year-olds to 17-year-olds (21.1 per 100 [average across all ages, 17.8 per 100]).[6] Thirty-three percent of a 1-year cohort of children presenting to a pediatric ED in children's hospital in Hawaii had injury complaints (trauma, burns, water-related events, or child abuse).[13] There can be significant differences between general EDs and pediatric EDs with respect to frequency of injury complaints in children; one analysis indicated that 41% of children in a general ED had injury complaints, compared to only 22% at a pediatric ED.[11]

| TABLE 2-1 | Prehospital Pediatric Emergencies |
|---|---|
| Injuries | Illnesses |
| • Motor vehicle crashes | • Seizures |
| • Falls | • Toxic/metabolic exposures |
| • Burns | • Cardiopulmonary problems |

| TABLE 2-2 | Pediatric Medical Admission Diagnoses |
|---|---|
| General ED | Pediatric ED |
| • Seizures | • Chronic disease |
| • Poisoning | • Abdominal pain |
| • Asthma | • Poisoning |
| • Abdominal pain | • Seizures |
| | • Asthma |

Source: Nelson DS, Walsh K, Fleisher G. Spectrum and frequency of pediatric illness presenting to a general community hospital emergency department. *Pediatrics.* 1992;90(1):5–10. Reprinted with permission.

Using mortality data, it appears that serious pediatric injuries are most frequently caused by motor vehicles, the child being either an occupant or a pedestrian. The exception would be among infants for whom homicide secondary to child maltreatment is most prominent. Occupant injuries are the most common cause of death among teenagers and young adults, whereas pedestrian and bicycle-associated motor vehicle crashes are the most common cause in children. Burns, submersion injury, and violent death from homicide and suicide are also extremely important mechanisms of injury-related death in childhood.[14]

One large study of pediatric injuries treated in Massachusetts EDs showed that sprains, lacerations, and contusions were the most common problems.[15] Another revealed that sprains, lacerations, fractures, and mild head injuries accounted for 90% of pediatric trauma in a general ED. Lacerations on the head and face accounted for 60% of all lacerations; the phalanx was the most common fracture site, followed by radius/ulna.[11]

### Illnesses

Respiratory diagnoses were the leading cause of illness-related ED visits for all age groups (0 to 20 years), accounting for 30% of visits.[6] Wheezing-related illness conditions were the most common noninjury complaints in the Hawaii children's hospital 1-year cohort, representing 14% of all presentations[13] In the comparative Massachusetts study, illness complaints varied significantly with ED type. In both the general and pediatric ED, however, fever and respiratory distress were the most frequent complaints. Upper respiratory infections (URI) and sore throat were more common in general ED pediatric patients than in pediatric ED patients, while fever, respiratory distress, abdominal pain, and gastroenteritis were more common in the pediatric ED.[11]

Respiratory illness is the leading reason for hospitalization of children. Asthma, pneumonia, and bronchiolitis together represent about one third of pediatric hospitalizations. Seizures and gastroenteritis are also important reasons for hospitalization. Deaths from illness during the neonatal period are most frequently due to congenital anomalies or birth-related conditions. The 2000 Vital Statistics revealed that the overall infant mortality rate fell to 6.9 deaths per 1000 live births, the lowest annual rate ever recorded in the US. However, infant death rates were strongly affected by race, with only 5.7 deaths per 1000 live births for whites, compared with 14.1 deaths per 1000 live births for blacks.[14] Deaths from illness during the neonatal period were most frequently due to congenital malformations, disorders related to prematurity, and low birth weight.[14] Most post neonatal noninjury mortality in childhood is secondary to sudden infant death syndrome (SIDS).[14] The overwhelming majority of unexpected pediatric (younger than 18 years) out-of-hospital cardiopulmonary arrests occur in children younger than 2 years, and most of those before age 1 are due to SIDS. Overall, pediatric death from illness is more common than from injury, but after age 12 months, injury is more likely.[14]

## Clinical Features

### Initial Assessment

The initial assessment has two parts: the visual and auditory general impression and the hands-on assessment of the ABCDEs. Using a developmentally appropriate approach will improve the sensitivity of the examination by adjusting the assessment technique to the expected growth and behavioral characteristics of the individual child.

Speedy assessment is essential to identify abnormal physiology and anatomy, to determine severity and urgency for intervention, and to guide general and specific treatment. For injury, the assessment is sometimes straightforward because the cause or mechanism of injury is usually known, the child's symptom is pain, and signs of obvious tissue deformity might identify the problem. The child still needs careful physical evaluation for physiologic problems and for less obvious but possibly serious injuries, particularly involving the brain or abdominal cavity. For illness, the assessment can be much trickier, especially in the infant, because onset, progression, and specific symptoms can be vague and signs of disease may be nonspecific.

A 21-month-old girl is brought to the emergency department after a 9-1-1 call. The mother explains that the child, who has a tracheostomy, has had copious secretions and has required more frequent suctioning and breathing treatments for 2 days. The child has severe cerebral palsy. The mother is anxious and demanding immediate hospitalization for the child. The child turns blue and becomes agitated whenever you approach but is easily consoled by the mother. There are no retractions or flaring. Her respiratory rate is 50 breaths/min and heart rate is 140 bpm. You are unable to obtain a blood pressure.

1. *How can the Pediatric Assessment Triangle be used to evaluate the severity of illness and urgency for care in a child with special health care needs?*

## Developing a General Impression: The Pediatric Assessment Triangle (PAT)

An approach to the initial assessment that represents the unique adaptations for children is the PAT. The PAT is a rapid, simple, and useful tool to assess children of all ages with all levels of illness and injury. The tool brings together the pediatric features of the first general impression, and it works for children with either illness or injury. Since the introduction of the PAT in the *Advanced Pediatric Life Support* (APLS) and *Pediatric Education for Prehospital Professionals* (PEPP) Courses, this pediatric evaluation tool has become a basic assessment model in national and international life support education.

The PAT is an easy way to begin the initial assessment of any child (Figure 2.1)[16] using only visual and auditory clues. Performing the PAT at the point of first contact with the patient will help identify key physiologic problems, establish a level of severity, and determine urgency for life support. It is based on listening and seeing and does not require a stethoscope, blood pressure cuff, cardiac monitor, or pulse oximeter. The PAT can be completed in 30 to 60 seconds. In reality, the PAT is a paradigm of the across-the-room assessment—an intuitive process for experienced pediatric providers.

Together, the three components of the PAT reflect the child's overall physiologic status, or

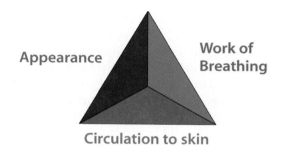

**Figure 2.1** Pediatric Assessment Triange (PAT).

the child's general state of oxygenation, ventilation, perfusion, and brain function. The components are: appearance, work of breathing, and circulation to skin. It is not a diagnostic tool; the PAT is an assessment tool that facilitates immediate physiologic evaluation by the clinician in emergency circumstances that require rapid life support decisions.

### Appearance

The child's general appearance is the most important thing to consider when determining how severe the illness or injury is, the need for treatment, and the response to therapy. Appearance reflects the adequacy of ventilation, oxygenation, brain perfusion, body homeostasis, and central nervous system (CNS) function.

There are many specific physical characteristics that help define a child's appearance. Some of the most important are summarized

| TABLE 2-3 | Characteristics of Appearance |
|---|---|

**The "Tickles" (TICLS) Mnemonic**

Characteristic

Features to look for

- **T**one

  Is she moving or vigorously resisting examination? Does she have good muscle tone? Or is she limp, listless, or flaccid?

- **I**nteractiveness

  How alert is she? How readily does a person, object, or sound distract her or draw her attention? Will she reach for, grasp, and play with a toy or exam instrument, like a penlight or tongue blade? Or is she uninterested in playing or interacting with the caregiver?

- **C**onsolability

  Can she be consoled or comforted by the caregiver? Or is her crying or agitation unrelieved by gentle reassurance?

- **L**ook/Gaze

  Does she fix her gaze on a face? Or is there a nobody-home, glassy-eyed stare?

- **S**peech/Cry

  Is her speech or cry strong and spontaneous? Or is it weak, muffled, or hoarse?

Adapted from: Dieckmann R, Brownstein D, Gausche-Hill M, eds. *Pediatric Education for Prehospital Professionals.* Sudbury, Ma: Jones and Bartlett Publishers, American Academy of Pediatrics; 2000:36.

in the "tickles" (TICLS) mnemonic: tone, interactiveness, consolability, look/gaze, and speech/cry (Table 2-3).[16] TICLS is an easy mnemonic to recall key physical characteristics of a child's appearance.

Identifying abnormal appearance might be a better way to detect subtle abnormalities in behavior that reflects underlying physiologic problems than adult-oriented neurologic scoring systems, such as the conventional AVPU scale or the Glasgow Coma Scale (GCS). Children with mild to moderate illness or injury can be alert on the AVPU and 15 (best score) on the GCS, and have an abnormal appearance.

### Techniques to Assess Appearance

Assess the child's appearance from the doorway. This is Step 1 in the PAT. Techniques for assessment of a conscious child's appearance include observing from a distance, allowing the child to remain in the caregiver's lap or arms, using distractions such as bright lights or toys to measure interactiveness, and kneeling down to be on eye level with the child. An immediate hands-on approach can cause agitation and crying and confuses the assessment. Unless a child is unconscious or obviously lethargic, get as much information as possible by observing before touching the child or taking vital signs.

One example of a child with a normal appearance might be an infant with good eye contact and good color who is reaching for a tongue blade. An example of an infant with a worrisome appearance might be a toddler who makes poor eye contact and is pale or mottled and listless (Figure 2.2).

Abnormal appearance can be due to lack of oxygen, ventilation, or brain perfusion. It can be the result of systemic problems such as poisoning, infection, or hypoglycemia. In another child, it can be due to acute brain injury from hemorrhage or edema, or to chronic brain injury from shaken baby syndrome. Regardless of what might be the cause, a grossly abnormal appearance establishes that the child is seriously ill or injured. Immediately begin life support efforts to increase oxygenation, ventilation, and perfusion while completing the hands-on assessment.

Although an alert, interactive child is usually not critically ill, there are some cases in which a child is critically ill or injured with-

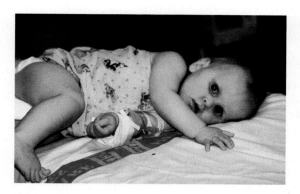

Figure 2.2 Abnormal appearance.

out having an abnormal appearance. Toxicologic or traumatic emergencies are good examples as follows:

- A child with a dangerous intoxication, such as from acetaminophen, iron, or cyclic antidepressants, might not show symptoms immediately after ingestion. Despite normal appearance, the child can develop deadly complications in the coming minutes or hours.

- A child with blunt trauma might be able to maintain adequate core perfusion despite internal bleeding by increasing cardiac output and systemic vascular resistance and might appear normal. When these compensatory mechanisms fail, the child might show rapid progression to decompensated shock.

Age differences are associated with important developmental differences in psychomotor and social skills. Therefore, normal or expected appearance and behavior vary by age group. Children of all ages engage their environment. For newborns, this occurs by energetic sucking and crying. For older infants, it occurs through smiling or tracking a light. For toddlers, it is by exploring and touching their surroundings. And for most adolescents, it is by talking. Knowing normal development for children of different age groups will guide the approach to children of all ages and will result in more accurate judgments about appearances. Table 2-4 summarizes important behavioral characteristics of children of different developmental ages and provides developmentally appropriate assessment techniques.

Although appearance reflects real illness or injury, it does not always show the cause of injury or illness. Appearance is the screening portion of the PAT. The other elements of the PAT—work of breathing and circulation to skin—provide more specific information about the type of physiologic derangement. They help to show the likely cause of system dysfunction while also providing additional clues about severity.

## Work of Breathing

Work of breathing is a more rapid indicator of oxygenation and ventilation than respiratory rate or chest sounds on auscultation—the traditional measures of breathing in adults. Work of breathing reflects the child's attempt to compensate for abnormalities in oxygenation and ventilation. Assessing work of breathing requires listening carefully for audible abnormal airway sounds and looking for signs of increased breathing effort. It is another hands-off evaluation method. Table 2-5 summarizes the key characteristics of work of breathing.

### Abnormal Audible Airway Sounds

Examples of abnormal airway sounds that can be heard without a stethoscope are snoring, muffled or hoarse speech, stridor, grunting, and wheezing. Abnormal airway sounds provide excellent anatomic and physiologic information about breathing effort and type and anatomic location of the breathing problem. They also help determine the severity of the problem.

Snoring, muffled or hoarse speech, and stridor suggest upper airway obstruction. The location in the upper airway where the obstruction exists determines the quality of the abnormal sounds. Snoring occurs if the oropharynx or hypopharynx is partially obstructed by the tongue and soft tissues. A gurgling sound suggests the presence of blood, secretions, or foreign body in the oropharynx or hypopharynx. Muffled or hoarse speech is abnormal vocalization, or expiratory sounds

| TABLE 2-4 | Behavioral Characteristics and Special Assessment Techniques | |
|---|---|---|
| Developmental Age | Behavioral Characteristics | Special Assessment Techniques |
| Neonate | Primitive reflexes only | Immediately assess airway, breathing, heart rate, and color. Because the neonate has no interactive behavior yet, focus assessment of appearance on muscle tone, spontaneous motor activity, and quality of cry. |
| Infant<br>Under 2 months | Physiologic responses<br>No separation anxiety | Obtain the pregnancy and delivery history, because manifestations of intrapartum or perinatal disease often manifest in this age. Signs of serious illness might be nonspecific, so a history of fussiness, feeding difficulty, or poor sleeping can be significant symptom of sepsis, metabolic abnormality, or a central nervous system problem. An episode of choking, apnea, loss of tone, or change in skin color might represent an apparent life-threatening event, or ALTE. Examine in any position. |
| 2–6 months | Social skills (smiles, tracks), motor skills (rolls over, sits, reaches), and vocalization | As infants develop a wider range of behaviors and become more interactive with the environment, TICLS as a measure of appearance becomes a more reliable indicator of disease and injury. Examine in any position and use distraction. Use calm, lilting speech to soothe and engage child. |
| 6–12 months | Socially interactive<br>Stranger/separation anxiety<br>Sits without support<br>Plays, babbles | Leave child on caregiver's lap. Anticipate stranger anxiety. Sit or squat at child's level. Offer toys and distractions (tongue blade, penlight). Examine toe-to-head. |
| Toddler | Fearless curiosity<br>Strong opinions, illogical<br>Egocentrism<br>Stranger/separation anxiety<br>Wide verbal variability | Approach gently and observe from the doorway. Leave the child on the caregiver's lap and get down to the child's level. Enlist the caregiver's assistance. Use distraction. Talk to the child about herself. Employ endless praise and reassurance. Explain procedures simply. Do the exam toe-to-head. |
| Preschooler | Magical, illogical thinkers<br>Misconceptions about illness and injury but logical<br>Fears of mutilation, loss of control, death, darkness, and being alone<br>Good language skills<br>Examine head-to-toe. | Speak directly to the child. Choose words carefully and clarify misconceptions. Use dolls or puppets for explanation. Allow the child to handle equipment and ask for her help. Set limits on behavior. Use games and distractions. Praise cooperation and avoid ridicule. |
| School-aged Child | Talkative, analytical<br>Understand cause and effect<br>Want involvement in care<br>Fears of separation, loss of control, pain, and physical disability | Speak directly to child and provide simple explanations. Anticipate questions and fears. Explain procedures and never lie. Respect privacy. Do not negotiate but provide options. Involve the child in the treatment. |
| Adolescent | Mobile, experimental, illogical<br>Understand cause and effect<br>Expressive<br>Fears of loss of independence, loss of control, body image | Explain everything. Encourage questions. Show respect and speak directly to patient. Be honest and nonjudgmental. Honor modesty and confidentiality. Do not succumb to provocation. Ask friends for assistance. |
| Child with Special Health Care Needs | Developmental age can be quite different than chronological age.<br>Child might represent mix of physical and emotional abnormalities. | Use understandable language and techniques. Do not assume the child is mentally impaired. Use information from caregiver and physician when possible. |

Adapted from: Dieckmann R, Brownstein D, Gausche-Hill M. eds. *Pediatric Education for Prehospital Professionals.* Sudbury, Ma: Jones and Bartlett Publishers, American Academy of Pediatrics; 2000:30–57.

| TABLE 2-5 | Characteristics of Work of Breathing |
|---|---|
| Characteristic | Features to Look for |
| Abnormal airway sounds | Snoring, muffled or hoarse speech; stridor; grunting; wheezing |
| Abnormal positioning | Sniffing position, tripoding, refusal to lie down |
| Retractions | Supraclavicular, intercostal, or substernal retractions of the chest wall; head bobbing in infants |
| Flaring | Nasal flaring |

Source: Dieckmann R, Brownstein D, Gausche-Hill M. eds. *Pediatric Education for Prehospital Professionals.* Sudbury, Ma: Jones and Bartlett Publishers, American Academy of Pediatrics; 2000:38. Reprinted with permission.

that occur when the child attempts to talk. Obstruction at or slightly above the level of the vocal cords or larynx produces these alterations in speech. Stridor is an inspiratory, high-pitched sound produced by obstruction at the level of the larynx or lower in the trachea and bronchi.

Obstruction of upper airway passages occurs in a variety of illnesses and injuries. Snoring or gurgling can be heard in a postictal child with posterior displacement of the tongue or in a child with a large tongue hematoma. Muffled or hoarse speech, or a "hot potato" voice, is common in the setting of peritonsillar abscess. Abnormal speech can also reflect a laryngeal fracture after blunt neck trauma. Stridor is most often from viral laryngotracheobronchitis (croup); foreign body aspiration is another cause in younger children.

Grunting is an instinctive mechanism to keep alveoli open for maximal gas exchange. Grunting involves exhaling against a partially closed glottis. It is a marker of alveolar lung disease or injury. This short, low-pitched sound is best heard at the end of the exhalation. Grunting is often present in children with moderate to severe hypoxia, and it reflects poor gas exchange because of fluid in the lower airways and air sacs. Some of the conditions that cause hypoxia and grunting are pneumonia, pulmonary contusion, and pulmonary edema.

Wheezing is the movement of air across partially blocked small airways. It is caused by lower airway obstruction, usually because of bronchoconstriction and edema from asthma or bronchiolitis. In the early phases of lower airway obstruction, wheezing is present during exhalation only and can be heard only by auscultation. As the obstruction increases and breathing requires more work, wheezing occurs during both inhalation and exhalation. With more obstruction, wheezing is audible without a stethoscope. Finally, if respiratory failure develops, work of breathing can diminish and the wheezing might not be heard at all. The most common cause of wheezing in childhood is asthma, although bronchiolitis, allergic reaction, and foreign objects in the lower airway are also possible etiologies, especially in infants and toddlers.

### Visual Signs

There are several useful visual signs of increased work of breathing. These signs reflect increased breathing effort by the child to improve oxygenation and ventilation. Examples of visual signs that represent instinctive actions to compensate for hypoxic stress are abnormal positioning, retractions, nasal flaring, and tachypnea.

Abnormal positioning is immediately evident from the doorway. There are several types of posture that indicate compensatory efforts to increase airflow. A child who is in the "sniffing" position is trying to line up the axes of the airways to open the airway and increase airflow. This position is usually the result of severe upper airway obstruction (Figure 2.3) from such conditions as retropharyngeal abscess, foreign body aspiration, or epiglottitis. The child who refuses to lie down or who leans forward on outstretched arms (tripod position) is trying to use accessory muscles to improve breathing (Figure 2.4). This sign is

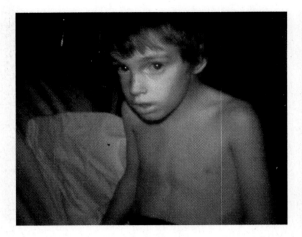

Figure 2.3 The sniffing position is an abnormal position and reflects upper airway obstruction.

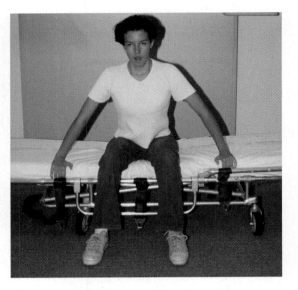

Figure 2.4 The abnormal tripod position indicates the patient's attempts to maximize accessory muscle use.

observed in children with severe bronchoconstriction from asthma or bronchiolitis. The sniffing position and the tripod position are abnormal and indicate increased work of breathing and severe respiratory distress.

Retractions are common physical signs of increased work of breathing. They represent use of accessory muscles to help breathing. Retractions are easily missed unless the clinician looks for them specifically after the child is properly exposed. Retractions are a more useful measure of work of breathing in children than in adults. This is because a child's chest wall is less muscular and thinner, and the inward excursion of skin and soft tissue between the ribs is visually more apparent. Retractions are a sign that the child is recruiting extra muscle power to try to expand the chest more fully and move more air into the lungs. They can be in the supraclavicular area (above the clavicle), the intercostal area (between the ribs), or the substernal area (under the sternum), as illustrated in Figure 2.5.

The amount and location of retractions reflect the severity and degree of hypoxia. A child with mild retractions in only one anatomic area, such as the intercostal area, is obviously not working as hard and does not have as severe a hypoxic insult as a child with deep retractions in more anatomic areas. When a child exhausts compensatory mechanisms and approaches respiratory failure, retractions can paradoxically decrease. This is an ominous

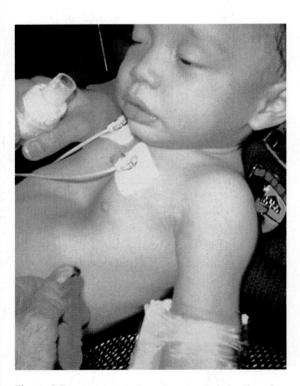

Figure 2.5 Retractions indicate increased work of breathing and can occur in the supraclavicular, intercostal, and substernal areas.

trend and signals impending respiratory arrest. Assisted ventilation is imperative.

One form of accessory muscle use in infants is head bobbing—the use of neck muscles to improve breathing during severe hypoxia. The child extends the neck while inhaling, then allows the head to fall forward while exhaling. This visual sign suggests moderate to severe hypoxia.

Tachypnea is another visual clue to increased work of breathing, but it can be deceptive. The specific, counted respiratory rate must be age adjusted for interpretation The range of normal respiratory rates in children is wide and is subject to great variability in emergency settings where pain, cold, and anxiety can cause mild to moderate tachypnea in the absence of hypoxia. In addition, tachypnea can reflect a physiologic response to metabolic acidosis and might not represent a primary respiratory abnormality at all. Respiratory rates that are too fast (greater than 60/min) or too slow (less than 12 to 20 breaths per min) might not be adequate to maintain minute ventilation. Remember, minute ventilation (MV) is equal to respiratory rate (RR) times tidal volume (TV), or $MV = RR \times TV$. Rates that are too slow will decrease MV as TV cannot be increased to compensate, and rates that are too fast result in a marked decrease in TV and therefore MV.

Nasal flaring is another form of accessory muscle use that reflects significantly increased work of breathing (**Figure 2.6**). Flaring is the exaggerated opening of the nostrils during labored breathing and indicates moderate to severe hypoxia. Inspect the face specifically to detect flaring, as it is easily missed.

### Techniques to Assess Work of Breathing
Step 2 in the PAT is assessing work of breathing. Begin by listening carefully from a distance for abnormal audible airway sounds, then looking for key visual signs. From the doorway, try to hear abnormal sounds. Then note if the child has abnormal positioning, especially the sniffing posture or tripoding. Next, have the caregiver uncover the chest of the child for direct inspection or have the child undress on the caregiver's lap. Look for the quality and location of intercostal, supraclavicular, and substernal retractions and note if there is head bobbing in infants. After examining for retractions, note if the respiratory rate is grossly increased. Last, inspect for nasal flaring.

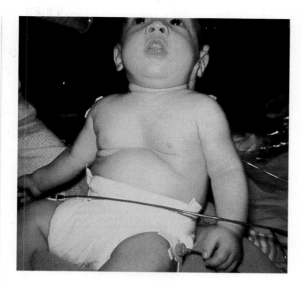

**Figure 2.6** Nasal flaring indicates increased work of breathing and moderate to severe hypoxia.

Children can have increased work of breathing because of abnormalities anywhere in their airways, air sacs, pleurae, or chest walls. However, assessing these auditory and visual characteristics together helps to show the type of problem and the degree of distress. The type of abnormal airway sound gives an important clue to the anatomic location of the illness or injury process, whereas the number and type of visual signs of increased work of breathing help in determining the degree of physiologic stress.

Combining assessment of appearance and work of breathing can also help establish the severity of the child's illness or injury. If a child readily compensates for hypoxic stress by increasing work of breathing, the brain is perfused with relatively normal levels of oxygen and carbon dioxide, so appearance is relatively normal. A child with normal appearance and increased work of breathing is in respiratory distress—a compensated physiologic state that describes most cases of respiratory illnesses and injuries of childhood. However, if increased work of breathing does not compensate for the hypoxic stress, the brain is perfused with blood with decreased oxygen content. If further decompensation occurs and breathing becomes increasingly inadequate, the brain experiences both decreased oxygen and increased

**Signs of Increased Work of Breathing**
- Abnormal airway positioning
- Retractions
- Nasal flaring
- Head bobbing
- Stridor
- Wheezing
- Grunting

| TABLE 2-6 | Characteristics of Circulation to Skin | |
| --- | --- | --- |
| **Characteristic** | **Features** | |
| • Pallor | • White or pale skin or mucous membrane coloration from inadequate blood flow | |
| • Mottling | • Patchy skin discoloration due to vasoconstriction | |
| • Cyanosis | • Bluish discoloration of skin and mucous membranes | |

Source: Dieckmann R, Brownstein D, Gausche-Hill M, eds. *Pediatric Education for Prehospital Professionals.* Sudbury, Ma: Jones and Bartlett Publishers, American Academy of Pediatrics; 2000:40. Reprinted with permission.

carbon dioxide. Hypoxia causes restlessness and agitation, and hypercapnia causes lethargy and diminished responsiveness. Hence, the patient's appearance in states of acute hypoxia and hypercapnia is distinctly abnormal. The combination of abnormal appearance and increased work of breathing indicates an uncompensated physiologic state that is termed respiratory failure. Finally, the combination of abnormal appearance and abnormally decreased work of breathing implies impending respiratory arrest.

## Circulation to Skin

The goal of rapid circulatory assessment is to determine the adequacy of cardiac output and the perfusion of vital organs. Heart rate, blood pressure, and cardiac auscultation—key indicators of circulatory function in adults—are not helpful in forming an accurate general impression in a child and, like respiratory rate, can be deferred to the ABCDE, hands-on phase of the initial assessment. The child's appearance is one indicator of perfusion, because inadequate perfusion of the brain will cause abnormal behavior. But abnormal appearance can be caused by many conditions other than decreased perfusion. For this reason, other signs of perfusion must be added to the appearance evaluation to assess the child's circulatory condition.

An important sign of perfusion in children is circulation to skin. When cardiac output is too low, the body compensates by increasing heart rate and by shutting down circulation to nonessential anatomic areas, such as the skin and mucous membranes, in order to preserve blood supply to the most vital organs (brain, heart, and kidneys). Therefore, in most children who have inadequate core perfusion, circulation to skin is dramatically diminished by intense neuromotor regulation. Hence, visual signs reflect the overall status of core circulation. Pallor, mottling, and cyanosis are visual indicators of reduced circulation to skin and mucous membranes. Table 2-6 summarizes these characteristics.

Pallor is usually the first sign of poor skin or mucous membrane perfusion. It can also be a sign of anemia or hypoxia. Mottling is caused by constriction of blood vessels to the skin and is another sign of poor perfusion (Figure 2.7).

Cyanosis is a blue discoloration of the skin and mucous membranes. Do not confuse acrocyanosis—blue hands and feet in a newborn or infant less than 2 months of age—with true cyanosis. Acrocyanosis is a normal finding when a young infant is cold, and it reflects vasomotor instability rather than hypoxia or shock (Figure 2.8). True cyanosis is a late finding of respiratory failure or shock. A hypoxic child is likely to show other physical abnormalities long before turning blue, including abnormal appearance and increased work of breathing. A child in shock will also have pallor or mottling. Never wait for cyanosis to begin supplemental oxygen. Acute cyanosis is

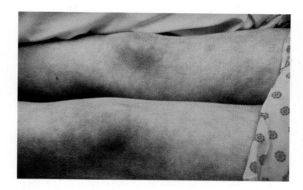

**Figure 2.7** Mottling is the result of constriction of blood vessels to the skin and can indicate poor perfusion.

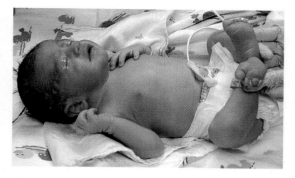

**Figure 2.8** Acrocyanosis. Source: Kattwinkel J, ed. *Textbook of Neonatal Resuscitation* 5th ed. Elk Grove, Ill: American Academy of Pediatrics and American Heart Association; 2006:A-4.

always a critical sign of either hypoxia and/or ischemia that requires immediate intervention with breathing support.

Abnormal circulation to skin in combination with normal appearance can suggest compensated shock. The abnormal appearance in compensated shock can be subtle, and some children seem remarkably alert. However, if the circulatory stress continues and compensatory mechanisms fail to compensate, the brain receives inadequate blood supply and appearance becomes abnormal. Poor motor tone, lack of interactiveness, restlessness, and listlessness are important indicators of disordered physiology. When observed in a child with abnormal circulation to skin, especially with a history of volume loss or blunt injury, these characteristics suggest perfusion failure or decompensated shock.

Another clue for the presence of shock is tachypnea without signs of increased work of breathing; this is called effortless tachypnea and represents the child's attempt to blow off extra carbon dioxide to correct the acidosis generated by poor perfusion. Effortless tachypnea is different from the rapid and labored respirations and increased work of breathing present with illnesses and injuries associated with primary oxygenation and ventilation problems.

**Techniques to Assess Circulation to Skin**

Step 3 in the PAT is evaluating circulation to skin. Be sure the child is exposed enough for visual inspection but not cold. Cold can cause false skin signs. In other words, the cold child can have normal core perfusion but abnormal circulation to skin. Cold circulating air temperature is the most common reason for misinterpretation of skin signs.

Inspect the skin and mucous membranes for pallor, mottling, and cyanosis. Look at the face, chest, abdomen, and extremities. Then, inspect the lips for cyanosis. In dark-skinned children, circulation to skin is sometimes more difficult to assess. The lips and mucous membranes in the mouth might be the best places to look.

## Using the PAT to Evaluate Severity and Illness or Injury

Combining the three components of the PAT can answer three critical questions: What is the most likely physiologic abnormality? How severe is the child's illness or injury? How fast do I have to intervene, and what type of general and specific treatment should I give?

The three elements of the PAT work together and allow rapid assessment of the child's overall physiologic stability, and allow the physician to form a general impression. For example, if a child is interactive and pink but has a few intercostal retractions, the general impression would be respiratory distress. In this PAT configuration, take time to approach the child in a developmentally appropriate manner to complete the initial assessment, including a careful hands-on ABCDE evaluation. On the other hand, if the child is limp with unlabored rapid breathing and pale or mottled skin, the PAT suggests decompensated shock. In this case, move rapidly through the initial assessment and begin resuscitation based on the ABCDEs. A child who has abnormal appearance but normal work of breathing and normal circulation to skin, could have an important and potentially dangerous combination of PAT characteristics suggesting a primary brain dysfunction or a major metabolic or systemic problem, such as postictal state, subdural hemorrhage, brain concussion, intoxication, hypoglycemia, or sepsis. Table 2-7 provides a summary of different PAT configurations with the general impression or physiologic state and potential emergency etiologies.

The PAT has two important advantages. First, it quickly gives the clinician critical information about the child's physiologic status before touching or agitating the child. This is important because it can be difficult to identify abnormal appearance, increased work of breathing, or decreased circulation to skin when a child is agitated and crying. Second, the PAT helps set priorities for the rest of the hands-on initial assessment. The PAT takes only seconds to complete, it identifies the need for lifesaving interventions, and it blends into the next phase of hands-on physical assessment.

The three components of the PAT—appearance, work of breathing, and circulation to skin—can be assessed in any order. Unlike the PAT, the ABCDEs of resuscitation must be done in order.

| TABLE 2-7 | PAT Configurations and Emergency Etiologies | | | |
|---|---|---|---|---|
| Appearance | Work of Breathing | Circulation to Skin | General Impression of Physiologic State | Examples of Etiologies |
| Abnormal | Normal | Normal | Primary brain dysfunction<br><br>Systemic problem | Shaken baby<br>Brain injury<br>Sepsis<br>Hypoglycemia<br>Intoxication |
| Normal | Abnormal | Normal | Respiratory distress | Mild asthma<br>Bronchiolitis<br>Croup<br>Community-acquired pneumonia<br>Foreign body aspiration |
| Abnormal | Abnormal | Normal | Respiratory failure | Severe Asthma<br>Pulmonary contusion<br>Penetrating chest injury |
| Normal | Normal | Abnormal | Compensated shock | Diarrhea<br>External blood loss |
| Abnormal | Normal | Abnormal | Decompensated shock | Severe gastroenteritis<br>Major burn<br>Major blunt injury<br>Penetrating abdominal injury |
| Abnormal | Abnormal | Abnormal | Cardiopulmonary failure | Cardiopulmonary arrest |

Adapted from: Dieckmann R, Brownstein D, Gausche-Hill M, eds. *Pediatric Education for Prehospital Professionals.* Sudbury, Ma: Jones and Bartlett Publishers, American Academy of Pediatrics; 2000:30–57.

A 7-year-old boy is hit by a car in front of his home. He was thrown 5 feet and had loss of consciousness. The boy did awake, but the father decided to take him to the physician's office when he noted the boy becoming sleepy.

In the office, the boy opens his eyes with a loud verbal stimulus but will not speak or interact. There are no abnormal airway sounds, but intercostal retractions and flaring are present. His skin is pale. Respiratory rate is 50 breaths/min, heart rate is 145 bpm, and blood pressure is 90 palp. The chest is clear with decreased tidal volume. The skin feels cool; capillary refill time is 4 seconds, and brachial pulse is present. Pupils are equal and reactive. He has a large frontal hematoma.

1. *Does this child's assessment suggest serious injury?*
2. *What actions are required by the physician in the office?*
3. *How should this child be transported to the emergency department?*

## Assessing the Pediatric ABCDEs

The initial assessment has two main parts: the PAT, and the hands-on physical assessment of the ABCDEs. The PAT provides the general impression of the pediatric patient. The PAT uses pediatric-specific observations in combination with the chief complaint to evaluate the efficacy of cardiopulmonary function, to establish a level of severity, and to determine urgency for care. The intent is to provide an objective overview of the child and an instant picture of the child's physiologic status.

The second part of the initial assessment is an ordered, hands-on, physical evaluation of the ABCDEs. It provides a prioritized sequence of life support interventions to reverse organ failure. As in adults, there is a specific order for treating life-threatening problems as they are identified, before moving to the next step. The steps are the same as with adults, but there are important pediatric differences in anatomy, physiology, and signs of distress. ABCDE assessment includes the following components:

- Airway
- Breathing
- Circulation
- Disability
- Exposure

## Airway

The PAT will usually identify the presence of airway obstruction. However, the loudness of the stridor or wheezing is not necessarily related to the amount of airway obstruction. For example, asthmatic children in severe distress might have little or no wheezing. Similarly, a child with an upper airway foreign body below the vocal cords could have minimal stridor. Abnormal airway sounds tell whether there is any amount of upper or lower airway obstruction.

### Techniques to Assess and Manage the Airway

If the airway is not open, perform manual airway-opening maneuvers such as the head tilt-chin lift, or the jaw thrust maneuver in a trauma patient. Maintain a neutral neck position. Suction frequently. Determine if the airway is maintainable or not maintainable with manual techniques and suction.

If positioning and suctioning do not establish a patent airway, consider airway obstruction. Perform age-specific obstructed airway techniques (back blow and chest thrusts for children <1 year of age; abdominal thrusts [Heimlich maneuver] for children ≥1 year of age), then consider direct laryngoscopy with Magill forceps. If airway obstruction continues, perform alternative airway access procedures using needle or surgical cricothyrotomy depending on the child's age, provider skill level, and available equipment (see Chapter 22, Emergency Medical Procedures).

If the airway is open, look for chest rise with breathing. If gurgling is present, suction carefully, because this means there is mucus, blood, or a foreign body in the mouth or airway.

## Breathing

### Respiratory Rate

Determine the respiratory rate per minute by counting the number of chest rises in 30 seconds, then doubling that number. Interpret the respiratory rate carefully. Normal infants might show periodic breathing, or stopping and starting breathing for less than 20 seconds. Therefore, counting for only 10 to 15 seconds can result in a respiratory rate that is too low.

Respiratory rates can be difficult to interpret. Rapid respiratory rates can simply reflect high fever, anxiety, pain, or excitement. As an example, for every degree in temperature elevation, the respiratory rate will increase by 2 to 5 respirations per minute. Normal rates, on the other hand, can occur in a child who has been breathing rapidly with increased work of breathing for some time and is now becoming fatigued. Finally, interpret respiratory rate based on what is normal for age. Table 2-8 shows the range of normal respiratory rate for age.

Recording several respiratory rates can be especially useful, and the trend is sometimes more accurate than the first documented rate. A sustained increase or decrease in respiratory rate is often significant. Use the respiratory rate in conjunction with other information about breathing.

Pay close attention to extremes of respiratory rate. A very rapid respiratory rate (more than 60/min for any age), especially with abnormal appearance or marked retractions, indicates respiratory distress and possibly respiratory failure. An abnormally slow respiratory rate is always worrisome because it might mean respiratory failure. Red flags are respiratory rates of less than 20/min for children younger than 6 years, and of less than 12/min for children younger than 15 years. A normal respiratory rate alone never determines that breathing is adequate. The respiratory rate must be interpreted with appearance, work of breathing, and air movement.

### Auscultation

Listen with a stethoscope over the midaxillary line to hear abnormal lung sounds in inhalation and exhalation, such as crackles and wheezing (Figure 2.9). Inspiratory crackles indicate alveolar disease. Expiratory wheezing indicates lower airway obstruction. Also evaluate air movement and effectiveness of work of breathing. A child with increased work of breathing and poor air movement might be in impending respiratory failure.

Table 2-9 lists abnormal breath sounds, their causes, and common examples of associated disease processes.

| TABLE 2-8 | Normal Respiratory Rate for Age |
| --- | --- |
| **Age** | **Respiratory Rate (breaths/min)** |
| Infant | 30–60 |
| Toddler | 24–40 |
| Preschooler | 22–34 |
| School-aged child | 18–30 |
| Adolescent | 12–16 |

Source: Dieckmann R, Brownstein D, Gausche-Hill M, eds. *Pediatric Education for Prehospital Professionals.* Sudbury, Ma: Jones and Bartlett Publishers, American Academy of Pediatrics; 2000:43. Reprinted with permission.

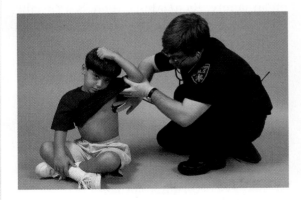

**Figure 2.9** Listen with a stethoscope over the midaxillary line to hear abnormal lung sounds.

| TABLE 2-9 | Interpretation of Breath Sounds | |
|---|---|---|
| **Sound** | **Cause** | **Examples** |
| Stridor | Upper airway obstruction | Croup, foreign body aspiration, retropharyngeal abscess |
| Wheezing | Lower airway obstruction | Asthma, foreign body, bronchiolitis |
| Expiratory grunting | Inadequate oxygenation | Pulmonary contusion, pneumonia, drowning |
| Inspiratory crackles | Fluid, mucus, or blood in the airway | Pneumonia, pulmonary contusion |
| Absent breath sounds despite increased work of breathing | Complete airway obstruction (upper or lower airway), physical barrier to transmission of breath sounds | Foreign body, severe asthma, hemothorax, pneumothorax Pleural fluid, pneumonia, or pneumothorax |

Source: Dieckmann R, Brownstein D, Gausche-Hill M, eds. *Pediatric Education for Prehospital Professionals.* Sudbury, Ma: Jones and Bartlett Publishers, American Academy of Pediatrics; 2000:44. Reprinted with permission.

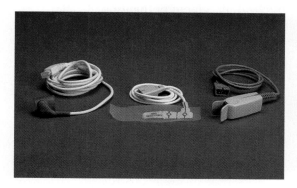

**Figure 2.10A** Various pulse oximeter probes wrap around or clip onto a digit or earlobe.

**Figure 2.10B** Pulse oximetry is an excellent tool for assessing the effectiveness of breathing.

## Oxygen Saturation

After determining the respiratory rate and performing auscultation, determine the child's oxygen saturation level. Pulse oximetry is an excellent tool to use in assessing a child's breathing (**Figure 2.10A**). **Figure 2.10B** illustrates the technique of placing a pulse oximetry probe on a young child. There are various anatomic locations for application of sensors, including fingers, toes, nose, and ear lobe.

A pulse oximetry reading above 94% saturation indicates that oxygenation is probably adequate. A reading below 90% in a child with 100% mask oxygen could be an indication for assisted ventilation. Be careful not to underestimate respiratory distress in a child with a reading above 94%. A child in respiratory distress or early respiratory failure might be able to maintain oxygenation by increasing work of breathing and respiratory rate. This child might not appear to be ill by pulse oximetry findings alone. Interpret oxygen saturation together with work of breathing. Table 2-10 summarizes circumstances in which pulse oximetry can be deceptive and underestimate the level of gas exchange abnormality.

### Measurement of Carbon Dioxide

Measurement of carbon dioxide ($CO_2$) is becoming increasingly available as a monitoring method in selected children. It can identify situations that can potentially result in hypoxia and help in the differential diagnosis of hypoxia. The common techniques include capnometry, capnography, and end-tidal $CO_2$

| TABLE 2-10 | Conditions Associated With Deceptive Pulse Oximetry |
|---|---|
| **Condition** | **Effect on $Sao_2$** |
| Inadequate signal | Abnormally low |
|   -Poor perfusion | |
|   -Patient movement | |
|   -Wrong probe | |
| Tachypnea | Abnormally high |
| Methemoglobinemia | Abnormally high |
| Cyanotic congenital heart disease | Abnormally low |
| Carboxyhemoglobin | Abnormally high |

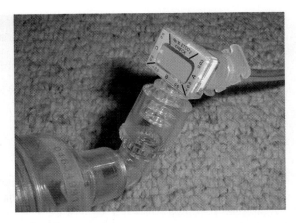

**Figure 2.11** End-tidal $CO_2$ detector device, with purple indicating a measurement <4 mm Hg.

detection. Capnometry suggests measurement or analysis of $CO_2$ production alone, without graphic waveform records. The devices usually provide a continuous, digitalized quantitative measurement. Digitalized colorimetric devices will have either a transcutaneous probe or an infrared sensor in a nasal adaptor or attached to a tracheal tube. Therefore, capnometry and capnography can be used on nonintubated and intubated children. Digital capnometers provide real-time measurements of exhaled $CO_2$ levels through the entire respiratory cycle and will display a digital readout of the inspired and end-tidal $CO_2$ concentrations, as well as the respiratory rate. Infrared sensors can be positioned either in the mainstream tubing or as a side stream of the oxygen delivery system.

A second option in intubated patients is a qualitative, colorimetric end-tidal $CO_2$ measurement. Colorimetric detectors are inexpensive detection devices attached to a tracheal tube; they read only the highest $CO_2$ concentrations at the end of expiration. They use a filter paper that changes color on contact with $CO_2$. Color readings include purple (<4 mm Hg $CO_2$) (Figure 2.11), tan (4 to 15 mm Hg $CO_2$), and yellow (>15 mm Hg $CO_2$) (Figure 2.12).[17] The filter paper begins as purple and should change to yellow with the exhalation phase as $CO_2$ contacts the filter paper. Lack of change of color from purple indicates either esophageal placement or that the patient is not

perfusing, as is the case in cardiopulmonary arrest. Tan represents either retained $CO_2$ in the stomach or states of poor perfusion with tracheal placement of the tube.

Measurement of $CO_2$ has variable value in respiratory assessment, but in selected cases allows better detection of potentially life-threatening problems than clinical judgment alone. It is extremely useful when the child has respiratory distress and is being treated in a monitored setting. The most important use of digital capnometry and capnography is its noninvasive ability to provide an instantaneous measurement of the level of $CO_2$ in the arterial blood.

Important applications of $CO_2$ measurement include:

- Procedural sedation—During procedural sedation, apnea and respiratory depression are important untoward effects of many sedation and analgesic agents. When ventilation decreases, $CO_2$ concentration at the sampling site will fall rapidly and can be instantaneously detected by capnometry or capnography. Therefore, $CO_2$ monitoring can serve as an apnea monitor in neonates, infants, and children and might identify respiratory depression before pulse oximetry or clinical assessment.
- Tracheal tube placement—$CO_2$ monitoring is probably the best way to detect esophageal intubation and displacement of a tracheal tube. $CO_2$ values less than 4 mm Hg indicate esophageal placement in patients with a

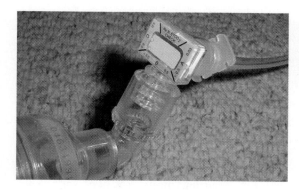

Figure 2.12 End-tidal $CO_2$ detector device, with yellow indicating a measurement >15 mm Hg.

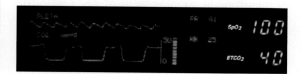

Figure 2.13A Capnograph monitor showing normal end-tidal $CO_2$ wave form. The upper wave form is the pulse oximeter signal ($Sp_{O_2}$). The lower wave form is the end-tidal $CO_2$ ($ETCO_2$) reading. The expected wave form is flat and near 0 during inhalation. During exhalation, the $CO_2$ rises rapidly to a plateau, which then falls rapidly as exhalation ends (forming a square wave). The numerical readout of 40 indicates the $CO_2$ measured during the latter part of exhalation (end tidal), which should correlate with $Pa_{CO_2}$ if pulmonary perfusion is good. If the $ETCO_2$ monitor is in line with an endotracheal tube, such a square wave pattern is a reliable indicator of tracheal intubation.

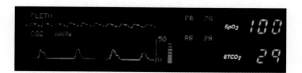

Figure 2.13B Capnograph monitor showing abnormal end-tidal $CO_2$ wave form. The lower wave form ($ETCO_2$) does not have the expected square wave pattern and indicates an abnormal reading. The numerical readout of 29 will not correlate with $Pa_{CO_2}$ since the wave form indicates a source other than normally perfused lungs. Possible causes of this abnormal wave form could be an esophageal intubation or tracheal intubation of poorly perfused lungs (e.g., during less-than-optimal CPR).

pulse. In addition to confirmation of the tracheal tube placement in the trachea, capnography can detect a total occlusion or accidental extubation.

- Monitoring of ventilation—Capnography is not only a reliable noninvasive monitor to predict $PaCO_2$ in awake infants and children who are breathing spontaneously, but also serves as a useful device to monitor $PaCO_2$ during mechanical ventilation of intubated children.

- Monitoring response to treatment—In severe airway obstruction from conditions such as asthma and croup, the shape of the capnogram is altered. With adequate treatment, the capnogram reverts to normal. Hence, capnography appears to be useful as a measure of response to therapy (Figure 2.13).

- Predicting survival in cardiopulmonary arrest—In the child in cardiopulmonary arrest, a persistent capnometry reading less than 4 mm Hg is highly associated with death. One pediatric study and several adult studies have demonstrated significant differences in capnometry readings between survivors and nonsurvivors of cardiopulmonary arrest.[18,19]

- Treatment of herniation syndrome— Capnometry can be helpful in early intracranial pressure regulation in the patient with head injuries. If a child with a unilateral blown pupil and brainstem herniation responds to above-normal ventilatory rates, note the capnometer reading at the time the pupil constricts and maintain minute volume at that level pending surgical intervention.

## Techniques to Assess and Manage Breathing

If the child is in respiratory distress, apply oxygen using an age-appropriate technique that delivers a desired oxygen concentration. If the child is in respiratory failure based on the PAT, assist ventilation with a bag-mask device and 100% oxygen. In selected cases, where the airway is potentially unstable, insert an airway adjunct, either a nasopharyngeal or oropharyngeal airway. Then, after appropriate preoxygenation and ventilation, when equipment and personnel are ready, perform tracheal intubation.

Most children do not require immediate assisted ventilation, and hands-on assessment of breathing is possible in most cases with the child on the caregiver's lap. First, count the respiration rate and interpret the rate for the child's age. Then, listen to the chest, using a nonthreatening approach that does not upset the child and prompt crying. Sometimes it is easier to have the caregiver apply the stethoscope to the chest wall. Next, determine oxygen saturation by pulse oximetry using a suitable probe to obtain a good waveform, and interpret the saturation level in the context of work of breathing. Finally, in selected circumstances, when capnometry or capnography is available in conjunction with pulse oximetry, use measurements of $CO_2$ to further evaluate effectiveness of ventilation.

## Circulation

The PAT provides important visual clues about circulation to skin. Add to these observations with more information from the hands-on evaluation of heart rate, pulse quality, skin temperature, capillary refill time, and blood pressure. In cases where there is potential physiologic instability, attach a cardiac monitor.

### Heart Rate

Guidelines often used to assess adult circulatory status—heart rate and blood pressure—have important limitations in children. First, normal heart rate varies with age, as noted in Table 2-11. Second, tachycardia can be an early sign of hypoxia or low perfusion, but it can also reflect less serious conditions such as fever, anxiety, pain, and excitement. Like respiratory rate, interpret heart rate within the overall history, the PAT, and entire initial assessment. A trend of increasing or decreasing heart rate can be quite useful and might suggest worsening hypoxia or shock or improvement after treatment. When hypoxia or shock becomes critical, heart rate falls, leading to frank bradycardia. Bradycardia (rate less than 60/min in children or less than 100/min in newborns) indicates critical hypoxia and/or ischemia. When the heart rate is above 180/min, a cardiac monitor is necessary to accurately determine heart rate.

### Pulse Quality

Feel the pulse to determine the heart rate. Normally, the brachial pulse is palpable inside or medial to the biceps (Figure 2.14). Note the quality as either weak or strong. If the brachial pulse is strong, the child is probably not hypotensive. If a peripheral pulse cannot be felt, attempt to find a central pulse. Check the femoral pulse in infants and young children, or the carotid pulse in an older child or adolescent. If no pulse is felt, listen for heart tones with a stethoscope over the heart, then count heart rate. Absence of a central pulse is an indication for CPR.

### Skin Temperature and Capillary Refill Time

Next, do a hands-on evaluation of circulation to skin. Is the skin warm or cool? With enough perfusion, the child's skin should be warm near the wrists and ankles. With decreasing perfusion, the line of separation from cool to warm advances up the limb.

Check capillary refill time at the kneecap, foot, toes, hands, or forearm. Be sure the child is not cold from exposure because skin signs

| TABLE 2-11 | Normal Heart Rate for Age |
| --- | --- |
| Age | Heart Rate (beats/min) |
| Infant | 100–160 |
| Toddler | 90–150 |
| Preschooler | 80–140 |
| School-aged child | 70–120 |
| Adolescent | 60–100 |

Source: Dieckmann R, Brownstein D, Gausche-Hill M, eds. *Pediatric Education for Prehospital Professionals.* Sudbury, Ma: Jones and Bartlett Publishers, American Academy of Pediatrics; 2000:45. Reprinted with permission.

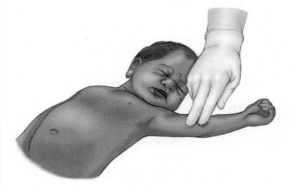

Figure 2.14 The anatomic position of the brachial pulse is medial to the biceps muscle.

will be deceptive. Normal capillary refill time is less than 2 to 3 seconds. The value of capillary refill time is controversial. Peripheral perfusion can vary in some children, and environmental factors such as cold room temperature can affect capillary refill time. Also, it might be difficult to accurately count seconds under critical circumstances. The capillary refill time is just one element of the assessment of circulation. It must be evaluated in the context of the PAT and other perfusion characteristics such as heart rate, pulse quality, and blood pressure.

Signs of circulation to the skin (skin temperature, capillary refill time, and pulse quality) are tools to assess a child's circulatory status.

### Blood Pressure

Blood pressure determination and interpretation can be difficult in children because of lack of patient cooperation, confusion about proper cuff size, and problems remembering normal values for age. Figure 2.15A depicts the different sizes of blood pressure cuffs, and Figure 2.15B demonstrates the technique for getting a correct blood pressure in the arm or thigh. Always use a cuff with a width of two thirds the length of the upper arm or thigh. Although technical difficulties reduce the reliability of a cuff blood pressure in patients younger than 3 years, make an attempt to determine a blood pressure in all patients.

Even if obtained accurately, blood pressure can be misleading. Although a low blood pressure definitely indicates decompensated shock, a normal blood pressure frequently exists in children with compensated shock. An easy formula for determining the lower limit of acceptable blood pressure by age is: minimal systolic blood pressure = 70 + [2 × age (in years)]. For example, a 5-year-old with a systolic blood pressure of 70 mm Hg is probably in decompensated shock. Table 2-12 shows approximate normal systolic blood pressure for age. High blood pressure is not a common clinical problem for children.

### Techniques to Assess and Manage Circulation

If a child is apneic and unresponsive based on the PAT, check for a carotid, femoral, or brachial pulse, if no pulse is present, begin CPR along

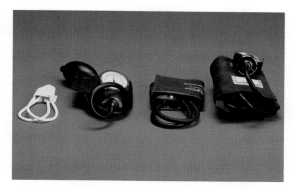

**Figure 2.15A** There are several different blood pressure cuff sizes: neonatal, infant, child, and adult.

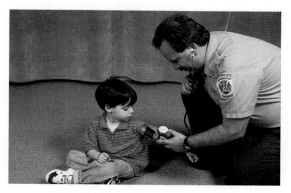

**Figure 2.15B** To obtain an accurate blood pressure reading, use a cuff that is two-thirds the length of the child's upper arm.

| TABLE 2-12 | Normal Blood Pressure for Age | |
|---|---|
| **Age** | **Minimal Systolic Blood Pressure (mm Hg)** |
| Infant | >60 |
| Toddler | >70 |
| Preschooler | >75 |
| School-aged child | >80 |
| Adolescent | >90 |

Source: Dieckmann R, Brownstein D, Gausche-Hill M, eds. *Pediatric Education for Prehospital Professionals.* Sudbury, Ma: Jones and Bartlett Publishers, American Academy of Pediatrics; 2000:47. Reprinted with permission.

with assisted ventilation. Attach a cardiac monitor and evaluate the rhythm. Then, obtain vascular access with an intraosseous needle, or an intravenous (IV) if a peripheral vein is visible, and begin drug administration based on the presenting rhythm. Sometimes, it is neces-

| TABLE 2-13 | Shock Types | | |
|---|---|---|---|
| | **Hypovolemic** | **Distributive** | **Cardiogenic** |
| Common causes | Vomiting | Sepsis | Myocarditis |
| | Diarrhea | Toxins | Supraventicular tachycardia |
| | Blood loss | Spinal cord injury | Left to right defects |
| | | Anaphylaxis | |
| Distinguishing clinical signs and symptoms | History | Fever | Crackles in lungs |
| | Cool skin | Ingestion history | Extreme tachycardia |
| | Thready pulses | Major trauma | Heart murmur |
| Treatment | Crystalloid | Crystalloid | Pressors |
| | Blood products | Pressors | Countershock |
| | | | Cardiotonic drugs |

sary to perform electrical countershock before vascular access if the rhythm is an unstable supraventricular or ventricular dysrhythmia.

When a child is in compensated or decompensated shock based on the PAT, immediately obtain vascular access before doing the hands-on assessment. However, many children are not physiologically unstable and deserve a comprehensive assessment of circulation before vascular access.

For most children, begin the circulatory assessment by determining heart rate. Apply a cardiac monitor and feel for a brachial or femoral pulse if the child is potentially unstable based on the PAT. Then, touch the skin at the kneecap to assess for color, temperature, and capillary refill time (CRT). Last, obtain a blood pressure using an appropriate-sized cuff and interpret the measurement based on the child's age.

When the assessment suggests a perfusion problem, distinguish the shock type, obtain vascular access, and deliver drugs, fluids, and sometimes blood products. Table 2-13 summarizes the different forms of shock. In children, hypovolemic shock or distributive shock from trauma or sepsis causes most perfusion problems. Boluses of isotonic fluids and/or blood products, and occasionally pressor drugs in severe sepsis, are the treatment priorities. Cardiogenic shock occurs rarely in children because of either an acquired condition such as myocarditis, a dysrhythmia, or a congenital condition such as a large ventricular septal defect (VSD). Treatment for these patients includes pressors, minimal fluids, and sometimes other cardiotonic drugs such as adenosine.

## Disability

Assessment of disability or neurologic status involves quick evaluation of the two parts of the central nervous system: the cerebral cortex and the brain stem. Assess neurologic status (controlled by the cortex) by looking at appearance as part of the PAT and at level of consciousness with the AVPU scale (Table 2-14). The Pediatric Glasgow Coma Scale, also called the Modified Glasgow Coma Scale, is a second option if the child is a trauma patient, although the Pediatric Glasgow Coma Scale has never been validated as a predictive instrument in children.

Evaluate the brainstem by checking the responses of each pupil to a direct beam of light. A normal pupil constricts after a light stimulus. Pupillary response can be abnormal in the presence of drugs, ongoing seizures, hypoxia, or impending brainstem herniation. Next, evaluate motor activity. Look for symmetrical movement of the extremities, seizures, posturing, or flaccidity.

### AVPU Scale

The AVPU scale (Table 2-14) is a conventional way of assessing level of consciousness in all patients with either illness or injury conditions. It categorizes motor response based on simple responses to stimuli. The patient is either alert, responsive to verbal stimuli, responsive only to painful stimuli, or unresponsive.

| TABLE 2-14 | AVPU scale | | |
|---|---|---|---|
| **Category** | **Stimulus** | **Response Type** | **Reaction** |
| Alert | Normal environment | Appropriate | Normal interactibility for age |
| Verbal | Simple command or sound stimulus | Appropriate | Responds to name |
| | | Inappropriate | Nonspecific or confused |
| Painful | Pain | Appropriate | Withdraws from pain |
| | | Inappropriate | Sound or motion without purpose or localization of pain |
| | | Pathological | Posturing |
| Unresponsive | No perceptible response to any stimulus | Pathological | |

Source: Dieckmann R, Brownstein D, Gausche-Hill M, eds. *Pediatric Education for Prehospital Professionals.* Sudbury, Ma: Jones and Bartlett Publishers, American Academy of Pediatrics; 2000:47. Reprinted with permission.

**Abnormal Appearance and the AVPU Scale**

The PAT and the AVPU scale are not the same. A child with altered level of consciousness on the AVPU scale will always have abnormal appearance in the PAT. Assessing appearance using the PAT might give an earlier indication of the presence of illness and injury. A child with a mild to moderate illness or injury can be alert on the AVPU scale but have an abnormal appearance.

The application of the AVPU scale method is controversial. It has not been well tested for effectiveness in children. However, there is no other easy way to assess disability in children. The more complicated Pediatric Glasgow Coma Scale (or Modified Glasgow Coma Scale) for neurologic injury involves memorization and numerical scoring tasks that can be hard to accomplish in critical situations. A recent study did demonstrate that, for pediatric blunt injury patients, inpatient mortality could be predicted using the unresponsive component of the AVPU scale, and the no motor response from the Glascow Coma Scale.[20]

**Techniques to Assess and Manage Disability**

With knowledge of the child's appearance from the PAT, perform another specific assessment of overall CNS function. Use either the AVPU scale or the pediatric Glasgow Coma Scale on trauma patients. Next, check both pupils for light reaction. Then, look for symmetrical or abnormal motor activity.

If the disability assessment demonstrates altered level of consciousness (ALOC), begin general life support/monitoring with oxygen, a cardiac monitor, and pulse oximetry. Then obtain vascular access, do a rapid bedside test for serum glucose, and begin isotonic fluid administration at a minimal infusion rate. Measure exhaled $CO_2$ if possible.

If the child has a brainstem herniation syndrome, begin assisted ventilation at a higher than normal rate for age and watch $CO_2$ levels. If pupillary constriction occurs, maintain ventilatory rate at the same frequency to sustain a measured $CO_2$ level. Begin drug therapy to reduce intracranial pressure. If the child begins seizing, administer anticonvulsant drugs.

**Exposure**

Proper exposure of the child is necessary for completing the initial physical assessment. The PAT requires that the caregiver remove part of the child's clothing to allow careful observation of the face, chest wall, and skin. Completing the ABCDE components of the initial assessment requires further exposure, as needed, to fully evaluate physiologic function and anatomic abnormalities. Be careful to avoid rapid heat loss, especially in a cold environment, with infants and children.

**Techniques to Assess and Manage Exposure**

Disrobe the child completely and look at the entire body, including the back. If the child is alert, be sensitive to modesty by exposing one body area at a time. Maintain a warm ambient environment, especially in infants and toddlers, by using an external heat source. Warm the IV fluids. In some patients undergoing prolonged resuscitation, attach a rectal probe to allow ongoing monitoring of core body temperature.

## Summary of Initial Assessment

The initial assessment has the goal of identifying abnormal physiology; it includes the general impression and the hands-on physical assessment of the ABCDEs. The PAT is the basis for the general impression. It includes characteristics of appearance, work of breathing, and circulation to skin and uses auditory and visual clues obtained from across the room. The rest of the initial assessment includes an evaluation of pediatric-specific indicators of cardiopulmonary or neurologic abnormalities. Although vital signs can be useful in the initial assessment, they can also be misleading. They must be examined carefully and looked at together with other parts of the initial assessment. Interventions might be necessary at any point in the ABCDE se-

### KEY POINTS

**Initial Assessment**

- Begin your assessment with the PAT.
- Form a general impression based on the PAT and begin management for patients in respiratory distress, respiratory failure, shock, or cardiopulmonary failure.
- Continue your assessment with the ABCDEs.
- Modify or add to management priorities based on findings of ABCDEs.

quence. After the initial assessment, additional assessment is also necessary.

## Focused History and Physical Examination

After completing the initial assessment and addressing immediate physiologic or anatomic abnormalities, perform additional assessment with a focused history and physical examination in stable patients, and by ongoing assessment of all patients. Dangerous signs and symptoms that are potentially life-threatening can escape detection in the initial assessment. Generally, the initial assessment is intended to detect immediate life-threatening problems that can compromise basic life functions. The comprehensive history and physical examination is intended to detect less immediate threats to life and have several specific objectives:

- Obtaining a complete history, including the mechanism of injury or circumstances of the illness
- Performing a detailed physical examination
- Establishing a clinical diagnosis
- Staging ancillary testing with laboratory investigations and imaging

**History**

To obtain a focused history, use the SAMPLE mnemonic, as suggested in Table 2-15. After getting the focused history, reassess the physical findings based on the additional information. Focus the physical examination on the anatomic areas of concern after obtaining the history from the child or caregiver (or both).

If a child has an apparently minor condition, such as low-grade fever, feeding difficulties, fussiness, or minor trauma, be careful not to overlook clues to possible dangerous underlying conditions (Table 2-16). Child maltreatment, ingestions, and early systemic infections or sepsis in infants, toddlers, or preschoolers are examples of conditions in which the child might not have any acute

## TABLE 2-15 Pediatric SAMPLE Components

| Component | Explanation |
|---|---|
| Signs/Symptoms | Onset and nature of symptoms or pain or fever<br>Age-appropriate signs of distress |
| Allergies | Known drug reactions or other allergies |
| Medications | Exact names and doses of ongoing drugs<br>Timing and amount of last dose<br>Timing and dose of analgesic/antipyretics |
| Past medical problems | History of pregnancy, labor, delivery<br>Previous illnesses or injuries<br>Immunizations |
| Last food or liquid | Timing of the child's last food or drink, including bottle or breast feeding |
| Events leading to the injury or illness | Key events leading to the current incident<br>Fever history |

Source: Dieckmann R, Brownstein D, Gausche-Hill M, eds. *Pediatric Education for Prehospital Professionals.* Sudbury, Ma: Jones and Bartlett Publishers, American Academy of Pediatrics; 2000:51. Reprinted with permission.

## TABLE 2-16 Potentially Dangerous Signs

| Sign or Symptom | Examples of Possible Etiologies |
|---|---|
| Lethargy | Sepsis, shaken baby, intoxication |
| Poor feeding, sleeping, or fussiness | Congestive heart failure, sepsis |
| Bilious vomiting | Midgut volvulus |
| Unusual odor | Intoxication, metabolic acidosis |
| Bruising, burns, unusual trauma | Child maltreatment |
| Petechiae | Sepsis |
| Nonfrontal hematoma of head | Intracranial hemorrhage |
| Bulging fontanel | Meningitis, encephalitis |
| Retinal hemorrhage | Shaken baby |
| Rhinorrhea after head trauma | Basilar skull fracture |
| Otorrhea | Basilar skull fracture |
| Postauricular bruising | Basilar skull fracture |
| Sweet breath odor | Ketosis |
| Drooling | Bacterial upper airway infection, foreign body |
| Stridor with crying | Laryngomalacia |
| Heart murmur | Ventricular septal defect, artrial septal defect, tetralogy of Fallot |
| Hip click | Congenital hip dislocation |
| Difficulty walking | Septic hip, occult fracture, sepsis, leukemia, slipped capital femoral epiphysis, or Legg-Calvé-Perthes disease |

alterations of anatomy or physiology, or the physical findings are not logically related to the complaint or history.

### Detailed Physical Examination

This physical evaluation must include all anatomic areas. Often this portion of the assessment is not possible because of lifesaving treatment priorities. Sometimes it is unnecessary because the problem has been fully evaluated in initial assessment, or the complaint and history are minor and in a specific location (e.g., earache, twisted ankle).

Use the toe-to-head sequence for the detailed physical examination of infants, toddlers, and preschoolers. This approach will gain the child's trust and cooperation and will increase the accuracy of the physical findings. Get the assistance of the caregiver in the detailed examination.

Note the following special anatomic characteristics of children when performing the comprehensive examination:

- General Observations—Observe the clothing for any unusual odors or for stains that might suggest a poison. Remove soiled or dirty clothing and save, and wash the skin with soap and water when there is time. If the infant or child vomits, note if the vomit contains bile or blood. Bile can suggest obstruction, and blood can suggest occult abdominal trauma or gastrointestinal bleeding.

- Skin—Inspect the skin carefully for rashes and for bruising patterns that may suggest maltreatment. Look for bite marks, straight line marks from cords or straps, pinch marks, or hand, belt, or buckle pattern bruises. Inspect for nonblanching petechiae or purpuric lesions, and look for any new lesions that occur during your physical examination and ongoing assessment.

- Head—The younger the infant or child, the larger the head in proportion to the rest of the body (Figure 2.16). In the infant, the large head sits atop a small and weak neck. Because of this, the head is very easily injured when deceleration occurs (such as in motor vehicle crashes).

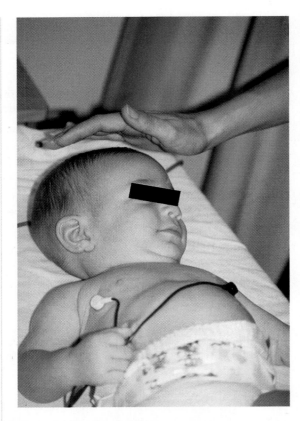

**Figure 2.16** The infant's head is disproportionately large compared to older children and adults.

Look for bruising, swelling, and hematomas. Significant blood can be lost between the skull and scalp of a small infant. The anterior fontanel in infants younger than 9 to 18 months can provide useful information about pressure within the central nervous system. A bulging and nonpulsatile fontanel can suggest meningitis, encephalitis, or intracranial bleeding. A sunken fontanel suggests dehydration.

- Eyes—A thorough evaluation of pupil size, reaction to light, and symmetry of extraocular muscle movements can be difficult to perform in infants. Gently rocking infants in the upright position will often get them to open their eyes. A colorful distracting object can then be used to look at eye movements. Retinal hemorrhages on ophthalmoscopic examination suggest possible subdural hematoma, often a marker of shaken baby syndrome or child maltreatment.

- Nose—Many infants prefer to breathe through their noses, as well as through their mouths, and when the nose is plugged with mucus, they are unable to breathe unless they are crying. The most common cause of respiratory distress in small infants is nasal obstruction from mucus. Gentle bulb or catheter suction of the nostrils can bring relief. In the toddler, foreign bodies are often the cause of nasal obstruction or unilateral discharge. Peas, beans, paper, plastic toys, and a myriad of small objects find their way into the toddler's nostrils. Leaking fluid (cerebrospinal fluid [CSF] rhinorrhea) after head trauma suggests a basilar skull fracture.

- Ears—Look for any drainage from the ear canals. Leaking fluid (CSF otorrhea) suggests a basilar skull fracture. Check for bruises behind the ear or Battle sign, another sign of basilar skull fracture. The presence of pus can indicate an ear infection or perforation of the eardrum.

- Mouth—Avoid looking in the mouth if the child has stridor. A partially obstructed airway in a child with stridor can become completely obstructed if touched. In the trauma patient, look for active bleeding and loose teeth. Note the smell of the breath. Many types of ingestions have specific odors, especially hydrocarbons. Acidosis can impart a sweet smell to the breath. Drooling suggests a bacterial infection of the upper airway, such as peritonsillar abscess or bacterial tracheitis, or a foreign body.

- Neck—Locate the trachea for midline positioning. Listen with a stethoscope over the trachea at the midline. This is a quick and easy way to tell the difference between the sounds of mucus in the mouth, nose, and pharynx versus wheezing and stridor.

- Chest—Reexamine the chest for penetrations, bruises, or rashes. If the child is injured, feel the clavicles and every rib for tenderness and/or deformity.

- Heart—Listen to the heart for murmurs or abnormal sounds, such as friction rubs or gallops.

- Back—Inspect the back for penetrations, bruises, or rashes. Percuss for tenderness.

- Abdomen—Inspect the abdomen for distention. Gently palpate the abdomen and watch closely for guarding or tensing of the abdominal muscles, which can suggest infection, obstruction, or intraabdominal injury. Note any tenderness or masses.

- Pelvis—Compress the pelvis, and feel for instability and tenderness.

- Extremities—Assess for symmetry. Compare both sides for color, warmth, size of joints, and tenderness. Put each joint through full range of motion while watching the eyes of the child for signs of pain. Check for a hip click in infants.

- Neurologic examination—Do a cranial nerve evaluation. Have children close and open their eyes, smile, and stick out their tongues. If cooperative, hold an object in front of their eyes and track eye movements up, down, left, and right. Doing some simple maneuvers such as lifting their arms and legs, shrugging their shoulders, pushing against resistance, and squeezing your hand can test some gross motor functions. Look for a pronator drift with the child's arms extended. If there is no injury and the patient is old enough, have the child walk and observe the gait; is it normal, wide based, or ataxic? Assess for reflexes, especially if the child complains of back pain or shows signs of motor weakness.

## Ongoing Assessment

Perform ongoing assessment of all patients to observe responses to treatment and to track the identified physiologic and anatomic problems. Sometimes the ongoing assessment identifies new problems. The ongoing assessment provides necessary guidance about continuing and modifying treatment.

After the initial assessment and resuscitation, perform a focused history and detailed examination on stable patients. Look for dangerous signs and symptoms not evident in the initial assessment. The additional assessment is more likely to detect anatomic problems that are not life-threatening than physiologic abnormalities. The more detailed nature of this portion of the physical assessment allows the clinician to develop a reasonable hypothesis for etiology or diagnosis, helps planning for imaging and ancillary laboratory testing, and assists with providing specific treatment. Last, always perform ongoing assessment to observe response to interventions and to guide changes in treatment.

## KEY POINTS

**Common Elements in the Ongoing Assessment:**

- PAT
- ABCDEs
- Repeat vital signs
- Reassessment of positive anatomic findings
- Review of the effectiveness and safety of treatment

## THE BOTTOM LINE

- Your assessment of an infant or child begins with the initial assessment: the PAT followed by the ABCDEs.
- Form a general impression that will drive your management priorities.
- Continue assessment with a focused history and detailed physical examination if your general impression of the child is stable, or once initial management steps have begun or stabilized a child in respiratory distress, respiratory failure, or shock.
- Perform ongoing assessment throughout the ED stay.

## Check Your Knowledge

1. All of the following are components of the PAT except:
   A. Appearance
   B. Circulation
   C. Heart rate
   D. Work of breathing

2. Abnormalities in which of the following components of the PAT would indicate a decompensated shock state?
   A. Appearance and circulation
   B. Appearance and work of breathing
   C. Circulation
   D. Work of breathing and circulation to skin

3. All of the following are techniques or signs of shock except:
   A. Effortless tachypnea, hyperpnea
   B. Interactiveness
   C. Pulse quality
   D. Work of breathing

4. You are about to assess an 8-month-old boy. Based on his developmental level, which of the following techniques would be helpful?
   A. Do your assessment from a standing position
   B. Examine head to toe
   C. Offer distractions
   D. Separate infant and mother

## References

1. Dieckmann RA. Epidemiology of pediatric emergency care. In: Dieckmann RA, Fiser DH, Selbst SM. *Illustrated Textbook of Pediatric Emergency and Critical Care Procedures*. St. Louis, Mo: Mosby; 1997:3–7.

2. McCraig LF, Ly N. National hospital ambulatory medical care survey: 2000 emergency department summary. *Vital and Health Statistics*. Hyattsville, MD: Dept. of Health and Human Services, Centers for Disease Control and Prevention, National Center for Health Statistics; April 22, 2002 Hyattsville, Md. Available at: http://www.cdc.gov/nchs/data/ad/ad326.pdf. *Accessed December 14, 2002.*

3. American College of Emergency Physicians. The role of the emergency physician in the care of children. *Ann Emerg Med.* 1990;19:435–436.

4. Fuchs S, Jaffe DM, Christoffel KK. Pediatric emergencies in office practice: prevalence and office preparedness. *Pediatrics.* 1989;83:1989.

5. Schweich PJ, DeAngelis C, Duggan AK. Preparedness of practicing pediatricians to manage emergencies. *Pediatrics.* 1991;88:223–229.

6. Weiss HB, Mathers LJ, Forjuoh SN, et al. *Child and Adolescent Emergency Department Visit Data Book*. Pittsburgh, Pa: Center for Violence and Injury Control, Allegheny University of the Health Sciences; 1997.

7. Friday GA, Khine H, Lin SL, Caliguiri LA. Profile of children requiring emergency treatment for asthma. *Annals Allergy, Asthma & Immun.* 1997;78:221–224.

8. Kallsen GW. Epidemiology of Pediatric Prehospital Emergencies. In: Dieckmann RA, ed. *Pediatric Emergency Care Systems: Planning and Management*. Baltimore, Md: Williams & Wilkins;1991:153–158.

9. Meador SA. Age-related utilization of advanced life support services. *Prehospital Disaster Med.* 1991;6(1):9–14.

10. Elixhauser A, Machlin SR, Zodet MW, et al. Health care for children and youth in the United States: 2001 annual report on access, utilization, quality and expenditures. *Ambulatory Pediatrics.* 2002;2:419–437.

11. Nelson DS, Walsh K, Fleisher G. Spectrum and frequency of pediatric illness presenting to a general community hospital emergency department. *Pediatrics.* 1992;90(1):5–10.

12. Johnson DW, Adair C, Brant R, et al. Differences in admission rates of children with bronchiolitis by pediatric and general emergency departments. *Pediatrics.* 2002;110(4).

13. Yamamoto LG, Wiebe RA, Wallace JM, Sia CC. The Hawaii EMSC project data. *Pediatr Emerg Care.* 1992;8(2):70–78.

14. Minino AM, Arias E, Kochanek KD, et al. Deaths: Final data for 2000. *National Vital Statistics Reports.* Sept 16, 2002;Vol 50(15) Available at: www.cdc.gov/nhcs/data/nvsr/nvusr50/nvsr_5015.pdf. Accessed December 14, 2002.

15. Gallagher SS, Finison K, Guyer B, et al. The incidence of injuries among 87,000 Massachusetts children and adolescents: results of the 1980–1981 statewide childhood injury surveillance system. *Am J Public Health.* 1984;74: 1340–1347.

16. Dieckmann R, Brownstein D, Gausche-Hill M, eds. *Pediatric Education for Prehospital*

# CHAPTER REVIEW

*Professionals*. Sudbury, Ma: Jones and Bartlett Publishers, American Academy of Pediatrics; 2000:30–57.

17. Ward KR, Yealy DM. Endtidal $CO_2$ monitoring in emergency medicine. Part 1. Basic principles. *Acad Emerg Med*. 1998;5:628–636.

18. Bhende MS, Thompson AE. Evaluation of an end-tidal $CO_2$ detector during pediatric cardiopulmonary resuscitation. *Pediatrics*. 1995;95:395–399.

19. Wayne MA, Levine RL, Miller CC. Use of end-tidal carbon dioxide to predict outcome in pre-hospital cardiac arrest. *Ann Emerg Med*. 1995;25:762–767.

20. Hannan EL, Farrell LS, Meaker PS, Cooper A. Predicting inpatient mortality for pediatric trauma patients with blunt injuries: a better alternative. *J Pediatr Surg*. 2000:35:155–159.

## CASE SUMMARY 1

A 6-month-old boy who has had persistent vomiting for 24 hours presents to the emergency department. The infant is lying still and has poor muscle tone. He is irritable if touched, and his cry is weak. There are no abnormal airway sounds, retractions, or flaring. He is pale and mottled. The respiratory rate is 45 breaths/min, heart rate is 170 beats per minute (bpm), and blood pressure is 50/palp. Air movement is normal, and breath sounds are clear to auscultation. The skin feels cool, and capillary refill time is 4 seconds. The brachial pulse is weak. His abdomen is distended.

1. *What are the key signs of serious illness in this infant?*
2. *How helpful are heart rate, respiratory rate, and blood pressure in evaluating cardiopulmonary function?*

This infant is severely ill. The PAT indicates poor appearance with diminished tone, poor interactiveness, and weak cry. These are important signals of weakened cardiopulmonary and/or neurologic function in an infant. Work of breathing is normal, although the respiratory rate is high, and circulation to skin is poor. The PAT establishes this child as a critical patient who requires aggressive resuscitation. However, the respiratory rate, heart rate, and blood pressure are possibly within the normal ranges for age. Therefore, use vital signs in the context of findings on PAT and the entire initial assessment. In this case, the PAT tells you that the child has an abnormal appearance and decreased skin circulation, which suggest shock.

The hands-on ABCDE phase of the assessment shows poor skin signs and diminished brachial pulse. These important physical findings confirm the PAT impression of shock. Furthermore, when you review the vital signs in the context of the initial assessment, you might identify that this child has effortless tachypnea, a physiologic attempt to clear acidosis generated by shock.

## CASE SUMMARY 2

A 21-month-old girl is brought to the emergency department after a 9-1-1 call. The mother explains that the child, who has a tracheostomy, has had copious secretions and has required more frequent suctioning and breathing treatments for 2 days. The child has severe cerebral palsy. The mother is anxious and demanding immediate hospitalization for the child. The child turns blue and becomes agitated whenever you approach but is easily consoled by the mother. There are no retractions or flaring. Her respiratory rate is 50 breaths/min, and heart rate is 140 bpm. You are unable to obtain a blood pressure.

**CASE SUMMARY 2 CONT**

1. *How can the Pediatric Assessment Triangle be used to evaluate the severity of illness and urgency for care in a child with special health care needs?*

The PAT is a good way to get a general impression of this child and to judge the degree of illness and urgency for care. Many other conventional assessment methods, such as history taking, auscultation, and blood pressure determinations, would be frustrating to attempt and possibly inaccurate in the first few minutes. The child's appearance is somewhat reassuring, with comfort in her mother's arms, and a vigorous cry. There are no retractions or flaring, so work of breathing is normal despite of a respiratory rate in the highest range for age. Circulation to skin is normal. With these PAT findings, it is highly unlikely that the child has a serious illness. The PAT provides the impression of a relatively well child and allows you to stand back and gain the confidence of the child and mother before rushing to a hands-on evaluation. Place this child in the mother's arms and allow the mother to keep the girl on her lap while you proceed with the evaluation. When the child is less agitated, approach gently to complete the initial assessment. Use a toe-to-head sequence.

The PAT is the important first phase of the initial assessment. It does not replace the hands-on assessment of the ABCDEs and vital signs. The PAT for this child should reassure you. Obtain information about the child's baseline neurologic and cardiopulmonary status from the mother or primary physician and use the physical assessment to compare the presenting condition with the established baseline.

**CASE SUMMARY 3**

A 7-year-old boy is hit by a car in front of his home. He was thrown 5 feet and had loss of consciousness. The boy did awake, but the father decided to take him to the physician's office when he noted the boy becoming sleepy.

In the office, the boy opens his eyes with a loud verbal stimulus but will not speak or interact. There are no abnormal airway sounds, but intercostal retractions and flaring are present. His skin is pale. Respiratory rate is 50 breaths/min, heart rate is 145 bpm, and blood pressure is 90/palp. The chest is clear with decreased tidal volume. The skin feels cool; capillary refill time is 4 seconds, and brachial pulse is present. Pupils are equal and reactive. He has a large frontal hematoma.

1. *Does this child's assessment suggest serious injury?*
2. *What actions are required by the physician in the office?*
3. *How should this child be transported to the emergency department?*

This child's appearance is grossly abnormal, with a serious mechanism of injury. The boy's lethargic appearance, increased work of breathing, and abnormal skin signs on the PAT suggest possible intracranial, chest, and abdominal injuries. The child might have concussion, hemorrhage, or brain edema in conjunction with a chest injury and abdominal hemorrhage. In this child, establishing a baseline neurologic status in the office will help clinicians at the hospital evaluate the trend of neurologic response. The initial assessment suggests an unstable patient who needs rapid treatment in the office with 100% $O_2$, crystalloid fluids, and immediate EMS transport to the hospital.

## chapter 3

# The Pediatric Airway in Health and Disease

**Phyllis Hendry Stenklyft, MD, FAAP, FACEP**
**Mary E. Cataletto, MD, FAAP**
**Brian S. Lee, MD**

## Objectives

1 Compare the anatomic and physiologic differences between adult and pediatric airways.

2 Discuss a general approach to pediatric airway emergencies, including the difficult airway.

3 Describe clinical features, diagnosis, and management of upper and lower airway obstruction and diseases of the lung.

## Chapter Outline

Introduction
Anatomic and Physiologic Responses to Airway Maneuvers
General Approach to Airway Emergencies

**Upper Airway Obstruction**
Croup
Foreign Body Aspiration
Retropharyngeal Abscess
Epiglottitis
Anaphylaxis

**Lower Airway Obstruction**
Bronchiolitis
Asthma

**Disease of Oxygenation and Ventilation and Disease of the Lungs**
Bronchopulmonary Dysplasia
Cystic Fibrosis
Pneumonia
Respiratory Failure

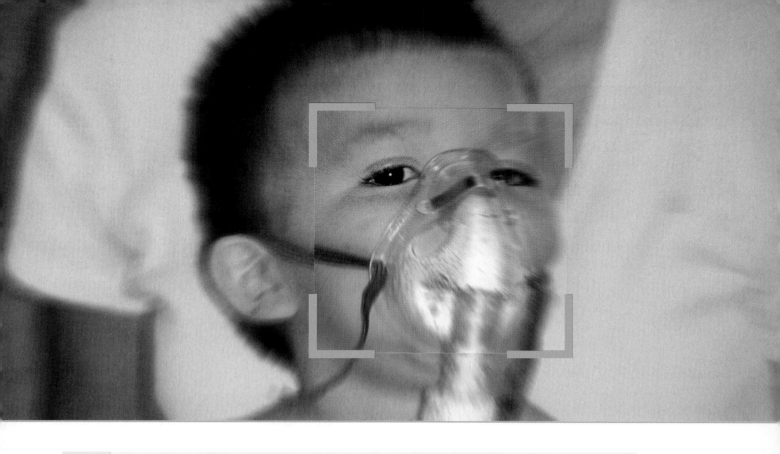

**CASE SCENARIO 1**

A 6-month-old boy presents to the emergency department with wheezing, severe retractions, and stridor. The infant has poor tone and is poorly responsive to his surroundings. He has intercostal retractions, and his color is pale. His vital signs include respiratory rate of 80 breaths per minute; a heart rate of 190 beats per minute (bpm); temperature (rectal) of 38.6°C; and oxygen saturation of 80% on room air. His mother reveals that he was born at 28 weeks' gestation and was intubated and mechanically ventilated for 6 weeks prior to hospital discharge. The patient also has Pierre Robin syndrome.

1. *How would you assess and categorize this patient's airway?*
2. *What special precautions would you take in planning airway management and possible intubation?*

## Introduction

The first step toward successful airway management is a thorough understanding of normal pediatric airway anatomy and physiology, differences between adult and pediatric airway anatomy and physiology, and anatomic airway anomalies that occur in children. The infant airway differs significantly from that of the adult; as a child becomes older, the airway becomes more comparable to adult anatomy. By 8 or 9 years of age, the airway is considered similar to the adult airway, with the exception of size. Table 3-1 provides a comparison of infant and adult airways.

These anatomic differences affect all the steps involved in airway management. For example, a small infant lying flat on a gurney might need a towel placed under the back of the shoulders to align the airway and correct for a forward flexion of the head and neck because of the prominent occiput. Also, a straight blade is preferred to a curved blade to accommodate the infant's anterior airway and large tongue. Certain congenital and acquired conditions predispose the airway to difficult management; some of these conditions are listed in Table 3-2.

There are numerous physiologic differences between adult and pediatric airways and

**TABLE 3-1  Comparison of Infant and Adult Airways[1-3]**

|  | Infant | Adult |
|---|---|---|
| Head | Large prominent occiput resulting in sniffing position | Flat occiput |
| Tongue | Relatively larger | Relatively smaller |
| Larynx | Cephalad position, opposite C2 and C3 vertebrae | Opposite C4 to C6 |
| Epiglottis | $\Omega$ shaped, soft | Flat, flexible |
| Vocal cords | Short, concave | Horizontal |
| Smallest diameter | Cricoid ring, below cords | Vocal cords |
| Cartilage | Soft, less calcified | Firm, calcified |
| Lower airway | Smaller, less developed | Larger, more cartilage |

**TABLE 3-2  Selected Conditions Associated With Difficult Intubation**

**Congenital Anomalies**
- Down syndrome — Large tongue, small mouth, frequent laryngospasm
- Goldenhar syndrome — Mandibular hypoplasia
- Pierre Robin syndrome — Large tongue, small mouth, mandibular anomaly
- Turner syndrome — Short neck

**Tumor/Mass**
- Cystic hygroma — Compression of airway
- Hemangioma — Hemorrhage

**Infection**
- Epiglottitis — Inability to visualize cords
- Croup — Airway irritability, edema below cords

**Cervical Spine Stabilization** — Prevents optimal head and neck positioning

**Upper Airway Obstruction**
- Angioneurotic edema — Difficulty visualizing cords
- Peritonsillar abscess

**Facial Trauma** — Difficulty opening mouth

**TABLE 3-3  Risks for Aspiration of Gastric Contents**

**Full Stomach**
- Children; less than 6 hours since last meal
- Infants; less than 4 hours since last meal

**Unknown History of Last Oral Intake**
- Trauma
  - Elevated ICP
  - Swallowed blood
- Delayed Gastric Emptying
  - Drugs
  - Diabetes
  - Infection/sepsis
- Intestinal Obstruction
- Esophageal Conditions
  - Reflux
  - Motility disorders
- Obesity
- Pregnancy
- Pain

respiratory systems. Children have increased rates of oxygen ($O_2$) consumption, increased chest wall compliance, lower lung compliance and elastic recoil, and diminished functional residual capacity, predisposing them to respiratory failure.[4]

Infants and young children are particularly susceptible to emesis and aspiration due to air swallowing during crying, diaphragmatic breathing, and a short esophagus. Recent oral intake is one of many causes of increased risk for gastric aspiration (Table 3-3). A history of most recent oral intake should be elicited for all patients, if possible, before proceeding with intubation. Because this history can be unobtainable in the critically ill child, all patients should be assumed to be in a nonfasting state.

## Anatomic and Physiologic Responses to Airway Maneuvers

Anatomical and physiological factors in children affect the performance of airway techniques. These factors include a flexible trachea, a prominent neck, soft tissue, a relatively large tongue for the oral cavity, a profound vagal response to stimulation of the posterior pharynx, and a dependence on diaphragmatic excursion for ventilation.

## Bag-Mask Ventilation

Bag-mask ventilation is a technique that requires proper hand placement on the mask and jaw and specific ventilation volumes and rates. Because of flexible tracheal rings, too much pressure on a mask with the thumb and index finger (C component of the E-C clamp) can result in flexion of the head on the neck and possible airway obstruction. Finger placement of the middle, ring, and fifth fingers must be on the angle of the jaw (E component of the E-C clamp) to avoid pushing on the submental soft tissue, which can result in the tongue being forced back into the posterior pharynx, causing airway obstruction (Figure 3.1). The Sellick maneuver (cricoid pressure) can be used to occlude the esophagus and limit gastric distention. Too much cricoid pressure can occlude or distort the airway anatomy. Insertion of a nasogastric tube will decompress the stomach but can induce emesis through stimulation of the oropharynx or by keeping the lower esophageal sphincter open. Maintaining appropriate ventilation rates and providing only the amount of ventilation volume that initiates chest rise (state "squeeze, release, release") are key steps to the proper technique of bag-mask ventilation. If too much volume at too high a pressure is delivered, gastric distention might impede diaphragmatic movement, resulting in hypoventilation.

## Laryngoscopy and Intubation

Direct laryngoscopy in a conscious patient is a noxious stimulus that can result in increased intracranial pressure (ICP), pain, emesis, hypoxemia, hypertension, and cardiac dysrhythmias (Figure 3.2). Bradycardia can develop due to a vagal reflex during laryngoscopy, as a

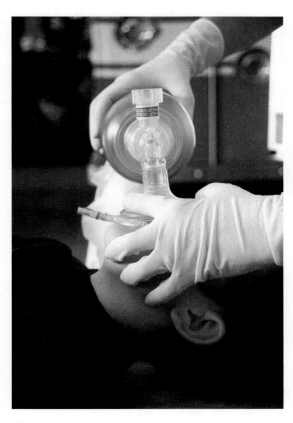

Figure 3.1 E-C clamp positioning for bag-mask ventilation.

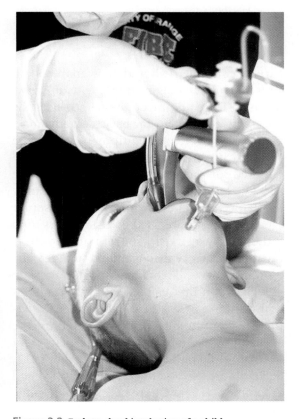

Figure 3.2 Endotracheal intubation of a child.

direct effect of succinylcholine or other medications, or as a result of hypoxemia. Infants are much more likely to develop bradycardia than are adults.

Intubation trauma can cause significant edema and obstruction of the airway. One millimeter of circumferential edema can result in a 16-fold increase in resistance in a 4 mm infant airway.

## General Approach to Airway Emergencies

Pediatric patients who need urgent or emergent airway management usually present with very little warning; therefore, advance preparation is a key element in the general approach to management. Advance preparation includes selection and stocking of appropriate airway and respiratory equipment, protocols for rapid sequence intubation (RSI) and difficult airway situations, training of physicians and staff in airway management, and routine practice, or "mock code," scenarios.

### Equipment

Airway equipment should be available in all sizes for children ranging from premature newborns to large adolescents. Table 3-4 lists the necessary equipment for basic and advanced airway management. Equipment should be carefully inventoried at regular intervals and checked for proper functioning. Alternative airway equipment should always be readily available, especially when neuromuscular blocking agents are used or risk factors for a difficult airway exist. Appropriate monitoring during airway management includes cardiorespiratory and blood pressure monitoring, as well as continuous pulse oximetry and ongoing clinical assessment. Colorimetric end-tidal carbon dioxide ($ETCO_2$) detectors are available for verifying tracheal tube placement in infants and children. Quantitative $ETCO_2$ detectors are used for ongoing monitoring and assessment (See Chapter 22, Emergency Medicine Procedures).

| TABLE 3-4 | Equipment for Basic and Advanced Pediatric Airway Management |
|---|---|

Uncuffed tracheal tubes in sizes 2.5 to 5.5

Cuffed tracheal tubes in sizes 6.0 to 9

Tracheal tube stylets

Laryngoscope handles in good working order

Laryngoscope blades
    Straight (Miller) in sizes 0 to 3
    Curved (Macintosh) in sizes 2 to 3

Oropharyngeal airways

Nasopharyngeal airways

Pediatric and adult Magill forceps

Nonrebreather oxygen masks (adult and pediatric)

Ventilation masks in all sizes for bag-mask ventilation

Self-inflating ventilation bags (450 to 1200 mL) with oxygen reservoir and positive end-expiratory pressure valve

Oxygen source

Suctioning source

Large-bore stiff suction tips (Yankauer)

Flexible suction catheters (French sizes 5 to 16)

Nasogastric tubes (French sizes 6 to 14)

Pulse oximeter

Cardiorespiratory monitor

Tracheostomy tubes

Tracheostomy surgical instrument set

14-Gauge needle catheter for needle cricothyrotomy or other commercially available set

Cricothyrotomy tray

End-tidal $CO_2$ monitor or detector

Laryngeal mask airway

Ideally, charts with age- and weight-related equipment sizes and RSI medication dosages should be available. Because there is little time to guess weights and find the correct-sized equipment during a true emergency, intubation equipment should be stocked in an age- or length-related manner with easy access. A pediatric resuscitation tape that relates patient length to weight and precalculates dosages and equipment size can be helpful during an emergency when weight and age cannot be determined accurately (Figure 3.3).[5]

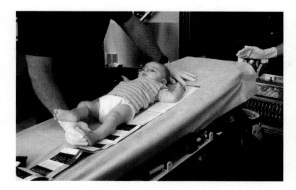

Figure 3.3 Length-based resuscitation tape.

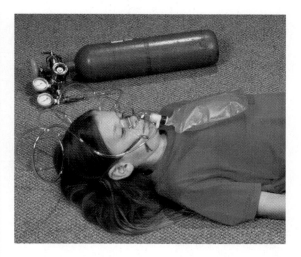

Figure 3.4 Child with partial nonrebreather mask.

## Basic Airway Management

Once it has been determined that an airway or respiratory problem exists, it is important to progress in a calm, step-wise manner beginning with basic airway skills and frequent reassessment. Before the application of advanced airway techniques, the airway should be assessed and the patient ventilated and oxygenated as needed. For the conscious, spontaneously breathing child, it is usually appropriate to allow the child to assume a position of comfort and to supply $O_2$ via nasal cannula or mask (Figure 3.4). If the child resists, a blow-by technique usually is well tolerated (Figure 3.5). In the unconscious child, the airway should be checked for obstruction. If noisy breathing and poor air flow result from obstruction, then the airway should be opened through either the chin lift/head tilt or jaw thrust maneuver. If cervical spine trauma is suspected, a jaw thrust maneuver is used, with great care taken to avoid movement of the neck. If opening the airway does not restore adequate ventilation, begin assisted ventilation with bag-mask ventilation. Place an oral or nasopharyngeal airway as needed to maintain the airway during bag-mask ventilation (Figures 3.6 and 3.7). (Refer to Chapter 22 to review the detailed procedure for bag-mask ventilation and other basic airway procedures.) Suctioning of the airway is often required to remove secretions, blood, or foreign material. Gastric inflation can be reduced by using the correct size of equipment and the proper technique for bag-mask ventilation, as well as by applying cricoid pressure or insert a

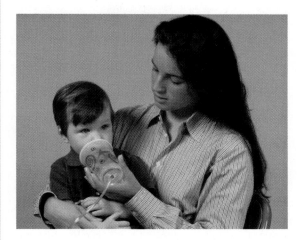

Figure 3.5 If the child resists application of a mask or nasal cannula, administer $O_2$ through a nonthreatening object such as a paper cup.

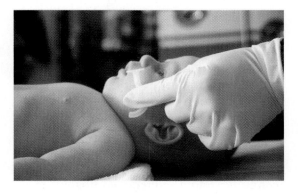

Figure 3.6 Measuring an oropharyngeal airway.

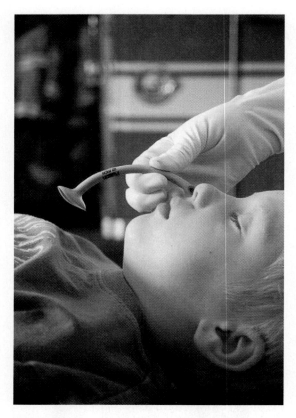

**Figure 3.7** Placing a nasopharyngeal airway in a child.

nasogastric tube. Ventilation with the bag-mask technique using high-flow $O_2$ should precede endotracheal intubation when the patient is hypoventilating to create an $O_2$ reserve for the time required to place the tracheal tube and reinitiate ventilation.[1–4]

## Advanced Airway Management

After basic airway measures have been accomplished, the patient should be reassessed for improvement or the need to progress to advanced airway techniques. The urgency of this progression will be determined by the condition of the patient, the skill of the provider, and the location of the care (out-of hospital, clinic, or emergency department). The next step in airway management after bag-mask ventilation is usually endotracheal intubation. This is commonly accomplished using the RSI technique. Rapid sequence intubation facilitates endotracheal intubation, reduces complications of the procedure, and has become a standard emergency department (ED)procedure for adult and pediatric intubation.[6–9]

If the patient is being adequately oxygenated and ventilated by the bag-mask ventilation technique, reassess the need for more advanced airway techniques. As in cases of children with a seizure, airway opening techniques and/or bag-mask ventilation might be all that is necessary to manage the airway. If the patient requires prolonged bag-mask ventilation or the health care provider is not skilled in endotracheal intubation or RSI, then the best course of action is to continue bag-mask ventilation until transfer to definitive care. Gausche et al found no difference in survival or outcome of children when comparing bag-mask ventilation and endotracheal intubation in the out-of-hospital setting (*JAMA* 2000;283:783–790).

The provider should be aware of advanced techniques such as the laryngeal mask airway (LMA), tracheal light, retrograde intubation, and cricothyrotomy (see Chapter 22). These techniques are rarely needed but may be necessary in cases of a failed difficult airway or unusual airway anatomy. Successful endotracheal intubation for adults and children occurs in tertiary and community ED settings in almost 100% of cases with two attempts. The need for a surgical airway is rare.[3,7,9] Chapter 22 reviews the procedures for endotracheal intubation, RSI, LMA, cricothyrotomy, and retrograde intubation.

Rapid sequence intubation is an important technique in the management of children requiring endotracheal intubation because it increases compliance with patient to the procedure and reduces subsequent complications. The following section will briefly review the rationale and general order of RSI. Rapid sequence intubation requires advance preparation.

## Rapid Sequence Intubation

The purpose of RSI is to rapidly induce unconsciousness and neuromuscular blockade in preparation for intubation. Rapid sequence intubation facilitates intubation and decreases aspiration, untoward physiologic responses, and psychological trauma associated with awake intubation. The procedure blunts the cardiovascular and ICP responses associated with intubations.[2–4,6,8]

Any patient requiring endotracheal intubation is a potential candidate for RSI. Rapid sequence intubation should be used with caution in the following conditions: significant facial edema, trauma, or fractures; distorted laryngotracheal anatomy; or airway anomalies.

A thorough knowledge of the medications used in RSI, technique of endotracheal intubation, and anatomy of the pediatric airway is essential before attempting intubation with RSI. Ideally, RSI should be attempted before the child develops cardiopulmonary compromise. Early initiation of RSI allows the physician to complete the procedure while the child still has some physiologic reserve.

The sequential steps for RSI are listed below. Health care personnel can perform many of the steps simultaneously. An appointed team leader must direct the sequence and medication selection. The history of the acute illness and the entire medical history influence the choice of medications used in RSI. Frequently, emergency airway scenarios do not allow time for a detailed history. The mnemonic AMPLE has been used to direct the history needed for RSI: A—Allergies; M—Medicines, drugs of abuse; P—Past medical problems, previous anesthesia; L—Last oral intake; E—Events, including prehospital course.

Steps of RSI:

1. Brief history and anatomical assessment
2. Preparation of equipment and medications
3. Preoxygenation
4. Premedication with adjunctive agents (atropine or lidocaine)
5. Sedation and induction of unconsciousness
6. Cricoid pressure (Sellick maneuver)
7. Neuromuscular blocking agent for muscle relaxation
8. Intubation
9. Confirmation of tracheal tube placement (clinical, pulse oximetry, and $CO_2$ detection)
10. Post-intubation care: Tracheal tube secured; chest radiograph; nasogastric tube placement, medical record or procedure note documentation

## The Difficult Airway

A crucial step in the evaluation of a child for RSI and emergency airway management is to determine if there are any features that would make bag-mask ventilation, endotracheal intubation, or cricothyrotomy difficult to achieve. An airway is usually labeled as "difficult" because the patient's normal anatomy is modified due to an acute insult or because the patient has a baseline abnormal airway and requires airway management for an unrelated cause. Clinically, the failed airway can be defined as one of two types: cannot intubate but can oxygenate with bag-mask ventilation, or cannot intubate and cannot oxygenate. The difficult, failed airway has been well described in the adult anesthesia and emergency medicine literature. Less is known about predicting and managing the difficult airway in the pediatric population. It has been estimated that 1% to 3% of patients present with difficult airways leading to difficult intubation under direct visualization. The anesthesia literature indicates that intubation is unsuccessful in 0.1% to 0.4% of patients who were assessed to have no risks for a difficult airway. These statistics do not adequately reflect the emergency medicine airway situation. The National Emergency Airway Registry (NEAR) is a multicenter, prospective emergency medicine–led registry. The pilot phase included 1,288 patients with an incidence of "rescue" cricothyrotomy of 1%.[3]

The most important factor in determining success or failure in airway management is the physician performing the procedure. The physician directing the airway management must attempt to recognize and predict the possibility of a difficult airway, choose the appropriate technique or equipment, have a comprehensive knowledge of the pharmacologic and technical skills for RSI, and be skilled in airway rescue techniques if the initial airway management fails.

In general, the difficult airway is predicted by looking at the patient's unique anatomic features; examining the airway, head, and neck; and assessing for airway obstruction, and cervical spine mobility. Mallampati et al classified airways based on the degree of visualization of the pillars, soft palate, and

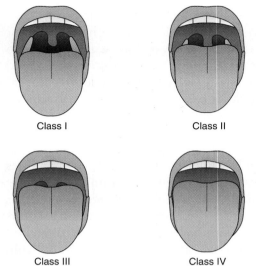

Class I          Class II

Class III          Class IV

**Figure 3.8** Mallampati grades.
Adapted from Walls RM, Luton RC, Murphy MF, Schneider RE. *Manual of Emergency Airway Management.* Lippincott Williams & Wilkins, 2000.

uvula.[10] The classification is an indication of the amount of space in the mouth to accommodate the laryngoscope and tracheal tube. There are four Mallampati grades, with Grade I indicating excellent oral access and Grade IV difficult access and intubation (Figure 3.8). The significance of the Mallampati score in infants and small children is unknown. The developers of the National Emergency Airway

Course have developed the "LEMON Law" for identification of the adult difficult airway as follows[3]:

L—Look externally

E—Evaluate the 3-3-2 Rule (3 fingers between the patient's teeth, 3 fingers at the space from the mentum to the hyoid bone, and 2 fingers between the thyroid notch and the floor of the mouth)

M—Mallampati grade

O—Obstruction

N—Neck mobility

Algorithms for management of the difficult airway have been published for adults but not specifically for pediatric patients, although some have been proposed as modifications of adult algorithms (Figure 3.9).

Selected conditions associated with the difficult pediatric airway are listed in Table 3-2. Once one of these risk factors has been identified, a step-wise approach should be taken, including calling for anesthesia or surgical assistance and considering other types of airway management, such as awake intubation, LMA, lighted stylet, or cricothyrotomy. Before starting any RSI procedure, it should be established that the patient can be effectively ventilated by the bag-mask ventilation technique and appropriate airway adjuncts, or an emergency airway tray should be readily available.

**CASE SCENARIO 2**

A 13-month-old boy is brought to the emergency department by paramedics. The mother had found him choking and gagging in the kitchen next to a container of spilled nuts. She immediately called 9-1-1. Paramedics note that the child's appearance is normal and alert, the work of breathing is increased with audible stridor and subcostal retractions, and his color is normal. Paramedics administer blow-by $O_2$ and transport the child to the emergency department. On arrival, the child is awake and alert and in moderate respiratory distress. The patient is placed immediately in a monitored bed. Vital signs are respiratory rate of 60/min, heart rate of 160/bpm, blood pressure of 88/56, temperature 37.1°C, and oxygen saturation 93%.

1. *What are your initial management priorities?*
2. *What diagnostic studies are necessary?*
3. *What are the possible complications to consider on initial evaluation?*
4. *What is the definitive management of this condition and disposition of the patient?*

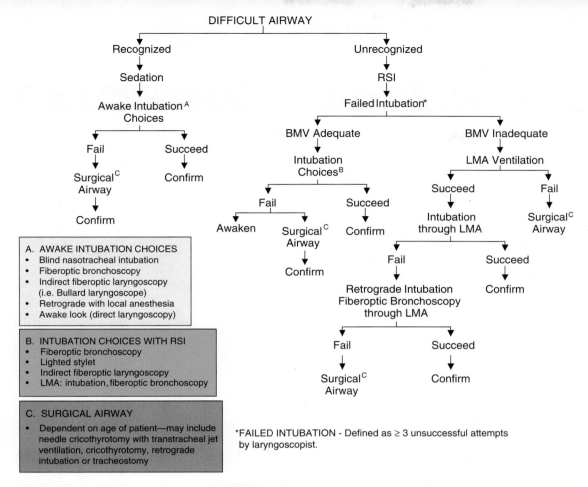

Figure 3.9 Algorithm for management of the difficult airway.
Adapted from Lee BS, Gausche-Hill M. *Pediatric Airway Management*. Clinical Pediatric Emergency Medicine, W. B. Saunders, 2001; 2:102.

# ■ Upper Airway Obstruction

## Croup

Laryngotracheobronchitis, commonly referred to as croup, is a frequent cause of upper airway obstruction in children. Most of these cases are caused by viral infection of the subglottic airway, producing a characteristic clinical syndrome consisting of a barky cough, stridor, and hoarseness.

Viral etiologies include parainfluenza virus[1–3] (accounting for more than two thirds of cases) and influenza A and B. Bacterial infections are much less common and include *Mycoplasma pneumoniae, Staphylococcus aureus, Streptococcus pyogenes,* and *Haemophilus influenzae.*[11,12]

## YOUR FIRST CLUE

### Classic Signs and Symptoms of Conditions Causing Upper Airway Obstruction

- Croup: Barking cough, hoarse voice, and stridor develop over several days.

- Foreign Body Aspiration: Choking, followed by stridor, and decreased breath sounds, develop rapidly over minutes.

- Retropharyngeal Abscess: Fever, neck pain/stiffness, drooling, and sore throat.

- Epiglottitis: Fever, drooling, sore throat, muffled voice, and absence of cough develop over hours to a day.

- Anaphylaxis: Angioedema, stridor, wheezing, and shock develop within minutes to hours.

| TABLE 3-5 | Clinical Croup Score* | | |
|---|---|---|---|
| | 0 | 1 | 2 |
| Cyanosis | None | In room air | In 40% $O_2$ |
| Inspiratory breath sounds | Normal | Harsh with rhonchi | Delayed |
| Stridor | None | Inspiratory | Inspiratory and expiratory or stridor at rest |
| Cough | None | Hoarse cry | Bark |
| Retractions and flaring | None | Flaring and suprasternal retractions | Flaring and suprasternal retractions plus subcostal and intercostal retractions |

*A score of ≥4 indicates moderately severe airway obstruction. A score of ≥7, particularly when associated with $Paco_2$ of >45 and $PaO_2$ of <70 (in room air), indicates impending respiratory failure.

## Epidemiology

The incidence of croup in the United States is approximately 3 to 5 per 100 children. Croup affects children 6 months to 6 years of age, with the incidence sharply declining after 6 years of age. Peak incidence occurs in the second year of life. Seasonally, most cases of croup occur during the fall and early winter.[12,13]

## Clinical Features

Prodromal symptoms mimic those of an upper respiratory infection. Typically these antecedent symptoms last 1 to 2 days. With the onset of croup, the more characteristic symptoms begin. Fever is present in about one half of the cases and tends to be low grade. Barky cough and stridor are seen in 90% or more of patients. Hoarseness and retractions are also common. Stridor is the hallmark of upper airway obstruction. In mild cases, stridor is evident only on auscultation with a stethoscope or with agitation. As the disease progresses and airway obstruction becomes more severe, stridor will be more audible and present during the inspiratory and expiratory phases.[12,13] A croup score for determining severity can be seen in Table 3-5. In general, duration of croup symptoms is 5 to 10 days.

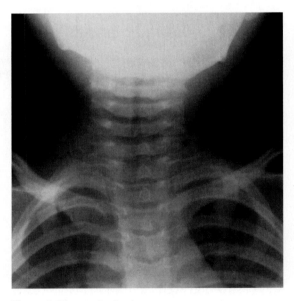

Figure 3.10 Steeple sign in croup.

## Diagnostic Studies

The diagnosis of croup is made clinically. The utility of laboratory studies and imaging is limited, and routine ancillary studies are not necessary. Plain radiographs of the neck might show a characteristic finding of subglottic narrowing referred to as the steeple sign (Figure 3.10).

## Differential Diagnosis

Epigolottitis, bacterial tracheitis, peritonsiliar abscess, uvulitis, foreign body (FB) aspiration, allergic reaction, and neoplasm are other etiologies of infectious and noninfectious upper airway obstruction that can present with symptoms similar to croup.

## Management

Mist or humidified $O_2$ has a theoretical benefit of moistening thick secretions and decreasing inflammation of the airway in croup. However, there are little data to support this hypothesis, and trials have not demonstrated significant benefit of this treatment.[12-14] If the child becomes more agitated by the mist device and the $O_2$ saturation level is normal, it should be discontinued.

Nebulized epinephrine should be promptly started in all patients with moderate to severe croup. Epinephrine acts at α- and β-adrenergic receptors causing vasoconstriction and improvement of mucosal edema, and bronchial smooth muscle relaxation.[15] Two formulations of epinephrine can be used for nebulization. The l-epinephrine dose is 0.5 mL/kg of a 1:1000 concentration to a maximum of 5 mL/dose. Racemic epinephrine, which contains both l- and k-isomers of epinephrine, is dosed as 0.05 mL/kg to a maximum of 0.5 mL of 2.25% solution with a saline diluent. Comparison of these two forms has not demonstrated a significant difference in efficacy.[16]

Steroids should be administered early in the management of moderate to severe croup. Nebulized budesonide and dexamethasone, given intramuscularly or orally, are the two corticosteroids that have been studied for the treatment of croup. There has been no significant difference in efficacy in comparison studies.[17,18] Dexamethasone is a long-acting corticosteroid with a half-life of 36 to 72 hours. Effective dexamethasone dosages of 0.15 mg/kg to 0.6 mg/kg per dose either orally or intramuscularly have shown similar benefits. The 0.6 mg/kg dose is more widely used in clinical practice.[13,19] Benefits of dexamethasone in the hospital setting include faster improvements in symptoms and croup scores, decreased incidence of endotracheal intubation in children admitted for croup, and

shorter hospital stays.[15,20] Safety and efficacy of dexamethasone in mild to moderate croup in the outpatient setting has been demonstrated by fewer return visits and lower hospitalization rates.[17,21,22] Budesonide has been studied mostly in the inpatient setting. A dose of 2 mg nebulized in saline solution has shown similar efficacy compared with dexamethasone.[17,18]

General indications for endotracheal intubation in respiratory failure should be used in the management of a child with severe croup. Endotracheal intubation or tracheostomy can be necessary in less than 6% of patients. Tracheal tube size should be one-half to one full size smaller than predicted by size and age to allow for subglottic edema and to reduce the risk of subglottic stenosis.[23]

In the past, treatment with nebulized racemic epinephrine was a criterion for admission to the hospital. This was due to the "rebound" effect with return of symptoms up to 2 hours after treatment with racemic epinephrine. This dogma was mostly driven by limited data from earlier studies with small sample sizes. Recent literature has refuted this practice and concluded that use of racemic epinephrine in the ED for outpatient management of croup is safe and effective. These studies recommended an observation period of 180 to 240 minutes in the ED prior to discharge, with documentation of periodic croup

---

### KEY POINTS

**Management of Croup**

- Begin cool mist as long as it does not increase agitation.
- Begin treatment with steroids: dexamethasone 0.15 to 0.6 mg/kg PO or IM, or budesonide 2 mg/2 mL saline nebulized.
- Begin epinephrine for signs of moderate to severe respiratory distress: racemic 0.05 mL/kg to a maximum of 0.5 mL of 2.25% in 2 mL of saline nebulized or l-epinephrine (1:1,000 solution) 0.5 mL/kg nebulized.
- Assist ventilation for signs of respiratory failure.

scores and reevaluation for return of symptoms. During observation, patients who experienced relapse of symptoms were hospitalized but did not have post-treatment croup scores that were worse than on presentation to the ED. There were no significant complications seen in patients discharged home. All of the patients included in the studies of outpatient treatment with racemic epinephrine also received intramuscular dexamethasone.[13,19]

Guidelines for disposition have been specifically addressed in only one prospective study. Criteria for discharge of patients home were a croup score less than 4, pulse oximetry higher than 90%, and adequate hydration. Hospital admission rates vary widely from 4% to 46%. The average length of hospitalization is 1 to 2 days.[12,13,17,19]

## Foreign Body Aspiration

Foreign body (FB) aspiration is one of the leading causes of accidental death in infants and young children, accounting for 150 to 300 annual fatalities in children in the United States.[24,25] Most cases are seen in the 1-to 2-year-old age group, accounting for up to two thirds of all cases.[26,27] Food items are the most commonly aspirated airway FBs in children (Figure 3.11).[28] Nuts, especially peanuts, are the most common foods aspirated into the respiratory tree, making up approximately one half of all FB cases.[24,29] During the period between 1972 and 1992, the US Consumer Product Safety Commission reported 449 deaths from

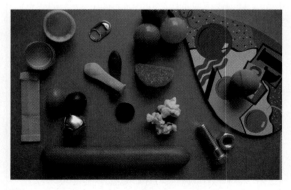

Figure 3.11 Examples of foreign bodies aspirated by children.

man made objects. The most common and most lethal non–food objects were balloons, including two fatalities secondary to blown-up latex gloves in physicians' offices. Under the Federal Hazardous Substances Act, a toy or object intended for young children must pass a test using a Small Parts Test Fixture (SPTF). The SPTF is a cylinder with a diameter of 3.17 cm and length of 5.71 cm. Any object that can fit inside the SPTF does not pass.[28] An empty toilet paper roll cut in half by length is a convenient household item with roughly the same dimensions.

## Clinical Features

The history and physical findings in FB aspiration can be quite variable. The following are signs and symptoms seen in children with documented FB aspiration listed in order by decreasing frequency: history of choking/ aspiration (22% to 88%), wheezing (40% to 82%), stridor (8% to 71%), cough (42% to 54%), decreased breath sounds on auscultation (51%), hoarseness (29%), respiratory distress (18%), cyanosis (3% to 29%), fever (17%), respiratory arrest (3%).[27,30] The incidence of patients who have no symptoms or physical findings on presentation ranges from 8% to 80%.[31] A history of choking is the most reliable predictor of FB aspiration and should prompt further evaluation and consideration for bronchoscopy.[29,32]

Sites of obstruction by FB are as follows: larynx (7%), trachea (14%), right mainstem bronchus (30%), left mainstem bronchus (23%), right bronchus (21%), left bronchus (5%).[30] Laryngotracheal FBs are the minority, but can be immediately life threatening and cause complete airway obstruction.

Delays in diagnosis and treatment can lead to pneumonia, obstructive emphysema, and bronchiectasis.[26] Delays in diagnosis as long as 4 months have been reported.[27] Mortality is uniformly a result of asphyxiation.[29] In rare cases in which FB lodges in the distal airways and bronchoscopy is unsuccessful, thoracotomy with incisional removal of the FB might be necessary.

## Diagnostic Studies

Radiographic studies, including standard chest radiograph, lateral decubitus, expiratory, lateral neck, and fluoroscopy, do not have very good sensitivity or specificity. Radiopaque FBs are seen in 6% to 15% of films. Other findings suggestive of lower airway FB include air trapping/ hyperinflation (38% to 63%), atelectasis (8% to 25%), pulmonary consolidation (1% to 5%), and barotrauma (7%) (**Figure 3.12**).[24,30] Fluoroscopy is diagnostic of FB when differential ventilation of the lungs causes mediastinal shifting during respiration. Normal plain films are seen in up to one in four cases of FB aspiration and should not lower the clinical suspicion of airway FB.

## Differential Diagnosis

The differential diagnosis for airway FB includes upper respiratory disorders, as listed previously, and lower airway disorders, including reactive airway disease and bronchiolitis.

## Management

In the setting of airway FB, most cases will present with partial airway obstruction. The goal of management in the ED is to support oxygenation and ventilation and to prevent and treat total airway obstruction. Rapid cardiopulmonary assessment is key in patients

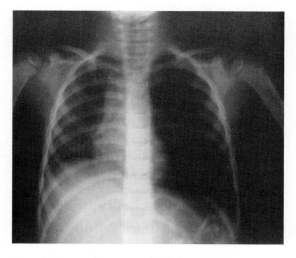

**Figure 3.12** Findings associated with foreign body aspiration.

with suspected airway FB. A multidisciplinary approach is vital, and airway specialists must be mobilized early.

The therapeutic modality of choice for lower airway FBs is bronchoscopy, preferably done in the operating room.[26] The FB retrieval rate approaches 100%[33] with bronchoscopy, the gold standard for diagnosis and treatment. In the absence of respiratory failure or imminent respiratory failure, the child should be left in a position of comfort, with supplemental $O_2$ as needed. All efforts should be made to limit agitation (i.e., intravenous (IV) access and unnecessary radiographs should be deferred) until the airway is secured using inhalational anesthesia in the operating room.

In the rare case of complete airway obstruction and respiratory failure, basic life support (BLS) measures should be started immediately. Airway positioning and bag-mask ventilation are the initial intervention. If bag-mask ventilation is adequate for ventilation, then the patient should be rapidly transported to the operating room for definitive therapy. If unable to ventilate with bag-mask ventilation, then five back blows and chest thrusts are done in infants younger than 1 year or five abdominal thrusts in children to attempt dislodgement of the impacted FB.[34] Direct laryngoscopy is the next step to attempt visualization of the FB and removal with Magill forceps. If BLS measures fail, options are limited in attempting to ventilate the patient. Orotracheal intubation can be attempted in an effort to dislodge the FB to a distal bronchus and ventilate one lung, or to intubate around the FB. Immediate surgical airway is another option via cricothyrotomy in the older child, tracheotomy, or needle cricothyrotomy with transtracheal jet ventilation in younger children and infants. The mortality rate among patients with FB aspiration and a failed airway attempt is extremely high.

Heliox has been described in a case report as an effective temporizing measure in a child with severe respiratory distress awaiting bronchoscopy. The helium-oxygen mixture is less dense than $O_2$ or room air and improves ventilation in cases of airway obstruction.[35]

## Retropharyngeal Abscess

Retropharyngeal abscess (RPA) is the most common deep space neck infection seen in children. The retropharyngeal space is a potential space containing lymph nodes, which drain the nasopharynx, adenoids, posterior nasal sinuses, and middle ear. Anatomically, the boundaries of the retropharyngeal space consist of the skull base superiorly, the mediastinum inferiorly, the visceral fascia anteriorly, the carotid sheaths laterally, and the prevertebral fascia posteriorly.[36]

Retropharyngeal abscess is most commonly caused by suppuration of the lymph nodes following infection of the pharyngeal structures, middle ear, and sinuses. Lymphatic drainage of these areas causes the lymph nodes in the retropharyngeal space to become infected with progression to cellulitis and abscess formation. Uncommon causes of RPA include trauma to the oropharynx caused by penetrating FBs, endoscopic procedures, and endotracheal intubation.[37]

### Epidemiology

Children younger than 6 years constitute more than 96% of RPA cases, with a peak incidence in 3-to-5 year-old children.[23,38] The incidence of RPA sharply declines after age 6 because the lymph nodes in the retropharyngeal space become obliterated and involute during this age. Older children and adults with RPA have a higher incidence of trauma, IV drug abuse, and iatrogenic causes.[39]

### Clinical Features

Fever, neck pain, and sore throat are the most common symptoms and are present in most cases of RPA. Hoarse voice, poor oral intake, drooling, cervical adenopathy, and stiff neck are also common symptoms. Frank obstructive symptoms such as stridor and sleep apnea are less common.[40] Physical findings can include a visible asymmetric pharyngeal bulge in up to half of the cases of RPA.

Complications in cases of RPA have become rare in the antibiotic era. Airway obstruction requiring endotracheal intubation or tracheotomy is rare in the pediatric population in contrast to the adult population.[41] In rare cases, RPA can rupture anteriorly into the airway, causing aspiration of pus. Septic jugular vein thrombosis presents with fever, rigors, tenderness, and swelling along the sternocleidomastoid muscle. Septic emboli can travel to distant organs, causing meningitis, lateral sinus thrombosis, pulmonary infarcts, and endocarditis. Diagnosis is confirmed by computed tomography (CT) or magnetic resonance imaging (MRI) of the neck. Carotid artery rupture can result in exsanguination, ipsilateral Horner syndrome, and palsies of cranial nerves 9 through 12. Mediastinitis presents with chest pain, dyspnea, sepsis, and shock and is usually confirmed by CT and MRI. Chest radiography might reveal widening of the mediastinum.[36] Untreated, mediastinitis has a mortality rate that approaches 100%. The overall complication risk and mortality rates associated with RPA are very low.[38] This likely represents early diagnosis, judicious use of antibiotics, and better diagnostic tools such as CT in evaluating RPA.

## Diagnostic Studies

Cultures of the purulent material from the abscess should be obtained to guide antimicrobial therapy. Group A β-hemolytic *Streptococcus* and *S aureus* are the most commonly cultured bacteria in pediatric neck infections.[37] Most deep neck abscesses are also polymicrobial, including anaerobic oral flora, most commonly the *Bacteroides* genus.

Plain radiographs of the neck with special attention to the prevertebral soft tissues are useful in evaluation of RPA (Figure 3.13). Normal prevertebral soft tissue dimensions on plain lateral radiograph of the neck are less than 7 mm at C2 and less than 22 mm at the level of C6.[36,42] Sensitivity of a plain radiograph for RPA indicated by thickening of the soft tissue is up to 88% to 100%.[23] The radiograph must be taken during inspiration and with the neck in extension to avoid false positives.

Computed tomography is the test of choice for evaluating deep neck abscesses and is approximately 90% accurate in diagnosing RPA. Computed tomography also identifies the stage of disease from cellulitis to phlegmon to organized abscess.[38] Complications of RPA, such as jugular vein thrombosis, mediastinitis, and carotid artery rupture, can also be diagnosed by CT.[37]

## Differential Diagnosis

Other infections of the deep neck spaces to consider in the differential diagnosis of RPA include abscess formation in the lateral pharyngeal space, submandibular and submental space, peritonsillar space, pretracheal space, and epidural space. Ludwig angina and vertebral osteomyelitis should also be included in the differential diagnosis.[36,40] Other less common causes of swelling and upper airway obstruction include superficial neck infections such as cervical adenitis/abscess, neoplasms, benign and malignant, congenital lesions such as cystic hygroma, thyroglossal duct cyst, and branchial cleft cysts.[37]

## Management

All patients with RPA should receive parenteral broad-spectrum antimicrobial coverage, including gram-positive coverage with a β-lactamase–resistant antibiotic and anaerobic coverage. Antibiotics should be started promptly in the ED when the diagnosis of deep neck infection is suspected. Fifteen percent to 50% of the cases of RPA are successfully treated with IV antibiotics alone.[42,43] Many reported cases could actually be retropharyngeal cellulitis and not true RPA.

Definitive management is the adequate drainage of pus from the retropharyngeal space. There is some controversy in the literature about the indications, timing, and type of procedure for drainage of RPA. Needle drainage has been highly successful in some trials in conjunction with antibiotic therapy. The advantage of needle aspiration is the avoidance of an open procedure and general anesthesia. Surgical incision and drainage is recommended as the definitive therapy for all cases of RPA by many head and neck surgeons.[43]

The endotracheal intubation rate in RPA is very low preoperatively. If airway obstruction is severe and the child is in danger of imminent respiratory failure, then endotracheal intubation should be performed emergently. As in most cases of upper airway obstruction, this is ideally done in the operating room. The general indicators for respiratory failure and intubation are the same for RPA as for other causes. The tracheotomy rate is 0% to 8% in children with RPA.[38,43]

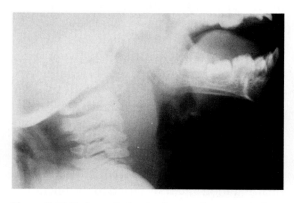

Figure 3.13 Radiograph showing increase in prevertebral soft tissue shadow associated with retropharyngeal infection.

## Epiglottitis

The incidence of epiglottitis has decreased dramatically in the past decade. Prior to the introduction of the *H influenzae* type b (Hib) vaccine in 1989, the peak incidence of epiglottitis occurred in young children between 1 and 5 years old. Incidence was approximately 10 per 100,000 before 1990. Since 1991, the incidence of Hib-associated epiglottitis in the pediatric population has approached zero. Hence, in the past decade, epiglottitis has become a disease seen predominantly in adults.[23,44-46]

### Clinical Features

Children with epiglottitis typically present with drooling, fever, respiratory distress, muffled voice, and toxic appearance in most cases. Prehospital respiratory arrest is almost always fatal and accounts for most of the mortality in this disease. Mortality of epiglottitis in children is approximately 2% secondary to airway obstruction.[44,45]

Airway obstruction is the most common and severe complication of epiglottitis. Deep neck infections and abscess of the epiglottis itself have been reported. Fewer than 10% will develop pneumonia during the course. Meningitis has not been reported as a complication in recent large retrospective reviews.[45,47]

### Diagnostic Studies

Blood cultures should be done routinely in suspected cases of epiglottitis after the patient's airway has been evaluated. Bacteremia with Hib is seen in more than one half of the cases of epiglottitis. Patients with positive blood cultures for Hib generally have a more severe clinical presentation and hospital course.[44,45] In the postvaccine era, other gram-positive cocci have been found in blood cultures, including Group A β-hemolytic *Streptococcus, S aureus,* and *S pneumoniae.*[46]

Most patients who can tolerate a radiographic examination will exhibit a swollen epiglottis on lateral radiograph of the neck, classically known as the "thumbprint" sign (**Figure 3.14**). Plain radiographs of the neck are normal in up to 20% of cases.[23] Leukocytosis is present

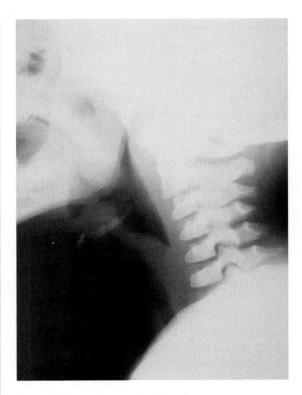

**Figure 3.14** Findings with epiglottitis.

in most cases of epiglottitis but its presence is not useful in clinical decision making.

### Differential Diagnosis

The differential diagnosis for epiglottitis includes pharyngitis, croup, bacterial tracheitis, and other upper airway disorders.

### Management

When the diagnosis of epiglottitis is suspected, efforts should primarily be directed at securing the airway. Patients in severe respiratory distress, complete or near-complete airway obstruction, should undergo endotracheal intubation immediately in the ED. Two-person bag-mask ventilation can be palliative. Preparations should be made in advance for surgical airway if orotracheal intubation fails. Patients with signs of airway obstruction but not in severe distress should be prepped for intubation in the operating room. The child should be left in a position of comfort with minimal agitation and transferred to the operating room for laryngoscopy and endotracheal intubation. Patients without respiratory com-

**The Management of Epiglottitis**

- Patient alert and able to maintain airway: Leave in position of comfort and transport to the operating room for airway management
- Patient not alert and with signs of respiratory failure: Begin bag-mask ventilation, attempt endotracheal intubation, consider laryngeal mask airway, cricothyrotomy, tracheostomy

promise or drooling, and minimal inflammation of the epiglottis on laryngoscopy, can be medically managed without endotracheal intubation in the pediatric intensive care unit (PICU). Laryngoscopy, direct or indirect, does not precipitate complete airway obstruction.[45] Tracheal tubes should be one to two sizes smaller than usually appropriate for the child's age and size.

Intravenous antibiotics should be started as soon as possible. Second- or third-generation cephalosporins are effective against *H influenzae* and also against the less common bacteria seen in epiglottitis. Other effective antibiotics include β-lactamase–resistant penicillins.[46]

# Anaphylaxis

Anaphylaxis is a potentially life-threatening condition that can occur through three basic mechanisms. Type 1 hypersensitivity, the most common etiology, occurs when an antigen binds circulating IgE from previous antigen exposure. Nonimmunologic direct action on mast cell degranulation is seen typically with contrast media, opiates, and physical stresses such as cold, vibration, or heat. Complement activation seen in hereditary angioedema (C1 esterase deficiency) can also cause anaphylaxis. All of these mechanisms have a common final pathway, which is activation and degranulation of mast cells and basophils causing release of chemical mediators such as histamine and other vasoactive and chemotactic factors.[39]

## Epidemiology

An estimated 29,000 anaphylactic reactions occur in the United States each year, with approximately 150 fatalities.[48] The mortality rate of anaphylactic reactions in children is less than 2%. Foods cause most anaphylactic reactions in children, with peanuts and other nuts being the most common antigens. Other common food triggers include shellfish, eggs, and milk. Another common cause of anaphylaxis in children is insect stings, especially from the Hymenoptera order (bees, yellow jacket, wasps, and fire ants). The most common medications implicated are antibiotics, such as penicillins and cephalosporins. Exercise-induced anaphylaxis is a less common form seen during exercise, frequently after ingestion of certain foods. Risk factors for anaphylaxis are atopic and include asthma, allergic rhinitis, atopic dermatitis, and prior allergy to a substance.[49,50]

## Clinical Features

Angioedema is most common in the face and lips. Hypopharyngeal or laryngeal edema is also common and leads to upper airway obstruction with symptoms of throat swelling, dyspnea, stridor, hoarseness, and dysphagia.[51] Lower airway involvement leads to bronchospasm, wheezing, dyspnea, and chest tightness. Cardiovascular effects include hypotension (often severe and refractory), arrhythmias, and cardiogenic and distributive shock. Cutaneous symptoms include generalized flushing from vasodilation, urticaria, and angioedema. Gastrointestinal tract

**Signs and Symptoms of Anaphylaxis**

- Upper Airway: angioedema, dyspnea, stridor, hoarseness, dysphagia
- Lower Airway: wheezing, dyspnea, chest tightness
- Cardiovascular: arrhythmias, shock
- Cutaneous: angioedema of face and lips, flushing, urticaria
- Gastrointestinal: nausea, vomiting, diarrhea, abdominal cramps/pain

involvement causes nausea, vomiting, diarrhea, and abdominal cramps secondary to intestinal smooth muscle contraction and bowel edema.[49]

## Diagnostic Studies

The diagnosis of anaphylaxis is made clinically. Routine laboratory studies or radiographic studies are not necessary in the diagnosis or management of anaphylaxis.

## Management

Epinephrine is the treatment of choice in anaphylaxis. Action of epinephrine is at the $\alpha$- and $\beta$-adrenergic receptors causing vasoconstriction, increasing cardiac inotropy and chronotropy, and bronchial smooth muscle relaxation. Dosage is 0.01 mL/kg of 1:1,000 solution to a maximum dose of 0.3 mL, repeat every 15 minutes as needed. Epinephrine can be given subcutaneously or intramuscularly; however, some authors suggest that intramuscular injection is the route of choice in anaphylaxis.[48]

H1 antagonist antihistamines, such as diphenhydramine, should be given intravenously to all patients with anaphylaxis. These medications are effective in treating the cutaneous symptoms of urticaria and itching. H2 antagonist antihistamines are also recommended. Bronchospasm is treated with nebulized $\beta_2$ agonists, such as albuterol. Parenteral corticosteroids are given routinely to patients with anaphylaxis.[39] Vasopressors should be started in cases of hypotension refractory to IV fluid resuscitation. Dopamine and/or norepinephrine is titrated to maintain adequate blood pressure.

Endotracheal intubation is seldom required in the management of anaphylaxis.[51] However, it is important to remember that respiratory arrest secondary to airway obstruction is the leading cause of death in fatal cases of anaphylaxis.[50,52] In addition to the general indications for endotracheal intubation in respiratory failure, patients in respiratory distress with signs of severe upper airway obstruction, lingual edema, hypopharyngeal edema, or laryngeal edema should be intubated early to avoid the dreaded scenario of complete airway obstruction with the inability to intubate or ventilate.

## KEY POINTS

**Management of Anaphylaxis**

- Administer epinephrine 0.01 mL/kg of 1:1,000 solution to a maximum of 0.3 mL SC or IM, repeat every 15 minutes as needed.
- Nebulized albuterol
- H1 and H2 antihistamines (IV)
- Solumedrol IV
- Consider epinephrine 1:10,000 or 1:100,000 solution IV only if patient is in cardiopulmonary failure.

## Disposition

There are no studies that specifically address disposition of patients with anaphylaxis from the ED. Patients with mild symptoms that resolve after medical therapy can be safely discharged home if asymptomatic after several hours of observation in the ED. Patients who present with moderate to severe anaphylaxis should be admitted to the hospital for observation after treatment in the ED. Biphasic reactions account for up to 50% of fatal cases.[50] In a large pediatric population, biphasic reactions were reported in 6% of patients admitted to the hospital, of which half were serious and required repeat administration of epinephrine and 1% required intubation. The asymptomatic interval varied widely, from 1 to 28 hours.[53]

Preventive measures are vital in the treatment of anaphylaxis. After an anaphylactic reaction, all patients should undergo skin testing to identify potential allergens. Medical bracelets are recommended for anaphylaxis patients to identify their serious allergies. Epinephrine self-injection kits should be prescribed to all patients with a history of anaphylaxis. Several studies have demonstrated the deficiencies in proper use of epinephrine injection kits.[54,55] A review of anaphylaxis deaths reported patients holding an unused kit in hand, use of an expired kit, and one case of a patient who died waiting for the prescription to be filled at a pharmacy.[52]

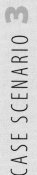

## CASE SCENARIO 3

A 6-month-old boy presents with acute respiratory distress preceded by a short history of upper respiratory tract symptoms and low-grade fever. He is irritable and feeding poorly. He is alert, but tachypneic, has nasal flaring and intercostal retractions, and is pale. His vital signs include a repiratory rate of 70/min, heart rate of 170 bpm, temperature of 38°C (rectal), and oxygen saturation 90% on room air. Diffuse bilateral wheezing is discovered on physical examination.

1. *What are your initial treatment priorities?*
2. *What diagnostic tests will be helpful?*

# ■ Lower Airway Obstruction

## Bronchiolitis

Respiratory syncytial virus (RSV) is the most common virus causing lower respiratory tract infection, primarily bronchiolitis, in infants.[56] The terms RSV and bronchiolitis are often used interchangeably. Most children have been infected by RSV before their second birthday.[57] Infants with prematurity and chronic pulmonary and congenital heart disease are at highest risk for severe disease (Table 3-6). Viral shedding generally lasts around 1 week; however, in infants with lower respiratory tract disease, it can last up to 4 weeks. Average incubation is 5 days.

Apnea can be the presenting manifestation of the infection; however, most infants with RSV present with an upper respiratory infection prodrome, followed by cough and wheezing. Hypoxia is most often due to ventilation/perfusion (V/Q) mismatch, although hypoventilation is seen as fatigue develops. Progression

| TABLE 3-6 | Risk Factors for Severe RSV Disease[56,57] |
|---|

- Prematurity
- Complex congenital heart disease
- Chronic lung disease
- Immunosuppression
- Neuromuscular disease
- Metabolic disorder

| TABLE 3-7 | Indications for Immunoprophylaxis with RSV-Immune Globulin Intravenous |
|---|---|

- Infants and children less than 2 years of age with chronic lung disease (CLD) who have required medical therapy for CLD within 6 months of anticipated RSV season. Some infants with severe disease benefit from prophylaxis for the first 2 years.
- Infants born at 32 weeks' gestation or earlier without CLD.
- Infants born at more than 28 weeks' gestation and who are less than 12 months of age at the start of RSV season.
- Infants born at 29 to 32 weeks' gestation and who are less than 6 months of age at the start of RSV season.
- Some infants born prematurely or with CLD who meet the criteria in the above requirements and who also have asymptomatic, acyanotic congenital heart disease.
- At this time, RSV-Immune Globulin Intravenous (IGIV) is contraindicated in infants with **cyanotic** congenital heart disease.

Source: American Academy of Pediatrics. Immunophylaxis: Report of the committee on infectious disease. *Redbook*. 2000; 25: 486. Reprinted with permission.

to respiratory failure and shunting can be seen with pneumonia and atelectasis. Immunoprophylaxis is recommended for infants at high risk[58] (Table 3-7). No vaccine is currently available.

Respiratory syncytial virus is a single-stranded RNA virus of the Paramyxoviridae family. Infection is spread by droplets and contact with contaminated surfaces. The eyes and nose are primary sites for inoculation.[57] Respiratory syncytial virus infections tend to occur in fall, winter, and spring in temperate climates. The most severe disease is seen in young infants, especially those younger than 6 weeks. Native Alaskan and American Indian infants have a disproportionately high hospitalization rate for RSV. The mortality rate in high-risk patients has been reported to be 2%.[57]

## Clinical Features

The clinical presentation of bronchiolitis varies by age. First infections are more likely to be symptomatic. Premature infants and infants with chronic lung disease, immunosuppression, or congenital heart disease are at increased risk for morbidity and mortality. Cough, nasal congestion, otitis media, and fever are commonly seen in these infants. Nonspecific findings can also be seen in this age group and include poor feeding and irritability. Apnea can be seen in infants, especially those born prematurely or who are younger than 6 weeks. Up to 70% of patients will have wheezing or rales with pneumonia. Hypoxia is common

to all infants hospitalized with RSV bronchiolitis. Increased work of breathing can manifest as tachypnea, tachycardia, grunting, flaring, supraclavicular and intercostal retractions, and head bobbing in infants. There can be clinical evidence of dehydration if the child has been feeding poorly during the illness.

The single most predictive factor for severe disease in a previously healthy infant is $O_2$ saturation lower than 95%. Other factors associated with severe disease include age younger than 3 months, gestational age younger than 34 weeks, toxic appearance, atelectasis, and tachypnea with respiratory rate

## YOUR FIRST CLUE

**Signs and Symptoms of Bronchiolitis**
- Cough
- Nasal congestion
- Otitis media
- Fever
- Tachypnea
- Tachycardia
- Increased work of breathing (grunting, flaring, supraclavicular and intercostal retractions, and head bobbing in infants)
- Hypoxia
- Apnea
- Apparent life-threatening event

greater than 70/min.[57] Diagnosis of bronchiolitis is generally made clinically, taking into account the clinical history, age of the child, time of year, and presence of other cases in the area. Testing for RSV is more frequently performed in those infants who present to the ED during peak RSV season.

## Complications

Complications of bronchiolitis include apnea, pneumonia, atelectasis, dehydration, respiratory failure, bacterial superinfection, and air leaks. Apnea is seen in up to 18% of infants with RSV, with the risk being higher in premature and young infants.

## Diagnostic Studies

The primary diagnostic studies for bronchiolitis include $O_2$ saturation measurements and chest radiograph. The chest radiograph classically shows hyperinflation (Figure 3.15). Pneumonia and atelectasis can also be seen. Arterial blood gas analysis is needed only in severe cases. Viral detection methods are available but do not usually change treatment or disposition, thereby making them unnecessary in the ED setting. Viral antigen detection is available for most of the viral agents that produce a clinical picture of bronchiolitis. Rapid antigen detection for RSV is widely available and is best performed on a nasopharyngeal aspirate. Positive detection of RSV is important in the disposition of chronically ill or immunosuppressed infants and febrile neonates.

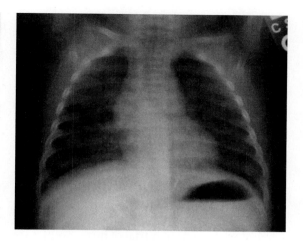

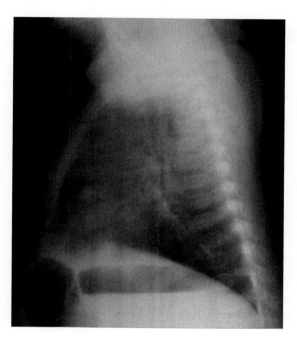

Figure 3.15 Findings of bronchiolitis.

## THE CLASSICS

**Chest Radiographic Findings in Patients With Bronchiolitis**
- Hyperinflation
- Peribronchial cuffing
- Pneumonia

## Differential Diagnosis

The differential diagnosis for bronchiolitis includes pneumonia, reactive airway disease, congestive heart failure, FB aspiration, congenital airway lesion, and viral upper respiratory infection.

## Management

General supportive care is the mainstay of management in bronchiolitis and includes antipyretics, suctioning, hydration (IV or orally), and ongoing clinical monitoring of vital signs and $O_2$ saturation. Supplemental $O_2$ and continuous pulse oximetry are used for infants with signs of respiratory distress and $O_2$ saturation levels lower than 95%. Mechanical ventilation is rarely necessary. Agitation can worsen hypoxemia and should be prevented.

The most controversial area of management is the use of bronchodilators such as albuterol.[59-61] It is often difficult to distinguish bronchiolitis from reactive airway disease with upper respiratory infection. A trial of bronchodilators (albuterol) is usually recommended. Studies have shown nebulized racemic epinephrine to be more effective than $\beta_2$ agonists.[62-63]

Ribavirin can be considered for hospitalized infants with severe disease and is administered as a continuous aerosol for 3 to 7 days. Ribavirin is potentially teratogenic; therefore, pregnant health care workers should be excused from caring for patients receiving this drug.[64] Heliox can also be considered for infants with severe disease.[65] The use of systemic or inhaled steroids has demonstrated no short- or long- term benefits in the acute phase of disease.[66] The only indications for antibiotics are in cases of a neonate with fever, pending cultures, or when the chest radiograph demonstrates findings consistent with pneumonia or superinfection.

Avoid exposing high-risk infants and children to infants and children with RSV. Nosocomial transmission can be high, and careful attention to standard infection control measures is critical to limit spread.

## KEY POINTS

**Management of Bronchiolitis**

- Supportive care is the mainstay of bronchiolitis treatment.
  - Correction of hypoxia and adequate hydration are basic tools that help to support infants with bronchiolitis.
  - Return to normal respiratory rates in an infant who has been working hard to breathe does not always indicate improvement.
  - It is important to assess the numbers in the context of the child because decreasing respiratory rates might also mean that the child is fatiguing and has impending respiratory failure.
- Nebulized albuterol and epinephrine can be tried, but studies show limited benefit.
- Corticosteroids can decrease duration of symptoms and length of stay, but benefit is not large.

**CASE SCENARIO 4**

A 5-year-old boy had an acute asthma episode at school during show-and-tell after a classmate brought in a new kitten. He was given albuterol by the school nurse but continued to have tachypnea and diffuse wheezing, and his mother was called to take him home. Wheezing continued despite two additional albuterol nebulizer treatments given consecutively at home. The mother brings him to the emergency department. On arrival, he is alert, shows increased work of breathing with nasal flaring and retractions, and has normal skin color. Vital signs are respiratory rate 50 breaths per minute; a heart rate of 130 bpm; a blood pressure of 120/80 mmHg; axillary temperature 36.6°C; pulse oximetry 89% on room air. He is acutely short of breath with poor air entry and no wheezing on auscultation of the chest.

1. *What are your priorities?*
2. *What is the significance of absent wheezing in this scenario?*

# Asthma

Asthma is a chronic inflammatory disease of the airways characterized by complete or partial reversible airway obstruction, increased mucus production, and airway edema. It is a common problem in childhood that affects approximately 7% of children in the United States, and accounts for more than 867,000 ED visits, acute care visits, and hospitalizations. Children younger than 4 years have the highest hospitalization and ED visit frequencies. In 1998, 246 children ages 0 to 17 years died from asthma.[67] Various aspects of the disease have been proposed to define asthma, including reversible airway obstruction, recurrent cough without clear evidence of airway narrowing, airway hyperresponsiveness, chronic airway inflammation, and altered T cell function.

Genetics and the environment have influential roles in the development of the phenotypic presentation. Exposure to cigarette smoke, urban and low income environments, and preteen obesity in girls have been associated with increased rates of asthma. About one third of asthmatic children seen in the ED are admitted to a hospital.[68] Rapid onset of symptoms (less than 3 hours) and history of prior intubation are risk factors for deterioration. Table 3-8 reviews important questions to ask about the history.

## Clinical Features

The principal presentations of asthma include cough, wheeze, chest congestion, and difficulty breathing. Correct diagnosis is sometimes difficult, especially before 12 months of age when 30% of children with lower respiratory tract illnesses can wheeze. Other respiratory conditions must be considered and excluded.

Decision making is guided by overall clinical impression and is influenced by judgment about the family's ability to care for the child in their environment. Infections are a frequent trigger in children and should be addressed. Ventilation/perfusion mismatch is the most common cause for hypoxia in asthma exacerbations. A complete physical examination should be done, with special emphasis on de-

| TABLE 3-8 | Abbreviated Asthma History for ED Patients |
| --- | --- |

**Present Episode**
- When did it start?
- Can you identify the trigger?
- What medications have you taken so far (include times)?
- How did you respond to those medications (peak expiratory flow rate [PEFR] and clinical response)?

**Asthma History**
- Baseline asthma: what medications do you usually take?
- How often do you wheeze, cough, or have shortness of breath?
- How often do you need to come to the ED? When was your last visit?
- How often were you hospitalized? Did you need to go to PICU?
- Have you ever been intubated?
- How often and when were you last on oral steroids?

**Other**
- Do you have any other medical problems?
- Do you take any other medications?
- Do you take any herbal remedies?

termining the mental status and work of breathing of the patient. Documentation should include the position of comfort, respiratory rate, quality of air exchange, presence or absence of grunting, nasal flaring, retractions, wheezes, rhonchi, and crackles. Crackles can also be heard with pneumonia, atelectasis, and heart failure. Pulsus paradoxus correlates with forced expiratory volume and asthma severity in adults; however, in children, it is often difficult to assess and therefore is of limited value.[69] Complications of asthma include recurrent episodes of atelectasis due to mucus plugging, pneumothorax, pneumomediastinum, and respiratory failure.

## Diagnostic Studies

Pulmonary function studies are a mainstay of asthma management because asthma is a disease primarily of small- and mid-sized airways. The F25–75 (mean flow rates over middle 50%

of vital capacity) is a sensitive indicator of airflow obstruction in children. Peak expiratory flow rate (PEFR) is more reflective of larger airways. The forced expiratory volume in 1 second ($FEV_1$) is also an indicator of airflow obstruction. Peak flow meters are often used as a guide in the ED but are insufficient alone to define the disease. Furthermore, they are very effort dependent; children younger than 5 years have a difficult time mastering the technique, and some older children require practice to perform accurately. Even under the best circumstances, the peak flow meter might not accurately reflect the degree of obstruction in all children.[68]

Pulse oximetry is an excellent monitoring adjunct to assist in determining baseline status and response to therapy. Keep in mind the various factors that will cause the oxyhemoglobin desaturation curve to shift. Accurate pulse oximetry values depend on adequate blood flow to the monitoring site. Indications for measurement of arterial blood gasses (ABGs) include $O_2$ saturation less than 90% on maximal $O_2$ therapy, no clinical improvement despite aggressive therapy, and mental status changes. Chest radiographs are not routinely recommended. Considerations for a chest radiograph include first episode of wheezing, fever, and crackles, and patients with clinical evidence of a right-to-left shunt or poor response to standard therapy.

## Differential Diagnosis

The differential diagnosis for asthma includes bronchiolitis, upper respiratory infection (URI), pneumonia, congestive heart failure, congenital airway anomalies, and FB aspiration.

## Management

Management pathways following the most recent National Institutes of Health guidelines[70,71] are presented in **Figure 3.16**, Tables 3-9 through 3-12, and Table 3-21.

Supplemental $O_2$ and clinical monitoring are appropriate for all patients with respiratory distress. At one time, $O_2$ saturation levels of lower than 91% in the ED were associated with the need for hospital admission. However, a more recent multicenter study[72] refutes this finding and concludes that $O_2$ saturation alone is inadequate to predict the need for admission. Measurement of ABGs should be considered in patients who require maximal $O_2$ therapy.

Short-acting bronchodilators are considered the main rescue therapy for asthma. Corticosteroids are recommended for moderate to severe exacerbations and for patients who respond poorly or incompletely to β-agonist therapy. Because asthma is an inflammatory disease, early treatment with corticosteroids can help ameliorate an asthma episode.

Asthma severity in the ED is categorized as mild, moderate, or severe. Mild exacerbations are associated with PEFR of 80% or greater predicted (or personal best). Albuterol may be given up to three times in the ED and oral or IV steroids administered if no immediate response (after one dose of inhaled β-agonist) or if there is a recent medication history of oral steroids. Moderate exacerbations are associated with a PEFR between 50% and 80% predicted (or personal best). Treatment includes that for mild exacerbations plus inhaled short-acting $\beta_2$-agonists every hour for 1 to 3 hours (provided the child shows improvement), systemic corticosteroids, and supplemental $O_2$ to keep $O_2$ saturations at 90% or greater. Severe exacerbations are associated with PEFR less than 50% predicted (or personal best). Treatment includes supplemental $O_2$ (to achieve $O_2$ saturation greater than 90%), nebulized bronchodilators, and an anticholinergic agent

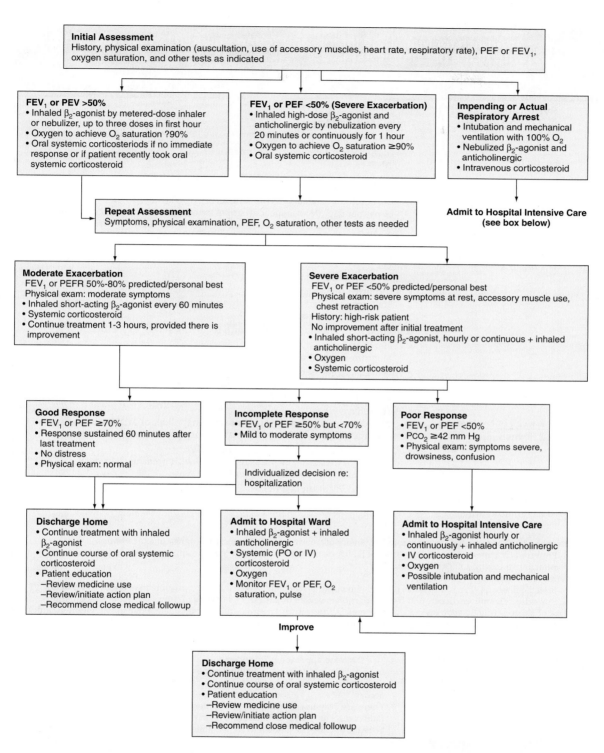

**Initial Assessment**
History, physical examination (auscultation, use of accessory muscles, heart rate, respiratory rate), PEF or $FEV_1$, oxygen saturation, and other tests as indicated

**$FEV_1$ or PEV >50%**
• Inhaled $\beta_2$-agonist by metered-dose inhaler or nebulizer, up to three doses in first hour
• Oxygen to achieve $O_2$ saturation ?90%
• Oral systemic corticosteriods if no immediate response or if patient recently took oral systemic corticosteroid

**$FEV_1$ or PEF <50% (Severe Exacerbation)**
• Inhaled high-dose $\beta_2$-agonist and anticholinergic by nebulization every 20 minutes or continuously for 1 hour
• Oxygen to achieve $O_2$ saturation ≥90%
• Oral systemic corticosteroid

**Impending or Actual Respiratory Arrest**
• Intubation and mechanical ventilation with 100% $O_2$
• Nebulized $\beta_2$-agonist and anticholinergic
• Intravenous corticosteroid

**Admit to Hospital Intensive Care (see box below)**

**Repeat Assessment**
Symptoms, physical examination, PEF, $O_2$ saturation, other tests as needed

**Moderate Exacerbation**
$FEV_1$ or PEFR 50%-80% predicted/personal best
Physical exam: moderate symptoms
• Inhaled short-acting $\beta_2$-agonist every 60 minutes
• Systemic corticosteroid
• Continue treatment 1-3 hours, provided there is improvement

**Severe Exacerbation**
$FEV_1$ or PEF <50% predicted/personal best
Physical exam: severe symptoms at rest, accessory muscle use, chest retraction
History: high-risk patient
No improvement after initial treatment
• Inhaled short-acting $\beta_2$-agonist, hourly or continuous + inhaled anticholinergic
• Oxygen
• Systemic corticosteroid

**Good Response**
• $FEV_1$ or PEF ≥70%
• Response sustained 60 minutes after last treatment
• No distress
• Physical exam: normal

**Incomplete Response**
• $FEV_1$ or PEF ≥50% but <70%
• Mild to moderate symptoms

**Poor Response**
• $FEV_1$ or PEF <50%
• $PCO_2$ ≥42 mm Hg
• Physical exam: symptoms severe, drowsiness, confusion

Individualized decision re: hospitalization

**Discharge Home**
• Continue treatment with inhaled $\beta_2$-agonist
• Continue course of oral systemic corticosteroid
• Patient education
  –Review medicine use
  –Review/initiate action plan
  –Recommend close medical followup

**Admit to Hospital Ward**
• Inhaled $\beta_2$-agonist + inhaled anticholinergic
• Systemic (PO or IV) corticosteroid
• Oxygen
• Monitor $FEV_1$ or PEF, $O_2$ saturation, pulse

**Admit to Hospital Intensive Care**
• Inhaled $\beta_2$-agonist hourly or continuously + inhaled anticholinergic
• IV corticosteroid
• Oxygen
• Possible intubation and mechanical ventilation

**Improve**

**Discharge Home**
• Continue treatment with inhaled $\beta_2$-agonist
• Continue course of oral systemic corticosteroid
• Patient education
  –Review medicine use
  –Review/initiate action plan
  –Recommend close medical followup

**Figure 3.16** Management guidelines for asthma.[71]

**TABLE 3-9**  **Stepwise Approach for Managing Infants and Young Children (5 years old and younger) with Acute or Chronic Asthma[71]**

| Classify Severity: Clinical Features Before Treatment or Adequate Control | | Medications Required To Maintain Long-Term Control |
|---|---|---|
| | **Symptoms/Day**<br>**Symptoms/Night** | **Daily Medications** |
| **Step 4**<br>Severe Persistent | Continual<br>Frequent | • Preferred treatment:<br>  - High-dose inhaled corticosteroids<br>    AND<br>  - Long acting inhaled β₂-agonists<br>    AND, If needed,<br>  - Corticosteroid tablets or syrup long term (2 mg/kg/day, generally do not exceed 60 mg per day). (Make repeat attempts to reduce systemic corticosteroids and maintain control with high-dose inhaled corticosteroids.) |
| **Step 3**<br>Moderate Persistent | Daily<br>> 1 night/week | • Preferred treatments:<br>  - Low-dose inhaled corticosteroids and long-acting inhaled β₂-agonists<br>    OR<br>  - Medium-dose inhaled corticosteroids.<br><br>• Alternative treatment:<br>  - Low-dose inhaled corticosteroids and either leukotriene receptor antagonist or theophylline.<br><br>If needed (particularly in patients with recurring severe exacerbations):<br>• Preferred treatment:<br>  - Medium-dose inhaled corticosteroids and long-acting β₂-agonists<br>• Alternative treatment:<br>  - Medium-dose inhaled corticosteroids and either leukotriene receptor antagonist or theophylline. |
| **Step 2**<br>Mild Persistent | > 2/week but < 1x/day<br>> 2 nights/month | • Preferred treatment:<br>  - Low-dose inhaled corticosteroids (with nebulizer or MDI with holding chamber with or without face mask or dry powder inhaler).<br><br>• Alternative treatment (listed alphabetically):<br>  - Cromolyn (nebulizer is preferred or MDI with holding chamber) OR leukotriene receptor antagonist. |
| **Step 1**<br>Mild Intermittent | ≤ 2 days/week<br>≤ 2 nights/month | • No daily medication needed. |

**Quick Relief**

All Patients

- Bronchodilator as needed for symptoms. Intensity of treatment will depend on severity of exacerbation.
  - Preferred treatment: Short-acting inhaled β₂-agonists by nebulizer or face mask and space/holding chamber
  - Alternative treatment: Oral β₂-agonists
- With viral respiratory infection
  - Bronchodilator q4–6h up to 24 hours (longer with physician consult); in general, repeat no more than once every 6 weeks
  - Consider systemic corticosteroid if exacerbation is severe or patient has history of previous severe exacerbations.
- Use of short-acting β₂-agonists >2 times a week in intermittent asthma (daily, or increasing use in persistent asthma) may indicate the need to initiate (increase) long-term control therapy.

**Step down**
Review treatment every 1 to 6 months; a gradual stepwise reduction in treatment might be possible.

**Step up**
If control is not maintained, consider step up. First, review patient medication technique, adherence, and environmental control.

**Note**

- The stepwise approach is intended to assist, not replace, the clinical decision-making required to meet individual patient needs.
- Classify severity: assign patient to most severe step in which any feature occurs.
- There are very few studies on asthma therapy for infants.
- Gain control as quickly as possible (a short course of systemic corticosteroids might be required); then step down to the least medication necessary to maintain control.
- Minimize use of short-acting inhaled β₂-agonists. Over-reliance on short-acting inhaled β₂-agonists (e.g., use of short-acting inhaled β₂-agonist every day, increasing use or lack of expected effect, or use of approximately one canister a month even if not using it every day) indicates inadequate control of asthma and the need to initiate or intensify long-term control therapy.
- Provide parent education on asthma management and controlling environmental factors that make asthma worse (e.g., allergies and irritants).
- Consultation with an asthma specialist is recommended for patients with moderate or severe persistent asthma. Consider consultation for patients with mild persistent asthma.

**Goals of Therapy: Asthma Control**

- Minimal or no chronic symptoms day or night
- Minimal or no exacerbations
- No limitations on activities; no school/parent's work missed
- Minimal use of short-acting inhaled β₂-agonist
- Minimal or no adverse effects from medications

## TABLE 3-10 Stepwise Approach for Managing Asthma in Adults and Children Older Than 5 Years: Treatment [71]

| Classify Severity: Clinical Features Before Treatment or Adequate Control | | | Medications Required to Maintain Long-Term Control |
|---|---|---|---|
| | Symptoms/Day<br>Symptoms/Night | PEF or FEV$_1$<br>PEF Variability | Daily Medications |
| **Step 4**<br>Severe Persistent | Continual<br>Frequent | ≤60%<br>>30% | • Preferred treatment:<br>  - High-dose inhaled corticosteroids<br>    AND<br>  - Long-acting inhaled β$_2$-agonists<br>    AND, if needed,<br>  - Corticosteroid tablets or syrup long term (2 mg/kg/day, generally do not exceed 60 mg/day). (Make repeat attempts to reduce systemic corticosteroids and maintain control with high-dose inhaled corticosteroids.) |
| **Step 3**<br>Moderate Persistent | Daily<br>>1 night/week | >60%–<80%<br>>30% | • Preferred treatment:<br>  - Low- to medium-dose inhaled corticosteroids and long-acting inhaled β$_2$-agonists.<br><br>• Alternative treatment (listed alphabetically):<br>  - Increase inhaled corticosteroids within medium-dose range<br>    OR<br>  - Low- to medium-dose inhaled corticosteroids and either leukotriene modifier or theophylline.<br><br>If needed (particularly in patients with recurring severe exacerbations):<br>• Preferred treatment:<br>  - Increase inhaled corticosteroids within medium-dose range and add long-acting inhaled β$_2$-agonists.<br>• Alternative treatment:<br>  - Increase inhaled corticosteroids within medium-dose range and add either leukotriene modifier or theophylline. |
| **Step 2**<br>Mild Persistent | >2/week but <1/day<br>>2 nights/month | ≥80%<br>20%–30% | • Preferred treatment:<br>  - Low-dose inhaled corticosteroids.<br>• Alternative treatment (listed alphabetically): cromolyn, leukotriene modifier, nedocromil, OR sustained release theophylline to serum concentration of 5–15 mcg/mL. |
| **Step 1**<br>Mild Intermittent | ≤2 days/week<br>≤2 nights/month | ≥80%<br><20% | • No daily medication needed.<br>• Severe exacerbations can occur, separated by long periods of normal lung function and no symptoms. A course of systemic corticosteroids is recommended. |
| **Quick Relief**<br>All Patients | | | • Short-acting bronchodilator: 2–4 puffs short-acting inhaled β$_2$-agonists as needed for symptoms.<br>• Intensity of treatment will depend on severity of exacerbation; up to 3 treatments at 20-minute intervals or a single nebulizer treatment as needed. Course of systemic corticosteroids might be needed.<br>• Use of short-acting β$_2$-agonists >2 times a week in intermittent asthma (daily, or increasing use in persistent asthma) may indicate the need to initiate (increase) long-term control therapy. |

 **Step down**
Review treatment every 1 to 6 months; a gradual stepwise reduction in treatment might be possible.

 **Step up**
If control is not maintained, consider step up. First, review patient medication technique, adherence, and environmental control.

### Goals of Therapy: Asthma Control

- Minimal or no chronic symptoms day or night
- Minimal or no exacerbations
- No limitations on activities; no school/work missed
- Maintain (near) normal pulmonary function
- Minimal use of short-acting inhaled β$_2$-agonist
- Minimal or no adverse effects from medications

**Note**

- The stepwise approach is meant to assist, not replace, the clinical decision-making required to meet individual patient needs.
- Classify severity; assign patient to most severe step in which any feature occurs (PEF is % of personal best; FEV$_1$ is % predicted).
- Gain control as quickly as possible (consider a short course of systemic corticosteroids); then step down to the least medication necessary to maintain control.
- Minimize use of short-acting inhaled β$_2$-agonists. Over-reliance on short-acting inhaled β$_2$-agonists (e.g., use of short-acting inhaled β$_2$-agonist every day, increasing use or lack of expected effect, or use of approximately one canister a month even if not using it every day) indicates inadequate control of asthma and the need to initiate or intensify long-term control therapy.
- Provide education on self-management and controlling environmental factors that make asthma worse (e.g., allergens and irritants).
- Refer to an asthma specialist if there are difficulties controlling asthma or if step 4 care is required. Referral can be considered if step 3 care is required.

## TABLE 3-11 Usual Dosages for Asthma Medications, Long-Term Control[71]

| Medication | Dosage Form | Adult Dose | Child Dose* | Comments |
|---|---|---|---|---|
| **Inhaled Corticosteroids** *(see Table 3-21, page 96.)* | | | | |
| **Systemic Corticosteroids** | | | (Applies to all three corticosteroids) | |
| Methylprednisolone | 2, 4, 8, 16, 32 mg tablets | 7.5–60 mg/day in single dose in AM or every other day as needed for control | 0.25–2 mg/kg/day in single dose in AM or every other day as needed for control | • For long-term treatment of severe persistent asthma, administer single dose in AM either daily or on alternate days (alternate-day therapy might produce less adrenal suppression). If daily doses are required, one study suggests improved efficiency and no increase in adrenal suppression when administered at 3 PM (Beam et al 1992). |
| Prednisolone | 5 mg tablets, 5 mg/5 cc, 15 mg/5 cc | Short-course "burst": to achieve control 40–60 mg/day as single or two divided doses for 3–10 days | Short-course "burst": 1–2 mg/kg/day, maximum 60 mg/day for 3–10 days | • Short courses or "bursts" are effective for establishing control when initiating therapy or during a period of gradual deterioration. |
| Prednisone | 1, 2.5, 5, 10, 20, 50 mg tablets; 5 mg/cc, 5 mg/5 cc | | | • The burst should be continued until patient achieves 80% PEF personal best or symptoms resolve. This usually requires 3–10 days but might require longer. There is no evidence that tapering the dose following improvement prevents relapse. |
| **Long-Acting Inhaled β$_2$-Agonists** | | | | • Should not be used for symptom relief or exacerbations. Use with corticosteroids. |
| Salmeterol | MDI 21 mcg/puff | 2 puffs q12h | 1–2 puffs q12h | • May use one dose nightly for symptoms. |
| | DPI 50 mcg/blister | 1 blister q12h | 1 blister q12h | • Efficacy and safety have not been studied in children <5 years old. |
| Formoterol | DPI 12 mcg/single-use capsule | 1 capsule q12h | 1 capsule q12h | • Each capsule is for single use only; additional doses should not be administered for at least 12 hours. |
| | | | | • Capsules should be used only with the Aerolizer inhaler and should not be taken orally. |

*Children ≤ 12 years old

*(continues)*

| Medication | Dosage Form | Adult Dose | Child Dose* | Comments |
|---|---|---|---|---|
| **Combined Medication** | | | | |
| Fluticasone/Salmeterol | DPI 100 mcg, 250 mcg, or 500 mcg/50 mcg | 1 inhalation bid; dose depends on severity of asthma | 1 inhalation bid; dose depends on severity of asthma | • Not FDA approved in children <12 years old. 100/50 for patient not controlled on low- to medium-dose inhaled corticosteroids. 250/50 for patients not controlled on medium- to high-dose inhaled corticosteroids. |
| **Cromolyn and Nedocromil** | | | | |
| Cromolyn | MDI 1 mg/puff Nebulizer 20 mg/ampule | 2–4 puffs tid-qid 1 ampule tid-qid | 1–2 puffs tid-qid 1 ampule tid-qid | • One dose prior to exercise or allergen exposure provides effective prophylaxis for 1–2 hours. |
| Nedocromil | MDI 1.75 mg/puff | 2–4 puffs bid-qid | 1–2 puffs bid-qid | • See cromolyn above. |
| **Leukotriene Modifiers** | | | | |
| Montelukast | 4 mg or 5 mg chewable tablet 10 mg tablet | 10 mg every evening | • 4 mg every evening (2–5 years old) 5 mg every evening (6–14 years old) 10 mg every evening (>14 years old) | • Montelukast exhibits a flat dose-response curve. Doses >10 mg will not produce a greater response in adults. |
| Zafirlukast | 10 or 20 mg tablet | 40 mg daily (20 mg tablet bid) | • 20 mg daily (7–11 years old) (10 mg tablet bid) | • For zafirlukast, administration with meals decreases bioavailability; take at least 1 hour before or 2 hours after meals. |
| Zileuton | 300 or 600 mg tablet | 2,400 mg daily (give tablets qid) | Not approved for use in children <12 years old. | • For zileuton, monitor hepatic enzymes (ALT). |
| **Methylxanthines** | | | | |
| Theophylline | Liquids, sustained-release tablets, and capsules | Starting dose 10 mg/kg/day up to 300 mg max; usual max 800 mg/day | Starting dose 10 mg/kg/day; usual max: • <1 year old: 0.2 (age in weeks) + 5 = mg/kg/day • ≥1 year old: 16 mg/kg/day | • Adjust dosage to achieve serum concentration of 5–15 mcg/mL at steady-state (at least 48 hours on same dosage). • Due to wide interpatient variability in theophylline metabolic clearance, routine serum theophylline level monitoring is important. • Many factors affect serum theophylline concentration, such as food, age, other illnesses, and medications. Check package inserts. |

*Children ≤12 years old

# TABLE 3-12  Medications for Asthma Exacerbations[71]

| Medication | Adult Dose | Child Dose* | Comments |
|---|---|---|---|
| **Short-Acting Inhaled β₂-Agonists** | | | |
| **Albuterol** | | | |
| Nebulizer solution (5 mg/mL, 2.5 mg/3 mL, 1.25 mg/3 mL, 0.63 mg/3 mL) | 2.5–5 mg every 20 minutes for 3 doses, then 2.5–10 mg every 1–4 hours as needed, or 10–15 mg/hour continuously | 0.15 mg/kg (minimum dose 2.5 mg) every 20 minutes for 3 doses, then 0.15–0.3 mg/kg up to 10 mg every 1–4 hours as needed, or 0.5 mg/kg/hour by continuous nebulization | Only selective β₂-agonists are recommended. For optimal delivery, dilute aerosols to minimum of 3 mL at gas flow of 6–8 L/min. |
| MDI (90 mcg/puff) | 4–8 puffs every 20 minutes up to 4 hours, then every 1–4 hours as needed | 4–8 puffs every 20 minutes for 3 doses, then every 1–4 hours inhalation maneuver; use spacer/holding chamber. | As effective as nebulized therapy if patient is able to coordinate. |
| **Bitolterol** | | | |
| Nebulizer solution (2 mg/mL) | See albuterol dose | See albuterol dose; thought to be half as potent as albuterol on a mg basis. | Has not been studied in severe asthma exacerbations. Do not mix with other drugs. |
| MDI (370 mcg/puff) | See albuterol dose | See albuterol dose | Has not been studied in severe asthma exacerbations. |
| **Levalbuterol** (R-albuterol) | | | |
| Nebulizer solution (0.63 mg/3 mL, 1.25 mg/3 mL) | 1.25–2.5 mg every 20 minutes for 3 doses, then 1.25–5 mg every 1–4 hours as needed, or 5–7.5 mg/hour continuously | 0.075 mg/kg (minimum dose 1.25 mg) every 20 minutes for 3 doses, then 0.075–0.15 mg/kg up to 5 mg every 1–4 hours as needed, or 0.25 mg/kg/hour by continuous nebulization | 0.63 mg of levalbuterol is equivalent to 1.25 mg of racemic albuterol for both efficacy and side effects. |
| **Pirbuterol** | | | |
| MDI (200 mcg/puff) | See albuterol dose | See albuterol dose; thought to be half as potent as albuterol on a mg basis. | Has not been studied in severe asthma exacerbations. |
| **Systemic (Injected) β₂-Agonists** | | | |
| **Epinephrine** 1:1,000 (1 mg/mL) | 0.3–0.5 mg every 20 minutes for 3 doses subcutaneous or IM | 0.01 mg/kg up to 0.3–0.5 mg every 20 minutes for 3 doses subcutaneous or IM | No proven advantage of systemic therapy over aerosol. |
| **Terbutaline** (1 mg/mL) | 0.25 mg every 20 minutes for 3 doses subcutaneous | 0.01 mg/kg every 20 minutes for 3 doses then every 2–6 hours as needed subcutaneous | No proven advantage of systemic therapy over |

*Children ≤ 12 years old

(continues)

TABLE 3-12 **Medications for Asthma Exacerbations (Continued)[71]**

| Medication | Dosages | | Comments |
|---|---|---|---|
| | Adult Dose | Child Dose* | |
| **Anticholinergics** | | | |
| Ipratropium bromide | | | aerosol. |
|   Nebulizer solution (0.25 mg/mL) | 0.5 mg every 30 minutes for 3 doses then every 2–4 hours as needed | 0.25 mg every 20 minutes for 3 doses, then every 2 to 4 hours | |
|   MDI (18 mcg/puff) | 4–8 puffs as needed | 4–8 puffs as needed | |
| **Ipratropium with albuterol** | | | |
|   Nebulizer solution (Each 3 mL vial contains 0.5 mg ipratropium bromide and 2.5 mg albuterol.) | 3 mL every 30 minutes for 3 doses, then every 2–4 hours as needed | 1.5 mL every 20 minutes for 3 doses, then every 2–4 hours | |
|   MDI (Each puff contains 18 mcg ipratropium bromide and 90 mcg of albuterol.) | 4–8 puffs as needed | 4–8 puffs as needed | |
| **Systemic Corticosteroids** | (Dosages and comments apply to all three corticosteroids.) | | |
| Prednisone<br>Methylprednisolone<br>Prednisolone | 120–180 mg/day in 3 or 4 divided doses for 48 hours, then 60–80 mg/day until PEF reaches 70% of predicted or personal best | 1 mg/kg q6h for 48 hours then 1–2 mg/kg/day (maximum = 60 mg/day) in two divided doses until PEF 70% of predicted or personal best | |

May mix in same nebulizer with albuterol. Should not be used as first-line therapy; should be added to $\beta_2$-agonist therapy. Dose delivered from MDI is low and has not been studied in asthma exacerbations.

Contains EDTA to prevent discoloration. This additive does not induce bronchospasm.

given every 20 minutes or continuously for 1 hour, as well as systemic corticosteroids.[71] When these measures are insufficient to control symptoms, additional forms of therapy can be considered. Examples for use in severe exacerbations include terbutaline infusions, magnesium sulfate, and Heliox.[73,74] Leukotriene modifiers are not advised for acute rescue therapy.

Evaluation of hydration is important in asthmatic patients. The route of hydration is determined by patient status. Respiratory distress, hypoventilation, and apnea are contraindications for oral hydration. Many children who have had a recent viral illness and respiratory symptoms will not have had adequate oral intake. Adequate hydration helps keep secretions less viscous.[73]

Pharmacotherapy for acute asthma exacerbations is reviewed in Table 3-12.[69]

Some important things to avoid include feeding the tachypneic child, because of the increased risk for aspiration; sedating the anxious child because respiratory difficulty might be a reflection of hypoxia; overhydration; routine use of mucolytics; and administering oral β-agonists during acute episodes, because they have a longer and more variable onset of action and more systemic side effects.

Routine use of antibiotics for asthma exacerbations has not been shown to be efficacious except when necessary for the treatment of co-morbid conditions. Combination of long-acting β-agonists with inhaled steroids is superior to doubling the dose of inhaled corticosteroids, but there are concerns about the safety of long-acting β-agonists in severe asthma.[70] Inhaled corticosteroids have known benefit in chronic asthma; however, their use in acute episodes is less clear and requires further study. Whether continuous albuterol is superior to intermittent doses remains controversial, with some studies finding no difference and others reporting decreased ED stays with continuous therapy during the acute ED phase. The combination of ipratropium bromide with albuterol is also controversial, with some studies reporting decreases in ED stays. Optimal dosing regimens for ipratropium are being evaluated.

Theophylline is no longer used routinely in pediatrics because of its narrow therapeutic range, toxicity profile, and effect on the lower esophageal sphincter, which has been associated with an increased risk for reflux. However, Reane et al[75] recently showed clinical improvement in children with severe status asthmaticus who were already on maximal medical therapy, suggesting that a reevaluation of theophylline in children with impending respiratory failure might be warranted.

Mechanical ventilation can be administered either invasively with endotracheal intubation or noninvasively with nasal continuous positive airway pressure (CPAP). Indications for intubation include apnea, coma, and respiratory failure.

## THE BOTTOM LINE

- Asthma is a chronic condition. It is best managed by a partnership among patient, physician, and family.
- Emergency management of the asthma patient should be followed by an asthma action plan individualized for each child and updated regularly by the primary care provider.
- It is incumbent on emergency physicians to expedite affiliation with a medical home for those patients who appear recurrently in the ED for steroid burst therapy.

## CASE SCENARIO 5

A 10-month-old infant born at 28 weeks' gestation presents to the ED 4 months after discharge from initial hospital neonatal intensive care unit (NICU) stay. He is on chronic home $O_2$ therapy and was stable until 2 days ago when he developed URI symptoms followed by increased respiratory rate and increased $O_2$ requirements. On presentation in the ED he is alert, shows signs of increase in work of breathing (nasal flaring and retraction), and his color is pale. Vital signs include a respiratory rate of 60 breaths per minute; heart rate of 160 bpm; temperature of 37.90°C; and $O_2$ saturation 88%. He has diffuse wheezing on examination without rales. Your initial management includes supplemental $O_2$ and nebulized albuterol therapy. His $O_2$ saturation improves to 95% with 4 L $O_2$ by nasal cannula. Further assessment shows a right otitis media and clear rhinorrhea on detailed physical examination.

1. *What is your differential diagnosis?*
2. *What are your management priorities?*

# ■ Disease of Oxygenation and Ventilation and Disease of the Lungs

## Bronchopulmonary Dysplasia

Bronchopulmonary dysplasia (BPD) is a severe form of chronic lung disease. Diagnosis is based on the following three criteria: mechanical ventilation in the neonatal period, continued need for supplemental $O_2$ at day 28 of life, and pulmonary insufficiency.[76] It is most commonly seen in very low birth weight infants. Other factors associated with increased incidence include meconium aspiration syndrome, congenital heart disease (e.g., PDA), perinatal infection (e.g., cytomegalovirus), persistent pulmonary hypertension, and high levels of ventilatory support. In all cases, there is a significant inflammatory response in the airways of these infants; most infants with BPD have neutrophils in tracheal aspirates at 11 to 15 days of life. In older infants with BPD, alveolar macrophages are the predominant cell. Up to 50% of infants with BPD require hospital readmission during the first year of life. Pulmonary infections, especially RSV, and increased frequency of wheezing have been reported in hospitalized infants. Immunoprophylaxis for RSV is indicated for specific groups of infants with BPD.

Lung function and radiographic findings can improve with age, but some children will have persistent abnormalities. Hyde et. al. developed prognostic criteria based on the radiographic appearance at day 28.[77] Type 1 infants have patchy or homogeneous opacification without coarse reticulation and generally improve over time. This group constitutes most infants with BPD. Type 2 infants have coarse reticulation, streaky densities, and areas of emphysema. This type has a less favorable prognosis.

Variations in diagnostic criteria, patient population, and early treatment practices have led to difficulties in defining epidemiology. Risk factors include prolonged $O_2$ exposure, mechanical ventilation, and immaturity.[76] Postdischarge pulmonary exacerbations can be complicated by sequelae of prolonged intubation (subglottic stenosis, granulomas, laryngomalacia, and tracheomalacia), which can add to the increase in airway resistance caused by acute airway infections such as RSV.

## Clinical Features

Signs and symptoms of BPD include increased respiratory rate at rest and often increased work of breathing manifested by retractions. The Harrison groove, a depression on the lower edge of the thorax at the insertion of the diaphragm (pear-shaped chest) caused by tug of the diaphragm, and sometimes seen in patients with severe dyspnea, can be a result of chronic increased work of breathing. Pulmonary complications of BPD are listed in Table 3-13. Cor pulmonale is seen in infants who are chronically hypoxemic. Other complications of BPD include feeding difficulties, gastroesophageal reflux, failure to thrive, and acute life-threatening events (ALTE).

### TABLE 3-13 Pulmonary Complications of BPD

- Cor pulmonale
- Right ventricular hypertrophy and enlargement of the main pulmonary artery reflecting pulmonary hypertension
- Atelectasis
- Segmental or subsegmental collapse
- Hyperinflation

Source: Greenough A. Chronic lung disease in the newborn, in: Rennie JM, Roberton NRC. *Textbook of Neonatology*, 3rd ed. New York, Ny: Churchill Livingstone; 1999: 608–622. Reprinted with permission.

| TABLE 3-14 | Radiographic Criteria for Initial Staging of BPD[78] |
|---|---|
| • Stage 1: day 1–3 | Similar appearance to RDS |
| • Stage 2: day 4–10 | Marked radiopacity |
| • Stage 3: day 10–20 | Development of a cystic pattern |
| • Stage 4: more than 28 days | Hyperexpansion; variable cardiomegaly; streaky densities and areas of emphysema |

## KEY POINTS

**Management of Infants with BPD[79]**

- Increasing supplemental $O_2$—titrate to keep $O_2$ saturation at 92% or higher
- Bronchodilators (see Table 3-12):
  - Albuterol (nebulized)
  - Ipratropium bromide (aerochamber and metered-dose inhaler [MDI])
- Corticosteroids (inhaled) (see Table 3-21):
  - Budesonide *or*
  - Fluticasone (aerochamber and MDI)
- Consider trial of diuretics in the following circumstances:
  - Sudden weight gain
  - Sudden deterioration
  - Consider antibiotics in the following circumstances:
  - High index of suspicion of bacterial disease
  - Immunodeficiency
  - Recurrent pattern of respiratory infection with frequent exacerbations

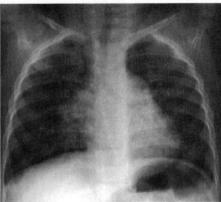
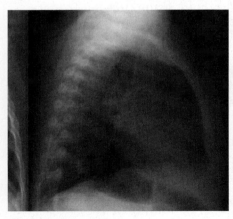

**Figure 3.17** Findings of bronchopulmonary dysphasia.

## Diagnostic Studies

A chest radiograph is important to making the diagnosis, with staging of BPD as reported by Northway et al.[78] Initial radiographic criteria for staging BPD are shown in Table 3-14. The chest radiograph in Figure 3.17 shows classic coarse reticulation with streaky densities and small cystic translucencies.

Comparison with previous radiographs is helpful in diagnosing pneumonia in this group of patients. Clinical findings must be correlated with radiographic changes.

## Management

If clinical or radiographic deterioration occurs in the patient with BPD, consider pulmonary infection. Management includes administering supple-

mental $O_2$ to keep $O_2$ saturation at 92% or higher, monitoring hemoglobin level, and obtaining a chest radiograph.[76] If wheezing is present, then a trial of a nebulized bronchodilator is indicated. Apnea is often the only manifestation of infection in patients with BPD. Measurement of ABGs is indicated to evaluate infants in severe respiratory distress. Look for change compared to baseline values. These infants often have little reserve and deteriorate rapidly. Send nasopharyngeal or tracheal secretions for viral studies, especially RSV, influenza, and adenovirus, to help determine the cause of the deterioration.

Patients requiring chronic $O_2$ supplementation are a particular challenge in emergency management because it is often difficult to assess the patient's change from baseline pulmonary status. Careful titration of supplemental $O_2$ is necessary to prevent the infant from retaining $CO_2$. Nebulized bronchodilator therapy and inhaled or systemic corticosteroids are often used; the efficacy of these therapies is controversial because bronchial smooth muscle might not be fully developed in infants. In cases where the child has shown excessive weight gain, diuretics can be added, and antibiotics are administered in cases of suspected bacterial infection.[79]

Indications for admission are found in Table 3-15 and include persistent tachypnea, hypoxia, inability to feed, new pulmonary infiltrates/pneumonia, or respiratory failure.

Management of infants with BPD can be difficult because too aggressive an approach can lead to further complications. Some important things to avoid in the management of patients with BPD include the following: agitation, because it can worsen hypoxia; oral feedings in infants with respiratory difficulty, because of increased risk of pulmonary aspiration; overhydration, because it can lead to pulmonary edema and worsen the degree of hypoxemia; overuse

of digoxin, because it can increase pulmonary vascular resistance; and the misconception that parents can be caregivers for a sick child 24/7. Consider hosptial admission if home support systems are inadequate or stressed.

| TABLE 3-15 | Indications for Admission in Patients with BPD |
| --- | --- |

- Respiratory rate greater than 70–80 bpm or a significant change from baseline
- Increasing hypoxia or hypercarbia/increased oxygen requirement
- Poor feeding associated with respiratory symptoms
- Apnea
- New pulmonary infiltrates

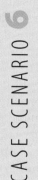

**CASE SCENARIO 6**

A 16-year-old boy who has been followed in the cystic fibrosis center in your hospital presents to the emergency department. He has been gradually losing weight and has been admitted for IV antibiotic therapy twice in the past 3 months. His lung function studies show a moderate to severe decrease in $FEV_1$. He presents today with acute onset of sharp chest pain radiating to the right shoulder. He is alert and anxious sitting in the tripod position; he is tachypneic and has no retractions; and his color is pale with perioral cyanosis. Vital signs include a respiratory rate of 40/min, heart rate of 15 bpm, and oxygen saturation of 80% on room air. Supplemental $O_2$ is delivered with a nonrebreather mask. Arterial blood gas analysis results are as follows: $FIO_2$, 0.6; pH, 7.4; $PCO_2$, 33; $PO_2$, 83; and $HCO_3$, 20.7. He is barrel chested, and breath sounds are significantly decreased on the right side. Hyperresonance is noted to percussion on the right side.

1. *What is the most likely cause of his chest pain?*
2. *What are your management priorities?*

## Cystic Fibrosis

Cystic fibrosis (CF) is the most common lethal genetic disease in the United States. It is a multisystem disease, associated with abnormalities of the CF transmembrane regulator (CFTR), which results in chronic sinopulmonary disease and pancreatic insufficiency.[80] Pulmonary disease progression is the major determinant of morbidity outside of the newborn period.[81] Average life expectancy as of 1999 is 30 years of age.[82]

Cystic fibrosis is an autosomal recessive disease, affecting approximately 30,000 people in the United States. The delta F 508 mutation is the most commonly seen. Frequency estimates in the United States are as follows: whites, 1:3200; blacks, 1:15,000; and Asians, 1:31,000.[80,82]

The main respiratory manifestation of CF is chronic cough, which becomes productive over time. Sputum is colonized early with *S aureus* and *H influenzae* and later with *Pseudomonas aeruginosa,* mucoid type.[82] It is typically thick and tenacious. During an exacerbation, some patients initially complain of fatigue, decreased appetite, and weight loss and later experience increased cough, congestion, and respiratory difficulty. Physical examination findings include fever, increased work of breathing (use of accessory muscles, tachypnea), and new or increased crackles on auscultation. Wheezing can also accompany exacerbations. Sputum is thick and purulent and is often blood streaked.[83] Recurrent infections are the rule rather than the exception in CF. New infiltrates can be seen with acute exacerbations. Bronchiectasis is the result of chronic and recurrent infections. Chronic hypoxemia associated with V/Q mismatch contributes to the development of pulmonary hypertension.

Most children are identified by age 4 years and can present with a history of chronic cough, recurrent episodes of wheezing, recurrent pneumonia, sinus disease, and failure to thrive. Approximately 70% are now identified in infancy.[80] Older children with more advanced disease can have the classic findings of barrel chest and digital clubbing along with failure to thrive. Pulmonary function testing provides a marker for clinical progression; $FEV_1$ has been used most frequently as a prognostic marker.[84]

Pneumothorax occurs in up to 23% of older patients with CF with advanced pulmonary disease. Initially this was believed to be a poor prognostic sign, but recent studies have not confirmed this. The recurrence rate is 50% to 70%. Management options consider whether the patient is a candidate for lung transplantation. A partial pleurectomy has a 95% success rate. Alternatives include intercostal drainage and chemical or limited surgical pleurodesis.[84]

Hemorrhage secondary to hemoptysis is uncommon in young children with CF. Blood-streaked sputum, however, is commonly observed in older children and is generally associated with an acute exacerbation. There is hypertrophy of bronchial vessels as the pulmonary disease progresses with more involved areas of bronchiectasis. Massive hemoptysis is believed to occur because of the increased pressure in the bronchial vasculature. By convention, significant hemoptysis is defined as the expectoration of 30 to 60 mL or more of fresh blood.

YOUR FIRST CLUE

**Signs, Symptoms, and Complications of Cystic Fibrosis**
- Chronic cough
- Decreased appetite/failure to thrive
- Weight loss
- Dyspnea
- Increased sputum production
- Recurrent pneumonia
- Recurrent sinusitis
- Hemoptysis
- Pneumothorax
- Respiratory failure

Respiratory failure and hypoxia develop in the child with CF as the pulmonary disease progresses with recurrent infections and the development of bronchiectasis and pulmonary fibrosis. Some children compensate by increasing their respiratory rate. With time they will develop dyspnea in addition to hypoxia, and gradual increases in $P_{CO_2}$ will be seen. Arterial blood gas analysis will reveal a compensated respiratory acidosis. Patients with advanced disease and chronic respiratory failure are poor candidates for ventilatory support. Patients with good initial pulmonary function who suffer an acute event that results in respiratory failure requiring ventilatory support have a better outcome.[84]

## Diagnostic Studies

Hyperinflation is an early finding on chest radiography. With time peribronchial cuffing, tram lines, recurrent infiltrates, fibrosis, and the formation of blebs and bullae are also seen (**Figure 3.18**). Cor pulmonale develops as the disease progresses. Diagnosis of tension pneumothorax is made clinically and can be confirmed with an upright PA chest film. Sputum cultures help guide antibiotic therapy for acute exacerbations. Pulmonary function studies are helpful in making determinations about invasive methods of ventilatory support but are usually unavailable in the ED. Chest CT with high resolution can

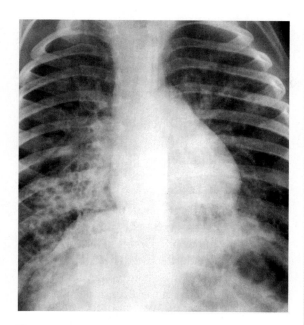

**Figure 3.18** Patient with cystic fibrosis.

be used to identify subpleural blebs and evaluate bronchiectasis. Magnetic resonance imaging and arteriography have been used to help identify sources of bleeding. Lipase, glucose, and sweat electrolytes also can be sent. The classic triad of findings consistent with CF includes chronic pulmonary disease, pancreatic insufficiency, and elevated sweat electrolytes.

## Management

Management strategies for acute pulmonary exacerbations, hemoptysis, and pneumothorax differ significantly.

### Acute Pulmonary Exacerbation

Oxygen should be administered to patients who are hypoxic. Some patients who are in the advanced stages of disease will have chronic respiratory failure. Consider respiratory drive when choosing $O_2$ therapy. If the patient is in moderate to severe respiratory distress or apneic, give 100% $O_2$ and be prepared to support ventilation if the event is thought to be acute and treatable. Initial antibiotic coverage is chosen from two independent categories to provide synergistic action against the more common CF organisms and to help delay the development of antibiotic resistance.[82] See Table 3-16 for recommendations. Therapy is continued for 2 to 3 weeks and may be done on an inpatient service combined with home IV therapy. Although home therapy is cost effective, studies suggest added benefits to hospitalization, including more aggressive respiratory

| TABLE 3-16 | Bacteria Associated with CF Pulmonary Exacerbations and Therapeutic Options | |
| --- | --- | --- |
| **Bacteria** | **First Choice** | **Alternative** |
| *S aureus* | Cephalothin Nafcillin | Vancomycin |
| *H influenzae, S aureus* | Ticarcillin clavulanate + gentamicin | Nafcillin + gentamicin |
| *S aureus, P aeruginosa* | Ticarcillin clavulanate + tobramycin | |
| *P aeruginosa* only | Ticarcillin + tobramycin | Tobramycin + ceftazidime, Piperacillin or imipenem |
| *P aeruginosa, B cepacia* | Ceftazidime + ciprofloxacin | Ceftazidime + chloramphenicol or TMP/SMX |
| *B cepacia* alone | Chloramphenical or TMP/SMX | |

Source: Ramsey BW. Drug therapy: Management of pulmonary disease in patients with cystic fibrosis. N Engl J Med. 1996; 335: 179–188. Reprinted with permission.

therapy than is feasible at home. In infants, endobronchial colonization is generally with *S aureus,* non typeable *H influenzae,* and gram-negative *Bacillus. Pseudomonas aeruginosa* becomes the predominant organism by age 10 years.[82] Antibiotic sensitivity profiles from sputum cultures, when available, are more accurate guides to therapeutic choices. Antibiotic doses should be adjusted for the volume of distribution and clearance rate seen in patients with CF. Although not all patients with CF will demonstrate bronchial reactivity, nebulized bronchodilators are often used in conjunction with chest percussion to facilitate pulmonary toilet.

Antibiotic selection can be difficult because of resistant organisms, limited antibiotic sensitivities, and impaired renal or hepatic function. Options should be discussed with the patient's pulmonologist or primary physician. Although intubation and mechanical ventilation are appropriate for patients with CF with an acute problem and reasonable chance for extubation, outcome in patients with advanced end-stage lung disease is uniformly poor.

Diuresis in patients with CF with cor pulmonale should be done with cautious monitoring of fluid and electrolyte status. Concerns include hypokalemia, hypochloremic metabolic alkalosis, and increased $P_{CO_2}$.

### Pneumothorax

Administer supplemental $O_2$ while preparing to place a chest tube. Needle aspiration is not indicated in this circumstance unless there is acute deterioration and shock.

### Hemoptysis

Initial management includes administering supplemental $O_2$ and sending a blood sample for type and crossmatch, complete blood count (CBC), and prothrombin time. Treatment options will depend on the degree of bleeding. For smaller amounts of bleeding in a stable patient, bed rest, antibiotics, and cough suppression might be sufficient. Fluids and blood are replaced as necessary by clinical evaluation. Vitamin K administration is recommended if the prothrombin time is elevated. For massive hemoptysis, stabilize the patient, intubate, and control bleeding to one lung or one lobe with Fogarty balloon tamponade. Persistent hemoptysis might require bronchial artery embolization or pulmonary resection. Chest percussion should be avoided in patients with hempotysis.[81,84]

## THE BOTTOM LINE

### Cystic Fibrosis

- Know the natural history of cystic fibrosis (CF).
- Anticipate pulmonary progression and be prepared to identify and treat complications promptly.
- A multidisciplinary team approach is helpful in long-term management of patients with CF.
- End-of-life decisions should be discussed in advance with the patient and family to avoid emotional decisions in the ED setting.

---

### CASE SCENARIO 7

A 2-year-old boy with asthma presents to the emergency department with a 1-week history of upper respiratory symptoms followed by increased cough and wheezing over the past 2 days. His mother has been giving him albuterol treatments every 4 hours at home without resolution or significant improvement. On arrival in the emergency department he is alert and in no acute distress and has audible wheezes; his color is normal. Vital signs include a respiratory rate of 40/min, heart rate of 150 bpm, temperature of 39°C (rectal), and oxygen saturation 93% on room air. Crackles are heard over the right anterior chest wall.

1. *What are your management priorities?*
2. *What study would be most useful to you in evaluating this child?*

# Pneumonia

Pneumonia is a common problem seen in EDs. It has an incidence of 4% per year in children younger than 5, 2% in children 5 to 9 years old, and 1% in children older than 9 years.[85] Viral agents are responsible for most pneumonias. Viral pneumonia has its peak incidence between ages 3 to 5 years. Boys are more frequently affected. Respiratory syncytial virus, parainfluenza types 1 and 3, and adenovirus are common etiologic agents for viral pneumonia. Viruses such as RSV have a seasonal pattern. Although bacterial causes are responsible for only a small percentage of childhood pneumonias, they result in higher mortality (2 to 3 times) and morbidity than viral pneumonia.[86]

Approximately 3 million children worldwide die each year from pneumonia.[86] Pneumococcal infection accounts for one fourth of these deaths.[87] In the United States, pneumococcal pneumonia accounts for more than 500,000 cases of pneumonia each year in children. *Pneumococcus* is the leading cause of community-acquired bacterial pneumonia and carries a risk for significant morbidity, including lobar consolidation, pleural effusion, necrotizing pneumonia, pneumatocele, and lung abscess.[86]

Etiologic considerations are based on the age of the child, immunization status, environment, exposures, and immunologic status. Common pathogens and treatment by age group are listed in Table 3-17.

## TABLE 3-17 Pathogens and Empiric Therapy in Pediatric Pneumonia

| Age | Bacterial Pathogens | Viral Pathogens | Other Pathogens | Empiric Therapy |
|---|---|---|---|---|
| <1 mo | Group B Streptococcus, Escherichia coli, Klebsiella, Pseudomonas, Listeria | Varicella, RSV | Chlamydia* | Ampicillin + aminoglycoside or ampicillin + cefotaxime* |
| 1–3 mo | H influenzae, S. pneumoniae, group A Streptococcus, pertussis, group B Streptococcus | RSV, parainfluenza, influenza, adenovirus | Chlamydia* | Ampicillin + cefotaxime* |
| 3 mo to 5 yr | S pneumoniae, H influenzae, S aureus, group A Streptococcus, pertussis | RSV, parainfluenza, influenza, enterovirus, rhinovirus | Chlamydia* | Cephalosporin or ampicillin + chloramphenicol or antistaphylococcal agent if course indicates* |
| >5 yr | S pneumoniae, H influenzae, group A Streptococcus | Parainfluenza, influenza, adenovirus, rhinovirus | Mycoplasma | Penicillin or ampicillin or cephalosporin or antistaphylococcal agent if course indicates or erythromycin if course suggests Mycoplasma |

*If *Chlamydia* is the suspected pathogen, erythromycin should be added to the treatment regimen.

| TABLE 3-18 | Risk Factors for Pneumonia |
|---|---|

- Young age
- Male
- Pollution
- Nutritional status
- Immunodeficiency
- Anatomic airway abnormalities
- Metabolic disease
- Socioeconomic factors

## Clinical Features

The diagnosis of pneumonia is made by integrating the clinical history and the physical examination and radiographic findings. Risk factors are listed in Table 3-18.[88] Viral pneumonia is often preceded by a prodromal phase including rhinorrhea and cough. These symptoms progress to increasing dyspnea and fever over days. Atypical pneumonias (*Mycoplasma pneumoniae*) generally share common clinical features with the viral pneumonias but can also present with acute symptoms. Bacterial pneumonias often have a more abrupt onset with fever, chest pain, cough, and dyspnea.

The history should include exposures at day care or school and travel history. Classic symptoms include cough, wheeze, dyspnea, fever, chest pain, malaise, vomiting, rhinorrhea, pharyngitis, and diarrhea. Tachypnea out of proportion to the fever should be noted. Physical examination findings can include cough, crackles, or decreased breath sounds. Wheezing might also be present, especially in those patients with a previous history of asthma. Abdominal pain can be seen with lower lobe pneumonia. Meningismus can be seen in upper lobe pneumonia, with pain radiating to the neck. Pulse oximetry might reveal decreased values, indicating the need for supplemental $O_2$. In patients with chronic lung disease, initial symptoms can be subtle and include fatigue, decreased appetite, weight loss, and increased sputum production.

Complications include secondary bacterial infections following viral pneumonitis, atelectasis, effusion, empyema, abscess, air leaks

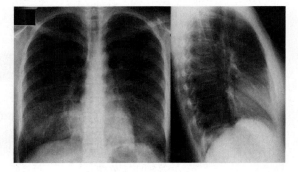

**Figure 3.19** Diffuse patchy infiltrates.

(pneumothorax, pneumomediastinum), hypoxia, respiratory failure, and dehydration (especially in young children).

## Diagnostic Studies

Although pneumonia can be diagnosed solely on clinical findings, most clinicians confirm their suspicions with a two-view chest radiography. If effusion is suspected, lateral decubitus views are helpful. Different patterns of pulmonary infection can be seen on radiographs as follows:

- Diffuse peribronchial thickening, often with hyperinflation from air trapping
- Diffuse, patchy interstitial pattern (Figure 3.19)
- Focal lobar consolidation (Figure 3.20).

Diffuse patchy infiltrates often with shaggy peribronchial infiltrates in the perihilar regions are commonly seen with viral infections, although

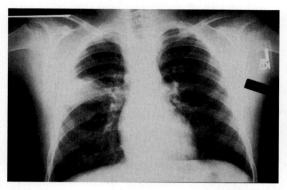

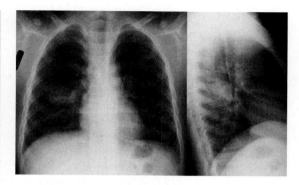

Figure 3.21 Round pneumonia.

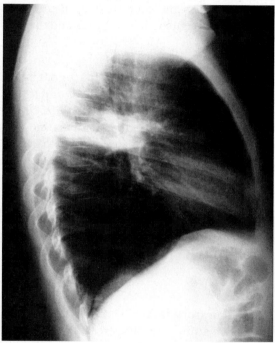

Figure 3.20 Focal infiltrates.

A CBC can be helpful in differentiating viral and bacterial infections. Sputum Gram stain and cultures and skin testing are rarely indicated in the ED setting. Pleurocentesis might be needed in severe cases with large effusions. Immunofluorescent detection or immunoassay for viral agents such as RSV, rapid antigen tests, serology with acute and convalescent titers, and cold agglutinins might be indicated in some patients, especially those with chronic illness or immunodeficiency. Single or continuous pulse oximetry is performed in most cases of suspected pneumonia.

## Differential Diagnosis

The differential diagnosis for pneumonia includes asthma, bronchiolitis, bronchitis, congestive heart failure, and upper respiratory

bacterial infections can also show a similar pattern. Lobar consolidation can be difficult to distinguish from atelectasis secondary to mucus plugging; however, signs of volume loss with shift of the trachea and unaffected lung to the atelectatic side are usually evident. Focal lobar consolidation sometimes presents as a "round" pneumonia and can be mistaken for a chest mass (Figure 3.21). Expiratory radiographs are often misinterpreted as pneumonia because normal vascular and airway markings will be accentuated if the lungs are underinflated when the film is taken at end expiration.

WHAT ELSE?

**Differential Diagnosis for Pneumonia**
- Asthma
- Bronchiolitis
- Bronchitis
- Congestive heart failure
- Upper respiratory infection

infection. History, clinical findings, and chest radiography can be helpful in distinguishing these disease processes from pneumonia.

## Management

For the previously well child with community-acquired pneumonia and no respiratory compromise, outpatient empiric therapy for the agents most commonly found in the particular age group is an appropriate initial treatment plan. It can be modified after evaluating the child's response to therapy. For the child in respiratory distress, supportive therapy (supple-mental $O_2$, antipyretics, bronchodilator therapy as indicated) is given in addition to IV antibiotics. Empiric antibiotics are listed in Table 3-17.[85,87,89]

Hospital admission should be considered for infants with lobar infiltrate, respiratory compromise, pleural effusion, dehydration, or failed outpatient management. Supportive care includes supplemental $O_2$, hydration, nutrition, and rest. Bronchodilators can be a useful adjunct to help facilitate pulmonary toilet. Children with significant effusions or empyema require thoracentesis for diagnosis and therapy.

---

**CASE SCENARIO 8**

An infant with acute respiratory distress is brought to the emergency department by his father. The boy was well until yesterday when he developed a runny nose and low-grade fever. This morning he is irritable, refuses his bottle and has vomited twice. On examination he is poorly responsive to his surroundings; he has marked increased work of breathing with stridor and intercostal retractions, and his color is pale to gray with circumoral cyanosis. Vital signs include a respiratory rate of 40/min, heart rate of 60 bpm, and oxygen saturation of 84% on room air. He has decreased air entry bilaterally and mild end-expiratory wheezes.

1. *What are your initial management priorities?*
2. *What is your differential diagnosis?*

---

## Respiratory Failure

Respiratory failure represents an inability of the body to adequately oxygenate and/or ventilate. It is more common in children than in adults. Certain anatomic factors predispose infants and young children to respiratory failure. These factors include smaller airway size, which increases airway resistance; circular chest wall configuration; more compliant chest wall; horizontal diaphragmatic insertion; and increased number of fatigue-prone type II muscle fibers in the infant diaphragm. Children younger than 3 months of age and children with neuromuscular disease, chronic lung disease, and complex congenital heart disease might have difficulty compensating by increasing respiratory work consistently over time. Monitoring of clinical status and pulse oximetry will help identify impending respiratory failure.

Respiratory failure is identified by pulmonary insufficiency, hypercarbia, and dyspnea. There are no absolute blood gas values that define this condition. Interpretation of ABGs will be made based on baseline blood gas status, altitude, and ongoing therapy.

### Clinical Features

Signs and symptoms of respiratory failure can be categorized as alterations in appearance, muscle tone, mental status, work of breathing, and color of the skin and perfusion. In early or probable respiratory failure (Type I—hypoxemia) a child can be anxious, tachypneic, tachycardic, and pale. As respiratory failure progresses to Type II (hypoxemia and hypercarbia), the mental status becomes more depressed, muscle tone is decreased, heart rate drops, and skin color becomes mottled or cyanotic. The progression can lead to cardiopulmonary failure with agonal respi-

**Signs and Symptoms of Respiratory Failure**

- **Mental status:** anxiety, restlessness, confusion, lethargy, coma
- **Skin:** cyanosis, pallor, diaphoresis
- **Breathing:** tachypnea → bradypnea → apnea
  - Nasal flaring, grunting
  - Use of accessory muscles
  - Dyspnea, paradoxical abdominal motion
- **Respiratory sounds:** stridor, wheezing, rales, or decreased breath sounds
- **Cardiac:** tachycardia, bradycardia, cardiac arrest

**TABLE 3-19   Normal Resting Respiratory Rates**

| Age | Rate (breaths/min) |
| --- | --- |
| Newborn | 30–60 |
| Infant (1–6 mo) | 30–50 |
| Infant (6–12 mo) | 24–46 |
| 1–4 yr | 20–30 |
| 4–6 yr | 20–25 |
| 6–12 yr | 16–20 |
| Older than 12 yr | 12–16 |

rations or apnea and decompensated shock. Finally, cardiopulmonary arrest occurs as all systems fail.

Respiratory distress is often the first clue to the development of respiratory failure. Infants and young children fatigue rapidly with acute respiratory infections and should be monitored appropriately.

## Diagnostic Studies

Arterial blood gases, cardiorespiratory monitoring, and pulse oximetry are the main diagnostic tools used in respiratory failure. Complications are usually the result of mechanical ventilation (barotrauma, pneumothorax) or progression to cardiopulmonary failure and arrest. Chest radiographs can help identify etiology.

Abnormal blood gas values are as follows:

- $Paco_2$ greater than 50 with acidosis (pH less than 7.25)
- $Paco_2$ greater than 40 with severe dyspnea
- $Pao_2$ less than 60 on $Fio_2$ 0.4

## Management

The key to management and prevention of respiratory failure is the recognition of early signs of respiratory distress. See Table 3-19 for normal ranges for respiratory rates. It is often difficult to determine the cause of respiratory failure in the ED. Management follows the guidelines for basic and advanced airway management discussed earlier in this chapter. Infants and children with more severe respiratory distress and impending or actual respiratory failure are usually separated from their parents; however, parents can have a very calming effect. Begin ventilatory support, when necessary to provide airway protection, administer pressure to improve oxygenation and to assist or control ventilation. Rapid sequence intubation is advantageous in children who are still aware of their surroundings and in those presumed or known to have increased ICP. Initial $O_2$ setting for children intubated and placed on mechanical ventilation should be 100%. The most frequent cause of hypoxemia in the clinical setting is V/Q mismatch. Other causes include hypoventilation, right-to-left shunt, and diffusion abnormality. Oxygen delivery systems are listed in Table 3-20. Adult respiratory distress syndrome can develop in children with acute respiratory failure.[90]

Standard precautions should be followed when handling respiratory secretions. Intravenous fluid therapy should be guided by the underlying cause and clinical assessment.

In children with end-stage lung disease (CF, interstitial lung disease), the benefits of mechanical ventilatory support should be carefully weighed. The child, old enough to participate in decision making, along with the

| TABLE 3-20 | Oxygen Delivery Techniques | |
|---|---|---|
| Device | Flow (L/min) | % Oxygen |
| Nasal prongs | 2–4 | 24–28 |
| Simple face mask | 6–10 | 35–60 |
| Face tent | 10–15 | 35–40 |
| Venturi mask | 4–10 | 25–60 |
| Partial rebreathing mask | 10–12 | 50–60 |
| Oxyhood | 10–15 | 80–90 |
| Nonrebreather mask | 10–12 | 90–95 |

family should have had the opportunity to discuss end-of-life care prior to the acute event that brought them to the ED. Blood gas values alone are insufficient to make the diagnosis of acute respiratory failure. Such an error might result in intubation of a compensated child with chronic lung disease.

Early identification and treatment are critical to improve outcome in the previously well child with acute respiratory failure. Care should be taken to address patient and family wishes regarding the initiation of ventilatory support when end-stage disease is present.

## TABLE 3-21 Asthma Medications for Long-Term Control: Inhaled Corticosteroids[71]

Estimated Comparative Daily Dosages for Children 12 Years Old and Younger

| Drug | Low Daily Dose | Medium Daily Dose | High Daily Dose |
|---|---|---|---|
| **Beclomethasone CFC** 42 or 84 mcg/puff | 84–336 mcg | 336–672 mcg | >672 mcg |
| **Beclomethasone HFA** 40 or 80 mcg/puff | 80–160 mcg | 160–320 mcg | >320 mcg |
| **Budesonide DPI** 200 mcg/inhalation | 200–400 mcg | 400–800 mcg | >800 mcg |
| Inhalation suspension for nebulization | 0.5 mg | 1 mg | 2 mg |
| **Flunisolide** 250 mcg/puff | 500–750 mcg | 1,000–1,250 mcg | >1,250 mcg |
| **Fluticasone MDI** 44, 110, or 220 mcg/puff | 88–176 mcg | 176–440 mcg | >440 mcg |
| **Fluticasone DPI** 50, 100, or 250 mcg/ inhalation | 100–200 mcg | 200–400 mcg | >400 mcg |
| **Triamcinolone acetonide** 100 mcg/puff | 400–800 mcg | 800–1,200 mcg | >1,200 mcg |

# Check Your Knowledge

1. Which of the following statements about bronchiolitis is correct?
   A. High-risk groups for severe bronchiolitis include infants with congenital heart disease and bronchopulmonary dysplasia
   B. Only 20% of children have been infected by RSV by their second birthday
   C. Oral corticosteroids are useful in reducing severity and need for admission
   D. Subsequent RSV infections are more severe than the initial infection

2. Treatment options for croup vary with severity of disease. All of the listed therapies have been shown to improve outcome in patients with croup except?
   A. Dexamethasone intramuscularly or intravenously
   B. Humidified oxygen
   C. L-epinephrine
   D. Racemic epinephrine

3. Which of the following statements about foreign body (FB) aspiration in children is correct?
   A. Bronchoscopy is the gold standard for diagnosis and treatment of FB aspiration.
   B. Chest radiographs are highly sensitive for determining the presence of FBs in the airways.
   C. Positive physical examination findings are always present after aspiration.
   D. Small toys as the most commonly aspirated item.
   E. The most common site of obstruction is the larynx.

4. Which of the following statements is correct regarding comparing infant and adult airway management?
   A. Adolescents are more likely to develop bradycardia
   B. Adults are more susceptible to air swallowing and emesis leading to aspiration
   C. Infants and children are more likely to experience oxygen desaturation
   D. RSI is not well tolerated by infants

# References

1. Berry FA, Yemen TA. Pediatric airway in health and disease. *Pediatr Clin North Am.* 1994;41: 153–180.
2. Perkin R, van Stralen D, Mellick LB. Managing pediatric airway emergencies: anatomic considerations, alternative airway and ventilation techniques, and current treatment options. *Pediatr Emerg Rep.* 1996;1(1):1–12.
3. Walls RM, Luten RC, Murphy MF, Schneider RE, eds. *Manual of Emergency Airway Management.* Philadelphia, Pa: Lippincott, Williams, & Wilkins; 2000.
4. Sullivan KJ, Kissoon N. Securing the child's airway in the emergency department. *Pediatr Emerg Care.* 2002;18:108–121.
5. Luten RC, Wears RL, Broselow J, et al. Length-based endotracheal tube and emergency equipment in pediatrics [published erratum appears in *Ann Emerg Med.* 1993:22:155]. *Ann Emerg Med.* 1992;21:900–904.
6. Gerardi M, Sacchetti A, Cantor R, et al. Rapid-sequence intubation of the pediatric patient. Pediatric Emergency Medicine Committee of the American College of Emergency Physicians. *Ann Emerg Med.* 1996;28:55–74.
7. Paston C, Sacchetti AD, Harris R. Infant and small child intubations in the community hospital emergency department. *Pediatr Emerg Care.* 1998;14:86.
8. Sacchetti A, Waxler J. Emergency endotracheal intubations: an update on the latest techniques. *Emerg Med Pract.* 2000;2(5):1–20.
9. Sakles JC, Laurin EG, Ranatappa AA, et al. Airway management in the emergency department: a one-year study of 610 tracheal intubations. *Ann Emerg Med.* 1998;31:325–332.
10. Mallampati SR, Gatt SP, Gugino LD, et al. A clinical sign to predict difficult tracheal intubation: a prospective study. *Can Anaesth Soc J.* 1985;32:429–434.
11. Malhotra A, Drilov LR. Viral croup. *Pediatr Rev.* 2001;22:5–11.

12. Wright RB, Pomerantz WJ, et al. New approaches to respiratory infections in children. *Emerg Med Clin North Am.* 2002;20:93–114.

13. Neto GM, Kentab O, Klassen TP, et al. A randomized controlled trial of mist in the acute treatment of moderate croup. *Acad Emerg Med.* 2002;9(9):873-879.

14. Bourchier D, Dawson KP, et al. Humidification in viral croup: a controlled trial. *Aust Paediatr J.* 1996:20:289–291.

15. Klasssen TP. Croup: a current perspective. *Pediatr Clin North Am.* 1999;46:1167–1178.

16. Waisman Y, Klein BL, et al. Prospective randomized double-blind study comparing L-epinephrine and racemic epinephrine aerosols in the treatment of laryngotracheitis (croup). *Pediatrics.* 1992;89:302–306.

17. Johnson DW, Jacobson S, et al. A comparison of nebulized budesonide, intramuscular dexamethasone, and placebo for moderately severe croup. *N Engl J Med.* 1998;339:498–503.

18. Klassen TP, Feldman ME, et al. Nebulized budesonide for children in mild to moderate croup. *N Engl J Med.* 1994;331:285–289.

19. Kunkel NC, Baker MD. Use of racemic epinephrine, dexamethasone and mist in the outpatient management of croup. *Pediatr Emerg Care.* 1996;12:156–159.

20. Kairys SW, Olmstead EM, et al. Steroid treatment of laryngotracheitis: a meta-analysis of the evidence from randomized trials. *Pediatrics.* 1989;83:683–693.

21. Cruz MN, Stewart G, et al. Use of dexamethasone in the outpatient management of acute laryngotracheitis. *Pediatrics.* 1995;96:220–223.

22. Geelhoed GC, Turner J, et al. Efficacy of a small single dose of oral dexamethasone for outpatient croup: a double-blind placebo-controlled clinical trail. *BMJ.*1996;313:140–142.

23. Schroeder LL, Knapp JF. Recognition and emergency management of infectious causes of upper airway obstruction in children. *Semin Respir Infect.* 1995;10:21–30.

24. Black RE, Johnson DG, et al. Bronchoscopic removal of aspirated foreign bodies in children. *J Pediatr Surg.* 1994;29:682–684.

25. Reilly JS, Cook SP, et al. Prevention and management of aerodigestive foreign body injuries in childhood. *Pediatr Clin North Am.* 1996;43: 1403–1413.

26. Friedman EM. Tracheobronchial foreign bodies. *Otol Clin North Am.* 2000;33:179–185.

27. Halvorson DJ, Mann C, et al. Management of subglottic foreign bodies. *Ann Otol Rhinol Laryngol.* 1996;105:541–545.

28. Rimell FL, Thome A. et al. Characteristics of objects that cause choking in children. *JAMA.* 1995;274:1763–1767.

29. Monetti S, Monetti C, et al. Eight years' experience with foreign-body aspiration in children: what is really important for a timely diagnosis? *J Pediatr Surg.* 1999;34:1229–1231.

30. Silva AB, Muntz JR, et al. Utility of conventional radiography in the diagnosis and management of pediatric airway foreign bodies. *Ann Otol Rhinol Laryngol.* 1998;107:834–838.

31. Reilly J, Thompson J, et al. Pediatric aerodigestive foreign body injuries are complications related to timeliness of diagnosis. *Laryngoscope.* 1997;107: 17–20.

32. Barrios JE, Gutierrez C, et al. Bronchial foreign body: should bronchoscopy be performed in all patients with a choking crisis? *Pediatr Surg Int.* 1997;12: 118–120.

33. Lee BS and Gausche-Hill M. Pediatric airway management. *Clin Pediatr Emerg Med.* 2001;2: 91–106.

34. 2005 International Consensus Conference on Cardiopulmonary Resuscitation and Emergency Cardiovascular Care Recommendations. 2005 international consensus on CPR and ECC science with treatment recommendations: part 6: pediatric basic and advanced life support. *Circulation.* 2005;112:III-73-III-90.

35. Brown L, Sherwin T, et al. Heliox as a temporizing measure for pediatric foreign body aspiration. *Acad Emerg Med.* 2002;9:436–437.

36. Weber AL, Sicilian A. CT and MR imaging evaluation of neck infections with clinical correlations. *Radiol Clin North Am.* 2000;38(5):941–968.

37. Nicklaus PJ, Kelley PE. Management of deep neck infection. *Pediatr Clin North Am.* 1996;43: 1277–1296.

38. Kirse DJ, Roberson DW. Surgical management of retropharyngeal space infections in children. *Laryngoscope.* 2001;111:1413–1423.

39. Kwong KY, Maalouf N, et al. Urticaria and angioedema: Pathophysiology, diagnosis and treatment. *Pediatr Ann.* 1998;27:719–724.

40. Gaglani MJ, Edwards MS. Clinical indicators of childhood retropharyngeal abscess. *Am J Emerg Med.* 1995;13:333–336.

41. Parhiscar A, Har-El G. Deep neck abscess: a retrospective review of 210 cases. *Ann Otol Rhinol Laryngol.* 2001;11:1051–1055.

42. Lee SS, Schwartz RH, et al. Retropharyngeal abscess: epiglottitis of the new millennium. *J Pediatr.* 2001;138:435–437.

43. Lalakea ML, Messner AH. Retropharyngeal abscess management in children: current practices. *Otol Head Neck Surg.* 1999;121:398–405.

44. Kickerson SL, Kirby RS, et al. Epiglottitis: a 9-year case review. *South Med J.* 1996;89: 487–490.

45. Mayo-Smith MF, Spinale JW, et al. Acute epiglottitis: an 18-year experience in Rhode Island. Chest. 1995;108:1640–1647.

46. Nakamura H, Tanaka H, et al. Acute epiglottitis: a review of 80 patients. *J Laryngol Otol.* 2001;115:31–34.

47. Kucera CM, Silverstein MD, et al. Epiglottitis in adults and children in Olmsted County, Minnesota, 1976–1990. *Mayo Clin Proc.* 1996;71:1155–1161.

48. Sampson HA. Food anaphylaxis. *Brit Med Bull.* 2000;56:925–935.

49. Kagy L, Blaiss MS. Anaphylaxis in children. *Pediatr Ann.* 1998;27:727–734.

50. Sampson HA, Mendelson L, et al. Fatal and near-fatal anaphylactic reactions to food in children and adolescents. *N Engl J Med.* 1992;327:280–284.

51. Shah UK, Jocobs IN. Pediatric angioedema: ten years' experience. *Arch Otol Head Neck Surg.* 1999;125:791–795.

52. Pumphrey RS. Lessons for management of anaphylaxis from a study of fatal reactions. *Clin Exp Allergy.* 2000;30:1144–1150.

53. Lee JM, Greenes DS. Biphasic anaphylactic reactions in pediatrics. *Pediatrics.* 2000;106: 762–766.

54. Gold MS, Sainsbury R. First aid anaphylaxis management in children who were prescribed an epinephrine autoinjector device (EpiPen). *J Allergy Clin Immunol.* 2000;106:171–176.

55. Sicherer SH, Forman JA, et al. Use assessment of self-administered epinephrine among food-allergic children and pediatricians. *Pediatrics.* 2000;105:359–362.

56. Krilov L. Recent development in the treatment and prevention of RSV infection. *Expert Opin Ther Patents.* 2002;12:441–449.

57. Staat MA. Respiratory syncytial virus infections in children. *Semin Respir Infect.* 2002;17:15–20.

58. American Academy of Pediatrics Committee on Infectious Diseases, Committee on Fetus and Newborn. Prevention of respiratory syncytial virus infections: indications for the use of palivizumab and update on the use of RSV-IGIV. *Pediatrics.* 1998;102:1211.

59. Dobson JV, Stephens-Groff SM, McMahon SR, Stemmler MM, Brallier SL, Bay C. The use of albuterol in hospitalized infants with bronchiolitis. *Pediatrics.* 1998;101:361.

60. Ngai P, Bye M. Bronchiolitis. *Pediatr Ann.* 2002;31: 90–97.

61. Kellner JD, Ohlsson A, Gadomski AM, Wang EE. Efficacy of bronchodilator therapy in bronchiolitis. A meta-analysis. *Arch Pediatr Adolesc Med.* 1996;150:1166.

62. Menon K, Sutcliffe T, Klassen TP. A randomized trial comparing the efficacy of epinephrine with salbutamol in the treatment of acute bronchiolitis. *J Pediatr.* 1995;126:1004.

63. Reijonen T, Korppi M, Pitkakangas S, Tenhola S, Remes K. The clinical efficacy of nebulized racemic epinephrine and albuterol in acute bronchiolitis. *Arch Pediatr Adolesc Med.* 1995;149:686.

64. American Academy of Pediatrics Committee on Infectious Diseases. *2000 Red Book.* 25th ed. Elk Grove, Il: American Academy of Pediatrics; 2000.

65. Martinon-Torres F, Rodriguez Nunez A, Martinez Sanchez J. Heliox therapy in infants with acute bronchiolitis. *Pediatrics.* 2002;109:68–73.

66. Berger I, Argaman Z, Schwartz S, et al. Efficacy of corticosteroids in acute bronchiolitis: short term and long term followup. *Pediatr Pulmonol.* 1998;26:162.

67. National Center for Health Statistics, Centers for Disease Control and Prevention, New Asthma Estimates: Tracking Prevalence, Health Care and Mortality. www.cdc.gov/nchs<http://www.cdc.gov/nchs, Oct 2001.

68. Smith S, Strunk RC. Acute asthma in the pediatric emergency department. *Pediatr Clin North Am.* 1999;46:1145–1165.

69. Baren J, Puchalski A. Current concepts in emergency department treatment of pediatric asthma. *Pediatr Emerg Med Rep.* 2002;105–112.

70. US Department of Health and Human Services; National Institutes of Health; National Heart, Lung, and Blood Institute; National Asthma Education and Prevention Program. *Quick Reference of the NAEPP Expert Panel Report: Guidelines for the Diagnosis and Management of Asthma–Update on Selected Topics 2002.* NIH Publication No. 02-5075, June 2003. (Updates the NAEPP *Expert Panel Report 2,* NIH Publication No. 97-4051.) Available at: www.nhlbi.nih.gov/guidelines/asthma/asthsumm.htm. Accessed March 2, 2006.

71. US Department of Health and Human Services; National Institutes of Health; National Heart, Lung, and Blood Institute; National Asthma Education and Prevention Program. *Expert Panel Report: Guidelines for the Diagnosis and Management of Asthma. Update on Selected Topics 2002.* NIH Publication No. 02-5075, June 2003:115-119, 122-123. (Updates the NAEPP *Expert Panel Report 2,* NIH Publication No. 97-4051.) Available at: www.nhlbi.nih.gov/guidelines/asthma/asthmafullrpt.pdf. Accessed March 2, 2006.

72. Keahey L, Bulloch B, et al. Initial oxygen saturation as a predictor of admission in children presenting to the emergency department with acute asthma. *Ann Emerg Med.* 2002;40:300–307.

73. Werner H. Status asthmaticus in children. *Chest.* 2001;119:1913.

74. Blitz M, Hughes R, et al. *Aerosolized magnesium sulfate for acute asthma.* Cochrane Database of Systemic Reviews. 2002.

75. Reane R, et al. Efficacy of intravenous theophylline in children with severe status asthmaticus. *Chest.* 2001:119:1480.

76. Greenough A. Chronic lung disease in the newborn. In: Rennie JM, Roberton NRC, *Textbook of Neonatology,* 3rd ed. New York, Ny: Churchill Livingstone; 1999:608–622.

77. Hyde I, English RE. The changing pattern of chronic lung disease of prematurity. *Arch Dis Child.* 1989;64:448–451.

78. Northway WH, Rosan RC, Porter DY. Pulmonary disease following respiratory therapy of hyaline membrane disease. *N Engl J Med.* 1967;276:357–368.

79. Nieveas FF, Chernick V. Bronchopulmonary dysplasia: an update for the pediatrician. *Clin Pediatr.* 2002;41:77.

80. Rosenstein B. What is a CF diagnosis? *Clin Chest Med.* 1998;19:423–441.

81. Ramsey BW. Management of pulmonary disease in patients with cystic fibrosis. *N Engl J Med.* 1996;335:179–188.

82. Rajan S, Saiman L. Pulmonary infections in patients with cystic fibrosis. *Semin Respir Infect.* 2002;17:47–56.

83. Marashall BC, Samuelson W. Basic therapies in cystic fibrosis: does standard therapy work? *Clin Chest Med.* 1998;19:487–503.

84. Aitken ML, Fiel SB, Stern RC. Cystic fibrosis: respiratory manifestations. In: Taussig LM, Landau LI et al. eds. *Pediatric Respiratory Medicine.* St Louis, Mo: Mosby; 1999:1009–1032.

85. Vaughan D, Katkin J. Chronic and recurrent pneumonias in children. *Semin Respir Infect.* 2002;17:72–84.

86. Miller MA, Ben Ami T, Daum R. Bacterial pneumonia in neonates and older children. In: Taussig LM, Landau Li, et al, eds. *Pediatric Respiratory Medicine.* St Louis, Mo: Mosby; 1999:595–664.

87. Tan TQ. Update on pneumococcal infections of the respiratory tract. *Semin Respir Infect.* 2002;17:3–9.

88. Denny FW. Acute lower respiratory tract infections. In: Taussig LM, Landau LI, et al, eds. *Pediatric Respiratory Medicine.* St Louis, Mo: Mosby; 1999:595–664.

89. Bradley JS. Old and new antibiotics for pediatric pneumonia. *Semin Respir Infect.* 2002;17: 57–64.

90. Bateman ST, Arnold JH. Acute respiratory failure in children. *Curr Opin Pediatr.* 2000;12:233–237.

CASE SUMMARY 1

A 6-month-old boy presents to the emergency department with wheezing, severe retractions, and stridor. The infant has poor tone and is poorly responsive to his surroundings. He has intercostal retractions, and his color is pale. His vital signs include respiratory rate of 80 breaths per minute; a heart rate of 190 beats per minute (bpm); temperature (rectal) of 38.6°C; and oxygen saturation of 80% on room air. His mother reveals that he was born at 28 weeks' gestation and was intubated and mechanically ventilated for 6 weeks prior to hospital discharge. The patient also has Pierre Robin syndrome.

1. *How would you assess and categorize this patient's airway?*
2. *What special precautions would you take in planning airway management and possible intubation?*

This airway is a potentially difficult one. The history of prematurity and previous intubation suggests the possibility of subglottic stenosis or other chronic changes. Pierre Robin syndrome includes micrognathia, mandibular hypoplasia, large tongue, and cleft soft palate. This syndrome is associated with difficult airway management due to inadequate visualization. In addition to underlying chronic or past medical problems, this patient is an infant with the clinical picture of bronchiolitis. The current disease state and age add the possibility of increased secretions and increased oxygen consumption.

Planning should take the previously stated risks into account. The first step is to ensure the infant can be adequately bag-mask ventilated. A nasal pharyngeal airway might be helpful in preventing airway obstruction from the large tongue. If airway management is done in the emergency department setting, then anesthesia and surgical backup should be notified. For RSI, only short-acting agents should be used in case intubation is unsuccessful. Laryngeal mask airway has been used successfully in this setting. A needle cricothyrotomy kit should be readily available. In an elective setting, a pediatric anesthesiologist is the best person to intubate this child.

CASE SUMMARY 2

A 13-month-old boy is brought to the emergency department by paramedics. The mother had found him choking and gagging in the kitchen next to a container of spilled nuts. She immediately called 9-1-1 Paramedics note that the child's appearance is normal and alert, the work of breathing is increased with audible stridor and subcostal retractions, and his color is normal. Paramedics administer blow-by $O_2$ and transport the child to the emergency department. On arrival, the child is awake and alert and in moderate respiratory distress. The patient is placed immediately in a monitored bed. Vital signs are respiratory rate of 60/min, heart rate 160/bpm, blood pressure 88/56, temperature 37.1°C, and oxygen saturation 93%.

1. *What are your initial management priorities?*
2. *What diagnostic studies are necessary?*
3. *What are the possible complications to consider on initial evaluation?*
4. *What is the definitive management of this condition and disposition of the patient?*

# CHAPTER REVIEW

Rapid cardiopulmonary assessment reveals an awake child with signs of airway obstruction but not in respiratory failure. Airway specialists are mobilized and an otolaryngologist and anesthesiologist are en route. The patient is started on supplemental blow-by oxygen, which he seems to tolerate well without further agitation. The patient is kept in a position of comfort and continuously monitored for deterioration.

No specific diagnostic studies are necessary in this patient. Intravenous access is deferred to prevent agitation. A portable chest radiograph is obtained, and the child remains calm during this procedure. The chest radiograph is normal.

The child is in danger of complete airway obstruction, and preparations for orotracheal intubation and needle cricothyrotomy are made. All appropriate equipment sizes and medication dosages are determined and ready at the patient's bedside.

The patient is rapidly transported to the operating room accompanied by the pediatric otolaryngologist. Preparations in the operating room have been made for rigid bronchoscopy and possible emergent tracheostomy. The child undergoes inhalation anesthesia, after which IV access is promptly established. Rigid bronchoscopy is performed with successful retrieval of a peanut from the subglottic airway. The patient is then transferred to the PICU for observation.

A 6-month-old boy presents with acute respiratory distress preceded by a short history of upper respiratory tract symptoms and low-grade fever. He is irritable and feeding poorly. He is alert but tachypneic, has nasal flaring and intercostal retractions, and is pale. His vital signs include a repiratory rate of 70/min, heart rate 170 bpm, temperature 38°C (rectal), and oxgen saturation 90% on room air. Diffuse bilateral wheezing is dicovered on physical examination.

1. *What are your initial treatment priorities?*
2. *What diagnostic tests will be helpful?*

Initial treatment priorities are to assess airway patency and position, administer humidified $O_2$, and give a trial of albuterol or another bronchodilator medication. The patient should be reassessed after each intervention.

Helpful diagnostic tests include a chest radiograph to look for classic hyperinflation and $O_2$ saturation readings. Viral cultures or rapid antigen detection for RSV should be considered if the patient is admitted or has chronic disease.

A 5-year-old boy had an acute asthma episode at school during show-and-tell after a classmate brought in a new kitten. He was given albuterol by the school nurse but continued to have tachypnea and diffuse wheezing, and his mother was called to take him home. Wheezing continued despite two additional albuterol nebulizer treatments given consecutively at home. The mother brings him to the emergency department. On arrival, he is alert, shows increased work of breathing with nasal flaring and retractions, and has normal skin color. Vital signs are a respiratory rate 50 breaths per minute; a heart rate of

130 bpm; blood pressure of 120/80 mmHg; axillary temperature 36.6°C; pulse oximetry 89% on room air. He is acutely short of breath with poor air entry and no wheezing on auscultation of the chest.

1. *What are your priorities?*
2. *What is the significance of absent wheezing in this scenario?*

This child is in acute respiratory distress. Leave the patient in a position of comfort and administer supplemental $O_2$. Begin treatment with a short-acting nebulized bronchodilator. Place an IV line and give solumedrol 2 mg/kg IV. Consider use of magnesium if the patient does not respond to albuterol and steroid treatment. Monitor the patient for the need for airway management.

Wheezing is a sound caused by airflow obstruction in the intrathoracic airways. Lack of this sound in a child having an acute asthma episode implies that the airflow is severely decreased. This is a more dangerous sign than audible wheezing.

A 10-month-old infant born at 28 weeks' gestation presents to the ED 4 months after discharge from initial hospital neonatal intensive care unit (NICU) stay. He is on chronic home $O_2$ therapy and was stable until 2 days ago when he developed URI symptoms followed by increased respiratory rate and increased $O_2$ requirements. On presentation in the ED he is alert, shows signs of increase in work of breathing (nasal flaring and retraction), and his color is pale. Vital signs include a respiratory rate of 60 breaths per minute; heart rate of 160 bpm; temperature of 37.90°C; and $O_2$ saturation 88%. He has diffuse wheezing on examination without rales. Your initial management includes supplemental $O_2$ and nebulized albuterol therapy. His $O_2$ saturation improves to 95% with 4 L $O_2$ by nasal cannula. Further assessment shows a right otitis media and clear rhinorrhea on detailed physical examination.

1. *What is your differential diagnosis?*
2. *What are your management priorities?*

Viral illnesses are common causes of acute pulmonary deterioration in infants with BPD. Respiratory syncytial virus is the most common of these and frequently results in hospitalization. Immunoprophylaxis for RSV is recommended for specific infants with chronic lung disease, and this child fulfills those criteria. Respiratory syncytial virus, influenza, and adenovirus should be considered. RSV is frequently associated with otitis media and pneumonia.

Assess airway, work of breathing, and circulation. The $O_2$ saturation will help you titrate the correct amount of $O_2$ the child will need. If the child is working hard to breathe, then give nothing orally, establish an IV line, and consider whether the child will need ventilatory support. Medication options have been described previously.

# CHAPTER REVIEW

A 16-year-old boy has been followed in the cystic fibrosis center in your hospital presents to the emergency department. He has been gradually losing weight and has been admitted for IV antibiotic therapy twice in the past 3 months. His lung function studies show a moderate to severe decrease in $FEV_1$. He presents today with acute onset of sharp chest pain radiating to the right shoulder. He is alert and anxious sitting in the tripod position; he is tachypneic and has no retractions; and his color is pale with perioral cyanosis. Vital signs include a respiratory rate of 40/min, heart rate of 150 bpm, and oxygen saturation of 80% on room air. Supplemental $O_2$ is delivered with a nonrebreather mask. Arterial blood gas analysis results are as follows: $FIO_2$, 0.6; pH, 7.4; $PCO_2$, 33; $PO_2$, 83; and $HCO_3$, 20.7. He is barrel chested, and breath sounds are significantly decreased on the right side. Hyperresonance is noted to percussion on the right side.

1. *What is the most likely cause of his chest pain?*
2. *What are your management priorities?*

Pneumothorax can be seen in up to 23% of patients with CF with moderate to severe pulmonary disease. Typically the onset is acute. Pain can radiate to the shoulder, and the patient might be acutely dyspneic. Acute-onset chest pain in a patient with CF should be addressed immediately.

Supplemental $O_2$ should be given immediately to all patients with respiratory distress. Pneumothorax greater than 10% should be treated with chest tube thoracostomy.

A 2-year-old boy with asthma presents to the emergency department with a 1-week history of upper respiratory symptoms followed by increased cough and wheezing over the past 2 days. His mother has been giving him albuterol treatments every 4 hours at home without resolution or significant improvement. On arrival in the emergency department he is alert and in no acute distress and has audible wheezes; his color is normal. Vital signs include a respiratory rate of 40/min, heart rate of 150 bpm, temperature of 39°C (rectal), and oxygen saturation 93% on room air. Crackles are heard over the right anterior chest wall.

1. *What are your management priorities?*
2. *What study would be most useful to you in evaluating this child?*

Fever and respiratory difficulty in a child with respiratory disease should raise the possibility of pneumonia. In this child priorities include administration of supplemental $O_2$ to keep saturations at 94% and IV access for hydration and administration of IV corticosteroids. Treatment with a short-acting bronchodilator and appropriate antibiotics is indicated by factors discussed previously.

Pulse oximetry and chest radiography will be most helpful in the evaluation. The $O_2$ saturation level will help guide $O_2$ therapy, and the chest x-ray will provide a diagnosis and need for further evaluation and treatment.

CASE SUMMARY 8

An infant with acute respiratory distress is brought to the emergency department by his father. The boy was well until yesterday when he developed a runny nose and low-grade fever. This morning he is irritable, refuses his bottle and has vomited twice. On examination he is poorly responsive to his surroundings; he has marked increased work of breathing with stridor and intercostal retractions, and his color is pale to gray with circumoral cyanosis. Vital signs include a respiratory rate of 40/min, heart rate of 60 bpm, and oxygen saturation of 84% on room air. He has decreased air entry bilaterally and mild end-expiratory wheezes.

1. *What are your initial management priorities?*
2. *What is your differential diagnosis?*

This case illustrates that a normal respiratory rate does not always signify that a child is breathing well. You would expect that an infant with this history would need to increase his respiratory rate to maintain adequate oxygenation and ventilation. A respiratory rate of 40 breaths per minute can also indicate that the infant is tiring. This finding, in conjunction with the other clinical findings, suggests respiratory failure. Management priorities include positioning the head, opening the airway, suctioning the airway, beginning bag-mask ventilation with 100% $O_2$ and preparing for RSI.

This is likely respiratory failure. Sepsis, occult trauma, and metabolic disease should be considered as possible etiologies, but this history is most consistent with croup, which develops over the course of a few days beginning with URI symptoms followed by inspiratory stridor and respiratory decompensation.

# chapter 4

# Cardiovascular System

Laura Fitzmaurice, MD, FAAP, FACEP
Michael J. Gerardi, MD, FAAP, FACEP

## Objectives

1 Present the clinical features and emergency management of cardiovascular disorders in children, including congenital and acquired heart disease, rhythm disturbances, cardiomyopathy, shock, and cardiac syncope.

## Chapter Outline

Introduction

**Congenital Heart Disease**

Cyanotic Heart Disease

Noncyanotic Heart Disease

Congestive Heart Failure

**Acquired Heart Disease**

Myocarditis

Acute Rheumatic Fever

Pericarditis

Bacterial Endocarditis

Kawasaki Disease

Rhythm Disturbances

Pulseless Arrest Rhythms

Cardiomyopathy

Postsurgical Complications

**Shock**

Hypovolemic Shock

Cardiogenic Shock

Distributive Shock

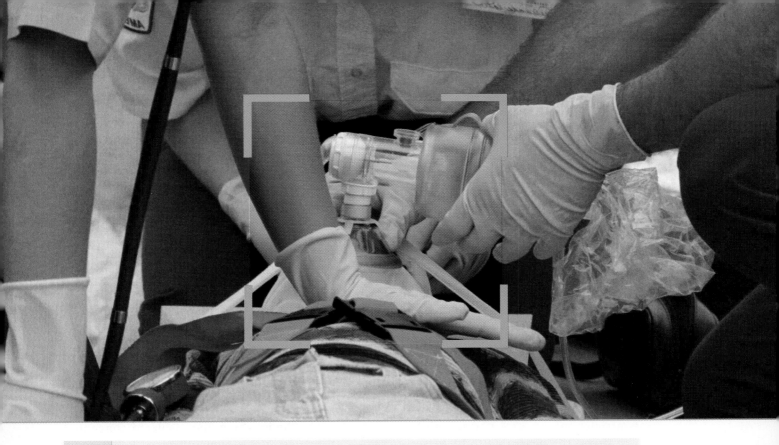

## CASE SCENARIO 1

A 10-day-old baby is brought to the emergency department by his mother. She tells the physician that he seems to be breathing fast and is not eating very well. He is a full-term baby delivered vaginally with a birth weight of 3.2 kg (7 lbs). He spent 2 days with his mother in the hospital and then was discharged after an uneventful circumcision. He has been slow to breastfeed since birth, but the mother became more alarmed when she noted that he would gasp and cry after sucking for a short time. He has about 3 or 4 wet diapers per day. He has no congestion or fever. He does not vomit with feedings and has had 2 yellow, seedy stools since passing meconium after birth. On initial exam he is pale, irritable, breathing fast, has nasal flaring, and is sweaty to touch. Vital signs show a respiratory rate of 70/min, heart rate of 170/min; blood pressure is 80/40 mmHg, temperature (rectal) of 37°C, and his weight is 2.9 kg. His lungs sound equal bilaterally with rales in both bases. Cardiac exam reveals a hyperactive precordium with a gallop rhythm. No murmurs are heard. The abdomen is distended with good bowel sounds, and his liver is palpated 4 cm below the right costal margin. Pulses feel weak in the lower extremities. The capillary refill is 3 to 4 seconds in the fingertips, and pulse oximeter reading is 90% on room air.

1. *What is your rapid assessment of this baby?*
2. *Based on this assessment, what are your treatment priorities?*
3. *What is the most likely etiology of the baby's condition?*
4. *What are acute and definitive treatment options?*
5. *What are some complications of this condition?*

## Introduction

It is important to recognize children with cardiovascular system (CVS) disorders from either a congenital anomaly or an acquired disease and be able to stabilize them and manage their acute problems. An understanding of normal CVS physiology in children and how it changes with growth and development is important to recognize the early signs and symptoms of CVS dysfunction.

## Background

Normal CVS function in pediatric patients is represented by normal vital signs (Table 4-1) and oxygen saturation, as well as the overall appearance of the child. A normal cardiac output is required to meet the body's needs; it is defined as the amount of blood that the heart pumps each minute and is calculated using a combination of heart rate and ventricular stroke volume. Many physiologic parameters such as the heart rate, stroke volume, mean arterial blood pressure, and vascular resistance affect the cardiac output. Stroke volume is the quantity of blood ejected from the heart with each contraction and is a function of the pumping action of the ventricle, which is dependent on preload, afterload, and contractility of the ventricle. Infants and young children rely mainly on the heart rate to increase cardiac output, as they have limited capacity to change stroke volume. Children older than 8 to 10 years develop the capacity of adults to change the stroke volume and heart rate to improve cardiac output. Oxygen delivery is the amount of oxygen delivered to the entire body per minute and is an essential component for adequate cardiac function. If the oxygen delivery falls for any reason, supplemental oxygen is required and/or the cardiac output must increase to maintain adequate oxygen delivery to the tissues. Oxygen delivery to the tissues is determined by the amount of blood flow through the lungs, the arterial oxygen content (dependent on oxygenation and hemoglobin concentration), and the cardiac output. Without adequate delivery, the metabolic demand of tissues is not met and shock (inadequate substrate delivery to meet metabolic demands) begins.

## ■ Congenital Heart Disease

Congenital heart disease has an incidence of 5 to 8 cases per 1,000 live births. Children of parents who have congenital heart disease have an increased incidence ranging from 5% to 15%. The most common isolated congenital heart lesion is a bicuspid aortic valve (most cases are asymptomatic and found on adult autopsies at a rate of 1% to 2%). Congenital heart disease lesions range from a small ventriculoseptal defect to a complex atrioventricular canal anomaly.[1–4] Typically, congenital heart lesions are divided into cyanotic and noncyanotic lesions. The child with a congenital anomaly usually does not show cardiovascu-

| TABLE 4-1 | Normal Vital Signs by Age | | |
|---|---|---|---|
| Age | Heart Rate | Respiratory Rate | Blood Pressure (Systolic) |
| Newborn | 90-180 | 40-60 | 60-90 |
| 1 mo | 110-180 | 30-50 | 70-104 |
| 3 mo | 110-180 | 30-45 | 70-104 |
| 6 mo | 110-180 | 25-35 | 72-110 |
| 1 yr | 80-160 | 20-30 | 72-110 |
| 2 yr | 80-140 | 20-28 | 74-110 |
| 4 yr | 80-120 | 20-26 | 78-112 |
| 6 yr | 75-115 | 18-24 | 82-115 |
| 8 yr | 70-110 | 18-22 | 86-118 |
| 10 yr | 70-110 | 16-20 | 90-121 |
| 12 yr | 60-110 | 16-20 | 90-126 |
| 14 yr | 60-100 | 16-20 | 92-130 |

Source: Shepherd™. Kansas City, Mo. Reprinted with permission.

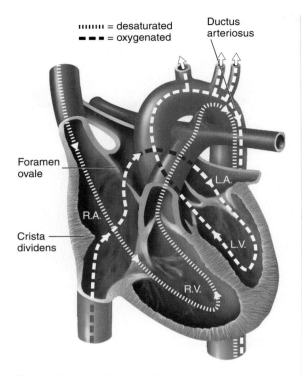

||||||| = desaturated
■ ■ ■ = oxygenated

Ductus arteriosus

Foramen ovale

Crista dividens

R.A.

L.A.

L.V.

R.V.

**Figure 4.1** Normal fetal circulation.

lar problems in utero, because the fetal/ maternal circulation, as a parallel pumping system, provides adequate support to help maintain growth. **Figure 4.1** provides a diagram of normal fetal circulation. The placental circulation is interrupted at birth, which increases the systemic arterial blood pressure. The newborn becomes hypoxic with the discontinuation of the placental flow relied on in utero. This causes an increase in blood pressure, heart rate, and the start of spontaneous respirations. The respirations help decrease pulmonary vascular resistance and increase the pulmonary blood flow. The pulmonary artery pressure decreases and there is an increase in pulmonary venous return and left atrial pressure, which closes the foramen ovale. Finally, the increase in systemic arterial pressure and decrease in pulmonary artery pressure cause flow through the ductus arteriosus to reverse. This initial rapid change slows down over the first 24 hours of life, and pulmonary artery pressures continue to decrease toward adult levels over the next 6 weeks of life. Some of this change

in pressure is aided by the anatomic structure of pulmonary vessels in the fetus and newborn, which have a thicker medial smooth muscle layer with increased vasoreactivity.[5–7]

In the normal fetal circulation, oxygenated blood returns from the placenta via the ductus venosus, mixing with some systemic venous return blood in the inferior vena cava (large broken line). This oxygenated blood partially mixes with deoxygenated systemic venous blood (small broken line) in the right atrium, but oxygenated blood is preferentially shunted through the foramen ovale to the left atrium and left ventricle where the most oxygenated blood is pumped to the cerebral and coronary circulations. The right ventricle pumps less oxygenated blood into the pulmonary artery. The pulmonary vascular bed is vasoconstricted, so most of the blood is shunted through the ductus arterious to mix with the systemic arterial circulation in the descending aorta (distal to the coronary and carotid arteries), thus delivering less oxygenated blood to the rest of the systemic arterial circulation.

## Cyanotic Heart Disease

Cyanotic heart disease (CHD) results from structural and flow anomalies that develop in utero. In children with structural congenital heart disease, the changes that occur at birth and the interruption of intrauterine flow place great stress on the infant's cardiovascular system. Oxygenation is not possible for the infant who relied on the extraneous shunting (in utero) received from the ductus arteriosus. The normal oxygen saturation on the right side is 70% to 75%, and on the left side it is 95% to 98%. The infant shunts deoxygenated blood into the systemic circulation; this is called right-to-left shunting. Some cyanotic heart disease conditions are highly dependent on shunting through the ductus arteriosus (e.g., transposition), in which case complete closure of the ductus is a terminal event. Cyanosis can present shortly after birth, when the ductus arteriosus begins to close. The lesions most commonly seen that are cyanotic in presentation include the five T's: (truncus arteriosus,

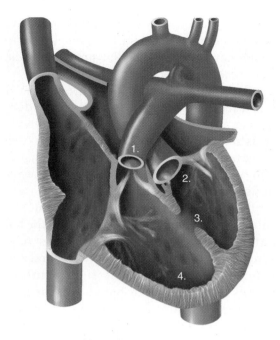

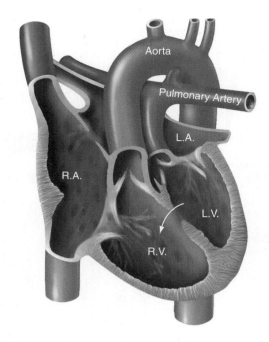

Figure 4.2  Tetralogy of Fallot: 1. pulmonic stenosis; 2. overriding aorta; 3. VSD; 4. RVH.

Figure 4.3  Transposition of the great vessels.

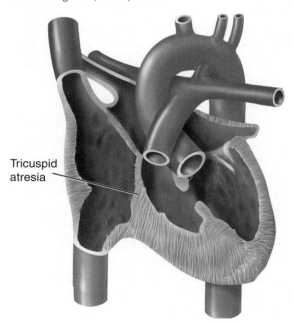

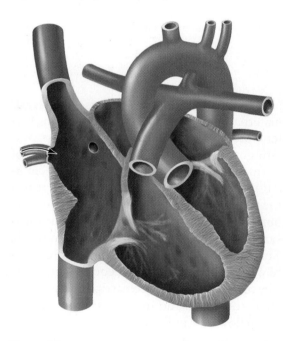

Figure 4.4  Tricuspid atresia.

Figure 4.5  Total anomalous pulmonary venous return.

tetralogy of Fallot (Figure 4.2), transposition of the great vessels (Figure 4.3), tricuspid atresia (Figure 4.4), and total anomalous pulmonary venous return (Figure 4.5)—along with severe aortic stenosis, hypoplastic left heart, and severe coarctation of the aorta.

## Clinical Features

Cyanosis as a presenting sign can be secondary to respiratory, cardiac, and hemoglobin disorders. Normal newborns will have cyanosis of the hands and feet. This is called acrocyanosis and is caused by cold stress and peripheral vaso-

**Signs and Symptoms of Cyanotic Heart Disease**

- Pediatric Assessment Triangle:
  - Appearance: Ranges in severity from cyanotic but active and vigorous to cyanotic with severe distress or lethargy (shock). Some patients might appear noncyanotic (normal) if the degree of right-to-left shunting is mild.
  - Work of breathing: Ranges in severity from normal (early, mild) to retractions/tachypnea/grunting (pulmonary edema or ductus dependent absence of pulmonary flow).
  - Circulation: Ranges in severity from cyanotic but well perfused to cyanotic with poor perfusion (shock).

Other signs and symptoms:

- Generalized cyanosis
- Tachypnea
- Respiratory distress
- Signs of shock
  - Poor distal perfusion
  - Cool extremities
  - Weak cry
  - Tachycardia

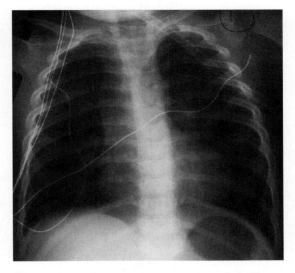

**Figure 4.6** Chest radiograph showing a boot-shaped heart in a patient with tetralogy of Fallot.

constriction. Generalized, or central cyanosis, is more ominous and is exacerbated by crying. The respiratory rate in children with cyanotic heart disease might not be as elevated as one would expect to see as with cyanosis caused by respiratory disorders. The baby can also have signs of shock with poor distal perfusion, cool extremities, weak cry, and a fast heart rate.

## Diagnostic Studies

To differentiate between the causes of cyanosis, apply 100% oxygen. In infants with respiratory and hemoglobin disorders, the $PaO_2$ will increase significantly. The child with a cyanotic heart disease from a significant right to left shunt will have a low $PaO_2$ to start, which will increase only slightly with 100% oxygen because deoxygenated blood bypasses the lungs and goes directly to the left side of the heart. This di-

lutes the fully oxygenated blood coming from the lungs with deoxygenated blood. The oxygen saturation of the resultant mixture will never reach 100% (hence, $PaO_2$ will never rise significantly above 100 mm Hg despite 100% inspired oxygen). This is called the hyperoxia test and can help to distinguish cyanotic heart disease from respiratory causes, although severe respiratory illness might also result in low oxygen saturation despite the application of oxygen. In children with CHD, a chest radiograph might show an abnormal cardiac shadow as well as decreased pulmonary vascularity (**Figure 4.6**). The ECG might show an abnormal axis, QRS, or ST segment changes. An echocardiogram will give the definitive diagnosis. Poor oxygen delivery can precipitate acidosis and shock, which require rapid intervention with support of the airway, breathing, and circulation (ABCs) as well as monitoring and inotropic drugs.

**Diagnostic Studies in Cyanotic Heart Disease**

- Hyperoxia test shows little to no improvement in oxygen saturation with the application of 100% oxygen.
- Chest radiograph might show typical boot-shaped heart of tetralogy of Fallot.

## Differential Diagnosis

The differential diagnosis for cyanotic congenital heart disease can be divided into those with increased pulmonary vascularity and those with decreased pulmonary vascularity. A special consideration in cyanotic congenital disease is ductal-dependent lesions such as transposition of the great vessels. If the ductus closes, blood flow to the lungs is completely interrupted because of the congenital anomaly.

---

### WHAT ELSE?

**Differential Diagnosis for Cyanotic Congenital Heart Disease**

- Increased pulmonary vascularity
  - Total anomalous pulmonary venous connection
  - Truncus arteriosus
  - Transposition of the great arteries
  - Complex lesions with intracardiac mixing and increased pulmonary blood flow
- Decreased pulmonary vascularity
  - Tetralogy of Fallot
  - Ebstein anomaly
  - All hypoplastic right heart defects
  - Complex lesions with intracardiac mixing and pulmonary stenosis/atresia

---

## Management

The primary focus of management in the ED and acute care setting is to optimize oxygenation and support cardiovascular function. The infant should be placed on high-flow oxygen via a nonrebreather face mask at 10 to 15 L/min and considered for elective intubation if significant respiratory distress is present. Cardiac, oxygen saturation, and blood pressure monitors are important for following response to therapy and as adjuncts in determining cardiac function. Intravenous (IV) access with maintenance fluid management can be started and baseline laboratory tests (hemoglobin/ hematocrit, electrolytes) should be obtained. Prostaglandin $E_1$ can be used to keep the ductus open after birth. It is infused at 0.05 to 0.1 mcg/kg per minute with an increase to 0.2 mcg/kg per minute over several minutes. Side effects of the infusion include apnea, pulmonary congestion, fever, hypotension, seizures, and diarrhea.[8–10] The infant should be considered for elective intubation if a prostaglandin infusion is started to secure the airway in case of apnea and to decrease the work of breathing. This can add stress to an already stressed heart. If the baby appears to be in shock, a fluid bolus can be started while monitoring the response to the fluid challenge to assess whether cardiac function worsens. The fluid bolus amount should be 10 mL/kg at a time due to the concern for iatrogenic overloading cardiac function. Diuretics might be needed to treat fluid retention. A dobutamine infusion (2 to 20 mcg/kg per minute) can be used to augment myocardial contractility. Dopamine and epinephrine can also be used to augment contractility, but they have other effects as well.

---

### KEY POINTS

**Management of Cyanotic Heart Disease**

- Provide 100% oxygen with a nonrebreather face mask or by tracheal intubation.
- Obtain IV access and obtain blood for laboratory analysis.
- Consider the administration of prostaglandin $E_1$.
- Administer a fluid challenge of normal saline 10 mL/kg.
- Obtain a chest radiograph and ECG.
- Obtain a pediatric cardiology consultation.
- Consider the administration of dobutamine to support blood pressure.

---

## Noncyanotic Heart Disease

Noncyanotic congenital heart diseases can present with signs of congestive heart failure and/or heart murmurs that are heard during physical exam.[11,12] They can be divided into left-to-right shunts and obstructive lesions. The left-to-right shunt lesions, which can show an increase in pulmonary circulation, include atrial septal defects, ventricular septal defects, and patent ductus arteriosus. Obstructive lesions include aortic stenosis, coarctation of the aorta, pulmonary stenosis, and mitral stenosis. Most of these patients present during the first 6 months of life when the shunt or obstruction overwhelms the cardiac compensation and function.

### Clinical Features

Clinical features include signs of congestive heart failure, such as tachypnea, tachycardia, diaphoresis, decreased feeding, hepatomegaly, various systolic flow murmurs, and gallop rhythms, depending on the specific lesion. The child might present with decreased activity or poor sleeping with respiratory distress.

### Diagnostic Studies

Diagnostic studies include chest radiography, ECG, and echocardiography. The chest radiograph will show an abnormal cardiac shadow or increased pulmonary vascular flow. The ECG can show an abnormal axis, QRS changes, ST segment changes, and chamber enlargement. The definitive test is two-dimensional echocardiography, which will define the abnormality and the degree of congestive heart failure.

### Differential Diagnosis

The differential diagnosis for noncyanotic congenital heart disease includes those entities that have increased pulmonary vascularity and those with normal pulmonary vascularity. The lesions with increased pulmonary vascularity include atrial septal defect, ventricular septal defect, patent ductus arteriosus, and atrioventricular septal defect (e.g., atrioventricular canal or endocardial cushion defect). The cardiac lesions with normal vascularity include aortic stenosis, pulmonary stenosis, and coarctation of the aorta. Symptomatic pulmonic stenosis can show pulmonary hypoperfusion.

---

## YOUR FIRST CLUE

**Signs and Symptoms of Noncyanotic Heart Disease**

- Pediatric Assessment Triangle:

  - Appearance: Ranges in severity—normal (early, mild), sweaty with feeding (early CHF), irritability (pulmonary edema), lethargic (shock).

  - Work of breathing: Ranges in severity—normal (early, mild), retractions/tachypnea/grunting (pulmonary edema).

  - Circulation: Ranges in severity—normal (early, mild), marginal perfusion (more severe), cyanosis (pulmonary edema), pallor, mottling (severe shock).

Other signs and symptoms:

- Hepatomegaly
- Heart murmur
- Gallop rhythm
- Decreased activity
- Poor sleeping

---

## WHAT ELSE?

**Differential Diagnosis of Noncyanotic Congenital Heart Disease**

- Lesions with increased pulmonary vascularity:

  - Atrial septal defect
  - Ventricular septal defect
  - Patent ductus arteriosus
  - Arterioventricular septal defect

- Lesions with normal vascularity:

  - Aortic stenosis
  - Pulmonary stenosis
  - Coarctation of the aorta

## Management

Management in the acute care setting begins with administration of oxygen for those children with respiratory distress and/or cardiovascular instability. Cardiac, oxygen saturation, and blood pressure monitors should be placed. IV access might be necessary to treat congestive heart failure (CHF). The drugs of choice for management of this condition would include diuretics and digoxin. Laboratory testing should include blood glucose and electrolytes.

## Congestive Heart Failure

CHF is a clinical syndrome in which the heart is unable to meet the hemodynamic demands and perfusion requirements of the body. The primary cause of CHF in infancy and childhood is from congenital heart disease. One possible uncommon congenital heart lesion is an anomalous left coronary artery that can cause an infant or child to present with a myocardial infarction. The etiology is an acute decrease in oxygen flow to the myocardium secondary to deoxygenated blood in the left coronary artery because it originates from the pulmonary artery. The infant typically presents with CHF, vomiting, and cardiomegaly at about 2 to 3 months of age. Other causes of CHF to consider include those of acquired heart disease such as myocarditis, endocrine and metabolic abnormalities, endocarditis, rheumatic fever and rheumatic heart disease, dysrhythmias, and pericardial effusions in older children. The typical problem is pulmonary overflow seen in children with large left-to-right shunts that can be exacerbated by infections such as respiratory syncytial virus (RSV). Children with cyanotic congenital heart disease can also develop overflow CHF. Other physiologic reasons for CHF are myocardial impairment, outflow obstructive lesions (usually on the left side), and rhythm abnormalities. With myocardial impairment, there is decreased cardiac output and passive venous congestion. The obstructive lesions and arrhythmias can cause CHF because of impaired ventricular function with resultant pulmonary venous congestion.

## Clinical Features

Children with CHF present with tachycardia and a gallop, tachypnea with rhonchi and wheezing, rales in the lung bases, pallor, and/or cool skin. The extremities will have decreased perfusion, and there might be peripheral edema. Capillary refill will be prolonged, and the lower extremities might be mottled. The abdominal exam might show hepatomegaly. If the cardiac problem has been present for a period of time, the child will present with growth failure and undernutrition.

## YOUR FIRST CLUE

**Signs and Symptoms of CHF**

- Pediatric Assessment Triangle:

  - Appearance: Ranges in severity—sweaty with feeding (early), irritability, lethargic (shock).

  - Work of breathing: Ranges in severity—degrees of retractions/tachypnea/grunting (pulmonary edema) to respiratory failure.

  - Circulation: Ranges in severity—pallor (mild hypoxemia), marginal perfusion (more severe), cyanosis (pulmonary edema), poor perfusion, mottling (severe shock).

Other signs and symptoms:

- Tachycardia
- Gallop rhythm
- Respiratory distress
- Wheezing or rales
- Hepatomegaly
- Peripheral edema
- Shock

## Diagnostic Studies

Diagnostic studies include chest radiography, which can show an enlarged cardiac shadow as well as pulmonary edema (Figure 4.7). An

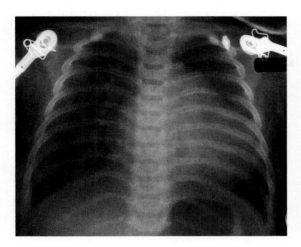

Figure 4.7A Chest radiograph showing cardiomegaly. Note the heart size is greater than 50% of the diameter of the chest. This is a 2-month-old with a VSD and DiGeorge syndrome with cardiomegaly, without pulmonary edema.

Source: Yamamoto LG. Seizure and VSD in 2–month-old infant. In: Yamamoto LG, Inaba AS, DiMauro R, eds. *Radiology Cases In Pediatric Emergency Medicine.* 1995: Volume 2, Case 2.

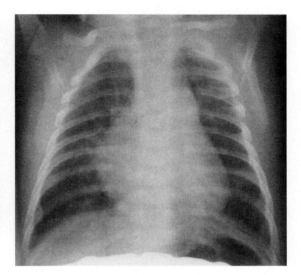

Figure 4.7C This is a 2–month-old with mild cardiomegaly and pulmonary edema.

Source: Matsuda JJ. Tachypnea in a 2–month-old. In: Yamamoto LG, Inaba AS, DiMauro R, eds. *Radiology Cases In Pediatric Emergency Medicine.* 1996: Volume 4, Case 3.

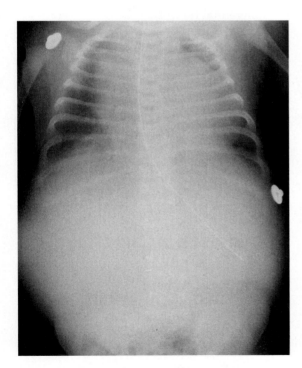

Figure 4.7B This is a 6-week-old with high output CHF and resultant severe cardiomegaly.

Source: Yamamoto LG. Respiratory distress and abdominal distention. In: Yamamoto LG, Inaba AS, DiMauro R, eds. *Radiology Cases In Pediatric Emergency Medicine.* 1995: Volume 3, Case 11.

ECG can show cardiac chamber dilation as well as ST segment changes and/or T-wave abnormalities. Arterial blood gas analysis or pulse oximetry and the hemoglobin/hematocrit will help determine oxygen delivery. Electrolytes (along with the hemoglobin/hematocrit) can estimate the degree of excess fluid, acidosis, and electrolyte imbalance that might need correction. An echocardiogram can be used to determine an underlying congenital cardiac lesion as a cause for CHF as well as how well the heart is pumping (contractility).

## Differential Diagnosis

The differential diagnosis includes all causes of cardiac failure that might be secondary to respiratory failure, such as infection, sepsis, or severe anemia (high output CHF). Primary cardiac causes of CHF are related to the abnormal anatomic flow and contractility.

## Management

Initial management in the ED begins with cardiorespiratory resuscitation and managing the ABCs. The goals of treatment include relief of pulmonary and systemic venous congestion, improvement of myocardial performance, and reversal of the underlying process. Humidified oxygen support is important, as is elevating the head and shoulders about 45 degrees to support pulmonary function. Cardiac, oxygen saturation, and blood pressure monitoring provide baseline information. Elective intubation might need to be considered in those children with respiratory distress who do not improve with initial management. Early IV access is important. Baseline electrolytes should be obtained since correcting electrolyte abnormalities is important to optimize cardiac function. Diuretics remain a mainstay of therapy for CHF. Diuretic therapy can be used to help increase renal perfusion and sodium delivery to the renal excretion sites, thus helping the body rid itself of excess free water. Furosemide is the most commonly used diuretic for this purpose and is given as an IV dose of 0.5 to 2 mg/kg. Nitroglycerin can cause vasodilatation, which might be useful to reduce the preload and afterload on the right and left ventricles. This decreases cardiac workload and helps the heart pump more efficiently. Digoxin is the most widely used drug for the treatment of heart failure in children. It increases the force and velocity of ventricular contraction. It is given as a loading dose (IV in the case of acute heart failure). The dosage is 25 to 50 mcg/kg IV/PO with a maintenance dose rate of 5 to 15 mcg/kg/day in two divided doses. It has a narrow therapeutic range so serum levels need to be monitored and the potassium should be kept in a normal range, since hypokalemia increases the potential for digoxin toxicity. Other inotropic agents that can be used include dopamine, dobutamine, and epinephrine, which are all infused as a titratable continuous drip. All three of these improve contractility and heart rate. Dobutamine is the most specific for improving contractility and increasing the heart rate. Dopamine and epinephrine also increase systemic vascular resistance, which increases the blood pressure, but excessive vasoconstriction can adversely affect visceral organ perfusion.

# Acquired Heart Disease

## Myocarditis

Myocarditis is an inflammatory disease of the myocardium that can result from direct infection of the myocardium (e.g., viral myocarditis), toxin production (e.g., diphtheria), or an immune response as a delayed sequela of an infection (postviral or postinfectious myocarditis). A common type of myocarditis is acute rheumatic fever (ARF).

**CASE SCENARIO 2**

A 10–year-old boy presents with a chief complaint of chest pain and shortness of breath. He has had 5 days of cold and cough symptoms. According to his mom, he has been lying around a lot and has missed 1 week of school. He is usually a very active child but complains that he is "just too tired" to play. He complains that his chest hurts, mostly with cough. He says that he has a hard time catching his breath whenever he gets up to walk around. He has had no medical problems or surgeries. He is in the fourth grade at school and had been the star basketball player until becoming ill. His only exposure to illness is his aunt, who was recently hospitalized for pneumonia. On initial presentation, he is a thin, pleasant boy who seems tired but talks in complete sentences without difficulty. He is tachypneic with mild retractions and is slightly pale in color, with dusky nail beds. His vital signs include a respiratory rate of 30/min, heart rate of 130/min, a blood pressure of 90/65 mmHg, and an oral temperature of 37.8°C. Oxygen saturation is 90% on room air. His weight is 36.4 kg (80 lbs). He is lying on the gurney with the head elevated. Capillary refill time is 4 to 5 seconds. His lungs have diminished breath sounds, with an occasional end expiratory wheeze with deep breaths. His heart sounds are present but faint without any murmurs. His abdomen is distended with a palpable liver and spleen.

1. *What is your initial assessment?*
2. *What are the treatment priorities?*
3. *What are the most likely etiologies based on this assessment?*
4. *What are initial and definitive treatment options?*
5. *What are the complications of this condition?*

## Clinical Features

Clinical features that might be present with myocarditis include fever, signs of CHF, dysrhythmias, muffled heart tones (i.e., distant heart sounds), and systolic murmurs.

## Diagnostic Studies

The primary tests to aid in diagnosis include a chest radiograph, ECG, blood cultures, and antibody titers. An echocardiogram is indicated to determine the area of enlargement of the heart as well as to assess contractility and to rule out any underlying congenital heart abnormalities.

## Differential Diagnosis

In working up the child, consider other causes of CHF, which can include sepsis, toxins, congenital heart disease, and metabolic abnormalities.

## Management

Management in the ED begins with the ABCs, followed by inotropic support for the heart, control of dysrhythmias, and treatment of CHF.

---

**YOUR FIRST CLUE**

**Signs and Symptoms of Myocarditis**

- Pediatric Assessment Triangle:
  - Appearance: Ranges in severity—normal (early, mild), sweaty with feeding (early CHF), irritability, lethargy (shock).
  - Work of breathing: Ranges in severity—normal (early, mild), retractions/tachypnea/grunting (pulmonary edema).
  - Circulation: Ranges in severity—normal (early, mild), marginal perfusion (more severe), cyanosis (pulmonary edema), poor perfusion (severe shock).

Other signs and symptoms:

- Fever
- Muffled heart tones
- Dysrhythmias
- Heart murmur
- Gallop rhythm
- Shock

## Acute Rheumatic Fever

Acute rheumatic fever (ARF) is perhaps the most common cause of acquired heart disease in children worldwide. In the United States, its incidence had decreased in most areas, but some areas have experienced a resurgence. ARF results from an immune response that occurs as a delayed sequela of a group A streptococcal infection.

### Clinical Features

The attack rate following this infection ranges from 0.3% to 3% (of those with an untreated streptococcal infection) and is most common in children 6 to 12 years old.[13–15] The rheumatic process affects multiple organs, with carditis being the most serious. The diagnosis is made using the Jones criteria (Table 4-2), which uses major and minor criteria with evidence of previous group A streptococcal infection. The major criteria include carditis, polyarthritis, chorea, erythema marginatum, and subcutaneous nodules (Figure 4.8).

Clinically, children present with one of the major Jones criteria. Migratory polyarthritis is the most common. The arthritis is not very impressive on inspection, but it is extremely tender and will render the patient nonambulatory if it involves any of the lower extremity joints. The arthritis will migrate from one joint to another, often with two or more joints involved simultaneously. Commonly involved joints include the knee, ankle, small foot joints (tarsals), elbow, wrist, shoulder, and small hand joints (carpals); however, any joint can be affected. Arthritis is distinguished from arthral-

| TABLE 4-2 | Jones Criteria for Guidance in the Diagnosis of Rheumatic Fever | |
|---|---|
| **Major** | **Minor** |
| Carditis | Fever |
| Migratory polyarthritis | Arthralgia |
| Chorea | Previous rheumatic fever/rheumatic heart disease |
| Erythema marginatum | Elevated ESR or CRP |
| Subcutaneous nodules | Prolonged PR interval |
| Diagnosis requires two major criteria or one major plus two minor. Additionally, there must be evidence of antecedent streptococcal infection for the diagnosis of rheumatic fever. An exception is chorea, which alone (no need for any minor criteria to be present) can make the diagnosis without evidence of streptococcal infection. | |

gia in that arthritis has objective findings of inflammation such as tenderness on palpation, tenderness with range of motion, visible swelling or redness, or limited range of motion. Arthralgia is only a subjective sense of joint pain without the above findings. Carditis will often present in an occult fashion unless chest pain or CHF is present. Fever might be the chief complaint. The most common manifestation of carditis is valvulitis. However, less specific manifestations of ARF carditis include myocarditis, second-degree and third-degree AV block, and pericarditis. Valvulitis most often involves mitral insufficiency (holosystolic murmur at the apex radiating to the axilla) and aortic insufficiency (diastolic murmur heart over the base). ARF valvulitis can result in chronic rheumatic heart disease. As the valves scar, they can develop elements of stenosis as well. Mitral and aortic insufficiency occur in acute rheumatic carditis, while mitral stenosis and aortic stenosis are complications of rheumatic carditis commonly seen in rheumatic heart disease (note the difference between acute rheumatic fever carditis and

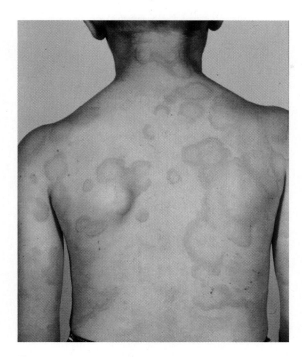

**Figure 4.8** Erythema marginatum in a child with ARF.

rheumatic heart disease). Sydenham chorea is a subacute presentation of rheumatic fever (i.e., it occurs longer after the initial streptococcal infection, so acute phase reactants might no longer be elevated), which manifests as choreiform movements. Subcutaneous nodules and erythema marginatum are rare major criteria that occur with ARF.

## Diagnostic Studies

Diagnostic studies include CBC, ESR, or CRP to look for Jones minor criteria of acute inflammation. Typically, the ESR and CRP are in the very high range. The CBC is nonspecific. An ECG can show a prolonged PR interval (first-degree AV block), which is a Jones minor criterion and is not indicative of carditis. However, if ECG signs of CHF or advanced-degree AV block are present, these findings are more suggestive of carditis. Chest radiograph can show CHF. Doppler echocardiography is the most sensitive indicator of valvulitis. Evidence of preceding group A streptococcal infection is required for the diagnosis. This can include an elevated streptococcal serology (antistreptolysin

O, or a multiple streptococcal antibody assay) or a positive throat culture for group A streptococci. A reliable history indicating a previous episode of scarlet fever might suffice, but streptococcal serology is more objective.

## Differential Diagnosis

Differential diagnosis includes other entities that have similar cardiac, CNS, and joint involvement such as Lyme disease, systemic lupus erythematosas (SLE), systemic arthritis, bacterial endocarditis and myocarditis.

## Management

Management priorities in the ED are to make a diagnosis when possible, and to hospitalize the patient for further management. Although the treatment for polyarthritis is NSAIDs, these patients are usually nonambulatory, making it difficult to discharge them to home. Additionally, the diagnosis of ARF has future consequences since penicillin prophylaxis is required until age 18 or for life (depending on risk of recurrence). Thus, establishing an accurate diagnosis as an inpatient is required to commit a patient to such long-term prophylaxis. Carditis might require corticosteroid treatment under the direction of a cardiologist. Congestive heart failure should be treated as noted in the CHF section.

## Pericarditis

Pericarditis is an acute or chronic inflammation of the pericardial sac with an increase in the pericardial fluid volume and pressure causing cardiac stroke volume reduction. The pericardium can be divided into two components: the visceral pericardium (or epicardium), and the parietal pericardium. The parietal pericardium surrounds the heart and limits the diastolic dimensions of the heart. It attaches along the great vessels and has minimal elasticity. The visceral pericardium covers the heart and great vessels with a delicate lining that also includes fat, coronary vessels, and nerves. Between these two layers is a fluid layer to help protect the heart and its contractility. The usual fluid volume in the pericardial sac is 10 to 30 mL. When there is a sudden increase in fluid, or constriction of the pericardial sac, this results in restriction of chamber-filling volume, which results in stroke volume reduction and hypotension (a process known as tamponade).[16–18] This increases the end diastolic pressure in the ventricle, which impairs ventricular filling and the ejection volume. The most common etiology is infectious, with approximately 30% resulting from a bacterial cause. The most common viral etiology is Coxsackie virus. Other causes include autoimmune disease, trauma, and neoplasms. A specific endpoint condition that can result from the acute or chronic inflammatory process is constrictive pericarditis. It is characterized by thickening of the pericardium adherent to the myocardium, causing restriction of the diastolic expansion of the ventricles. The most common cause of constrictive pericarditis is tuberculosis. Other bacterial causes of pericarditis include pneumococci, staphylococci, and *Haemophilus influenzae* pericarditis.

## Clinical Features

Clinically, the child might present with chest pain and respiratory distress. The child who has altered cardiac function from either an increase in pericardial fluid or constriction of the pericardial sac will present with signs of CHF as well as a precordial "knock" or rub (like the sound of shoes walking on snow).

The classic signs include exercise intolerance, fatigue, jugular venous distention, lower extremity edema, hepatomegaly, poor distal pulses, diminished heart tones, and pulsus paradoxus.

## Diagnostic Studies

An ECG can show ST segment elevation in multiple leads (Figure 4.9) or show signs of tamponade while showing low-voltage QRS complexes or electrical alternans (Figure 4.10). A chest radiograph can show a normal or enlarged cardiac silhouette. There is a pleural effusion in 50% of cases. A two-dimensional echocardiogram is the gold standard for diagnosis and can differentiate between possible causes for the cardiac enlargement and impairment. Magnetic resonance imaging (MRI) or computed tomography (CT) can be used to determine pericardial thickness but are not needed for acute diagnostic testing unless there is difficulty in obtaining a clear picture with echocardiography.

## Differential Diagnosis

The differential diagnosis includes the various causes of pericarditis including infectious (viral and bacterial), as well as autoimmune, rheumatic, systemic lupus erythematosus, and juvenile rheumatoid arthritis. Other causes to consider include traumatic hemopericardium, dysrhythmias, and toxicologic abnormalities.

## Management

The management priorities in the acute care setting are pain control, oxygenation support, and definitive management of the pericarditis. The child should be supported with head and shoulders elevated. Humidified oxygen should be given while monitoring for dysrhythmias. Oxygen saturation will help recognize deterioration. Once the diagnosis of pericarditis is made, the pericardial sac should be tapped for fluid (pericardiocentesis) for diagnostic and/or therapeutic reasons. The child should be placed on anti-inflammatory medication and antibiotics. Emergency pericardiocentesis might be necessary if acute tamponade is present.

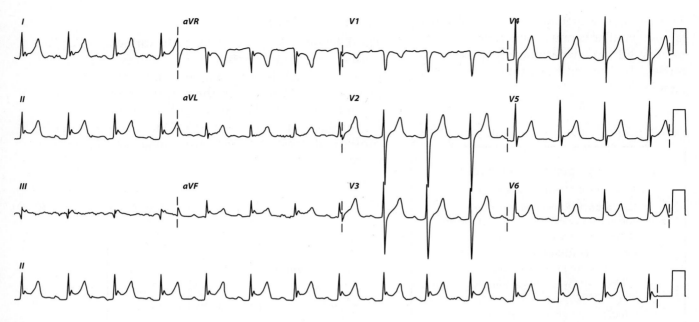

**Figure 4.9** ECG demonstrating ST-segment elevation in multiple leads consistent with pericarditis.

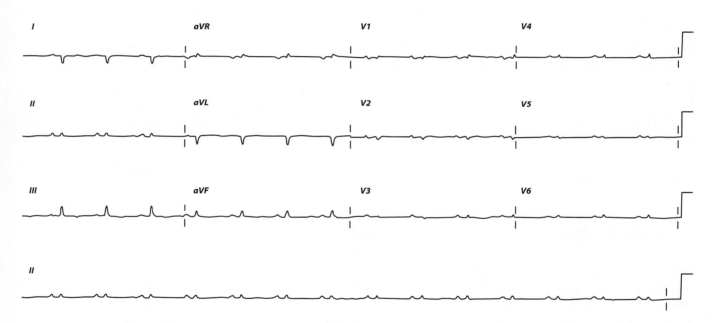

**Figure 4.10** Low voltage QRS complexes.

## THE BOTTOM LINE

- Obtain echocardiography to distinguish pericardial effusion from dilated heart, and to determine the degree of constriction and contractility compromise.

## Bacterial Endocarditis

Endocarditis, although uncommon, is increasing in incidence, mostly because children are surviving congenital heart disease with artificial valves and patches, as well as an increased frequency of patients with central lines for various therapies. Endocarditis is an infection of the endothelial surface of the heart, with a propensity for the valves. Endocarditis can be caused by many different organisms, though 90% of cases are caused by Gram-positive cocci. Although alpha streptococcus (e.g., *Streptococcus viridans*) is the most common organism involved, infections with *Staphylococcus aureus, Streptococcus pneumoniae,* or group A β-hemolytic streptococci can be more virulent.

## Clinical Features

Patients typically present with fever, tachycardia, and signs of cardiac failure or dysrhythmia with a history of recent cardiac surgery or indwelling vascular catheter. Other signs include myalgias, heart murmur or petechiae, septic emboli, or splenomegaly. They can present with signs indistinguishable from myocarditis with poor cardiac contractility and inadequate perfusion with cool extremities, or symptoms similar to pericarditis, with pain in addition to CHF.

## Diagnostic Studies

In a child with suspected endocarditis, obtain laboratory tests, including CBC, ESR, or CRP and blood cultures as well as a chest radiograph and an ECG. The echocardiogram is the diagnostic gold standard and will help determine cardiac function as well as differentiate from congenital lesions or shunts. Laboratory evaluation will show elevated acute phase reactants (ESR and CRP), and a blood culture is usually positive. Echocardiography can show the nidus (e.g., vegetation) of infection but is only 80% sensitive.[19] A rhythm strip can show PVCs.

## Differential Diagnosis

Congenital cardiac lesions with bacteremia, myocarditis, and pericarditis should be considered as direct cardiac causes. In addition, septic emboli from IV drug use or indwelling catheter sepsis should be considered.

---

### WHAT ELSE?

**Differential Diagnosis of Bacterial Endocarditis**

- Bacteremia
- Myocarditis
- Occult congenital heart disease
- Central line catheter sepsis
- IV drug use

---

### YOUR FIRST CLUE

**Signs and Symptoms of Bacterial Endocarditis**

- Pediatric Assessment Triangle:
  - Appearance: Ranges from tired, with flushed skin and tachycardia, to pale, diaphoresis, and poor perfusion.
  - Work of breathing: Ranges from slightly tachypneic (early stages) to tachypneic with diaphoresis (in shock).
  - Circulation: Cutaneous signs of septic emboli can be visible; pale or mottled skin might be present.

Other signs and symptoms:

- Fever
- Heart murmur
- Splinter hemorrhages
- Petechiae
- Splenomegaly

## Management

Treatment involves stabilization of respiratory and cardiac function with oxygen and fluid management. Antibiotics should be started as quickly as possible after two or three sets of blood cultures have been obtained. Penicillin and gentamicin are the drugs of choice in patients who are not allergic to penicillin-based antibiotics. Vancomycin is a penicillin alternative that is empirically preferable because it provides coverage for resistant staphylococci and other resistant organisms. Antibiotic prophylaxis is appropriate for high-risk patients (those with congenital heart disease, cardiac surgery, valvular abnormalities) undergoing dental procedures or other procedures associated with an increased risk of bacteremia. Indwelling catheters, which might be harboring bacteria, should be removed.

## THE BOTTOM LINE

- Often a nonspecific presentation and a difficult diagnosis to make in the emergency department.
- Consider bacterial endocarditis in patients at risk with a fever.
- Consider endocarditis in any patient with fever and a heart murmur.
- Heart murmur of valvular involvement can be difficult to hear.
- Administer empiric antibiotic treatment when suspected.

## Kawasaki Disease

Mucocutaneous lymph node syndrome (MLNS) was first described by Kawasaki in 1967. The etiology is unknown, but it is seen most often in children younger than 5 years, during the winter and spring months. Boys are more susceptible than girls. There is also a predilection for Asian and black children.

### Clinical Features

Clinically, the child with Kawasaki disease presents with a history of fever for 5 days or more. The diagnostic criteria are the presence of conjunctivitis, cervical lymphadenopathy, erythematous mouth and pharynx and/or red, cracked lips and strawberry tongue, maculopapular exanthem (called polymorphous, which means that it can have many different patterns), and swelling of the hands with erythema of the palms (Figure 4.11A and Figure 4.11B).

These patients might present with cardiac abnormalities that present in similar manner to children with decreased myocardial contractility, myocarditis, or coronary insufficiency. The child might present or go on to develop CHF and shock with chest pain. Without treatment,

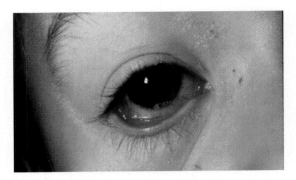

Figure 4.11A  Conjunctivitis.

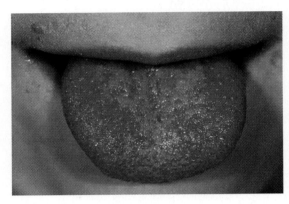

Figure 4.11B  Strawberry tongue, a sign of Kawasaki disease. Source: Habif TP, ed. *Clinical Dermatology: A Color Guide to Diagnosis & Therapy*. 4th Ed. St Louis, Mo: Mosby; 2004. Copyright 2004, Elsevier. Reprinted with permission.

## YOUR FIRST CLUE

**Signs and Symptoms of Kawasaki Disease**

- Pediatric Assessment Triangle:
  - Appearance: Fussy but alert.
  - Work of breathing: Mild tachypnea due to fever. Occasionally, severe respiratory distress due to myocarditis or myocardial infarction.
  - Circulation: Flushed skin or signs of shock with pallor or mottled skin.

Other signs and symptoms:

- Red, cracked lips
- Strawberry tongue
- Conjunctivitis
- Cervical lymphadenopathy
- Rash
- Swelling of hands and feet
- Chest pain

15% to 20% of children with Kawasaki disease will develop coronary artery aneurysms within 1 to 3 weeks from the onset of illness, which can eventually lead to a myocardial infarction or ischemia-induced dysrhythmias. A child who presents with a myocardial infarction might have more nonspecific findings than an adult. These patients can present with nausea, vomiting, and abdominal pain. They can be diaphoretic and crying, or asymptomatic.

## Diagnostic Studies

There are no specific laboratory tests to diagnose Kawasaki disease, but there might be an elevated white blood cell count, elevated platelet count, and an elevation of acute phase reactants (ESR and CRP). An ECG can show nonspecific ST segment and T-wave changes consistent with strain. A chest radiograph, if abnormal, will show some cardiac enlargement. Group A streptococci infection can mimic many of the signs of Kawasaki disease; therefore, a throat swab for rapid group A streptococci analysis and throat culture should be taken. Once other disease processes are ruled out, the child should undergo echocardiography to examine the coronary arteries.

## THE CLASSICS

**Diagnostic Studies in Kawasaki Disease**

- Elevated ESR and CRP
- Thrombocytosis
- Echocardiography might reveal coronary aneurysms.

## Differential Diagnosis

The differential diagnosis includes viral or rickettsial exanthems such as measles, Epstein-Barr virus infection, Rocky Mountain spotted fever, scarlet fever, leptospirosis, and toxic shock syndrome. Other diagnoses to consider are Stevens-Johnson syndrome, drug reaction (e.g., serum sickness), and juvenile rheumatoid arthritis. Consider the diagnosis of Kawasaki disease if any of the preceding conditions is also considered as a diagnostic possibility.

## WHAT ELSE?

**Differential Diagnosis for Kawasaki Disease**

- Rocky Mountain spotted fever
- Epstein-Barr virus exanthem
- Measles
- Other viral exanthem
- Stevens-Johnson syndrome
- Serum sickness
- Leptospirosis
- Toxic shock syndrome

## Management

The child with Kawasaki disease will need IV fluid support and cardiac monitoring. Once Kawasaki disease is thought to be the diagnosis, the patient should be hospitalized and treated with aspirin and intravenous immune globulin (IVIG). Early IVIG treatment reduces the risk of developing coronary aneurysms. A cardiology consult should be obtained for echocardiography and followup for potential future problems. The initial dose for aspirin is 80 to 100 mg/kg per day orally divided into equal 6-hour dosing until the patient is afebrile for 2 to 3 days. Then the dose for aspirin is 3 to 5 mg/kg orally once a day for 6 to 8 weeks. IVIG is begun as an infusion at a dose of 2 mg/kg given over 12 hours. IVIG can cause hypotension as well as nausea, vomiting, and seizures. Cardiac monitoring is essential.[20,21]

## KEY POINTS

**Management of Patients with Kawasaki Disease**

- Place cardiorespiratory monitor.
- Obtain IV access.
- Obtain blood for CBC, ESR, and CRP.
- Begin IVIG and aspirin therapy.
- Obtain cardiology consultation for echocardiography.

## Rhythm Disturbances

Pediatric patients have three basic types of pathologic rhythm disturbances, which include fast pulse (tachyarrhythmia), slow pulse (bradyarrhythmia), and absent pulse (pulseless) (Table 4-3). These can be further divided into seven classifications based on their anatomic function. Dysrhythmias might be the cause of impaired cardiac function leading to cardiac arrest. Occult dysrhythmias (e.g., prolonged QT syndrome, Wolff-Parkinson-White syndrome) might present with intermittent severe symptoms (e.g., palpitations or sudden death).

### Clinical Features

Clinical features of dysrhythmias are usually nonspecific. The child might present with fatigue or syncope, but most patients are asymptomatic on presentation. Hypoxemia is one of the most frequent causes of bradyarrhythmias, so the child might have cyanosis or respiratory problems as the presenting complaint. Children with tachyarrhythmias usually present with chest or abdominal pain and/or a feeling of the heart racing, and a complaint of not being able to catch their breath. Infants with tachyarrhythmias can present with nonspecific symptoms such as vomiting and irritability.

### Diagnostic Studies

An ECG is the initial diagnostic test to document the dysrhythmia, followed by ongoing cardiac monitoring, and a followup ECG to

| TABLE 4-3 | Classification of Rhythm Disturbances |
|---|---|

**Fast Rhythms**

- Supraventricular tachycardia
- Ventricular tachycardia

**Slow Rhythms**

- Sinus bradycardia
- Heart blocks

**Absent Pulses**

- Ventricular fibrillation
- Pulseless ventricular tachycardia
- Asystole
- Pulseless electrical activity

## YOUR FIRST CLUE

**Signs and Symptoms of Dysrhythmias**

- Pediatric Assessment Triangle:
  - Appearance: Ranges in severity from normal (sufficient cardiac output) to distress/lethargic (CHF or inadequate cardiac output).
  - Work of breathing: Ranges in severity from normal, depending on adequacy of cardiac output, and varying degrees of CHF.
  - Circulation: Ranges in severity—normal color (sufficient cardiac output) to pale, mottled, and cyanosis. Marginal perfusion (insufficient cardiac output, CHF), poor perfusion (severe shock).

Other signs and symptoms:

- Fatigue
- Irritability
- Vomiting
- Chest or abdominal pain
- Palpitations
- Respiratory distress
- Shock

document the effect of any antidysrhythmia agent on establishment of a normal heart rhythm. In addition, monitoring blood pressure will help in determining if the dysrhythmia is affecting cardiac function. Once it is determined which of the basic types of rhythm disturbances exists and whether the child is asymptomatic or needs treatment, examination of the ECG will help in differentiating between the various types of fast and slow rhythms. To discriminate between types of fast rhythms, look at the QRS complex width as well as P wave presence when determining the origin of the dysrhythmia, as well as any aberrant conduction problem. Both the PR interval and beat-to-beat pacing will help differentiate various slow rhythms.

The ECG of patients with Wolff-Parkinson-White syndrome will demonstrate a very short PR interval and a classic delta wave. These patients are at risk for recurrent paroxysmal supraventricular tachycardia (SVT). Other conditions predisposing to paroxysmal SVT might not be as evident on an ECG done when the patient is non-symptomatic, requiring long term (Holter) ECG rhythm monitoring to capture the intermittent abnormal rhythm. Patients with prolonged QT interval will have a prolonged corrected QT (QTc) interval. Many QTc intervals are in the borderline prolonged range. Patients with prolonged QTc intervals should be referred to a cardiologist because they are at risk for sudden death.

## Management

The management goal in the ED for any dysrhythmia is to make sure that all reversible causes are addressed, beginning with maintaining oxygenation and ventilation. Thinking of the six H's and five T's mnemonic for reversible causes of dysrhythmias and shock (as updated in 2005) will help treat any underlying cause and prevent cardiac arrest. The six H's are hypovolemia, hypoxia, hydrogen ion (acidosis), hypo-/hyperkalemia, hypoglycemia, and hypothermia. The five T's are toxins, tamponade (cardiac), tension pneumothorax, thrombosis (coronary or pulmonary), and trauma (hypovolemic, increased ICP) (Table 4-4).[22] Obtain IV access to administer antidysrhythmia medications. If, however, the rhythm is unstable supraventricular or ventric-

| TABLE 4-4 | Reversible Causes of Dysrhythmias and Shock, or Cardiorespiratory Arrest (updated 2005) |
|---|---|
| **Six H's** | **Five T's** |
| Hypovolemia | Toxins |
| Hypoxia | Tamponade (cardiac) |
| Hydrogen ion (acidosis) | Tension pneumothorax |
| Hypo-/hyperkalemia | Thrombosis (coronary or pulmonary) |
| Hypoglycemia | |
| Hypothermia | Trauma |

Source: ECC Committee, Subcommittees, and Task Forces of the American Heart Association. 2005 American Heart Association guidelines for cardiopulmonary resuscitation and emergency cardiovascular care: part 7.2: management of cardiac arrest. *Circulation.* 2005;112(Suppl I):IV-59.

ular tachycardia and requires cardioversion, the nonpharmacologic maneuvers might take precedence over IV access.

## Bradydysrhythmias

For bradydysrhythmias, consider hypoxia as a cause first and immediately support the airway, ventilation, and oxygenation. Chest compressions should be started for a heart rate less than 60/min with poor perfusion. The drug of choice for symptomatic bradydysrhythmias is epinephrine IV/IO at 0.01 mg/kg (0.1 mL/kg of 1:10,000 solution) or tracheal (endotracheal) 0.1 mg/kg (0.1 mL/kg of 1:1,000 solution). Repeat dose of epinephrine every 3 to 5 minutes. If bradycardia persists or transiently responds, consider an epinephrine infusion. Atropine can be used to treat a bradydysrhythmias if there is a suspicion of vagal stimulation or cholinergic drug toxicity. The recommended dose is 0.02 mg/kg, with a minimum dose of 0.1 mg and a maximum single dose of 0.5 mg in a child and 1 mg in an adolescent. This can be repeated in 5 minutes to a maximum total dose of 1 mg in a child and 2 mg in an adolescent. Atropine can be administered tracheally (endotracheally) without IV access. Cardiac pacing can also be considered in those cases of bradycardia from a congenital or acquired heart disease that has caused a complete heart block or sinus node dysfunction (Figure 4.12).

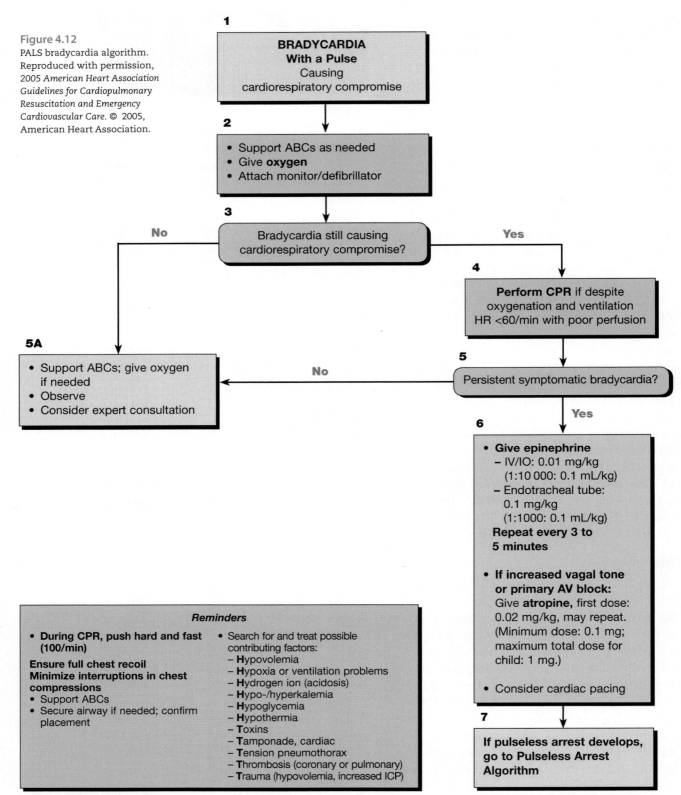

**Figure 4.12**
PALS bradycardia algorithm. Reproduced with permission, *2005 American Heart Association Guidelines for Cardiopulmonary Resuscitation and Emergency Cardiovascular Care.* © 2005, American Heart Association.

**1**
**BRADYCARDIA**
**With a Pulse**
Causing
cardiorespiratory compromise

**2**
- Support ABCs as needed
- Give **oxygen**
- Attach monitor/defibrillator

**3**
Bradycardia still causing cardiorespiratory compromise?

**No**

**Yes**

**4**
**Perform CPR** if despite oxygenation and ventilation HR <60/min with poor perfusion

**5A**
- Support ABCs; give oxygen if needed
- Observe
- Consider expert consultation

**No**

**5**
Persistent symptomatic bradycardia?

**Yes**

**6**
- **Give epinephrine**
  - IV/IO: 0.01 mg/kg (1:10 000: 0.1 mL/kg)
  - Endotracheal tube: 0.1 mg/kg (1:1000: 0.1 mL/kg)
  **Repeat every 3 to 5 minutes**

- **If increased vagal tone or primary AV block:** Give **atropine,** first dose: 0.02 mg/kg, may repeat. (Minimum dose: 0.1 mg; maximum total dose for child: 1 mg.)

- Consider cardiac pacing

**7**
If pulseless arrest develops, go to Pulseless Arrest Algorithm

***Reminders***

- **During CPR, push hard and fast (100/min)**
**Ensure full chest recoil**
**Minimize interruptions in chest compressions**
- Support ABCs
- Secure airway if needed; confirm placement

- Search for and treat possible contributing factors:
  – **H**ypovolemia
  – **H**ypoxia or ventilation problems
  – **H**ydrogen ion (acidosis)
  – **H**ypo-/hyperkalemia
  – **H**ypoglycemia
  – **H**ypothermia
  – **T**oxins
  – **T**amponade, cardiac
  – **T**ension pneumothorax
  – **T**hrombosis (coronary or pulmonary)
  – **T**rauma (hypovolemia, increased ICP)

## Tachydysrhythmias

Sinus tachycardia is not a dysrhythmia, but rather a response by the body to increased cardiac output, so the underlying cause should be identified and treated. Common causes include hypoxemia, hypovolemia, hyperthermia, fever, toxins/poisons/drugs, pain, and anxiety. Supraventricular tachycardia (SVT) is the most common tachydysrhythmia in children and can produce cardiovascular compromise. The heart rate is usually greater than 220/min but can reach as high as 300/min. Usually the QRS interval is narrow, or normal (<0.08 seconds). The cause is most commonly a reentry mechanism from an accessory pathway. It usually occurs quickly and without a history of volume loss, pain, or fever to suggest sinus tachycardia. In many instances, it might be difficult to distinguish between sinus tachycardia and SVT (Table 4-5). If the child is stable and has good perfusion, the treatment of choice is mechanical vagal interventions; If this is unsuccessful, then adenosine IV is recommended (Figure 4.13). Vagal maneuvers include an ice bag to the face (most applicable to infants and young children), or Valsalva maneuvers such as blowing into a straw or bearing down (most applicable in older cooperative children). Carotid massage and eyeball pressure are poor vagal maneuvers that are potentially harmful and should not be attempted. Adenosine is administered in a dose of 0.1 mg/kg as a rapid IV bolus (maximum initial dose 6 mg). This dose can be doubled on the second attempt to 0.2 mg/kg and increased again to 0.4 mg/kg up to a maximum of 12 mg if initial doses are unsuccessful in converting the rhythm. The rapidity of the adenosine bolus can be an important factor. If a peripheral vein is used, adenosine is most rapidly infused by a fast push followed by an immediate flush of the IV line as close to the IV insertion site as possible. If SVT persists and the child remains hemodynamically stable, expert consultation is advised, but amiodarone _or_ procainamide may be considered. Do not use both. If the child has poor perfusion, then synchronized cardioversion of the rhythm is the treatment of choice (Figure 4.13). Attempts to start an IV should occur concomitantly or should be deferred, rather than delaying cardioversion. The cardioversion dose is 0.5 to 1 J/kg, which can be increased to 2 J/kg if the initial attempt is unsuccessful. A baseline ECG and another after electrical or chemical cardioversion should be done to help determine the etiology and assess treatment effectiveness. Ideally, a rhythm strip should be running continuously during rhythm conversion attempts.

## Ventricular Tachycardia

Ventricular tachycardia (VT) is a rare dysrhythmia in pediatrics but is often life threatening.[23] Differentiating VT from SVT is important to initiate the appropriate treatment and prevent deterioration. In VT, typically the heart rate can go as high as 200/min and the QRS com-

| TABLE 4-5 Comparison of Sinus Tachycardia and Supraventricular Tachycardia | |
|---|---|
| **ST** | **SVT** |
| • History of underlying problem such as fever, dehydration, injury, pain | • History incompatible with ST (no history of dehydration, fever) or nonspecific |
| • P waves present | • P waves absent |
| • Heart rate varies with activity | • Heart rate does not change with activity |
| • Variable R-R interval with respirations | • Constant R-R interval with respirations |
| | • Abrupt rate changes (with conversion) |
| • Infants: HR <220/min | • Infants: HR >220/min |
| • Children: HR <180/min | • Children: HR >180/min |

Source: Hazinski MF, Zaritsky AL, Nadkarni VN et al, eds. *PALS Provider Manual*. Dallas, Tx: American Heart Association; 2002: 202. Reprinted with permission.

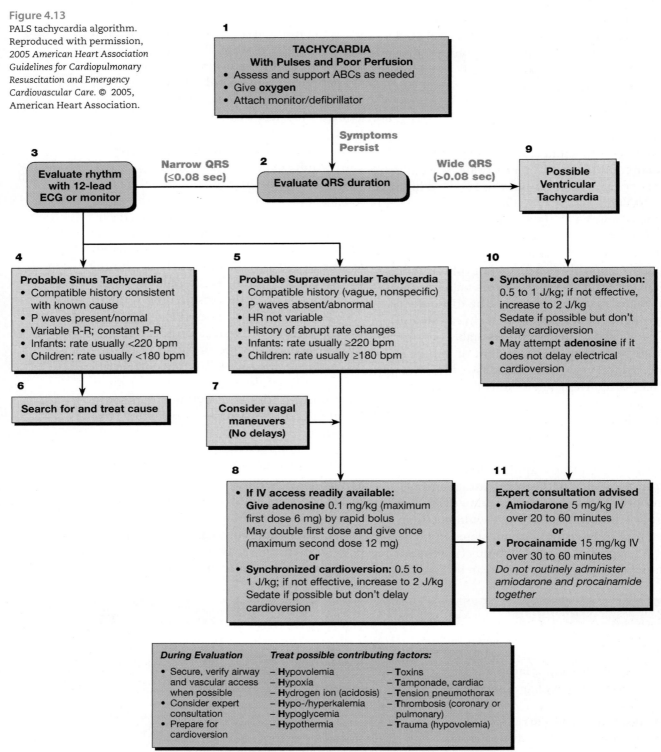

Figure 4.13
PALS tachycardia algorithm.
Reproduced with permission,
*2005 American Heart Association
Guidelines for Cardiopulmonary
Resuscitation and Emergency
Cardiovascular Care.* © 2005,
American Heart Association.

**1**

**TACHYCARDIA**
**With Pulses and Poor Perfusion**
• Assess and support ABCs as needed
• Give **oxygen**
• Attach monitor/defibrillator

**Symptoms Persist**

**3**

**Evaluate rhythm with 12-lead ECG or monitor**

**Narrow QRS (≤0.08 sec)**

**2**

**Evaluate QRS duration**

**Wide QRS (>0.08 sec)**

**9**

**Possible Ventricular Tachycardia**

**4**

**Probable Sinus Tachycardia**
• Compatible history consistent with known cause
• P waves present/normal
• Variable R-R; constant P-R
• Infants: rate usually <220 bpm
• Children: rate usually <180 bpm

**5**

**Probable Supraventricular Tachycardia**
• Compatible history (vague, nonspecific)
• P waves absent/abnormal
• HR not variable
• History of abrupt rate changes
• Infants: rate usually ≥220 bpm
• Children: rate usually ≥180 bpm

**10**

• Synchronized cardioversion: 0.5 to 1 J/kg; if not effective, increase to 2 J/kg Sedate if possible but don't delay cardioversion
• May attempt **adenosine** if it does not delay electrical cardioversion

**6**

**Search for and treat cause**

**7**

**Consider vagal maneuvers (No delays)**

**8**

• If IV access readily available: Give **adenosine** 0.1 mg/kg (maximum first dose 6 mg) by rapid bolus May double first dose and give once (maximum second dose 12 mg)
**or**
• Synchronized cardioversion: 0.5 to 1 J/kg; if not effective, increase to 2 J/kg Sedate if possible but don't delay cardioversion

**11**

**Expert consultation advised**
• **Amiodarone** 5 mg/kg IV over 20 to 60 minutes
**or**
• **Procainamide** 15 mg/kg IV over 30 to 60 minutes
*Do not routinely administer amiodarone and procainamide together*

| *During Evaluation* | *Treat possible contributing factors:* | |
|---|---|---|
| • Secure, verify airway and vascular access when possible | – **H**ypovolemia | – **T**oxins |
| | – **H**ypoxia | – **T**amponade, cardiac |
| | – **H**ydrogen ion (acidosis) | – **T**ension pneumothorax |
| • Consider expert consultation | – **H**ypo-/hyperkalemia | – **T**hrombosis (coronary or pulmonary) |
| | – **H**ypoglycemia | |
| • Prepare for cardioversion | – **H**ypothermia | – **T**rauma (hypovolemia) |

© 2005 American Heart Association

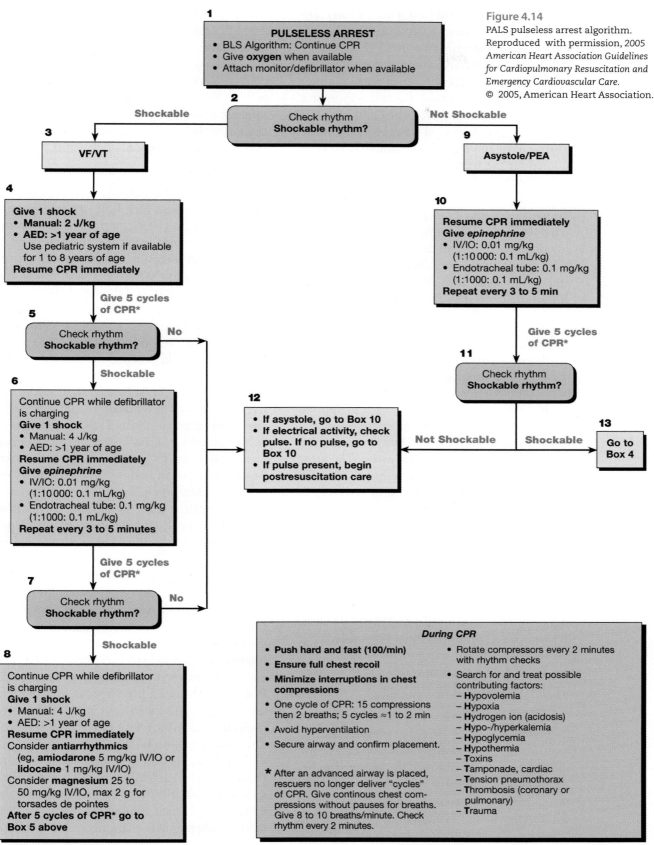

**1**

**PULSELESS ARREST**
- BLS Algorithm: Continue CPR
- Give **oxygen** when available
- Attach monitor/defibrillator when available

Figure 4.14
PALS pulseless arrest algorithm.
Reproduced with permission, *2005
American Heart Association Guidelines
for Cardiopulmonary Resuscitation and
Emergency Cardiovascular Care.*
© 2005, American Heart Association.

**2**

Check rhythm
**Shockable rhythm?**

Shockable ← → Not Shockable

**3**

**VF/VT**

**9**

**Asystole/PEA**

**4**

**Give 1 shock**
- **Manual: 2 J/kg**
- **AED: >1 year of age**
  Use pediatric system if available
  for 1 to 8 years of age
**Resume CPR immediately**

Give 5 cycles
of CPR*

**10**

**Resume CPR immediately**
**Give** *epinephrine*
- IV/IO: 0.01 mg/kg
  (1:10 000: 0.1 mL/kg)
- Endotracheal tube: 0.1 mg/kg
  (1:1000: 0.1 mL/kg)
**Repeat every 3 to 5 min**

Give 5 cycles
of CPR*

**5**

Check rhythm
**Shockable rhythm?**  → No

Shockable

**11**

Check rhythm
**Shockable rhythm?**

**6**

Continue CPR while defibrillator
is charging
**Give 1 shock**
- **Manual: 4 J/kg**
- **AED: >1 year of age**
**Resume CPR immediately**
**Give** *epinephrine*
- IV/IO: 0.01 mg/kg
  (1:10 000: 0.1 mL/kg)
- Endotracheal tube: 0.1 mg/kg
  (1:1000: 0.1 mL/kg)
**Repeat every 3 to 5 minutes**

**12**

- **If asystole, go to Box 10**
- **If electrical activity, check
  pulse. If no pulse, go to
  Box 10**
- **If pulse present, begin
  postresuscitation care**

Not Shockable ← → Shockable

**13**

Go to
Box 4

Give 5 cycles
of CPR*

**7**

Check rhythm
**Shockable rhythm?**  → No

Shockable

**8**

Continue CPR while defibrillator
is charging
**Give 1 shock**
- **Manual: 4 J/kg**
- **AED: >1 year of age**
**Resume CPR immediately**
Consider **antiarrhythmics**
  (eg, **amiodarone** 5 mg/kg IV/IO or
  **lidocaine** 1 mg/kg IV/IO)
Consider **magnesium** 25 to
  50 mg/kg IV/IO, max 2 g for
  torsades de pointes
**After 5 cycles of CPR* go to
Box 5 above**

***During CPR***

- **Push hard and fast (100/min)**
- **Ensure full chest recoil**
- **Minimize interruptions in chest
  compressions**
- One cycle of CPR: 15 compressions
  then 2 breaths; 5 cycles ≈1 to 2 min
- Avoid hyperventilation
- Secure airway and confirm placement.

- Rotate compressors every 2 minutes
  with rhythm checks
- Search for and treat possible
  contributing factors:
  – **H**ypovolemia
  – **H**ypoxia
  – **H**ydrogen ion (acidosis)
  – **H**ypo-/hyperkalemia
  – **H**ypoglycemia
  – **H**ypothermia
  – **T**oxins
  – **T**amponade, cardiac
  – **T**ension pneumothorax
  – **T**hrombosis (coronary or
    pulmonary)
  – **T**rauma

**\*** After an advanced airway is placed,
  rescuers no longer deliver "cycles"
  of CPR. Give continous chest compressions without pauses for breaths.
  Give 8 to 10 breaths/minute. Check
  rhythm every 2 minutes.

© 2005 American Heart Association

**Rhythm Disturbances** 131

plex is wide. Most children with VT have underlying heart disease, either congenital or acquired. If a child with VT is hemodynamically stable, cardiology consultation is recommended. If VT is confirmed, consider the use of amiodarone _or_ procainamide. Do not administer these two drugs together. If the child has poor perfusion, synchronized cardioversion is the treatment of choice. Amiodarone may be considered for the treatment of hemodynamically unstable VT (Source: 2005 International Consensus Conference on Cardiopulmonary Resuscitation and Emergency Cardiovascular Care Recommendations. 2005 international consensus on CPR and ECC science with treatment recommendations: part 6: pediatric basic and advanced life support. _Circulation._ 2005;112:III-73-III-90). (Figure 4.14).

## Pulseless Arrest Rhythms

Cardiopulmonary arrest is the endpoint when the body's compensation mechanisms have been overwhelmed and are unable to overcome dysfunction in respiratory and cardiac systems. In pediatrics, the most common primary cause is respiratory failure, but impaired cardiac output can also lead to arrest. The most common rhythm in an out-of-hospital arrest is asystole, and the likelihood of recovery is less than 1%.[24,25] Other pulseless arrest rhythms include ventricular fibrillation, pulseless ventricular tachycardia, and PEA.

### Clinical Features

The child presents with no pulse but might have pulseless electrical activity (PEA). Other signs are cool extremities and cyanotic skin. There is no respiratory effort. The underlying cause might not be evident on initial exam, but looking for signs of trauma is important when trying to find an etiology.

### Diagnostic Studies

Body temperature, ECG, cardiorespiratory monitoring, and blood pH will help determine the cardiac status and provide prognostic indicators for successful resuscitation. A poor prognosis is indicated by PEA or asystole in the absence of four H's and four T's, and/or the presence of severe acidosis (pH < 6.9). A bedside glucose (rapid test), arterial blood gas analysis, and electrolytes are important to guide resuscitation.

Once the resuscitation has begun, consider potentially reversible causes. Again, the mnemonic of four T's and four H's includes tamponade, toxins/poisons/drugs, tension pneumothorax, thromboembolism, and hypoxemia, hypovolemia, hypothermia, and hyper/hypokalemia.

### Management

For cardiopulmonary arrest, the first priority is the ABCs. Ventilate with 100% oxygen via bag-mask and begin chest compressions. Monitor the cardiac activity or the effectiveness of chest compressions (measure blood pressure, perfusion, and oxygen saturation) and assess the rhythm. While doing CPR, prepare for intubation and IV/IO access. After endotracheal intubation, chest compressions should be performed at a rate of 100 compressions per minute, and ventilation should proceed without pauses for compressions at a rate of 8 to 10 ventilations per minute. Caution must be exercised not to deliver too many ventilations at the expense of chest compressions (Source: ECC Committee, Subcommittees, and Task Forces of the American Heart Association. 2005 American Heart Association guidelines for cardiopulmonary resuscitation and emergency cardiovascular care: part 11: pediatric basic life support. _Circulation._ 2005;112(Suppl I):IV-161). If the rhythm shows PEA or asystole, administer epinephrine and resume CPR. Epinephrine may be repeated every 3 to 5 minutes. High-dose epinephrine may be considered in β-blocker overdose (Source: 2005 International Consensus Conference on Cardiopulmonary Resuscitation and Emergency Cardiovascular Care Recommendations. 2005 international consensus on CPR and ECC science with treatment recommendations: part 12: Pediatric advanced life support. _Circulation._ 2005;112:IV-167-IV-187). If at any time there is electrical activity, check pulse. If present, begin postresuscitation care. If absent, continue CPR; follow asystole pathway. If the rhythm shows VF or VT, defibrillate at 2 J/kg and resume CPR immediately. After 5 cycles (2 minutes) of CPR, check rhythm. If shockable, continue CPR while defibrillator is charging and give a dose of epinephrine, then defibrillate with 4 J/kg. If epinephrine cannot be given prior to shock, resume CPR and administer the drug during CPR. After 5 cycles of CPR, check rhythm. If shockable, continue CPR and defibrillate at 4 J/kg, then resume CPR. Consider amiodarone or lidocaine, and administer while CPR is provided for 5 cycles, then check rhythm. If torsade de pointes is present, consider magnesium during CPR. If rhythm is still shockable, repeat CPR-drug-shock cycle with epinephrine and 4 J/kg defibrillation energy dose.

Termination of resuscitation is a critical issue. Studies show little to no meaningful survival if spontaneous circulation has not returned after 30 minutes of resuscitation or after 2 doses of epinephrine have been delivered.[26–28] Few children survive out-of-hospital cardiopulmonary arrest, and fewer will have a normal neurologic recovery.[26,29] When asked, parents wish to be present during the resuscitation of their child, and it often can help parents with the grieving process.[30,31]

## THE BOTTOM LINE

- Management for patients with dysrhythmias is driven by presence or absence of poor perfusion.

- Sinus tachycardia is not an arrhythmia, but its etiology must be determined.

- Provide oxygenation and ventilation for all patients in cardiopulmonary arrest as the primary etiology is respiratory failure.

- Once resuscitation has begun, evaluate and treat reversible cause of cardiopulmonary arrest.

- Family presence during resuscitation should be encouraged by ED staff.

## Cardiomyopathy

The danger of cardiomyopathies is that these conditions can lead to sudden death. Hypertrophic cardiomyopathy (formerly called idiopathic hypertrophic subaortic stenosis), which can be inherited, and other cardiomyopathies predispose otherwise healthy appearing children to life-threatening dysrhythmias. These children might have a family history of sudden death, syncope (with or without exercise), and a systolic murmur that increases with certain specific maneuvers. The heart murmur is often a harsh crescendo/decrescendo murmur with an associated $S_4$ and will increase with standing from the squatting position and Valsalva maneuver. The murmur is heard best at the left sternal border and apex and does not radiate to the carotids, distinguishing it from an aortic stenosis murmur. Chronic cardiomyopathies might cause chronic CHF.

### Diagnostic Studies

Diagnostic studies include ECG, chest radiograph, and echocardiogram. The ECG can be nonspecifically abnormal in up to 95% of all cases of hypertrophic cardiomyopathy, which might include signs of left ventricular hypertrophy and ST-T changes. The chest radiograph is often normal. Echocardiography reveals asymmetric septal hypertophy in 90% of cases.

## YOUR FIRST CLUE

**Signs and Symptoms of Cardiomyopathy**

- Pediatric Assessment Triangle:

  - Appearance: Healthy and normal appearing; sudden collapse; chronic cardiomyopathies possibly leading to chronic CHF with varying degrees of distress and failure to thrive.

  - Work of breathing: Normal, unless chronic CHF is present.

  - Circulation: Normal; patients at risk for sudden cardiac arrest.

  Other signs or symptoms:

- Family history of sudden death
- Heart murmur
- Dysrhythmia
- Syncope with exercise

### Differential Diagnosis

The differential diagnosis is that of benign and malignant murmurs, left ventricular hypertrophy due to exercise, and vasovagal syncope.

## Management

A child who presents with exercise-induced syncope should be withdrawn from any and all significant physical activity pending a cardiology evaluation. A child who presents with a clinical course suggesting cardiovascular instability (e.g., a murmur or palpitations), should be admitted for observation in a monitored bed and undergo an urgent evaluation by a cardiologist (ECG, echocardiogram, and exercise stress testing).

---

### THE BOTTOM LINE

**Cardiomyopathy**
- Exercise-induced syncope or syncope associated with cardiac signs and symptoms warrants a cardiology evaluation.
- The child should be instructed to not exercise until cleared by cardiology.

---

## Postsurgical Complications

Postsurgical problems in children who have had cardiac surgery can include rhythm disturbances, infections (including endocarditis or bacteremia), and pulmonary edema. Most acute problems will be seen while recovering from the surgical procedure.[32–34] However, after discharge, most will still have some pulmonary edema secondary to thoracostomy tube removal and the healing process of the surgical procedure. They might have an acute deterioration during the home recovery stage. If the surgical procedure involved accessing the interior of the heart, the child is also at risk for new dysrhythmias after the surgical procedure while the tissue heals, especially if this is near or over the electrical conduction pathways. Other postsurgical complications include those that occur in multiple-step procedures in which a palliative shunt is placed, which might clot or become dysfunctional. In this case, the child might present with symptoms reflective of the original cardiac lesion.

### Clinical Features

Clinically, these patients present with specific features related to their underlying problem but all might look pale and will have a midsternotomy scar. Febrile children can be tired and tachycardic as well as tachypneic. They can have either bounding pulses or decreased pulses in the distal extremities. Signs of CHF can be present in those with pulmonary edema as well as cardiac shunt malfunction.

---

### YOUR FIRST CLUE

**Signs and Symptoms of Postsurgical Cardiac Complications**
- Pediatric Assessment Triangle:
  - Appearance: Ranges in severity—normal (good functional surgical repair), sweaty with feeding, failure to thrive (CHF), irritability (pulmonary edema), lethargic (shock), sudden decompensation (clot formation within a shunt or disruption of surgical repair).
  - Work of breathing: Ranges in severity—normal (good functional repair), retractions/tachypnea/grunting (pulmonary edema).
  - Circulation: Ranges in severity—normal (good functional repair), cyanosis (palliative or inadequate surgical repair), poor perfusion (shock, sudden decompensation).

Other signs and symptoms
- History of congenital heart disease and cardiac surgery
- Presence of sternotomy or thoracotomy scar
- Fatigue
- Fever
- Respiratory distress
- Dysrhythmia

---

## Differential Diagnosis

The differential diagnosis is primarily that of problems with the heart itself secondary to the surgical procedure versus the usual childhood illnesses and injuries. The febrile child might have an infection obtained in the hospital or at home. Table 4-6 summarizes the common palliative and definitive surgical procedures typically performed for the listed cyanotic heart disease conditions.

## Management

These patients require stabilization of airway, ventilation, and circulation. Oxygen saturation monitoring with humidified oxygen administration is the first step. Cardiac and blood pressure monitoring will help detect dysrhythmias and determine cardiovascular stability. An ECG should be obtained to determine the exact rhythm. A chest radiograph might show pulmonary edema or an abnormal cardiac shadow, which should be compared to the postsurgical chest radiograph if possible. An echocardiogram might be indicated if there is concern of pericardial fluid, abnormal cardiac contractility, or an alternation in the surgical repair.

An IV should be placed for fluid management. Depending on the clinical presentation and diagnostic testing, the child might need an intervention for a dysrhythmia or pulmonary edema. The child might require pericardiocentesis. Consultation should be made with the pediatric cardiac surgeon for any postsurgical problems. Information on the type of repair and potential complications with their management can be found on an Emergency Information Form (EIF). Ask the patient's family if an EIF is available or note if the patient has a Medic-Alert bracelet. If so, contact the MedicAlert Foundation for additional information.

### THE BOTTOM LINE

**Postsurgical Cardiac Complications**

- Obtain rapid history and assess children in shock or respiratory distress for congenital heart disease and postsurgical complications.
- Utilize the EIF to gather information, contact specialists, and guide therapy.
- Obtain rapid echocardiography and cardiology consultation for definitive diagnosis and cardiac function determination.

## ■ Shock

Shock is a condition in which the tissue perfusion of nutrients and oxygen is inadequate to meet the metabolic demands of the body. It can be divided into four major types: hypovolemic, cardiogenic, distributive, and septic (Table 4-7). The end result is inadequate functional cardiac output to meet the perfusion demands of the body. Early recognition is important to prevent tissue damage and progression to cardiopulmonary arrest. The goals of the initial assessment are to determine if this is a compensated shock or decompensated shock. Compensated shock occurs when the vital organs continue to be perfused by compensatory mechanisms and the blood pressure is normal when measured. These compensatory mechanisms are triggered by receptors for pressure (carotid body), volume (right atrium), and chemical aberrations (pH in aortic arch). Shock triggers catecholamine release, which results in

### KEY POINTS

**The Management of Postsurgical Cardiac Complications**

- Start cardiorespiratory monitoring.
- Provide supplemental oxygen.
- Obtain IV access.
- Arrhythmia management.
- CHF management.
- Obtain ECG and chest radiograph.
- Contact cardiologist or cardiac surgeon.

| TABLE 4-6 | Common Palliative and Definitive Surgical Procedures Typically Performed for the Listed Cyanotic Heart Disease Conditions* |
|---|---|

### Total Anomalous Pulmonary Venous Return

- Obstructive lesion
  - Balloon atrial septostomy
  - Complete repair later
  - Patches and anastomotic procedures to reroute blood flow

### Tetralogy of Fallot

- Palliative repair
  - Blalock-Taussig—subclavian artery to pulmonary artery
  - Potts—descending aorta to left pulmonary artery
  - Waterston—ascending aorta to right pulmonary artery
- Surgical repair
  - Closure of the ventriculoseptal defect
  - Relief of the pulmonic stenosis

### Transposition of the Great Vessels

- Surgical repair today
  - Arterial switch operation—Jatene operation
- Surgical procedures that are no longer performed
  - Mustard or Senning procedure (intracardiac baffle that diverts blood to the correct side)

### Tricuspid Atresia

- Palliative surgery for relief of hypoxemia
  - Less than 1 month of age
    - Central aortopulmonary shunt
    - Modified Blalock-Taussig shunt
  - 1–6 months of age
    - Modified Blalock-Taussig shunt
  - Greater than 6 months of age
    - Modified Blalock-Taussig shunt
    - Bidirectional Glenn anastomosis
  - Surgical repair
    - Staged modified Fontan procedure

### Truncus Arteriosus

- Surgical closure
  - Closure of the ventriculoseptal defect
  - Right ventricle-pulmonary artery connection with aortic homograft (Rastelli repair) or conduit with a semilunar valve

### Hypoplastic Left Heart

- Surgical palliation—Norwood operation
  - First stage
    - Connecting the main pulmonary arterial trunk to the ascending aorta and aortic arch
    - Dividing the ductus arteriosus
    - Modified Blalock-Taussig shunt
  - Second stage
    - Bidirectional cavopulmonary (superior vena cava and pulmonary arteries) connection (Glenn)
    - Closing the aortopulmonary window
- Modified Fontan procedure—cavopulmonary isolation procedure (anastomosis of the inferior vena cava to the pulmonary arteries)
  - Completed at 12–18 months of age
- Transplant protocol

### Coarctation of the Aorta

- Surgical closure
- Dividing the ductus

*This table does not address surgical repair of mixed cardiac lesions.

reduction in the vagal tone and an increase in heart rate and contractility. Decompensated shock occurs when these compensatory mechanisms have become overwhelmed and are inadequate, causing hypotension. In the pediatric patient, the blood pressure usually does not drop until the later stages of physiologic decompensation. Aggressive resuscitation might reduce the risk of multiple organ failure by reducing the time of hypoperfusion. If the resuscitation is not successful, the child will have irreversible shock secondary to organ failure and can progress to cardiopulmonary arrest.

## Hypovolemic Shock

Hypovolemic shock is the most common type of shock seen in infants and children. Shock results from a decrease in intravascular volume. This loss can be from loss of blood, plasma, or water, which decreases the preload for cardiac output. Some of the more common causes of hypovolemic shock include dehydration and injuries resulting in blood loss. The history is important to determine the volume of fluid loss by assessing input and output over the course of the illness. If a recent weight is known, it can be compared to the presentation weight to help quantify the fluid deficit.

### Clinical Features

The child might present with early signs of shock that can be readily measured, such as fast heart rate, normal or low blood pressure, pulses that are weaker in the distal versus central areas of the body, and/or prolonged capillary refill times. Other signs include evidence of end-organ hypoperfusion, such as decreased responsiveness to the environment, pale or cyanotic skin color with coolness distally, and decreased urine output.

### Diagnostic Studies

After the initial physical exam, a quick test for glucose and electrolytes is indicated. The degree of acidosis, as well as other electrolyte abnormalities, will help determine severity. A CBC count should be obtained to assess for anemia.

| TABLE 4-7 | Classification and Etiologies of Shock |
|---|---|

- *Hypovolemic:* Dehydration, blood loss from injuries
- *Cardiogenic:* Congenital heart disease or acquired heart disease
- *Distributive:* Anaphylaxis, spinal cord injury
- *Septic\*:* Infection

\*Might have hypovolemia, cardiac dysfunction, and distributive components.

### Management

The type of shock must be determined in order to select the proper resuscitation options. Sometimes, the underlying cause cannot be determined until the patient has been stabilized. Some causes of hypovolemia to consider include volume depletion from vomiting/diarrhea, excess insensible water loss (heat stroke), urinary loss (diabetes insipidus or mellitus), and bleeding (both internally and/or externally) from trauma.

The goals for management are to improve tissue perfusion and decrease acidosis. The first priority is to administer oxygen, initiate cardiorespiratory monitoring, and keep the child warm. IV or IO access should then be established. Volume-expanding crystalloids (normal saline or lactated Ringer's) should be given in a bolus of 20 mL/kg as fast as possible and repeated after reassessing the child if there are still signs of inadequate perfusion. If bleeding has caused the hypovolemic shock, the hemorrhage must be controlled. Blood is the resuscitation fluid of choice (given in 10 mL/kg aliquots of packed red blood cells until stable). Volume-expanding IV crystalloid solution can be substituted in 20 mL/kg boluses until blood is available.

## Cardiogenic Shock

Cardiogenic shock is a state of poor myocardial function and contractility. There can be an impaired ejection of blood due to an impedance to outflow or a decrease in myocardial contractility. There might also be an intrinsic electrical conduction abnormality that causes an inadequate heart rate and cardiac output. The important concept to consider is that fluids alone will not definitively improve this state of shock and will impair cardiovascular function over time, because the problem is not one of inadequate filling pressures but rather a decrease in moving the fluid. Most children who present with cardiogenic shock have an underlying congenital heart condition, but this can be the acute presentation of an acquired heart condition such as myocarditis.

### Clinical Features

The child presents with signs of tachycardia, tachypnea, pale or cyanotic color to the nailbeds, with prolonged capillary refill. In addition, rales and/or rhonchi, a gallop rhythm, and hepatomegaly might be present. In the case of a conduction abnormality, the child will have a paradoxically low heart rate despite the presence of other signs of shock on exam.

### Diagnostic Studies

Diagnostic testing includes a chest radiograph and an ECG, which might reveal an underlying cardiac abnormality with an enlarged heart shadow and chamber enlargement, low ECG voltages, and possibly ST-T wave changes. An echocardiogram might be needed to differentiate between a structural abnormality and a functional contractility problem.

### Differential Diagnosis

Determining a cardiogenic etiology of shock can be difficult, but this is important because it modifies the resuscitation strategy. Those that cause an outflow obstruction include coarctation of the aorta, aortic stenosis, and pulmonary embolus. A child with decreased contractility might have a history of asphyxia, acquired myocarditis, or myocardial infarction. The causes of conduction problems to consider include sick sinus syndrome, pacemaker failure, complete heart block, hypoxemia, hyperkalemia, and digitalis or tricyclic antidepressant toxicity.

### Management

The priority in the ED is to maintain airway, ventilation, and perfusion. Administer humidified oxygen. Cardiorespiratory monitoring is started and IV/IO access established. Despite the possibility of fluid overload in cardiogenic shock, give volume-expanding crystalloid solution at a lower volume (e.g., 10 mL/kg) and/or at a slower rate, and monitor the response to prevent worsening of cardiac function while trying to treat the underlying cause of shock. Inotropic agents such as dopamine, dobutamine, or epinephrine should be started to improve the contractility and support the heart rate. Dobutamine, more specifically, augments contractility and heart rate (β-1 effects), but it might initially cause hypotension because of a lack of α receptor activity, leading to a relative decrease in systemic vascular resistance. Dopamine and epinephrine increase systemic vascular resistance in addition to the β-1 effects. Inamrinone (formerly known as amrinone) or milrinone (both type III phosphodiesterase inhibitors) might be needed as well. They cause relaxation of vascular muscle and vasodilation.

## Distributive Shock

Distributive shock is caused by inappropriate vasodilation with a maldistribution of blood flow and increased vascular capacity.[35–38]

### Clinical Features

In septic shock, the child might present with tachycardia, tachypnea, warm skin with flushing, and stronger central versus distal pulses. During this period of "warm shock," the clues of cardiovascular instability are primarily erratic changes in blood pressure and pulse strength. Patients will eventually continue to deteriorate toward decompensated shock without prompt treatment, and they often require inotropic agents to support the cardiovascular system. Anaphylaxis can be associated with angioedema, urticaria, stridor, hoarseness, wheezing, respiratory distress, arrhythmias, and shock. Spinal cord injury can produce hypotension due to a loss of sympathetic tone. It can also result in apnea or diaphragmatic breathing. The classic finding of neurogenic shock is hypotension without tachycardia or vasoconstriction.

### Diagnostic Studies

Radiographs should be taken if indicated for infection or traumatic injury. The history and physical exam will help to differentiate the various causes of distributive shock and point to the type of testing most appropriate, while keeping the ABCs stable.

### Differential Diagnosis

Distributive shock can result from any process resulting in venodilation, such as drug or toxins, spinal trauma, sepsis, or anaphylaxis.

### Management

Although septic shock is commonly considered distributive shock, it has components of hypovolemia, cardiac dysfunction, and maldistribution of blood flow and deserves recognition as a unique form of shock. The first priority in the management of septic shock is volume expanding fluids. Epinephrine and/or dopamine might be needed early to reverse the maldistribution of blood flow. Cardiac dysfunction with impaired ejection fraction is common with septic shock and might need inotropic support to improve myocardial contractility.

If a metabolic acidosis is present, early intubation and ventilatory support will help to reduce metabolic demands. Appropriate antibiotics should be given as soon as possible.

If a spinal cord injury is suspected, management includes spinal immobilization and IV fluids. If blood pressure does not improve after a fluid bolus, vasopressors might be indicated. Methylprednisolone should be given within 8 hours of injury. Management of anaphylaxis includes epinephrine (SC, IM), albuterol, antihistamines, and corticosteroids with IV fluid resuscitation. If hypotension is refractory to IV fluids, vasopressor support is indicated.

## Check Your Knowledge

1. Which newborn anatomic structure closes at birth or shortly thereafter to help with the transition from the intrauterine to extrauterine environment?
   A. Coronary sinus
   B. Ductus arteriosus
   C. Pulmonary artery
   D. Ventricular septum

2. Which of the following is a common cyanotic congenital heart lesion?
   A. Patent ductus arteriosus
   B. Tetralogy of Fallot
   C. Pulmonary stenosis
   D. Ventricular septal defect

3. Which of the following drugs can be a lifesaver in a newborn with CHF secondary to closure of the ductus arteriosus?
   A. Digoxin
   B. Dopamine
   C. Furosemide
   D. Prostaglandin $E_1$

4. Which of the following is a major criterion of the Jones criteria for the diagnosis of ARF?
   A. Arthralgias
   B. Elevated white blood cell count
   C. Erythema marginatum
   D. Positive ASO titer

## References

1. Gillum RF. Epidemiology of congenital heart disease in the United States. *Am Heart J.* 1994;127(4 Pt 1):919–927.
2. Clark ED. Pathogenetic mechanism of congenital cardiovascular malformations revisited. *Semin Perinatol.* 1996:20(6):465–472.
3. Hoffman JL. Incidence of congenital heart disease: I. Postnatal incidence. *Pediatr Cardiol.* 1995;16(3):103–113.
4. Opitz J, Yost HJ, Clark EB. Chapter 55. Heart formation: evolution and developmental field theory. In: Clark EB, Nakazawa M, Takao A, eds. *Etiology and Morphogenesis of Congenital Cardiovascular Disease: Twenty Years of Progress in Genetics and Developmental Biology.* Armonk, Ny: Futura Publishing; 2000:311–321.
5. Teitel DF, Iwamoto HS, Rudolph AM. Changes in the pulmonary circulation during birth-related events. *Pediatr Res.* 1990;27:372–378.
6. Teitel DF, Iwamoto HS, Rudolph AM. Effects of birth-related events on central blood flow patterns. *Pediatr Res.* 1987;22:557–566.
7. Townsend SF, Rudolph CD, Rudolph AM. Changes in ovine hepatic circulation and oxygen consumption at birth. *Pediatr Res.* 1989;25:300–304.
8. Hammerman C, Aramburo MJ, Bui KC. Endogenous dilator prostaglandins in congenital heart disease. *Pediatr Cardiol.* 1987; 8(3):155–159.
9. Calder AL, Kirker JA, Neutze JM, Starling MB. Pathology of the ductus arteriosus treated with prostaglandins: comparisons with untreated cases. *Pediatr Cardiol.* 1984;5(2):85–92.
10. Silove ED. Administration of E-type prostaglandins in ductus-dependent congenital heart disease. *Pediatr Cardiol.* 1982;2(4): 303–305.
11. Rein AJ, Omokhodion SI, Nir A. Significance of a cardiac murmur as the sole clinical sign in the newborn. *Clin Pediatr.* 2000;39(9):511–520.
12. Klewer SE, Samson RA et al. Comparison of accuracy of diagnosis of congenital heart disease by history and physical examination versus echocardiography. *Am J Cardiol.* 2002;89(11):1329–1331.
13. Ayoub EM. Resurgence of rheumatic fever in the United States: the changing picture of a preventable disease. *Postgrad Med.* 1992;92:133–142.
14. Dajani AS, Bisno AL, Ching KJ et al. Prevention of rheumatic fever: a statement for health professionals by the Committee on Rheumatic Fever, Endocarditis, and Kawasaki Disease of the Council on Cardiovascular Disease in the Young, American Heart Association. *Circulation.* 1988; 78:1082–1086.
15. Johnson DR, Stevens DL, Kaplan EL. Epidemiologic analysis of group A streptococcal erotypes associated with severe systemic infections, rheumatic fever or uncomplicated pharyngitis. *J Infect Dis.* 1992;166:374–382.
16. Holt JP. The normal pericardium. *Am J Cardiol.* 1970;26:455–463.
17. Tamburro RF, Ring JC, Womback K. Detection of pulsus paradoxus associated with large pericardial effusions in pediatric patients by analysis of the pulse-oximetry waveform. *Pediatrics.* 2002; 109(4):673–677.
18. Levine MJ. Implications of echocardiographically assisted diagnosis of pericardial tamponade in contemporary medical patients: detection before hemodynamic embarrassment. *J Am Coll Cardiol.* 1991;17:59–65.

# CHAPTER REVIEW

19. Ferrieri P, Gewitz MH et al. Unique features of infective endocarditis in childhood. *Pediatrics.* 2002;109(5):931–943.

20. Sundel RP. Update on the treatment of Kawasaki disease in childhood. *Curr Rheumatol Rep.* 2002;4(6):474–482.

21. Lang B, Duffy CM. Controversies in the management of Kawasaki disease. *Best Pract Res Clin Rheumatol.* 2002;16(3):427–442.

22. 2005 International Consensus Conference on Cardiopulmonary Resuscitation and Emergency Cardiovascular Care Recommendations. 2005 international consensus on CPR and ECC science with treatment recommendations: part 6: pediatric basic and advanced life support. *Circulation.* 2005;112:III-73-III-90.

23. Alexander ME, Berul CI. Ventricular arrhythmias: when to worry. *Pediatr Cardiol.* 2000; 21(6):532–541.

24. Kochanek PM, Clark RS, Ruppel, RA, Dixon CE. Cerebral resuscitation after traumatic brain injury and cardiopulmonary arrest in infants and children in the new millennium. *Pediatr Clin North Am.* 2001;48(3):661–681.

25. Hickey RW, Zuckerbraun, NS. Pediatric cardiopulmonary arrest: current concepts and future directions. *Pediatr Emer Reports.* 2003;8(1):1–12.

26. Young KD, Seidel JS: Pediatric cardiopulmonary resuscitation: a collective review. *Ann Emerg Med.* 1999;33:195–205.

27. Sirbaugh PE, Pepe PE, Shook JE et al. A prospective, population-based study of the demographics, epidemiology, management, and outcome of out-of-hospital pediatric cardiopulmonary arrest. *Ann Emerg Med.* 1999;33: 174–184.

28. Zaritsky A, Nadkarni V, Getson Kuehl K. CPR in children. *Ann Emerg Med.* 1987;16:1107–1110.

29. Gausche M, Lewis RJ, Stratton SJ et al. Effect of out-of-hospital pediatric endotracheal intubation on survival and neurological outcome: a controlled clinical trial. *JAMA.* 2000;283:6:783–790.

30. Boie ET, Moore GP, Brummett C, Nelson DR. Do parents want to be present during invasive procedures performed on their children? A survey of 400 parents. *Ann Emerg Med.* 1999;34:70–74.

31. Meyers TA, Eichhorn DJ, Guzzetta CA. Do families want to be present during CPR? *J Emerg Nurs.* 1998;24:400–405.

32. Turley K, Mavroudis C, Ebert PA. Repair of congenital cardiac lesions during the first week of life. *Circulation.* 1982;66(2 PT 2):1214–1219.

33. Jenkins KJ, Gauvreau K, Newburger J et al. Consensus-based method for risk adjustment for surgery for congenital heart disease. *J Thoracic Cardiovas Surg.* 2002;123(1):110–118.

34. Armstrong BE. Congenital cardiovascular disease and cardiac surgery in childhood: acyanotic congenital heart defects and interventional techniques. *Curr Opin Cardiol.* 1995;10(1):68–77.

35. Butt W. Pediatric critical care—septic shock. *Pediatr Clin North Am.* 2001;48(3):601–625.

36. Bone RC. Pathophysiology of sepsis. *Ann Intern Med.* 1991;115:457–469.

37. Carcillo JA, Davis AL, Zaritsky A. Role of early fluid resuscitation in pediatric septic shock. *JAMA.* 1991;266:1242–1245.

38. Saez-Llorens X, McCracken GH. Sepsis syndrome and septic shock in pediatrics: current concepts of terminology, pathophysiology, and management. *J Pediatr.* 1993;123:497–508.

A 10-day-old baby is brought to the emergency department by his mother. She tells the physician that he seems to be breathing fast and is not eating very well. He is a full-term baby delivered vaginally with a birth weight of 3.2 kg (7 lbs). He spent 2 days with his mother in the hospital and then was discharged after an uneventful circumcision. He has been slow to breastfeed since birth, but the mother became more alarmed when she noted that he would gasp and cry after sucking for a short time. He has about 3 or 4 wet diapers per day. He has neither congestion nor a fever. He does not vomit with feedings and has had 2 yellow, seedy stools since passing his meconium after birth. On initial exam he is pale, irritable, breathing fast, has nasal flaring, and is sweaty to touch. Vital signs show a respiratory rate of 70/min, heart rate of 170/min; blood pressure is 80/40 mmHg, temperature (rectal) of 37°C, and his weight is 2.9 kg. His lungs sound equal bilaterally with rales in both bases. Cardiac exam reveals a hyperactive precordium with a gallop rhythm. No murmurs are heard. The abdomen is distended with good bowel sounds, and his liver is palpated 4 cm below the right costal margin. Pulses feel weak in the lower extremities. The capillary refill is 3 to 4 seconds in the fingertips, and pulse oximeter reading is 90% on room air.

1. *What is your rapid assessment of this baby?*
2. *Based on this assessment, what are your treatment priorities?*
3. *What is the most likely etiology of the baby's condition?*
4. *What are acute and definitive treatment options?*
5. *What are some complications of this condition?*

---

This baby is in respiratory distress and has compensated shock. Place the baby on humidified oxygen and start cardiac and oxygen saturation monitoring. Oxygen administration results in an improvement in the oxygen saturation to 99%. An IV should be started with normal saline or lactated Ringer's fluids at a 10 mL/kg bolus for shock, possibly caused by ineffective pumping of the heart. Examine the pulses in all extremities for color, temperature, and strength. Measure the blood pressure. Assess the precordium for activity and listen for murmurs, arrhythmias, and gallop rhythms. Prepare for intubation in case the respiratory status deteriorates. Obtain a chest radiograph and an ECG. Electrolytes and/or arterial blood gas analysis will be helpful to determine the degree of acidosis.

The most likely etiology is CHF from congenital heart disease. Oxygen and fluids should be started initially. Then, consider the possibility of starting Prostaglandin $E_1$ ($PGE_1$) as an IV infusion of 0.05 to 0.1 mcg/kg per minute if deterioration occurs, until the specific congenital heart lesion is determined. $PGE_1$ might be held if the infant is stable until the echocardiogram is done and a cardiologist is expected to arrive soon. After the IV is started and fluids are being given, administer furosemide (0.5 to 1 mg/kg). $PGE_1$ and digoxin can be used to help improve flow dynamics and contractility in ductal-dependent lesions and in CHF, respectively. If the blood pressure and perfusion do not improve, the next step will be to use inotropic agents such as a dobutamine infusion at 2 to 20 mcg/kg per minute, or an epinephrine infusion at 0.1 to 1.5 mcg/kg per minute can be started. An echocardiogram will need to be obtained for definitive diagnosis and management.

# CHAPTER REVIEW

CASE SUMMARY 1 CONT.

The baby is in CHF and the underlying etiology is important to determine the proper management. If the CHF is not addressed, the baby will fall further into shock and become decompensated, leading to cardiorespiratory arrest and death.

The baby was diagnosed with coarctation of the aorta with the coarctation at the level of the ductus, which made systemic flow ductal dependent. The chest radiograph revealed moderate cardiomegaly with increased pulmonary vascular markings. An echocardiogram gave the definitive diagnosis. After medical management with $PGE_1$, diuretics, and inotropes, as well as IV fluids for the acidosis, the baby was in a stabilized condition and was scheduled for surgical repair.

CASE SUMMARY 2

A 10-year-old boy presents with a chief complaint of chest pain and shortness of breath. He has had 5 days of cold and cough symptoms. According to his mom, he has been lying around a lot and has missed 1 week of school. He is usually a very active child but complains that he is "just too tired" to play. He complains that his chest hurts, mostly with cough. He says that he has a hard time catching his breath whenever he gets up to walk around. He has had no medical problems or surgeries. He is in the fourth grade at school and had been the star basketball player until becoming ill. His only exposure to illness is his aunt, who was recently hospitalized for pneumonia. On initial presentation, he is a thin, pleasant boy who seems tired but talks in complete sentences without difficulty. He is tachypneic with mild retractions and is slightly pale in color, with dusky nail beds. His vital signs include a respiratory rate of 30/min, heart rate of 130/min, a blood pressure of 90/65 mmHg, and an oral temperature of 37.8°C. Oxygen saturation is 90% on room air. His weight is 36.4 kg (80 lbs). He is lying on the gurney with the head elevated. Capillary refill time is 4 to 5 seconds. His lungs have diminished breath sounds, with an occasional end expiratory wheeze with deep breaths. His heart sounds are present but faint without any murmurs. His abdomen is distended with a palpable liver and spleen.

1. *What is your initial assessment?*
2. *What are the treatment priorities?*
3. *What are the most likely etiologies based on this assessment?*
4. *What are initial and definitive treatment options?*
5. *What are the complications of this condition?*

This child is in respiratory distress and cardiogenic shock. He needs immediate oxygen support as well as cardiac and oxygen saturation monitoring. His oxygen saturation increases to 98% on 15 L/min of oxygen by nonrebreather mask.

He most likely has an acquired cardiac problem. He had a respiratory illness during the winter months, so he might have had influenza or another viral illness that is now causing a secondary myocarditis. He could also have a congenital heart lesion that had been asymptomatic until this illness, possibly an anomalous coronary artery or valvular disease. Pericarditis could also be present but would be somewhat unusual, as he does not complain of chest pain.

CASE SUMMARY 2 CONT.

He needs gentle diuretic therapy, afterload reduction, and possibly inotropic support. He needs an echocardiogram performed to determine whether he has an intrinsic cardiac lesion, muscle hypertrophy, or fluid in the pericardial sac impeding filling and/or contractility. Without treatment to keep him from progressing into cardiogenic shock, he will deteriorate to a point that cardiac arrest is imminent either from decompensated shock or a fatal dysrhythmia.

Chest radiography revealed an enlarged heart, and an echocardiogram showed poor cardiac contractility. Myocarditis was diagnosed. He was maintained on inotropes and pressor agents and recovered to a point that he could be discharged 2 weeks later. He needs to be followed for years to assess the degree to which he regains his baseline cardiac function.

# chapter 5

# Central Nervous System

Daniel J. Isaacman, MD, FAAP, FACEP
Jennifer L. Trainor, MD, FAAP
Steven G. Rothrock, MD, FAAP, FACEP

## Objectives

1 List the causes of altered level of consciousness (ALOC) in the pediatric patient.

2 Develop a systematic approach to the emergency department management of the child with ALOC.

3 Recognize the unique presentation of meningitis and encephalitis at different ages.

4 Describe proper evaluation and management for meningitis and encephalitis.

5 Understand the causes of potential morbidity and mortality associated with these disease processes.

6 Identify and differentiate neurologic signs and symptoms that may lead to life-threatening consequences or permanent neurological damage.

7 Describe proper evaluation and management for serious neurologic conditions.

8 Define simple and complex febrile seizures, epilepsy, and status epilepticus.

9 Describe the evaluation and management of children with febrile and afebrile seizures.

10 Describe the initial stabilization and management of children in status epilepticus.

11 Describe the complications of prolonged status epilepticus.

## Chapter Outline

Altered Level of Consciousness

Meningitis

Encephalitis

Headache

Weakness

**Seizures**

Febrile Seizures

Afebrile Seizures

Status Epilepticus

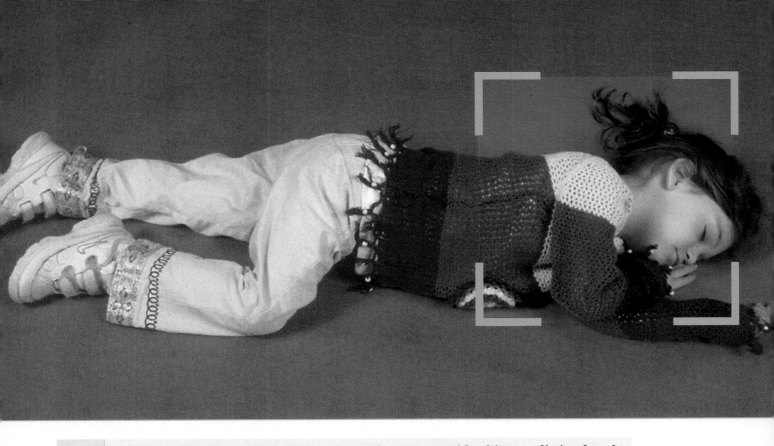

A 2-year-old boy presents to the emergency department with a history of being found sleeping in the garage. His parents were unable to awaken him. He was last seen 30 minutes earlier when his mother let him out to play in the backyard. On examination, the child is somnolent but responds to deep pain. His airway is open and respirations are unlabored. Vital signs include a respiratory rate of 36 breaths per minute, a heart rate of 116 beats per minute (bpm), blood pressure of 98/64, and temperature of 38.0°C. Oxygenation saturation measured by pulse oximetry is 98% on room air. Further examination reveals no focal deficits.

1. *What is the most important initial intervention in this patient?*
2. *What are possible etiologies?*
3. *What should you include in the management and evaluation?*

A 3-month-old boy is brought in by his mother, who says that he is "fussy and not acting right." He was found to be sleepy after returning from a visit to his aunt's home. He is cranky during the examination yet otherwise lethargic. The patient is afebrile with a respiratory rate of 20 breaths per minute, a heart rate of 74 bpm, a blood pressure of 110/70, and the pupils are 4 mm bilaterally and briskly reactive. The only abnormality on examination is a small 2-cm hematoma on the occiput, which, according to his mother, was sustained in a fall from a couch.

1. *What are your concerns for this patient?*
2. *What should be done immediately?*

# Altered Level of Consciousness

The child presenting with ALOC represents one of the most difficult diagnostic and management problems in pediatric emergency medicine. The gravity of the situation, the need to react quickly to avoid irreversible damage, and the wide array of possible diagnoses call for a calm and orderly approach to the problem at hand. The initial management includes immediate attention to the ABCs of resuscitation (Airway, Breathing, Circulation) to sustain life and prevent loss of existing brain function.

## Clinical Features

Four pathophysiologic variables help determine the nature of any lesion affecting the brain, the functional level of involvement, and the rate and extent of progression of the disease process. These variables include the pattern of respiration, the size and reactivity of the pupils, spontaneous and induced eye movements, and motor responses.

### Respiratory Pattern

Control of ventilation is governed by centers located in the lower pons and medulla and modulated by cortical centers located mainly in the forebrain. Respiratory abnormalities signify either metabolic derangement or neurologic insult in those areas. Several characteristic patterns exist (and are presented in order of rostrocaudal involvement). Postventilation apnea is generally characterized by brief periods of apnea lasting 10 to 30 seconds, followed by voluntary deep breathing. It is generally representative of forebrain involvement. Cheyne Stokes respirations constitute a breathing pattern in which phases of hyperpnea regularly alternate with apnea. The depth of breathing waxes in a smooth crescendo and then, once a peak is reached, wanes in an equally smooth decrescendo. Cheyne Stokes respirations usually imply dysfunction of structures deep within both cerebral hemispheres or in the diencephalon. This pattern of ventilation commonly occurs in metabolic encephalopathy. Central neurogenic hyperventilation is manifested by sustained regular and rapid respirations despite a normal $PaO_2$ and a low $PaCO_2$. This rare and serious finding points to midbrain dysfunction. Apneustic breathing is characterized by brief inspiratory pauses lasting 2 to 3 seconds, often alternating with end-expiratory pauses. Clinically, this pattern is characteristic of pontine infarction but occasionally can be seen in anoxic encephalopathy or severe meningitis.

### Eye Findings

The eye examination tells much about the level of the lesion and the prognosis of the patient. Specific eye evaluations include pupillary size and responsiveness, spontaneous and induced eye movements, and results of funduscopic examination.

#### Pupillary Signs

The pupillary reactions, constriction and dilatation, are controlled by the sympathetic and parasympathetic nervous system. Because brainstem areas controlling consciousness are adjacent to those controlling the pupils, pupillary changes are often informative. Additionally, because pupillary pathways are relatively resistant to metabolic insult, the presence or absence of a reaction to light is the single most important physical finding to distinguish structural from metabolic disease. Most metabolic conditions affecting the central nervous system (CNS) lead to constricted pupils that remain reactive to light. Pupillary findings are invalid if eye-altering medications have been accidentally ingested or therapeutically administered.

Pupillary responses to structural lesions depend on the primary disturbance site and on secondary effects of increased intracranial pressure (ICP). Pressure transmitted laterally and downward, generally from mass lesions, can cause a unilaterally fixed and dilated pupil from pressure exerted by the medial aspect of the temporal lobe (uncus) on the third cranial nerve. Transtentorial herniation occurs when pressure forces are exerted on the brainstem and transmitted symmetrically downward. The pupils are initially small, but as herniation continues, the pupils may become asymmetric, then fixed and dilated (Figure 5.1).

#### Induced Eye Movements

Two specific eye maneuvers are helpful in evaluating the comatose child. The oculocephalic, or doll's eye reflex, is performed by holding the

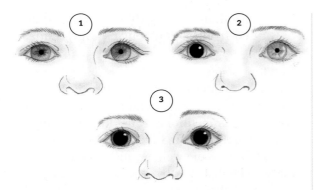

Figure 5.1 Transtentorial herniation sequence.

eyelids open and briskly rotating the head from side to side. This test is contraindicated in any child when cervical spine injury is a possibility. The normal, or positive, doll's eye response is conjugate deviation of the eyes contrary to the direction in which the head is turned. The stimulus for this reflex involves either the vestibular system, the proprioceptive afferents in the neck, or both.

The oculovestibular reflex is evaluated by caloric testing. This test is performed by elevating the patient's head to 30 degrees and slowly injecting 50 mL of ice cold water through a catheter placed in the external auditory canal. This technique causes vestibular stimulation. In the normal awake patient with brainstem intact, the response to ice water testing is nystagmus, with the slow component toward the irrigated ear and the fast nystagmus away from the irrigated ear. In the unconscious patient whose brainstem is intact, the fast nystagmus is abolished and the eyes move toward the stimulus and remain tonically deviated for a minute or more before slowly returning to the midline. The test is contraindicated if tympanic membranes are not intact or there is suspicion of basilar skull fracture.

Deviation of the eyes at rest is also of great diagnostic significance. With cerebral lesions, conjugate deviation is noted toward the side of the lesion, whereas with brainstem lesions, conjugate deviation is away from the lesion. The setting sun sign, characterized by downward deviation of the eyes, is associated with upper midbrain lesions and hydrocephalus.

Third nerve paralysis generally causes the eye to point downward and outward.

### Funduscopic Examination

A brief ophthalmoscopic examination should be performed to assess the presence or absence of papilledema or retinal hemorrhages. Papilledema is a late sign of increased ICP and merits efforts aimed at its control. Retinal hemorrhages, thought to be highly suggestive of abuse, have also been rarely reported to occur via other mechanisms.[1-4]

### Motor Examination

The motor examination of the comatose patient consists of eliciting various responses to stimuli, either auditory or physical. Muscle strength, tone, and deep-tendon reflexes should be assessed for normality and symmetry. The ability of the patient to localize, as well as the presence or absence of abnormal posturing, also helps assess the severity of involvement. Decorticate posturing (flexion of the upper extremities with extension of the lower extremities) suggests involvement of the cerebral cortex and subcortical white matter with preservation of brainstem function. Decerebrate posturing (rigid

## YOUR FIRST CLUE

**Signs of ALOC**

- Poor responsiveness to environmental cues
- Abnormal pattern of respiration, signifying metabolic derangement or neurologic insult
- Size and reactivity of the pupils: Poorly reactive, unequal, or fixed pupils implying structural lesion
- "Setting sun" pupils pointing downward, implying midbrain lesion or hydrocephalus
- Papilledema: Increased intracranial pressure (ICP)
- Retinal hemorrhages: Diffuse axonal injury—shaken baby syndrome
- Spontaneous and induced eye movements
- Nonpurposeful motor responses

extension of the arms and legs) generally represents added brainstem involvement, usually at the level of the pons.

The flaccid patient with no response to painful stimuli has the gravest prognosis and generally has suffered injury deep into the brainstem.

## Diagnostic Studies

Laboratory evaluation of the patient with altered mental status can be divided into the routine and the specific. Suggested laboratory tests for the patient with altered mental status of undetermined etiology include complete blood cell (CBC) count, electrolytes, blood urea nitrogen (BUN), creatinine, and immediate bedside and serum glucose. When a metabolic cause for coma is suspected, liver function testing, serum ammonia, measured and calculated serum osmolality, and toxicology screens should be considered. Arterial blood gas analysis is useful in monitoring the adequacy of ventilation and oxygenation. Focal abnormalities or signs of increased ICP generally mandate a computed tomography (CT) scan once the patient is stabilized. In the patient who remains an enigma, a stat electroencephalogram (EEG) should be considered because some forms of status epilepticus have little to no motor component and are therefore not clinically obvious. Performance of a lumbar puncture for suspected meningitis can be done if no signs of increased ICP are present. Additional laboratory tests to consider, when clinically indicated, include blood alcohol level, thyroid function tests, blood lead level, blood culture, skeletal survey, and barium or air contrast enema.

## Differential Diagnosis

The etiologic possibilities are diverse. The mnemonic AEIOU TIPS has been a useful method for organizing the diagnostic possibilities.

### A

#### Alcohol

Alcohol is more commonly encountered in adolescents than younger pediatric patients. However, alcohol is not an infrequent cause of accidental ingestion in the young child. Young children can exhibit ALOC at serum levels less than 100 mg/dL and can also be obtunded from concurrent hypoglycemia.

#### Abuse

Child abuse must be considered in any child presenting in a coma, particularly when the history and physical examination findings are not consistent. The practitioner must look for subtle physical signs of trauma, including bruising, cranial tenderness or swelling, and retinal hemorrhages. The shaken baby syndrome can result in ALOC without external signs of physical abuse.[5]

### E

#### Electrolytes

Any condition that causes abnormal fluid losses can result in ALOC due to abnormalities in electrolytes such as sodium, potassium, calcium, and magnesium. Disorders such as adrenal insufficiency and the syndrome of inappropriate antidiuretic hormone can also result in ALOC.

#### Encephalopathy

Reye syndrome is a consideration in any child who presents with a history of pernicious vomiting leading to altered mental status, particularly when there is a history of an antecedent varicella or flu-like illness treated with salicylates. Since 1980, when the association between Reye syndrome and aspirin use was first reported, there has been a sharp decline in the reported incidence of this disease.[6–7] Recent studies have suggested that many cases previously diagnosed as Reye syndrome might represent inborn errors of metabolism not previously recognized.[8,9]

Lead encephalopathy, while unusual, continues to be a concern in the pediatric age group, particularly in children living in older buildings where lead paint might still be present. Children can develop rapid rises in blood lead levels after ingestion of loose paint chips or by mouthing items contaminated with lead paint, dust, and soil. An antecedent history of fatigue, vomiting, or abdominal pain in a child living in an older dwelling should alert the practitioner to the possibility of this diagnosis. Screening tests include blood lead, free erythrocyte protoporphyrin, and CBC. Occasionally, radiopaque lead chips will be found on abdominal radiography. Treatment involves chelation therapy.[10]

## I

### Infection

Meningitis and encephalitis are more common in pediatric patients than in adults. Infections outside the CNS, particularly sepsis, can also cause ALOC if associated with cerebral hypoperfusion.

## O

### Overdose Ingestion

Ingestion is always a strong consideration in the young child with an unexplained alteration in consciousness. A complete history of medications in the household should be obtained early in the evaluation of these patients.

## U

### Uremia

Hemolytic uremic syndrome is a multisystem disorder characterized by a prodromal phase of gastroenteritis or upper respiratory infection followed by acute onset and rapid progression of renal failure, microangiopathic hemolytic anemia, and thrombocytopenia. Other causes of chronic renal impairment in childhood can also lead to uremic encephalopathy.

## T

### Trauma

Trauma is a major cause of ALOC. It is the leading cause of death in the first 4 decades of life. Head injuries, chest injuries leading to hypoxia, and blood loss leading to shock all have significant effects on the level of consciousness.

## I

### Insulin/Hypoglycemia

Although known diabetics are obviously at risk for accidental insulin overdose, occasionally toddlers will ingest another family member's oral hypoglycemia agent, or ingest alcohol or other medications that can cause hypoglycemia. Ketotic hypoglycemia, probably the most common cause of hypoglycemia in childhood, is actually a diagnosis that compromises a number of disease processes. Children with this problem are often young (18 months to 5 years) and often have histories of low birth weight. Attacks are episodic, most likely to occur in the morning and after prolonged fasting, and are frequently associated with ketonuria. Hypoglycemia episodes, resulting from an inappropriate response to a prolonged fasting state, respond promptly to the administration of glucose. Recently an overlap in the symptomatology between ketotic hypoglycemia and glycogen synthase deficiency has been described.[11]

### Intussusception

Intussusception, caused by the prolapse of a portion of small intestine into an adjacent loop, has been known to present with mental status changes prior to the development of abdominal findings. In the child younger than 3 years with unexplained ALOC, intussusception should be entertained. Direct a careful history at any antecedent vomiting, abdominal pain, or blood in the stool, and repeated examinations of the abdomen with stool testing for blood.[12] A recent association between intussusception and the administration of tetravalent rotavirus vaccine has resulted in suspension of its administration.[13]

### Inborn Errors of Metabolism

These are important disorders to keep in mind, particularly when the onset of symptoms is early in life. Presenting signs include vomiting, seizures, hypoglycemia, and/or metabolic acidosis. Blood ammonia levels are helpful, and urine screens for organic and/or amino acids are often diagnostic.

## P

### Psychogenic

Although factitious ALOC is rare in young children, it is worth considering in older children and adolescents. Careful neurologic examination will often reveal abnormalities inconsistent with an organic etiology.

## S

### Seizures

Postictal states are common causes of ALOC, and an actively seizing infant can appear to be in a coma until close observation reveals continued subtle seizure activity. At times seizure activity is completely occult clinically and can be diagnosed only with an EEG.

### Stroke, Shock, and Other Cardiovascular Causes

Cardiovascular abnormalities such as arteriovenous malformations can present in childhood, resulting in CNS symptomatology including ALOC. Poor brain perfusion caused by hypovolemia can lead to altered sensorium in the presence of an otherwise normal CNS.

### Shunt

Patients with ventriculoperitoneal or ventriculoatrial shunts can present with ALOC when the shunt is blocked or infected. Patients are often lethargic and complain of headache and might have difficulty looking upward (sundowning). Rapid evaluation of the shunt is necessary.

## Management

### Initial Assessment

The initial task is to assess the adequacy of the patient's airway, degree of ventilation, and circulatory status. Patients with a history of trauma should be immobilized with the neck positioned in the midline. A bedside glucose should be obtained.

### Airway and Breathing

Ensure the patency of the airway while protecting the cervical spine if there is a possibility of cervical spine trauma. Open the airway using the chin-lift (if no trauma is suspected) or jaw-thrust maneuver. Avoid hyperextension of the neck so as not to occlude the airway in an infant. Insert a nasal airway as needed (if no basilar skull fracture is suspected); oral airways are best avoided in lightly comatose and conscious patients because of the risk of inducing vomiting and aspiration. Provide supplemental oxygen ($O_2$). If the child is apneic or has respiratory failure, assist ventilatory efforts with bag-mask ventilation or intubation. Intubation will be necessary if the patient has an inadequate gag reflex. If respirations are present but noisy, suction and inspect for foreign material. Mild hyperventilation to a $PaCO_2$ of 30 to 35 mm Hg is indicated if there are signs of increased ICP.[14]

### Circulation (Cardiovascular Status)

The patient's skin perfusion and capillary refill best estimate circulatory status. Take the patient's pulse and blood pressure, and place the child on a monitor. Achieve venous or intraosseous access, draw diagnostic blood specimens, and perform a rapid estimate of blood sugar. The state of hydration as indicated by physical examination should dictate the fluid selection and rate. Shock should be treated as described previously (Chapter 4, Cardiovascular System). Check $O_2$ saturation by pulse oximetry. Only after the ABCs are addressed should attention be directed to the neurologic and general examinations.

### Disability (Neurologic Status)

Perform an objective evaluation of the child's level of consciousness using either the AVPU system or the Glasgow Coma Scale. (See Chapter 9, Trauma.) Note pupillary size and reactivity. Look for evolving signs of increased ICP, such as alterations in vital signs (including Cushing triad of bradycardia, hypertension, and irregular respirations), pupillary responses, respiratory pattern, or ophthalmoscopic examination. Treat patients with clinical evidence of increased ICP as detailed in Chapter 9, Trauma. Save a tube of blood for later laboratory study. Infuse glucose 0.5 to 1 g/kg IV (2 to 4 mL/kg of D25 solution) for documented hypoglycemia. If the child improves, a continuous infusion of 10% dextrose should be initiated at the child's maintenance rate. If intravenous (IV) access cannot be obtained, administer glucagon intramuscularly (<20 kg, 0.5 mg; >20 kg, 1 mg/dose). Infuse naloxone (birth to 5 years, 0.1 mg/kg IV >5 years or 20 kg, 2 mg IV) to reverse a potential narcotic-induced mental status alteration.

### Exposure

Remove the patient's clothing and other items that hinder full evaluation, and replace them as needed after adequate examination.

## Secondary Assessment

Once the immediate life-threatening concerns have been addressed, an abbreviated focused history should be obtained. The practitioner should determine if the child has had any chronic or recent illness, antecedent fever, rash, pernicious vomiting, or trauma. Explore any recent exposure to infection, medications, or intoxicants. Immunization, medical, and family histories should be obtained when time permits. Be alert for any inappropriate responses and delays in seeking care that would arouse the suspicion of child abuse.

The observations in the secondary assessment should attempt to uncover signs of occult infection, trauma, or toxic or metabolic derangements. Important areas to evaluate include the fundi, extraocular movements, anterior fontanel, and the neck for bruits and stiffness. Many afebrile toddlers with altered mental status have unknown ingestions. Signs suggestive of a specific toxidrome should be explored as outlined in Chapter 8, Toxicological Emergencies.

## Disposition

The previously described approach might delineate a specific cause of ALOC. When a presumptive diagnosis is confirmed, carry out specific management. Definitive therapy can be initiated in the ED. Admit or transfer any patient to a pediatric intensive care unit who does not respond to therapeutic intervention and who will require ongoing monitoring or intensive therapy, or in whom the diagnosis is still in question after the initial management.

In general, the prognosis of the pediatric coma patient is much better than his or her adult counterpart. Particularly in relation to traumatic etiologies, age seems to be a major independent factor affecting morbidity and mortality. Most of the data regarding prognosis of children with hypoxic ischemic brain injury have been related to victims of near-drowning or cardiopulmonary arrest. Predictors of poor outcome include long (>25 min) duration of cardiac arrest, blood glucose higher than 250 mg/dL, unresponsiveness on arrival, Glasgow Coma Scale score lower than 8 on arrival, pH lower than 7.10 on presentation, or duration of coma greater than 24 hours.[15–21] Nevertheless, physicians can be cautiously optimistic about the potential for recovery in most children presenting with significant altered mental status.

## KEY POINTS

**Management of ALOC**

- Assess and treat abnormalities in oxygenation and ventilation.
- Place on a monitor.
- Obtain vascular access.
- Obtain blood for laboratory evaluation and test for glucose level.
- Begin specific therapy based on likely differential diagnosis.

---

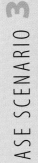

**CASE SCENARIO 3**

A 3-month-old girl presents with fever, fussiness, and poor feeding. She is irritable and difficult to console but is breathing comfortably on her own and maintaining a good airway. Vital signs include a respiratory rate of 36 breaths per minute, heart rate of 120 bpm, a blood pressure of 90/58 torr, temperature of 39.2°C, and oxygen saturation of 98% on room air. Her fontanel appears full and her neck appears supple. Capillary refill time is 2 seconds. The remainder of the examination is nonfocal.

1. Which examination findings in this child are consistent with the diagnosis of meningitis?
2. What is the most important therapy to deliver at this time?
3. What are possible complications?

# Meningitis

Meningitis, an infection of the meninges that surround the brain and spinal cord, remains a significant cause of morbidity and mortality in childhood. Despite major advances in the prevention of serious bacterial infection caused by *Haemophilus influenzae* type B (Hib) and *Streptococcus pneumoniae* in the past decade, cases of meningitis continue to occur.

## Epidemiology

The greatest risk for meningitis occurs in the first year of life. Over this time, the bacteriology of the disease shows great change. During the neonatal period, infants are at greatest risk of meningitis from infection with *Escherichia coli* and other Gram-negative organisms, group B-*Streptococcus*, and *Listeria monocytogenes*. At approximately 4 to 6 weeks of age, *S pneumoniae, Neisseria meningitidis,* and *H influenzae* infections become more prevalent. The peak age-specific incidence for these pathogens occurs at 6 to 8 months of age, the time at which the immunity afforded by passively acquired maternal IgG antibodies disappears.

The rates of meningitis due to infection with *H influenzae, N meningitidis,* and *S pneumoniae* in children younger than 5 years are quite similar in North America, Europe, and Asia. Exceptions are lower rates of Hib disease in East Asia and higher rates of pneumococcal and Hib disease in Alaska natives and in Africa.[22] Since the licensure of the Hib vaccine, this distribution has changed dramatically. (See Table 5-1.) Although *H influenzae* is still a consideration in the unimmunized population, vaccination has dramatically lowered its overall incidence. The recent adoption of pneumococcal vaccination should dramatically alter the contribution from *S pneumoniae* in the coming years.

Socioeconomic conditions have a major impact on the incidence and distribution of meningitis. Poverty, overcrowding, limited access to health care, and the low educational level of caregivers are all associated with an increase in the incidence of meningitis. Exposure to cigarette smoke has recently been demonstrated to increase the risk of bacterial menin-

| TABLE 5-1 | Incidence of Meningitis (Most to Least) |
|---|---|
| **1986 (pre-Hib)** | **1994-1995 (post-Hib)** |
| *H influenzae* | *S pneumoniae* |
| *S pneumoniae* | *N meningitidis* |
| *N meningitidis* | Group B strep |
| Group B strep | *L monocytogenes* |
| Other | *H influenzae* |

Adapted from: Wegner JD, Hightower AW, Facklam RR et al. Bacterial meningitis in the United States 1986: report of a multistate surveillance study. *J Infect Dis* 1990;162:1316–1323; and Schuchat A, Robinson K, Wegner JD et al. Bacterial meningitis in the United States in 1995. *N Engl J Med* 1997;337:970–976.

gitis. Carriers of Hib, pneumococcus, and meningococcus have been found to be more common among both active and passive smokers, thus increasing the risk to household and other close contacts.[22,23]

## Clinical Features

The clinical presentation of patients with meningitis generally involves some combination of fever, irritability, and/or lethargy and, in children older than 18 months, nuchal rigidity. Although some overlap in the signs and symptoms exists between patients with bacterial meningitis and those with aseptic meningitis, in general children with aseptic meningitis appear less ill. Other characteristics suggestive of aseptic meningitis include the time of the year (enteroviral cases cluster during the late spring and summer months), the presence of photophobia or other signs of enteroviral disease, and a high prevalence of enteroviral disease in the community.

Bacterial meningitis generally presents with fever, irritability (or lethargy), and neck stiffness. In infants younger than 3 months, clinical signs can be particularly subtle, thus arguing for a high index of suspicion for this disease in febrile infants in this age group.

It is important to realize that children younger than 18 months might not have the neck musculature adequately developed to manifest nuchal rigidity, and thus this sign is unreliable in this age group. In children older than 18 months, physical findings become more reliable. Patients generally have headache, vomiting, and neck pain, and almost all manifest nuchal rigidity. Other signs and symptoms occuring with some regularity include anorexia, nausea, headache, vomiting, focal neurologic signs, and seizures.[24]

On physical examination, alterations in the level of consciousness can be highly variable, extending from extreme lethargy and/or coma to combativeness and irritability. Kernig sign (inability to extend the legs with the hips flexed) and Brudzinski sign (flexion of the neck causes flexion at the hip, knee, or ankle) are indicative of meningeal irritation, but their absence does not exclude the presence of meningitis. A bulging or tense fontanel in an infant suggests increased ICP but can be present in infants with febrile illnesses without meningitis. Petechiae or purpura, hallmarks of meningococcal disease, can also be seen with other infections caused by *S pneumoniae* and *H influenzae*. Approximately 25% of children with meningococcal infections will have a maculopapular rash preceding the development of petechiae or purpura.

Focal neurologic signs might be detected on presentation and are primarily associated with increased ICP or impaired cerebral blood flow. Third and sixth cranial nerve palsies, with accompanying pupillary dilatation and impaired lateral gaze, are indicative of increased ICP and should trigger immediate efforts to lower ICP. Ataxia and hearing loss might be noted, because inflammation and infection involving the inner ear affect hearing and balance. Papilledema, generally a later finding, is often suggestive of a complication such as a venous sinus thrombosis, subdural empyema, or brain abscess.[24,25]

Seizures are noted in up to 20% of children during the initial presentation or early in the course and tend to occur more frequently

in patients with meningitis caused by *S pneumoniae* or *H influenzae*. Eighty percent of these seizures have complex features (focal seizure, multiple seizures in 24 hours, duration >15 minutes), while children with meningitis who have seizures and no complex features almost uniformly have other features diagnostic of meningitis.[26]

A search for an underlying condition should always be considered in children presenting with bacterial meningitis. As many as 20% of children with bacterial meningitis will have some predisposing condition for developing this serious infection. Etiologies to consider include the presence of a ventriculoperitoneal shunt, an underlying malignancy, head trauma with resultant cerebrospinal fluid (CSF) leak, splenic dysfunction, or other immunodeficiency states.

## Diagnostic Studies

The diagnosis of meningitis is made with culture of the spinal fluid. Fluid should be obtained for cell count and differential, glucose and protein, and culture. Classically, bacterial infection yields a high white blood cell count with marked polymorphonuclear predominance, elevated protein levels, and low glucose. Profiles characteristic of normal CSF, and CSF with bacterial and viral meningitis are shown in Table 5-2. Recently, a significant amount of overlap between the CSF profile in bacterial meningitis and aseptic meningitis has been noted, making early differentiation more challenging.[27] Cytocentrifugation of the CSF can enhance the ability of the clinical microbiology laboratory personnel to detect bacteria on Gram-stained specimens.

Since the decline in invasive infections caused by Hib, the clinical usefulness of rapid antigen detection in CSF or other body fluids has come into question. Rarely does a positive result alter therapy. Times when latex agglutination should be considered include cases of partially treated meningitis, or those cases in which the Gram stain was consistent with meningococci, in which case clarifying the serotype quickly can have implications for providing meningococcal vaccine (types A and C). Latex agglutination of urine is to be avoided because of the very high occurrence of false-positives.

Polymerase chain reaction (PCR) of CSF has been used to detect microbial deoxyribonucleic acid (DNA) in patients with bacterial meningitis. Primers are available for simultaneous detection of the most common organisms, including *S pneumoniae, N meningitidis,* and *H influenzae.*[28] At present, rapid detection via PCR is not readily available at most centers. Another, perhaps more useful, application of PCR is documentation of the presence of specific viral gene products presence in CSF. In this situation, PCR results are often more rapid than culture, offering the possibility of earlier diagnosis of equivocal cases, which might lead to shortened hospital stays. A commercially available PCR for enterovirus is available in some countries.[29]

Other laboratory tests that should be obtained in the patient with suspected meningitis include blood culture, serum glucose, and electrolytes. Hypoglycemia resulting from poor intake and increased metabolic demand and hyponatremia from syndrome of inappropriate antidiuretic hormone secretion (SIADH) are important complications to consider.

## Differential Diagnosis

Although the constellation of irritability and high fever should always prompt consideration for meningitis, other entities can present with similar profiles. Infants and young children with cervical adenitis can present with fever and an inability to move the head, generally with accompanying head tilt or difficulty in turning the head from side to side rather than difficulty with flexion and extension. Children with retropharyngeal cellulitis can also pres-

| TABLE 5-2 | Common CSF Findings | | |
|---|---|---|---|
| | Normal* | Bacterial | Viral |
| Appearance | Clear | Clear to cloudy | Clear |
| Cell count (WBCs/mm³) | <10 | >100–20,000 | >10–500 |
| Differential (% PMNs) | 0 | >90 | 0–30† |
| Glucose (mg/dL) | 50–90 | <40 | 50–90 |
| Protein (mg/dL) | 15–45 | 100–500 | 50–100 |
| Gram stain (bacterial) | Negative | Positive | Negative |

*In the neonatal period, these normal values can vary as follows: cell count, <22 WBCs/mm³ with <60% PMNs; glucose, 34–119 mg/dL; and protein, 20–170 mg/dL.

†Can be predominantly polymorphonuclear neutrophil leukocytes (PMNs) early in the course of the illness.

ent as irritable with frank nuchal rigidity, often with accompanying poor oral intake or severe dysphagia. Other disease entities to consider include sinusitis, mastoiditis, CNS tumors/ abscesses, and encephalitis. Muscular torticollis, while often leading to difficulty with head movement, is generally distinguished from meningitis due to the lack of irritability and the absence of fever. Acute dystonia, often linked with the administration of phenothiazines or other anticholinergic agents, is often associated with characteristic muscular rigidity and, again, the absence of fever. Children with subarachnoid hemorrhages will generally have a history of trauma and severe headache and are less likely to present with fever than those with meningitis. Other conditions capable of producing meningismus include severe pharyngitis, arthritis, osteomyelitis of the cervical spine, and upper lobe pneumonia.

## WHAT ELSE?

**Differential Diagnosis of Neck Stiffness**
- Cervical adenitis
- Retropharyngeal abscess, cellulitis
- CNS tumors
- Encephalitis
- Pharyngitis
- Torticollis
- Cervical spine trauma

## Management

Successful management of bacterial meningitis involves rapid institution of antibiotic therapy and careful monitoring for potential complications.[30] Once the diagnosis of bacterial meningitis has been entertained and CSF is collected, antibiotic therapy should be started. In cases in which the diagnosis is suspected and the child is deemed too unstable to undergo lumbar puncture, or there is a delay due to a needed CT scan, empiric antibiotic therapy should be administered. Initial antibiotic coverage is often empiric with subsequent therapy guided by Gram stain and culture results. Infants in the first 4 to 6 weeks of life should be treated with ampicillin and cefotaxime or ampicillin and gentamicin to cover for Gram-negative enteric organisms, group B streptococci, and *Listeria monocytogenes*. In children older than 4 to 6 weeks, local resistance patterns to *S pneumoniae* should dictate the use of single (cefotaxime or ceftriaxone) or double (vancomycin plus cefotaxime or ceftriaxone) antibiotic coverage for Gram-positive meningitis until the organism and its sensitivities are known. Gram-negative infection in this age group should be covered adequately with cefotaxime or ceftriaxone.

The role of corticosteroids in the treatment of bacterial meningitis continues to be a source of considerable debate. The theoretical goal of steroid use in meningitis is to decrease meningeal inflammation and thus lower the incidence and severity of cerebral edema and resultant brain injury. Although existing data suggest a clear-cut reduction in sensorineural hearing loss in patients with *H influenzae* meningitis, disease from infection with this organism is now rare. No clear-cut benefit is demonstrable for dexamethasone in protecting against neurologic deficits from infection with all other organisms. Some experts have expressed concern that the use of corticosteroids might decrease the CSF penetration of some antimicrobials such as vancomycin, thus

## KEY POINTS

**Management of Suspected Bacterial Meningitis**
- Assess and treat abnormalities in oxygenation or ventilation.
- Monitor.
- Obtain blood samples for laboratory evaluation and bedside glucose testing.
- Obtain CT scan as indicated.
- Perform lumbar puncture.
- Begin antibiotic therapy based on age (<4 to 6 weeks, cefotaxime or gentamicin plus ampicillin; >4 to 6 weeks, cefotaxime or ceftriaxone +/− vancomycin).
- Treat complications.
- Admit patient.

offering a potential disadvantage with the use of steroids in cases of penicillin-resistant pneumococcal meningitis.

## Complications

The patient with meningitis is at risk for a number of serious and life-threatening complications. Bacterial meningitis with accompanying bacteremia can lead to a systemic inflammatory response with septic shock, respiratory distress syndrome, and disseminated intravascular coagulation. Intracranial complications can have devastating results. Familiarity with the most common complications allows the clinician to anticipate the development of complications and thereby institute immediate interventions as needed.

### Increased Intracranial Pressure

Acute bacterial meningitis can be associated with increased ICP, which can result in cerebral herniation or other life-threatening complications. Cerebral edema, whether vasogenic, cytotoxic, or interstitial in origin, is the major element contributing to raised ICP. Increases in ICP result in decreased cerebral perfusion pressure, with accompanying impairment in autoregulation of cerebral blood flow. Raised ICP should be anticipated, identified, and treated promptly. Some of the clinical signs of increased ICP are ALOC, a dilated or poorly reactive pupil, abnormalities of ocular motility, and the Cushing triad of hypertension, bradycardia, and irregular respirations.

Several methods are available to reduce ICP. Simple measures such as elevating the bed to 30 degrees and positioning the head midline should be routinely adopted. Intratracheal suctioning and endotracheal (ET) intubation can precipitate a significant rise in ICP, which can be minimized by prior administration of lidocaine. Antipyretic agents should be administered to reduce additional metabolic demand of core temperatures above 38°C. Mild hyperventilation can be used to decrease the $PaCO_2$ to 30 to 35 mm Hg, which results in cerebral vasoconstriction and reduced cerebral blood volume. The effectiveness of this approach beyond 24 hours might be minimal. Hyperosmolar agents such as mannitol decrease ICP by transiently raising the osmolarity of the intravascular space and pulling water from brain tissues into the extracellular intravascular compartment. When other modalities have failed to control ICP, high-dose barbiturate therapy might be useful.

### Seizures

Seizures frequently complicate bacterial meningitis. Approximately 20% to 30% of children with bacterial meningitis have a seizure before admission or at some time during their hospital course. Seizures can occur early or late in the course of the illness or manifest as a late complication after apparent recovery. Hypoglycemia and electrolyte (especially sodium) abnormalities must be excluded as causes of seizures. Early, brief seizure activity might not warrant initiation of anticonvulsant therapy. Prolonged or recurrent seizures require aggressive treatment, as outlined later in this chapter.

### Syndrome of Inappropriate Antidiuretic Hormone Secretion

Infections of the CNS can result in increased secretion of antidiuretic hormone (ADH) from the posterior pituitary gland. The result of this is retention of body water, hyponatremia, and expansion of the extracellular fluid space. The reported incidence of syndrome of inappropriate antidiuretic hormone secretion (SIADH) in bacterial meningitis varies greatly. It is also important to note that central diabetes insipidus has also been reported in children with CNS infections.

It is important to recognize that hyponatremia can result from dehydration or SIADH and as a result of administration of excessive free water. Analysis of serum and urinary electrolytes is essential to differentiate the various causes of hyponatremia. Because SIADH is the inappropriate secretion of ADH, one generally sees excess conservation of free water with resultant low serum osmolality, concentrated urine, and urinary osmolarity and sodium values inappropriately high in the face of such low serum levels. The circulatory compromise caused by intravascular volume depletion and cerebral edema secondary to SIADH are associated with significant neurologic morbidity and mortality. Thus efforts to normalize serum sodium and total body water content are imperative.

### Subdural Effusion/Empyema

The pathogenesis of subdural effusion in meningitis remains poorly understood. Clinical features include persistent or recurrent fever, seizures, and a variety of neurologic abnormalities. Whether these features are secondary to the effusion or due to meningeal inflammation is unclear. The overall incidence of subdural effusion ranges from 15% to 40%. It seems that young age, low peripheral white blood cell count, and high CSF levels of protein are associated with a higher likelihood of developing effusion. Because most subdural effusions resolve spontaneously, a noninvasive approach in an otherwise improving patient is appropriate. In those patients in whom the effusion has been related to a clinical deterioration or in whom a subdural empyema is suspected, subdural evacuation should be performed.

# Encephalitis

Encephalitis is an inflammation of the brain; meningoencephalitis is an inflammation of the brain and meninges, usually due to an infectious agent. Encephalitis is usually caused by viruses (e.g., enterovirus, herpes, arboviruses). Arboviruses (e.g., eastern and western equine, St. Louis, West Nile) are the most common worldwide causes of encephalitis. Arboviruses are zoonoses with mosquito or tick vectors that transmit the virus to humans. Because common vertebrate reservoirs include birds (eastern and western equine, St. Louis, West Nile), horses (equine viruses) and rodents (California equine), an early clue to an epidemic can be disease first noted in the animal population.[31,32]

Multiple human herpes viruses have been identified as causative agents in CNS infections. Herpes simplex 2 is a leading cause of severe encephalitis in neonates with a mortality rate that approaches 80%. In older children, herpes virus 1 is the most common cause of nonepidemic encephalitis in the United States. Other viruses in the herpes class (varicella zoster) and cytomegalovirus (CMV) usually require an immunocompromised host for infection to occur.[33–35]

After herpes viruses, enteroviruses are the most common cause of encephalitis in the United States. Compared to herpes simplex encephalitis, enterovirus infection more commonly causes global encephalitis with generalized neurologic depression. In contrast to most viruses that are cleared by cell-mediated immune mechanisms, enterovirus infections are cleared by antibody-mediated immunity. For this reason, agammaglobulinemic children can have a more chronic encephalitis or meningoencephalitis following enteroviral infection.[36] Other rare causes include rabies virus, protozoa, bacteria (e.g., spirochetes), *Mycoplasma, Rickettsia, Chlamydia,* and fungi.[32,33]

## Clinical Features

Neonates are at particular risk for herpes simplex 2 encephalitis (HSE). These cases are acquired through vaginal delivery regardless of whether the mother is symptomatic. Neonatal HSE typically develops 2 to 30 days after delivery, with lethargy, poor feeding, irritability, tremors, or seizures. Vesicular lesions can manifest at the presenting part (scalp or buttocks). Other physical examination findings include temperature instability, a bulging fontanel, pyramidal tract signs, seizures, and systemic signs of infection (e.g., jaundice, respiratory distress, bleeding, or shock).[33–35]

Infants and older children present in one of two manners. Encephalitis can be the major manifestation of the disease, with prominent neurologic signs and symptoms. Classic features include the triad of fever, headache, and an ALOC. Other prominent features can include psychiatric symptoms, seizures, vomiting, focal weakness, photophobia, movement disorders, or memory loss. A history of wild mammal or bat exposure can indicate rabies, while rodent exposure can indicate lymphocytic choriomeningitis, and cat scratch disease can occur following exposure to kittens. Measles-mumps-rubella immunization in immunocompetent children excludes these viruses as causative agents. Immunocompromised patients (e.g., HIV, cancer) are at risk for parasitic (e.g., toxoplasmosis) and specific viral (e.g., CMV) encephalitides.[32,33]

Typical physical examination findings include altered mentation, elevated temperature, dysphasia, ataxia, hemiparesis, cranial nerve deficits, visual field loss, or papilledema. Skin examination might reveal vesicles in herpes virus infections, maculopapular rashes in enteroviral infections, or petechiae in *Rickettsia* infection. Prominent motor involvement can indicate a poliovirus infection; limbic system involvement might indicate a rabies virus, while the presence of aphasia, anosmia, or temporal lobe seizures can indicate a herpes virus infection.[32,33]

In contrast to patients presenting with prominent systemic and neurologic features, some cases present with features of the underlying disease (e.g., mononucleosis, varicella,

## YOUR FIRST CLUE

**Signs and Symptoms of Encephalitis**

- ALOC
- Fever
- Headache
- Psychiatric symptoms
- Seizures
- Vomiting
- Focal weakness
- Photophobia
- Movement disorders
- Dysphasia
- Ataxia
- Hemiparesis
- Cranial nerve deficits
- Visual field loss
- Papilledema
- Rash

mumps, roseola, HIV). In these cases, the diagnosis can usually be made based on the presenting clinical features with subsequent secondary encephalitis found on further evaluation when neurologic symptoms manifest.

## Diagnostic Studies

Magnetic resonance imaging (MRI) of the brain is the preferred diagnostic imaging study if encephalitis is highly suspected and the patient is clinically stable. Typical findings of herpes encephalitis in children include hypointensity on T1 weighted sequences and hyperintensity on T2 weighted sequences within the medial temporal and inferior frontal lobes.[37] With contrast, enhancement of the meninges, cortex, and white matter can occur.[37] Basal ganglia calcification also may be seen.[35] Epstein-Barr viral infections can show demyelinating lesions that clear quickly.[38] Although a CT scan of the head is often obtained to exclude mass or bleeding, this test is often normal in encephalitis. Occasionally, CT shows temporal or frontal lobe attenuation changes, petechial hemorrhages, or edema. Congenital CMV encephalitis can show intracranial calcification, cerebral dysgenesis, or other degenerative findings on CT and MRI, while these tests are often normal in acquired CMV, EBV, and varicella zoster encephalitis.[39] CT with contrast or MRI is required to diagnose lesions of toxoplasmosis.[40]

CSF analysis in viral encephalitis usually shows a lymphocytosis or monocytosis, elevated protein content, and normal or slightly low glucose.[39] An elevated CSF red blood cell count also can be found in herpes virus encephalitis. Six percent to 15% of patients with HSV-1 encephalitis have completely normal CSF studies.[32,41] Children with encephalitis due to other types of viruses (e.g., CMV, Epstein-Barr virus, human herpes virus 6 and 7) usually have normal CSF or mild elevation in protein or white blood cell counts.[39]

Polymerase chain reaction of CSF is the gold standard for diagnosing HSV encephalitis, with sensitivity of 95%.[42] Polymerase chain reaction for enterovirus infection also approaches 100%.[36] Polymerase chain reaction of CSF also can be diagnostic in cases of varicella, CMV, EBV, and human herpes virus 6 and 7.[41,42] Polymerase chain reaction of saliva is the best test for detecting rabies virus infection. Culture of CSF, conjunctivae, skin, or mucosal vesicular lesions will yield the HSV virus in half of neonatal cases, while cell culture of urine or saliva is nearly 100% in congenital CMV encephalitis. Varicella can be cultured from skin vesicles in most cases. Cultures are generally not useful for Epstein Barr virus, human herpes virus 6 and 7, and many arboviruses. Acute phase sera can be tested for IgM via enzyme linked immunosorbent assay (ELISA) in patients with arboviral infections (e.g., eastern and western equine, California, St. Louis).[32,33]

An EEG in a child with encephalitis usually shows slowing of background activity and occasional diffuse or focal seizure activity.[41] In herpes virus infection, the EEG might show periodic high-voltage spike wave activity in the temporal lobes and slow wave complexes every 2 to 3 seconds in up to 81% of cases.[32,41] This pattern also can occur with other viruses.[41]

## THE CLASSICS

**Diagnostic Features of Encephalitis**

- CSF Profile: lymphocytosis or monocytosis, elevated protein content, and normal or slightly low glucose; can be completely normal
- MRI: hypointensity on T1 weighted sequences and hyperintensity on T2 weighted sequences within the medial temporal and inferior frontal lobes (herpes); enhancement of the meninges, cortex, and white matter; demyelination; basal ganglia calcifications
- CT: normal; temporal or frontal lobe attenuation changes, petechial hemorrhages or edema
- EEG: slowing of background; focal spikes in temporal lobe (herpes)

Brain biopsy is a final resort for diagnosing encephalitis. This testing is invasive and often reserved for deteriorating patients in whom the diagnosis of encephalitis is uncertain or in whom identification of a specific pathogen is needed.

### Differential Diagnosis

A number of life-threatening disorders must be considered in patients who present with a clinical picture of encephalitis. Hypoglycemia and hypoxia can be excluded with immediate bedside tests. Other metabolic disorders (e.g., inborn metabolic errors, hepatic encephalopathy, uremia) require measurement of ammonia or specific metabolic byproducts. Sepsis, systemic bacterial infections, bacterial meningitis, viral (aseptic) meningitis, and intracranial abscesses, masses, and bleeding can cause similar symptoms. CT, MRI, lumbar puncture, radiography, or blood cultures might be required to distinguish between these possibilities. Toxins that cause fever and an altered mental status can be confused with encephalitis (e.g., amphetamines, anticholinergics, arsenic, cocaine, LSD, phencyclidine, phenothiazines, salicylates, theophylline, and thyroxine). Clues to a toxin-induced encephalopathy include the presence of other classic toxidrome features (e.g., anticholinergic symptoms, sympathomimetic symptoms with cocaine or amphetamines, respiratory alkalosis with salicylate toxicity). Other considerations in patients with clinical features of encephalitis include postinfectious disease (e.g., acute cerebellar ataxia), nonconvulsive status, vasculitis, stroke, and acute confusional migraines.

## WHAT ELSE?

**Differential Diagnosis of Encephalitis**

- Metabolic disorders
- Sepsis
- Meningitis
- Intracranial abscesses, masses, and bleeding
- Toxins

## Management

Most patients with encephalitis present with altered mental status, seizures, focal neurologic deficits, or ill appearance. Apply a cardiac monitor and pulse oximeter, and obtain venous access. Perform a bedside glucose test, and immediately treat any life-threatening complications (e.g., seizure, airway compromise, hypoxia, hyperthermia, shock).

Neuroimaging should precede lumbar puncture in all patients with impaired consciousness, signs of increased ICP, focal neurologic signs (or inability to perform reliable neurologic and ophthalmoscopic examination), impending shock, or suspected bleeding diathesis (e.g., petechiae). Although MRI is more accurate at diagnosing encephalitis, CT without contrast will identify tumors, masses, or bleeding that precludes performing a lumbar puncture. For patients who undergo neuroimaging, administer broad-spectrum IV antibiotics after appropriate bacterial cultures are obtained (urine, blood) until bacterial meningitis is excluded. For patients with probable herpes virus infection (i.e., obvious vesicles), prompt administration of acyclovir 10 mg/kg IV for infants and children and 20 mg/kg IV for neonates is indicated.[32]

If neuroimaging does not reveal an obvious alternative cause for symptoms, no signs of increased ICP are present, and there are no contraindications, perform a lumbar puncture.

Send CSF for Gram stain, glucose protein, cell count, and differential. If Gram stain is negative and features strongly suggestive of bacterial meningitis (i.e., CSF white blood cell count >1,000 cells/mm$^3$) are not present, send PCR and cultures for enteroviral and herpes virus infections. Obtain concurrent cultures from vesicles, mucous membranes, and urine for herpes and enterovirus. Specialized testing (e.g., ELISA for arboviruses, antibody titers for *Mycoplasma pneumonia*, monospot) might be required depending on the clinical presentation.[42] Admit patients, with instructions for continuous cardiorespiratory monitoring (e.g., intensive care or stepdown unit).

## KEY POINTS

**Management of Encephalitis**

- Apply a cardiac monitor and pulse oximeter.
- Obtain venous access.
- Send blood and urine samples to the laboratory for diagnostic testing and bacterial culture.
- Perform a bedside glucose test.
- Perform CT of the head or MRI (if immediately available).
- Obtain lumbar puncture and send for analysis, bacterial culture, and polymerase chain reaction testing.
- Administer antibacterials and acyclovir.
- Admit patient to monitored bed.

---

**CASE SCENARIO 4**

A 3-year-old boy presents to his physician after his parents witness episodes of "clumsiness" with repeated falling. He has had no headache, fever, or neck pain. Initial assessment reveals an alert, playful child with no increased work of breathing and pink extremities. Vital signs include a respiratory rate of 20 breaths per minute; heart rate of 118 bpm, blood pressure of 90/60, and temperature of 37°C. On further examination, pupils are 5 mm bilaterally, briskly reactive, but with vertical nystagmus. Strength is equal and 5/5 in all extremities. He is unsteady while walking, with his feet placed wide apart.

1. *What is the most appropriate imaging study for this patient?*

A 13-year-old boy presents with a sudden onset of excruciating headache. He has not been ill recently, does not have a history of headaches, and has no recent history of fever or trauma. Family history is negative for migraines. Vitals signs include a respiratory rate of 20 breaths per minute, heart rate of 98 bpm, blood pressure of 106/68, and a temperature of 37.0 C. Examination reveals an uncomfortable white male teenager complaining of severe headache. Neurologic examination is nonfocal and remarkable only for terminal neck flexion tenderness. No papilledema is noted.

1. What is the appropriate management strategy for this patient?

# Headache

## Clinical Features and Differential Diagnosis

Headache is a common complaint in children, with frequent headaches occurring in 2.5% of children by 7 years of age and another third having occasional headaches. By age 15, 16% have frequent and more than half have infrequent headaches.[43] Headaches account for 1.3% of pediatric visits to the ED.[44–46] Important disorders that require identification include aneurysms, tumors, bleeding, infection, and increased ICP from any cause.

Parents are often concerned that a headache is a harbinger of a tumor or mass. Many studies have found that cancerous mass is a rare cause of headache (3 per 100,000) in children.[47] This might account for the fact that it typically takes four or more physician visits before a brain tumor is considered as the cause of a headache in a child.[48] Children with isolated headache and no associated neurologic symptoms rarely have significant CT abnormalities.[49–52] Several clues should raise the suspicion of a brain tumor. Prospective studies have found that sleep-related headache (worse with lying down or on arising in the morning), absence of family history, vomiting, confusion, abnormal neurologic examination, absence of vision symptoms, and headache duration less than 6 months are independent predictors of intracranial mass lesions.[52,53]

Most children with brain tumors have additional symptoms indicating intracranial pathology, and nearly all children with brain tumors and headache have signs of intracranial disease.[47,53] The Childhood Brain Tumor Consortium evaluated 3,291 children with brain tumors and found that 62% had headaches. More than 99% of these children had another symptom prior to their first hospitalization, including vomiting in 72% to 86%; personality, speech, or school problems in 81% to 87%; weight loss in 66% to 79%; difficulty walking (if 2 years old or older) in 77% to 92%; upper extremity weakness in 63% to 79%; seizures in 6% to 23%; and diplopia (if older than 4 years) in 60% to 63%, depending on whether the tumor was infratentorial or supratentorial.[56] Physical examination abnormalities were present in 98% with supratentorial and 99% with infratentorial tumors. Lethargy or confusion was present in 72% to 77%, papilledema in 65% to 81%, and head tilt in 50% to 76%.[47]

Nontraumatic brain hemorrhage and intracranial vascular malformations are rare but important causes of headache in children. The most common causes of spontaneous intracranial bleeding in children are arteriovenous malformations (AVMs), arteriovenous fistulas (AVFs), systemic hematologic disorders (e.g., thrombocytopenia, hemophilia), tumors, and aneurysms.[54–56] Acute onset headache and vomiting are the most prominent symptoms occurring in most these patients.[54–56] Up to 20% with subarachnoid bleeding have mild warning leaks manifesting 1 to 2 weeks prior to the acute bleed. Of these, 41% have been recently seen by a physician and the diagnosis missed.[57] During the acute hemorrhage, nearly one half of all patients have an altered level of consciousness (GCS <15), one third have seizures, with hemiparesis, aphasia, and vision symptoms each occurring in a minority of patients.[54-57]

Systemic disease with neurologic manifestations can be important causes of headache in children. Hypertensive encephalopathy occurs in the setting of severe hypertension (diastolic above 95th percentile for age) with breakdown of cerebral autoregulation or vasospasm and associated neurologic symptoms. Almost all children will have headache, seizures, or vision changes.[58] Children with hypertensive encephalopathy usually have renally mediated hypertension, although occasional cases are due to coarctation of the aorta, pheochromocytoma, or neuroblastoma.[58] Examination is performed to identify the cause of hypertension (e.g., drugs, Wilms tumor, renal disease, coarctation, phakomatosis, hyperthyroidism) and the presence of complications (e.g., CNS bleeding, renal failure, congestive heart failure).[58] Cranial CT in hypertensive encephalopathy can be normal or occasionally reveal reversible white matter hypodensity, ventricular compression, or sulcal and cisternal obliteration.[58] Associated intracranial bleeding can be present. Typical MRI findings include widespread focal increased white matter and cortical T2 weighted signals, especially within the occipital lobe.[58]

A multitude of systemic diseases can cause headaches. Although meningitis and encephalitis are relatively common intracranial infections with prominent headache, intracranial abscesses are rare. Intracranial abscess occurs most commonly in patients with cyanotic heart disease and partially or untreated sinus and otologic infections.[59] Headache, vomiting, ALOC, and fever are prominent symptoms with focal deficits occurring in a minority of patients.[59] Other systemic diseases causing neurologic manifestations with headache include vasculitides (e.g., Henoch-Schönlein purpura), systemic infections (e.g., tick-borne disease), toxin exposure (e.g., car-

bon monoxide, lead), and environmental (e.g., high altitude) exposures. Evaluation in these cases involves identification and treatment of the underlying disorder while searching for intracranial complications (bleed or infection).

## Diagnostic Studies

All children with headache require a thorough systemic and neurologic examination to identify features associated with serious disease. If serious disorders are suspected, CT with contrast will identify most tumors, while MRI is particularly suited for identification of posterior fossa masses (brainstem and cerebellum). CT with contrast and MRI will identify abscesses, while CT without contrast is required if intracranial bleeding is suspected.[59] Importantly, 98% of patients with subarachnoid bleeding will have an abnormal CT if performed within 12 hours of symptoms. The accuracy of CT drops as the time from symptom onset extends beyond 12 hours. For this reason, lumbar puncture must be performed following CT to identify blood or xanthochromia if a subarachnoid hemorrhage is suspected.[56,60,61] A nonbleeding aneurysm or AVM might not be identified on typical CT or MRI.[56,60,61] If these disorders are suspected, MR angiography or formal angiography is required. Aneurysm, AVM, and intracranial bleeding require prompt neurosurgical evaluation.

### Increased Intracranial Pressure

Two important subpopulations who present with headache include children with increased ICP and ventricular shunt malfunction or infection.

Children with increased ICP present with a variety of complaints. Infants with ICP manifest features specific to an intracranial process (e.g., a bulging fontanel, large head circumference, seizures, upward gaze paralysis [setting sun sign]) or nonspecific symptoms (e.g., irritability, altered mentation, vomiting, failure to thrive). One author analyzed symptoms in 107 children with measured progressive hydrocephalus mostly due to spina bifida, meningitis, or hemorrhage.[62] After children with ventricular shunts were excluded, half with elevated ICP had no symptoms; 33% had headache or irritability, and 16% had vomiting.[62] The most common signs were increased head size in 76%, a tense fontanel in 65%, splayed cranial sutures in 39%, scalp vein distention in 33%, and neck rigidity in 14%.[62] Older children can present with headache, vomiting, mental status changes, or focal neurologic findings (e.g., altered walking, cranial nerve deficits).[63] Clearly, the cause of increased ICP, the acuity of onset, and the underlying age and condition of the patient are important determinants of presenting features.

Signs of increased ICP vary with the location and magnitude of pressure. Cerebral mass lesions can manifest as focal weakness or altered behavior, while cerebellar and brainstem lesions can affect gait and balance. As pressure increases, the possibility of herniation of parts of the brain to adjacent areas rises. Uncal herniation (medial temporal lobe) in a downward direction through the tentorium compresses the third cranial nerve, leading to ipsilateral pupillary dilation. Continued downward pressure compresses the pyramidal tract, causing contralateral weakness. Central herniation occurs when both hemispheres and basal nuclei have herniated downward through the tentorium with resulting altered mental status, respiratory abnormalities, and bilateral corticospinal tract compression with bilateral weakness. Less frequent herniation syndromes include cingulate herniation (herniation of the cingulated gyrus laterally under the falx cerebri) and posterior fossa herniation (cerebellum herniates upward through the tentorium or downward through the foramen magnum). If unabated, herniation is followed by coma and cardiopulmonary arrest.[63]

### Ventricular Shunt Disorders

Ventricular shunts have been used routinely for the past 50 years to successfully treat hydrocephalus.[64] Ventricular shunt placement is the most common neurosurgical procedure performed in children, and most pediatric health care workers will see children with these devices. The two major complications following this procedure are shunt obstruction and shunt infection.

Symptoms and signs of shunt obstruction are usually related to increased ICP (e.g., altered mentation, headache, vomiting, seizures, altered gait, cranial nerve deficits including decreased upward gaze, and papilledema).[65] Additionally, ventriculoperitoneal shunt malfunction can manifest as abdominal pain, bowel obstruction, or an abdominal mass.[64] Identification of shunt malfunction requires plain films of the skull (AP and lateral) and of the areas of the body containing the shunt in addition to cranial CT. Identification of increased ICP in patients who are shunted can be difficult. Up to 24% of CT scans will be interpreted as normal, unchanged, or having smaller ventricles.[66,67] Even if there is no acute CT abnormality, neurosurgical evaluation is mandatory when shunt obstruction is suspected.

Most shunt infections occur near the time of their placement, with 70% occurring within 2 months and 80% within 6 months.[64] Clinical features of shunt infection differ depending on the type of shunt present. Ventriculoperitoneal shunt infections typically manifest with fever, shunt malfunction, or abdominal pain.[68,69] Less frequent features include meningismus (only one third of cases), headache, irritability, and feeding difficulty.[64,68] Shunt malfunction can coexist. Inflammation along the course of the shunt is highly specific for shunt infection.[68] Children with ventriculoatrial shunt infection have fever in most cases, with irritability or headache in half of all cases.[64,68] Less common presentations include renal insufficiency due to shunt nephritis (due to antigen antibody complex deposition within the renal glomeruli), septic pulmonary emboli, cardiac tamponade, septal perforation, vena cava obstruction, mycotic aneurysms, and endocarditis. Initial evaluation of patients with suspected shunt infection involves exclusion of shunt obstruction radiographically. Cerebrospinal fluid is withdrawn in a sterile manner from the shunt reservoir and sent for cell count, Gram stain, and culture to exclude infection.

## Management

Apply cardiac telemetry and a pulse oximeter to monitor cardiopulmonary status. Patients with significantly altered mental status are at risk for aspiration and rapid deterioration; therefore, control their airways with endotracheal intubation as appropriate. Immediate neurosurgical consultation is required for patients with increased ICP amenable to surgery (e.g., AVM, mass, bleeding, shunt obstruction). Intracranial infections (e.g., abscess, cavernous sinus thrombosis) require IV antibiotics against common pathogens (e.g., third-generation cephalosporins if nonimmunocompromised). Shunt infection usually requires external ventricular drainage or externalization of shunt, and empiric antibiotics effective against *Staphylococcus aureus* and *Staphylococcus epidermidis* (vancomycin or nafcillin and an aminoglycoside, or rifampin) until culture results can further direct therapy.[64,69]

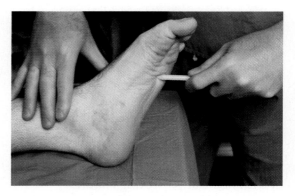

**Figure 5.2** Normal downgoing plantar reflex (negative Babinski sign).

## Weakness

### Clinical Features and Differential Diagnosis

Weakness can be divided into the primary location of strength loss (proximal or distal muscles) or into the anatomical cause of weakness (upper or lower motor neuron). Upper motor neuron disease affects the cerebral cortex or the spinal cord. Lower motor neuron disease affects the motor unit, which includes the anterior horn cells of the spinal column, the nerves (axons) connecting to the muscle, the neuromuscular junction, and the muscle.[70]

Examples of upper motor neuron diseases affecting the cerebrum include stroke, bleeding, degenerative disorders, and birth-related trauma such as cerebral palsy. Patients with cerebral disease can manifest with associated encephalopathy, seizures, or evidence of diminished higher cognitive function. Deep tendon reflexes are increased, and spasticity, hypertonicity, and a Babinski reflex (dorsiflexion of the great toe) can be present (**Figure 5.2**). Hemiplegia or weakness involving one side of the body usually occurs with cerebral insults (e.g., stroke). Facial weakness, if present, is ipsilateral to the weakness in the extremities, with dysphasia often a prominent feature when the dominant hemisphere is affected (e.g., middle cerebral artery occlusion). Occasionally, strokes affect the posterior cerebral artery, causing cerebellar symptoms (e.g., vertigo, ataxia) in addition to hemiplegia.[70–72]

Hemiplegia is the most common presenting feature of stroke in children and requires a thorough evaluation for underlying disease.[73] Important causes include disorders affecting the vasculature, heart, and blood, and inherited diseases associated with intracranial anomalies.[74] Identification of underlying disease will influence management.

In contrast, acute spinal cord lesions produce flaccid paralysis, with absent deep tendon reflexes, absent Babinski reflexes, and associated bowel and bladder incontinence or urinary retention. After the acute spinal cord insult, flaccidity is replaced by spasticity, and deep tendon reflexes become hyperactive. Often, a distinct sensory level can identify the site of the lesion. The term paraplegia is used to describe partial or complete loss of strength in the lower extremities, while quadriplegia describes loss of strength in the upper and lower extremities. Although most cases of paraplegia and quadriplegia are related to spinal cord disease, rare cases are related to cerebral disease (e.g., cerebral palsy).[74–75]

Transverse myelitis, epidural abscesses, tumors, spontaneous bleeding, infarction, and trauma can lead to acute spinal cord dysfunction. Acute onset of symptoms is typical of bleeding, infarction, and trauma. Children with transverse myelitis and epidural abscesses often develop back pain and fever and a more gradual onset of symptoms followed by an

| TABLE 5-3 | Differentiating Lower Motor Neuron Weakness | | | |
|---|---|---|---|---|
| | Anterior Horn Cell | Peripheral Nerve (Axon) | Neuromuscular Junction | Muscle |
| Muscle atrophy | ↑↑↑ | ↑ | — | ↑↑ |
| Fasciculations | ↑↑↑ | — | — | — |
| Sensory deficit | — | ↑ | — | — |
| Reflexes | Normal or ↓ | Normal or ↓ | Normal | Normal, ↓ in late disease |
| CK levels | Normal or ↑ | Normal | Normal | ↑↑ |
| Examples | Polio Amyotrophic lateral sclerosis Spinal muscular atrophy | Guillain-Barré Organophosphates Lead toxicity Diphtheria | Myasthenia Botulism Tick paralysis | Muscular dystrophy Periodic paralysis ↓or ↑K Myositis |

↑ = prominent (or hyperactive reflexes), ↓ = diminished, — = not present

acute onset of weakness. As with acute stroke, identification of the underlying disease will influence management.[57]

Features of lower motor neuron disease differ depending on the site of the lesion. (See Table 5-3.) Most children with acute or chronic flaccid limb weakness have a disorder of the motor unit.[76] Sensory changes are an important distinguishing characteristic that can be present in a peripheral neuropathy. Distal weakness preceding proximal weakness also is prominent. Neuromuscular junction disorders (e.g., botulism, myasthenia) exert an early effect on bulbar muscles (e.g., ocular muscles, swallowing), while muscular disorders (e.g., muscular dystrophy, myopathies) typically cause weakness in proximal large muscles, with leg weakness often manifesting before upper extremity weakness. Motor neuron (anterior horn cell) disorders cause profound weakness, prominent fasciculations, and atrophy.[71,74–76]

## Diagnostic Studies

CT and MRI are used to evaluate cerebral disease, and MRI is best for defining spinal cord lesions. Underlying disorders require identification and management (e.g., hypoglycemia, reversal of coagulopathy in hemophilia, exchange transfusion for stroke due to sickle cell disease). Evaluation of lower motor neuron lesions involves distinguishing among the various causes based on their clinical presentation. Serum creatine kinase (CK) is often elevated in muscle disorders. More formal testing (e.g., EMG, nerve conduction studies, and muscle biopsy) might be required to accurately differentiate among causes of lower motor neuron weakness.[74,76]

## Management

Neurologic assessment proceeds in an orderly manner with a goal of first identifying and then treating any disorder that can lead to life-threatening respiratory failure (Guillain-Barré, botulism), seizures (electrolyte abnormalities, intracranial mass, or bleeding), or predispose to sepsis or hypotension. At this point, consider airway management or support respirations, supply $O_2$ if needed, and apply a cardiac monitor and pulse oximeter to children at risk for deterioration.

Next, disorders that can cause irreversible neurologic deficits must be identified (e.g., spinal cord compression, expanding intracerebral mass), followed by disorders that are treatable. CT or MRI can be used to identify lesions amenable to surgery. Specific agents that can improve outcome include steroids (for CNS, spinal cord edema), anticholinesterases (myasthenia), and electrolyte or glucose replacement therapy.

# ■ Seizures

A seizure is the clinical manifestation of an abnormal and excessive electrical discharge from neurons in the brain. Although this definition is narrow, the clinical spectrum of illness associated with seizures is wide. Children with seizures present from infancy through adolescence. Their diagnosis, management, and treatment will vary widely depending on age, presence of preexisting neurologic abnormalities, and presence or absence of acute coexisting illness. A carefully performed history and physical examination are critical to making the diagnosis, distinguishing among the various etiologies, and directing evaluation and management.

## Febrile Seizures

### Epidemiology

Febrile seizures are the most common convulsive disorder of childhood. Approximately 3% to 5% of children will experience a febrile seizure before their fifth birthday, with the peak onset in the second year of life.[77,78] Approximately two thirds of the patients are male, with a median age of onset of 19 to 23 months. The risk of febrile seizure increases when there is a history of febrile seizures in first degree relatives, as does the risk of recurrence.[79]

## Clinical Features

By definition, febrile seizures occur in children 6 months to 5 years of age who do not have evidence of intracranial infection or known seizure disorder. Eighty percent of these seizures are simple (generalized, lasting less than 15 minutes, occurring only once in a 24-hour period), carry few risks of complications, and have excellent short- and long-term prognoses. Children whose seizures have focal features, last more than 15 minutes, or occur more than once in a 24-hour period are classified as having complex febrile seizures. Children with complex febrile seizures have higher rates of recurrent febrile seizures and epilepsy than do children with simple febrile seizures.[79]

The seizure will be the first sign of febrile illness in approximately 25% to 50% of cases. Most febrile seizures occur during the first 24 hours of illness. Children with febrile seizures often have high mean temperatures (39.6°C). According to a multicenter retrospective review of 455 patients with first-time simple febrile seizures, the most common associated infectious illnesses were otitis media (34%), upper respiratory infection (12%) or viral syndrome (6%), and pneumonia (6%). Urinary tract infection (3%), gastroenteritis (2%), varicella (2%), and bronchiolitis (1%) were identified in a smaller subset of patients. Thirty-four percent of patients had no infectious diagnosis identified at the time of ED discharge, presumably because they were so early in the course of their illness.[80]

In this data set, bacteremia occurred in 1.3% of children in whom blood cultures were drawn. Other retrospective series also performed after the advent of the H influenzae vaccine have demonstrated similar rates of bacteremia: 2.1% in a younger patient population (2 to 24 months) from a single institution,[81] and 2.9% in children younger than 6 years with simple or complex febrile seizures from a different single center tertiary care institution.[82]

## YOUR FIRST CLUE

### Signs and Symptoms of Simple Versus Complex Febrile Seizures

**Simple**
- <10–15 minutes duration
- Generalized; nonfocal neurologic exam
- No recurrence in 24 hours

**Complex**
- >15 minutes duration
- Focal seizure or focal neurologic examination
- Repeated seizures within 24 hours

## Diagnostic Studies

The cornerstone of diagnosis remains a carefully performed history and physical examination. The body of evidence to date indicates that routine diagnostic evaluation of children with simple febrile seizure is not indicated.[83] Children who have been pretreated with antibiotics, who have focal seizures, or whose seizure occurs after several days of illness should be carefully evaluated to rule out meningitis and other significant bacterial infections.

In patients whose level of consciousness has not returned to baseline or who are lethargic or irritable, lumbar puncture should be performed to exclude meningitis (see earlier section). In addition, children younger than 6 months are outside the usual age group susceptible to febrile seizures. This group probably warrants a more careful evaluation with attention to metabolic derangements, possible underlying neurologic disorders, as well as meningitis or encephalitis. Febrile seizure is infrequently the sole sign of viral meningitis. In a comprehensive retrospective review of patients with bacterial meningitis, seizure was never the sole presenting sign.[84] The threshold for performing lumbar puncture varies based on individual patient characteristics, the accessibility of followup care, and the clinician's comfort level with infants and young children.

An EEG is not indicated for evaluation either in the ED or as an outpatient. CT or MRI should be reserved for the child with a focal seizure, focal neurologic findings, history of head trauma, or failure to return to baseline neurologic status.

### Differential Diagnosis

Children with chills associated with high fevers can be mistakenly identified as having had a febrile seizure. A careful history, with a demonstration of the rhythmic movements associated with clonic seizures in comparison with the tremulous nature of chills by the clinician, can help distinguish between these two entities. Children with febrile seizures are a distinct patient group from children with epilepsy who have intercurrent febrile illnesses. Fever is known to lower the seizure threshold in such children. These children might require additional anticonvulsant medication during febrile illnesses, unlike children with febrile seizures.

### Management

Antibiotics are not indicated unless there is a focus of infection documented on physical examination or by laboratory evaluation. Anticonvulsants have no role in the treatment of simple febrile seizures.[85] In a single study, oral diazepam prophylaxis was shown to be effective in decreasing the recurrence rate of febrile seizures in a select high-risk population.[86] This success was not reproduced in other studies, largely due to noncompliance. The practice of using around-the-clock acetaminophen and/or ibuprofen does not prevent febrile seizures and can contribute to parental fever phobia.

## Afebrile Seizures

### Epidemiology

Between 25,000 and 40,000 children per year in the United States will experience a first afebrile seizure.[87] Epilepsy is characterized by recurrent unprovoked seizures and is not diagnosed until the patient has two or more afebrile seizures. The overall incidence of epilepsy in childhood is between 4 and 9 per 1,000 from population-based studies. The reported percentage of children who go on to have epilepsy after a single afebrile seizure varies between 29% and 82%,

based on the cohort cited and whether the patient population was studied prospectively or retrospectively. In population-based studies, more children with developmental delay or learning disability develop epilepsy in comparison with children with normal development.[88]

### Clinical Features and Differential Diagnosis

Seizures can be divided into categories based on motor and sensory involvement, as well as presence or absence of alteration of consciousness. (See Table 5-4.) A careful history of the event will often give clues to the seizure type and help distinguish seizures from other paroxysmal events such as breath-holding spells, gastroesophageal reflux (GER) with apnea, vasovagal syncope, arrhythmias, and pseudoseizures. (See Table 5-5.) Although there can be substantial overlap between behavioral descriptors of seizure and nonseizure events, in one prospective study, 13 descriptors were found to differentiate between seizure and nonseizure events. They include jerking/twitching, stiffening, changes in breathing, staring off, biting or chewing the tongue, glassy eyes, unresponsiveness, mumbling or slurring words, eyes/head turned to one side, and lack of memory of the event. All of these were significantly more common in patients with seizures.[89] When in doubt as to the nature of the event, a broader workup might be necessary.

### WHAT ELSE?

**Differential Diagnosis of Seizures**
- Breath-holding spells
- Vasovagal syncope
- GER with apnea
- Arrhythmia

### Diagnostic Studies

Routine laboratory investigation in children older than 6 months has not been shown to be helpful in elucidating the cause of seizures or influencing their management. In the absence of a history of illness, vomiting and/or

**TABLE 5-4    Categorization of Seizures**

| Generalized Seizures | Description |
|---|---|
| • Tonic-clonic | Rhythmic stiffening and jerking of trunk and extremities |
| • Tonic | Stiffening without jerking of trunk and extremities |
| • Atonic | "Drop attacks" |
| • Absence | Staring or brief loss of consciousness without postictal depression |
| • Myoclonic | Sudden, brief muscle jerks, either unilateral or bilateral |
| • Infantile spasms | Cluster of sudden, tonic contractions of head, trunk, and extremities ("Salaam") |
| **Partial seizures** | |
| • Simple partial seizure | Motor, somatosensory, or autonomic symptoms without alteration of consciousness during or after seizure |
| • Complex partial seizure | Motor or autonomic symptoms with altered level of consciousness; often preceded by aura and followed by postictal depression; might generalize |

Adapted from Reuter D, Brownsten D. Common emergent pediatric neurologic problems. *Emerg Med Clin North Am.* 2002; 20(1):155–176.

**TABLE 5-5    Outline for Seizure Assessment**

| Associated Factors | Ictal Symptoms | Postictal Symptoms |
|---|---|---|
| Age | Aura—subjective sensations | Amnesia for events |
| Family history | Behavior—mood or behavior change prior to the seizure | Confusion |
| Developmental status | | Lethargy |
| Behavior | Vocal—cry or gasp, slurring of words, garbled speech | Sleepiness |
| Health at seizure onset—fever, acute illness symptoms, sleep deprivation | Motor—head eye turning or deviation, posturing, jerking, stiffening, automatisms, focality | Headaches and muscle aches |
| | | Transient focal weakness (Todd's paralysis) |
| Exposure to trauma or toxins | Respiration—change in breathing pattern, apnea, cyanosis | Nausea or vomiting |
| | Autonomic—papillary dilatation, drooling, change in respiratory or heart rate, incontinence, pallor, vomiting | |
| | Loss of consciousness, inability to understand or speak | |

Source: Hirtz D, Ashwal S, Berg A et al. Practice parameter: evaluating a first nonfebrile seizure in children. *Neurology.* 2000;55(5):616–623. Reprinted with permission.

diarrhea, or suspected ingestion, they are not indicated.[87] In infants younger than 6 months, hyponatremia and hypocalcemia are known precipitants of seizures. Hypoglycemia is strongly associated with seizure activity at any age in association with ingestion of alcohol, oral hypoglycemic agents, and insulin admin-istration. A rapid assay for glucose is helpful in a child who is actively seizing, or who is in the immediate postictal period. Otherwise, laboratory testing should be reserved for children based on individual clinical circumstances or a failure to return to baseline alertness. Toxicology screening should be considered if there is any question of intentional or unintentional toxin exposure. There is no evidence to indicate that lumbar puncture should be routinely performed on the child with an afebrile seizure. In children with persistent alteration of mental status of unknown etiology or meningeal signs, lumbar puncture should be considered for the evaluation of meningitis or encephalitis (see earlier section). Head imaging should be performed prior to lumbar puncture if signs of elevated ICP (Cushing triad: bradycardia, hypertension, and irregular respirations) are present.[87]

For children with known epilepsy who are currently taking antiseizure drugs, consider measuring drug level to determine compliance and therapeutic concentrations. Nontrough levels have limited diagnostic value to the treating neurologist unless they clearly show toxic levels or absence of drug.

In a child with new-onset seizure, an EEG can be helpful in neurologic followup to help differentiate seizure from nonseizure events, determine seizure type or epilepsy syndrome, and better define the risk for recurrent seizures. It is not necessary to perform the EEG as part of the initial ED evaluation in an otherwise well child. In fact, if it is performed shortly after the seizure (<48 hours), the EEG might show diffuse postictal slowing without prognostic significance. The absence of abnormal EEG findings does not exclude the diagnosis of seizure, nor does the presence of an abnormal EEG in isolation confirm that a seizure occurred.[87]

Although abnormalities in neuroimaging can be found in up to one third of children with first-time afebrile seizures, in well-designed studies, only 2% revealed clinically significant findings that contributed to clinical management. In most of these cases, either the seizure was focal or the child had specific clinical findings in addition to the seizure, which prompted the evaluation. In their practice parameter, "Evaluating the First Nonfebrile Seizure in Children," the American Academy of Neurology, the Child Neurology Society, and the American Epilepsy Society do not recommend routine neuroimaging in these children.[87] They recommend emergency neuroimaging only for children with focal postictal deficits not rapidly resolving (Todd paralysis) or those who fail to return to neurologic baseline several hours after the incident. Nonurgent MRI should be considered in several patient groups: children younger than 1 year, those with focal seizures, and children with unexplained neurologic abnormalities or undiagnosed cognitive or motor impairments. Children in whom head trauma is suspected or known represent a separate patient group and should undergo emergent imaging as outlined in Chapter 9, Trauma.[87]

## Management

In a child with new-onset seizure who is not actively seizing in the ED, no treatment is indicated at the time of the evaluation. Appropriate consultation with a pediatric neurologist and outpatient followup care should be arranged for all children suspected of having a first-time seizure. If the episode represents a recurrent seizure in a child who has previously been evaluated with EEG and who is not on antiseizure drugs, neurologic consultation with a consideration for therapy should occur. If an epileptic child on antiseizure therapy has breakthrough seizures, compliance and acute illness history should be carefully reviewed. Decisions regarding alteration of current therapy should be made in consultation with the patient's pediatric neurologist. During febrile illnesses, many children with known epilepsy will have an increase in seizure frequency. One successful approach to this patient population has been to prescribe rectal diazepam to break the seizure cluster.[87] It can be used either in the ED or at home by the parents in a commercially available rectal gel preparation (Diastat).

Children who have an obvious precipitant to the seizure should be managed in accordance with the underlying injury or illness process. Table 5-6 indicates common causes of toxin-mediated seizures and any specific recommendations unique to the toxicologic agent. Benzodiazepines remain the drugs of first choice in terminating seizure activity in children. They are effective, potent, act rapidly, and are easily administered in the field and in the ED. (See Table 5-7.) Recurrent seizures should be managed as in the status epilepticus (SE) pathway outlined in Figure 5.3.

## TABLE 5-6 Mnemonic for Toxin-Induced Seizures. OTIS CAMPBELL

| Toxic Substance | Antidotes, Special Instructions (initial drug of choice—benzodiazepine) |
|---|---|
| Organophosphates | Atropine, pralidoxime |
| Tricyclic antidepressants | |
| Isoniazid | Pyridoxine (gm/gm INH ingested); might not respond to antiseizure drugs |
| Insulin | Glucose |
| Sympathomimetics | |
| Camphor, Cocaine | |
| Amphetamines | |
| Methylxanthines (theophylline, caffeine) | Use pentobarbital if no response |
| PCP, Propoxyphene, Phenol, Propranolol | |
| Benzodiazepine withdrawal, Botanicals | |
| Ethanol withdrawal | Magnesium sulfate |
| Lithium | |
| Lidocaine | AVOID PHENYTOIN 2°; arrhythmia risk |
| Lindane | |
| Lead | BAL, CaEDTA |

Source: Erickson TB, Aks SE, Gussow L, Williams RH. Toxicology update: A rational approach to managing a poisoned patient. *Emergency Medicine Practice,* August 2001, Vol 6, Number 8. Reprinted with permission.


## TABLE 5-7 Drugs Used to Terminate Status Epilepticus*

| Drug | Dose | Max Dose | Onset of Action | Duration of Action | Rate |
|---|---|---|---|---|---|
| Lorazepam | 0.05–0.1 mg/kg IV | 4 mg | 2–3 min | 12–24 hrs | ≤ 2 mg/min |
| Diazepam | 0.1–0.3 mg/kg IV 0.5 mg/kg PR | 10 mg | 1–3 min | 5–15 min | ≤ 2 mg/min |
| Midazolam | 0.05–.15 mg/kg IV/IM | 6 mg | 2–3 min (IV) 10–20 min (IM) | 30–60 min (IV) 1–2 hrs (IM) | ≤ 2 mg/min |
| Phenytoin | 20 mg/kg IV | 1,000 mg | 10–30 min* | 12–24 hrs | ≤ 1 mg/kg/min ≤ 50 mg/min |
| Fosphenytoin | 15–20 mg/kg PE⁻ IV/IM | 1,000 mg | 10–30 min* | 12–24 hrs | ≤ 3 mg/kg/min ≤ 150 mg/min |
| Phenobarbital | 20 mg/kg IV | 1,000 mg | 10–20 min | 1–3 days | ≤ 1–2 mg/kg/min ≤ 100 mg/min |

*After infusion.

PE⁻=Phenytoin Equivalents.

Adapted from: Pellock JM. Status epilepticus in children: update and review. *J Child Neurol.* 1994;9(suppl):2S27–2S35; Hanhan UA, Fiallos MR, Orlowski JP. Status epilepticus. *Pediatr Clin North Am.* 2001;48(3):1–12; and Haafiz A, Kissoon N. Status epilepticus: current concepts. *Pediatr Emerg Care.* 1999;15(2):119–129.

**Stabilize the Patient (0–10 minutes)**
  Evaluate the airway (position, suction)
  Provide 100% oxygen by face mask
  Assess ventilation and support as needed (consider oral or nasal airway)
  Measure and monitor vital signs
  Establish vascular access
  Obtain blood for rapid glucose assay and other specimens as indicated by history and physical
  Control hyperthermia (rectal acetaminophen 15 mg/kg)

**Begin Therapy (10–45 minutes)**
  1) Glucose 0.5 g/kg if hypoglycemic (2 mL/kg D25, 5 mL/kg D10)
  2) Lorazepam 0.10 mg/kg IV, max 4 mg/dose, may repeat × 1 in 5–10 minutes
     OR
  Diazepam 0.1–0.3 mg/kg IV, max 10 mg/dose, may repeat × 1 in 5 minutes
     OR if no IV access
  Diazepam 0.5 mg/kg per rectum, max 20 mg
  FOLLOWED BY
  IF CHILD:
  3) Fosphenytoin 20 mg/kg IV or IM, 3 mg/kg/min, max 1,000 mg
  OR
  Phenytoin 20 mg/kg IV, 1 mg/kg/min, max 1,000 mg
  IF NEONATE:
  4) Phenobarbital 20 mg/kg IV, 1 mg/kg/min. BE PREPARED TO VENTILATE.
  5) If seizure activity continues 10 minutes after infusion of phenobarbital in a neonate, consider repeated doses of phenobarbital at
     10 mg kg dose, up to a maximum of 40 mg/kg.
  6) If seizure activity continues after 2 doses of benzodiazepine and an appropriate antiepileptic drug load, move to therapy for refractory
     SE.

**Initiate Therapy for Refractory Status Epilepticus (>45–60 minutes)**
  1) Rapid sequence intubation and mechanical ventilation.
  2) Consider continuous EEG monitoring.
  3) Optimal placement in critical care ICU setting with consideration for central venous pressure monitoring, especially if using
     pentobarbital.
  4) Midazolam drip 0.2 mg/kg IV load, followed by 1 mcg/kg/min drip, increase 1 mcg/kg/min every 15 minutes until burst suppression
     OR
  Pentobarbital drip 5–15 mg/kg IV load, followed by 0.5–5 mg/kg/hr infusion
     OR
  Propofol drip 1–3 mg/kg IV load, followed by 2–10 mg/kg/hr drip
     OR
  Valproic Acid 15–20 mg/kg IV load over 1–5 min, may repeat q 10–15 minutes to max of 40 mg/kg or 5 mg/kg/hr infusion

**Figure 5.3** Management Protocol for Status Epilepticus.

Adapted from: Pellock JM. Status epilepticus in children: update and review. *J Child Neurol.* 1994;9(suppl):2S27–2S35; Hanhan UA, Fiallos MR, Orlowski JP. Status epilepticus. *Pediatr Clin North Am.* 2001;48(3):1–12; and Haafiz A, Kissoon N. Status epilepticus: current concepts. *Pediatr Emerg Care.* 1999;15(2):119–129.

## Status Epilepticus

### Epidemiology

Every year in the United States, approximately 120,000 individuals will experience status epilepticus (SE). More than half of these will be children. One third of the episodes will be the initial event in a patient with new-onset epilepsy. One third will occur in children with established epilepsy, and one third will occur as isolated events at the time of an acute in-sult.[91] Up to 70% of children with epilepsy presenting before 1 year of age will experience an episode of SE in their lifetimes.[92]

Historically, high rates of mortality have been associated with SE, especially in the adult population. However, more recent reports indicate that the mortality rate related to the prolonged seizure per se in children is probably only 1% to 3%.[92,93] Seizure duration of greater than 1 hour, especially in association with hypoxia, has been associated with permanent neurologic injury and increasing rates of mortality.[94]

## Clinical Features

As defined by the World Health Organization in its *Dictionary of Epilepsy*, SE is "a condition characterized by an epileptic seizure that is sufficiently prolonged or repeated at sufficiently brief intervals so as to produce an unvarying or enduring epileptic condition."[95] Practically speaking, and for the purposes of most research studies, it is defined by continuous or repetitive seizure activity of at least 30 minutes' duration. However, almost all self-limited seizures stop within 5 minutes; therefore, the Working Group on Status Epilepticus of the Epilepsy Foundation of America recommends that any patient with seizure duration of longer than 10 minutes have anticonvulsant therapy initiated.[96] By extension, any child presenting to the ED actively seizing should be considered to be in SE at that point and managed accordingly. The earlier the attempt to control the seizure, the easier it will be to stop.

## Diagnostic Studies

Diagnostic studies should be tailored to rapidly determine metabolic, toxicologic, or neurologic derangements that might have precipitated SE. (See Table 5-8.) Rapid bedside assay for glucose is indicated in all patients. Children with a variety of seizure precipitants can become hypoglycemic with ongoing seizure activity. Depending on the clinical scenario, serum levels of sodium, calcium, and phosphorus are indicated for children with ongoing seizure activity. Tests of renal and hepatic function can be useful. Antiseizure drug levels might be helpful in a child with known epilepsy if found to be toxic or drastically subtherapeutic. Specific serum toxicologic levels should be directed by the history, including the presence of drugs in the home or surroundings that are known to cause seizures. A urine toxicology screen, usually only available for drugs of abuse, has a rapid turnaround time in most institutions and might influence management. If head trauma is suspected based on the history or physical examination, emergency CT scan of the head is indicated.

| TABLE 5-8 | Precipitants of Status Epilepticus |
|---|---|
| Precipitants | Children <16 y, % |
| Fever/infection (non-CNS) | 35.7 |
| Medication change | 19.8 |
| Unknown | 9.3 |
| Metabolic | 8.2 |
| Congenital | 7.0 |
| Anoxia | 5.3 |
| CNS infection | 4.8 |
| Trauma | 3.5 |
| Cerebrovascular | 3.3 |
| Ethanol/drug-related | 2.4 |
| Tumor | 0.7 |

Adapted from: DeLorenzo RJ, Towne AR, Pellock JM, Ko D. Status epilepticus in children, adults and the elderly. *Epilepsia*. 1992;33(suppl 4):S15–S25.

## Differential Diagnosis

Differential diagnosis of SE includes complex febrile seizures, toxic ingestion or drug withdrawal, intercurrent febrile illness or subtherapeutic antiseizure levels in a child with known epilepsy, meningitis or encephalitis, intracranial injury, or progressive neurodegenerative disorder. Many authors have categorized children with SE into five broad categories: cryptogenic (idiopathic), remote symptomatic, febrile, acute symptomatic, and progressive encephalopathy.[97] Figure 5.4 lists the relative frequency of different etiologies in a pediatric cohort of patients with SE.

## Management

Management of this life-threatening condition mandates the usual resuscitative measures prior to specific therapy for seizures. Airway, breathing, and circulation, as in any other emergent situation, should be assessed first. Much of the morbidity and mortality associated with SE can be attributed to hypoxia and its ensuing complications. The hypoxia associated with SE is multifactorial. Impairment of mechanical ventilation secondary to tonic-clonic activity, increased salivation, increased tracheobronchial

Cryptogenic (idiopathic) (25%–40%): no apparent cause; neurologically normal children; possibly first unprovoked seizure in a child with idiopathic epilepsy

Remote symptomatic (10%–25%): a child with known CNS insult in the past; intraventricular hemorrhage, cerebral palsy, trauma, meningitis

Febrile (20%–30%): sole etiology is temperature >38.4°C; some classify as "acute symptomatic"

Acute symptomatic (25%–50%): a child with an acute illness (trauma, meningitis, hypoxia, hyponatremia) OR a child in whom anticonvulsants have been discontinued or decreased in a child known to have seizures (physician directed, noncompliance)

Progressive neurologic disorder (2%–6%): neurodegenerative disorders, neurocutaneous syndromes (neurofibromatosis, Sturge-Weber, tuberous sclerosis)

**Figure 5.4** Distribution of status epilepticus in children. Adapted from: Maytal J, Shinnar S, Moseh SL, Alvarez LA. Low morbidity and mortality of status epilepticus in children. *Pediatrics.* 1989;83(3):323–331.

secretions, and increased $O_2$ consumption by tissues all contribute. The combination of seizure activity and hypoxia in turn causes a decrease in brain ATP activity, a decrease in glucose, and an increase in lactic acidosis. Acidosis and hypoxia superimposed on ongoing seizure activity lead to impaired cardiovascular function, decreased cardiac output, and hypotension. The acidosis of SE is mixed respiratory and metabolic. The metabolic component is primarily due to the buildup of lactic acid secondary to impaired tissue oxygenation and perfusion in the face of increased metabolic needs and energy expenditure.[96]

In the first 30 minutes of seizure activity, there is massive catecholamine release and sympathetic discharge. This results in an increase in heart rate, blood pressure, central venous pressure, cerebral blood flow, and serum glucose. After 30 minutes of generalized tonic-clonic activity, blood pressure begins to drop, and cerebral blood flow, although still increased above baseline, drops to the point where it might be unable to supply adequate substrate and $O_2$ to meet increased cerebral metabolic demands. This results in impaired cortical oxygenation.[96]

Systemic effects of prolonged seizure activity include increase in body temperature, decrease in serum glucose, increase in serum potassium level, and elevations in creatine phosphokinase. As a result of muscle breakdown, myoglobinuria and acute renal failure can ensue.[96]

The mainstays of management involve continuous attention to the ABCs of resuscitation to prevent systemic and cerebral hypoxia. The goals are to maintain adequate vital function to prevent systemic complications, terminate the seizure activity as quickly as possible while minimizing morbidity from treatment, and evaluate and treat the underlying cause of SE.[96]

The risk of respiratory failure is high throughout the entire resuscitation and can be due to the seizure activity itself, the medications used to terminate seizures, and postictal hypoventilation. Proper position of the patient supine on the bed with the head in midline or left lateral decubitus positioning to prevent aspiration of emesis is essential. The use of a neck/shoulder roll for airway positioning, a jaw-thrust maneuver, or the placement of an oral or nasal airway are often all that is needed to open an obstructed upper airway. One hundred percent $O_2$ via a nonrebreather mask should be initiated in all patients. Suction equipment and an appropriately sized bag-mask device should be immediately available at the bedside.

Next, an IV line should be placed and blood drawn as previously outlined. If hypoglycemia is documented, 0.5 to 1 g/kg of glucose should be given as a bolus, either as 2 to 4 mL/kg of D25, or 5 to 10 mL/kg of D10. Glucagon can be given via the intramuscular route if no IV access has been established.[96] Tubes of blood can be drawn and set aside in case further evaluation is required.

After the initial resuscitative measures have been accomplished, specific therapy aimed at terminating seizure activity and preventing its recurrence should begin. (See Table 5-7.) Benzodiazepines are the first-line drugs for the treatment of SE. As a class, they act rapidly and are highly effective. Most children will stop seizing with 1 or 2 doses. All benzodiazepines cause some degree of respiratory depression, which can be reduced by slowing infusion rates and waiting appropriate intervals before giving additional doses. Lorazepam and diazepam have rapid onsets of action, with median times to end of seizure of 2 and 3 minutes, respectively. Lorazepam has a much longer duration of action secondary to its smaller volume of distribution and produces less respiratory depression. Effective brain levels can continue for 12 to 24 hours. For these reasons it is favored as the initial treatment of SE in most centers.[91]

In the absence of intravenous access, rectal diazepam (Diastat) can be initiated at a dose of 0.5 mg/kg. Respiratory depression is not commonly seen via this route, probably because of slightly slower absorption, which makes this a good medication to use at home and in the field to safely terminate seizure clusters or SE. Diazepam is rapidly redistributed, and seizures can recur in 15 to 20 minutes.[91] Therefore, when diazepam is used for SE, it should be immediately followed by a long-acting AED such as fosphenytoin.[95]

Fosphenytoin is a phosphate-ester prodrug of phenytoin, that has several advantages over the parent compound. In contrast to phenytoin, it is compatible with any IV solution and can be administered with dextrose.[91] The side effect profile has been substantially improved by withdrawal of the ethylene glycol base used as a diluent for phenytoin. This decreases the possibility of arrhythmias associated with phenytoin. In addition, it is not tissue toxic and can even be given via the intramuscular route if necessary. In addition, it can be given at triple the maximal rate of phenytoin.[96] In neonates, phenobarbital should be substituted for fosphenytoin, as it has a higher likelihood of terminating seizure activity in this age group. It should be dosed at 20 mg/kg and given at maximal rate of 0.5 to 1 mg/kg per minute. The combination of a benzodiazepine plus phenobarbital in a neonate carries a significant risk of respiratory depression and apnea. Hypotension can also occur. Respiratory and hemodynamic support should be immediately available.

If seizure activity continues for an additional 5 to 10 minutes, a second dose of benzodiazepine should be given.[91,96,97] The managing physician should remain alert to the possible ongoing need for airway intervention, as cumulative doses of benzodiazepines carry higher rates of respiratory depression. If the child has had 1 or 2 ap-

propriate doses of benzodiazepine plus loading with either fosphenytoin or phenobarbital and seizure activity has persisted, the child should be considered to be in refractory SE. Most of these patients will need to be paralyzed, intubated, and mechanically ventilated. They require careful monitoring (including continuous EEG monitoring) in a critical care setting.

Refractory SE can be very difficult to terminate, and there is no consensus as to the optimal management of these patients. Figure 5.3 outlines the various pharmacologic interventions currently in favor. Larger prospective studies need to be done using these drugs to better define the optimal management strategy for the pediatric patient. Pentobarbital, a short-acting barbiturate, has been used for some time to terminate SE. However, there are significant complications associated with the ongoing use of this drug, including hypotension, myocardial depression, low cardiac output, and delayed neurologic recovery.[91,96] For these reasons, many centers have switched to treating refractory SE with the water-soluble benzodiazepine midazolam as a continuous infusion. It is lipophilic at physiologic pH, has a rapid onset of action, and quickly passes the blood-brain barrier. The major advantage of midazolam is the absence of significant cardiovascular depression, especially in comparison with pentobarbital. It is unclear why patients who have not previously responded to other benzodiazepines respond to midazolam, but small initial studies show promising success rates.[96,98,99]

Propofol is another highly effective, lipid-soluble drug. It is a nonbarbiturate anesthetic with hypnotic and anticonvulsant properties, a rapid onset of action, and quick recovery times. A few case reports and small studies have reported cessation of seizure activity or inducement of burst suppression after a propofol bolus followed by continuous infusion. Known side effects include bradycardia, apnea, and hypotension with rapid infusion. It has less cardiorespiratory depression than pentobarbital. Some case reports have described unexplained acidosis, and further study of this drug is warranted.[96]

The newest drug in the armamentarium for refractory SE is valproic acid. It has been recently approved by the US Food and Drug

Administration for use in SE. The drug is known to be effective in partial and generalized epilepsy syndromes in childhood. It can be administered IV as a bolus of 15 to 20 mg/kg and used as a continuous infusion at a rate of 5 mg/kg per hour. In one study involving 41 children, SE was successfully terminated in 78% of cases. Two thirds of the patients responded within 6 minutes of the initial bolus. The biggest advantage of valproic acid is that it is significantly less sedating than the other drugs mentioned and has an excellent cardio-vascular profile. Clinical trials to date have been limited.[96]

Children with SE should be transferred to a facility capable of providing pediatric critical care. These patients belong in a critical care unit where they can be monitored for the development of cerebral and systemic complications of SE. Consultation with a pediatric neurologist is essential in the ongoing management and follow-up care of these patients.

## KEY POINTS

### Management of Seizures

- ABCs (airway, breathing, circulation).
- Cardiorespiratory and pulse oximetry monitoring.
- Obtain vascular access.
- Perform rapid glucose test and treat hypoglycemia.
- Terminate seizure.
- Evaluate and treat underlying cause.

## THE BOTTOM LINE

### Central Nervous System Disorders

- Rapid identification of CNS disorders requires a thorough history and physical examination along with diagnostic testing.
- A common complication of CNS disorders is respiratory failure, which must be recognized and treated.
- Seizures are common presenting complaints for CNS disorders, and parents must be given anticipatory guidance on how to handle seizure recurrences.

## Check Your Knowledge

1. A child presents to the ED with lethargy after consuming 3 oz of his mother's perfume. Which of the following studies is the most helpful bedside test for the evaluation of this patient's altered mental status?
   - A. Hemoglobin
   - B. Serum electrolytes
   - C. Serum glucose
   - D. Toxicology screen

2. Of the following options, which is the best method for acutely lowering increased ICP?
   - A. Hyperoxygenation
   - B. Intravenous steroids
   - C. Midline positioning of the neck
   - D. Mild hyperventilation

3. All of the following are common complications of bacterial meningitis except:
   - A. Acute renal failure
   - B. Seizures
   - C. SIADH
   - D. Subdural effusion

4. All of the following are criteria of simple febrile seizures except:
   - A. Age 6 months to 5 years
   - B. Associated with no neurologic deficit
   - C. Fever greater than 40°C
   - D. Lasting less than 15 minutes

## References

1. Christian CW, Taylor AA, Hertle RW, Duhaime A. Retinal hemorrhages caused by accidental household trauma. *J Pediatr.* 1999;135:125–127.
2. Mei-Zahav M, Uziel Y, Raz J, Ginot N, Wolach B, Fainmesser P. Convulsions and retinal haemorrhage: should we look further? *Arch Dis Child.* 2002;86(5):334–335.
3. Gilliland MG, Luckenbach MW. Are retinal hemorrhages found after resuscitation attempts? A study of the eyes of 169 children. *Am J Forensic Med Pathol.* 1993;14(3):187–192.
4. Odom A, Christ E, Kerr N et al. Prevalence of retinal hemorrhages in pediatric patients after in-hospital cardiopulmonary resuscitation: a prospective study. *Pediatrics.* 1997;99:E3.
5. Duhaime AC, Christina CW, Rorke LB, Zimmerman RA. Nonaccidental head injury in infants—"the shaken baby syndrome." *N Engl J Med.* 1998;338:1822–1829.
6. Belay ED, Bresee JS, Holman RC, Khan AS, Shahriari A, Schonberger LB. Reye's syndrome in the United States from 1981 through 1997. *N Engl J Med.* 1999;340(18):1377–1382.
7. Monto AS. The disappearance of Reye's syndrome—a public health triumph. *N Engl J Med.* 1999;340(18):1423–1424.
8. Orlowski JP. Whatever happened to Reye's syndrome? Did it ever really exist? *Crit Care Med.* 1999;27(8):1582–1587.
9. Gauthier M, Guay J, Lacroix J, Lortie A. Reye's syndrome: a reappraisal of diagnosis in 49 presumptive cases. *Am J Dis Child.* 1989;143:1181–1185.
10. Kim D, Buchanan S, Noonan G, McGeehin M. Treatment of children with elevated blood lead levels. *Am J Prev Med.* 2002;22(1):71.
11. Rutledge SL, Atchison J, Bosshard NU, Steinmann B. Case report: liver glycogen synthase deficiency—a cause of ketotic hypoglycemia. *Pediatrics.* 108;2001:495–497.
12. Birkhahn R, Fiorini M, Gaeta TJ. Painless intussusception and altered mental status. *Am J Emerg Med.* 17(4);1999:345–347.
13. American Academy of Pediatrics, Committee on Infectious Diseases (1999–2000). Possible association of intussusception with rotovirus vaccination. *Pediatrics.* 1999;104:575.
14. Mazzola CA, Adelson PD. Critical care management of head trauma in children. *Crit Care Med.* 2002;30:S393–401.
15. Jacinto SJ, Gieron-Korthals M, Ferreira JA. Predicting outcome in hypoxic-ischemic brain injury. *Pediatr Clin N Am.* 2001;48:647–660.
16. White JR, Farukhi Z, Bull C et al. Predictors of outcome in severely head-injured children. *Crit Care Med.* 2001;29(3):534–540.
17. Levi L, Guilburd JN, Bar-Yosef G et al. Severe head injury in children—analyzing the better outcome over a decade and the role of major improvements in intensive care. *Childs Nerv Syst.* 1998;14(4–5):195–202.
18. Prasad MR, Ewing-Cobbs L, Swank PR, Kramer L. Predictors of outcome following traumatic brain injury in young children. *Pediatr Neurosurg.* 2002;36(2):64–74.
19. Mandel R, Martinot A, Delepoulle F et al. Prediction of outcome after hypoxic-ischemic encephalophathy: a prospective clinical and electrophysiologic study. *J Pediatr.* 2002;141(1):45–50.

20. Luerssen TG, Klauber MR, Marshall LF. Outcome from head injury related to patient's age: a longitudinal prospective study of adult and pediatric head injury. *J Neurosurg.* 1988;68: 409–416.

21. Margolis LH, Shaywitz BA. The outcome of prolonged coma in childhood. *Pediatrics.* 1980; 65:477–483.

22. Gold R. Epidemiology of bacterial meningitis. *Infect Dis Clin N Amer.* 1999;13:515–526.

23. Kaplan S. Clinical presentations, diagnosis, and prognostic factors of bacterial meningitis. *Infect Dis Clin N Amer.* 1999;13:579–594.

24. Lipton JD, Schafermeyer RW. Evolving concepts in pediatric bacterial meningitis—Part I: pathophysiology and diagnosis. *Ann Emerg Med.* 1993;22(10):1602–1615.

25. Lipton JD, Schafermeyer RW. Evolving concepts in pediatric bacterial meningitis—Part II: current management and therapeutic research. *Ann Emerg Med.* 1993;10:1616–1629.

26. Green SM, Rothrock SG, Clem KJ. Can seizures be the sole manifestation of meningitis in febrile children? *Pediatrics.* 1993;93:527–534.

27. Negrini B, Kelleher K, Wald E. Cerebrospinal fluid findings in aseptic versus bacterial meningitis. *Pediatrics.* 2000;105:316–319.

28. Corless CE, Guiver M, Borrow R et al. Simultaneous detection of Neisseria meningitidis, Haemophilus influenzae, and Streptococcus pneumoniae in suspected cases of meningitis and septecemia using real-time PCR. *J Clin Microbiol.* 2001;39:1553–1558.

29. Robinson CC, Willis M, Meagler A et al. Impact of rapid polymerase chain reaction results on management of pediatric patients with enteroviral meningitis. *Pediatr Infect Dis J.* 2002;21: 283–286.

30. Rauf S, Roberts N. Supportive management in bacterial meningitis. *Infec Dis Clin N Am.* 1999;13:647–659.

31. Horga MA, Fine A. West Nile virus. *Pediatr Infect Dis J.* 2001;20:801–802.

32. Whitley RJ, Gnann JW. Viral encephalitis: familiar infections and emerging pathogens. *Lancet.* 2002;359(9305):507–513.

33. Cherry JK, Shields WD. Encephalitis and meningoencephalitis. In: Feigin RD, Cherry JD, eds. *Textbook of Pediatric Infectious Disease.* 4th ed. Philadelphi, Pa: WB Saunders; 1998:457–468.

34. Pritz T. Herpes simplex encephalitis. *eMed J.* 2001;2:1–11. Available at: www.emedicine.comemergtopic 247.htm.

35. Ressler JA, Nelson M. Central nervous system infections in the pediatric population. *Neuroimaging Clin N Am.* 2000;10:427–443.

36. Rotbart HA. Enteroviral infections of the central nervous system. *Clin Infect Dis.* 1995;20:971–981.

37. Leonard JR, Moran CJ, Cross DT III, Wippold FJ II, Schlesinger Y, Storch GA. MR imaging of herpes simplex type 1 encephalitis in infants and young children: a separate pattern of findings. *AJR.* 2000;174:1651–1655.

38. Shian WJ, Chi CS. Epstein-Barr virus encephalitis and encephalomyelitis: MR findings. *Pediatr Radiol.* 1996;26:690–693.

39. Bales JF. Human herpesviruses and neurological disorders of childhood. *Semin Pediatr Neurol.* 1999;6:278–287.

40. Abgrall S, Rabaud C, Costagliola D. Incidence and risk factors for toxoplasmic encephalitis in human immunodeficiency virus-infected patients before and during the highly active antiretroviral therapy era. *Clin Infect Dis.* 2001;33: 1747–1755.

41. Bales JF. Viral infections of the central nervous system. In Berg BO (ed). *Principles of Child Neurology.* New York, Ny: McGraw Hill; 1996: 839–858.

42. Rajnik M, Ottolini MG. Serious infections of the central nervous system: encephalitis, meningitis, and brain abscess. *Adolesc Med.* 2000;11:401–425.

43. Linder SL, Winner P. Pediatric headache. *Med Clin North Am.* 2001;85:1037–1053.

44. Burton LJ, Quinn B, Pratt-Cheney JL, Pourani M. Headache etiology in a pediatric emergency department. *Pediatr Emerg Care.* 1997;13:1–4.

45. Lewis DW, Qureshi F. Acute headache in children and adolescents presenting to the emergency department. *Headache.* 2000;40:200–203.

46. Lewis DW. Headache in the pediatric emergency department. *Semin Pediatr Neurol.* 2001;8:46–51.

47. Childhood Brain Tumor Consortium. The epidemiology of headache among children with brain tumor. *J Neuro-Oncol.* 1991;10:31–46.

48. Edgeworth J, Bullock P, Bailey A, Gallagher A, Crouchman M. Why are brain tumors still being missed? *Arch Dis Child.* 1996;74:148–151.

49. Chu ML, Shinnar S. Headaches in children younger than 7 years of age. *Arch Neurol.* 1992; 49:79–82.

50. Forsyth R, Farrell K. Headache in childhood. *Pediatr Rev.* 1999;20:39–45.

51. Maytal J, Bienkowski RS, Patel M, Eviatar L. The value of brain imaging in children with headaches. *Pediatrics.* 1995;98:413–416.

52. Medina LS, Pinter JD, Zurakowski D, Davis RG, Kuban K, Barnes PD. Children with headaches: clinical predictors of surgical space-occupying lesions and the role of neuroimaging. *Radiology.* 1997;202:819–824.

53. Rossi LN, Vassella F. Headache in children with brain tumors. *Childs Nerv Syst.* 1989;5:307–309.

54. Al-Jarallah A, Al-Rifai MT, Riela AR, Roach ES. Nontraumatic brain hemorrhage in children: etiology and presentation. *J Child Neurol.* 2000;15: 284–289.

55. Lin CL, Loh JK, Kwan AL, Howng SL. Spontaneous intracerebral hemorrhage in children. *Kaohsiung J Med Sci.* 1999;15:146–151.

56. Livingstonn JH, Brown JK. Intracerebral haemorrhage after the neonatal period. *Arch Dis Child.* 1996;61:538–544.

57. Jakobsson KE, Saveland H, Hillman J et al. Warning leak and management outcome in aneurysmal subarachnoid hemorrhage. *J Neurosurg.* 1996;85:995–999.

58. Wright RR, Mathews KD. Hypertensive encephalopathy in childhood. *J Child Neurol.* 1996;11:193–196.

59. Giannoni C, Sulek M, Friedman EM. Intracranial complications of sinusitis: a pediatric series. *Am J Rhinol.* 1998;12:173–178.

60. Sames TA, Storrow AB, Finkelstein JA, Magoon MR. Sensitivity of new generation computed tomography in subarachnoid hemorrhage. *Acad Emerg Med.* 1996;3:16–20.

61. Sidman R, Connolly E, Lemke T. Subarachnoid hemorrhage diagnosis: lumbar puncture is still needed when the computed tomography scan is normal. *Acad Emerg Med.* 1996;3:827–831.

62. Kirkpatrick M, Engleman H, Minns RA. Symptoms and signs of progressive hydrocephalus. *Arch Dis Child.* 1989;64:124–128.

63. Fenichel GM. Increased intracranial pressure. In: Fenichel GM, ed. *Clinical Pediatric Neurology: A Signs and Symptoms Approach.* 3rd ed. Philadelphia, Pa: WB Saunders; 1997:91–117.

64. Key CB, Rothrock SG, Falk JL. Cerebrospinal fluid shunt complications: an emergency medicine perspective. *Pediatr Emerg Care.* 195;11: 265–273.

65. Garton HJL, Kestle JRW, Drake JM. Predicting shunt failure on the basis of clinical symptoms and signs in children. *J Neurosurg.* 2001;94:202–210.

66. Cantrell P, Fraser F, Pilling D, Carty H. The value of baseline CT head scans in the assessment of shunt complicationis in hydrocephalus. *Pediatr Radiol.* 1993;23:485–486.

67. Iskandar BJ, McLaughlin C, Mapstone TB, Grabb Pa, Oakes WJ. Pitfalls in the diagnosis of ventricular shunt dysfunction radiology reports and ventricular size. *Pediatrics.* 1998;101:1031–1036.

68. Kontny U, Hofling B, Gutjahr D et al. CSF shunt infections in children. *Infection.* 1993; 21:89–92.

69. Whitehead WE, Kestle JRW. The treatment of cerebrospinal fluid shunt infections. *Pediatr Neurosurg.* 2001;35:205–210.

70. Andersson PB, Rando TA. Neuromuscular disorders of childhood. *Curr Opin Pediatr.* 1999;11: 497–503.

71. Berg BO. The clinical evaluation. In Berg BO, ed. *Principles of Child Neurology.* New York, Ny: McGraw Hill; 1997:5–22.

72. Fenichel GM. The hypotonic infant. In: Fenichel GM, ed. *Clinical Pediatric Neurology: A Signs and Symptoms Approach.* 3rd ed. Philadelphia, Pa: WB Saunders; 1997:153–175.

73. Nagaraja D, Verma A, Tahy AB, Kumar MV, Jayakumar PN. Cerebrovascular disease in children. *Acta Neurol Scand.* 1994;90:251–255.

74. Fenichel GM. Hemiplegia. In: Fenichel GM, ed. *Clinical Pediatric Neurology: A Signs and Symptoms Approach.* 3rd ed. Philadelphia, Pa: WB Saunders; 1997:253–266.

75. Fenichel GM. Paraplegia and quadriplegia. In: Fenichel GM, ed. *Clinical Pediatric Neurology: A Signs and Symptoms Approach.* 3rd ed. Philadelphia, Pa: WB Saunders; 1997:267–283.

76. Fenichel GM. Flaccid limb weakness in childhood. In: Fenichel GM, ed. *Clinical Pediatric Neurology: A Signs and Symptoms Approach.* 3rd ed. Philadelphia, Pa: WB Saunders; 1997:176–203.

77. Verity CM, Golding J. Risk of epilepsy after febrile convulsions: a national cohort study. *BMJ.* 1991;303:1373–1376.

78. Nelson K, Ellenberg J. Prognosis in children with febrile seizures. *Pediatrics.* 1978;61:720–727.

79. Trainor JL. Evaluating and treating the child with a febrile seizure. *Clin Ped Emerg Med.* 1999;1:13–20.

80. Trainor JL, Hampers LC, Krug SE, Listernick R. Children with first-time simple febrile seizures are at low risk of serious bacterial illness. *Ac Emerg Med.* 2001;8:781–787.

81. Shah SS, Alpern ER, Swerling L et al. Low risk of bacteremia in children with febrile seizures. *Arch Pediatr Adolesc Med.* 2002;156:469–472.

82. Teach S, Geil P. Incidence of bacteremia, urinary tract infections, and unsuspected bacterial meningitis in children with febrile seizures. *Ped Emerg Care.* 1999;15:9–12.

83. Provisional Committee on Quality Improvement Subcommittee on Febrile Seizures. Practice parameter: the neurodiagnostic evaluation of the child with a first simple febrile seizure. *Pediatrics.* 1996;97:769–772, 773–765.

84. Green SM, Rothrock SG, Glem KJ et al. Can seizures be the sole manifestation of meningitis in febrile children? *Pediatrics.* 1993;92:527–534.

85. Committee on Quality Improvement, AAP et al. Practice parameter: long-term treatment of the child with simple febrile seizures. *Pediatrics.* 1999;103(6)1–7.

# CHAPTER REVIEW

86. Knudsen FU. Recurrence risk after first febrile seizure and effect of short-term diazepam prophylaxis. *Arch Dis Child.* 1985;60:1045–1049.

87. Hirtz D, Ashwal S, Berg A et al. Practice parameter: evaluating a first nonfebrile seizure in children. *Neurology.* 2000;55(5): 616–623.

88. Verity CM, Ross EM, Golding J. Epilepsy in the first 10 years of life: findings of the child health and education study. *Brit J Med.* 1992;305:857–861.

89. Williams J, Grant M, Jackson M et al. Behavioral descriptors that differentiate between seizure and nonseizure events in a pediatric population. *Clin Pediatr.* 1996;243–49.

90. Reuter D, Brownstein D. Common emergent pediatric neurologic problems. *Emerg Med Clin North Am.* 2002;20(1):155–176.

91. Pellock JM. Status epilepticus in children: update and review. *J Child Neurol.* 1994;9(suppl): 2S27–2S35.

92. Hauser WA. Status epilepticus: epidemiologic considerations. *Neurology.* 1990;40(suppl 2):9–13.

93. DeLorenzo RJ, Pellock JM, Towne AR, Boggs JG. Epidemiology of status epilepticus. *J Clin Neurophysiol.* 1995;12(4):316–325.

94. DeLorenzo RJ, Towne AR, Pellock JM, Ko D. Status epilepticus in children, adults and the elderly. *Epilepsia.* 1992;33(suppl. 4):S15–S25.

95. Gastauf H, ed. *Dictionary of Epilepsy. Part I: Definitions.* Geneva, Switzerland: World Health Organization, 1973.

96. Hanhan UA, Fiallos MR, Orlowski JP. Status epilepticus. *Pediatr Clin North Am.* 2001;48(3): 1–12.

97. Maytal J, Shinnar S, Moseh SL et al. Low morbidity and mortality of status epilepticus in children. *Pediatrics* 1989; 83(3):323–331.

98. Pellock JM. Use of midazolam for refractory status epilepticus in pediatric patients. *J Child Neurol.* 1998;13:581–587.

99. Igartua, J, Silver P. Maytal J, Sagy M. Midazolam coma for refractory status epilepticus in children. *Crit Care Med* 1999;27:1–10.

## CASE SUMMARY 1

A 2-year-old boy presents to the emergency department with a history of being found sleeping in the garage. His parents were unable to awaken him. He was last seen 30 minutes earlier when his mother let him out to play in the backyard. On examination, the child is somnolent but responds to deep pain. His airway is open and respirations are unlabored. Vital signs include a respiratory rate of 36 breaths per minute, a heart rate of 116 beats per minute (bpm), blood pressure of 98/64, and temperature of 38.0°C. Oxygenation saturation measured by pulse oximetry is 98% on room air. Further examination reveals no focal deficits.

1. What is the most important initial intervention in this patient?
2. What are possible etiologies?
3. What should you include in the management and evaluation?

The initial management of this patient should include attention to his airway. As he is breathing well on his own, $O_2$ should be provided for support to maximize $O_2$ delivery to the tissues. The child described in this case is of toddler age—the age of exploration. Leading causes of altered mental status at this age include infection, poisonings, and trauma. Because he was well appearing with no prodrome and no history of fever, infection becomes less likely. Because the child was found in the garage, a search for the possible toxins in that area should be undertaken. To that end, tests assessing any potential metabolic derangement and hypoglycemia might be helpful. The vital signs in this patient are normal, the neurologic examination is nonfocal, and the laboratory values show a metabolic and anion gap (serum sodium minus the sum of chloride plus bicarbonate) acidosis, thus narrowing the differential to methanol, ethanol, and ethylene glycol. Because oxalate crystals are seen in the urine and are associated with ethylene glycol, a major ingredient found in antifreeze, poisoning by this substance is the most likely diagnosis.

CASE SUMMARY 2

A 3-month-old boy is brought in by his mother, who says that he is "fussy and not acting right." He was found to be sleepy after returning from a visit to his aunt's home. He is cranky during the examination yet otherwise lethargic. The patient is afebrile with a respiratory rate of 20 breaths per minute, a heart rate of 74 bpm, a blood pressure of 110/70, and the pupils are 4 mm bilaterally and briskly reactive. The only abnormality on examination is a small 2-cm hematoma on the occiput, which, according to his mother, was sustained in a fall from a couch.

1. What are your concerns for this patient?
2. What should be done immediately?

This patient has an unexplained hematoma on the occiput and an acute alteration in mental status. Head injury, either accidental and unwitnessed or nonaccidental, should be at the top of your list. The vital signs, while normal for an adult, are abnormal for an infant: the blood pressure is too high and the pulse is too low. The combination of a high blood pressure, a low pulse, and irregular respirations (Cushing triad) is a finding compatible with increased ICP. Coupled with an altered mental status, this presentation requires immediate intervention. This patient should be electively intubated, making sure not to use pharmacologic agents that raise ICP. Routine hyperventilation for long-term control is contraindicated, but mild hyperventilation is still recommended for acute increases in ICP. Once stabilized, a good secondary assessment should be done, including a good ophthalmoscopic examination to look for retinal hemorrhages. A CBC, urinalysis, and liver function test should be done because occult intra-abdominal injury with resultant blood loss can accompany these injuries. A CT scan of the head without contrast will be helpful in finding any acute or chronic subdurals, or both.

CASE SUMMARY 3

A 3-month-old girl presents with fever, fussiness, and poor feeding. She is irritable and difficult to console but is breathing comfortably on her own and maintaining a good airway. Vital signs include a respiratory rate of 36 breaths per minute, heart rate of 120 bpm, a blood pressure of 90/58 torr, temperature of 39.2°C, and oxygen saturation of 98% on room air. Her fontanel appears full and her neck appears supple. Capillary refill time is 2 seconds. The remainder of the examination is nonfocal.

1. Which examination findings in this child are consistent with the diagnosis of meningitis?
2. What is the most important therapy to deliver at this time?
3. What are possible complications?

The infant is manifesting many of the classic aspects of an acute presentation of bacterial meningitis. The patient is irritable, highly febrile, and has a bulging fontanel. The fact that the patient has a supple neck should not dissuade the examiner from the overall impression of meningitis. Children younger than 18 months frequently lack sufficient neck musculature to manifest nuchal rigidity. Because the patient is well oxygenated and at present has stable vital signs, the most pressing intervention is the rapid delivery of intravenous antibiotics. With a Gram-positive organism with morphology consistent with *S pneumoniae* on Gram stain, cefotaxime or ceftriaxone, and vancomycin, should be started. Potential complications of meningitis include seizures, SIADH, and increased ICP.

# CHAPTER REVIEW

A 3-year-old boy presents to his physician after his parents witness episodes of "clumsiness" with repeated falling. He has had no headache, fever, or neck pain. Initial assessment reveals an alert, playful child with no increased work of breathing and pink extremities. Vital signs include a respiratory rate of 20 breaths per minute; blood pressure of 90/60 heart rate of 118 bpm, and temperature of 37°C. On further examination, pupils are 5 mm bilaterally, briskly reactive, but with vertical nystagmus. Strength is equal and 5/5 in all extremities. He is unsteady while walking, with his feet placed wide apart.

**1.** *What is the most appropriate imaging study for this patient?*

Neurologic evaluation revealed that this boy had normal pupils with normal extraocular movements. His fundi could not be examined due to poor cooperation. Vertical nystagmus was present when he looked up to the right. He had 5/5 equal strength in all of his extremities. He walked with a tilt to the right and a wide-based gait. Due to his abnormal neurologic examination, a cranial CT was ordered and revealed a midline posterior fossa tumor.

A 13-year-old boy presents with a sudden onset of excruciating headache. He has not been ill recently, does not have a history of headaches, and has no recent history of fever or trauma. Family history is negative for migraines. Vitals signs include a respiratory rate of 20 breaths per minute, heart rate of 98 bpm, blood pressure of 106/68, and a temperature of 37.0 C. Examination reveals an uncomfortable white male teenager complaining of severe headache. Neurologic examination is nonfocal and remarkable only for terminal neck flexion tenderness. No papilledema is noted.

**1.** *What is the appropriate management strategy for this patient?*

Due to the excruciating headache, the boy received an immediate noncontrast CT. As his examination showed terminal neck flexion tenderness, he was empirically started on cefotaxime 50 mg/kg IV prior to the CT scan. CT revealed a large subarachnoid hemorrhage confirmed by lumbar puncture, which yielded 53,000 red blood cells and only 41 white blood cells with a negative Gram stain. Cultures of CSF were negative for 48 hours. A cerebral aneurysm from the posterior aspect of the circle of Willis was detected by cerebral angiography. Neurosurgical consultation was arranged, and definitive clipping of the aneurysm was conducted.

**CASE SUMMARY 6**

A 2-year-old previously healthy child with a generalized clonic seizure is brought to the emergency department by EMS. The parents estimate that he had been having a seizure for 5 minutes prior to arrival of the paramedics at the scene. Paramedics noted that the child was having a generalized seizure and was blue around the lips. The patient was placed on 100% $O_2$ by face mask, and a rapid assay for glucose was 80 mg/dL. Rectal diazepam was administered and the child continues to seize on arrival in the emergency department.

1. *What is the most important initial intervention for this patient?*
2. *What medications can be used to stop the seizure?*
3. *What are some of the possible etiologies of this child's seizure?*

The most important intervention in a seizing child is assessment of the ABCs. This includes opening the airway, suctioning, applying 100% $O_2$, and placing the child on cardiac monitors. Then, there are several drugs that can be used initially to stop the seizure, including rectal diazepam, IV lorazepam, or IV diazepam. The workup should be based on further history and physical examination. Possible etiologies include infection, toxins, metabolic causes (e.g., hypoglycemia), trauma, or tumor.

**CASE SUMMARY 7**

A 26-month-old boy is brought to the emergency department by his parents after a generalized clonic seizure at home. The child had been previously healthy and, other than feeling a little warm before the seizure, had not been ill. The seizure lasted 5 minutes, and the parents report that he turned pale. The parents are not aware of any trauma or ingestion. The child slept on the ride to the hospital, awoke at triage, and is crying vigorously as you approach. Vital signs include a respiratory rate of 32 breaths per minute, heart rate of 170 bpm, blood pressure of 95/65, and temperature of 39.8°C. The history reveals that the child has had no previous seizures and has a normal developmental history. Upper respiratory symptoms started the day of presentation. His physical examination reveals clear rhinorrhea, an erythematous pharynx without exudates, and clear lungs. He is alert and playing with toys on the bed.

1. *What is the most appropriate initial intervention?*
2. *What is the most appropriate diagnostic evaluation at this time?*
3. *What is appropriate counseling for the parents?*

In a child who has had a seizure but is now awake, the most important aspect is a detailed and complete history and physical examination. Because these are unremarkable, the most likely diagnosis for this patient is a simple febrile seizure. Diagnostic studies should be those that can provide a clue to the etiology of the fever. Appropriate counseling for the parents includes instructions on what to do in the event of a recurrent seizure, explanation of the risks of recurrent seizures and epilepsy, and reassurance of the benign nature of simple febrile seizures.

# chapter 6

# Metabolic Disease

Nicole Glaser, MD
Gregory M. Enns, MB, ChB
Nathan Kuppermann, MD, MPH, FAAP

## Objectives

1 Describe the epidemiology, clinical features, and emergency management of diabetes mellitus, adrenal insufficiency, syndrome of inappropriate secretion of antidiuretic hormone, water intoxication, and diabetes insipidus.

2 Describe the fluid and electrolyte problems associated with these conditions.

3 Discuss the clinical features and emergency management of metabolic diseases of the newborn and young child.

## Chapter Outline

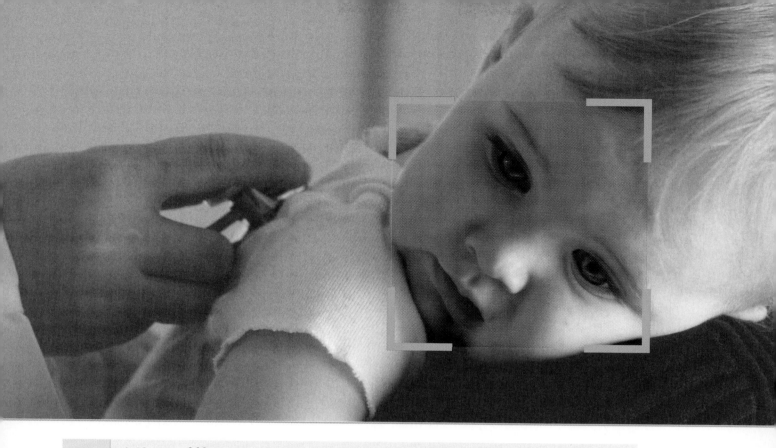

**CASE SCENARIO 1**

A 10-year-old boy presents to the emergency department with altered mental status and a 2-week history of polyuria and weight loss. He complains of abdominal pain. On examination, he appears lethargic, has a respiratory rate of 36 breaths per minute, a heart rate of 150 beats per minute (bpm), a blood pressure of 80, and a temperature of 37.9°C. Pulse oximetry is 97% on room air. He has dry mucous membranes, a normal abdominal examination, and a neurologic examination remarkable only for lethargy. Bedside rapid glucose measurement is above the upper limit of the glucose meter (>500 mg/dL).

1. What therapeutic actions must be taken immediately?
2. What laboratory tests would you order?
3. What is the most important potential complication?

## Introduction

The emergency management of endocrine and metabolic disorders presents diagnostic and therapeutic challenges. Many of these disorders, such as congenital adrenal hyperplasia and inborn errors of metabolism, occur relatively infrequently. Nonetheless, rapid and appropriate intervention is necessary to prevent complications. Awareness of key clinical and laboratory findings that differentiate endocrine and metabolic disorders from other entities with similar presenting features is essential.

## Diabetic Ketoacidosis

Diabetic ketoacidosis (DKA) is the most important complication of type 1 diabetes mellitus (DM1) (Figure 6.1). DKA occurs when insulin concentrations are low relative to the concentrations of counter-regulatory hormones, particularly glucagon. This imbalance results in hyperglycemia along with the breakdown of fat to form ketone bodies, eventually resulting in acidosis. DKA occurs in 25% to 40% of children with new onset of DM1, and repeat hospital visits for DKA occur in

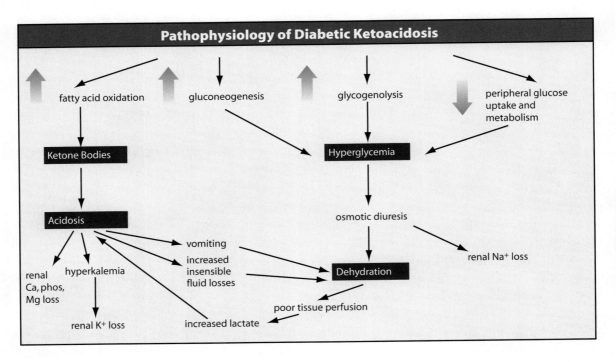

**Pathophysiology of Diabetic Ketoacidosis**

fatty acid oxidation

gluconeogenesis

glycogenolysis

peripheral glucose uptake and metabolism

Ketone Bodies

Hyperglycemia

Acidosis

osmotic diuresis

renal Ca, phos, Mg loss

hyperkalemia

vomiting

increased insensible fluid losses

Dehydration

renal Na+ loss

renal K+ loss

increased lactate

poor tissue perfusion

**Figure 6.1** Diabetic ketoacidosis.
Source: Behrman RE, Kliegman RM. *Nelson Essentials of Pediatrics,* 4th Edition. Philadelphia, Pa: W.B. Saunders; 2002:185. Reprinted with permission.

children with known DM1 at a rate of 8 to 15 episodes per 100 person-years.[1,2] This depends on how DKA is defined, but it is less common than in the past because a greater emphasis is now placed on tighter glucose control. Causes of DKA in children with known DM1 include episodes of intercurrent illness (31%) and presumed omission or incorrect administration of insulin injections (69%); bacterial infections (13%) are less common causes of DKA in children.[3]

## Clinical Features

DKA is characterized by hyperglycemia and elevated serum ketone concentrations resulting in acidosis. Inadequate insulin concentrations allow the partial oxidation of fatty acids to form ketone bodies. This process then results in acidosis with an elevated anion gap. The hyperglycemia results in osmotic diuresis with polyuria, polydipsia, and eventual dehydration. Presenting features of DKA include a history of polyuria, polydipsia, nausea, and vomiting. Abdominal pain and intestinal ileus are common features and can mimic an acute abdomen. In a patient with clinical signs of dehydration, the pres-

ence of polyuria helps differentiate DKA from gastroenteritis and other causes of dehydration. Acidosis results in compensatory tachypnea, and a characteristic fruity (acetone) breath odor can often be detected. Because the hyperosmolar state allows for the relative preservation of intravascular volume, signs of dehydration can be less obvious than in dehydrated patients with more normal serum osmolality. Alterations in mental status can range from disorientation to depressed consciousness. This alteration of mental status is typically due to dehydration

## YOUR FIRST CLUE

**Signs and Symptoms of DKA**

- History of polyuria, polydipsia, weight loss, nausea, and vomiting
- Signs of dehydration
- Breath with fruity odor
- Abdominal pain
- Tachypnea
- Lethargy

and acidosis but can also reflect more serious underlying pathology. Rarely, children with DKA present to the ED with clinically apparent cerebral edema,[4] as well as cerebral infarctions or thromboses.

## Complications

Complications of DKA typically occuring during treatment include hypokalemia and hypoglycemia. Hypocalcemia, hypophosphatemia, and hypomagnesemia can also occur but are much less common. Of the more serious complications of DKA, clinically apparent cerebral edema is the most frequent, occurring in approximately 1% of DKA episodes. Cerebral edema is the most important diabetes-related cause of mortality in children with DM1.[5]

Although cerebral edema can occur prior to hospital treatment of DKA, this complication more typically occurs several hours after initiation of therapy. The clinical presentation of cerebral edema can take different forms. Typically, patients with cerebral edema complain of headache and exhibit alterations in mental status. As this condition progresses, signs of increased intracranial pressure and/or impending cerebral herniation can develop. These include obtundation, papilledema, pupillary dilation or anisocoria, blood pressure variability, bradycardia, and apnea.

Other complications of DKA are rare, but include cerebral infarctions or thrombosis, acute renal tubular necrosis leading to renal failure, pancreatitis, and intestinal necrosis.

## Diagnostic Studies

DKA is defined by hyperglycemia (serum glucose concentration generally >200 mg/dL), acidosis (venous pH generally <7.25 or serum bicarbonate <15 mEq/L), and the presence of ketones in the serum or urine. Electrolyte abnormalities also occur as a result of urinary losses and shifts due to acidosis. High serum concentrations of potassium are often found early in the course of DKA but might be normal or low if the ketoacidotic state is prolonged. Intracellular potassium concentrations, however, are characteristically depleted, as are total body concentrations of sodium, phosphate, calcium, and magnesium. Although to-

---

## THE CLASSICS

**Laboratory Findings in DKA**
- Hyperglycemia
- Metabolic acidosis
- Ketonemia or ketonuria

---

tal body sodium is depleted, the degree of depletion is less than that suggested by the measured serum sodium measurement, because the measured sodium concentration is also artificially depressed due to hyperglycemia. Blood urea nitrogen (BUN) concentrations are usually elevated due to prerenal azotemia. The white blood cell count is often elevated and frequently left-shifted as a result of the ketoacidotic state alone.[3] It is generally unnecessary to search for a source of infection beyond performing a careful physical examination unless fever or other specific signs of infection are present.

## Differential Diagnosis

The presenting symptoms and signs of DKA can initially be confused with gastroenteritis or other gastrointestinal disorders that present with vomiting and abdominal pain. Infections such as pneumonia, meningitis, and urinary tract infections also rarely present with metabolic acidosis, tachypnea, and altered mental status, or can be a cause for the development of DKA. The history of polyuria despite clinical dehydration, absence of diarrhea, and presence of tachypnea with fruity breath odor, however, should differentiate DKA from these other entities even before laboratory tests are ordered. DKA must also be differentiated from hyperglycemic hyperosmolar nonketotic coma (HHNK), which presents with severe hyperglycemia (serum glucose concentration >600 mg/dL, and often >1,000 mg/dL), profound dehydration, and a depressed level of consciousness, but mild or no ketosis. HHNK can in fact represent one extreme in a continuum of presentations of DKA, although HHNK is rare in children. It occurs more frequently in patients with type 2 rather than type 1 diabetes and in children with neurological abnormalities that lead to abnormal thirst mechanisms or limited access to liquids.

## Management

Therapeutic measures for the treatment of DKA include replacement of fluid deficits, correction of acidosis and hyperglycemia via insulin administration, replacement of depleted electrolytes, and monitoring for complications.

## Fluid Replacement

Optimal fluid management for DKA has been a subject of great controversy, mainly due to theoretical concerns about the role of fluid administration in contributing to cerebral edema. Available evidence, however, does not confirm a primary role for fluid administration in causing this complication. Recent evidence suggests that children who present with low partial pressures of arterial carbon dioxide ($Paco_2$) and high BUN and those treated with bicarbonate are at higher risk for cerebral edema. Fluid administration does not appear to have a significant role after adjusting for these factors.[4] Appropriate restoration of perfusion and hemodynamic stability, therefore, should not be compromised by theoretical concerns associated with fluid administration.

The average degree of dehydration in children with DKA is approximately 7%; therefore, most children with DKA should not manifest signs of severe dehydration. If there is evidence of poor perfusion or significant hypovolemia, however, the clinician should administer an intravenous fluid bolus of 20 mL/kg of isotonic fluid (normal saline (NS) or lactated Ringers (LR)) over 30 to 60 minutes to restore intravascular volume and renal perfusion. More rapid administration of fluids is indicated if signs of shock are present. NS or LR fluid boluses can be repeated if necessary to restore perfusion, but care should be taken to avoid overly rapid replacement of fluid deficits. If there is no overt clinical evidence of hypovolemia or hypoperfusion, intravenous fluid management should be less aggressive, and deficits should be replaced gradually. Once perfusion has been restored, 1/2–3/4 normal saline (3/4 NS must be made by the pharmacy or nursing staff by adding 37 mEq of NaCl to one liter of 1/2 NS) can be used to replace the remaining deficit (to avoid hyperchloremia with excessive NS infusion). The rate of fluid infusion should be calculated such that the remaining fluid deficit is replaced over a 48-hour period, in addition to maintenance fluids.

## Hyperglycemia

Insulin should be administered via continuous intravenous infusion at a dosage of 0.1 U/kg per hour. An initial intravenous bolus of 0.1 U/kg of insulin is sometimes given before the initiation of the continuous infusion, but this practice is controversial and little data exist to determine whether the initial bolus is beneficial (or potentially harmful). Therefore, this initial insulin bolus should be considered optional. When serum glucose concentrations fall below 250 to 300 mg/dL during treatment, glucose should be added to the intravenous fluids to ensure that hypoglycemia does not occur. The insulin infusion rate generally should not be decreased until the severity of acidosis has diminished (serum bicarbonate concentration >17 mEq/L).

## Acidosis

The acidosis in DKA is due primarily to two factors: the production of ketone bodies due to relative insulin deficiency, and the accumulation of lactate due to dehydration. Insulin treatment promotes the metabolism of ketone bodies and halts further ketone production. The administration of intravenous fluids treats the dehydration. This therapeutic combination is generally sufficient for the correction of acidosis. In the past, bicarbonate administration has been a therapeutic option of great controversy. Recent studies, however, have suggested an association between bicarbonate therapy and cerebral edema.[4] This association was maintained after adjusting for markers of disease severity and potential confounding factors such as the degree of acidosis and hyperglycemia. Bicarbonate therefore should be avoided unless there is symptomatic hyperkalemia or the acidosis is severe enough to cause hemodynamic instability not responsive to other therapeutic measures.

### Electrolyte Imbalances

Regardless of the serum potassium concentration at presentation, total body potassium is depleted in patients with DKA. With treatment of DKA, serum potassium concentrations can decrease rapidly as insulin and fluid therapy improve the state of acidosis and potassium shifts to the intracellular space. Therefore, once adequate urine output is established and normal or low serum potassium levels are confirmed, potassium should be added to the intravenous fluids. Potassium replacement should be given as a mixture of potassium chloride and potassium phosphate at a concentration of 30 to 40 mEq/L. Although severe hypophosphatemia occurs rarely in children with DKA, the consequences can be devastating. Therefore, it seems prudent to administer part of the potassium as a phosphate, although thorough study of this issue is lacking.

### Monitoring and Treating Complications

Glucose concentrations should be measured hourly using a bedside glucose monitor while the patient has moderate to severe acidosis (serum bicarbonate concentration <17 mEq/L) (Figure 6.2). A reasonable rate of decline in the serum glucose concentration is <100 mg/dL per hour. With the initial infusion of intravenous fluids and restoration of renal perfusion, however, glucose concentrations might decrease more rapidly. Electrolyte concentrations should be measured every 3 to 4 hours, or more frequently if severe abnormalities are present.

Careful monitoring is essential for early detection of complications of DKA, particularly cerebral edema. Neurologic and mental

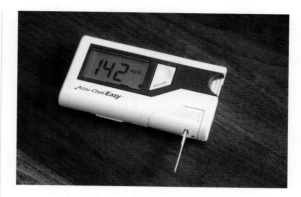

**Figure 6.2** Bedside glucose monitor.

status should be checked hourly. Although the effectiveness of cerebral edema treatment interventions in this setting is unclear, patients who have deterioration in mental status generally should be treated for presumed cerebral edema and subsequently evaluated using computed tomography or magnetic resonance imaging. It is commonly believed that early treatment with hyperosmolar agents such as mannitol in patients with DKA and cerebral edema can be beneficial, but clinical data are lacking.[6] Because the potential adverse effects of mannitol in this setting are relatively minor, mannitol should be strongly considered. Glucocorticoids are of unclear usefulness for DKA-related cerebral edema. Greater hyperventilation has been shown to be associated

## KEY POINTS

### Management of DKA and Its Complications

- Hypovolemia: 20 mL/kg NS followed by $\frac{1}{2}$–$\frac{3}{4}$ NS to replace deficit over 48 hours.

- Hyperglycemia: Insulin at 0.1 U/kg/hr.

- Acidosis: Avoid bicarbonate administration.

- Hypokalemia: 30–40 mEq/L as mixture of potassium chloride and potassium phosphate.

- Hypoglycemia: Monitor glucose and electrolytes frequently.

- Cerebral edema: Mannitol, controlled hyperventilation.

with a greater likelihood of adverse outcome of DKA-related cerebral edema; therefore, aggressive therapeutic hyperventilation probably should be avoided.[6]

## Hypoglycemia in Diabetic Children

Although mild episodes of hypoglycemia are a relatively frequent occurrence in children with DM1, severe hypoglycemic events (with associated loss of consciousness or seizure) are uncommon, occurring at a rate of approximately 5 to 19 events per 100 patient-years.[1,2,7] Risk factors for severe hypoglycemia include younger age, lower hemoglobin A1c values, underinsurance, and higher daily insulin dose.[1,7] Causes of severe hypoglycemia include missed meals, exercise, and errors in insulin dosing. In almost 40% of such episodes, however, no cause can be determined.[7]

### Clinical Features

Diabetic patients with hypoglycemia can present with seizures, loss of consciousness, combativeness, or other mental status alterations. Alterations in mental status such as irritability, combativeness, lethargy, or disorientation might persist for prolonged periods after serum glucose concentrations have been restored to normal. Other neurologic deficits, such as hemiplegia or aphasia, might also occur following such episodes and can likewise persist for many hours.[8]

### Diagnostic Studies and Management

In a diabetic patient with altered mental status, glucose concentration should be assessed rapidly with a bedside glucose meter. Hypoglycemia (<40 to 60 mg/dL) should be corrected as rapidly as possible with an intravenous infusion of 0.5 gm/kg of dextrose. This can be accomplished by infusing 5 mL/kg of D10 in an infant, 2 mL/kg of D25 in a toddler, or 1 mL/kg of D50 in older children (the product of the mL/kg and the D% should equal 50). In the event that intravenous access cannot be established rapidly, glucagon (1 mg) can be given via intramuscular injection. If neurologic or mental status abnormalities persist for prolonged periods after correction of hypoglycemia, other possibilities should be considered, such as toxicologic causes as well as other intracranial pathology.

## Hypoglycemia in Nondiabetic Children

Hypoglycemia can result from excessive insulin production (insulinoma, hyperinsulinism) or decreased concentrations of counter-regulatory hormones (deficiencies of growth hormone, cortisol, or both). Hypoglycemia can also result from inborn metabolic errors that impair gluconeogenesis, glycogenolysis, or fatty acid oxidation. Unsuspected hypoglycemia can be found when patients present to the emergency department with episodes of acute illness. A recent study revealed that a substantial percentage (28%) of these patients had previously undiagnosed fatty acid oxidation defects (19%) or endocrine disorders (9%).[9]

### Clinical Features

Infants with hypoglycemia can present with jitteriness, poor feeding, lethargy, hypotonia, hypothermia, apneic episodes, or seizures. Symptoms of hypoglycemia in infants might also be subtle and less obvious than those in older children. In older children, symptoms of hypoglycemia include headaches; vision changes; mental status changes such as confusion, lethargy, irritability, or anxiety; and seizures. Adrenergic symptoms such as palpitations, sweating, pallor, and tremulousness are usually also present. Hypoglycemia should be considered in all patients presenting with unexplained alterations in mental status, seizure, or loss of consciousness, and a routine bedside test for hypoglycemia should be part of pediatric resuscitation procedures.[10]

### Diagnostic Studies

If hypoglycemia is suspected, a rapid glucose test should be performed using a bedside blood

**Signs and Symptoms of Hypoglycemia**
- Infants: Jitteriness, poor feeding, lethargy, hypotonia, hypothermia, apnea, seizures.
- Children: Headaches, altered mental status, diaphoresis, pallor, palpitations, tremulousness, seizure.

**Differential Diagnosis of Hypoglycemia**
- Toxins (oral hypoglycemic agents, β-blockers, ethanol)
- Hypopituitarism
- Adrenal insufficiency
- Fatty acid oxidation defects
- Hyperinsulinism
- Ketotic hypoglycemia
- Sepsis

glucose meter. A glucose concentration <50 mg/dL should be considered abnormal and treated. If the bedside test reveals a low glucose concentration, a confirmatory venous sample should be sent to the laboratory for measurement with greater accuracy. Treatment for hypoglycemia, however, should not be delayed while awaiting results. At the time that the confirmatory sample is drawn, an additional serum sample (enough for special studies) should be obtained for future measurement of hormone concentrations and other biochemical measures. It is essential that this sample be drawn at the time of the hypoglycemic event. Without information from this sample, it is usually impossible to determine the cause of the hypoglycemic episode. If hypoglycemia is confirmed, the measurements to be obtained on the initial sample include serum insulin, cortisol, and growth hormone concentrations, as well as serum ketones, lactate, and free fatty acid concentrations.[11] A toxicologic evaluation for ethanol, salicylates, propranolol, and oral hypoglycemic agents should also be considered. Remaining serum from the initial sample should be stored for additional biochemical testing if necessary. Finally, a urine sample should also be obtained and tested for ketones and reducing substances. An additional sample of urine should likewise be stored for future testing.

## Differential Diagnosis

There are many possible causes of hypoglycemia, and a discussion of all etiologies is beyond the scope of this chapter. Among the more frequent causes (in patients without diabetes mellitus) are toxic ingestions (oral hypoglycemic agents, β-blockers, ethanol), sepsis, hypopituitarism, adrenal insufficiency, fatty acid oxidation defects, hyperinsulinism, and ketotic hypoglycemia. Analysis of the initial serum sample will differentiate among many of these entities and will indicate whether additional analyses are necessary to investigate less frequent causes of hypoglycemia.

## Management

Hypoglycemia should be corrected as rapidly as possible with an intravenous infusion of 0.5 g/kg of glucose (dextrose). This can be accomplished by infusing 5 mL/kg of D10 in an infant, 2 mL/kg of D25 in a toddler, and 1 mL/kg of D50 in older children (the product of the mL/kg and the D% should equal 50). Subsequently, an intravenous infusion of 10% dextrose at 1.5 times maintenance rates should be provided to maintain glucose concentrations in the normal range and reverse the catabolic state. If adrenal insufficiency is known or strongly suspected and adequate samples have been set aside for further study, intravenous hydrocortisone should be given (50 mg for children younger than 4 years and 100 mg for children older than 4 years).

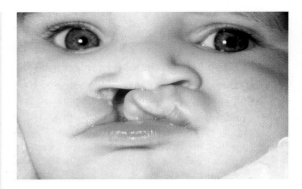

**Figure 6.3** Midline facial malformation.

# Adrenal Insufficiency/ Congenital Adrenal Hyperplasia

Adrenal insufficiency can be primary (resulting from processes directly affecting the adrenal gland) or secondary (resulting from deficiency of adrenocorticotropic hormone [ACTH]). In either primary or secondary adrenal insufficiency, the clinical manifestations result from lack of adequate production of cortisol. In primary adrenal insufficiency, additional symptoms and electrolyte abnormalities result from the lack of mineralocorticoids. Congenital adrenal hyperplasia (CAH) is the predominant cause of adrenal insufficiency in infants, with a prevalence of 1 in 10,000 births. In older children, acquired adrenal insufficiency is uncommon and can result from a variety of conditions.

## Clinical Features

The clinical manifestations of adrenal insufficiency differ depending on the age of the patient and whether the adrenal insufficiency is primary (CAH, Addison disease) or secondary (hypopituitarism, pituitary suppression by exogenous glucocorticoids). Infants with adrenal insufficiency typically present with poor feeding and poor weight gain, vomiting, and lethargy. On physical examination, infants might manifest hypotension and tachycardia.

Hyperkalemia can result in cardiac arrhythmias. Depending on the infant's karyotype and the specific metabolic defect, the genitalia of infants with CAH might appear ambiguous or normal. In the most common type of CAH (21 hydroxylase deficiency), female infants will manifest ambiguous genitalia, but male infants have normal genitalia. Infants of both sexes with CAH can be hyperpigmented, particularly in the genitalia, due to high concentrations of ACTH. Infants with secondary adrenal insufficiency due to hypopituitarism might manifest midline facial malformations and male infants might have a microphallus (**Figure 6.3**).

In older children, adrenal insufficiency typically presents with a history of fatigue, anorexia, weight loss, and postural hypotension. Patients might complain of chronic or acute abdominal pain. Patients with secondary adrenal insufficiency also might have a history of neurosurgical procedures, central nervous system (CNS) tumors, congenital malformations causing hypopituitarism, or a history of prolonged use of glucocorticoid medications. Adrenal insufficiency causing hypoglycemia has been reported even in patients using inhaled glucocorticoid preparations.[12] On physical examination, patients are typically hypotensive and have tachycardia. Abdominal tenderness can be present and might mimic an acute abdomen. Hyperpigmentation (due to high concentrations of ACTH) can be present in primary, but not in secondary, adrenal insufficiency.

**Signs and Symptoms of Adrenal Insufficiency**

- Infants: Poor feeding, underweight, vomiting, lethargy, hypotension, tachycardia, and +/− hyperpigmentation, or ambiguous genitalia.

- Children: Fatigue, weight loss, postural hypotension, +/− hyperpigmentation, and abdominal pain.

- Other clues: History of CNS surgery or tumors, or prolonged corticosteroid or glucocorticoid use.

**Classic Laboratory Findings in Adrenal Insufficiency**

- Primary adrenal insufficiency: Hyperkalemia, hyponatremia, hypoglycemia, and acidosis.

- Secondary adrenal insufficiency: Hypoglycemia.

## Diagnostic Studies

Laboratory evaluation in patients with primary adrenal insufficiency typically reveals hyperkalemia, hyponatremia, hypoglycemia, and acidosis. If hyponatremia is present, an immediate urine sodium should be obtained; a high value would indicate the presence of inappropriate salt wasting, which would narrow the differential substantially to syndrome of inappropriate secretion of antidiuretic hormone (SIADH), adrenal insufficiency, salt-losing nephropathy, and sodium-wasting drugs. Not all patients manifest all of these laboratory abnormalities, however, and the diagnosis cannot be excluded based on the absence of one or more of these findings. BUN and creatinine concentrations can be elevated due to dehydration. In secondary adrenal insufficiency, hyperkalemia and hyponatremia are absent due to preservation of aldosterone production, and hypoglycemia might be the main biochemical abnormality.

If adrenal insufficiency is suspected, a serum sample for measurement of cortisol and ACTH should be drawn prior to glucocorticoid therapy for diagnostic purposes. When CAH is suspected, serum 17-hydroxyprogesterone concentration should also be measured.

## Differential Diagnosis

Most of the symptoms of adrenal insufficiency are nonspecific and can suggest other, more common diagnoses. Adrenal insufficiency in infants might be confused with other illnesses that present with lethargy, vomiting, poor weight gain, hypotension, and tachycardia. These include infections (e.g., sepsis), gastrointestinal disturbances (e.g., pyloric stenosis), congenital heart disease, other metabolic disorders (e.g., inborn errors of metabolism), hematologic disorders (e.g., methemoglobinemia), neurologic diseases (e.g., infantile botulism), or child abuse with intracranial hemorrhage. The presence of hyperkalemia, hyponatremia, and acidosis, as well as ambiguous genitalia (when present) and hyperpigmentation serve to differentiate CAH from these other entities. In older children, mild symptoms of primary adrenal insufficiency might be confused with mononucleosis or anorexia nervosa. More severe symptoms can suggest infections (e.g., sepsis), hematologic disease, or an acute abdomen. Again, the presence of hyperpigmentation and the characteristic laboratory abnormalities serve to differentiate these entities. Secondary adrenal insufficiency can be even more difficult to differentiate from other entities because of the lack of hyperpigmentation and the lack of specific laboratory features other than hypoglycemia. In these cases, a history of CNS tumors, neurosurgical procedures, or congenital CNS malformations, or a history of prolonged exogenous glucocorticoid usage must be relied on to suggest the diagnosis.

## Management

Adrenal insufficiency is treated acutely with fluid resuscitation, administration of dextrose to correct hypoglycemia, and the administration of glucocorticoids. An initial fluid bolus of normal saline (20 mL/kg) should be given rapidly and repeated as necessary to restore perfusion. Following the initial bolus(es), a continuous infusion of normal saline with dextrose (D5 NS) should be given. Intravenous hydrocortisone should be administered immediately (50 mg for children younger than 4 years and 100 mg for children older than 4 years). Hydrocortisone can also be administered by intramuscular injection if there are delays in achieving intravenous access. Symptomatic hyperkalemia or hyperkalemia resulting in ECG changes should be treated with calcium gluconate to reverse the membrane effects of hyperkalemia, then sodium bicarbonate and glucose with insulin to promote the movement of potassium into cells. Albuterol aerosol, which also promotes movement of potassium to the intracellular space, can be considered, but its beta effect can promote arrhythmias.

# Diabetes Insipidus

Diabetes insipidus (DI) is caused by a lack of production of antidiuretic hormone (ADH) (central DI) or resistance to the effect of antidiuretic hormone (nephrogenic DI). The lack of the antidiuretic effect leads to an inability to concentrate urine and large urinary losses of free water, resulting in polyuria and polydipsia symptoms. If patient is denied access to water or the thirst sensation is abnormal, hypernatremia and dehydration will result. Nephrogenic DI generally presents in infancy, but central DI can occur at any age and might be secondary to CNS tumors, meningitis or encephalitis, head trauma, post neurosurgery, or in the setting of other conditions that affect the CNS, including histiocytosis and leukemia.[13]

## Clinical Features

Characteristic symptoms of DI are intense polyuria and polydipsia. Older children, who generally have an intact sense of thirst and access to fluids, typically present without any significant abnormalities on physical examination. Infants, however, frequently present with poor weight gain, poor growth, hyperthermia, and signs of dehydration.

## Diagnostic Studies

Because they do not have unlimited access to fluids, infants generally will manifest hypernatremia and hyperosmolality at presentation. The urine is inappropriately dilute (<300 mOsm/L), establishing the diagnosis. Older children usually do not manifest hypernatremia or hyperosmolality unless their fluid intake is restricted or their thirst mechanism is abnormal. For these children, a carefully monitored water deprivation study is often necessary to establish the diagnosis. CNS imaging and laboratory testing are necessary to search for the cause of DI.

## Differential Diagnosis

Similar symptoms of polyuria and polydipsia occur most commonly in diabetes mellitus but can also occur in psychogenic polydipsia. Patients with hypercalcemia or hypokalemia can also have impaired urinary concentrating ability.

## Management

Patients without hypernatremia and dehydration do not require acute intervention for DI but should undergo evaluation to determine the underlying cause. Patients with hypernatremic dehydration and hyperosmolality should be treated with fluid resuscitation. This includes an initial 20 mL/kg fluid infusion of NS to restore perfusion, followed by subsequent slow correction due to concerns of cerebral edema with overly aggressive free water replacement. An endocrinologist should arrange for further diagnostic testing and initiation of treatment as soon as possible.

# Syndrome of Inappropriate Secretion of Antidiuretic Hormone

The syndrome of inappropriate (i.e., excessive) secretion of antidiuretic hormone

(SIADH) is characterized by hyponatremia and low serum osmolality. These features occur in the absence of dehydration or volume depletion and are associated with inappropriately elevated urine sodium concentration and urine osmolality. SIADH can occur in a variety of clinical settings, most frequently CNS disorders such as meningitis or encephalitis, cerebral hemorrhage, head trauma, or following neurosurgical procedures. Less commonly, SIADH can be due to pharmacologic agents, neoplasms outside of the CNS, or other causes.[14] Iatrogenic hyponatremia due to excessive ADH action can also be seen in patients treated with desmopressin acetate (DDAVP) who drink excessive amounts of fluids.

## Clinical Features

Patients with SIADH frequently will not manifest symptoms of hyponatremia until the serum sodium concentration falls below 120 mEq/L. Below this level, symptoms might include anorexia, nausea, vomiting, lethargy, irritability, or confusion. With severe hyponatremia, seizures or coma can occur.

### YOUR FIRST CLUE

**Signs and Symptoms of SIADH**
- Hyponatremia in association with head trauma, cerebral hemorrhage, or other intracranial pathology.
- Absence of clinical signs of dehydration.
- Signs of hyponatremia (nausea, vomiting, altered level of consciousness, seizure).

## Diagnostic Studies

A diagnosis of SIADH is supported by the finding of hyponatremia (serum sodium concentration below 130 mEq/L), along with elevated urine osmolality (>100 mOsm/L) and urine sodium concentration (>18–20 mEq/L). BUN concentrations are typically normal or low. Apparent hyponatremia due to abnormalities in the measurement of serum sodium concentration caused by hyperlipidemia or hyperproteinemia should be excluded as well as hyponatremia due to the osmotic effect of hyperglycemia.

### THE CLASSICS

**Laboratory Findings in Patients With SIADH**
- Hyponatremia (<130 mEq/L).
- High urine osmolality (>100 mOsm/L).
- Inappropriately high urine sodium concentration (>18–20 mEq/L).

## Differential Diagnosis

Other causes of hyponatremia include water intoxication, hyponatremic dehydration, adrenal insufficiency, renal failure, diuretic use, nephrotic syndrome, cirrhosis, congestive heart failure, severe hypothyroidism, cystic fibrosis, and the cerebral salt-wasting syndrome. Many of these diagnoses can generally be excluded based on the absence of signs of dehydration and absence of edema, lack of hyperkalemia, low or normal BUN and creatinine concentrations, and inappropriately elevated urine osmolality and urine sodium concentration. The cerebral salt-wasting syndrome is partic-

### WHAT ELSE?

**Differential Diagnosis of SIADH**
- Water intoxication
- Hyponatremic dehydration
- Adrenal insufficiency
- Renal failure
- Diuretic use
- Nephrotic syndrome
- Hypothyroidism
- Cystic fibrosis
- Cerebral salt-wasting syndrome
- Congestive heart failure
- Cirrhosis

ularly important to exclude because it occurs in clinical settings similar to those in which SIADH is frequent.[14] Cerebral salt-wasting is characterized by renal sodium and fluid loss. Signs of dehydration and hypovolemia are generally present, and BUN concentrations are typically elevated, helping to differentiate this syndrome from SIADH.

## Management

Patients with mild or no symptoms should be treated with restriction of fluids alone. Patients with severe neurologic symptoms (extreme lethargy, coma, or seizures) should be treated with 3% saline (3% sodium chloride) solution to raise the serum sodium concentration to a level of approximately 125 mEq/L. The correct dosage of 3% saline can be calculated by assuming that 12 mL/kg of 3% saline will increase the serum sodium concentration by 10 mEq/L. The minimal dosage required to achieve a serum concentration of 125 mEq/L should be infused over a 1-hour period. Serial serum sodium measurements, which take approximately 1 hour, can significantly compromise the clinician's ability to titrate 3% saline, because an excessive amount might have been given by the time the test results are available. Rapid bedside serum sodium testing is preferable. Treatment with 3% saline solution should continue only until neurologic symptoms improve. Further treatment can then be accomplished with fluid restriction. Rapid correction of hyponatremia should be avoided because of the risk of central pontine myelinolysis. A careful search for an underlying cause for SIADH is necessary if the cause is not known.

## Water Intoxication

Water intoxication occurs most frequently in infants when daily water intake is excessive in relation to their daily intake of sodium. This situation occurs most frequently because of inappropriate dilution of infant formulas or misguided supplemental feedings of solute-free water.[15,16] Excess water ingestion during infant swimming lessons has also been a cause of this condition. Less commonly, water intoxication can be seen in patients with psychiatric illness and psychogenic polydipsia, or as a manifestation of child abuse.

### Clinical Features

Clinical manifestations of water intoxication result from hyponatremia. Infants typically present with poor feeding, vomiting, and lethargy. Hypothermia and edema might also be present. With severe hyponatremia, seizures can occur and might be prolonged. It has been suggested that hypothermia can be a specific marker for hyponatremia in infants with a new onset of seizures.[16]

## KEY POINTS

**Management of SIADH**

- Restrict fluids in patients with mild or no symptoms.
- Treat with 3% saline (3% sodium chloride) only in patients with extreme lethargy, coma, or seizures.
- Obtain urine sample to test for osmolarity and/or urine sodium when hyponatremia is found.
- Rapid correction of hyponatremia should be avoided to prevent central pontine myelinolysis.

## YOUR FIRST CLUE

**Signs and Symptoms of Water Intoxication**

Signs and symptoms of hyponatremia with a history of inappropriate dilution of infant formula or water intake include:

- Poor feeding
- Vomiting
- Lethargy
- Seizures
- Hypothermia

## Diagnostic Studies

Hyponatremia (serum sodium concentration <130 mEq/L) is present, and the urine is dilute. Serum potassium, urea nitrogen, and creatinine concentrations are typically normal, and patients are not acidotic, which helps exclude other causes of hyponatremia. Apparent hyponatremia due to abnormalities in the measurement of serum sodium concentration caused by hyperlipidemia or hyperproteinemia, and hyponatremia caused by the osmotic effect of hyperglycemia, should also be excluded.

## Differential Diagnosis

The differential diagnosis of hyponatremia is extensive and includes renal failure, diuretic use, renal tubular defects (renal tubular acidosis), SIADH, adrenal insufficiency (CAH, Addison disease), cystic fibrosis, nephrotic syndrome, cirrhosis, and congestive heart failure. Hyponatremia can also occur in infants or children with gastrointestinal fluid and electrolyte losses when these losses are replaced with free water or other fluids deficient in sodium. This scenario differs, however, from classic water intoxication in that clinical and laboratory features of dehydration are present and the urine is concentrated. A careful history, including feeding practices, and the finding of dilute urine should suggest the diagnosis of water intoxication.

## Management

For infants who are asymptomatic or have mild symptoms of hyponatremia, reinstitution of normal daily sodium and fluid intake is generally all that is required. For infants with severe manifestations of hyponatremia (extreme lethargy, seizures, or coma), treatment with 3% saline solution should be initiated with caution.

**CASE SCENARIO 2**

A 14-month-old girl presents to the emergency department with a one-day history of tactile fever, loss of appetite, and intermittent emesis. This morning, she did not seem interested in her usual breakfast and seemed sleepier than usual. On examination, she has respirations of 40 breaths per minute, a heart rate of 170 bpm, blood pressure of 80/40, and a temperature of 36.0°C. She appears lethargic and has mildly dry mucous membranes and no obvious source of infection. Bedside rapid glucose measurement reveals a blood glucose of 20 mg/dL.

1. *What therapeutic measures must be taken immediately?*
2. *What laboratory tests would you order?*
3. *What complications can occur as part of the disease process and secondary to therapeutic intervention?*

# Metabolic Disease of the Newborn and Young Child

More than 300 human disorders involving various biochemical pathways have been identified (**Figure 6.4**). Because inborn errors of metabolism are individually rare, there is a tendency to consider the possibility of such disorders as a last resort, after more common causes of distress have been excluded. However, the aggregate incidence of inborn errors of metabolism is relatively high, with as many as one child in every 1,000 births being affected. When a child with a metabolic disorder has an acute catastrophic presentation, appropriate therapy must be started immediately because of the high risk of morbidity or mortality if treatment is delayed. Therefore, the physician must consider these disorders in all children who have nonspecific features of distress on initial presentation. Specialized metabolic laboratory testing is required to make a definitive diagnosis of an inborn error of metabolism. Even simple tests, however, such as the measurement of blood gases, glucose, electrolytes, CBC, lactate, and ammonia, and the evaluation of urine for ketones and reducing substances, can provide valuable clues to the presence of an inborn error of metabolism.[17]

## Clinical Features

Most of these disorders are inherited as autosomal recessive traits, although X-linked, maternal (mitochondrial), and autosomal dominant (rarely) inheritance can occur.[18] A detailed family history might reveal the existence of consanguinity or an affected relative with a similar illness, and, therefore, can be of great diagnostic importance. Special attention should be given to familial occurrence of stillbirths, unexplained early deaths, neurologic diseases, developmental regression, or delayed development of any degree or severity. A history of maternal illness in pregnancy can also provide a clue to the presence of an inborn error of metabolism in a child. For example, acute fatty liver of pregnancy might occur in a heterozygous mother carrying a homozygous fetus affected with various fatty acid oxidation disorders.[19]

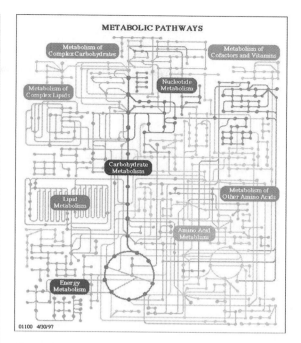

**Figure 6.4** Metabolic pathways.

In general, the onset of symptoms of metabolic disease is postnatal, appearing after an interval of apparent good health, and following an uneventful pregnancy. This interval might be as short as a few hours or as long as several days, months, or even longer. The child might do well until subjected to an event that causes catabolism (infection, fasting, dehydration) or an excessive load of protein or carbohydrates. If the child is exposed to such a stressor, he or she can become seriously ill very suddenly, and can present as a baby with sudden infant death of unexplained etiology. The absence of a normal period, however, does not exclude metabolic disease from diagnostic consideration. Neonatal distress from asphyxia or complications of prematurity can constitute the environmental stress that unmasks an underlying inborn error of metabolism.

Symptoms associated with inborn errors of metabolism tend to be nonspecific. Neonatal irritability and feeding difficulties, associated with uncoordinated sucking and swallowing, might be present. Other gastrointestinal symptoms, including intermittent vomiting, dehydration, and failure to thrive, can also occur. In mildly affected children, symptoms can disappear only to recur in days, weeks, or months. More severely affected infants have inexorable progression from lethargy to coma, to episodic apnea and death if left untreated. Generalized or partial seizures occur in some instances. Various other neurologic symptoms might also be present, including developmental regression, tone abnormalities, tremulousness, lethargy, and a weak cry. The EEG might suggest nonspecific diffuse encephalopathy.

Most inherited metabolic diseases are not associated with specific abnormal physical findings. Nevertheless, certain aspects of the physical examination should be emphasized. Hepatomegaly can be seen in carbohydrate disorders (galactosemia, glycogen storage disease, hereditary fructose intolerance), peroxisomal disorders, tyrosinemia, lysosomal storage disorders, inborn errors of bile acid metabolism, neonatal hemochromatosis, some forms of congenital lactic acidosis, and organic acidemias and fatty acid oxidation defects that might have a Reye-like syndrome presentation. Abnormal, brittle hair can occur in some urea cycle defects (argininosuccinicaciduria, citrullinemia), holocarboxylase synthetase deficiency, and Menkes syndrome (pili torti). An unusual odor has been noted in several metabolic disorders, including tyrosinemia (rancid butter), branched-chain ketoaciduria (maple syrup), isovaleric acidemia or multiple acyl-CoA dehydrogenase deficiency (sweaty feet), and 3-methylcrotonyl-CoA carboxylase deficiency (cat-like urine odor). Ketosis accompanies many of these conditions and will cause the sweet odor of ketone bodies in the urine.

## Diagnostic Studies

The specialized investigations needed to confirm the presence of an underlying metabolic disorder, such as detailed amino acid, organic acid, and acylcarnitine analyses, are performed at only a handful of medical centers. Nevertheless, a diagnosis can at least be suspected, and an inborn error of metabolism disease category reasonably hypothesized, on the basis of simple studies and the clinical presentation.[19] Blood gases, electrolytes, glucose, lactate, ammonia levels, and basic urinalysis often provide the first clues to the existence of an inborn error of metabolism. Because an intercurrent infection might be the stressor that causes symptoms to appear for the first time, a CBC should be obtained and blood and urine cultures strongly considered. Children with urea cycle defects can have normal routine laboratory test results (with the exception of marked hyperammonemia), although a mild respiratory alkalosis might be present. Hyperammonemia can also be seen in organic acidemias and fatty acid oxidation defects. Organic acidemias also feature severe metabolic acidosis with marked anion gap. However, in fatty acid oxidation disorders, hypoketotic hypoglycemia is the general rule, because proper function of the fatty acid oxidation cycle is required for the production of ketone bodies.

Because diagnostic metabolites can disappear or become less apparent after the initiation of therapy, metabolic studies should be obtained as soon as possible (immediately before initiating fluid bolus or other therapy, if possible), although results of such testing typically are not available immediately. Specific metabolic investigations include quantitative

---

## YOUR FIRST CLUE

**Signs and Symptoms of Inborn Errors of Metabolism**

- History of consanguinity
- Irritability
- Feeding difficulties
- Lethargy
- Hypotonia
- Vomiting
- Signs of dehydration
- Failure to thrive
- Hepatomegaly
- Unusual odor
- Brittle hair

---

plasma amino acids, carnitine levels, acyl-carnitine profile, and analysis of urine for organic acids and reducing substances. If the local laboratory does not handle such specimens regularly, collecting and freezing ($-20°C$) blood and urine samples for later distribution to specialist laboratories under the guidance of a metabolism expert might be the key to establishing a diagnosis. Specific enzymatic or DNA tests are often required to make a precise diagnosis.

Many inborn errors of metabolism are associated with high mortality. Blood (5 cc heparinized plasma for metabolic studies and 10 cc whole blood collected in an ethylenedi-amine tetra-acetic acid (EDTA) tube for DNA isolation) and urine specimens should be collected and frozen at $-20°C$ for further metabolic analysis from all children who die unexpectedly from unknown causes. In states that store the newborn screening card, the neonatal blood spot can also be retrieved for further metabolic analysis by tandem mass spectrometry. If an autopsy is performed, portions of muscle, heart, and liver should be snap frozen immediately for possible future analysis. Bile can also be analyzed for the presence of fatty acid oxidation disorders.[20] A skin, diaphragm, and/or lung biopsy also should be obtained for establishing a fibroblast cell line for possible future enzymatic or DNA analyses. With an established diagnosis, the family can obtain accurate genetic counseling for future pregnancies, and additional at-risk family members can be identified.

## Differential Diagnosis

Because the signs and symptoms of inborn errors of metabolism are nonspecific, other causes of acute distress in children, including infection, toxins, trauma, congenital structural brain abnormalities, or cardiopulmonary dysfunction, must be considered in the differential diagnosis. Unless an inborn error is suspected, the condition might be misdiagnosed as having hypoxic-ischemic encephalopathy, intraventricular hemorrhage, sepsis, heart failure, or a gastrointestinal illness such as pyloric stenosis or intestinal obstruction. Therefore, a high index of suspicion is important, because the physician must initiate appropriate therapy without delay (and without a final diagnosis in hand) to decrease morbidity and mortality. In addition, a concomitant acquired disorder can obscure the diagnosis of an inherited metabolic disease. For example, neutropenia can occur in organic acidemias, leading to an increased susceptibility of bacterial infection. The underlying disorder might be missed if an infection is also present and focus is directed solely towards antimicrobial therapy. *Escherichia coli* sepsis frequently supervenes in neonates with galactosemia, and the typical jaundice, liver failure, and vomiting that accompany that disorder might wrongly be ascribed solely to sepsis as well. Other acquired conditions that can complicate the presentation of a metabolic disorder include pulmonary hemorrhage or primary respiratory alkalosis that might occur in urea cycle defects.

---

### THE CLASSICS

**Laboratory Findings in Children With Inborn Errors of Metabolism**

- Hyperammonemia
- Elevated lactate
- Metabolic acidemia
- Ketosis
- Nonketotic (or hypoketotic) hypoglycemia

---

### WHAT ELSE?

**Differential Diagnosis of Inborn Errors of Metabolism**

- Infection
- Toxins
- Trauma
- Congenital structural brain abnormalities
- Shock
- Reye syndrome

---

## Management

Rapid assessment, establishment of vascular access, and administration of appropriate fluids (with dextrose) are priorities in managing patients with inborn errors of metabolism in acute crisis. Dehydration and hypoglycemia should be treated with boluses of NS and dextrose solutions, respectively. Maintenance intravenous fluids should then be started to prevent recurrence of hypoglycemia and hypovolemia and stop the catabolic spiral. Administration of 10% dextrose (with electrolytes based on the child's weight) at 1.5 times maintenance is usually adequate. General supportive measures (maintenance of oxygenation and acid/base balance, treatment of infection) should, of course, be provided. Intravenous carnitine (100 mg/kg) may be beneficial in certain organic acidemias and fatty acid oxidation disorders but is usually used after consultation with a metabolic specialist. The child might need immediate admission to an intensive care unit for further monitoring and other procedures (e.g., hemodialysis).

In children who are already known to have an inborn error of metabolism, the importance of listening closely to the history provided by the parents or regular caregiver must be stressed. A child with a metabolic disorder can appear relatively well but might decompensate rapidly. If such a child is not maintaining adequate fluid and caloric intake, or "does not seem to be his usual self," or both, the metabolic specialist should be contacted, and intravenous fluids with dextrose should be administered even in the absence of documented hypoglycemia or other markers of metabolic imbalance. The goal in such cases is to provide therapy in a timely manner to prevent a metabolic crisis.

## KEY POINTS

### Management of Patients With Inborn Errors of Metabolism

- Measure serum glucose, ammonia, and lactate in infants and children with lethargy.
- Obtain urinalysis (evaluate for infection or ketones).
- Begin fluid resuscitation with normal saline for dehydration.
- Treat hypoglycemia.
- Contact metabolic specialist immediately once diagnosis is suspected.

## THE BOTTOM LINE

### Issues in the Diagnosis and Management of Inborn Errors of Metabolism

- Maintain a high index of suspicion, especially in the presence of hypoglycemia, metabolic acidosis, ketosis, or hyperammonemia.
- Although specialized tests are needed to arrive at a final diagnosis, simple laboratory studies often provide the first clues to the presence of an inborn error of metabolism.
- Early detection and treatment are essential.

## Check Your Knowledge

1. All of the following are associated with increased risk of cerebral edema in a child with DKA except:
   A. High BUN concentration at presentation
   B. High serum glucose concentration at presentation
   C. Low $P_{CO_2}$ at presentation
   D. Treatment with sodium bicarbonate

2. All of the following are clues to the presence of adrenal insufficiency except:
   A. Acanthosis nigricans
   B. Ambiguous genitalia
   C. Hyperpigmentation
   D. Midline facial defects and microphallus

3. SIADH should be treated with which of the following:
   A. Administration of hydrocortisone
   B. Administration of oral sodium and/or normal saline
   C. Administration of 3% saline if the sodium concentration is <130 mEq/L
   D. Fluid restriction unless the patient is seizing or severely lethargic/comatose

4. Which of the following statements regarding hypernatremia in patients with DI is correct?
   A. Never occurs in infants with DI because of high fluid intake
   B. Occurs in all patients with DI
   C. Rare in older children with DI and normal thirst mechanisms
   D. Should be treated with 3% sodium chloride solution

## References

1. Rewers A, Chase HP, Mackenzie T, et al. Predictors of acute complications in children with type 1 diabetes. *JAMA*. 2002;287: 2511–2518.

2. Levine B, Anderson BJ, Butler DA, et al. Predictors of glycemic control and short-term adverse outcomes in youth with type 1 diabetes. *J Pediatr*. 2001;139:197–203.

3. Flood RG, Chiang VW. Rate and prediction of infection in children with diabetic ketoacidosis. *Am J Emerg Med*. 2001;19:270–273.

4. Glaser N, Barnett P, McCaslin I, et al. Risk factors for cerebral edema in children with diabetic ketoacidosis. *N Engl J Med*. 2001;344(4): 264–269.

5. Edge JA. Cerebral edema during treatment of diabetic ketoacidosis: are we any nearer finding a cause? *Diabetes Metab Res Rev*. 2000;16: 316–324.

6. Marcin JP, Glaser N, Barnett P, et al. Factors associated with adverse outcomes in children with diabetic ketoacidosis-related cerebral edema. *J Pediatr*. 2002;141(6):793–797.

7. Davis EA, Keating B, Byrne GC, Russell M, Jones TW. Hypoglycemia: incidence and clinical predictors in a large population-based sample of children and adolescents with IDDM. *Diabetes Care*. 1997;20:22–25.

8. Pocecco M, Ronfani L. Transient focal neurologic deficits associated with hypoglycemia in children with insulin-dependent diabetes mellitus. *Acta Paediatr*. 1998;87:542–544.

9. Weinstein DA, Butte AJ, Raymond K, Korson MS, Weiner DL, Wolfsdorf JI. High incidence of unrecognized metabolic and endocrinologic disorders in acutely ill children with hypoglycemia. *Pediatr Res*. 2001;49:88A.

10. Losek JD. Hypoglycemia and the ABCs (sugar) of pediatric resuscitation. *Ann Emerg Med*. 2000;35(1):43–46.

11. Lteif AN, Schwenk WF. Hypoglycemia in infants and children. *Endocrinol Metabol Clin*. 1999; 28(3):620–646.

12. Drake AJ, Howells RJ, Shield JPH, et al. Symptomatic adrenal insufficiency presenting with hypoglycemia in children with asthma receiving high-dose inhaled fluticasone propionate. *BMJ*. 2002;324:1081–1083.

13. Maghnie M, Cosi G, Genovese E, et al. Central diabetes insipidus in children and young adults. *N Engl J Med*. 2000;343:998–1007.

14. Albanese A, Hindmarsh P, Stanhope R. Management of hyponatremia in patients with acute cerebral insults. *Arch Dis Child*. 2001;85: 246–251.

15. Bruce RC, Kliegman RM. Hyponatremic seizures secondary to oral water intoxication in infancy: association with commercial bottled drinking water. *Pediatrics*. 1997;100(6):E4.

16. Farrar HC, Chande VT, Fitzpatrick DF, Shema SJ. Hyponatremia as the cause of seizures in infants: a retrospective analysis of incidence, severity and clinical predictors. *Ann Emerg Med*. 1995;26:42–48.

# CHAPTER REVIEW

17. Enns G, Packman S. Diagnosing inborn errors of metabolism in the newborn: laboratory investigations. *NeoReviews.* 2001;2:e192–200.
18. Enns G, Packman S. Diagnosing inborn errors of metabolism in the newborn: clinical features. *NeoReviews.* 2001;2:e183–191.
19. Matern D, Hart P, Murtha AP, et al. Acute fatty liver of pregnancy associated with short-chain acyl-coenzyme A dehydrogenase deficiency. *J Pediatr.* 2001;138:585–588.
20. Rinaldo P, Matern D, Bennett MJ. Fatty acid oxidation disorders. *Annu Rev Physiol.* 2002;64:477–502.

## CASE SUMMARY 1

A 10-year-old boy presents to the emergency department with altered mental status and a 2-week history of polyuira and weight loss. He complains of abdominal pain. On examination, he appears lethargic, has a respiratory rate of 36 breaths per minute, a heart rate of 150 bpm, a blood pressure of 80, and a temperature of 37.9°C. Pulse oximetry is 97% on room air. He has dry mucous membranes, a normal abdominal examination and a neurologic examination remarkable only for lethargy. Bedside rapid glucose measurement is above the upper limit of the glucose meter (>500 mg/dL).

1. What therapeutic actions must be taken immediately?
2. What laboratory tests would you order?
3. What is the most important potential complication?

This child is hypotensive, mainly due to dehydration. Immediate volume resuscitation with boluses of normal saline (20 mL/kg) should be administered to restore perfusion. An insulin infusion should be initiated as soon as possible after intravenous fluid therapy has been initiated.

A reasonable set of initial laboratory tests would include serum electrolytes, a venous blood gas (because $PCO_2$ is a predictor of cerebral edema), and a urine specimen for ketones. Complete blood cell counts are not usually helpful.[3]

Clinically apparent cerebral edema occurs in approximately 1% of children with DKA. Frequent neurologic monitoring is indicated.

CASE SUMMARY 2

A 14-month-old girl presents to the emergency department with a one-day history of tactile fever, loss of appetite, and intermittent emesis. This morning, she did not seem interested in her usual breakfast and seemed sleepier than usual. On examination, she has respirations of 40 breaths per minute, a heart rate of 170 bpm, blood pressure of 80/40, and a temperature of 36.0°C. She appears lethargic and has mildly dry mucous membranes and no obvious source of infection. Bedside rapid glucose measurement reveals a blood glucose of 20 mg/dL.

1. *What therapeutic measures must be taken immediately?*
2. *What laboratory tests would you order?*
3. *What complications can occur as part of the disease process and secondary to therapeutic intervention?*

The child is hypoglycemic and mildly hypotensive. Resuscitation with boluses of 2 mL/kg D25 (or 5 mL/kg D10) to normalize blood glucose should be started without delay, followed by administration of volume (normal saline bolus of 20 mL/kg) until perfusion is restored. Fluids consisting of D10 + sodium chloride 40 mEq/L (roughly D10 1/4 NS) at 1.5 times maintenance should then be started if the child weighs <20 kg (1/2 normal saline may be used for children weighing >20 kg). Appropriate potassium supplementation (usually 1–2 mEq for each 100 mL delivered) is added as needed. Electrolytes must be monitored closely.

Initial studies include electrolytes, glucose, blood gas, CBC, blood and urine cultures, and urine for ketones. Most of the samples can be obtained from the intravenous catheter immediately before fluid resuscitation therapy is initiated. The finding of nonketotic (hypoketotic) hypoglycemia is a clue to the presence of an underlying fatty acid oxidation defect. Metabolic disorders might be unmasked by an infection severe enough to cause catabolism, but an obvious infection or clear exacerbating factor is not always present. Because of the risk of multiorgan system failure, measurement of liver enzymes, BUN, creatinine, and CPK levels can also be helpful. Metabolic studies include lactate, ammonia, plasma amino acids, carnitine levels, acylcarnitine profile, and urine organic acids. Simply freezing aliquots of serum and urine and contacting a metabolic specialist for further guidance with respect to specialized testing is an appropriate alternative if your laboratory does not routinely handle such specimens.

Fatty acid oxidation disorders can progress to multi organ system failure (Reye-like syndrome). Seizures, cardiomyopathy, liver failure, and kidney failure might supervene. There is a significant risk of death.

Secondary to therapeutic interventions, cerebral edema of unclear pathogenesis might occur in some inborn errors of metabolism. Potentially, this complication can also occur if a high rate of relatively dilute dextrose solution (e.g. D5) is used. Therefore, close monitoring of fluid resuscitation and neurologic status is imperative.

# chapter 7

# Environmental Emergencies

Dee Hodge III, MD

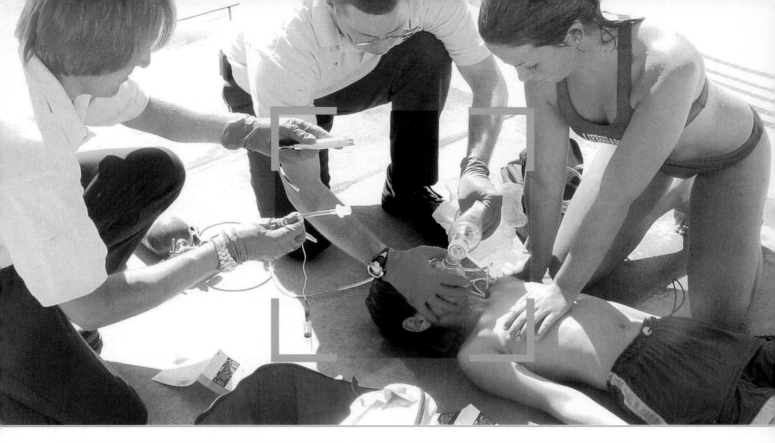

**CASE SCENARIO 1**

A 4-year-old boy is brought to the emergency department after being bitten by a spider a few hours previously at his family's camp site. The child says that the spider was dark but cannot remember any identifying marks. On examination his respiratory rate is 26/min, heart rate is 130 beats per minute (bpm), blood pressure is 100/60, and his temperature is 37°C. He is calm but complaining of pain in the bite area. His right forearm is swollen and erythematous, with two small marks at the center of the wound. His hand is pink, pulses are 2+, and he is able to move his fingers. The remainder of the examination is normal.

1. *What is the differential diagnosis of this spider bite?*
2. *What signs or symptoms would help distinguish the type of spider bite?*
3. *What studies are needed?*
4. *What treatment is necessary?*

## Introduction

Environmental emergencies have become more common as children and adults participate in outdoor activities such as camping, mountain climbing, skiing/snowboarding, hiking, and just enjoying nature. Unfortunately, some of these activities can result in injuries such as envenomations by snakes and spiders, or body temperature disturbances including hyperthermia and hypothermia.

In addition, submersion injuries, which include drowning, have been the second leading cause of unintentional death in young children for a number of years. This chapter will address the diagnosis and treatment of these problems.

## ■ Envenomations

### Snake Bites

In 2001, more than 6,000 snake bites were reported to the American Association of Poison Control Centers, with 26% of them occurring in children.[1] The bites causing the most concern are those that involve the venomous snakes, such as those in the Crotalidae (pit vipers) and Elapidae (coral snakes) families.

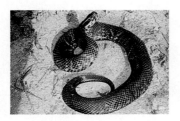
A. Cottonmouth

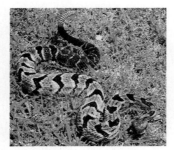
B. Rattlesnake

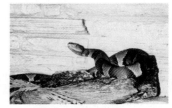
C. Copperhead

**Figure 7.1** Pit vipers.

## Pit Vipers

Pit viper (Crotalidae) envenomation is a rare but important cause of morbidity and mortality in the United States (Figure 7.1). The pit viper family includes rattlesnakes, water moccasins (cottonmouth), and copperheads.

The severity of envenomation varies widely with the species; however, any member of the pit viper family found in North America is capable of inflicting significant damage that requires treatment.

### Clinical Features

Pit viper venoms differ in the relative amounts of their component parts, including myonecrotic enzymes, cardiotoxins, nephrotoxins, hemotoxins, and neurotoxins. Due to these differences, clinical presentations can vary. Envenomation results in extensive capillary leak and local tissue necrosis.

After a major envenomation, the release of vasodilatory compounds, hypovolemia from the loss of integrity of the capillary endothelium, and bleeding can all contribute to the rapid development of circulatory shock.

### Assessment

As in all emergencies, first consider respiratory and circulatory systems (airway, breathing, circulation, the ABCs). In the absence of immediate life-threatening symptoms, demographic variables and physical findings should be considered to assess the severity of the bite. Information regarding the size and species of the snake (if possible), circumstances related to the bite, number of bites inflicted, first aid methods used, time of the bite, and transport time required should be obtained. The severity of the bite should be staged (Table 7-1). In as many as 20% of bites, there is no venom injected ("dry bites").

| TABLE 7-1 Envenomation Staging |
| --- |
| • No Envenomation <br> Occurs in approximately 20% of strikes; no venom has been released, and only fang marks are present. <br><br> • Mild Envenomation <br> Fang mark or marks are present, with edema and tissue necrosis confined to the surrounding area. No clinical or laboratory evidence of systemic effects is present. <br><br> • Moderate Envenomation <br> Edema, bullae, or ecchymoses extending beyond the immediate area of the bite to include a large part of the extremity. Tender adenopathy might be present, depending on the site of the bite. Clinical or laboratory evidence of systemic venom effects might be present, depending on the species. <br><br> • Severe Envenomation <br> Rapid extension of edema, bullae, or ecchymoses involving the entire extremity; shock demonstrated by tachycardia, hypotension, poor perfusion, or change in level of consciousness; elevation of prothrombin time, or creatine kinase; depression of platelet count or fibrinogen. Bites on the thorax, the head, and neck should be assumed to be severe. |

### Management

First aid includes reassurance of the child and caregivers. If the child can be kept quiet, the spread of toxins throughout the body can be lessened. Transportation for definitive medical care should be accomplished as soon as possible. Venom extraction kits based on suction are not harmful and can remove a small amount of the venom if used within 5 minutes of envenomation. Incision of the wound, local ice, electric shock therapy, and venous or arterial tourniquets are not recommended. The caregivers will be anxious even if the child has no envenomation. For many snake bites in children, reassurance, careful observation, serial measurements, and supportive care are all that is necessary.[2]

Place an intravenous line and initiate correction of hypovolemia with 20mL/kg crystalloid. Give a second saline bolus of 20 mL/kg if needed. The persistence of hypotension mandates invasive monitoring and inotropic support in addition to administration of antivenin.

Institute basic and advanced life support as indicated. Obtain appropriate laboratory studies, including a CBC count, prothrombin time, fibrinogen degradation products, platelet count, blood urea nitrogen (BUN), creatine kinase (CK), and urinalysis. Maintain the extremity at heart level. For moderate to severe bites, start a second intravenous line, obtain blood for transfusion, and cross-match before starting infusion of antivenin.

In all snake bites, cleanse the wound area and follow tetanus prophylaxis guidelines. Recent studies question the use of antibiotics in preventing secondary infection. There is a low incidence of infection after pit viper bites, and current evidence does not support the use of prophylactic antibiotics.[3] Administer analgesia as needed for pain. Do not use sedatives, ice, tourniquets, or aspirin.

Measure the extremity circumference at a marked location and recheck every 15 to 30 minutes for 6 hours; after that, check at least every 4 hours for a total of 24 hours. Progression of edema beyond the site of the bite might warrant the use of antivenin even after 12 hours. Repeat the laboratory studies every 6 hours; if significant changes occur, treat the patient with antivenin.[1]

## Use of Crotalidae Antivenin

In moderate to severe envenomations, administer antivenin (**Figure 7.2**). Copperhead bites are often treated without antivenin, but diamondback rattlesnake envenomations are very dangerous and require antivenin therapy. As many as 75 vials of the polyvalent antivenin

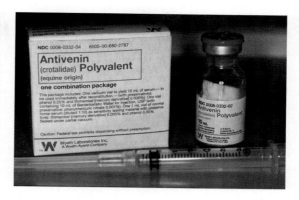

**Figure 7.2** Antivenin.

have been used in a child bitten by a rattlesnake. There are currently two antivenins available. The older polyvalent antivenin, Antivenin Crotalidae Polyvalent (ACP), is derived from horse serum. Acute and delayed hypersensitivity reactions are a risk when using ACP. The newer Crotalidae polyvalent immune Fab antivenin (crotaline Fab, CroFab) is ovine derived, with a much lower risk of both acute and delayed hypersensitivity reactions.[4–8]

The polyvalent antivenin initial dose is based on the envenomation ranking as follows:

- No envenomation: No skin testing, no antivenin
- Mild envenomation: Skin testing followed by 5 vials
- Moderate envenomation: Skin testing followed by 10 vials
- Severe envenomation: Skin testing followed by 15 vials

The improved specificity and small molecular weight of Fab antivenin allow for a different dosing. The dosing schedule is shown in Table 7-2. However, it is important to note that, for both types of antivenin, the dose for children is no different from the dose for adults. Antivenin dosing is based on the severity of the envenomation, not the patient's size or weight.

If acute hypersensitivity reaction occurs, mild symptoms of urticaria, itching, and flushing are treated with a decrease in the antivenin infusion rate and with diphenhydramine. Serious anaphylactic reactions require discontinuation of antivenin, followed

| TABLE 7-2 | Pit Viper Envenomation: How to Use CroFab Antivenin |
| --- | --- |

**Initial Dosing**

- 4 to 6 vials intravenous (IV) over 1 hour (reconstitute each vial with 10 mL sterile water and dilute total planned dose in 250 mL normal saline; start infusion slowly while observing for a reaction)

**Reassessment**

- Reassess coagulation 1 hour after IV CroFab
- Reassess swelling 1 hour after IV CroFab
- Reassess other systemic parameters 1 hour after IV CroFab
- Repeat 2 to 6 vials IV if continued progression (reassess after each dose and repeat if envenomation syndrome continues to progress)

**Further Dosing After Control of Envenomation Syndrome**

- Choice:
    - A. Fixed dosing with 2 vials every 6 hours for 3 doses, or
    - B. 2 to 6 vials only if signs of envenomation progression recur (Note: patients that did not have coagulopathy initially are at lower risk for recurrence)
- Reassess every 2 to 5 days after discharge until 20 days after the envenomation

## KEY POINTS

**Management of Pit Viper Envenomation**

- Provide supportive care and continuous cardiorespiratory monitoring.
- Do not incise the wounds, apply ice, use tourniquets, or administer aspirin.
- Obtain IV access, send blood to the laboratory for diagnostic studies, and begin fluid resuscitation for signs of hypovolemia.
- Administer analgesics and sedation as needed.
- Cleanse the wound and provide tetanus prophylaxis.
- Measure the extremity circumference at a marked location and maintain the extremity at heart level and immobile.
- Administer antivenin in moderate to severe envenomation.
- Asymptomatic patients can be discharged home after 12 hours of observation.
- Admit patients requiring treatment with antivenin.

by airway control, as needed, and treatment with epinephrine.

### Disposition

Asymptomatic patients should be observed and followed with careful measurements for more than 12 hours. If laboratory studies are normal, the patient who remains stable, can be discharged from the emergency department after the 12-hour observation period. Patients receiving antivenin need careful, continuous monitoring. It is reasonable to initiate antivenin therapy in a monitored setting such as an emergency department (ED). In patients requiring further antivenin for continued progression of symptoms or those with severe envenomations with systemic manifestations, admission to a pediatric intensive care unit is indicated. All patients should have a followup appointment at 5 days, with those receiving antivenin seen again in another 5 to 15 days, for the possible development of serum sickness. These symptoms typically are responsive to diphenhydramine and corticosteroid therapy.

### Coral Snakes

There are only two species of coral snake (Elapidae) in the United States: the Eastern (found in the southeast) and the Sonoran (found in Arizona and New Mexico) (Figure 7.3). Together, they account for only approximately 1% of the snakebites in the United States. They are 2 feet long and have a black snout. In North America, wide red and black circumferential bands alternate with a thin yellow band, resulting in the mnemonic verse: "Red on yellow, kill a fellow; red on black, venom lack."

### Clinical Features

The snake has two fangs, which leave two punctures less than 1 cm apart. There is only mild pain and minimal edema. Within 4 hours, paresthesia and weakness are followed by diplopia and bulbar signs, such as dysphagia and dysphoria. Respiratory failure can develop.

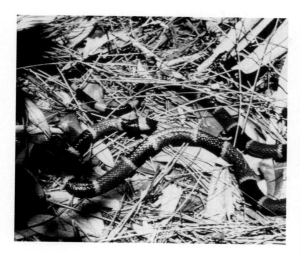

**Figure 7.3** Coral snake.

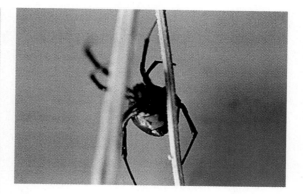

**Figure 7.4** Black widow spider.

## Management

Local measures are of no help. Supportive care should be provided as indicated. There is a specific antivenin for the Eastern variety, which tends to be more toxic, but none for the Sonoran. Unlike pit viper bites, the antivenin (3 to 5 vials in 250 mL of normal saline) is recommended for any patient with a documented bite because it is more difficult to monitor the progression of symptoms. Patients should be admitted to a pediatric intensive care unit, and, on discharge, should be followed up closely after treatment for serum sickness symptomatology.

---

### KEY POINTS

**Management of Coral Snake Envenomation**

- Provide supportive care.
- Provide antivenin for any patient with a bite from the eastern coral snake.

---

## Spider Bites

In 2001, more than 16,000 spider bites were reported to the American Association of Poison Control Centers, with more than 5,000 bites occurring in children. Fortunately, only 1,300 of these were by poisonous spiders.[1]

## Black Widow Spider

The female of the genus *Latrodectus* is noted for her red hourglass configuration on the ventral side of the abdomen and her ability to envenomate human contacts (**Figure 7.4**). The fangs of the smaller male spiders are unable to penetrate human skin. The venom of these spiders consists of peptides that are capable of causing release of acetylcholine at the myoneural junction, thus producing excessive muscle contraction. Norepinephrine also is released by the venom.

### Clinical Features

Black widow spider bites present as known exposures in the pediatric patient or, more commonly, as an unknown problem with an unusual constellation of symptoms. Consider black widow spider envenomation in a child presenting with a sudden onset of irritability and muscle rigidity, particularly of the abdominal musculature, and with perspiration and elevation of vital signs, especially hypertension. Systemic symptoms usually have their onset between 30 and 90 minutes after the bite and peak in 3 to 12 hours. Other supportive findings include muscle rigidity in one or more extremities, respiratory distress from diaphragmatic muscle paralysis, and periorbital swelling not associated with other signs of angioedema. Rarely, convulsions can occur.[9] Given the extreme irritability of bitten children and the rigidity of their abdominal musculature, the possibility of central nervous system infection or an acute intra-abdominal process must be considered.

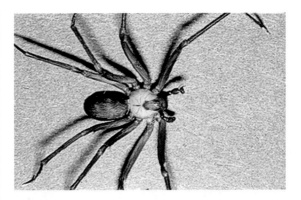

**Figure 7.5** Brown recluse spider.

Differentiation of these diagnoses might require a CBC count, abdominal radiographs, and lumbar puncture. If a history of contact with a black widow spider is obtained, those tests might not be necessary. Arterial blood gas analysis might be indicated in children with suboptimal respirations.

### Management

Patients requiring advanced life support or the administration of antivenin should be admitted to a tertiary care facility. Antivenin typically is reserved for younger patients with severe symptoms, such as intractable pain, marked hypertension, or seizures. Initially, administer benzodiazepines (diazepam 0.1 to 0.2 mg/kg every 2 to 4 hours, or lorazepam, 0.05 to 0.1 mg/kg every 4 to 8 hours) for muscle spasms, and opiates (morphine 0.1 to 0.2 mg/kg IV) for pain. This therapy might ease the muscle rigidity and spasms, but efficacy is variable. Calcium gluconate, which has been advocated in the past, has been shown to be ineffective in as many as 96% of patients. Antivenin should be considered in patients with hypertension, tachycardia, or symptoms unresponsive to narcotic and benzodiazepine therapy. Antivenin provides a rapid improvement in symptoms, but it is horse serum derived and carries a risk of hypersensitivity reaction. One vial (2.5 mL) of antivenin (Lyovac) is diluted with 50 to 100 mL of normal saline and infused over 30 to 60 minutes.[9,10] Most patients have a relatively benign course and can be managed with inpatient observation in a monitored setting.

## Brown Recluse Spider

The brown recluse spider (*Loxosceles reclusa*) is a brown spider common in the southern and midwestern United States. It is 1 to 5 cm long and has a characteristic violin or fiddle-shaped area on the dorsal cephalothorax (**Figure 7.5**). The venom contains calcium-dependent enzyme sphingomyelinase D, which has a direct lytic effect on red blood cells. After cell wall damage, an intravascular coagulation process causes a cascade of clotting abnormalities and local polymorphonuclear leukocyte infiltration, culminating in a necrotic ulcer.

### Clinical Features

The clinical response to loxoscelism ranges from a cutaneous irritation or necrotic arachnidism to a disseminated intravascular coagulation-like life-threatening systemic re-

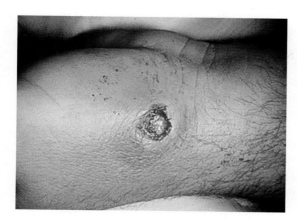

Figure 7.6 Brown recluse spider bite.

**Signs and Symptoms of Brown Recluse Spider Envenomation**

- Dull blue-gray macule, surrounded by erythema and a ring or halo of pallor
- Fever
- Nausea
- Vomiting
- Rash
- Headache
- Muscle pain
- Arthralgia
- Hemolysis
- Shock

action. Baseline coagulation studies can be predictive of the systemic reaction. There have been two reported pediatric deaths between 1998 and 1999.[1] Signs and symptoms of envenomation most often are localized to the bite area (Figure 7.6). Typically, there is little pain at the time of the bite. Within a few hours, the patient will experience itching, swelling, erythema, and tenderness over the bite. Classically, erythema surrounds a dull blue-gray macule circumscribed by a ring or halo of pallor. Within 3 to 4 days, the wound forms a necrotic base with a black eschar. Within 7 to 14 days, the wound develops a full necrotic ulceration. One third of patients develop central necrotic lesions. Ten percent develop deep necrotic ulcers from 1 to 30 cm in diameter that can take up to a month to heal. Systemic symptoms occur in up to 40% of victims. Signs and symptoms start 12 to 72 hours after the bite and include fever, nausea, vomiting, diffuse rash, headache, muscle pain, arthralgia, hemolysis, thrombocytopenia, shock, and renal failure.[11,12]

**Management**

No specific therapy has been proved effective in the treatment of brown recluse envenomation. The wound should be cleaned and tetanus immunization updated. The involved extremity should be immobilized to reduce pain and swelling. Early application of ice lessens the local wound reaction; heat will exacerbate the symptoms. Antibiotic treatment is indicated for secondary wound infections only. Antihistamines

might be beneficial. Dapsone has been used in limited studies and has not been shown to change the outcome. Dapsone use carries a risk of methemoglobinemia and hemolysis, and its use cannot be recommended for pediatric patients. Early excisional treatment can cause complications such as recurrent wound breakdown and hand dysfunction. Delayed closure and skin grafting might be necessary once the necrotic process has subsided several weeks later. For those with systemic involvement, treat symptoms and aggressively manage shock and renal failure if present. [11,12]

**KEY POINTS**

**Management of Brown Recluse Spider Bite**

- Local wound care.
- Tetanus prophylaxis.
- Immobilize the affected extremity.
- Apply ice to reduce pain.
- Administer antihistamines.

## CASE SCENARIO 2

A 12-year-old boy is running track when he collapses. The coach runs to him, finds him delirious but breathing, and calls 9-1-1. On arrival at the emergency department, the patient is drowsy and nauseated. His respiratory rate is 16, heart rate is 84, blood pressure is 90/60, and tympanic temperature is 39°C. He remembers his name but not the date or the events leading to his emergency department visit. His skin is hot and sweaty, but the remainder of his physical examination is normal.

1. *Does this child exhibit signs and symptoms of heat exhaustion or heat stroke?*
2. *Is the tympanic temperature measurement accurate?*
3. *What are the treatment priorities for this patient?*

# Body Temperature Disturbances

Body temperature usually is maintained between 36°C and 37.5°C through a balance of heat-generating and heat-dissipating processes. The thermostat regulating temperature is lodged within the preoptic nucleus of the anterior hypothalamus; that center senses the temperature of the perfusing blood and emits nerve signals that ultimately result in heat production or loss. As a consequence, body temperature normally is modulated within a very narrow range. ED equipment must include devices for recording extremes of body temperature.

## Thermoregulation

Heat is generated in many ways as follows:

- As a byproduct of basal metabolism: Approximately 960 calories of heat per square meter of surface area are produced this way each day.
- As a consequence of the actions of catecholamines and thyroxine on cellular processes: For example, some of the additional heat produced during exercise is due to the excess catecholamines released.
- As a result of muscular activity: Shivering, in particular, generates heat.
- As a byproduct of an increase in temperature itself: By accelerating chemical reactions, increases in temperature result in additional heat production.

In contrast, heat is lost from the body surface as follows:

- Radiation: Transfer to the environment in the form of infrared heat waves. This type of heat loss is dependent on the difference of temperature between the environment and the body surface. For example, when one person stands very close to another but does not touch, one can feel the heat from the other body. This thin rim of heat surrounding bodies is the heat lost by radiation. Approximately 55% of heat loss occurs via radiation.
- Conduction: Transfer by direct contact with another surface. When a person places a hand on a cold surface, the hand begins to get cold because of heat loss through conduction. This accounts for only 2% to 3% of heat loss. This can increase up to 5 times with wet clothing and 25 times with submersion in cold water.
- Convection: Conduction to air, which then is carried away by wind currents. Heat is also lost when the air heated by close proximity to the body is removed through air movement. Normally, this accounts for 12% of heat loss.
- Evaporation: Heat is lost through conversion of a liquid (sweat or moisture from the lungs) to a gas. Insensible losses account for 30% of heat loss. Greater losses occur in cool, dry environments. Each day, 360 calories of heat per square meter of surface area is lost via evaporation of water from skin surface and lungs. It is important to note that radiation,

conduction, and convection prove ineffective when the ambient temperature exceeds 37°C. Only evaporation allows heat wastage in such extreme conditions. Even evaporation fails to dissipate heat effectively when the humidity exceeds 90% to 95%. When the hypothalamus detects an increase in blood temperature, cutaneous vasodilation and sweating ensue, blood flow to the surface increases, and more heat is lost. Sweating dissipates heat through evaporation. Conversely, when the preoptic nucleus senses a decrease in blood temperature, nerve signals are emitted that result in peripheral vasoconstriction and shivering. Because less blood reaches the periphery, more heat is conserved, and shivering produces an additional heat load.

## Hyperthermia

Heat-related syndromes are more common in the hot, humid months. They are implicated in an average of 381 deaths in the United States annually. The majority of deaths are in the elderly, but approximately 4% occur in children younger than 14 years.[13] Heat illness is a spectrum of disease that can range from the minor self-limiting syndromes of heat edema and prickly heat to the potentially fatal heat stroke. It is imperative to recognize serious heat illness syndromes and treat them promptly to prevent death or serious morbidity.

Factors that predispose a patient to heat illness are age (infants and the elderly), obesity, dehydration, abnormalities of the skin, drugs, lack of acclimatization, fatigue, excessive or restrictive clothing, fever and infection, and a previous episode of heat stroke. Some medications (e.g., succinylcholine) are associated with rare syndromes that result in hyperthermia. Malignant hyperthermia is characterized by severe hyperthermia, muscle rigidity, and autonomic dysfunction after exposure to certain anesthetics. A similar syndrome can occur after exposure to neuroleptic medications such as butyrophenones and phenothiazines.

Infants and small children are at increased risk of serious heat illness because of poorly developed thermoregulatory mechanism. With an increased interest in outdoor sports and competitive athletics, older children and adolescents are more at risk for thermal illness. Practitioners therefore should have a good understanding of the clinical manifestations and treatment of heat illness, and prevention of thermal injury should be an important focus in caring for an athlete.[14]

### Pathophysiology

The body at rest, with no mechanism for cooling, generates sufficient heat to cause an increase in temperature of 1°C per hour. Exercise or hard work will increase heat production 12-fold. Body temperature also rises secondary to external sources, when air temperature exceeds body temperature, or when there is a large radiant head load (e.g., bright sunlight, hot tub, sauna).

When the body is faced with an increase in heat load either from an increase in metabolism (e.g., exercise) or from the environment (e.g., sauna, direct sunlight), the hypothalamus triggers the heat-losing mechanism, including vasodilation and sweating through the sympathetic nervous system. Cardiac output increases, as do heart rate, stroke volume, and systemic venous pressure. Large amounts of blood are shunted to the surface to aid in heat dissipation. The individual body's ability to lose heat has a maximal rate. Once this rate is exceeded, the core body temperature will rise.

Young children have less efficient thermoregulation than adults. The temperature at which children begin to sweat is higher than that in adults. They produce more heat for a given exercise than do adults and have a lower rate of sweating. Their body surface area per weight is higher, thereby making them more susceptible to the extremes of environmental temperature. Children also have a slower rate of acclimatization. Acclimatization is a physiologic adaptive process to hot environments that occurs over time. The time required varies but approximates exercising for 100 minutes per day for 10 days (14 days in children). Acclimatization is thought to occur via activation of the renin-angiotensin-aldosterone system. Eventually, there will be a small increase in temperature for the same workload and a decrease in cardiac output, cutaneous blood flow, and energy expenditure. There is also an increase in extracellular and plasma volumes.

## Minor Heat Illnesses

### Heat Edema

Heat edema is a minor heat illness in which the hands and feet become edematous. Heat edema usually occurs within the first days of exposure to a hot environment. The pathophysiology is thought to be secondary to cutaneous vasodilatation and possibly an increase in antidiuretic hormone secretion. Heat edema is self limited, and treatment consists of moving the patient to a cooler environment.

### Heat Cramps

Heat cramps are severe cramps of heavily exercised muscles that occur after exertion. They usually occur in patients who have sweated in large amounts and imbibed hypotonic fluids. It is important not to confuse heat cramps with the muscle rigidity of malignant hyperthermia or neuroleptic malignant syndrome, which can be fatal if unrecognized. The pathophysiology of cramps is uncertain but thought to be due to decreased sodium, secondary to dilution with hypotonic oral solutions. Management consists of removing the patient from the heat stress and providing rest and oral fluids (electrolyte drinks, not salt tablets) or IV fluids and salt replacement (normal saline).[15]

### Heat Syncope

Heat syncope is a syncopal episode during heat exposure occurring in unacclimatized people in the early stages of heat exposure. There is a decrease in vasomotor tone, venous pooling, and hypotension, with mild dehydration. Heat syncope is self limited, and treatment consists of moving the patient to a cooler environment. The patient should regain consciousness once supine or placed in the Trendelenburg position. IV saline, lactated Ringer's, or oral electrolyte fluids should be administered.

## Major Heat Illnesses

### Heat Exhaustion

Heat exhaustion is a precursor to heat stroke and must be differentiated from other illnesses, especially heat stroke. The symptoms of heat exhaustion include a temperature up to 39°C, malaise, headache, nausea, vomiting, irritability, tachycardia, and dehydration. Mental function remains intact. Liver function tests (SGOT, SGPT, LDH) are not significantly elevated.

In heat exhaustion, vasodilatation with blood shunted toward the periphery occurs. Sweating increases, thereby causing water and sodium loss. There is a decrease in central circulating blood volume. A compensatory increase in heart rate and stroke volume occurs, as well as a decrease in renal blood flow. Temperature-regulatory mechanisms remain intact.

Management of heat exhaustion initially consists of moving the patient to a cool environment. IV fluids should be administered to treat dehydration. Initially, 20 mL/kg normal saline or lactated Ringer's should be infused, and then projected losses should be replaced. Laboratory studies should include a CBC count, electrolytes, BUN, creatinine, liver function tests, and urinalysis. Vital signs should be followed closely. The patient should be observed in the ED until normal or hospitalized for observation. If at any time there is doubt, the patient should be treated for heat stroke. Long-term sequelae usually do not occur. Patients who are discharged should avoid heat stress for 24 to 48 hours.

## YOUR FIRST CLUE

**Signs and Symptoms
of Heat Exhaustion**
- Environmental exposure
- Temperature less than 39°C
- Sweating
- Headache
- Malaise
- Nausea, vomiting
- Tachycardia
- Intact mental status

## Heat Stroke

Heat stroke is a life-threatening emergency in which normal thermoregulatory mechanisms are no longer functioning. Patients with exposure to heat stress usually present with rectal temperatures of greater than 41°C and an altered mental status that can range from bizarre behavior to seizures and coma.

There are two types of heat stroke: exertional and nonexertional (classic). Exertional heat stroke can be found in the unacclimatized athlete. The patient usually has a rapid onset of severe prostration with headache, ataxia, syncope, seizures, and coma. Tachycardia, tachypnea, and hypotension are present. The sweating mechanism usually is intact. Nonexertional or classic heat stroke is of slower onset and more common in infants and the elderly. Marked dehydration usually is present. Symptoms include anorexia, nausea, vomiting, malaise, dizziness, confusion, seizures, coma, tachycardia, tachypnea, and hypotension. Sweating can be absent.

In heat stroke, all temperature regulation is lost. A precipitous rise in core body temperature occurs, leading to pathologic changes in every organ. The extent of the damage is dependent on the body temperature, exposure time, workload, tissue perfusion, and individual resistance. Some patients exhibit myocardial damage with an elevation of CK-MB, cerebral edema, intravascular coagulation and thrombocytopenia, hepatocellular degeneration, cholestasis, acute tubular necrosis, interstitial nephritis, or myoglobinuria.[16]

### Management

Initial management of the patient with heat stroke begins like the management of all other patients: airway, breathing, and circulation. Cooling, the cornerstone of therapy, should be promptly initiated. Remove the patient's clothing and move to an air-conditioned room if possible. Optimal cooling should be greater than 0.1°C per minute. Stop cooling at 39°C. The rectal temperature should be monitored continuously.

Methods of cooling vary in their effectiveness and practicality. One of the most effective and practical ways to cool a patient is to continuously spray water over the body surface and create air movement with fans. Ice packs can be applied to the groin and axillae. The use of peritoneal lavage, ice enemas, and ice gastric lavage has not been well studied in humans.[17–19] Cold intravenous solutions add little to the cooling process and can cause arrhythmias. Cold inhaled oxygen has been studied in the animal model and found to be ineffective. Submersion in cold water has been used by the military with excellent success but may be impractical in an unstable patient. Antipyretics are ineffective in the patient with heat stroke.

Laboratory evaluation includes a CBC count, electrolytes, BUN, creatinine, glucose, calcium, liver function tests, coagulation studies, CK-MB, arterial blood gas analysis, urinalysis, and a blood culture (if sepsis is suspected).

Simultaneous with cooling, IV lines should be placed. Start fluid replacement with a saline bolus of 20 mL/kg of normal saline or lactated Ringer's and repeat as needed to maintain perfusion and urine output. A central venous line and Foley catheter should be placed for fluid monitoring. Hypoglycemia should be treated with 0.5 to 1 g/kg dextrose, given as 2 to 4 mL/kg 25% dextrose, or for older children 1 to 2 mL/kg of 50% dextrose.

Once initial treatment of the patient has started, consider a differential diagnosis. Head trauma, cerebrovascular accident (CVA), thyroid

---

## YOUR FIRST CLUE

**Signs and Symptoms of Heat Stroke**

- Temperature higher than 39°C
- Change in mental status
- Dehydration
- Nausea
- Vomiting
- Headache
- Ataxia
- Syncope
- Seizures
- Coma

storm, malignant hyperthermia, neuroleptic malignant syndrome, drug ingestion, or heat exhaustion with syncope can all be precipitating or coexisting conditions.

Heat stroke complications are numerous. If seizures occur, they should be treated with benzodiazepines and then phenobarbital. Hypotension that is unresponsive to fluids and cooling should be treated with inotropes such as dopamine or dobutamine. Incipient renal failure can be treated with furosemide and mannitol. Dysrhythmias can be seen in those with heat stroke and can include a variety of abnormalities. Cooling usually controls these abnormalities. Unfortunately, no treatment exists for central nervous system and thermoregulatory control abnormalities.

Prognosis of the patient with heat stroke is dependent on the duration of coma, severity of coagulopathy, severity of liver function abnormalities, duration of high temperature, and presence of a preexisting illness.[16]

### Prevention

Heat stroke can be prevented by educating parents and coaches about its dangers. It is recommended that exertion be avoided during the warmest daytime hours (10:00 AM to 4:00 PM) in hot weather, especially when the temperature is greater than 80°F and humidity approaches 70%. Light clothing should be worn, and adequate intake of an electrolyte solution should be consumed before exercise. Athletes should take frequent breaks during exercise for fluid replacement with electrolyte solutions (like Gatorade) and not wait until they are thirsty. Salt supplements in the form of salt pills should not be used.[14] Athletes and those working outdoors should limit the duration and intensity of activity until acclimated over a period of 10 to 14 days. Symptoms of heat illness should be recognized early, and the athlete or worker should be moved to a cool environment.

## Hypothermia

Hypothermia is defined as a core temperature of less than 35°C (95°F). Neonates are predisposed to the development of hypothermia because of their underdeveloped thermoregulatory system, relatively large body surface-to-body mass ratio, and decreased subcutaneous fat. The neonate is most prone to hypothermia immediately after delivery due to conduction and evaporative heat losses (from being covered with amniotic fluid and placed on a cool surface.) It is important to dry and cover the neonate to prevent heat loss. Infants and young children can develop hypothermia from a simple exposure to cold while wearing inadequate clothing for the environmental conditions. Hypothermia can occur in all seasons. Most cases of accidental hypothermia in children are associated with near-drowning accidents in cold or icy water environments.

Factors found to predispose individuals to the development of hypothermia include the following:

- Endocrine or metabolic derangements (hypoglycemia, hypothyroidism)
- Infection (meningitis, sepsis)
- Intoxication (alcohol, opiates)
- Intracranial pathology (traumatic, congenital, other)
- Submersion injury
- Environmental exposure
- Dermatologic (burns)
- Iatrogenic (cold IV fluids, exposure during treatment)

Mortality from hypothermia is related directly to the associated underlying disorder and is highest for submersion injury.

## Pathophysiology

When the core body temperature begins to drop, the preoptic anterior hypothalamus senses blood cooling and immediately initiates sympathetic neurogenic signals, causing an increase in muscle tone and metabolic rate. This is most evident in the shivering reflex, which is an attempt by the body to increase heat production through involuntary muscle contraction. Heat production can be increased to approximately four times the normal rate by these mechanisms. Neonates lack the ability to shiver. The sympathetic nervous system also causes cutaneous vasoconstriction, thereby shunting blood toward the vital organs and defending against further heat loss. As the body cools, the metabolic rate is reduced, reflected by a decrease in $CO_2$ production and slowing of the heart rate. Situations that create heat loss through convection and conduction, such as high winds or wet clothes, greatly accelerate the development of hypothermia. The most profound effects occur during submersion in cold water; in this environment, rapid heat loss is intensified by movement. Apnea and asystole can occur very quickly.

## Clinical Features

The clinical findings of progressive hypothermia in children and adolescents depend on the degree of hypothermia, which can be categorized as mild, moderate, or severe.

### Mild Hypothermia (32° to 35°C) (89.6° to 95°F)

The patient might exhibit slowing of mental status, which produces slurred speech and mild uncoordination. Inappropriate judgment or behavior might be the only manifestations of mild hypothermia. The shivering reflex is preserved in this temperature range.

### Moderate Hypothermia (28° to 32°C) (82.4° to 89.6°F)

This temperature range leads to a progressive decrease in the level of consciousness. Coma is likely at temperatures of less than 30°C. The patient appears cyanotic and will develop tissue edema. Shivering is replaced by muscle rigidity. Respiratory activity might be difficult to detect, and pulses are frequently difficult to palpate. Blood pressure is decreased or unobtainable. The classic ECG change of an Osborn (J) wave might be apparent (Figure 7.7).

### Severe Hypothermia (<28°C) (<82.4°F)

The patient is comatose with dilated and unresponsive pupils. It might be impossible to detect any vital signs, and the distinction between

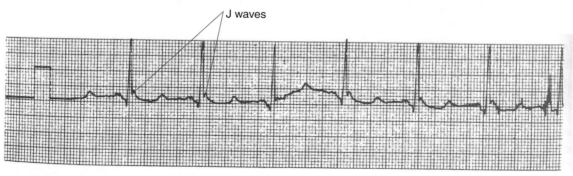

J waves

**Figure 7.7** Classic ECG change of a J wave.

death and profound hypothermia can be difficult to make. Respiratory arrest and ventricular fibrillation occur in older patients at temperatures of less than 28°C.

## Management

As with all severely ill or injured patients, the hypothermic patient must be assessed from head to toe, with particular attention paid to assessment of vital functions, followed immediately by resuscitation as indicated. No prospective controlled studies comparing the various rewarming modalities have been done in humans. The following recommendations are therefore based on clinical experience.

---

### KEY POINTS

**Management of Hypothermia**
- Provide supportive care and cardiorespiratory monitoring and begin rewarming.
- Provide continuous temperature monitoring with either a rectal or an esophageal probe for patients with moderate to severe hypothermia.
- Begin passive rewarming for patients with mild hypothermia.
- Begin active rewarming for patients with moderate to severe hypothermia.
- Admit patients to a monitored setting.

---

### Methods of Rewarming

There are two types of rewarming: passive and active. Passive rewarming involves the use of warm blankets. Passive rewarming is useful only for the mildest cases. Active external techniques are widely used. These include hot packs, heating lamps, forced air external warmers, and plumbed pads. These techniques rewarm the periphery before the core and therefore can promote complications (afterdrop, rewarming shock, and ventricular fibrillation). It should be noted that forced air rewarming using a device such as the Bair Hugger (Augustine Medical, Eden Prairie, Mn) has shown some success in patients with moderate to severe hypothermia and intact circulation.[20]

Active core rewarming involves the use of a number of invasive techniques, as follows, in order of increasing effectiveness:

- Intubate the patient and increase the humidifier temperature on the ventilator to 44°C. This is a very effective method of core rewarming.
- Heat IV fluids to 40° to 42°C and deliver through a fluid warmer. Only a fluid warmer capable of delivering large volumes with rapid heating and special insulated tubing can provide the rates and temperatures required by hypothermia patients. Devices such as the Hotline warmer (Level 1, Inc. Rockland, Mass) meet these criteria. Other methods include keeping IV fluid bags in a blanket warmer or heating them rapidly in a microwave oven. The bag should be shaken well to distribute warmth evenly. These methods can be used as an alternative. There is substantial heat loss through the tubing, and by the time the fluids reach the patient there is little active rewarming.
- Perform gastric lavage with a nasogastric tube or rectal lavage with an enema tube using warmed electrolyte solutions heated to 40° to 44°C.
- Perform peritoneal lavage with warmed electrolyte solutions heated to 40° to 42°C. Lavage is carried out with a standard peritoneal lavage kit.
- In severe cases, perform open thoracotomy with mediastinal irrigation.
- Extracorporeal blood rewarming with a modified form of cardiopulmonary bypass is the fastest method of restoring body temperature and cardiac output, but this technique often is not readily available.

### Treatment of Mild Hypothermia

Mild hypothermia can be treated with passive rewarming if the patient is stable and no underlying pathology is causing the hypothermia. Patients with core temperatures of greater than 32°C usually are conscious, with spontaneous cardiac activity, unless the hypothermia is associated with other significant illness or traumatic injury such as submersion. Mildly hypothermic patients who respond well to rewarming might not warrant laboratory assessment.

### Treatment of Moderate to Severe Hypothermia

As with all ill or injured patients, the hypothermic patient must be assessed from head to toe, with particular attention to the ABCs. Securing the airway and ensuring adequate ventilation are the first concerns. This should be followed by an assessment of heart rate and blood pressure. At temperatures of less than 30°C, the myocardium is resistant to defibrillation and pharmacologic agents. If the patient has a nonperfusing rhythm, along with monitor evidence of ventricular fibrillation or ventricular tachycardia, then defibrillation should be attempted only once. If unsuccessful, CPR should be continued until the patient's temperature is greater than 30°C, when repeat defibrillation should be performed.

All moderately or severely hypothermic patients need continuous temperature monitoring with either a rectal or an esophageal probe. If a rectal probe is used, be sure any cold feces are removed before probe placement. These patients must be treated aggressively with active rewarming, warm humidified oxygen, warmed IV fluids, and various lavage techniques. Patients with moderate to severe hypothermia might have large amounts of fluid sequestration. Rewarming the victim must be accompanied by fluid resuscitation to prevent cardiovascular collapse. An initial fluid bolus of 20 mL/kg in the form of crystalloid is indicated. Insert an indwelling (Foley) catheter to monitor urinary output. Unless needed, defer insertion of a central venous pressure line until a core temperature of 30°C is obtained to prevent precipitation of ventricular fibrillation. The goal should be to raise the core temperature 1° to 2°C per hour.

With rewarming, peripheral vasodilation occurs and the cold extremities are perfused. This causes the circulating blood to become colder as it passes through the cold extremity and then returns to the central organs, leading to a phenomenon known as core temperature afterdrop. Core temperature afterdrop can cause additional problems with mental status, breathing, and particularly, cardiac dysrhythmias. These effects usually are transient; nevertheless, rewarming of cold extremities with hot packs should be avoided.

The cold myocardium is resistant to defibrillation and drugs. If initial treatment fails to establish a rhythm, CPR must continue until a core temperature of greater than 30°C is reached. At this point, if a perfusing cardiac rhythm has not been established, follow standard life support drug protocols in an attempt to restore a viable cardiac rhythm.

In moderate to severe hypothermia, laboratory studies should include serum electrolytes, blood gases and pH, hemoglobin, white blood cell count, and tests for renal and hepatic function. In profoundly hypothermic patients, thought must be given to the presence of an underlying disease process that predisposes the patient to hypothermia development, such as endocrine disturbances, drug and alcohol intoxication, and trauma. It is important to exclude hypoglycemia by measuring the blood glucose, and blood and urine samples also should be taken for toxicology screening. The presence of any underlying head or spinal cord injury should be excluded, and the possibility of sepsis as a cause of the hypothermia must be addressed in younger children. Resuscitation efforts should continue until the body temperature is greater than 32°C (greater than 90°F) for at least 30 minutes. Children have a remarkable ability to withstand hypothermia, particularly submersion, through induction of the diving reflex, which results in shunting of blood to the brain and heart; this process is thought to contribute to intact survival after submersion in very cold water (less than 5°C).

## Disposition

Admit all patients with core hypothermia for observation. Children who present with core temperatures of less than 32°C, altered mental status, or multi–organ system failure should be admitted to the intensive care unit for continuous cardiac monitoring until rewarming is accomplished. Underlying problems frequently will be discovered during the observation period. Children with core temperatures as low as 14°C have survived with full neurologic recovery.

## Submersion Injury

Drowning is the second major cause of unintentional injury in children aged 1 to 14 years.[21] In addition, for every child who drowns, four children are hospitalized for submersion injuries.[22] The incidence of submersion injuries is highest in boys younger than 5 years; the next highest incidence is in boys between 15 and 19 years.[21]

Drowning can be defined as suffocation by submersion (totally covered) or immersion (partially covered) in any liquid medium (usually water).[23] The term near-drowning implies survival of at least 24 hours after the incident. However, near-drowning is an inaccurate term, as some of these patients die after the 24-hour period. For this section, the term submersion injury will be used to describe drowning, whether involving pools, natural or manmade bodies of freshwater, saltwater, or domestic sites (bathtubs and buckets).

The relative availability of different types of bodies of water and the climate, geography, and socioeconomic setting determine the most likely site of submersion for each community. In North America, unfenced swimming pools represent a major water risk to the unsupervised child younger than 5 years. Although absent adult supervision is a factor in most pediatric submersions, the victim might have predisposing medical conditions such as seizures, alcohol or drug ingestion (especially in preadolescents and adolescents), and trauma, both accidental and nonaccidental

(e.g., suicide, child abuse, homicide). The possibility of child abuse must be considered in home submersion injuries, such as in bathtubs or water pails. In the absence of child abuse, a history of diving or trauma-associated injury is rare.[21,24-26]

### Pathophysiology

Prolonged submersion results in global hypoxic injury. The responses of vital end organs to hypoxia and the resulting acidosis follow specific timelines (Table 7-3). Loss of consciousness occurs rapidly. Aspiration of water, which occurs in 90% of drowning victims, causes surfactant washout with subsequent atelectasis. Aspiration and the pulmonary response to hypoxia (reflex-mediated pulmonary hypertension with intrapulmonary shunting) increase the ventilation/perfusion mismatch and oxygen requirement. Myocardial hypoxia results in cardiac arrest within minutes of the submersion. Laryngospasm prevents aspiration in 10% of cases and results in "dry" drowning.

In the child who has been severely asphyxiated, vital organs begin to fail and cerebral edema, gastrointestinal bleeding, acute respiratory distress syndrome, and myocardial failure develop. Central nervous system hypoxia is the most common cause of death after a successful cardiac resuscitation. Acute respiratory distress syndrome is common in submersion victims in intensive care units.[23] The delayed immersion syndrome in victims who initially appear to have minimal injury is an uncommon, delayed acute respiratory dis-

## TABLE 7-3 Timeline of Common Organ System Response to Severe Submersion

| System | Symptoms and Signs at Scene | Symptoms and Signs Hours Later |
|---|---|---|
| Cardiac | Cardiac arrest | Myocardial failure |
| Central nervous system | Loss of consciousness | Cerebral edema (6–12 hrs) |
| Pulmonary | Hypoxia, pulmonary edema | Acute respiratory distress syndrome (can develop at 24 hrs) |
| Gastrointestinal | None | Mucosal sloughing, diarrhea, third spacing of fluids resulting in hypovolemia (6–12 hrs) |
| Renal | None | Renal failure, oliguria/anuria, electrolyte imbalance (6–12 hrs) |

tress syndrome-like response to hypoxia that can occur up to 24 hours after submersion.[27,28]

Although uncommon, coagulopathies or renal failure can develop after hypoxia. Myoglobinuria or hemoglobinuria also may precipitate renal failure. Fluid absorption leading to fluid shifts and electrolyte changes is not a significant problem for the submersion victim.

The outcome for submersion victims generally is either intact survival or death, and outcome usually can be predicted in the field.[29–31] Most victims who resume spontaneous ventilations in the field, become responsive, have a sinus rhythm, and have been submerged for less than 5 minutes survive without neurologic sequelae. For victims submerged in waters 5°C or warmer who present in cardiac arrest, aggressive prehospital care can result in return of spontaneous circulation within 10 minutes and intact survival.[32] For victims submerged in nonicy waters (greater than 5°C), the most reliable predictors for death or severe neurologic sequelae include the following:

- Submersion longer than 25 minutes
- Resuscitation longer than 25 minutes
- Pulseless cardiac arrest on arrival in the ED
- Unresponsiveness on arrival at the hospital
- Elevated blood glucose level
- Hypothermia

Less reliable outcome predictors in the ED are absence of spontaneous respirations, fixed pupils, and pH greater than 7.1.[32]

On occasion, children submerged in icy waters (less than 5°C) have survived neurologically intact despite prolonged (longer than 60 minutes) submersions and resuscitations. Such rapidly induced hypothermia might provide cerebral protection. These anecdotal survivals and the death-like state induced by severe hypothermia led to the belief that all hypothermic victims should be warmed before cessation of resuscitation. However, data suggest that hypothermia after nonicy but cold water (greater than 5°C) immersion does not provide a protective benefit. Almost all case reports of miraculous survival have followed submersion in icy waters. Knowing the temperature of the immersion water might be helpful to the practitioner faced with the dilemma of determining whether the victim's hypothermia is due to rapid cooling or prolonged circulatory arrest.

## Clinical Features

Direct assessment of the ABCs and initiation of critical support are primary. Initial signs and symptoms usually reflect cardiopulmonary and cerebral hypoxic injury. Hypothermia might not be recognized unless a rectal temperature is obtained along with other vital signs. A thermometer capable of measuring temperatures significantly below the normal range is needed to assess the hypothermic patient accurately. Because occult injury to the head, cervical spine, or other areas might be present, all submersion victims should be assessed thoroughly for evidence of other trauma. Evaluate all submersion victims for possible abuse or nonaccidental trauma with a social/family evaluation. Evaluate for other precipitating causes of submersion injury.

An altered mental status might be due to a combination of cerebral hypoxia and underlying disease processes. Consider drug ingestion, intracranial injury, or a postictal state. Obtain a blood alcohol level and drug screen on all preadolescents and adolescents, and blood pH and oxygen saturation on all victims. Further assessment of respiratory status is dictated by the patient's condition. Hematocrit and electrolytes usually are normal.

Repeated assessment of the victim's pulmonary status for evolving sequelae is key. Aggressive, expectant care is the rule. Never underestimate how much near-drowning patients can deteriorate regardless of how well they appear (Figure 7.8). However, for those patients who arrive in the ED awake, alert, and fully responsive, prognosis is very good. If these children have a normal chest x-ray and arterial blood gases on arrival, again in 6 hours, are asymptomatic, and have no supplemental oxygen requirement, they can be considered for discharge after observation of 6 to 8 hours.

## Management

The goal of therapy is reversal of hypoxia. Appropriate aggressive airway management in the field is essential for submersion victims. The usual basic and advanced cardiac life support measures should be applied. Management interventions are described in Tables 7-4 and 7-5.

Positive pressure ventilation and 100% oxygen are provided to ensure best outcome. Many apneic, unresponsive victims will respond to basic life support efforts to ventilate and will breathe and awaken at the scene. Considerable amounts of water are usually swallowed, and vomiting is likely. Nasogastric tube insertion and gastric evacuation should be accomplished early in the resuscitation.

Recent studies support the use of standard basic and advanced cardiac life support guidelines.[33] However, many submersion victims are also hypothermic. (See Hypothermia section.) At temperatures of less than 30°C, the myocardium is resistant to defibrillation and pharmacologic agents. If the patient has a

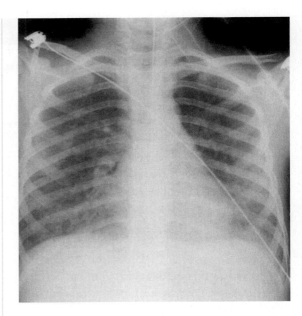

**Figure 7.8** An abnormal chest radiograph after a submersion.

| TABLE 7-4 | Managing the Responsive Patient |
|---|---|

**Prehospital**

- Assess ABCs; provide oxygen if any signs of respiratory distress.
- Stabilize cervical spine if diving or significant fall.
- Remove wet clothing; provide blankets.
- Monitor for developing respiratory distress.
- Transport.

**Emergency Department**

- Assess ABCs and oxygen saturation; monitor ECG.
- Clear cervical spine.
- Rule out underlying comorbidity, especially drugs, alcohol, and possible child abuse.
- Monitor glucose level.
- Assess rectal temperature.
- Admit for any oxygen requirement; observe for delayed oxygen requirement.

nonperfusing rhythm along with monitor evidence of ventricular fibrillation or ventricular tachycardia, defibrillation should be attempted only once. If unsuccessful, CPR should be continued until the patient's temperature is above

30°C, when repeat defibrillation should be performed.

Consideration should be given to warming the hypothermic victim to greater than 32°C before the decision to cease efforts is made. Rewarming definitely should be attempted if the victim was submerged in icy water less than 5°C. When there is no return of spontaneous circulation, the decision to cease resuscitation is a clinical judgment based on the victim's submersion duration, response to resuscitation, duration of the resuscitation, and whether the submersion waters were icy or nonicy. After 25 minutes of resuscitation, survival is very unlikely in the victim submerged in nonicy (greater than 5°C) waters. No predictors exist for the submersion victim in icy (less than 5°C) waters.

Routine use of antibiotics is not recommended, but an exception can be considered for children who were submerged in grossly contaminated water (e.g., sewage). Dexamethasone has no value in the acute care setting and does not improve respiratory distress outcomes.

## TABLE 7-5  Managing the Unresponsive Patient

### Prehospital

- Assess ABCs; ensure cervical spine control; bag-mask ventilate with 100% oxygen; intubate; insert orogastric or nasogastric tube.
- Initiate rhythm-appropriate electrical interventions and medication; CPR.
- Obtain vascular access; use normal saline to keep open.
- Remove wet clothing.
- Reassess airway and breathing.
- Transport to facility that can provide emergency pediatric care.

### Emergency Department

- Continue CPR until return of spontaneous circulation or physician decides that resuscitation cannot be accomplished.
- Stabilize and evaluate cervical spine.
- Assess ABCs; tracheal tube placement; obtain chest radiograph and arterial blood gases; pass orogastric or nasogastric tube; monitor oxygen saturation and ECG; assess rectal temperature with a thermometer capable of detecting hypothermia.
- Place patient requiring ventilatory support on a respirator; use positive end-expiratory pressure (5–10 cm $H_2O$); repeat arterial blood gas determination as indicated.
- Ensure vascular access; check glucose using glucose oxidase reagent strip; monitor blood pressure; run fluid to keep open unless treating shock.
- Electrical intervention for ventricular dysrhythmias.
- Initiate rewarming for hypothermic patients.
- Evaluate neurologic status; obtain serum glucose and treat if indicated; consider drug screening; assess and treat hypothermia.
- Admit to a pediatric intensive care unit.

## Prevention

One way to reduce the number of submersion injuries is by prevention. Because most young victims drown in swimming pools, four-sided pool fencing and adequate, constant supervision are needed. Older children often drown during risk-taking behavior, so swimming lessons (for those older than 5 years), use of personal flotation devices, and avoidance of alcohol and drugs are recommended.[22] Another often forgotten site of drowning is the household tub or buckets of water. If anything interrupts bath time (such as the telephone or doorbell), an infant or child should be taken out of the tub. In addition, all water should be removed from containers such as 5-gallon buckets or pails immediately after use.[22]

## THE BOTTOM LINE

- Environmental emergencies are a diverse group of conditions resulting from environmental insults, each with unique signs, symptoms, and management.
- Recognition of symptoms and consideration of an environmental etiology of the clinical features will result in early diagnosis and appropriate management.
- Prevention is key in reducing injuries.

# CHAPTER REVIEW

## Check Your Knowledge

1. An 11-year-old boy is playing football on a hot, humid afternoon in August. During the second quarter, he comes out of the game complaining of headache and feeling "sick to my stomach." While on the sideline he vomits once. The coach notes that he is sweating profusely. This child is most likely suffering from which of the following conditions?
   A. Heat cramps
   B. Heat exhaustion
   C. Heat stroke
   D. Heat syncope

2. On arrival in the ED, the child described in question #1 is noted to have a pulse of 110 and a temperature of 39°C. He is alert and oriented and is vomiting as you enter the room. Which of the following interventions is the most appropriate at this point?
   A. Give acetaminophen 15 mg/kg per rectum
   B. Place patient in tub of ice water
   C. Start an IV of normal saline at 20 mL/kg and obtain CBC, electrolytes, BUN, and creatinine
   D. Start an IV of normal saline at 20 mL/kg and start ice water enemas

3. An 8-month-old is found abandoned in a dumpster on a cool fall evening. He is brought by police to the ED. On examination, the infant is lethargic with poor tone. The pulse is 60, the respiratory rate is 10, and the temperature is 30°C. There are no signs of trauma. Which of the following methods is the best way to rewarm this patient?
   A. Forced air rewarming device
   B. Warm blankets plus heat lamps
   C. Warm humidified $O_2$ by ET tube
   D. Warmed oxygen by ET tube plus IV fluids heated to 40°C

4. Which of the following differentiates coral snake envenomations from pit viper envenomations?
   A. Degree of pain and edema
   B. Response to antivenin therapy
   C. Signs of neurologic involvement
   D. Small number of patients who require antivenin therapy

## References

1. Litovitz TL, Klein-Schwartz W, Rodgers Jr. GC et al. 2001 Annual report of the American Association of Poison Control Centers toxic exposure surveillance system. *Am J Emerg Med* 2002;20:391–452.

2. Lawrence WT, Giannopoulos A, Hansen A. Pit viper bites: rational management in locales in which copperheads and cottonmouths dominate. *Ann Plast Surg.* 1996;36:276–285.

3. LoVecchio F, Klemens J, Welch S et al. Antibiotics are rarely required following rattlesnake envenomation. *Ann Emerg Med.* 1999 (abstract);89:874–876.

4. Bond GR. Controversies in the treatment of pediatric victims of Crotalinae snake envenomation. *Clin Pediatr Emerg Med.* 2001;2:192–202.

5. Dart RC, Seifert SA, Boyer LV et al. A randomized multicenter trial of Crotalinae polyvalent immune Fab (ovine) antivenom for the treatment of Crotaline snakebite in the United States. *Arch Inter Med.* 2001;161(16):2030–2036.

6. Dart RC, McNally J. Efficacy, safety and use of snake antivenom in the United States. *Ann Emerg Med.* 2001;37:181–188.

7. Dart RC, Seifert SA, Carroll L et al. Affinity-purified, mixed monospecific crotalid antivenom ovine Fab for the treatment of crotalid venom poisoning. *Ann Emerg Med.* 1997;30:33–39.

8. Offerman SR, Bush SP, Moynihan JA, Clark RF. Crotaline Fab antivenom for the treatment of children with rattlesnake envenomation. *Pediatrics.* 2002;110:968–971.

9. Clark RF, Wethern-Kestner S, Vance MV et al. Clinical presentation and treatment of black widow spider envenomation: a review of 163 cases. *Ann Emerg Med.* 1992;21:782–787.

10. O'Malley GF, Dart RC, Juffner EF. Successful treatment of latrodectism with antivenin after 90 hours. *N Engl J Med.* 1999;340:657.

11. Erickson T, Hryhorczuk DO, Lipscomb J et al. Brown recluse spider bites in an urban wilderness. *J Wilderness Med.* 1990;1:258–264.

12. Wright SW, Wrenn KD, Murray L et al. Clinical presentation and outcome of brown recluse spider bite. *Ann Emerg Med.* 1997;30:28–32.

13. Centers for Disease Control: heat-related illnesses and deaths—Missouri, 1998 and United States 1979–1996. *MMWR*. 1999;48:469–472.

14. American Academy of Pediatrics, Committee on Sports Medicine. Climatic heat stress and the exercising child and adolescent (RE9845). *Pediatrics*. 2000;106:158–159.

15. Squire DL. Heat illness. Fluid and electrolyte issues for pediatric and adolescent athletes. *Pediatr Clin North Am*. 1990;37:1085–1109.

16. Bouchama A, Knochel JP. Heat Stroke. *N Engl J Med*. 2002;346(35):1978–1988.

17. Costrini A. Emergency treatment of exertional heatstroke and comparison of whole body cooling techniques. *Med Sci Sports Exerc*. 1990;22:15–18.

18. Harker J, Gibson P. Heat stroke: a review of rapid cooling techniques. *Intensive Crit Care Nurs*. 1995;11:198–202.

19. White JD, Kamath R, Nucci R et al. Evaporation versus iced peritoneal lavage treatment of heatstroke: comparative efficacy in a canine model. *Am J Emerg Med*. 1993;11:1–3.

20. Steele MT, Nelson MJ, Sessler DI et al. Forced air speeds rewarming in accidental hypothermia. *Ann Emerg Med*. 1996;27:479–484.

21. Brenner RA, Trumble AC, Smith GS, Kessler EP, Overpeck MD. Where children drown, United States 1995. *Pediatrics*. 2001;108(1):85–89.

22. American Academy of Pediatrics, Committee on Injury and Poison Prevention. Drowning in infants, children and adolescents. *Pediatrics*. 1993;92:292–293.

23. Orlowski JP, Szpilman D. Drowning: rescue, resuscitation, and reanimation. *Pediatr Clin NA* 2001;48:627–646.

24. Pearn J, Nixon J, Wilkey I. Freshwater drowning and near-drowning accidents involving children: a five-year total population study. *Med J Aust*. 1976;2:942–946.

25. Pearn JH, Wong RY, Brown J et al. Drowning and near-drowning involving children: a five-year total population study from the City and County of Honolulu. *Am J Public Health*. 1979;69:450–454.

26. Quan L, Gore EJ, Wentz KR et al. Ten-year study of pediatric drownings and near-drownings in King County, Washington: lessons in injury prevention. *Pediatrics*. 1989;83:1035–1040.

27. Modell JH. Drowning. *N Engl J Med*. 1993;328:253–256.

28. Weinstein MD, Krieger BP. Near-drowning: epidemiology, pathophysiology, and initial treatment. *J Emerg Med*. 1996;14(4):461–467.

29. Graf WD, Cummings, P, Quan L et al. Predicting outcome in pediatric submersion victims. *Ann Emerg Med*. 1995;26:312–319.

30. Habib DM, Tecklenburg FW, Webb SA, Anas NG, Perkin RM. Prediction of childhood drowning and near-drowning morbidity and mortality. *Pediatr Emerg Care*. 1996;12:255–258.

31. Quan L, Kinder D. Pediatric submersions: prehospital predictors of outcome. *Pediatrics*. 1992;90:909–913.

32. Suominen PK, Korpela RE, Silfvast TGO, Olkkola KT. Does water temperature affect outcome of nearly drowned children? *Resuscitation*. 1997;35:111–115.

33. American Heart Association, Guidelines 2000 for cardiopulmonary resuscitation & emergency cardiovascular care. Submersion or near-drowning. *Circulation* 2000;102 (suppl 1): 1–233 – 1–236.

## Additional Reading

Banner W. Bites and stings in the pediatric patient. *Curr Probl Pediatr*. 1988;18:1–69.

Baum CR. Environmental emergencies. In: Fleisher GR, Ludwig S eds. *Textbook of Pediatric Emergency Medicine*, 4th ed., Baltimore, Md: Williams & Wilkins; 2000:943–963.

Bracker MD. Environmental and thermal injury. *Clin Sports Med*. 1992;11:419–436.

Corneli HM. Hot topics in cold medicine: controversies in accidental hypothermia. *Clin Pediatr Emerg Med*. 2001;2:179–191.

Cruz NS, Alvarez RG. Rattlesnake bite complications in 19 children. *Pediatr Emerg Care*. 1994;10:30–33.

Diekema DS, Reuter DG. Arthropod bites and stings. *Clin Pediatr Emerg Med*. 2001;2:155–167.

Erickson T, Herman BE, Bowman MJ. Snake envenomations. In: Strange GR, Ahrens WR, Lelyveld S et al, eds. *Pediatric Emergency Medicine: A Comprehensive Study Guide*. 2nd ed. New York, Ny: McGraw-Hill; 2002:676–679.

Erickson T, Herman BE, Bowman MJ. Spider bites. In: Strange GR, Ahrens WR, Lelyveld S et al, eds. *Pediatric Emergency Medicine: A Comprehensive Study Guide*. 2nd ed. New York, Ny: McGraw-Hill; 2002:680–685.

Hoffman JL. Heat-related illness in children. *Clin Pediatr Emerg Med*. 2001;2:203–210.

Jolly BT, Ghezzi, KT. Accidental hypothermia. *Emerg Med Clin North Am*. 1992;10:311–327.

Lavelle JM, Shaw KN. Near drowning: is emergency department cardiopulmonary resuscitation or intensive care unit cerebral resuscitation indicated? *Crit Care Med*. 1993;21:368–273.

Rowin ME, Christensen D, Allen EM. Pediatric drowning and near-drowning. In: Rogers MC, Nichols DG, eds. *Textbook of Pediatric Intensive Care.* 3rd ed., Baltimore, Md: Williams & Wilkins; 1996:875–892.

Shields CP, Sixmith DM. Treatment of moderate-to-severe hypothermia in an urban setting. *Ann Emerg Med.* 1990;19:1093–1097.

Simon HB. Hyperthermia. *N Engl J Med.* 1993;329(7):483–487.

Sterba JA. Thermal problems: prevention and treatment. In: Bennett PB, Elliott DH, eds. *The Physiology and Medicine of Diving.* 4th ed. London; WB Saunders: 1993.

Strange GR. Heat and cold illness. In: Strange GR, Ahrens WR, Lelyveld S et al, eds. *Pediatric Emergency Medicine: A Comprehensive Study Guide.* 2nd ed. New York, Ny: McGraw-Hill; 2002:703–714.

Sullivan JB, Wingert WA, Norris RL. North american venomous reptile bites. In: Auerbach PS, ed. *Wilderness Medicine: Management of Wilderness and Environmental Emergencies.* 3rd ed. St. Louis, Mo: Mosby; 1995:680–709.

Tanen DA, Ruha AM, Graeme KA et al. Epidemiology and hospital course of rattlesnake envenomations cared for at a tertiary referral center in central Arizona. *Acad Emerg Med.* 2001;18:517–574.

Tek D, Olshaker J. Heat illness. *Emerg Med Clin North Am.* 1992;10:299–310.

Wingert WA, Chan L. Rattlesnake bites in southern California and rationale for recommended treatment. *West J Med.* 1988;148:37–44.

Wintemute GH. Childhood drowning and near-near drowning in the United States. *Am J Dis Child.* 1990;144:663–669.

# CHAPTER REVIEW

A 4-year-old boy is brought to the emergency department after being bitten by a spider a few hours previously at his family's camp site. The child says that the spider was dark but cannot remember any identifying marks. On examination his respiratory rate is 26/min, heart rate is 130 beats per minute (bpm), blood pressure is 100/60, and his temperature is 37°C. He is calm but complaining of pain in the bite area. His right forearm is swollen and erythematous, with two small marks at the center of the wound. His hand is pink, pulses are 2+, and he is able to move his fingers. The remainder of the examination is normal.

1. *What is the differential diagnosis of this spider bite?*
2. *What signs or symptoms would help distinguish the type of spider bite?*
3. *What studies are needed?*
4. *What treatment is necessary?*

This child shows no signs of severe envenomation at time of presentation, a few hours after the bite occurred. The spiders that should be considered include the black widow spider, brown recluse spider, and many other nonvenomous spiders. The least likely in this group is black widow envenomation, as the child lacks muscle rigidity, hypertension, and irritability. The signs of brown recluse envenomation can include itching, swelling, erythema, and tenderness of the bite. The classic description is that the bite has erythema surrounding a dull blue gray macule with surrounding pallor. Other spider bites are likely to result in local reactions that can include erythema, swelling, itching, and tenderness.

No specific laboratory tests or studies will discriminate between bites. However, with severe brown recluse envenomation, one could have low platelets and evidence of hemolysis. The specific treatment is symptomatic care, with some period of observation to ensure the symptoms do not change. This patient does not require crotaline Fab, but should have the arm elevated, and an ice pack applied to the bite.

A 12-year-old boy is running track when he collapses. The coach runs to him, finds him delirious but breathing, and calls 9-1-1. On arrival at the emergency department, the patient is drowsy and nauseated. His respiratory rate is 16, heart rate is 84, blood pressure is 90/60, and tympanic temperature is 39°C. He remembers his name but not the date or the events leading to his emergency department visit. His skin is hot and sweaty, but the remainder of his physical examination is normal.

1. *Does this child exhibit signs and symptoms of heat exhaustion or heat stroke?*
2. *Is the tympanic temperature measurement accurate?*
3. *What are the treatment priorities for this patient?*

CASE SUMMARY 2 CONT.

Based upon the history of altered level of consciousness, there is a concern that this child could be suffering from heat stroke. The tympanic temperature of 39°C is the upper limit of normal for heat exhaustion, but a tympanic temperature does not give the core temperature in hyperthermia or hypothermia. A rectal temperature is required to determine core temperature. In addition, the presence of sweating should not deter you from the diagnosis of heat stroke. The treatment priorities for both heat exhaustion and heat stroke include attention to the ABCs. Cooling the body is the cornerstone of therapy, followed by IV fluids.

CASE SUMMARY 3

A 7-year-old girl jumped off a diving board at a local pool and did not resurface. She was pulled from the pool by lifeguards and given mouth-to-mouth resuscitation. When the EMTs arrived, she was breathing on her own. She was immobilized on a backboard, a cervical collar was placed, and she was given oxygen by face mask. In the emergency department, respiratory rate is 30, her heart rate is 124, blood pressure is 100/70, and temperature is 35°C. She is crying, but responds to questions. Her physical examination reveals a hematoma on the top of her head that is painful to touch. She is able to grasp with both hands and wiggle and feel her toes. The remainder of her examination is normal.

1. *What are the treatment priorities for this patient?*
2. *What is an effective way to warm this patient?*
3. *What findings would mandate that this patient be admitted to the hospital?*

The treatment priorities for this patient remain airway and cervical spine stabilization, breathing, and circulation. Her oxygen saturation should be measured, and she should be placed on a cardiac monitor. Since her respiratory rate is elevated, she could be developing respiratory distress, so she requires oxygen and careful monitoring of her respiratory status. Her temperature is low, so she should be warmed by removing wet clothing and applying warm blankets, warm IV fluid, and/or warm humidified oxygen. If the trauma evaluation was negative, reasons to admit this child to the hospital may include an oxygen requirement and an abnormal chest radiograph initially or after 6 hours of ED observation.

# chapter 8

# Toxicology: Ingestions and Smoke Inhalation

Timothy B. Erickson, MD, FACEP, FACMT

## Objectives

1 Explain the general management principles for ingestions and toxic exposures.

2 Identify methods used to minimize drug absorption.

3 Describe the specific therapies, including antidotes, for common poisonings.

4 Identify the available resources for consultation for managing the child with poisoning or toxin exposure.

5 Describe the ways smoke can be toxic.

6 Discuss the clinical progression of inhalation toxicity.

7 Describe the steps in evaluation and management of the patient exposed to smoke and who may have carbon monoxide poisoning.

## Chapter Outline

General Evaluation and Management of Ingestions

**Specific Ingestions**
  Acetaminophen
  Ethanol
  Methanol and Ethylene Glycol
  Anticholinergic Agents
  Caustics
  Clonidine
  Cyanide
  Cyclic Antidepressants
  Hydrocarbons
  Iron
  Opioids
  Organophosphates
  Salicylates
  Selective Serotonin Reuptake Inhibitors
  Gamma hydroxybutyrate
  Ecstasy
  Overall Management Issues

Additional Routes of Exposure

Smoke Inhalation

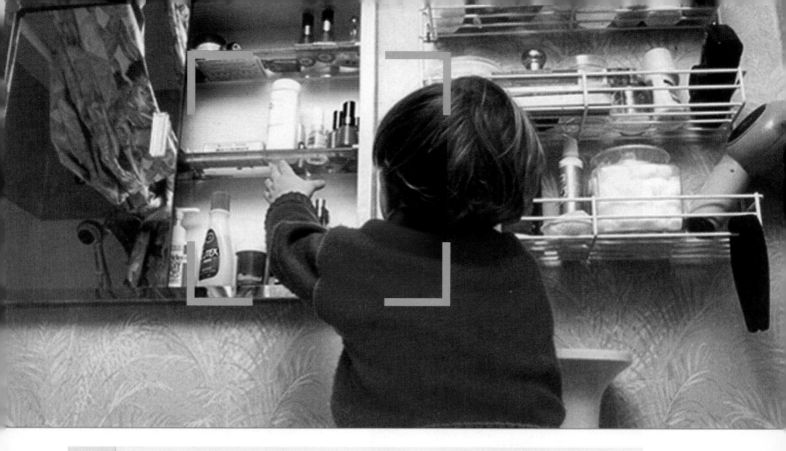

**CASE SCENARIO 1**

A 2-year-old boy presents to the emergency department with his frantic parents, who had found him unresponsive in the bathroom with pills and empty bottles "scattered all over the floor." The child is normally healthy.

The child is lethargic with no response to stimuli, with shallow and slow respirations but no cyanosis. Vital signs include a respiratory rate of 8 breaths per minute, a pulse of 70 beats per minute (bpm), blood pressure of 80/40 mmHg, and temperature of 35.6°C. Focused physical examination reveals pupils that are 4 mm each and reactive to light, a supple neck, clear lungs, nontender abdomen with no masses, normoactive bowel sounds, extremities with good pulses, and no focal neurologic deficits. There is no evidence of trauma.

1. *What are the initial management priorities in this child?*
2. *What antidotes should be administered?*
3. *What further history is important in this case?*

## General Evaluation and Management of Ingestions

Poisoning continues to be a preventable cause of morbidity and mortality in children and adolescents. It is imperative that pediatricians, family physicians, emergency physicians, and pediatric emergency physicians be familiar with the general approach to the poisoned child as well as the latest treatment methods available.[1]

Poisoning can occur from ingestion, dermal absorption, or inhalation of toxins, with ingestions being the most common exposure (Figure 8.1). Although many pediatric patients present with a history of a specific toxic exposure, others present with unexplained signs or symptoms and no history of poisoning.[2, 3]

### Epidemiology

Since the early 1960s, there has been a 95% decline in the number of pediatric poisoning deaths. Child-resistant product packaging, increased parental awareness of potential household toxins, a national toll-free poison

235

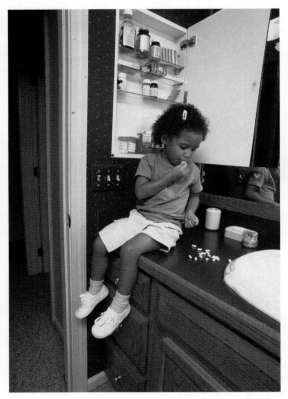

A.

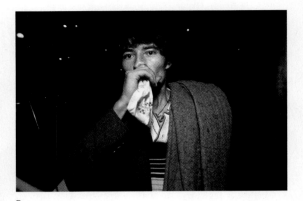

B.

Figure 8.1  A. Ingestion. B. Inhalation of toxins.

control telephone number, and advances in emergency and critical care medicine have all helped to reduce morbidity and mortality.[4] More than 60% of calls received by regional poison centers in the United States involve children younger than 17 years.[5] Most exposures in this group are accidental and result in minimal toxicity. The highest morbidity and mortality rates occur in adolescent and adult patients, but younger children also can be severely affected.[4, 5]

## Clinical Features

Toxins cause damage to the body by a variety of mechanisms. Toxins can act at a cellular level (e.g., cyanide) or affect a specific organ system, such as the brain (e.g., narcotics, hypnotic sedatives, major tranquilizers), autonomic nervous system (e.g., organophosphates), lung (e.g., hydrocarbons, paraquat), gastrointestinal tract (e.g., caustics, corrosives), liver (e.g., acetaminophen), or blood (e.g., heavy metals). The range of pathologic processes that can be caused by noxious agents is great.

If possible, attempt to identify the specific poison. Obtain a detailed history from the patient, family members, friends, rescuers, or bystanders. It is important to identify the ingested substance or substances, the amount and time of ingestion, presence of allergies or underlying diseases, and any first aid treatment that has already been administered. Family, friends, or police might need to search the home for the toxin. Examine clothing and personal effects for ingestants and MedicAlert identification.

Perform a brief physical examination, concentrating on neurologic and cardiopulmonary status. Identify distinct toxic syndromes if present (Table 8-1). The physical examination and vital signs can help identify particular groups of toxins. Hypertension suggests cocaine, amphetamines, phencyclidine, sympathomimetic overdose, or sedative or narcotic withdrawal; hypotension suggests β-blocker, sedative-hypnotic, or narcotic drugs. Tachycardia can be present in ingestions of the same drugs that cause hypertension; bradycardia can be associated with digitalis, β-blockers, calcium channel antagonists, clonidine, or hypothermia. Fever can be produced by salicylates, anticholinergics, or withdrawal from alcohol or narcotics. Respirations are depressed with sedative-hypnotics and narcotics but increased in cases of pulmonary aspiration (hydrocarbons), pulmonary edema (smoke inhalation, narcotics, salicylates), and metabolic acidosis (ethylene glycol, methanol, salicylates). Pupil size (Table 8-2) and skin signs (Table 8-3) also can help identify the class of ingested agent.

| TABLE 8-1 | Toxic Syndromes—Classic Signs and Symptoms |
|---|---|
| **Toxin** | **Syndrome** |
| Opioids | Respiratory failure |
| | Coma |
| | Miosis |
| Cyclic antidepressants | Coma |
| | Convulsions (seizures) |
| | Cardiac dysrhythmias |
| | QRS greater than 100 milliseconds |
| Organophosphates cholinergics | Diarrhea, diaphoresis |
| | Urination |
| | Miosis |
| | Bronchorrhea, bronchospasm, bradycardia |
| | Emesis, vomiting |
| | Lacrimation |
| | Fasciculations |
| | Salivation |
| Anticholinergic agents | Flushing ("red as a beet") |
| | Dry skin and oral mucosa ("dry as a bone") |
| | Hyperthermia ("hot as a hare") |
| | Delirium ("mad as a hatter") |
| | Mydriasis ("blind as a bat") |
| | Tachycardia |
| | Urinary retention |
| Sympathomimetic agents | Mydriasis |
| | Anxiousness |
| | Tachycardia |
| | Hypertension |
| | Hyperthermia |
| | Diaphoresis |

| TABLE 8-2 | Toxic Pupillary Findings |
|---|---|

**Miosis (COPS)**
C—Cholinergics, clonidine
O—Opiates, organophosphates
P—Phenothiazines, pilocarpine, pontine bleed
S—Sedative-hypnotics

**Mydriasis (AAAS)**
A—Antihistamines
A—Antidepressants
A—Anticholinergics, atropine
S—Sympathomimetics (cocaine, amphetamines)

| TABLE 8-3 | Toxic Skin Signs |
|---|---|

**Diaphoretic skin (SOAP)**
S—Sympathomimetics
O—Organophosphates
A—ASA (salicylates)
P—PCP (phencyclidine)

| **Red Skin** | Carbon monoxide, boric acid |
|---|---|
| **Blue Skin** | Cyanosis, methemoglobinemia |

With an assessment of mental status based on the Glasgow Coma Scale or AVPU (alert, responds to verbal stimuli, responds to painful stimuli, unresponsive) system, quantify the level of consciousness. Always consider other causes of altered mental status, such as metabolic imbalance or trauma, and rule them out through appropriate evaluation.

## Diagnostic Studies[6]

Patients with central nervous system (CNS) or cardiopulmonary compromise require cardiac monitoring. If cardiac rhythm disturbances are present or the patient is known to have ingested a cardiotoxic poison (e.g., tricyclic antidepressant or digitalis), obtain a 12-lead ECG and closely monitor the blood pressure.

If the level of consciousness is altered or respiratory problems are present, obtain a chest radiograph. Aspiration pneumonitis or noncardiogenic pulmonary edema can be present. Certain medications such as iron, other heavy metals, and enteric-coated capsules, might be seen on abdominal radiographs.

Serum electrolyte and arterial blood gas determinations can provide valuable information about possible toxic or metabolic processes. If the arterial blood gas reveals a metabolic acidosis, calculation of the anion gap ($Na^+ - [Cl^- + CO_2]$) can provide valuable information. A normal anion gap of 8 to 12 mEq/L can result from loss of bicarbonate (diarrhea) or the addition of chloride. An increased anion gap greater than 12 mEq/L is suggestive of the presence of organically active acids, which can occur with several toxins (salicylates, iron, isoniazid, methanol, ethylene glycol, toluene, cyanide) or metabolic problems (diabetic ketoacidosis, lactic acidosis).[4]

An osmolar gap (measured osmoles–calculated osmoles) of greater than 10 will be present in patients who have ingested ethanol, methanol, isopropanol, or ethylene glycol. Calculated osmoles are derived from the formula $2Na^+$ + glucose/18 + blood urea nitrogen (BUN)/2.8 + ethanol/4.[4]

Toxicology screening of blood and urine rarely contributes to the acute management. There might be academic or forensic indications for obtaining these studies, in which case they can be ordered on a routine turnaround time. A negative toxicology screen does not rule out the possibility of a toxin. If a particular drug or class of drugs is suspected, communicate this to the laboratory. Serum levels of specific drugs might be available to guide management or predict prognosis. Examples include acetaminophen, aspirin (ASA), digoxin, ethanol, ethylene glycol, iron, lead, lithium, and theophylline.

## Management

Management is based on the following four general principles:

- Provision of supportive care pediatric assessment triangle, (PAT) ABCs (airway, breathing, circulation)
- Prevention or reduction of absorption
- Enhancement of excretion
- Administration of antidotes

### Initial Assessment

In the initial assessment, the physician must determine rapidly whether a child is in respiratory failure or shock.

Treat the patient, not the poison. Attention to the standard ABCs of resuscitation, as well as the PAT, are always the first priority. Evaluate the appearance, work of breathing, and circulation to the skin. Derangements should be treated with oxygen, support of ventilation, specific therapy, and fluid resuscitation as indicated. The PAT is followed by the ABCDEs (airway, breathing, circulation, disability, exposure). Assess the glucose level using a bedside glucose oxidase reagent strip and administer glucose (0.5 to 1 g/kg as 2 to 4 mL/kg of 25% dextrose in water, or for older children, as 1 to 2 mL/kg of 50% dextrose in water) by intravenous push if indicated. Naloxone can be used for any child in a coma at a dose of 0.1 mg/kg; it is also acceptable to administer 2 mg for a child older than 5 years.

### Prevention or Reduction of Absorption[7–11]

Syrup of ipecac-induced emesis is no longer advocated in the health care setting for the treatment of the acutely poisoned patient. Gastric lavage is indicated only if the patient arrives less than 1 hour after ingestion of a potentially life-threatening toxin, massive ingestions, or for those substances that do not bind to charcoal. First-line treatment for significant ingestions consists of a single dose of activated charcoal in water. Mixing the charcoal in soda or juice makes it more palatable for children. The dose is 1 to 2 g/kg in children younger than 6 years and 50 to 100 g in adolescents or adults. A nasogastric tube might be required for complete administration. There are no contraindications for its use; however, it is ineffective for a small group of substances (Table 8-4). Hyperosmolar adjunctive cathartics (e.g., sorbitol, magnesium citrate) are contraindicated in children younger than 6 years because of the potential risk for fluid and electrolyte imbalance.

Whole bowel irrigation can be accomplished through the rapid administration of polyethylene glycol electrolyte lavage solution (Colyte, GoLYTELY) via nasogastric tube.[12] It irrigates out the contents of the gastrointestinal tract and is indicated for the ingestion of significant amounts of iron or delayed-release pharmaceuticals. The rate of administration is 500 mL/hr for preschoolers and 1 to 2 L/hr for teenagers and adults. The end point is a clear rectal effluent that takes several hours. This

| TABLE 8-4 | Substances Not Absorbed by Activated Charcoal |

**PHAILS**

P—Pesticides

H—Hydrocarbons

A—Acids, alkali, alcohols

I—Iron

L—Lithium

S—Solvents

procedure is contraindicated in patients with ileus, obstruction, perforation, or significant gastrointestinal hemorrhage.

## Enhancement of Excretion

Several techniques aimed at enhancing excretion can be used, and each is indicated in only a few situations.

### Ion Trapping

In theory, acidification and alkalinization of the urine enhance the excretion of weak bases and weak acids. The former should be avoided altogether because of the risks of acidemia and exacerbation of rhabdomyolysis. Urinary alkalinization should be considered for significant salicylate and phenobarbital poisonings.

### Neutral Diuresis

Urine flow can be increased through the administration of excess intravenous (IV) crystalloid and should be considered for significant lithium or bromide poisonings. Pulmonary edema, cerebral edema, and renal failure are contraindications for this technique.

### Multiple-Dose Charcoal

Multiple-dose charcoal might be indicated with drugs that undergo enterohepatic or enteroenteric recirculation (e.g., phenobarbital, theophylline, carbamazepine). In theory, this technique enhances the excretion of toxins by using the gastrointestinal epithelium as a dialysis membrane (gastrointestinal dialysis). In smaller children, overzealous administration should be avoided to prevent iatrogenic complications such as charcoal aspiration and bowel obstruction.

### Hemodialysis

This technique is indicated for methanol, ethylene glycol, significant salicylate, phenobarbital, theophylline, and lithium poisonings.

### Charcoal Hemoperfusion

This technique is rarely indicated. It is used most commonly in significant theophylline poisoning.

## Administration of Antidotes

Antidotes and antagonists are available for only a small number of poisonings and are not intended for indiscriminate use. Use antidotes carefully, particularly in the pediatric patient with an unknown overdose, because overuse can complicate an initial presentation by producing other forms of poisoning. In weighing the benefits and risks of administering a specific antidote, consider the patient's clinical status, appropriate laboratory values, expected pharmaceutical action of the toxin, and possible adverse reactions associated with the antidote. Specific antidotes are listed in Table 8-5.

| TABLE 8-5 | Antidotes |
| --- | --- |
| Poison | Antidote |
| • Acetaminophen | N-Acetyl-L-cysteine (NAC) (oral or IV) |
| • Anticholinergics | Physostigmine |
| • Anticholinesterase insecticides | Atropine, 2-PAM |
| • Benzodiazepines | Flumazenil |
| • β-blockers | Glucagon, isoproterenol |
| • Carbon monoxide | Oxygen |
| • Cyanide | Cyanide antidote kit |
| • Cyclic antidepressants | Sodium bicarbonate |
| • Digoxin | Digoxin specific Fab fragments |
| • Ethylene glycol | Ethanol, 4-MP (fomepizole) |
| • Iron | Deferoxamine |
| • Isoniazid | Pyridoxine |
| • Lead | Succimer, BAL, calcium EDTA |
| • Mercury | BAL, DMSA |
| • Methanol | Ethanol, 4-MP |
| • Methemoglobinemia | Methylene blue |
| • Opioids | Naloxone |

A 16-year-old girl presents to the emergency department 3 hours after ingesting two handfuls of extra-strength acetaminophen. She complains of nausea and vomiting. She has no significant past medical history.

The patient is alert, but has a depressed affect and makes poor eye contact. She has no increased work of breathing, and her skin color is normal. Vital signs include a respiratory rate of 20 breaths per minute, pulse of 110 bpm, blood pressure of 130/60 mmHg, and temperature of 37.3° C. Focused examination reveals that her pupils are 3 mm bilaterally reactive to light; she has a supple neck, no heart murmurs, and clear lungs. Her abdomen is tender to touch in the epigastric region, but there is no guarding, and no peritoneal signs. She has good symmetrical pulses and no focal neurologic deficits.

1. What is the primary target organ of acetaminophen poisoning?
2. What diagnostic laboratory data should be obtained?
3. Does this patient meet the criteria for antidote therapy?

# ■ Specific Ingestions

## Acetaminophen

### Clinical Features

Acetaminophen is the most commonly used drug for analgesia and antipyresis in children. Ingestions most often are seen in children younger than 6 years, but overdose also can be associated with suicide attempts in adolescents. Toxicity is unlikely in children younger than 6 years because they usually ingest nontoxic amounts. Ingestions in older children and multiple dosing in younger children by well-meaning parents are potentially serious, and careful assessment and management are necessary to ensure a good outcome.[13,14]

Acetaminophen is absorbed rapidly after ingestion, with peak plasma levels at less than 1 hour. The drug is metabolized in the liver, with 2% excreted unchanged in the urine. In older children, 94% is metabolized to the glucuronide and sulfate conjugates, and 4% is metabolized through the cytochrome oxidase P-450 system (which produces a reactive metabolite). When the glutathione stores are less than 30% of normal, the highly reactive metabolite binds to hepatic macromolecules, and hepatic damage ensues.

The clinical course has been divided into four stages as follows:

- **Stage 1.** This stage consists of the first 24 hours after ingestion. Young children might vomit; older children can have nausea, vomiting, generalized malaise, and diaphoresis. The mean onset of symptoms is 6 hours after the ingestion, with 60% of patients symptomatic by 14 hours. Liver enzymes and prothrombin times are normal.

- **Stage 2.** Patients are asymptomatic during the second 24 hours (quiescent phase). Liver enzymes can become elevated.

- **Stage 3.** In serious overdoses, the peak of symptoms and abnormalities is seen 48 to 96 hours after the ingestion. Serum aspartate transaminase (AST) concentrations can be as high as 20,000 to 30,000 IU/L. An elevated prothrombin time is considered the best laboratory guide to the severity of hepatic encephalopathy. Death can occur in this stage from hepatic failure or coagulopathy.

- **Stage 4.** Approximately 7 to 8 days after ingestion, hepatic abnormalities are almost resolved in survivors. Recovery is complete, and hepatic sequelae are not expected.

## Diagnostic Studies

Draw blood samples to determine acetaminophen levels from patients with potentially serious overdoses. After a single acute ingestion, blood is drawn up to 4 hours after ingestion to determine acetaminophen level. If more than 4 hours have passed, draw blood immediately. Once the plasma level has been determined, plot it on the Rumack-Matthew nomogram to determine whether the level is toxic in relation to time (Figure 8.2).[14] If the level cannot be determined within 8 hours of ingestion, initiate treatment with N-Acetyl-L-cysteine (NAC) after consultation with the poison center. If the time and amount of ingestion are unknown, determination of acetaminophen level is still recommended with subsequent blood drawn at 4-hour intervals to determine the half-life of the drug. A prolonged elimination half-life of more than 3 hours is indicative of hepatic damage or delayed absorption. It is also important to follow laboratory parameters in a case of serious poisoning; these include prothrombin time, AST, ALT, and bilirubin, as well as electrolytes, blood urea nitrogen, and creatinine.

## Differential Diagnosis

Acetaminophen poisoning usually does not present with altered mental status within the first 24 hours after ingestion. Consider the possibility that patients presenting with CNS depression have a multiple-drug overdose. Interpret histories with caution, particularly in the adolescent. It often is difficult to distinguish between toxic and nontoxic overdoses by history alone. With any potential acetaminophen ingestion, any other over-the-counter medications and pain relievers such as salicylates (aspirin) and nonsteroidal anti-inflammatory agents (ibuprofen) should be considered in the differential diagnosis.

## Management

After a brief assessment, administer activated charcoal in water (or mixed with a cathartic if older than 6 years) if less than 4 hours have elapsed since the ingestion. Activated charcoal binds well to acetaminophen and can lessen a

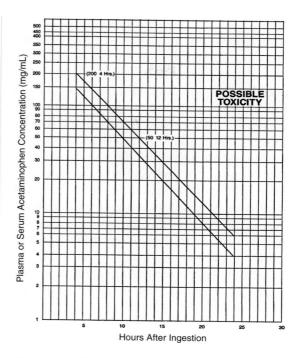

**Figure 8.2** Rumack-Matthew nomogram for estimating severity of acute acetaminophen poisoning. The time coordinator refers to time of ingestion. Serum levels drawn before 4 hours might not represent peak levels.

Source: Rumack BH, Matthew H. Acetaminophen poisoning and toxicity. *Pediatrics.* 1975;55:871–876. Adapted with permission.

potentially hepatotoxic ingestion. In the older child, a relatively large dose, such as 100 g, might be required because of the large amount of acetaminophen typically ingested. In practice, the concern of charcoal absorbing orally administered NAC and diminishing its bioavailability has been overstated. Routine doses of both agents can be administered if indicated.

Oral NAC is available as a 20% concentrate. It has a strong smell of sulfur, which is generally unacceptable to children. Dilute the concentrate to a 5% concentration (i.e., if starting with a 20% concentrate, dilute 3:1). The taste might be improved by mixing it with orange juice or carbonated beverages. Use a cup with a cap and hole for a straw to avoid the smell. The initial dose of NAC is 140 mg/kg with subsequent doses of 70 mg/kg at 4-hour intervals for 17 doses.

IV NAC is licensed in the United States, Europe, and Canada.[15] Currently there are two

IV protocols: 20 hours and 48 hours. In the 20-hour protocol, it is given as three separate infusions: 150 mg/kg over the first 60 minutes, 50 mg/kg over the next 4 hours, and 100 mg/kg over the next 16 hours. Administration of the first infusion over 60 instead of 15 minutes decreases the risk for adverse reactions such as flushing, itching, and hives. The advantages of IV therapy are a shorter protocol, no concern that vomiting or charcoal will decrease the bioavailability of the antidote, and ease of administration. It is not unusual for patients receiving IV NAC to develop hives, requiring treatment with antihistamines. Most patients (99%) recover within 1 week if managed appropriately. Patients requiring careful monitoring might be managed best in a pediatric tertiary care center.

## Ethanol[16,17]

Ethanol poisoning is more likely to occur in an older child; however, it can also occur in a toddler. In addition to alcohol-containing beverages such as beer, wine, and hard liquor, children have access to cologne and perfume (40% to 60% ethanol), mouthwash (containing up to 75% ethanol), and numerous over-the-counter and prescription medications containing ethanol (Figure 8.3). Characteristic breath odor and serum levels make the diagnosis. Mixed drug/ethanol toxicity frequently confounds the clinical picture. A blood ethanol level of 100 mg/dL is considered sufficient to cause intoxication. Levels approaching 500 mg/dL can be lethal. In general, treatment is supportive and sometimes includes assisted ventilation. Due to low hepatic glycogen stores, small children are extremely prone to hypoglycemia when intoxicated with ethanol. Intoxication in combination with hypoglycemia can markedly impair mental status.

## Methanol and Ethylene Glycol[16,17]

### Clinical Features

Very small volumes of methanol or ethylene glycol are potentially life-threatening. These toxic alcohols are commonly found in windshield washer fluid and antifreeze products and other widely available commercial and household

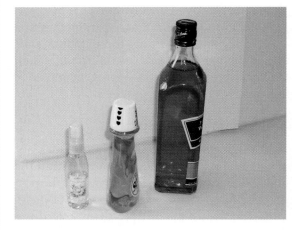

Figure 8.3 Common sources of ethanol.

---

**CASE SCENARIO 3**

A 3-year-old boy is discovered by his father drinking "some blue fluid from a jug" in the garage. Thirty minutes later, on examination in the emergency department, the child is sleepy but cries easily when awakened. He has no increased work of breathing, and his color is normal. His vital signs include respiratory rate of 32 breaths per minute, heart rate of 80 bpm, blood pressure of 80/40 mmHg, and temperature of 36.1°C. The remainder of his examination is noncontributory, and the father says that he is normally healthy.

1. *What is the differential diagnosis?*
2. *Is gastric decontamination indicated?*
3. *Is there a role for antidote therapy?*

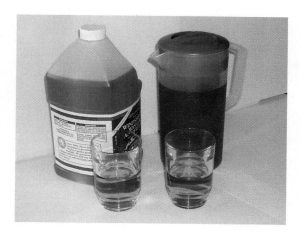

**Figure 8.4** The bright colors make toxins highly attractive to children.

products that are brightly colored and highly attractive to young children (Figure 8.4).

Both methanol and ethylene glycol produce an altered mental status with inebriation and CNS depression. Both induce an osmolar gap and severe anion gap metabolic acidosis. Methanol can eventually lead to blindness, and ethylene glycol can cause acute renal failure. Both act through the production of toxic metabolites, which can be blocked by ethanol through a competitive inhibition of the alcohol dehydrogenase enzyme.

### Diagnostic Studies

Laboratory studies should be sent for CBC count, serum electrolytes, renal function (BUN/creatinine), arterial blood gas, serum osmolality, serum ethanol, ethylene glycol, methanol, and isopropanol levels.

### Differential Diagnosis

When considering the possibility of methanol poisoning, the clinician should also consider ethylene glycol poisoning. In addition, isopropanol and ethanol poisoning should be included in the differential, because each can create an osmolar gap; however, they do not generally produce a profound metabolic acidosis.

### Management[18]

Along with acid/base, fluid, and electrolyte monitoring, traditional management consists of suf-ficient ethanol therapy to produce a serum concentration of 100 mg/dL. The usual dose is 0.6 g/kg infused over 30 to 40 minutes. Oral ethanol can be used if IV ethanol is not readily available. During the infusion of an ethanol drip, the child's glucose levels should be monitored to avoid hypoglycemia. Treatment of methanol and ethylene glycol poisoning has been recently revolutionized by the introduction of the antidote 4-MP (4-methylpyrazole, or fomepizole),[19] which competitively inhibits the alcohol dehydrogenase enzyme. Unlike ethanol therapy, 4-MP does not potentiate sedation or induce profound hypoglycemia, and it can be safely administered in children. In patients with significant acidosis or peak serum methanol and ethylene glycol levels of greater than 50 mg/dL, nephrology consultation for extracorporeal intervention with hemodialysis is indicated. Folate (up to 50 mg q4h) is a therapeutic cofactor for methanol, and thiamin (up to 100 mg) serves a similar function for ethylene glycol.

## Anticholinergic Agents

### Clinical Features

Anticholinergic poisoning can be caused by jimsonweed, deadly nightshade, potato leaves, and a number of medications, including antihistamines, benztropine, atropine, phenothiazines, and tricyclic antidepressants (Figure 8.5). Most overdoses involving drugs with anticholinergic actions do not result in a pure anticholinergic syndrome; this is especially so for cyclic anti-

---

## YOUR FIRST CLUE

**Signs and Symptoms of Anticholinergic Poisoning**

- "Red as a beet" (flushing)
- "Blind as a bat" (pupillary mydriasis)
- "Dry as a bone" (dry skin, decreased oral secretions)
- "Hot as a hare" (febrile)
- "Mad as a hatter" (delirium)

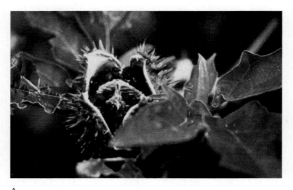

A.

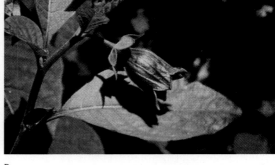

B.

Figure 8.5 A. Jimsonweed. B. Deadly nightshade.

depressants because the life-threatening toxicity is due to direct myocardial depression.

### Diagnostic Studies

Routine laboratory studies should include CBC count, serum electrolytes, BUN, creatinine, and glucose. If the patient demonstrates seizures or hyperthermia, a creatinine phosphokinase (CPK) and urine myoglobin should be obtained to rule out rhabdomyolysis. With any moderate to severe overdose, a 12-lead ECG is indicated. Routine toxicology screens usually do not include detection of antihistamines.

### Differential Diagnosis

If the child is hyperthermic, bacteremia or sepsis should be considered. Other drugs that can cause hyperthermia include nicotine, antidepressants, sympathomimetics, and antihistamines (mnemonic NASA).[20] With delirium or acute mental status changes, consider other drug ingestions, metabolic causes, or head trauma. If the patient is tachycardic, other drugs such as the sympathomimetic agents (cocaine, amphetamines, PCP) should be ruled out.

### Management

Treatment is mainly supportive. With the exception of tricyclic antidepressants, in severe pure anticholinergic poisoning, consider using the antidote physostigmine. Indications include severe agitation, profound hyperthermia, hallucinations, or uncontrollable seizures. Physostigmine is administered in a dose of 0.5 mg IV to a young child and 1 to 2 mg IV

to an adolescent over 2 to 3 minutes. An alternative therapy would be IV administration of a benzodiazepine such as diazepam in a similar clinical scenario.[21]

## Caustics

### Clinical Features

Caustics are chemicals that cause tissue injury on contact (Figure 8.6). These agents account for approximately 5% of all accidental toxic exposures, with small children most frequently affected. Agents such as drain cleaners, lye, Clinitest tablets, oven cleaners, automatic dishwasher detergents, toilet bowel cleaners, and button batteries are examples of caustic substances. Alkali burns cause liquefaction necrosis and injury that penetrates deep into the tissues, predominantly in the esophagus. Acid burns cause coagulation necrosis, primarily in the stomach, with severe injury to superficial gastric mucosa. The exposed child might present with excessive crying, refusal to eat or drink, drooling, oropharyngeal burns, stridor, vomiting, and abdominal pain. If severe, the patient might have acute respiratory distress, airway edema, and shock.

### Diagnostic Studies

Laboratory studies should include a CBC count, serum electrolytes, renal function tests, coagulation profile, and glucose. Pulse oximetry and a chest radiograph are indicated in any

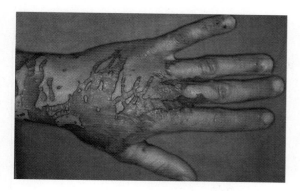

**Figure 8.6** Caustics cause tissue injury on contact.

child with respiratory symptoms. Patients with abdominal pain should have an abdominal radiograph to assess for gastrointestinal perforation and diagnostic free air. Endoscopy will determine the extent of the injury, guide management, and determine prognosis.

### Differential Diagnosis

Identification of the specific caustic agent, whether acid or alkali, its volume, concentration, and pH, is critical in determining an agent's potential toxicity. As with any child in respiratory or upper airway distress, infections such as epiglottitis, pharyngeal abscess, and tracheitis must be considered. In addition, foreign body aspiration must be ruled out.

### Management

Initial treatment might include immediate dilution with water or milk. If possible, a regional poison center (1-800-222-1222) should be contacted for instructions regarding proper dilution in the home. Often, well-meaning caregivers give too large a volume of milk or water, causing gastric distention and vomiting. Children with oral burns or a definite history of significant ingestion should be considered for esophagoscopy within 12 hours of the injury. After ingestion of liquid drain cleaners, esophageal burns can occur without the presence of oropharyngeal burns. Gastric evacuation is contraindicated, and charcoal provides no benefit. Depending on the degrees of second-degree esophageal

burns, corticosteroids and antibiotics might be indicated.[22]

## Clonidine

### Clinical Features

Clonidine is a centrally acting antihypertensive agent. It stimulates $\alpha_2$-adrenergic receptors in the brain, which makes it effective in lowering blood pressure. It primarily is prescribed for patients with chronic hypertension and narcotic patients in detoxification programs. It is packaged in very small tablets (0.1 mg, 0.2 mg, and 0.3 mg) that can be hard for the elderly to see and easy for a child to swallow (**Figure 8.7**). Clonidine also is available in patch form, which can still contain the drug after use. A child can obtain a toxic dose simply by sucking on the patch.

Symptoms of ingestion are low blood pressure, altered mental status, miosis, and respiratory depression.[23] Children present with respiratory rates, blood pressure, and pulse rates less than 50% of normal for their age groups. The child who ingests massive quantities of clonidine can present with initial hypertension, usually lasting less than 1 hour. As the brain perceives the hypertension, the central sympatholytic downregulating effects begin to dominate and the patient becomes hypotensive. Antihypertensive drugs should not be used because of the transient nature of the hypertension.

### Diagnostic Studies

If the child is manifesting signs and symptoms of toxicity such as CNS depression, laboratory studies should include a CBC count, serum electrolytes, renal functions, and glucose. Pulse oximetry and chest radiography are indicated in any child with respiratory symptoms. If the child is demonstrating cardiovascular toxicity marked by hypotension and bradycardia, an ECG should be obtained and the child placed on continuous cardiac monitoring.

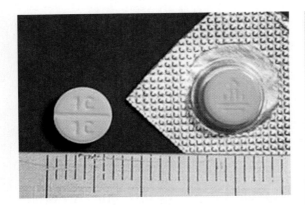

Figure 8.7 In tablet form, clonidine can be difficult to see and easy for children to swallow.

## Differential Diagnosis

Children with clonidine overdose resemble those with narcotic poisoning, with symptoms including miotic pupils, CNS depression, bradycardia, and hypotension. Other medications that can cause bradycardia include propranolol, anticholinesterase drugs, calcium channel blockers, ethanol, and digoxin (mnemonic PACED).[20]

## Management

Treatment is straightforward and supportive. Stimulation of a child with altered mental status often will increase heart and respiratory rates. Apply oxygen by face mask. Place the child in a Trendelenburg position. Obtain IV access, and be prepared to administer a 20 mL/kg bolus of lactated Ringer's or normal saline. Inotropic drugs seldom are required but, if necessary, are effective. If the respiratory rate does not improve, begin bag-mask ventilation. A few children will require intubation and mechanical ventilation until the drug effects wear off, usually within 24 hours.

Because children with clonidine overdose resemble those with narcotic poisoning, including small pupils, naloxone has been used. In the patient with known clonidine ingestion, naloxone is of little use because it is not necessary in milder cases; it will not correct the severe cases and might sufficiently lighten them so that hypertension is aggravated; and it is of no help in the hypotensive stage. Although naloxone can transiently increase the respiratory rate, it rarely obviates the need for ventilatory support in more severe overdoses. The symptomatic child will have to be observed in the hospital for 12 to 36 hours because the clonidine half-life is 12 to 16 hours.

## Cyanide[24,25]

### Clinical Features

Poisoning with cyanide can occur through dermal exposures or ingestion of silver polish, laetrile, certain insecticides, specific masticated fruit seeds, and acetonitrile-containing nail cosmetics (nail glue removers). Pulmonary exposure appears frequently in home fires (i.e., cyanide gas released from burning synthetic materials); suspect this in smoke inhalation victims. Death can occur within 1 to 15 minutes. Survivors who reach the emergency department can manifest seizures, profound acidosis, shock, or coma. Flushing often is a unique sign, and cyanosis is a relatively late finding. The characteristic smell of bitter almonds is detected in some cases.

### Diagnostic Studies

Cyanide blood levels can be obtained, but the results are never available emergently and therefore have little clinical applicability. Arterial blood gases, serum electrolytes, and a serum lactic acid level can be helpful in the acute setting because cyanide induces a profound elevated anion gap metabolic acidosis. Once the cyanide antidote kit has been administered, serial methemoglobin levels should be monitored. If the patient was involved in a fire, a carbon monoxide level should be obtained.

## Differential Diagnosis

If the child is a fire victim, carbon monoxide poisoning should be ruled out. Other toxic causes of elevated anion gap acidosis include aspirin, iron, ethylene glycol, and methanol poisoning. In addition, diabetic ketoacidosis and sepsis should be considered.

## Management

Begin rapid treatment with 100% oxygen, ventilatory assistance, and administration of the cyanide antidote kit (amyl nitrite, sodium nitrite, followed by thiosulfate). Keep in mind that the ampule of sodium nitrite in the commercially available cyanide antidote kits is an adult dose; if that dose is rapidly given to a child, it could cause profound hypotension, severe methemoglobinemia, and death. The dose of sodium nitrite for a child is 10 mg/kg, or 0.33 mL of 3% solution of sodium nitrite per kilogram of body weight. A slower rate of infusion will also help prevent hypotension. Sodium thiosulfate is administered intravenously in a 25% solution at a pediatric dose of 1.6 mL/kg (400 mg/kg) up to 50 mL (12.5 g) over 10 minutes.

# Cyclic Antidepressants

## Clinical Features

Mechanisms of cyclic antidepressant toxicity include direct myocardial (quinidine-like) depression, inhibition of norepinephrine uptake, and anticholinergic activity. Ingestion can produce significant CNS and life-threatening cardiovascular toxicity. Findings include combativeness, delirium, coma, seizures, hypotension, and dysrhythmia. A clinical hallmark of cyclic antidepressant poisoning is that the child might appear clinically stable soon after ingestion, only to rapidly deteriorate within the first 2 hours of presentation. Seizures are a poor prognostic sign because seizures induce acidosis, exacerbating the cardiotoxic effects of the cyclic antidepressant. Following an unintentional tricycle antidepressant (TCA) ingestion, children are often initially asymptomatic.[26]

## Diagnostic Studies

In all suspected cases of TCA toxicity, obtain an ECG immediately. A QRS duration of greater than 100 milliseconds is a risk factor for dysrhythmia.[27] Specific serum levels for cyclic antidepressants have little clinical applicability guiding management but might help document the presence of the drug in a child with an unknown ingestion. Also, some of the newer urine toxicology tests can qualitatively screen for the presence of cyclic antidepressants. Serial arterial blood gases should be obtained to guide clinical management of the patient's acid-base status.

## Differential Diagnosis

The clinician should also consider other anticholinergic drugs, such as diphenhydramine and other antipsychotic agents such as phenothiazines and lithium. The differential diagnosis can include other cardiotoxic drugs such as cocaine, digitalis, carbamazepine, and calcium channel antagonists.

## Management

Treat hypotension with a crystalloid challenge of 20 mL/kg of Ringer's lactate or normal saline; if unsuccessful, proceed to the use of pressors. The drug of choice for the patient with a dysrhythmia is IV sodium bicarbonate.[28] A wide QRS interval is an early indication for its use. Alkalinization via hyperventilation also is efficacious. The goal is blood pH 7.45 to 7.55. Physostigmine has no role in cyclic antidepressant overdose, despite the anticholinergic properties; the potent cardiotoxic properties of cyclic antidepressants prevent its use.

Symptomatic patients require an intensive care unit setting; however, long periods of monitoring of asymptomatic patients are not required. For patients with a normal level of consciousness, vital signs, and normal ECG from the outset, a 6-hour period of continuing normality of these parameters is sufficient. Those with an abnormality in any of these three require at least a 24-hour observation period in a monitored setting.

---

## KEY POINTS

**Management of Antidepressant Ingestion**
- Fluid resuscitation at 20 mL/kg
- Sodium bicarbonate for wide QRS interval
- No physostigmine!
- 24-hour monitoring for alteration in mental status, vital signs, or ECG

---

## Hydrocarbons

### Clinical Features

Hydrocarbons are found as solvents, fuels, and additives in household cleaners and polishes. The major toxicity of such compounds stems from their low surface tension and vapor pressure, which allow them to spread over large surface areas, such as in the lungs, leading to a chemical pneumonitis. Young children usually ingest hydrocarbons accidentally, while adolescents often abuse hydrocarbons as volatile inhalants (model glue) and paint solvents (toluene).[29]

Patients who ingest hydrocarbons might choke, cough, and gag as the product is swallowed, and vomit soon afterward. Aspiration of the product at the time of the initial swallowing can cause aspiration pneumonitis. It has been shown that the mere presence of the substance in the hypopharynx can cause chemical pneumonitis by spreading to contiguous surfaces in the airway. In addition to the pulmonary findings, there can be transient associated CNS symptoms secondary to systemic absorption of some of the hydrocarbons. Rarely, hepatic, renal, or myocardial injury occurs.

The amount of a hydrocarbon that has been ingested by a child often is difficult to quantify. Less than 1 mL of some compounds, such as mineral seal oil, when aspirated directly into the trachea, can produce severe pneumonitis and eventual death. Other compounds are difficult to aspirate and are not well absorbed from the gastrointestinal tract. Generally, compounds such as asphalt or tar, lubricants (e.g., motor oil, household oil, heavy greases), and liquid petrolatum are not toxic when ingested.

Adolescents who abuse hydrocarbons can acutely suffer CNS toxicity, which is manifested by euphoria, disinhibition, disorientation, and hallucinations. These patients are also at risk for chemical pneumonitis and life-threatening cardiotoxicity. Tragically, inhalant abuse is on the rise, as is mortality from its use. Chronic abuse can result in renal complications and lasting neurocognitive impairment.

### Diagnostic Studies

Following hydrocarbon ingestion, pulse oximetry and serial chest radiographs are indicated for the child demonstrating respiratory symptoms to rule out hypoxia and aspiration pneumonitis. In an adolescent abusing a volatile substance, an ECG and continuous cardiac monitoring should be obtained. In addition, serum electrolytes, renal function, and the patient's acid-base status should be followed.

### Differential Diagnosis

In any child with a history of hydrocarbon ingestion, it is important to identify the agent because this can have implications for management and prognosis. In a child with respiratory symptoms, pneumonia, reactive airway disease, and foreign body ingestion should be ruled out. Other chemicals causing respiratory compromise, such as insecticides (organophosphates), herbicides (paraquat), and pulmonary irritants (chlorine gas), should be considered. In an adolescent abusing volatile substances, the chance concomitant use of other illicit drugs such as cocaine, amphetamines, opioids, and marijuana should be addressed.

## Management

Asymptomatic children with a normal physical examination should be observed for 4 to 6 hours in the emergency department. If they remain well, they can be discharged with appropriate instructions to return if fever, tachypnea, or cough develops.

Treatment of hydrocarbon pneumonitis consists of supportive care. Antibiotics should not be used prophylactically. The use of corticosteroids in the treatment of aspiration from hydrocarbons has been associated with increased morbidity and is not recommended.

Inducement of emesis with syrup of ipecac or decontamination with gastric lavage is also contraindicated. Charcoal administration is not indicated unless the ingested compound contains a dangerous additive that has the potential for systemic toxicity. Other hydrocarbon compounds, including gasoline, kerosene, charcoal lighter fluid, and mineral spirits, are unlikely to produce systemic symptoms after ingestion.

Treatment for adolescents under the influence of volatile hydrocarbons includes supportive care measures and standard cardiac life support measures as indicated. Because of the cardiac sensitization of the volatiles, some experts caution against the overuse of cardiac stimulants such as epinephrine and advocate the use of β-blockers for ventricular tachydysrhythmias. However, this theory is underreported and requires further study.

# Iron[30]

## Clinical Features

Fortunately, over the past decade the pediatric mortality rate associated with iron poisoning has declined with heightened public awareness and improved child-proof packaging enforced by the FDA (Figure 8.8).

The lethal dose of elemental iron is 200 to 250 mg/kg, although gastrointestinal symp-

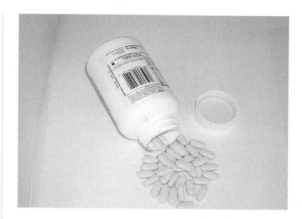

Figure 8.8 Adult multivitamins are a potential cause of iron poisoning.

toms can be seen at doses of 15 to 30 mg/kg. When calculating the ingested dose, remember that the elemental iron per unit dose is only a fraction of the total milligram weight of the tablet. Ferrous sulfate, the most commonly ingested product, is 20% elemental iron; ferrous fumarate has 32% elemental iron, and ferrous gluconate has only 10%. The toxic dose is not absolute, and fatal reactions have been reported with ingestions of only 75 mg/kg. Therefore, all ingestions should be considered potentially dangerous. Significant toxicity, however, is uncommon at amounts less than 60 mg/kg. All patients who have ingested significant amounts of iron develop gastrointestinal symptoms within 6 hours.

For iron-poisoned patients, the acute pathophysiology and clinical picture have been classified into four stages, as follows:

- **Gastrointestinal Stage.** The first signs of iron toxicity are gastrointestinal; early symptoms include vomiting, rapid onset of diarrhea, colicky abdominal pain, and gastrointestinal hemorrhage. Iron directly damages the gastrointestinal mucosa and can lead to massive fluid loss and hemorrhage. The gastrointestinal effects can contribute to systemic hypovolemia by the third spacing of the fluid in the small bowel.

- **Relative Stability Stage.** The gastrointestinal signs and symptoms might ameliorate before the onset of overt shock. In such instances, there is a stage of relative stability. This does not last longer than 6 to 12 hours, and patients are not really symptom free during this time. Careful assessment will yield evidence of decreased perfusion and acidosis.

- **Shock Stage.** The third stage is characterized by circulatory failure, profound shock, and acidosis. Shock, the most common cause of fatality in iron poisoning, has a complex etiology that includes hypovolemic, distributive, and cardiac depressant factors. The chief causes of the acidosis are the hydrated unbound circulating iron and lactic acidosis secondary to shock.

- **Hepatotoxicity Stage.** Hepatotoxicity occurs within the first 48 hours. Earlier onsets correlate with increased severity. This is the second most common cause of mortality.

Gastrointestinal scarring is a late manifestation of iron poisoning, occurring 2 to 6 weeks after ingestion. Typically, it presents as gastric outlet obstruction, but any portion of the small intestine can be involved.

## Diagnostic Studies

Prompt clinical assessment coupled with early abdominal radiographs and timely serum iron levels are the mainstay of the management of the iron-poisoned patient (Table 8-6). A negative radiograph in a symptomatic patient does not exclude iron ingestion. Reasons for a negative radiograph can be that the iron was not ingested; or the ingested iron has dissolved or was absorbed; a liquid iron preparation was ingested; or a pediatric multivitamin-plus-iron pharmaceutical with a very small amount of iron per tablet was ingested. The latter pharmaceutical is associated with only mild symptoms. Serum iron levels, if obtained promptly, often correlate with the likelihood of developing symptoms. Usually, iron levels of less than 350 mcg/dL, when drawn 2 to 6 hours after ingestion, predict a benign course. Patients with levels in the range of 350 to 500 mcg/dL often show mild stage I symptoms but rarely develop serious complications. Levels of more than 500 mcg/dL suggest signif-

---

| TABLE 8-6 | Management of the Iron-poisoned Patient |
| --- | --- |

- Assess stability of patient's condition, and stabilize if required.
- History: How much? When? Type of iron salt? Enteric coated? Symptoms?
- Determine serum iron level.
- Obtain abdominal radiograph to corroborate ingestion. Three planes are required to rule out drug concretions or adherence to gastric wall. Consider gastrotomy for presence of concretions, gastric wall adherence, or a potentially fatal amount of iron in the stomach.
- If radiograph suggests greater than 30 mg/kg elemental iron in a child or greater than 1 g in an adolescent, begin whole bowel irrigation with polyethylene glycol electrolyte lavage solution. Patients with negative radiographs do not require gastrointestinal decontamination. If asymptomatic, they will remain so; if symptomatic, it is too late for it to be of benefit.
- Chelate the symptomatic patient with deferoxamine.
- Admit to intensive care unit for shock or decreased level of consciousness.

---

icant risk for stage III manifestations. However, serum iron determination is not always available on a stat basis.

CBC, serum electrolytes, BUN, creatinine, glucose, and liver function tests should also be obtained. An arterial blood gas analysis can be helpful, as an elevated anion gap acidosis can occur.

## Differential Diagnosis

Other toxins causing gastrointestinal irritation and vomiting should be considered, such as salicylates, theophylline, and colchicine. Other hepatotoxins such as acetaminophen, arsenic, carbon tetrachloride, and Amanita phalloides mushrooms should be added to the differential list of potential poisons. Other medications besides iron that are visible (radiopaque) on x-ray include choral hydrate, heavy metals (mercury), phenothiazines, enteric-coated pills (salicylates), and sustained-release medications (theophylline). Use the mnemonic CHIPES for an easy memory tip.[20]

## Management

The amount of iron ingested is often hard to quantify, and minimal safe levels are not well established. Although controversial, syrup of ipecac might still have a role in large iron ingestions witnessed in the home setting; however, its' use in the emergency department is not recommended. Gastric lavage has little benefit more than 1 hour after ingestion. In addition, the diameter of the gastric evacuation tube used in a child often is too small to allow removal of significant pill fragments and concretions. Iron is not adsorbed to charcoal. Whole bowel irrigation is considered the technique of choice with large ingestions. Gastrotomies have been performed with massive overdoses. Intragastric complexing with bicarbonate, phosphate, or deferoxamine should be avoided because these approaches are ineffective and can be dangerous.

Patients arriving with severe early symptoms of iron toxicity, including vomiting, diarrhea, gastrointestinal bleeding, depressed sensorium, or circulatory compromise require urgent, intensive treatment. The first priority is obtaining venous access. Simultaneously, blood should be drawn for CBC count, blood glucose, electrolytes, BUN, liver function tests, serum iron, and typing and cross-matching. The total iron-binding capacity (TIBC) level often is inaccurate in the setting of iron poisoning and not useful in the management of an acute overdose. Patients in shock should be supported with normal saline or lactated Ringer's solution and blood transfusions if indicated. These patients often are very acidotic and require large amounts of sodium bicarbonate. Specific chelation therapy with IV deferoxamine should be started immediately in all severely poisoned patients. Careful attention should be paid to hydration states because fluid-depleted patients treated with deferoxamine are at risk for hypotension, anaphylaxis, and acute renal failure.

Chelation therapy with parenteral deferoxamine enhances the excretion of iron. Indications for chelation are the presence of symptoms or a serum iron concentration of greater than 350 mcg/dL. The IV dose of deferoxamine is 15 mg/kg per hour up to a maximum of 6 g/day. Indications for cessation of chelation are the absence of symptoms and resolution of acidosis or when the maximal dose has been given. The classic "vin rose" urine color change will result if iron-binding stores are saturated and free iron is complexed with deferoxamine. Although this finding can be helpful in diagnosing toxicity, its results often are subtle; therefore, an absent color change does not rule out significant iron poisoning.

Further problems can include hypotension, profound metabolic acidosis, hypoglycemia or hyperglycemia, anemia and colloid loss due to gastrointestinal hemorrhage (after equilibration), renal shutdown due to shock, and hepatic failure with an associated bleeding diathesis. The maintenance of an adequate urine output is critical to prevent renal failure and promote excretion of the iron-deferoxamine complex. If renal failure occurs, chelation can be continued with concurrent extracorporeal removal, with charcoal hemoperfusion favored over hemodialysis for removal of the iron-deferoxamine complex.

# Opioids

## Clinical Features

Opioid agents include heroin, codeine, morphine, meperidine, propoxyphene, methadone, and diphenoxylate-atropine (Lomotil).[31] The classic triad of opioid overdose is decreased level of consciousness, depressed respirations, and pinpoint pupils (Figure 8.9). In massive overdoses, noncardiogenic pulmonary edema can occur. Overdoses with meperidine can cause seizures, whereas overdose with propoxyphene can cause cardiotoxicity.

## YOUR FIRST CLUE

**Signs of Opioid Ingestion**
- Decreased level of consciousness
- Decreased respirations
- Pinpoint pupils

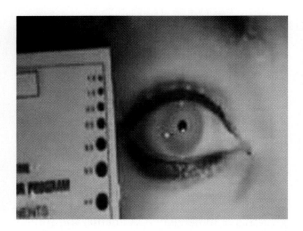

**Figure 8.9** Pinpoint pupils (<1 mm) are part of the classic triad of opioid overdose. This image depicts near-pinpoint pupils. Source: National Institute on Chemical Dependency (http://www.ni-cor.com/ni-corsignsandsymptomsofalcoholismanddrugaddiction.html)

## Diagnostic Studies

In a pediatric patient presenting with a suspected opioid overdose, a CBC count, serum electrolytes, and glucose should be obtained. The patient should have continuous cardiac monitoring with pulse oximetry measured. If in respiratory distress, a chest radiograph should be obtained to rule out aspiration pneumonitis or noncardiogenic pulmonary edema. A standard urine toxicology screen will qualitatively detect most opioids such as heroin.

## Differential Diagnosis

The differential diagnosis of a child presenting with respiratory and CNS depression should include sedative-hypnotic agents (benzodiazepines and barbiturates), ethanol, and any of the other toxic alcohols. A patient with pinpoint pupils might have also been exposed to clonidine, phenothiazines, or organophosphate insecticides, or could be suffering from a pontine hemorrhage. If an adolescent patient is under the influence of heroin, other illicit drugs should be considered.

## Management

The primary treatment of opioid ingestion includes airway stabilization and the administration of the pure opioid antagonist naloxone. If given rapidly, intubation can generally be avoided. Any patient with suspected opioid toxicity or any patient with altered mental status of unknown etiology should receive a trial of an IV bolus of naloxone (0.1 mg/kg, or 2 to 4 mg for children older than 5 years). If needed, naloxone can be continued intravenously via continuous infusion. In addition, the antidote can be administered via the tracheal tube, subcutaneously, or intralingually with a comparable onset of action. Diphenoxylate, propoxyphene, and methadone overdoses sometimes require very large doses of naloxone and prolonged therapy. Some sources recommend the IV administration of a longer-acting opioid antagonist such as nalmefene for those narcotic agents with a longer pharmacologic half life ($T1/2$).[32]

# Organophosphates[33]

## Clinical Features

Organophosphates permanently inactivate acetylcholinesterase, leading to an accumulation of acetylcholine at the neuromuscular junction.

Vomiting usually is the initial symptom. Other associated symptoms, such as pinpoint pupils, muscle fasciculation, and wheezing, also can be present. Toxicity can mimic gastroenteritis, asthma, seizures, or heat exhaustion. These symptoms usually are seen clinically as a result of toxic exposures of organophosphate and carbamate insecticides. The most serious symptoms for these patients are overwhelming bronchorrhea and even respiratory failure.

> ### WHAT ELSE?
>
> **Differential Diagnosis for Opioids**
> - Sedative-hypnotics
> - Ethanol/toxic alcohols

## Diagnostic Studies

Laboratory studies in symptomatic patients include electrolytes for patients with vomiting and diarrhea, along with a chest radiograph and arterial blood gas analysis for any child with severe respiratory distress. Organophosphates will cause depression of the red blood cell (true) cholinesterase and plasma (pseudo) cholinesterase activity. Levels can be obtained, but the long turnaround time (particularly for the true cholinesterase level) usually makes this test obsolete in the emergent care of the critically ill child.

## Differential Diagnosis

The differential diagnosis for a child with suspected organophosphate poisoning includes carbamate insecticide toxicity, herbicide poisoning (paraquat), hydrocarbon ingestion and aspiration, as well as nerve or chemical warfare agent poisoning. Nontoxic causes of respiratory distress such as pneumonia, reactive airway disease, and foreign body aspiration should be ruled out.

## Management

In moderate to severe poisoning, the treatment priority is maintenance of the airway, accomplished through intubation. Atropine can be injected intravenously at 0.5 to 1 mg doses or more until the airway has become sufficiently dry that ventilation is no longer impaired. Large doses (10 mg or more) of atropine might be required for satisfactory clinical response. With organophosphate insecticide poisoning, a cholinesterase regenerator such as pralidoxime chloride (2-PAM, Protopam) might be required. The dosing includes a 25 mg/kg IV loading dose over 5 to 30 minutes, then 10 mg/kg/hour or repeat loading every 1 to 2 hours dose for 1 to 2 doses until muscle weakness is relieved, then at 10 to 12 hour intervals if cholinergic signs recur. This drug is not indicated in carbamate insecticide poisoning. When managing these patients, skin decontamination is essential, as is protection of the staff from dermal absorption (i.e., gloves and protective clothing must be worn).

## Salicylates[34]

### Clinical Features

The usual signs and symptoms of acute salicylate ingestion are nausea, vomiting, hyperventilation, hyperpyrexia, tinnitus, oliguria, disorientation, coma, convulsions, and hyperglycemia (hypoglycemia in the young child). Less common manifestations include respiratory depression, pulmonary edema, acute tubular necrosis, hepatotoxicity, and syndrome of inappropriate secretion of antidiuretic hormone (SIADH).

**Signs and Symptoms of Salicylate Poisoning**

- Nausea and vomiting
- Hyperventilation
- Hyperpyrexia
- Tinnitus
- Oliguria
- Disorientation or coma
- Seizures
- Hyperglycemia
- Pulmonary edema
- Acute tubular necrosis
- SIADH
- Liver failure

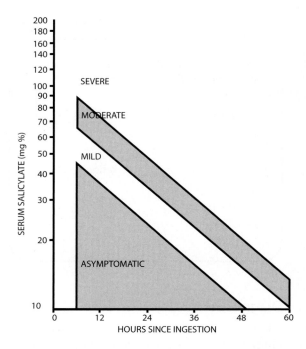

**Figure 8.10** Done nomogram for salicylate poisoning. The Done nomogram should be used with the following cautions: The patient has taken a single acute ingestion and is not suffering from chronic toxicity and has not ingested a delayed-release aspirin preparation; and the blood level to be plotted on the nomogram was drawn more than 6 hours after ingestion.

Source: Done AK. Salicylate intoxication: significance of measurements of salicylate in blood in cases of acute ingestion. *Pediatrics.* 1960;26:800. Adapted with permission.

## Diagnostic Studies

In any child with a suspected aspirin overdose, arterial blood gases should be measured. Although the classic blood gas interpretation in acute salicylism is a mixed respiratory alkalosis/metabolic acidosis, children with salicylate poisoning can rapidly develop metabolic acidosis not preceded by respiratory alkalosis. Serum electrolytes, BUN, creatinine, serum glucose, serum ketones, and an acetaminophen level should also be determined.

In acute ingestions, serum salicylate levels are prognostic and are usually drawn approximately 6 hours postingestion. They have less use in chronic salicylism. The Done nomogram (Figure 8.10), although historically known to determine the severity of a salicylate overdose, actually has very limited use clinically. This nomogram should be used only in patients with a single acute overdose. Serum levels in patients with chronic toxicity or ingestions of enteric-coated preparations should not be plotted. The ultimate decision to treat should be predicated on symptomatology rather than the Done nomogram result.

Because of the potential for delayed salicylate toxicity and formation of gastric concretions, more than one salicylate level is recommended to ensure a declining trend. Generally, ingestions of less than 150 mg/kg are mild; 150 to 300 mg/kg, moderate; 300 to 500 mg/kg, serious; and greater than 500 mg/kg, severe.

## Differential Diagnosis

In any pediatric patient with suspected aspirin toxicity, poisoning with other pain relievers such as acetaminophen and nonsteroidal anti-inflammatory agents should be considered.

In addition, because salicylate poisoning impairs glucose metabolism and results in ketosis, diabetic ketoacidosis (DKA) should be ruled out. Other pharmaceutical agents that cause elevated anion gap metabolic acidosis (iron and isoniazid-INH) should also be considered.

## Management

Management includes the general principles for all ingestions. Monitor potassium levels carefully because they are usually low. For moderate and severe ingestions, an IV line should be established, and 5% dextrose in water with 50 mEq/L of sodium bicarbonate given at a rate of 10 to 15 mLq/kg over 1 to 2 hours. The goal of alkalinization is to maintain urine pH greater than 7; however, this will not be accomplished without aggressive potassium supplementation. Arterial blood gas analysis helps determine the degree of acidosis. If the pH is less than 7.15, an additional 1 to 2 mEq/kg bicarbonate can be given over 1 to 2 hours. Avoid rapid bicarbonate administration because it may lead to relative CNS acidosis and seizures. Severe, persistent acidosis might require 1 to 2 mEq/kg bicarbonate every 2 hours. Hemodialysis or hemoperfusion may be necessary in unresponsive acidosis (pH less than 7.1), renal failure, noncardiogenic pulmonary edema, seizures, or progressive deterioration after trials of standard therapy. The salicylate level is not useful as the only criterion for dialysis unless it is over 80 mg/dL in an acute ingestion. The threshold for dialysis is lower for chronically poisoned patients because the toxicity is more severe, and generally, serum levels are less impressive than in the acute overdose.

## KEY POINTS

### Management of Salicylate Ingestions
- IV fluid resuscitation and sodium bicarbonate administration.
- Monitor and replace potassium as needed.
- Hemodialysis or hemoperfusion for salicylate level greater than 80 mg/dL, renal failure, severe metabolic acidosis, pulmonary edema, seizures.

# Selective Serotonin Reuptake Inhibitors

## Clinical Features

Selective serotonin reuptake inhibitors (SSRI) such as fluoxetine (Prozac), sertraline (Zoloft) and herbal St. John's Wort are popular antidepressants currently available and widely prescribed. In therapeutic doses, SSRIs are relatively safe and were originally designed in response to the high incidence of adverse effects and deaths attributed to cyclic antidepressants. However, in large overdoses, or in combination with other medications, SSRIs can cause significant morbidity and mortality in the pediatric patient.

Acute oral overdose can be associated with nausea and vomiting, dizziness, tremors, lethargy, and CNS depression. Seizure activity and death have been reported with doses well over 100 times the recommended therapeutic dose. Most adverse side effects are associated with coingestions or secondary to hyperthermia by a drug-drug interaction known as the serotonin syndrome. This syndrome is similar in presentation to the neuroleptic malignant syndrome (NMS) but milder in presentation with less associated mortality. Pharmacologically, it results from serotonin excess as opposed to dopamine depletion, as is the case with NMS.

## Differential Diagnosis

The differential diagnosis of SSRI ingestion should be cyclic antidepressants. If hyperthermia develops, anticholinergics and antihistamines should be added to the list of possibilities.

## Management

Most accidental pediatric SSRI overdoses result in only mild toxicity. Treatment of SSRI toxicity includes supportive care, airway management, and gastric decontamination with activated charcoal. If the serotonin syndrome is diagnosed or suspected, cooling measures and benzodiazepines usually suffice.

## γ-Hydroxybutyrate

γ-hydroxybutyrate (GHB) was synthesized in 1960 and first used as an anesthetic agent and for the treatment of sleep disorders, as it induces REM sleep. However, its use was halted when the drug was found to induce seizure activity. An erroneous study in the 1970s reported that GHB might stimulate growth hormone production; therefore, the drug became popular in the body-building community. In addition, due to its euphoric and mind-altering effects, it has become a very popular drug of abuse with adolescents in the party scene. The Drug Enforcement Administration (DEA) has classified GHB as a federally controlled substance like marijuana. It has also been tragically used in date rape due to its rapid onset and amnestic properties. Currently, it is under FDA investigation for clinical use in narcolepsy.

GHB is a colorless, odorless liquid or gel (Figure 8.11). As a powder, it has a salty taste. Its onset of action is rapid, and it is obtainable on the street and over the Internet and can be easily produced in the home. One of the precursors of GHB, γ-butyrolactate (GBL), has also gained recent popularity.

### Clinical Features

GHB ingestion results in drowsiness, dizziness, and disorientation within 15 to 30 minutes. High doses can result in a depressed respiratory drive, bradycardia, and anesthesia. The hallmark of GHB toxicity is marked agitation with stimulation despite apnea and hypoxia.

### Differential Diagnosis

Included in the differential for a GHB overdose are opiates, sedative-hypnotics including barbiturates, benzodiazepines, and chloral hydrate (the original "Mickey Finn"), calcium channel blockers, clonidine, and ethanol.

### Management

Treatment involves airway protection if necessary (often, the patient will suddenly awaken in 4 to 6 hours and extubate). Atropine can be used for profound bradycardia. Activated charcoal can be administered following recent ingestions for gastric decontamination; however, do not give patients with respiratory failure oral medication. There is no proven antidote for GHB, although some anecdotal reports claim that physostigmine can reverse the effects of GHB. Currently, this practice is not widely supported in the literature.

## Ecstasy

### Clinical Features

Ecstasy (3,4, methylenedioxymethamphetamine) is a designer amphetamine that has become one of the most widely abused drugs in the adolescent patient population (Figure 8.12). The pharmacologic effects are a blend of sympathomimetic amphetamine stimulation with the hallucinogenic effects of mescaline. The

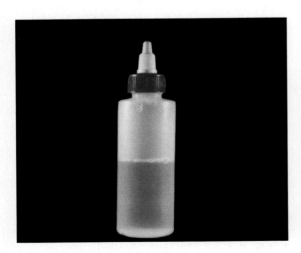

**Figure 8.11** GHB.

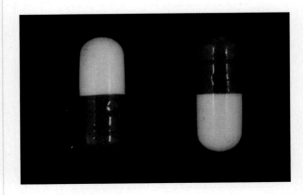

**Figure 8.12** Ecstasy.

drug is extremely popular at "rave" parties and at dance clubs.

Following ingestion, the onset of action is 30 to 90 minutes; plateau effects are achieved in 2 to 3 hours. The drug is abused because (in therapeutic doses) it induces extreme euphoria, increased energy, feelings of belonging, heightened sensations, empathy, music appreciation, fear dissolution, and bright, intense visual perceptions.

Negative toxic effects of ecstasy include bruxism, trismus, short-term memory loss, confusion, headaches, vertigo, ataxia, vomiting, depression, and psychological addiction. Major complications include profound hyperthermia, hypertension, seizures, dehydration, hypernatremia and hyponatremia, hepatic and renal failure, rhabdomyolysis, myocardial infarction, and intracranial hemorrhage.

### Differential Diagnosis

The drugs that could be confused with ecstasy ingestion include other amphetamines, LSD, and phencyclidine (PCP).

### Management

The treatment of symptomatic patients is supportive care, airway management, rapid cooling, along with liberal doses of benzodiazepines for tachycardia, hypertension, and agitation. For gastric decontamination of recent ingestions, activated charcoal is recommended. Toxicology urine screens that are marketed to detect amphetamines can be negative after ecstasy and designer amphetamine use.

## Overall Management Issues

Consultation with a local or regional poison center can often provide helpful input in making the decision regarding disposition. After being observed for 4 to 6 hours, some patients who have ingested potentially toxic substances and are asymptomatic or minimally affected can be discharged with appropriate instructions for return if necessary. Because repeat ingestions occur in 10% to 50% of children, all discharged patients and their families should be given instructions about poison prevention

techniques. Children with significant toxic ingestions or potential intoxication with substances that have delayed effects (sustained-release products) require admission to the hospital. The specific ingestion and degree of physiologic alteration determine whether treatment in a pediatric intensive care unit is warranted. A conservative approach is also recommended for toxins that can cause potential mortality in small doses (e.g., camphor, benzocaine, lomotil, chloroquine, methyl salicylates).[5,35–37] All patients with intentional overdoses should undergo psychiatric assessment.

## Additional Routes of Exposure[38]

Hazardous chemical exposure includes direct contact with the skin or eye or inhalation of noxious gases (Figure 8.13). The risk of skin exposure is chiefly from acid or alkali burns due to direct contact. However, systemic toxicity is possible in situations involving lipophilic substances. Eye exposure is a local injury concern, not systemic toxicity. Inhalation exposures are discussed in detail in Chapter 18, Preparedness for Acts of Nuclear, Biological, and Chemical Terrorism. Health care workers must be careful to avoid personal exposure to toxic chemicals. Appropriate protective clothing is indicated.

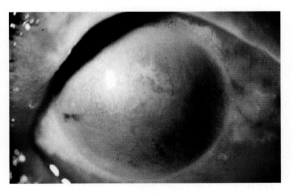

**Figure 8.13** Injury caused to the eye by hazardous chemical exposure.

## Ophthalmic and Cutaneous Exposure

Assessment consists of direct inspection of the body part for evidence of caustic or corrosive damage. Copious irrigation of exposed areas with water or saline solution should be initiated immediately, preferably at the scene. Chemical burns are managed as thermal burns. Irrigation of caustic eye injuries should be copious and started as early as possible. Adequacy of irrigation can be judged by checking pH of the tears when acidic or basic compounds have resulted in eye injury. Followup management of eye exposures is dependent on the results of the fluorescein examination after irrigation. A negative result requires no interventions; ophthalmologic consultation should be considered for any positive finding.

---

**CASE SCENARIO 4**

A 5-year-old boy was in an apartment fire but escaped with burns to his feet. In the emergency department he is frightened, but able to speak in full sentences. His respiratory rate is 30 breaths per minute, heart rate is 120 bpm, blood pressure is 100/70, and his temperature is 37.6°C. Physical examination reveals no carbonaceous sputum and no stridor or wheezing. He has partial-thickness burns to the soles of his feet, with good distal pulses and color.

1. *What is the most significant physical examination finding in this child?*
2. *What is the most important therapy for this patient?*

---

## Smoke Inhalation

### Background[39]

Smoke inhalation is a leading cause of morbidity and mortality in burn victims. Exposure to noxious substances in the atmosphere can directly injure the respiratory apparatus or can indirectly produce systemic intoxication (**Figure 8.14**). The nature of the resulting illness depends on the source, intensity, and duration of exposure. Offending agents range from single, well-defined chemicals such as hydrogen cyanide, which produces severe systemic toxicity when inhaled, to the airborne products of a residential fire, a complex matrix of organic and inorganic chemicals, heated atmospheric gases, and the gaseous products of incomplete combustion.

Smoke contains four categories of environmental threat: heat, asphyxiants (chiefly carbon monoxide and hydrogen cyanide), particulate matter, and pulmonary irritants.

### Heat

Upper airway burns are often encountered in victims of closed-space fire and can occur whenever

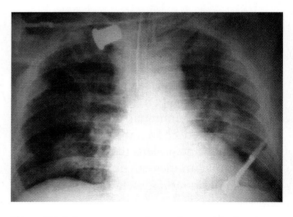

**Figure 8.14** Exposure to noxious substances in the atmosphere can directly injure the airway, bronchi, and lungs.

the temperature of inhaled gas exceeds 150°C. However, thermal injury distal to the vocal cords is quite unusual because the temperature of inhaled smoke decreases rapidly as it passes down the respiratory tree; thus, direct thermal injury to the lung is uncommon. However, significant burns of the supraglottic region or vocal cords frequently produce edema sufficiently severe to result in upper airway obstruction. In contrast, the latent heat of steam is sufficiently high that burns of the distal airway and lung do occur with this toxic inhalation.

### Asphyxiants

Asphyxiants include carbon monoxide (CO), which is produced by the incomplete combustion of hydrocarbons such as wood and paper, and hydrogen cyanide (HCN), a byproduct of combustion of nitrogen-containing polymers such as wool or silk. Hydrogen sulfide ($H_2S$) is a physical asphyxiant that produces hypoxemia through displacement of oxygen from the atmosphere. The characteristic odor of cyanide is that of burned almonds, whereas that of sulfides is rotten eggs.

CO is the most frequently encountered asphyxiant. This colorless, odorless compound has an affinity for hemoglobin (Hb) approximately 250 times greater than that of oxygen. Binding of CO to Hb diminishes the oxygen-carrying capacity of blood by a proportion equal to the percentage of carboxyhemoglobin (COHb) and shifts the oxyhemoglobin dissociation curve to the left. In addition, there is evidence that CO interferes with cellular oxygen metabolism at the mitochondrial level. Dissolved oxygen is not affected by CO; therefore, the measured $PaO_2$ can be normal even when the oxygen saturation (percentage of Hb bound to oxygen) is profoundly depressed.[40]

Venous CO concentrations up to 5% are found in normal individuals. Concentrations of 20% often produce significant neurologic symptoms, but a single level might not correlate with clinical manifestations. Concentrations of greater than 60% frequently are associated with death or neurologic morbidity. In a particular patient, however, specific COHb levels are less important in management than the history of exposure and condition of the patient.

In addition to household fires, children can be exposed to many other sources of CO, including poorly repaired motor vehicles and those left running while parked, and malfunctioning or inappropriate household heaters. In rare instances, children are exposed to other asphyxiants such as HCN or $H_2S$ after environmental catastrophes or while playing in an industrial area.

### Particulate Matter

Particulate matter consists mainly of carbon. Large particles (i.e., greater than 5 $\mu$m) are deposited in the trachea or bronchi, and those less than 1 $\mu$m reach the pulmonary alveoli. Although carbon per se is physiologically inert, it can be coated with toxic chemical products of combustion such as acrolein, hydrochloric acid, or aromatic hydrocarbons. In addition, inhalation of carbon dust has been shown to produce airway hyperreactivity.

### Pulmonary Irritants

Pulmonary irritants include a heterogeneous group of compounds including ammonia, sulfur oxides, nitrogen oxides, halogen acids (e.g., HCl), chlorine gas, aldehydes (e.g., acrolein), ketones, and phosgene. These chemicals present both as gases or bound to the surface of small particles and can incite pulmonary edema and mucosal injury.

## Clinical Features

Inhalation injury should be considered in any child who is exposed to fire or presents with a burn injury (other than scald). History of exposure in an enclosed space or physical features such as facial burns, singed nasal hairs, carbonaceous deposits in the pharynx, stridor, or hoarseness suggest the possibility of upper airway injury. Although respirations might be unlabored initially, laryngeal edema is progressive in the smoke inhalation patient and is not at its peak until 2 to 8 hours after injury.

The presentation of pulmonary injury ranges in severity from mild wheezing, rales, and rhonchi to frank respiratory failure with cyanosis. After a patient's exposure to fire, an altered sensorium, particularly with loss of consciousness, should be assumed to indicate CO poisoning and central nervous system hypoxia. Concurrent traumatic closed-head injury should remain in the differential diagnosis until excluded.

Non–fire-related toxic inhalation also chiefly involves CO. CO poisoning should be considered in any child with nausea, vomiting, or headache, with or without altered sensorium, when there is no other obvious etiology. Typical presentations include a child who is found unconscious in a home in which a charcoal grill is used for heating, a child who begins to vomit and becomes somnolent while riding in the back seat of an automobile in poor repair, or a child living in a kerosene-heated home. Not infrequently, the child with occult CO toxicity presents with a nonfebrile flu-like illness and improves considerably while under care in the ED. The symptoms subside after removal of the child from exposure to a faulty car exhaust or a toxic home environment. Multiple patients from the same locale suggest CO poisoning as well. Even when all victims are exposed to similar amounts of CO, children are often more severely affected. A high index of suspicion for CO toxicity must be maintained to prevent recurrent toxicity or even death.

## YOUR FIRST CLUE

**Signs and Symptoms of Smoke Inhalation**
- Facial burns
- Carbonaceous sputum
- Stridor

**CO Poisoning**
- Nausea
- Vomiting
- Headache
- Decreased level of consciousness
- Multiple patients with similar symptoms

## Diagnostic Studies[41]

The diagnostic evaluation of the child after inhalation injury focuses on assessment of airway patency, baseline pulmonary function, and determination of CO poisoning. Children who present with a history consistent with exposure to fire or CO intoxication require determination of CO level (usually expressed as percent COHb). In most hospitals, this determination is performed with cooximetry, which also indicates the percentage of methemoglobin. This can be run on a venous or arterial sample. Although pulse oximetry is very useful in the evaluation of oxygen saturation, this technique does not detect the presence of COHb or other abnormal hemoglobins and should never be depended on for this purpose. In fact, the oxygen saturation is falsely elevated with CO poisoning.

In room air, the half-life of COHb is approximately 4 hours. It decreases to 60 to 90 minutes when the child receives an $F_{IO_2}$ of 1.0 and 15 to 30 minutes under hyperbaric conditions (3 atmospheres). Because burn victims are generally treated with oxygen ($F_{IO_2} = 1$) at the scene of the fire and en route to the hospital, significant toxicity can be manifest even when COHb levels are low at the time of presentation. A normal COHb level at the time of admission does not exclude CO poisoning if the history or physical findings suggest that condition to be present.

The chest radiograph is an essential baseline diagnostic study, particularly when exposure occurs in a fire. It initially can be normal but eventually will reveal bilateral patchy and confluent areas of opacification. Other appropriate laboratory studies include a CBC count, urinalysis, and serum electrolytes, BUN, creatinine, and liver function tests. An ECG should be performed to establish a baseline and to detect the presence of myocardial ischemia or infarction.

## Management

Care of the child with inhalation injury follows the usual ABC emergency sequence. In addition to administration of oxygen ($F_{IO_2} = 1$) and routine measures to assess and secure the airway, after stabilization, children at risk of upper airway thermal injury (facial, oral, or pharyngeal burns, hoarseness, stridor) require urgent bronchoscopy to evaluate for life-threatening airway obstruction. Of course, when airway edema appears to be evolving or signs of obstruction are severe, immediate intubation is required and can prevent catastrophic loss of airway patency.

Aggressive fluid administration, consistent with appropriate burn resuscitation parame-

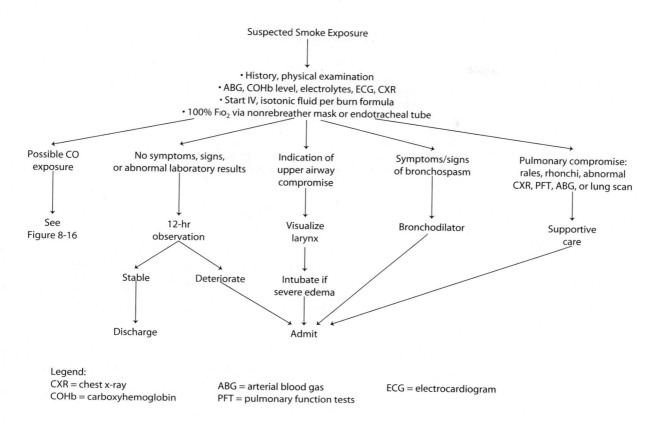

**Figure 8.15** General guide for management of children exposed to smoke.
Source: Thom SR. Smoke inhalation. *Emerg Med Clin North Am.* 1989;7(2):371–387. Adapted with permission.

ters, does not increase the risk of pulmonary edema in the patient with combined burn and inhalation injury. Fluids should not be restricted in an effort to limit the progression of airway and pulmonary compromise.

Diagnostic and management algorithms are presented in **Figures 8.15** and **8.16**. Oxygen is the initial treatment of choice for most other sequelae of toxic inhalation. As noted previously, oxygen reduces the half-life of COHb, thereby accelerating the rate at which levels decease.[42,43] Oxygen ($F_{IO_2} = 1$) is administered until the COHb concentration is less than 5% and the patient has fully regained normal neurologic function.

In cases of CO poisoning, there is a significant residual tissue burden of CO that remains bound to cellular cytochrome systems and myoglobin even when the blood COHb concentration has returned to normal. Treatment with 100% oxygen under hyperbaric conditions (e.g., 2 to 3 atmospheres) can accelerate the rate of tissue

## KEY POINTS

**Management of CO Poisoning**

- Assess and treat abnormalities in ABCs.
- Provide 100% oxygen.
- Determine COHb level.
- Provide hyperbaric oxygen treatment for neurologic symptoms, COHb level greater than 25%, and pregnant women.

decontamination.[44,45] Therefore, when the history suggests exposure to CO, children who are found unconscious at the scene of the exposure and those with neurologic dysfunction at the time of presentation should be referred to a hyperbaric facility even if the blood COHb concentration has returned to normal.[46] When profound neurologic dysfunction exists at the fire scene, there is a strong probability that CO intoxication is

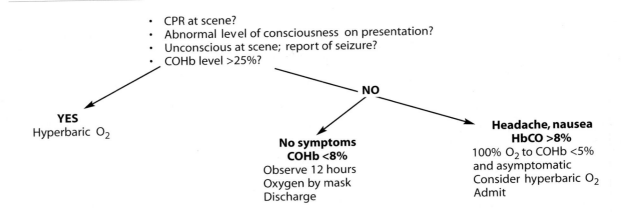

**Possible CO Exposure**

- ABCs (CPR if needed)
- 100% oxygen
- Cooximetry (to measure COHb) with arterial blood gas (to measure acidosis)
- Chest radiographs, monitor

- CPR at scene?
- Abnormal level of consciousness on presentation?
- Unconscious at scene; report of seizure?
- COHb level >25%?

**YES**
Hyperbaric O₂

**NO**

**No symptoms
COHb <8%**
Observe 12 hours
Oxygen by mask
Discharge

**Headache, nausea
HbCO >8%**
100% O₂ to COHb <5%
and asymptomatic
Consider hyperbaric O₂
Admit

**Figure 8.16** Guide for known or suspected CO poisoning.
Source: Thom SR. Smoke Inhalation. *Emerg Med Clin North Am.* 1989; 7(2):371–387. Adapted with permission.

implicated (perhaps in concert with hypoxemia). In this context, direct referral to a cooperating hyperbaric facility from the fire scene might be appropriate before determination of COHb concentration. There are studies suggesting that early application of hyperbaric oxygen can be lifesaving or reduce the possibility of severe neurologic injury. In addition, all children, even if neurologically intact, with a measured COHb level of greater than 25% and all pregnant women should be referred to such a facility.

The decision to refer to a hyperbaric facility will depend on locally available facilities and the stability of the patient. In many communities, hyperbaric chambers capable of permitting critical care during hyperbaric conditions are available. After the initial resuscitation and stabilization, assisted ventilation and hemodynamic support need not prevent hyperbaric treatment. Every emergency department should develop referral agreements and protocols with local and regional hyperbaric centers. Some recent sources question the overall efficacy of hyperbaric oxygen therapy in the setting of CO poisoning and argue that 100% normobaric oxygen administration is a more practical and superior treatment option.[43,47]

Suspected exposure to HCN is treated as described earlier for cyanide.[48,49] The treatment for $H_2S$ is the same except that thiosulfate is not needed. Management of other sequelae of inhalation injury follows standard principles of care. Respiratory failure is treated with assisted ventilation, including positive end-expiratory pressure, as indicated. A bronchodilator might be of value, but empiric use of antibiotics or a corticosteroid is discouraged.

## THE BOTTOM LINE

- Consider toxins as a cause for sudden changes in mental status or other physiologic features.
- Management focuses on the assessment and treatment of abnormalities in ABCs, identification of the toxin, and administration of an antidote.

## Check Your Knowledge

1. Activated charcoal will adsorb all of the following medications except:
   A. Ferrous sulfate
   B. Phenobarbital
   C. Salicylates
   D. Theophylline
   E. Verapamil

2. A high anion gap metabolic acidosis would be anticipated in each of the following toxic ingestions except:
   A. Ethylene glycol
   B. Iron
   C. Isopropanol
   D. Methanol
   E. Salicylates

3. A comatose adolescent patient with an acute exposure to an unknown toxin should receive all of the following therapeutic interventions except:
   A. Dextrose
   B. Flumazenil
   C. Intravenous normal saline solution
   D. Naloxone
   E. Oxygen

4. A mother brings her 2-month-old daughter to be checked for CO poisoning, because their detector had sounded. The infant has normal vital signs and is sleeping. The mother complains of a headache. While waiting for the blood gas results, you place both mom and infant on 100% oxygen. Assuming the levels are slightly elevated (10%), an appropriate amount of time on 100% oxygen for treatment would be:
   A. 15 to 30 minutes
   B. 60 to 90 minutes
   C. 180 minutes
   D. 240 minutes

## References

1. American Academy of Pediatrics, Committee on Injury and Poison Prevention. *Handbook of Common Poisonings in Children*. 3rd ed. Elk Grove Village, Il: American Academy of Pediatrics; 1994.

2. Fine JS, Goldfrank LR. Update in medical toxicology. *Pediatr Clinic North Am.* 1992;39:1031–1051.

3. Henretig FM. Special considerations in the poisoned pediatric patient. *Emerg Med Clin North Am.* 1994;12:549–567.

4. Erickson T. General principles of poisoning: diagnosis and management. In: Strange GR, Ahrens WR, Lelyveld S, et al, eds. *Pediatric Emergency Medicine: A Comprehensive Study Guide.* (2nd ed). New York, Ny: McGraw-Hill; 2002:559–565.

5. Litovitz T, Manoguerra A. Comparison of pediatric poisoning hazards: an analysis of 3.8 million exposure incidents. A report from the AAPCC. *Pediatrics.* 1992;89:999–1006.

6. Osterloh JD. Utility and reliability of emergency toxicologic testing. *Emerg Med Clin North Am.* 1990;8:693–723.

7. Ford M, Delaney K. Initial approaches to the poison patient. In: Ford M, Delaney K, Ling L, Erickson T (eds). *Clinical Toxicology.* Philadelphia, Pa: Harcourt-WB Saunders; 2001:4.

8. Kulig K, Initial management of ingestions of toxic substances. *N Engl J Med.* 1992;326:1677–1681.

9. Merigian KS, Woodard M, Hedges JR et al. Prospective evaluation of gastric emptying in the self-poisoned patient. *Am J Emerg Med.* 1990;8:479–483.

10. American Academy of Clinical Toxicology; European Association of Poison Centres and Clinical Toxicologists position statements on gastric lavage, activated charcoal, syrup of ipecac, cathartics, and whole bowel irrigation. *J Toxicol Clin Toxicol.* 1999;37:463–474.

11. Schnell LR, Tanz RR. The effect of providing ipecac to families seeking poison-related services. *Pediatr Emerg Care.* 1993;9:36–39.

12. Tenenbein M. Whole bowel irrigation in iron poisoning. *J Pediatr.* 1987;111:142–145.

13. Heubi JE, Barbacci MB, Zimmerman HJ. Therapeutic misadventures with acetaminophen: hepatotoxicity after multiple doses in children. *J Pediatrics.* 1998;132:22.

14. Rumack BH. Acetaminophen overdose in young children. Treatment and effects of alcohol and other additional ingestants in 417 cases. *Am J Dis Child.* 1984;138:428–433.

15. Perry HE, Shannon MW. Efficacy of oral versus intravenous N-acetylcysteine in acetaminophen overdose: results of an open-label clinical trial. *J Pediatr* 1998;132:149.

16. Erickson T. Toxic alcohols. In: Strange GR, Ahrens WR, Lelyveld S et al, eds. *Pediatric Emergency Medicine: A Comprehensive Study*

# CHAPTER REVIEW

*Guide.* (2nd Ed). New York, Ny: McGraw-Hill; 2002:569–573.

17. Erickson T. Toxic alcohol poisoning: when to suspect and keys to diagnosis. *Consultant.* 2000;40:1845–1856.

18. Barceloux DG, Krenzolok, Olson K et al: American Academy of Clinical Toxicology Ad Hoc Committee. Guidelines on the treatment of ethylene glycol poisoning. *J Toxicol Clin Toxicol.* 1999;37:537–560.

19. Brent J, McMartin K, Phillips S et al. Fomepizole for the treatment of ethylene glycol poisoning. *N Engl J Med.* 1999;340:832–838.

20. Erickson TB, Aks SE, Gussow L, Williams RH. Toxicology update: a rational approach to managing the poisoned patient. *Emerg Med Practice.* 2001;3(8);1–28.

21. Burns MJ, Linden CH, Graudins A et al. A comparison of physostigmine and benzodiazepines for the treatment of anticholinergic poisoning. *Ann Emerg Med.* 2000;35:374–381.

22. Anderson KD, Rouse TM, Randolph JG. A controlled trial of corticosteroids in children with corrosive injury of the esophagus. *N Engl J Med.* 1990;323:637–640.

23. Maloney MJ, Schwam JS. Clonidine and sudden death. *Pediatrics.* 1995;96:1176–1177.

24. Chin RG, Caldern Y. Acute cyanide poisoning: a case report. *J Emerg Med.* 2000;18:441–445.

25. Yen D, Tsai J, Wang LM et al. The clinical experience of acute cyanide poisoning. *Am J Emerg Med.* 1995;13:524–528.

26. McFee RB, Mofenson HC, Caraccio TR. A nationwide survey of the management of unintentional low dose tricyclic antidepressant ingestions involving asymptomatic children: implications for the development of evidence-based clinical guideline. *Clin Toxicol.* 2000;38:15–19.

27. Boehnert MT, Lovejoy FH. Value of the QRS duration versus the serum drug level in predicting seizures and ventricular arrhythmias after an acute overdose of tricyclic antidepressants. *N Engl J Med.* 1985;313:474–479.

28. McCabe JL, Cobaugh DJ, Menegazzi TR. Experimental tricyclic antidepressant toxicity: a randomized, controlled comparison of hypertonic saline solution, sodium bicarbonate, and hyperventilation. *Ann Emerg Med.* 1998;32:329–333.

29. Esmail A, Meyer L, Pottier A et al. Deaths from volatile substance abuse in those under 18 years: results from a national epidemiologic study. *Arch Dis Child.* 1993;69:356.

30. Morris CC. Pediatric iron poisonings in the United States. *South Med J.* 2000;93:352–358.

31. McCarron MM, Challoner RR, Thompson GA. Diphenoxylate-atropine (Lomotil) overdose in children: an update. *Pediatrics.* 1991;87:694–700.

32. Chumpa A. Nalmefene hydrochloride. *Pediatr Emerg Care.* 1999;15:141–143.

33. Aaron CK. Organophosphates and carbamates. In: Ford M, DeLaney KA, Ling L, Erickson T (eds). *Clinical Toxicology.* Philadelphia, Pa: WB Saunders; 2001:819–828.

34. Notarianni L. A reassessment of the treatment of salicylate poisoning. *Drug Safety.* 1992;7:292–303.

35. Koren G. Medications which can kill a toddler with one tablet or teaspoonful. *J Clin Toxicol.* 1993;31:407–41.

36. Liebelt EL, Shannon MW. Small doses, big problems: a selected review of highly toxic common medications. *Pediatr Emerg Care.* 1993;9:292–297.

37. Morelli J. Pediatric poisonings: the 10 most toxic prescription drugs. *Am J Nurs.* 1993;93:26–29.

38. Kirk MA, Cisek J, Rose SR. Emergency department response to hazardous materials incidents. *Emerg Med Clin North Am.* 1994;12:461–481.

39. Carvajal HF, Griffith JA. Burns and inhalation injuries. In: Fuhrman BP, Zimmerman JJ, eds. *Pediatric Critical Care.* 2nd ed. St Louis, Mo: Mosby-Year Book; 1998:1198–1210.

40. Ernst A, Zibrak JD: Carbon monoxide poisoning. *N Engl J Med.* 339:1603–1608, 1998.

41. Tomaszewski C. Carbon monoxide. In: Ford M, Delaney K, Ling L, Erickson T (eds). *Clinical Toxicolog.,* 1st ed. Philadelphia, Pa: WB Saunders; 2001:657–667.

42. Meert KL, Heidemann SM, Sarnaik AP. Outcome of children with carbon monoxide poisoning treated with normobaric oxygen. *J Trauma.* 1998;44:149–154.

43. Tighe SQ: Hyperbaric oxygen in carbon monoxide poisoning. 100% oxygen is the best option. *Br Med J.* 2000;321:110–111.

44. Hampson NB, Dunford RG, Kramer CC et al. Selection criteria utilized for hyperbaric oxygen treatment of carbon monoxide poisoning. *J Emerg Med.* 1995;13:227–231.

45. Tibbles PM, Edelsberg JS. Hyperbaric-oxygen therapy. *N Engl J Med.* 1996;334:1642–1648.

46. Rudge FW: Carbon monoxide poisoning in infants: treatment with hyperbaric oxygen. *South Med J.* 1993:86:334.

47. Scheinkestel CD, Bailey M, Myles PS et al. Hyperbaric or normobaric oxygen for acute carbon monoxide poisoning: a randomised controlled clinical trial. *Med J Austrl.* 1999;170: 203–210.

48. Kirk MA, Gerace R, Kilig KW. Cyanide and methemoglobin kinetics in smoke inhalation victims treated with the cyanide antidote kit. *Ann Emerg Med.* 1993;22:1413–1418.

49. Shusterman D, Alexeef G, Hargis C et al. Predictors of carbon monoxide and hydrogen cyanide exposure in smoke inhalation patient. *Clin Toxicol.* 1996;34:61–71.

CASE SUMMARY 1

A 2-year-old boy presents to the emergency department with his frantic parents, who had found him unresponsive in the bathroom with pills and empty bottles "scattered all over the floor." The child is normally healthy.

The child is lethargic with no response to stimuli, with shallow and slow respirations but no cyanosis. Vital signs include a respiratory rate of 8 breaths per minute, a pulse of 70 beats per minute (bpm), blood pressure of 80/40 mmHg, and temperature of 35.6°C. Focused physical examination reveals pupils that are 4 mm each and reactive to light, a supple neck, clear lungs, nontender abdomen with no masses, normoactive bowel sounds, extremities with good pulses, and no focal neurologic deficits. There is no evidence of trauma.

1. *What are the initial management priorities in this child?*
2. *What antidotes should be administered?*
3. *What further history is important in this case?*

On initial presentation, the greatest concern should be the status of the child's airway. Bag-mask ventilation was begun and vascular access obtained. The rapid glucose assessment demonstrated a reading of 20. The child's mental status and respiratory drive dramatically improved with intravenous dextrose administration, obviating the need for further assisted ventilation and intubation. The child was given activated charcoal by nasogastric tube because the specific toxin ingested was unknown. Baseline laboratory test results were all within normal limits. Serum acetaminophen, salicylate, and iron levels were negative. A urine toxicology screen for the standard drugs of abuse was also negative. Further history from the parents revealed the child had no history of diabetes mellitus or glucose disturbances. Among the many toxins available in the bathroom, it was determined that the child had most likely drunk from a previously full bottle of mouthwash, which contained ethanol and mint flavoring. The child's ethanol level returned with a serum level of 180 mg/dL. After close observation in the pediatric intensive care unit, with fluid and glucose supplementation, the child recovered uneventfully and was discharged home 48 hours after initial presentation.

CASE SUMMARY 2

A 16-year-old girl presents to the emergency department 3 hours after ingesting two handfulls of extra-strength acetaminophen. She complains of nausea and vomiting. She has no significant past medical history.

The patient is alert, but has a depressed affect and makes poor eye contact. She has no increased work of breathing, and her skin color is normal. Vital signs include a respiratory rate of 20 breaths per minute, pulse of 110 bpm, blood pressure of 130/60 mmHg, and temperature of 37.3° C. Focused examination reveals that her pupils are 3 mm bilaterally reactive to light; she has a supple neck, no heart murmurs, and clear lungs. Her abdomen is tender to touch in the epigastric region, but there is no guarding, and no peritoneal signs. She has good symmetrical pulses and no focal neurologic deficits.

1. What is the primary target organ of acetaminophen poisoning?
2. What diagnostic laboratory data should be obtained?
3. Does this patient meet the criteria for antidote therapy?

The patient's 4-hour acetaminophen level was measured at 300 mcg/mL, which is consistent with potential hepatotoxicity on the nomogram. As a result, oral NAC therapy was initiated, which the patient promptly vomited. The patient's vomiting subsided after metoclopramide therapy. Laboratory test results indicate normal LFTs and coagulation studies and a positive urine pregnancy test. The patient admitted she overdosed on acetaminophen when she learned of her untimely pregnancy. Despite the positive pregnancy test, the NAC therapy was continued for a full 17 doses because the minimal risk of fetal toxicity from the antidote is greatly outweighed by the benefits of properly treating the mother's acetaminophen-induced hepatoxicity. The patient recovered medically, but was transferred to a psychiatric ward, with an obstetrical consultation for initiation of prenatal care. Seven months later, the patient delivered a healthy full-term baby.

A 3-year-old boy is discovered by his father drinking "some blue fluid from a jug" in the garage. Thirty minutes later, on examination in the emergency department, the child is sleepy but cries easily when awakened. He has no increased work of breathing and his color is normal. His vital signs include respiratory rate of 32 breaths per minute, heart rate of 80 bpm, blood pressure of 80/40 mmHg, and temperature of 36.1°C. The remainder of his examination is noncontributory, and the father says that he is normally healthy.

1. What is the differential diagnosis?
2. Is gastric decontamination indicated?
3. Is there a role for antidote therapy?

Because this child presented within an hour of ingesting a potentially life-threatening toxin, gastric lavage was performed with return of bluish-tinged stomach contents. The child's laboratory test results were consistent with a mild metabolic acidosis, with an elevated osmolar gap. The ethanol level was zero, and levels for ethylene glycol, methanol, and isopropanol were sent to an outside reference lab. Because of the high suspicion for a toxic alcohol ingestion, the child received an appropriate dose of intravenous bicarbonate (indicated for a serum pH below 7.20) and the antidote 4-MP. The renal service was consulted for possible hemodialysis. The serum methanol level reported 12 hours later was 25 mg/dL. All other toxic alcohol levels were normal. The child's acidosis subsided and repeat methanol level 6 hours later was 5 mg/dL. An ophthalmology consultation was obtained, and the child recovered uneventfully with no vision impairment.

CASE SUMMARY 4

A 5-year-old boy was in an apartment fire but escaped with burns to his feet. In the emergency department he is frightened, but able to speak in full sentences. His respiratory rate is 30 breaths per minute, heart rate is 120 bpm, blood pressure is 100/70, and his temperature is 37.6°C. Physical examination reveals no carbonaceous sputum and no stridor or wheezing. He has partial-thickness burns to the soles of his feet, with good distal pulses and color.

1. What is the most significant physical examination finding in this child?
2. What is the most important therapy for this patient?

Although the child's burns could have caused severe pain, the priority remained his airway. The lack of respiratory distress, stridor, or wheezing were important, but did not diminish concerns of delayed pulmonary injury. The child required 100% oxygen by face mask, COHb level, ABG, and a chest radiograph. Careful monitoring of his respiratory status continued while he received initial burn care.

# chapter 9

# Trauma

Joseph J. Tepas III, MD, FAAP, FACS
Mary E. Fallat, MD, FACS, FAAP
Thomas M. Moriarty, MD, PhD

## Objectives

1 Describe unique anatomic and physiologic characteristics of the pediatric age group that affect response to injury and management.

2 Define concepts of the primary and secondary surveys and systematically discuss patient evaluation using these tools.

3 Establish and discuss management priorities based on life-threatening injuries identified in the primary survey.

4 Discuss the identification and initial treatment of life-threatening injuries to major organ systems.

5 Review relevant issues of injury prevention.

## Chapter Outline

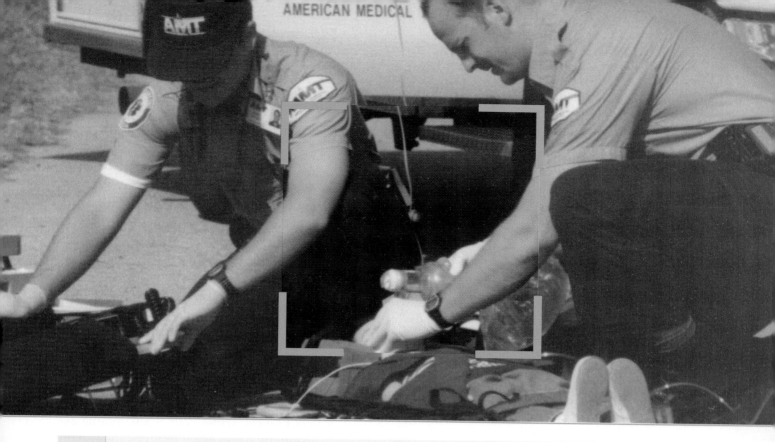

A 5-year-old boy is struck by a car while crossing the street. Paramedics find the boy unconscious and lying in the middle of the street about 15 feet from the vehicle. They begin an initial assessment using the Pediatric Assessment Triangle, as follows: appearance is unconscious, not responsive to surroundings; work of breathing is tachypneic, with no retractions; and circulation signs include a pale and diaphoretic color. The paramedics stabilize the cervical spine, administer 100% oxygen by face mask, and attempt intravenous (IV) access en route to the hospital. An IV is placed in the right antecubital fossa, and 50 mL of normal saline is infused prior to arrival.

On arrival in the emergency department the patient's airway is open; increased secretions are noted, and the trachea is midline. There is symmetric chest wall motion and poor tidal volume. No retractions are noted, and breath sounds are equal. The child's color is pale; skin signs show diaphoresis. There is no jugular venous distention, and capillary refill time is 4 seconds. The heart rate is 160, with a thready peripheral pulse quality. Blood pressure is 75/palp. The abdomen is distended and tense on palpation, and the pelvis is stable. The rectal area is normal and negative for occult blood. The patient is still unconscious. There is no spontaneous eye opening. He responds to painful stimuli with flexor posturing. Pupils are at midposition and 4 mm bilaterally sluggish reaction to light. He has a contusion on the forehead, an abrasion on the left arm with swelling at the level of the elbow, an abrasion on the left flank, and deformity on the left femur.

1. *What is the physiologic status of this child?*
2. *What are your initial management priorities?*
3. *Does this patient meet an indication for surgery?*

## Introduction

Trauma remains a major threat to the children of our world and is responsible for more than half of all childhood deaths in the United States. As infectious diseases and malnutrition become more effectively treated, injury is emerging as a major cause of pediatric mortality throughout the world.[1,2] Effective care of the seriously injured child is rooted in thorough understanding of the basic principles of advanced life support. The unique characteristics and needs of the child as a victim of injury mandate that these principles be focused into thorough, accurate, expeditious, and effective treatment. The purpose of this chapter is to describe the process of initial assessment and resuscitation of the injured child. What is accomplished in the minutes and hours after injury will define survival in terms of quality of life or precipitate avoidable disaster measurable in years of misery and impairment. The core of the process is injury recognition, intervention, anticipation of response, and continuous reassessment. Injury recognition requires an understanding of the epidemiology of childhood injury patterns. Intervention demands experience and training in life support. Anticipation of response and reassessment are the products of training and protocol. Each of these critical areas will be addressed in detail.

## Pathophysiologic and Anatomic Considerations

Children often respond differently to injury than adults do. Young children in particular might not be able to describe symptoms or localize pain. The common association of polysystem injury seen in children makes this inability to communicate both a challenge and a threat. The challenge requires experience and great patience on the part of the examining physician to reassure the anxious or uncooperative child while avoiding the threat of subtle or missed injury. Regardless of mechanism, every organ system of the injured child should be considered deranged until proved otherwise. Deranged conceptually addresses both organs directly damaged by the injuring agent and organ systems affected indirectly by the body's response to the injured organs.

Children clearly are not just small adults. They differ from adults in size but also in anatomy and physiology. A child's head occupies a larger relative body surface area and mass than does the head of an adult. Not surprising, head injuries in children are extremely common and account for a great percentage of serious morbidity and mortality. Over 80% of fatalities recorded in the National Pediatric Trauma Registry (NPTR) are the result of traumatic brain injury.[3]

There are age-specific differences in epidemiology, pathology, and outcome of traumatic brain injury.[4] The central nervous system of children younger than 3 years is in a state of dynamic development. The increase in head circumference during the first years of life reflects tremendous brain volume expansion. By the age of 6 months, the weight of the brain has doubled; by 2 years of age, it has reached 80% of adult weight. During this period, ongoing myelination, synapse formation, dendritic arborization, increasing neuronal plasticity, and biochemical changes take place. Injury to the developing brain can arrest these processes and produce deficits that become apparent only at a later stage of development.

The head is a major source of heat loss and contributes to the child's increased sensitivity to thermoregulatory stress. Occipital prominence decreases from birth until about 10 years of age and is responsible for relative neck flexion and a more anterior position of the airway in small children. The cranial sutures are open at birth and gradually fuse by 18 to 24 months of age; palpation of the anterior and posterior fontanels can be an important source of information. The ability of the cranial sutures to spread can also dissipate some of the adverse effects of increased intracranial pressure.

The type of injury varies with the age of the child. Child abuse is a major cause of severe head injury in infants. In some studies, 95% of all injuries resulting in intracranial hemorrhage in children younger than 1 year are due to child abuse.[4] Children who are ambulatory and younger than 5 years are likely to sustain head injuries as a result of falls at home; those older than 5 years are more likely to be involved as pedestrians or cyclists in collisions with motor vehicles. At any age, head trauma can be sustained by passengers in motor vehicle crashes.

A child's neck is shorter and supports a relatively greater mass than does the neck of an adult. Distracting forces more frequently disrupt the upper cervical vertebrae or their ligamentous attachments. Active growth centers and incomplete calcification make radiological assessment especially challenging. Half of children with cervical spinal cord injury have absolutely no abnormality on any mode of diagnostic imaging (spinal cord injury without radiographic abnormality, or SCIWORA),[5] emphasizing the importance of an accurate and thorough initial physical examination. Because the young child has a short, fat neck, evaluation of neck veins and tracheal position can be difficult.

The younger the child, the more the position of the larynx is cephalad and anterior. The epiglottis is tilted nearly 45 degrees in a child and is more floppy than that of an adolescent or adult (Table 9-1). In an adult patient, the glottis (or the level of the true vocal cords) is the narrowest portion of the upper airway and therefore the limiting factor in tracheal tube size. In the child younger than 8 years, the cricoid cartilage is the narrowest portion of the airway and also the site of abundant loose columnar epithelium. This epithelium is more susceptible to pressure necrosis, which can stimulate exuberant scar tissue, which can lead to stenosis. The size of the tracheal tube thus becomes a critical consideration.

In children, the thorax is more pliable than in adults. The ribs are more cartilaginous and therefore more flexible. There is much less overlying muscle and fat to protect the ribs and underlying structures, so blunt force applied to the chest is more efficiently transmitted to underlying tissues. This is clinically relevant because apparently normal external findings can mask significant internal derangement, such as a pulmonary contusion or pneumothorax. The diaphragm inserts at a nearly horizontal angle in a newborn and maintains this angle until approximately 12 years of age. This is in contrast to the oblique insertion of the diaphragm in an adolescent or adult. Children are diaphragmatic, or belly-breathers, which means they are dependent on effective diaphragmatic excursion for adequate ventilation. In addition, the diaphragmatic muscle is much more distensible in the child. A child's mediastinum is very mobile and therefore subject to sudden, wide excursions. As a result, a simple pneumothorax can become a life-threatening tension pneumothorax literally within seconds.

A child's abdomen is less well protected by overlying ribs and muscle. Viscera are more prone to injury (Figure 9.1). Seemingly insignificant forces can cause serious internal injury. Although the connective tissue and

| TABLE 9-1 | Comparison of Infant and Adult Airways | |
| --- | --- | --- |
| | **Infant** | **Adult** |
| Head | Large prominent occiput, resulting in sniffing position | Flat occiput |
| Tongue | Relatively larger | Relatively smaller |
| Larynx | Cephalad position, opposite C2 and C3 vertebrae | Opposite C4 through C6 |
| Epiglottis | Ω Shaped, soft | Flat, flexible |
| Vocal cords | Short, concave | Horizontal |
| Smallest diameter | Cricoid ring, below cords | Vocal cords |
| Cartilage | Soft, more flexible | Firm, stiffer |
| Lower airways | Smaller | Larger, more cartilage |

suspensory ligaments of the child are more elastic and can absorb more energy, the paucity of insulating fat allows more potential motion of these organs at impact. Significant internal injury therefore can be manifest by minimal external evidence.

Bone growth in children occurs at the epiphyses, or growth plates, of the long bones. These areas and the epiphyseal-metaphyseal junction are sites of relative weakness. In most cases, the ligamentous structures near the epiphyseal region actually are stronger than the growth plate itself; this explains the frequency of epiphyseal fractures seen in children. Because of the implications of disturbances of the growth plate, a separate classification system (Salter-Harris) has evolved for these injuries. In addition to the potential impact of fractures of the growth plate on long-term bony growth, changes in blood flow to the extremity can result in significant limb length discrepancy. Pediatric and adult differences in anatomy and physiology that have an effect on trauma management are outlined in Table 9-2.

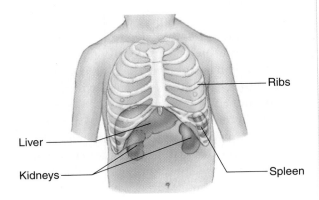

**Figure 9.1** Viscera in a child's abdomen are more prone to injury as they are less well protected by overlying ribs and musculature.

| TABLE 9-2 | Pediatric and Adult Differences in Anatomy and Physiology |
| --- | --- |

**Central Nervous System:**
- Pediatric brain in state of dynamic development.
  - Myelin is in process of forming.
  - More gray matter.
- Head is a source of heat loss.
- Pediatric skull has expandable sutures until 18–24 months of age.
- Prominent occiput causes the head to flex forward on the neck.
- Short/fat neck makes assessing for JVD and tracheal deviation challenging.

**Cervical Spine:**
- Neck supports greater weight, making cervical spine fractures and injury more likely in higher cervical spine.
- Cervical spine fractures are uncommon/more likely a ligamentous injury.
- Spinal cord injury without radiographic abnormality (SCIWORA) = 50% of children with spinal cord injury.

**Airway:**
- Larynx is more anterior and cephalad.
- Cricoid is narrowest portion of the airway versus the vocal cords.
- Epiglottis is floppy and Ω-shaped.

**Respiratory:**
- Pliable chest wall implies great force needed to break ribs and force transmitted to lungs and other intrathoracic structures.
- Horizontal insertion of the diaphragm and dependence of diaphragm for breathing.
- Mobile mediastinum can result in rapid transition from pneumothorax to tension pneumothorax.

**Abdominal:**
- Anterior placement of intra-abdominal organs and less subcutaneous fat make them more susceptible to injury.

**Skeletal:**
- Long bones with growth plates that fracture can result in extremity length discrepancies.

# Assessment and Management

Aggressive management of the airway and breathing is the foundation of pediatric trauma resuscitation. Data from the NPTR reflect the primacy of brain injury as the main driver of mortality and morbidity in childhood. Effective initial management of traumatic brain injury mandates airway control to support precise ventilation and adequate oxygenation. Only 6% of 92,000 cases registered in the NPTR initially presented with a systolic blood pressure ≤ 90 mm Hg. Mortality in this group was 18% and represented 42% of all children who died of their injuries. Severe shock must be aggressively treated with rapid intubation and ventilatory control, rapid resuscitation with isotonic crystalloid, and restoration of red cell mass to deliver adequate oxygenation. Children in coma without shock need identical airway control and confirmation that volume resuscitation and red cell mass are adequate to support neuronal oxygenation.

Trauma management begins with the same initial assessment of the child presented in Chapter 2, Pediatric Assessment. It includes all of the elements of the Pediatric Assessment Triangle (**Figure 9.2A and Figure 9.2B**):

- Appearance (mental status and muscle tone) suggests the level of consciousness.
- Work of breathing (increased, labored, or decreased) indicates the adequacy of ventilation and oxygenation.

- Circulation (skin and mucous membrane color) reflects the adequacy of oxygenation and perfusion.

The absence of immediate evidence of circulatory abnormalities neither guarantees hemodynamic stability nor excludes multisystem injury.[6]

Priorities for care of the seriously injured child are as follows:

Perform a rapid physical examination and check vital signs to identify all hemodynamic, neurologic, and anatomic abnormalities. Tools immediately available in the resuscitation area should include:

- Pulse oximetry
- Abdominal ultranography (FAST)
- Portable radiologic imaging
- Treat any immediate life-threatening disturbances.
- Perform airway management and obtain vascular access.
- Begin fluid resuscitation based on clinical assessment of circulatory status.
- Rapidly identify any injuries requiring surgical intervention.
- Reexamine the patient for non–life-threatening injuries and initiate therapy for these conditions.

The process by which these goals are achieved is continuous but can be divided conceptually into three phases: assessment, stabilization, and initiation of definitive management.

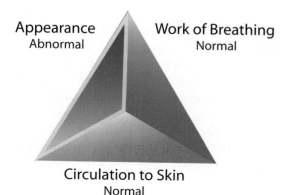

**Figure 9.2A** Pediatric assessment triangle in isolated head injury.

Appearance
Abnormal

Work of Breathing
Normal

Circulation to Skin
Normal

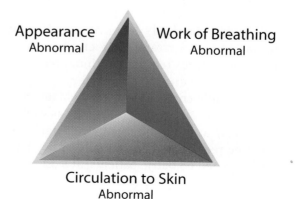

**Figure 9.2B** Pediatric assessment triangle in multisystem injury.

Appearance
Abnormal

Work of Breathing
Abnormal

Circulation to Skin
Abnormal

## Primary and Secondary Surveys

The primary survey and initial resuscitation usually require the first 5 to 10 minutes and focus on treating immediate threats to life. The secondary survey continues and broadens the scope of treatment based on a more thorough process of physical examination and appropriate diagnostic testing. Ideally, this phase should be completed within the first hour so definitive care or safe transport can begin. Life-threatening disorders must be recognized promptly and corrected before treatment of less-threatening problems. The sequence for evaluation is always the same. If sufficient expert personnel are available for assistance, many of these tasks can be done simultaneously.

The primary survey consists of an initial assessment of the status of the patient's airway, oxygenation, ventilation, circulation, and overall neurologic status. Primarily, it is a physiologic survey of the patient's vital systems. It is not uncommon to encounter serious physiologic alterations in the course of the primary survey, necessitating interruption of the course of the survey to perform resuscitative phases of care.

In contrast, the secondary survey (focused history and detailed physical examination) is a timely, directed evaluation of each body area, usually performed in a head-to-toe manner; the secondary survey is an anatomic survey in which the physician attempts to define the presence, type, and severity of injury to each anatomic area. The secondary survey essentially begins the child's definitive care. It is important to understand that children with multiple injuries require continual reassessment. The secondary survey must be performed while continuing to reevaluate all of the elements of the primary survey as well as the effects of initial intervention. Vital signs must be reevaluated continually on all seriously injured pediatric patients, at least every 5 minutes during the course of the primary survey and every 15 minutes during the remainder of the evaluation.

## Primary Survey

The steps in the primary survey include assessment of the following:

- Airway, with cervical spine stabilization
- Breathing and emergency treatment of immediately life-threatening chest injuries
- Circulation, with external control of hemorrhage
- Disability (neurologic screening examination)
- Exposure and thorough examination

The most important goals during the primary survey and resuscitative phase should be accomplished within 5 to 10 minutes (Table 9-3).

### Airway and Cervical Spine

The highest priority is establishment of a patent airway with adequate ventilation. Until cervical spine injury is excluded, the cervical spine must be protected, especially during airway manipulation. Lateral cervical spine radiographs are obtained as rapidly as feasible, but must not be permitted to delay or interfere with emergency airway management or rapid assessment and management of shock.

Some children with cervical spinal cord injury have symptoms of transient paresthesia, numbness, or paralysis but show no radiographic abnormality. This can occur in any child with a significant injury above the level of the clavicles, including children with head injuries, any child struck by a motor vehicle, a child involved in a high-speed motor vehicle crash, and any unconscious patient who has sustained significant trauma. Adequate stabilization can be accomplished with gentle but firm longitudinal support until a cervical immobilization device or semirigid collar can be provided. Even in cases in which the initial cervical radiographs are normal, stabilization must be maintained if neurologic injury is suspected on the basis of the history or physical examination. Cervical spine precautions may be discontinued if three views of the cervical spine are normal, if the child is awake, reliable, and asymptomatic, and if there is no evidence of a neurologic abnormality.

| TABLE 9-3 | Goals of the Primary Survey and Resuscitative Phase |
| --- | --- |

**ASSESSMENT**

**Airway**
- Obstruction

**Breathing and ventilation**
- Decreased rate
- Decreased breath sounds
- Decreased excursion

**Circulation**
- Neck vein distention
- Distant heart sounds
- Tachycardia
- Hemorrhage

**THERAPY**

**Airway**
- Relieve obstruction with jaw thrust
- Use of oral airway
- Endotracheal intubation
- Needle cricothyrotomy

**Ventilation**
- Provide 100% oxygen
- Treat apnea with intubation/ventilation
- Stabilize flail thorax with positive pressure ventilation
- Aspiration of tension pneumothorax
- Nasogastric tube to relieve gastric dilatation
- Chest tube insertion for hemothorax/pneumothorax

**Circulation**
- Apply pressure to control hemorrhage
- Two large-bore (14- to 18-gauge) intravenous catheters
- Intraosseous infusion if needed
- Normal saline or lactated Ringer's at 20 mL/kg for volume replacement
- Relieve pericardial tamponade
- Thoracotomy when indicated (rare)

## Airway

To open the airway of a child who does not have a suspected neck or spine injury, the head is placed in the sniffing position, with the neck slightly flexed on the chest and the head slightly extended on the neck (**Figure 9.3**). This position is easily accomplished by placing a folded towel or the rescuer's hand under the victim's neck.

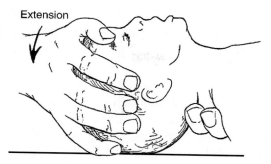

Extension

**Figure 9.3** Head positioning in the pediatric patient with trauma. The "sniffing position" is optimal, but spine stabilization must be maintained with all airway maneuvers.

To open the airway of a child with a possible neck or spine injury, the head is placed in the neutral position, with cervical spine elements fully aligned, using bimanual cervical spine stabilization. In infants and young children, the prominence of the occipital region can force the neck into slight flexion when the patient is placed supine, and it might be necessary to place a 1/2-inch to 1-inch layer of padding beneath the torso. Maintain cervical spine stabilization during the course of any airway maneuvers if cervical injury or neurologic abnormality has not been ruled out, and immobilize the neck with an extrication collar once the airway is controlled. The mandible is relaxed in the unconscious patient. Posterior displacement of the tongue will therefore produce airway obstruction. This is treated with the jaw-thrust maneuver, which is accomplished by placing hands at the angles of the mandible and applying gentle forward pressure. Remove any foreign matter present in the airway quickly with gentle suction. Neonates are preferential nasal breathers, so relieve nasal obstruction quickly through gentle suction to allow spontaneous ventilation.

### Endotracheal Intubation

Indications for endotracheal intubation in the trauma patient are as follows:
- Inability to ventilate the child using bag-mask ventilation
- Need for prolonged control of the airway, including prevention of aspiration in a comatose child
- Need for controlled ventilation in a patient with a serious head injury

- Flail chest
- Shock unresponsive to volume infusion

When intubation is necessary, proper preparation is an absolute requirement. The critical first step is preoxygenation with 100% oxygen. Gentle suction will usually clear the oropharynx of secretions and foreign matter. Unless contraindicated, emergency intubation of the child should always be accomplished using the oral approach. The acute angle of the posterior nasopharynx, anterior, and cephalad position of the larynx, necessity for additional tube manipulation, and probability of causing or increasing pharyngeal bleeding due to prominent adenoids/tonsils make nasotracheal intubation unacceptably hazardous in trauma situations. Oral endotracheal intubation in the pediatric trauma patient begins by maintaining inline stabilization of the cervical spine with the head and neck in neutral position. A complete review of the procedure can be found in Chapter 22, Critical Procedures.

If airway obstruction prevents adequate ventilation, there might be a direct injury to the larynx or trachea. In this unusual circumstance or in any situation in which effective ventilation is impossible, the preferred method for airway control is needle cricothyrotomy. A 14-gauge catheter-over-the-needle placed through the cricothyroid membrane and high or jet $O_2$ flow of 15 L/min can provide 30 to 40 minutes of temporary oxygenation (Figure 9.4).

### Breathing and Emergency Treatment of Immediate Life-Threatening Chest Injuries

The signs and symptoms of potentially serious airway and chest injury can be subtle, and children can deteriorate rapidly after injury. Administer supplemental oxygen to all pediatric major trauma victims in the initial stages of care, even if they have no apparent airway or breathing difficulty. Supplemental oxygen given via face mask at a flow rate of 12 L/min is well tolerated by most children.

In assessing the adequacy of the pediatric airway, remember the adage, "Look, listen, and feel." Once the airway has been opened, look at both sides of the thorax to determine whether there is symmetric chest wall rise. Children have small tidal volumes, and chest wall movement can be subtle. Carefully note suprasternal, intercostal, or subcostal retractions that can indicate increased work of breathing and respiratory distress. After tracheal tube insertion, listen for breath sounds on both sides of the chest (Figure 9.5). Breath sounds can be transmitted easily through the chest wall and adjacent structures in small children, and it is dangerous to rely solely on breath sounds to determine adequacy of ventilation. Use an end-tidal $CO_2$ monitor and confirm tracheal tube position with a chest radiograph.

In addition to assessing the adequacy of bilateral chest wall movement, it is important to confirm that the patient's respiratory rate is sufficient to provide oxygenation and ventilation. Any child who is hypoxic ($SaO_2$ <90%) or tachypneic needs additional respiratory support and careful evaluation for injury. A child in respiratory distress with unilateral absent breath sounds and tracheal deviation should be suspected of having a tension pneumothorax. Signs of poor perfusion are often present as the mediastinal structures are shifted to the opposite side due to the expanding pneumothorax.

Needle thoracostomy using a 14-gauge angiocath, followed immediately by tube thoracostomy (20 to 30 Fr, depending on patient size) can be lifesaving and is indicated without a preliminary chest radiograph (Figure 9.6). The unstable child with an open pneumothorax should have an impermeable dressing with three sides occluded placed directly over the wound (Figure 9.7). Cardiac tamponade is associated with penetrating trauma to the parasternal area. Signs of cardiac tamponade

## YOUR FIRST CLUE

**Signs and Symptoms of a Tension Pneumothorax**

- Respiratory distress
- Unilateral decreased or absent breath sounds
- Tracheal deviation
- Signs of poor perfusion (late)

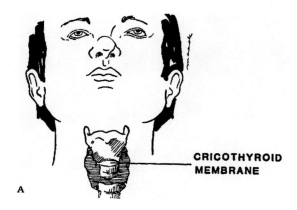

Figure 9.4A Locate the cricothyroid membrane.

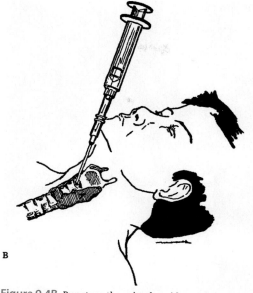

Figure 9.4B Puncture the cricothyroid membrane with a catheter-over-the-needle or commercially available cricothyrotomy device.

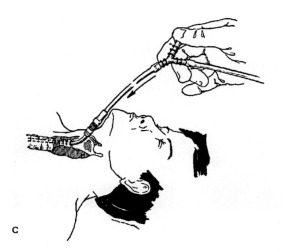

Figure 9.4C Pass the catheter into the membrane and remove the needle. Attach a Y-connector for instillation of oxygenation.

Figure 9.4D Surgical cricothyrotomy can be performed and an endotracheal tube placed to keep the airway open.

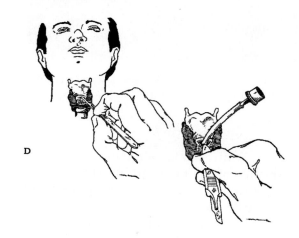

include hypotension, distended neck veins, and muffled heart sounds.

Children suspected of having cardiac tamponade should undergo immediate pericardiocentesis. A child with a penetrating injury to the chest who develops cardiac arrest on arrival or during resuscitation might benefit from an emergency thoracotomy if an appropriately trained and credentialed physician is present. See Chapter 22, Critical Procedures, for an outline of how to perform needle and tube thoracostomy, emergency department thoracotomy, and pericardiocentesis.

### Circulation

During the primary survey, the major goals of circulatory assessment and treatment are as follows:

- Assessment of the overall circulatory status of the injured patient
- Diagnosis and control of both external and internal hemorrhage
- Immediate intervention to provide appropriate vascular access and circulatory support

Circulatory assessment should include evaluation of the "3 P's." Circulatory effi-

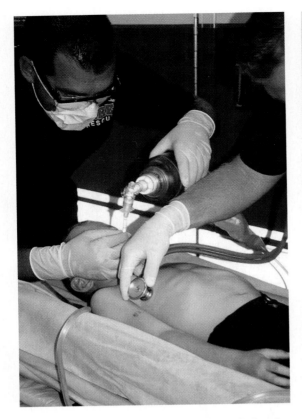

Figure 9.5 After tracheal tube insertion, listen for breath sounds on both sides of the chest.

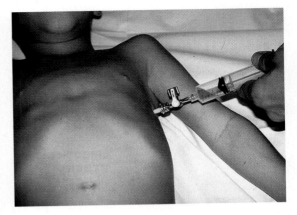

Figure 9.6 Needle thoracostomy can be performed prior to a chest radiograph to treat suspected tension pneumothorax.

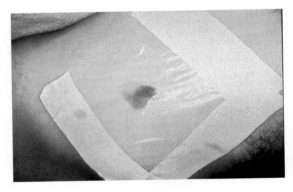

Figure 9.7 Cover chest wounds with an occlusive dressing taped on three sides.

ciency is directly dependent on the performance of the myocardium (pump), the integrity of the vascular system (pipes), and the sufficiency of circulating volume (prime). The most common threat to the pump is ischemia from hypovolemia or direct contusion. Disruption of the pipes can be catastrophic, which usually leads to immediate exsanguination, or subtle, subclinical ooze from a broken bone or damaged abdominal viscus. It is the latter that is most common and poses avoidable threat to effective neuronal oxygenation by gradually replacing oxygen-carrying erythrocytes with crystalloid resuscitation solutions. This is the reason that assessment of the prime is so critical to effective resuscitation.

Crystalloid bolus is an essential first step in restoring lost circulatory volume. In the absence of frank shock, which is the case in 94% of injured children, continued fluid man-

YOUR FIRST CLUE

**Signs and Symptoms of Cardiac Tamponade**

- Penetrating trauma to the parasternal area
- Distended neck veins
- Muffled heart sounds
- Poor perfusion/hypotension

agement must represent a judicious balance between effective oxygenation via adequate red cell mass and avoidable fluid overload by inappropriate volumes of crystalloid.

The time to address this issue is at immediate assessment. Management of brain injury is

**TABLE 9-4    Usual Ranges for Awake Heart Rate and Blood Pressure for Children**

| Age | Heart Rate (beats/min) | Blood Pressure (mm Hg) |
|---|---|---|
| Neonate | 85–205 | 60–80 by palpation |
| 1 yr | 100–130 | 80/40 to 105/70 |
| 5 yr | 80–110 | 80/50 to 110/80 |
| 10 yr | 70–100 | 90/55 to 130/85 |
| 15 yr | 60–80 | 95/60 to 140/90 |
| Adult | 60–80 | 100/60 to 140/90 |

much more effective if the first 48 hours are not complicated by inadequate fluid resuscitation or by having to diurese excessive fluid from the cerebral and pulmonary interstitium. Palpation of the pulse for quality (ie, weak or strong), rate, and regularity remains a reliable initial clinical assessment tool. Capillary refill in and of itself is not a reliable indicator of perfusion, but when combined with heart rate and pulse quality can be a valuable adjunct in the detection of hypoperfusion.[7] Capillary refill time should be less than 2 seconds and is generally assessed by gentle compression of the nailbeds.

Tachycardia is one of the first signs of hypovolemia and is a compensatory mechanism by the body to respond to decrease of circulating blood volume. Tachycardia is also the result of pain and anxiety; however, it will be more prolonged in children without adequate resuscitation. Hypotension eventually will occur, when compensatory mechanisms fail, resulting in bradycardia followed by cardiopulmonary arrest. The younger the child, the more fixed is the stroke volume and the more dependent is cardiac output on heart rate. Be familiar with the usual heart rates for children by age (Table 9-4). A weak and thready pulse is an indication of cardiovascular instability and impending cardiovascular collapse.

The assessment of perfusion is the basis for the early diagnosis and recognition of shock. Measures of circulatory adequacy include assessment of central nervous system status as a relative indicator of brain perfusion and urine output as an indicator of renal perfusion. Because central nervous system injuries are common in children, traumatic coma can cloud assessment of perfusion. Urine output is an accurate measure of renal perfusion, but it is of little benefit in very early patient assessment. Output should be maintained at 1 mL/kg per hour.

### Vascular Access

While circulatory status is being assessed, reliable vascular access must be established. The choices for vascular access include the following:

- Percutaneous peripheral venous cannulation with large-bore lines placed at one or two sites
- Intraosseous infusion
- Peripheral venous cutdown

Percutaneous central venous access is reserved for situations in which other routes have failed. In the setting of trauma resuscitation, the femoral approach is preferred, using the Seldinger technique for placement of at least a 5 French cannula. When a peripheral line cannot be placed, intraosseous fluid infusion is a valuable method to provide temporary circulatory access. Although intraosseous access is technically easier to obtain in children younger than 6 years old, it can be used at any age. There are also adult intraosseous access devices commercially available. The anterior tibial marrow can be cannulated quickly and used as an infusion site for fluids and medications (Figure 9.8). Complications are rare and usually involve subcutaneous infiltration of fluid or leakage from the puncture site after the needle has been removed. More serious complications, such as compartment syndrome, tibial fracture, osteomyelitis, and subcutaneous infections, have been reported. However, these occur mainly when the intraosseous infusion is maintained for extended periods of time, hypertonic fluids are infused, or evidence of limb edema is ignored.

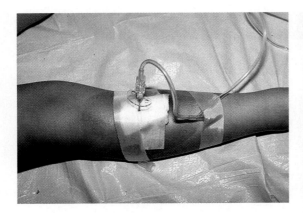

Figure 9.8 Intraosseous needle in the anterior tibia for rapid vascular access.

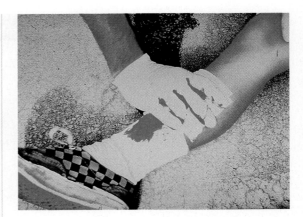

Figure 9.9 Apply direct pressure on all bleeding wounds.

Intraosseous infusion must never be used in a fractured extremity. Whenever this means of access is used, it is to be regarded as a temporizing measure while attempts at direct vascular access are continued.

The best sites for peripheral venous cutdown are the basilic vein near the antecubital fossa, the saphenous vein at the ankle, or the saphenofemoral junction at the groin. The lower extremity and groin sites have the advantage of being distant from the sites of airway manipulation and cardiopulmonary resuscitation. In patients with major intra-abdominal vascular injury or hemorrhage, an upper extremity vein is preferred. The external jugular vein is usually inaccessible in a trauma patient as a result of airway manipulation and cervical spine stabilization. The basilic vein at the elbow is, therefore, a good alternative. This vein lies lateral and superior to the medial epicondyle of the elbow. See Chapter 22, Critical Procedures, for an outline of steps to perform intraosseous needle placement and venous cutdown.

### Hemorrhage Control

Systematic assessment of the entire body surface is necessary to ensure all areas of external hemorrhage are evaluated and treated. Although information regarding the magnitude of blood loss at the scene can be misleading, obtain this information from paramedical personnel who were at the scene and learn what measures were used to control the bleeding. Any laceration can result in significant bleeding, but scalp and facial

## KEY POINTS

**Management of External Hemorrhage**
- Apply direct manual pressure over bleeding sites with sterile dressings.
- Maintain direct pressure with either manual pressure or pressure dressings.
- Ensure that pressure dressings do not occlude distal pulses.
- Elevate the bleeding areas to decrease the amount of blood loss.
- Do not blindly clamp vessels.

wounds are particularly prone to profuse hemorrhage. Begin measures to decrease external bleeding by applying direct pressure over bleeding sites with sterile dressings (Figure 9.9). Once pressure has been applied, maintain it with either manual pressure or pressure dressings. Ensure that pressure dressings do not occlude distal pulses. Elevate the bleeding areas to decrease the amount of blood loss. In most cases, the combination of direct pressure and elevation will arrest external hemorrhage.

In virtually every area of the body except the scalp, major nerves are in proximity to major blood vessels. Blind clamping of vessels can therefore result in peripheral nerve damage. Hemostats should only be used to clamp spurting vessels on the hair-bearing areas of the scalp.

Recognition of internal bleeding requires astute observation, a thorough physical examination, and attention to the subtle changes that sometimes occur with major internal hemorrhage. Life-threatening internal hemorrhage can occur in five body areas: chest, abdomen, retroperitoneum, pelvis, and thigh. Be alert to pain or swelling in any of the areas; this might be the first objective indication of internal hemorrhage.

### Shock and Circulatory Failure

During the initial phase of care of the trauma patient, shock nearly always is hypovolemic in nature. Other causes of shock include cardiac tamponade, tension pneumothorax, and spinal cord injury. Rapid hemorrhage, in contradistinction to catastrophic exsanguination, proceeds along a predictable process that begins with tachycardia, progresses to clinical signs of sluggish peripheral circulation with decreasing pulse pressure, and evolves into deepening obtundation. The high incidence of traumatic brain injury in children confuses the last of these findings, because this can be a primary cause of decreased level of consciousness. Regardless of the presence of potential brain injury, any child who is tachycardic and has a falling systolic pressure and poor peripheral perfusion has lost at least 25% of normal blood volume. This child needs immediate restoration of circulating volume with isotonic crystalloid and possibly transfusion of O negative blood. When blood loss exceeds 25% to 30% of total blood volume, compensatory vasoconstriction can fail abruptly and catastrophically. Hypotension, confusion, decreased urine output, and acidosis can emerge rapidly. At this point, irreversible vascular collapse can be imminent.

Patients with hypotension might have lost 25% of their total blood volume and probably have injuries that will cause these losses to continue. They usually require multiple boluses of fluid. Although these boluses can transiently restore circulating volume, they add red cell dilution to exsanguination and soon undermine rather than improve oxygen delivery. When more than two crystalloid boluses are required, immediate transfusion therapy is usually necessary.

### Volume Replacement

Normal saline or lactated Ringer's (LR) solution is the fluid of choice for initial resuscitation of the pediatric trauma victim. In the face of evolving cerebral edema, excess free water is to be avoided. Fluid replacement is divided into two phases: initial therapy and total replacement. When necessary, fluids are administered rapidly via intravenous push with a 60-mL syringe. Three-way stopcocks should be in line so larger volumes of fluid can be administered in as short a period of time as possible. Vital signs are evaluated carefully before and after bolus therapy. If vital signs do not improve immediately, more volume is given.

The following guidelines are only for initiation of therapy. If a child does not respond appropriately, suspect internal hemorrhage and look for other causes of refractory shock. Typically, approximately 3 mL of crystalloid replacement will be required to replace each milliliter of shed blood. Bolus infusion of 20 mL/kg (NS or LR) should be initiated for all patients who have sustained significant trauma or have signs of compensated or decompensated shock. If the initial bolus produces no improvement, it should be immediately repeated with another 20 mL/kg. If there is still no improvement, type-specific red cells should be immediately transfused and urgent surgical intervention considered.

If crystalloid bolus produces a sustained improvement in pressure and perfusion, NS or LR should be infused at 5 mL/kg per hour for several hours. If the child remains stable, the intravenous infusion rate should be adjusted to maintenance levels listed below, and normal saline or LR solution can be replaced by standard fluid maintenance solutions. Below are listed maintenance fluid volume requirements by weight.

- weight = 10 kg: 100 mL/kg per 24 hours
- weight = 10 kg to 20 kg: 1000 mL plus 50 mL/kg above 10 kg per 24 hours

- weight = >20 kg: 1500 mL plus 20 mL/kg above 20 kg per 24 hours

### Monitoring Fluid Resuscitation

It is critical to assess and record accurately the initial indicators of circulatory status (pulse, respirations, blood pressure, pulse pressure, and mental status). Follow these findings closely to track response to intervention.

### Pneumatic Antishock Garment

The pneumatic antishock garment (PASG) is no longer recommended for the treatment of shock. It might have some benefit in patients with unstable pelvic and lower extremity fractures; however, it might be no more effective than a properly applied external pelvic compression wrap.

## Disability

### Glasgow Coma Scale

The Glasgow Coma Scale (GCS) score is useful for the neurologic assessment of a trauma patient and also has predictive value for outcome. It involves an assessment of three components of neurologic function: eye opening, motor response, and verbal response. It can be used to assess both verbal and nonverbal children. Age-related modifications are listed in Table 9-5.

### AVPU

A rapid neurologic evaluation is part of the primary survey. This neurologic evaluation should include assessment of only pupillary response, patient's level of consciousness, and any local-

---

**TABLE 9-5    Pediatric Glasgow Coma Scale**

**Modified Glasgow Coma Scale**

| Child | Infant |
|---|---|
| **EYES:** | |
| 4  Opens eyes spontaneously | Opens eyes spontaneously |
| 3  Opens eyes to speech | Opens eyes to speech |
| 2  Opens eyes to pain | Opens eyes to pain |
| 1  **NO RESPONSE** | **NO RESPONSE** |
| _____ = Score (Eyes) | |
| **MOTOR:** | |
| 6  Obeys commands | Spontaneous movements |
| 5  Localizes | Withdraws to touch |
| 4  Withdraws | Withdraws to pain |
| 3  Flexion | Flexion (decorticate) |
| 2  Extension | Extension (decerebrate) |
| 1  **NO RESPONSE** | **NO RESPONSE** |
| _____ = Score (Motor) | |
| **VERBAL:** | |
| 5  Oriented | Coos and babbles |
| 4  Confused | Irritable cry |
| 3  Inappropriate words | Cries to pain |
| 2  Incomprehensible words | Moans to pain |
| 1  **NO RESPONSE** | **NO RESPONSE** |
| _____ = Score (Verbal) | |

_____ = Total Score (Eyes, Motor, Verbal) Scores will range from 3 to 15.

Source: James HE, Anas NG, and Perkin RM. *Brain Insults in Infants and Children.* Orlando, Fl: Grune & Stratton; 1985. Reprinted with permission.

izing finding such as paralysis or paresis of an extremity. A simple method for evaluating level of consciousness involves the mnemonic AVPU:

A- Alert
V- Responds to verbal stimuli
P- Responds to painful stimuli
U- Unresponsive

A more in-depth neurologic assessment should be performed during the secondary survey.

### Exposure and Examination

The child's clothing must be removed completely to allow full assessment of injury and a complete examination. A small child can become hypothermic quickly after exposure. A radiant warmer, warming blanket, or air convection unit might be required to maintain the child's temperature at 36° to 37°C. This part of the primary survey should include the log roll to examine the back and spine, assessment of the perineum for signs of injury, and a rectal examination to assess rectal tone and for the presence of blood in the rectal vault. If there are signs of urethral injury, such as blood at the meatus, a quick retrograde urethrogram should be obtained before passing an indwelling bladder catheter. Urine present in the bladder at the time of the insertion usually was produced before injury and does not reflect current output. If there are no signs of urethral injury, an indwelling urinary catheter should be placed on any moderately to severely injured trauma patient to assess for hematuria and to monitor urine output.

A nasogastric tube (or orogastric tube if there is evidence of midfacial or a basilar skull fracture) should be placed in every multiply injured child whose level of consciousness precludes accurate evaluation. For practical purposes this includes children with a GCS score less than or equal to 9, for whatever reason. Children with signs and symptoms of traumatic brain injury who are obtunded but not comatose will often become severely agitated when any invasive maneuver is attempted. In these patients, the benefit of relevant information or therapeutic effect must be balanced against the risk of additional injury from avoidable agitation. Similar clinical judgment should

## KEY POINTS

**Critical Steps in the Management of the Pediatric Trauma Patient**

**Primary Survey**

- Airway: open with jaw thrust; suction; secure if respiratory failure or decompensated shock

- Breathing: add supplemental oxygen; assist ventilation if respiratory failure; needle or tube thoracostomy for pneumothorax

- Circulation: compress and elevate external bleeding sites; obtain vascular access (peripheral, central, intraosseous); fluid resuscitate with 20 mL/kg normal saline or LR solution; begin packed red cells if >40 mL/kg of crystalloid is needed to maintain perfusion

- Disability: assess level of consciousness; pupillary response; motor response; calculate Glasgow Coma Scale score

- Exposure: remove clothing; keep infant or child warm

guide timing of insertion of a urinary catheter. If there is suspected urethral injury, as is often associated with a pelvic fracture, complete integrity of the urethra must be confirmed by urethrogram before a bladder catheter is placed.

## Secondary Survey

The secondary survey is a more comprehensive evaluation of each body area proceeding from head to toe. It should answer the following questions:

- Is an injury present in the anatomic area under evaluation?

- If so, what type of injury is present, and which organ is injured?

- What is the anatomic and physiologic derangement of each organ?

- What is the appropriate definitive care for the injury?

- What is the priority of therapy for this injury compared with other injuries identified in the secondary survey?

The components of the secondary survey are:

- History (SAMPLE)
- Complete examination
- Laboratory studies
- Radiographic studies
- Problem identification

During this phase, complete the history and perform a thorough physical examination. Pay attention to the adequacy of cervical stabilization obtained during the primary survey and continue aggressive resuscitation.

**Focused History**

The history is actually best obtained from the EMS service that transported the patient unless key witnesses are available. In most states, the EMS service is required to leave a run sheet, which becomes a permanent part of the hospital record. This document should contain event history and details of how the patient was found and his or her initial physiologic status. The history should include the mechanism of injury, time, status at the scene, changes in status, and patient complaints. Obtain a focused history using the mnemonic SAMPLE:

S- Signs and symptoms (What hurts?)
A- Allergies
M- Medications
P- Past illnesses
L- Last meal
E- Events preceding the injury
(What happened?)

The child's parents can be quite useful, not only for the history, but also in assessment of the child's interactions with them. Ask if immunizations are up-to-date.

**Detailed Physical Examination**

Head

Begin the secondary survey with an evaluation of the eyes, including conjunctiva, pupillary size and reaction, retinal appearance, and vision, if possible. Examine the face for evidence of maxillofacial trauma by palpating bony prominences. Check the dentition. Examine the scalp carefully for lacerations or underlying soft tissue injury. Suspect basilar skull fracture if the Battle's sign or raccoon eyes are present or if hemotympanum or cerebrospinal fluid rhinorrhea or otorrhea is apparent. Check for symmetric voluntary movement and neurologic function of the facial muscles.

Neck

Examine the neck for subcutaneous emphysema, abnormal tracheal position, hematoma, or localized pain. Palpate the cervical spine for step-offs, swelling, or tenderness. Neck vein distention also should be assessed.

Chest

Reevaluate the chest visually for adequacy of respiratory excursion, asymmetry of chest wall motion, or the presence of a flail segment. After observation, carefully palpate the chest for tenderness or crepitus and auscultate the lung fields and cardiovascular system.

Abdomen

Examine the abdomen next; it is important to remember that specific diagnoses usually are not immediately possible. Examination of the abdomen includes inspection for ease of movement with respiration, bruises, seatbelt marks, tire marks, and lacerations; auscultation of bowel sounds; and gentle palpation for localized findings. Observe and palpate the flanks. The abdomen might need to be examined several times to make an accurate assessment.

Pelvis

Compress the pelvis bilaterally to evaluate for tenderness or instability. If stable, palpate bony prominences of the pelvis to assess for tenderness. Carefully examine the perineum for laceration, hematoma, or active bleeding. Check the urethral meatus for blood.

Rectum

A rectal examination is necessary if not already completed; evaluate the integrity of the wall, displacement or distortion of the prostate, sphincter muscle tone, and occult gastrointestinal hemorrhage.

Extremities

Examine the extremities for signs of fracture, dislocation, abrasion, contusion, or hematoma formation. Note bony instability, and perform a neurovascular evaluation.

Back

Examination of the back should not be neglected. With the neck immobilized, if spinal injury or paralysis has not been excluded, gently roll the patient to examine the entire back and spine.

### Skin

Examine thoroughly for evidence of contusions, burns, and petechiae, as in traumatic asphyxia.

### Neurologic

Perform an in-depth neurologic examination, including motor, sensory, and cranial nerves, as well as level of consciousness. Examine the fundi. Check the nose again for cerebrospinal fluid (CSF) rhinorrhea.

## Diagnostic Studies

For the child with severe injury and an uncertain circulatory status, the first laboratory study should be a type and cross-match of blood for possible transfusion. If immediate transfusion is necessary, O negative blood should be infused. Do not exacerbate injury severity and physiologic stress in the bleeding child by delaying transfusion until cross-matched blood is available! Laboratory assessment of any injured child is highly individualized and driven by clinical judgment, suspected injuries, and anticipated critical care therapy. At a minimum, hematocrit or hemoglobin, white blood cell count, glucose, and urinalysis are needed; serial determinations can be helpful in the seriously injured child.

For any critically ill trauma patient, obtaining a rapid chest and anterior-posterior pelvic films is a priority to assess for injuries resulting in blood loss. A cervical spine radiographic series is required if a neck injury is suspected or if the child cannot be fully evaluated clinically but can be delayed in the critical patient. Other radiographs are obtained as directed by physical findings and history. More sophisticated studies for severely injured children usually include computed tomography of the head and abdomen.

Continuously monitor and frequently reevaluate the patient. A high index of suspicion and constant vigilance for signs of deterioration or the development of new problems will allow early diagnosis and management of ongoing pathophysiology.

It is important that those involved with emergency treatment of seriously injured children understand the principles of care and pri-orities of treatment in multiple trauma. The person who performs the initial evaluation and stabilization should retain full responsibility for therapy until direction of the child's total care is accepted by another qualified provider. One physician with appropriate credentials and experience must serve as the trauma team leader.

## YOUR FIRST CLUE

### Critical Signs and Symptoms in the Pediatric Trauma Patient

- Tension pneumothorax: tachypnea, hypoxemia, hypotension, +/− JVD, +/− absent breath sounds

- Pericardial tamponade: tachypnea, hypoxemia, hypotension, +/− JVD, muffled heart sounds

- Shock:
  - Compensated: decreased peripheral pulses, tachycardia, cool extremities, normal or increased blood pressure
  - Decompensated: absent peripheral pulses, tachycardia or bradycardia, delayed capillary refill, hypotension

- Basilar skull fracture: Battle's sign, raccoon eyes, hemotympanum, CSF otorrhea or rhinorrhea

- Increased intracranial pressure: headache, vomiting, altered level of consciousness, bulging fontanel (infant), papillary dilation, cranial nerve deficit, seizure, abnormal posturing, respiratory irregularity, bradycardia

- Spinal injury: altered level of consciousness, abnormal neuromotor or neurosensory examination, report of neurologic abnormality at any time after injury, neck or back tenderness, crepitus or pain on palpation or movement, limitation of neck or back motion, or unexplained hypotension

- Neurogenic shock: hypotension with warm, flushed skin, and spinal shock (decreased deep tendon reflexes, decreased sensory level, flaccid sphincters, and hypotonia)

- Traumatic asphyxia: Petechiae of the head and neck, subconjunctival hemorrhages, and occasionally, depressed level of consciousness

This is especially critical for coordination of consultative support, orchestration of therapy, and ensuring that the transition from initial assessment to definitive therapy is a seamless continuum of communication and care. One of the most common problems identified by performance improvement screening is inadequate, inaccurate, or missing documentation of critical information. Initial assessment and all resuscitation procedures must be immediately and completely recorded. Such records are essential in monitoring improvement or deterioration. Frequently, in the chaotic press of emergency care, important data and observations are overlooked; this can be avoided by adequate planning and assignment of record-keeping to experienced personnel.

## Central Nervous System Injuries

The goal of emergency care of traumatic brain injury is the prevention of secondary cerebral insults. Bruce et al[8] demonstrated that children have an exaggerated cerebrovascular response to injury compared with adults. Children are prone to develop diffuse brain swelling more readily. Brain insults can oc-cur at the time of impact due to damage sustained as a result of direct trauma to the skull and intracranial structures. These injuries include scalp lacerations and skull fractures, as well as traumatic neuronal and vascular injuries. Primary injuries sustained at the time of impact are rarely influenced by therapeutic interventions; however, secondary brain injury can occur as a result of the ongoing pathophysiologic derangements. Failure to recognize and treat respiratory failure and shock can further exacerbate brain injury.[9] Overzealous hydration can also contribute to cerebral swelling and secondary brain damage (Figure 9.10). The final common pathway leading to secondary brain injury is increased intracranial pressure (ICP) and decreased cerebral perfusion pressure (CPP). Maintenance of adequate CPP relies on maintenance of a normal blood pressure with appropriate volume expansion and inotropic support when necessary, as well as maneuvers to maintain ICP within normal limits.

### Determinants of Cerebral Perfusion Pressure

CPP is calculated as the mean arterial pressure (MAP) minus ICP. Increased ICP is the most

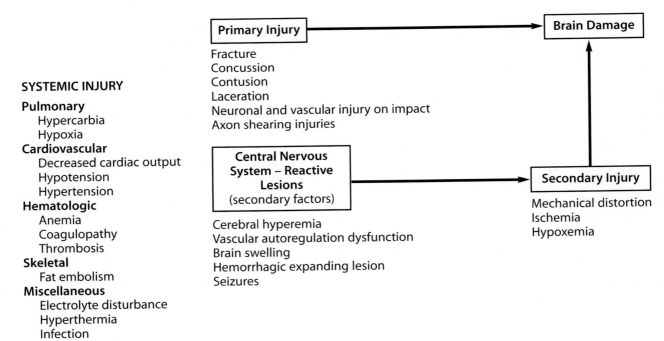

Figure 9.10 Dynamics of traumatic brain damage.

common cause of decreased CPP in the head-injured child older than 1 year; this occurs because of the unyielding nature of the cranial vault and relative low compliance of the intracranial contents. The intracranial cavity contains CSF, brain, and cerebral blood.

Intracranial volume (IC vol) is represented by the following formula:

$$IC\ vol = CSF\ vol + Blood\ vol + Brain\ vol$$

Under normal circumstances, the intracranial volume is maintained relatively constant because of compensatory adjustments in these three components. As such, ICP is kept relatively constant (<15 mm Hg) and fluctuates minimally with the Valsalva maneuver, respiration, pulse, and position. Once the compliance of the intracranial vault is exceeded, however, small changes in volume can cause massive increases in ICP (Figure 9.11).

## Buffering Mechanisms

### Cerebrospinal Fluid

The CSF is an important early buffer for the maintenance of ICP. The CSF is approximately 10% of the intracranial volume, and most is displaced easily into the spinal subarachnoid space when intracranial volume increases. With further increase in brain swelling, the ventricular system is compressed. This causes further displacement of CSF, which again diminishes the intracranial CSF volume. When CSF volume is almost totally displaced, intracranial compliance is diminished. At this point, minimal changes in intracranial volume can produce marked and sustained rises in ICP. In most cases, patients presenting with increased ICP have exhausted the CSF compensatory mechanism, so therapy to decrease ICP relies on other mechanisms, including manipulation of cerebral blood volume.

### Cerebral Blood Volume

Blood is approximately 8% of the intracranial volume. Most of the cerebral blood is in thin-walled venous capacitance vessels. Extrinsic pressure from a mass lesion can displace blood from these vessels. However, cerebral blood flow (CBF) can be increased in response to head trauma in childhood. This global increase in CBF (cerebral hyperemia) can occur shortly after injury. Although the underlying reasons for this increase in CBF and intracranial blood volume are unknown, it is well established that CBF is responsive to changes in $PaCO_2$ and $PaO_2$ (Figures 9.12 and 9.13).

Hypocarbia of 25 to 30 mm Hg reduces cerebral blood volume by approximately 50% from baseline levels at $PaCO_2$ of 40 mm Hg. This is important because children with severe head injury can hypoventilate and become hypercapnic, with resultant cerebral hyperemia. The $CO_2$ response is the rationale for hyperventilating the child with severe head injury and increased ICP. However, recent evidence suggests that prolonged hyperventilation to $PaCO_2$ levels of less than 35 mm Hg offers little benefit, and that levels of less than 25 mm Hg are potentially hazardous as a result of reduction

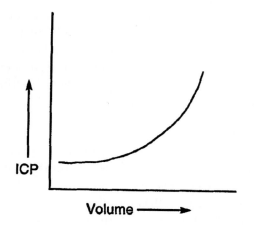

**Figure 9.11** Relationship of expanding intracranial volume to intracranial pressure.

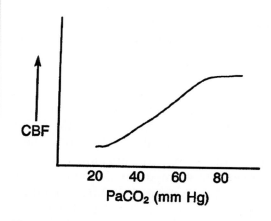

**Figure 9.12** Relationship of $PaCO_2$ to cerebral blood flow.

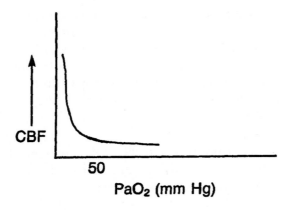

**Figure 9.13** Relationship of hypoxemia to increase in cerebral blood flow.

in global CBF achieved mainly by decreasing flow to undamaged brain tissue.[10] Seizure activity or hyperthermia increases cerebral metabolic rate and oxygen demand and can potentiate neuronal injury if metabolic demands are not met.

### Brain

The brain parenchyma occupies approximately 80% of the intracranial volume. It is minimally compressible and contributes very little to the intracranial volume-buffering system. In children with no significant underlying brain lesions, rapid recovery will occur if CPP is maintained within normal limits. However, in children with diffuse impact injuries, initial control of hyperemia will maintain a normal ICP, but delayed elevation of ICP can occur as the result of progression of cellular edema. Control of this edema can be achieved in part through avoidance of overhydration. Water restriction is no longer recommended because its salutary effects on ICP can be countered by untoward effects on MAP, thereby decreasing ICP.

### Comprehensive Neurologic Examination

A neurologic flow sheet facilitates an objective and serial recording of the patient's status. This is best accomplished initially using the Glasgow Coma Scale (Table 9-5) or the AVPU system. The three variables that correlate best with the degree of coma are adjusted to reflect their relative importance: motor (6), verbal (5), and eye opening (4). When recording motor response as an indication of the functional state of the brain as a whole, the best or highest response from any limb is recorded. However, any difference between the responsiveness of one limb and that of another can indicate focal brain damage, and for this purpose, the worst (most abnormal) response also should be noted. For motor response, it is best to pinch the medial aspect of each arm or leg, or apply pressure to a nail bed with a pencil. This can result in either flexion or extension of the elbow. If flexion is observed, stimulation (e.g., sternal rub) is applied to the head and neck or trunk above the nipple line to test for localization. Raising the hand above the chin in response to supraorbital pressure is a localizing response. The eye-opening response to speech does not necessarily require a command to open the eyes.

The neurologic examination includes an assessment of the cranial nerves, eyes, brainstem, motor system, sensory system, and cerebellum. The cranial nerves are a system of 12 nerves that exit the cranium without traversing the spinal cord. The olfactory nerve (CN I) is one of the most commonly involved in traumatic injuries, but this is usually of little clinical significance. The abducens (CN VI), facial (CN VII), and vestibulocochlear (CN VIII) nerves are most commonly involved in craniofacial trauma, due to their relatively long intraosseous course through the skull. Injuries to these nerves are frequently seen in association with skull fractures, particularly temporal bone fractures. Assessment of acute facial nerve injuries, especially peripheral injuries, should include specialty evaluation (otorhinolaryngology, plastic surgery, or neurosurgery). Hearing loss is common in children who have sustained skull fractures. This should be excluded with audiometric evaluations on a nonurgent basis in all children with moderate or severe traumatic brain injuries and/or basilar skull fractures.[11]

### Eyes

Eye examination is a crucial component of the neurologic examination. This examination includes the eye opening response as part of the GCS score, as well as pupillary size and reactivity, the light reflex, movement of the extraocular muscles, and examination of the fundus. Pupillary size and reactivity are controlled by cranial nerves II (optic, afferent limb) and III (oculomtor efferent limb), sympathetic fibers (via carotid artery), and parasympathetic fibers (via CN III). The most significant ocular finding in the trauma setting is an evolving unilateral cranial nerve III palsy, presenting as pupillary dilation and lateral deviation of the eye. This is a sign of uncal herniation, in which the cranial nerve is compressed by brain swelling against the brainstem at the level of the tentorial notch. Further swelling can result in brainstem compression and death.

A normal light reflex is a brisk pupillary constriction to light shone in the eye. An absent light reflex can be indicative of brainstem dysfunction, second or third cranial nerve injury, or retinal detachment. Light shone into one eye produces constriction of both eyes. This is the consensual reflex, and its absence might be due to interruption of the afferent limb of cranial nerve II, brainstem relay, or efferent limb of cranial nerve III.

Ophthalmoscopic examination is especially important in the setting of suspected child abuse. Retinal hemorrhages are frequently seen in cases of shaken baby syndrome. Papilledema is a late finding of elevated ICP. The absence of papilledema does not exclude the presence of raised ICP.

Brainstem reflex disturbances are indicative of severe traumatic brain injury. They include: pupillary response, cranial nerves II and III; doll's eye, cranial nerves III, VI, and VIII; corneal reflexes, cranial nerves V and VII; and gag reflex, cranial nerves IX and X. Testing of these reflexes is part of the brain death evaluation. All reflexes must be absent before the patient can be declared brain dead. Other components of the brain death evaluation include a failed apnea test and a GCS score of 3 after the presence of hypothermia and toxic substances has been excluded.

## Motor

The motor system examination consists of testing the power, reflexes, and tone of the major muscle groups. Hyperactive reflexes are indicative of an upper motor neuron injury (spinal cord), and hypoactive reflexes imply a lower motor neuron injury (peripheral nerve). Muscle tone is increased (spasticity) or decreased (flaccidity) in upper or lower motor neuron injuries, respectively. Upper motor neuron injuries are usually accompanied by a Babinski reflex.

The sensory system examination is perhaps less important than the motor system in the setting of acute traumatic brain injury. An isolated sensory loss is usually found in spinal cord or peripheral nerve injuries.

Cerebellar examination primarily consists of testing coordination of movement and balance.

## Management

Tables 9-6 and 9-7 are suggested guidelines for obtaining a head CT scan and practice guidelines for children with minor head trauma, respectively. Neurologically intact children who have sustained a mild traumatic brain injury (TBI) can be discharged home from the ED (Table 9-8). Instructions concerning head injury observation and precautions should be given to all parents prior to discharge from the ED (Table 9-9). Table 9-10 summarizes recommendations for return to sports activities after head trauma in children.[12,13] However, if intracranial pathology is detected on CT or MRI, the child should refrain from sports activity for the remainder of the season and discouraged from a future return to contact sports.

The child with a moderate TBI (GCS score of 8 to 12) presents in a less acute manner than one with a severe TBI, but the consequences of these injuries remain substantial in terms of the patient's short- and long-term disabilities. All patients with moderate TBI are admitted and at least one head CT scan is obtained. A neurosurgery consultation is obtained. The patient is closely observed with serial neurologic examinations for at least 24 hours. The family is given adequate information on head injuries, and at least one followup appointment with a neurosurgeon is advisable, usually within 2 weeks of injury. Parents of all children who sustain a TBI should be educated about postconcussive syndrome (Table 9-9) and the possible neurobehavioral consequences of a head injury.

## TABLE 9-6　Indications for Obtaining a CT Scan of the Head

**Absolute indications:**
- Penetrating injury
- GCS score of <15
- Focal neurologic deficit
- Posttraumatic seizures
- Persistent vomiting
- Extensive facial injury
- Signs of basilar skull fracture
- Calvarial skull fracture in patients younger than 2 years

**Relative indications:**
- History of change in level of consciousness
- Alcohol or drug intoxication
- Suspected child maltreatment
- Unreliable or inadequate history of injury
- Age <2, unless injury is trivial and witnessed by reliable adult
- Postconcussive amnesia
- Severe headache
- Calvarial skull fracture in patients 2 years old and older

Other suspicious findings (e.g., cranial bruit, violent mechanism of injury with other deaths), at discretion of any of the services involved in the care of the child

Adapted from: Kosair Children's Hospital Pediatric Trauma Manual, Louisville, Ky.

## TABLE 9-8　Criteria for Discharge From Emergency Department in Neurologically Intact Children

- Brief or no loss of consciousness*
- Loss of consciousness more than 24 hours prior to admission
- History compatible with only minor injury
- Asymptomatic, with a GCS score of 15
- Normal radiographic findings
- Reliable caregivers, informed about warning signs of neurologic deterioration
- Easy access to hospital should there be any deterioration

*The period "brief" is controversial and not well defined in the literature. Judgment should be used in individual cases.

Adapted from: American Academy of Pediatrics. The management of minor closed head injury in children. *Pediatrics.* 1999;104:1407–1415; and Mitchell KA, Fallat ME, Raque GH, Hardwick VG, Groff DB, Nagaraj HS. Evaluation of minor head injury in children. *J Pediatr Surg.* 1994;29:851–854.

## TABLE 9-7　American Academy of Pediatrics Practice Guidelines for Children With Minor Head Trauma (2–20 Years of Age)*

- Children with minor head injury and no loss of consciousness (LOC) without other symptoms—no need for CT
- Children with minor head injury and brief LOC (<1 minute), with associated symptoms—consider CT or observation
- Children with minor head injury and LOC, with or without associated symptoms—obtain CT

*Includes children with GCS=15, normal neurologic exam, no evidence of skull fracture

Source: American Academy of Pediatrics Practice Guideline: The Management of Minor Head Injury in Children. *Pediatrics.* 1999;104:1407–1415.

## TABLE 9-9　Instructions to Parents or Caregivers for Home Observation of Children Who Have Sustained Head Trauma

Immediately bring the child to the emergency department if any of the following signs or symptoms appears within the first 72 hours after discharge:
- Any unusual behavior
- Disorientation as to name and place
- Unusual drowsiness and sleepiness
- Inability to wake child from sleep
- Increasing headache
- Seizures, twitching, or convulsions
- Unsteadiness on feet
- Clear or bloody drainage from ear or nose
- Vomiting more than two or three times
- Blurred or double vision
- Weakness or numbness of face, arms, or legs
- Fever
- Stiff neck

## TABLE 9-10 Summary of Recommendations for Return to Sports Activities After Head Trauma in Children

**Return to play (same day)**

1. Signs and symptoms cleared within 15 minutes or less, both at rest and exertion.
2. Normal neurologic evaluation.
3. No documented loss of consciousness.

**Delayed return to play (not same day)**

1. Signs and symptoms not cleared in 15 minutes at rest or with exertion.
2. Documented loss of consciousness.
3. Any new headache in the first 48–72 hours should preclude play.

**Delayed return to play (loss of consciousness)**

1. Every athlete with concussion should be evaluated by a physician.
2. Loss of consciousness precludes return to play that day.
3. Symptoms lasting more than 15 minutes, or delayed onset of symptoms such as headache, dizziness, or confusion with rest or exertion should preclude play that day.
4. Deterioration of physical or mental status after initial trauma such as increasing headache, dizziness, nausea, and/or vomiting warrants transport to an emergency department for evaluation.
5. Persistence of symptoms for longer than 15 minutes after concussion should preclude play for 7 days.
6. If additional symptoms occur, or a second concussion occurs, consider no sports activity until asymptomatic for 1 month.

**CT evaluation shows pathology on CT**

1. If intracranial pathology is detected on CT or MRI, no sports activity for the remainder of the season and the athlete is discouraged from future return to contact sports.

Sources: Centers for Disease Control and Prevention. Sports-related recurrent brain injuries–United States. *MMWR Morb Mortal Wkly Rep.* 1997;46:224-227. Wojtys EM, Hovda D, Landry G, et al. Concussion in sports. *Am J Sports Med.* 1999;27(5):676-687.

# Cranial and Intracranial Injuries

## Skull Fractures

Skull fractures can involve the cranial vault or base. They are described as open if associated with an overlying scalp laceration, and as closed if not. Open skull fractures are usually treated with surgical debridement, especially if there is a depressed skull fracture and the underlying dura or brain is lacerated.[14]

### Linear Skull Fractures

Most skull fractures that occur in children are linear and extend across the cranial vault. These children frequently are asymptomatic except for swelling and tenderness over the fracture site. In younger children, even if the external signs are minimal but a skull fracture is suspected, radiographic evaluation should be undertaken for documentation. This is usually best accomplished by CT scan to identify the extent of fracture as well as assess the status of underlying intracranial contents.

### Depressed Skull Fractures

Depressed skull fractures usually are more obvious on physical examination. They are commonly the result of significant traumatic force acting on a small cross-sectional area (e.g., a blow from a hammer). Depressed skull fractures can be associated with underlying brain injury and, occasionally, dural tears. Depressed fractures can in some instances be compound or comminuted. Neurosurgical evaluation is mandatory in all cases.

### Basilar Skull Fractures

Basilar skull fractures involve the basal portion of the skull and can occur in the anterior, middle, or posterior cranial fossa. These fractures usually are characterized by periorbital subcutaneous hemorrhages (raccoon eyes), CSF rhinorrhea, or otorrhea, cranial nerve palsies, hemotympanum, or postauricular ecchymosis (Battle sign). These signs might appear at the initial assessment but also develop during stabilization; hence, serial examinations are important. In the young child, the dura closely adheres to the basilar skull and can lead to meningeal tears in basilar fractures. Children with CSF rhinorrhea or otorrhea should be evaluated by a neurosurgeon. Initial definitive treatment entails inpatient bed rest with the head of the bed elevated. Children whose cervical spines have not been cleared will require reverse Trendelenburg positioning. Over 95% of these injuries will heal spontaneously with this therapy. Antibiotic treatment is not needed. Any child who is suspected of having an anterior fossa basilar skull fracture is at risk for intracranial penetration with nasogastric tubes, so orogastric intubation is preferred for gastric decompression.

## Concussions

A concussion is a transient state of neuronal dysfunction resulting from trauma. It can manifest as transient confusion or loss of consciousness. In the infant and young child, there is a characteristic concussion syndrome seen minutes to hours after a fall. Consciousness rarely is lost; however, the child becomes pale, very sleepy, and might begin to vomit. Examination usually reveals a pale infant or child with tachycardia, clammy skin, normal blood pressure, no evidence of focal neurologic deficit, and a soft fontanel. The level of consciousness varies from spontaneous movements of all extremities to deep stupor with responses to pain only. These symptoms and signs usually subside rapidly. Occasionally, however, hospitalization and judicious administration of intravenous fluids will be necessary for 24 hours. This is mandatory if the GCS score falls below 15. An older child might present with irritability and vomiting. Amnesia of the events leading to the trauma (retrograde amnesia) or posttraumatic (antegrade) amnesia is fairly common in older children. The length of the posttraumatic amnesia usually correlates with the severity of head injury.

## Diffuse Axonal Injury

Diffuse axonal injury in children younger than 1 year commonly occurs as a result of child maltreatment due to shaken baby syndrome. Pathologically, there is tearing of the anterior bridging veins, petechial hemorrhage in the white matter and deep gray structures with shearing of myelin and axons, contusions of the corpus callosum, subarachnoid hemorrhage, and acute intracranial hypertension. These children often are brought to medical attention after hours of coma and usually have sustained several previous but less severe injuries. On examination, there often is no evidence of external trauma but perhaps some bruising or pinch marks on the upper arms. Infants present in several ways, including deep coma with decorticate posture or flaccidity,

fixed dilated pupils, and apnea or bradycardia. They can sometimes be aroused by painful stimulation, move all extremities, and breathe well spontaneously. In severe cases, the fontanel is full and tense. In almost all cases, retinal hemorrhages can be detected on ophthalmoscopic examination.[15]

Diffuse axonal injury in the older child can result from primary impact injury. Pathologically, this is due to areas of disruption of the blood-brain barrier and small intracranial hemorrhages, but it also can be due to significant contusions and lacerations as a result of shearing forces. More commonly, a pattern is seen of bilateral diffuse swelling produced by vasodilatation and hyperemia after trauma. This swelling is produced mainly by an increase in intracerebral blood volume; however, redistribution of blood from the subarachnoid and pial vessels into the intraparenchymal regions is a contributory factor. A child with a deteriorating neurologic status after a period of lucency is more likely to have generalized cerebral swelling than intracranial hemorrhage, but significant brain edema can be superimposed on this hyperemia. This is likely to occur in children who present in immediate deep coma, suggesting a significant degree of neuronal injury at impact. This primarily is due to white matter edema caused by disruption of the blood-brain barrier and can cause an increase in ICP not adequately controlled through hyperventilation. Treatment of diffuse axonal injury is primarily directed toward control of cerebral swelling and elevated ICP.

## Epidural Hematoma

Epidural hematomas are relatively rare (less than 3%), even in severe trauma in children. Epidural hematomas in adults commonly originate from a hemorrhaging middle meningeal artery that quickly separates the meningeal dura layer from the inner table of the skull. In children, however, most epidural hematomas are due to meningeal and diploic vein hemorrhage. These hematomas occasionally occur in the posterior cranial fossa due to a bleeding deep venous sinus. In contradistinction to the adult, the dura matter in the young child is tightly adherent to the skull. This factor probably is responsible for the varying and occasional subacute presentation of epidural hemorrhages in children. Epidural hematomas are true surgical emergencies, although small venous epidural hematomas can be managed conservatively.

In the infant and young child, an epidural hematoma usually results from a high fall onto a hard surface or a motor vehicle crash. Acute epidural hematoma in infancy can be associated with anemia and shock because a large amount of blood can accumulate in the head. This is due to the greater compressibility of the brain and the expandable nature of the cranial vault when cranial sutures have not yet fused. If an associated skull fracture is present, the hematoma can decompress into the subperiosteal galea with an even greater blood loss. This is an exception to the general rule that shock does not result from head injury alone.

Children younger than 5 years with epidural hematomas rarely present with the classic pattern of a lucid period followed by rapid neurologic deterioration occurring within hours of injury. The period of lucidity usually is not a totally asymptomatic interval but simply stabilization or an improvement in the level of consciousness. Many children at this age never become deeply unconscious but present within 48 hours of injury with papilledema, bradycardia, continued moderate lethargy, and sometimes recurrent vomiting over several days. These signs signify increased ICP and impending transtentorial herniation. Cranial vault fractures occur in only approximately 50% of children with epidural hemorrhages. In a child, epidural hemorrhage also can occur in the posterior cranial fossa after occipital trauma, resulting in nuchal rigidity, cerebellar signs, vomiting, and continued impaired consciousness. The outcome from epidural hematomas relies on prompt recognition and treatment. Figure 9.14 demonstrates the CT findings of a child with an epidural hematoma.

## Subdural Hematoma

Posttraumatic subdural hemorrhages are an important source of neurologic morbidity in children. Subdural hematomas occur 5 to 10 times more frequently than bleeding in the epidural

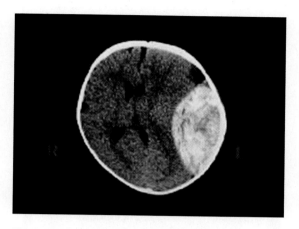

Figure 9.14 CT findings of a child with epidural hematoma.

space and tend to occur in infants more often than in older children. These hemorrhages are almost exclusively venous in origin, mostly due to cerebral bridging vein disruption between the dura and brain. In a young infant, the onset of symptoms can be relatively slow due to the relative plasticity of the skull. Infants can present with nonspecific symptoms such as vomiting, irritability, and low-grade fever. Some infants, however, will not present with symptoms until the subacute or chronic phase of subdural collection. In the subacute phase, the subdural blood organizes into a hemorrhagic cyst over several weeks and expands in size due to the osmotic pressure of red blood cell breakdown products. The usual presentation is that of a child with an enlarged head and no history of trauma. Occasionally, infants present with focal or generalized seizures. Physical examination reveals an irritable, lethargic baby with a bulging fontanel, "sunsetting" eyes, retinal and preretinal hemorrhages, and hypertonic musculature. Older children with subdural bleeding tend to present more acutely with symptoms and signs of increased ICP and impending transtentorial herniation. Figure 9.15 demonstrates CT findings of a child with a subdural hematoma.

## Cerebral Contusions

Brain contusions are commonly seen in deceleration injuries, where brain substance momentum exceeds the suddenly stationary cranium as occurs in high-speed automobile

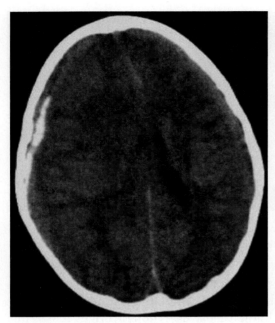

Figure 9.15 CT findings of a child with subdural hematoma.

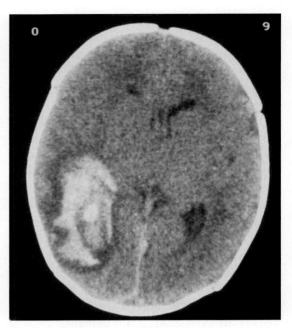

Figure 9.16 CT findings of a child with intracerebral hemorrhage.

crashes. The brain is subjected to shear stresses that result in varying degrees of brain tearing, contusion, and frank intracerebral hematoma formation. Cerebral edema is almost universally associated with intracerebral contusions. These injuries tend to occur near the tips (rostral extent) of the frontal and temporal lobes. A temporal lobe contusion is potentially lethal because of its close proximity to the brainstem, where swelling can quickly result in lateral herniation and death. Larger intraparenchymal hematomas frequently require surgical evacuation. Figure 9.16 demonstrates CT findings of a child with intracerebral hemorrhage.

## Brainstem Injuries

The brainstem is subject to shear injuries and compression by a swollen, adjacent traumatized brain. Differences in pressure between the supratentorial and infratentorial compartments will place stresses on brainstem tissue as the pressure dissipates between these compartments. If the brainstem moves through the tentorial notch (central herniation), tearing of vessels within the brainstem causes intraparenchymal hematomas known as Duret lesions or hemorrhages. This is a lethal condition.

## Intracranial Hypertension and Herniation

Intracranial hypertension is common in children with severe head injury, even in the absence of a mass lesion. The ICP can be elevated early or become elevated after several days because of persistent or uncontrollable cerebral hyperemia or vasogenic or cytotoxic cerebral edema. Symptoms of increased ICP occur only after the compensatory mechanisms for maintaining normal ICP have been exhausted. Early symptoms and signs of increased ICP include headache, vomiting, altered mental status, respiratory irregularity, and abnormal posturing. Prompt therapy should be instituted to avoid further increases in ICP, decreased CPP, or brain herniation (Figure 9.17). The diagnosis of elevated ICP should be established well before the onset of the late manifestations of hypertension, bradycardia, and pupillary dilatation. Herniation of the brain can take place at any of three anatomic sites: tentorial incisura, inferior edge of the falx cerebri, and foramen magnum. The most common herniation is a central transtentorial herniation of diffusely swollen cerebral hemispheres. When this occurs, the diencephalon and upper brainstem are compressed initially, causing deterioration in level of con-

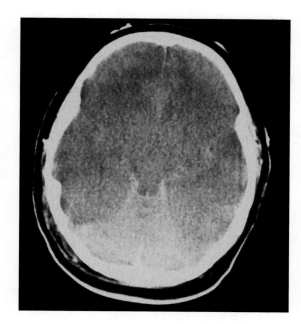

**Figure 9.17** Head injury with subarachnoid hemorrhage, diffuse cerebral edema, and impending herniation.

sciousness, respiratory irregularity, pupillary dilatation, upward gaze limitation, and progressive hypertonia. With continued caudal progression, decorticate posturing, pupillary dilatation, and hyperventilation develop. Basilar artery compression and brainstem ischemia also will develop and lead to further deterioration.

## Seizures

Seizures have been reported in some series in as many as 10% of children seen in emergency departments after experiencing head trauma. Posttraumatic seizures can be temporally divided into those of immediate, early, and late onset. An immediate seizure occurs within seconds of impact and can represent a traumatic depolarization of the cortex. This seizure can occur with mild trauma, is brief, and has no prognostic significance.

Early seizures account for approximately 50% of posttraumatic seizures; they take place within the first week of the traumatic event and usually are due to focal brain injury. Young children are more susceptible to the development of early posttraumatic seizures within the first 24 hours after trauma. Apparently equivalent numbers of patients have generalized or focal seizures, and 10% to 20% develop

status epilepticus. Approximately 25% of children with early seizures continue to have seizures after the first week.

Late posttraumatic epilepsy probably reflects cortical scarring. The severity of head injury, dural laceration, and intracranial hemorrhage are factors that determine whether late-onset seizures occur. Approximately 5% of hospitalized patients with head trauma develop late posttraumatic seizures. The long-term prognosis is worse in these patients because as many as 75% will develop a chronic seizure disorder.

Initial therapy for seizures can include a short-acting anticonvulsant (0.1 to 0.3 mg/kg diazepam 0.05 to 0.1 mg/kg lorazepam), followed by a long-acting anticonvulsant (20 mg/kg phenytoin). Phenytoin should be infused at a rate no faster than 1 mg/kg per minute or 50 mg/min, whichever is the slower rate. Fosphenytoin can be infused much faster, at rates up to 150 mg of phenytoin equivalents per minute. Prophylactic anticonvulsant therapy also might be indicated if extensive cortical lesions are evident on examination or CT scan. One week of therapy is common practice with focal lesions or blood on CT scan.

## Extracranial Head Injuries

### Scalp Injuries

Scalp injuries are fairly common. The scalp is very vascular, and scalp lacerations can be a source of major hemorrhage. If direct pressure does not control the hemorrhage, either infiltration of lidocaine with epinephrine (maximum 7 mg/kg) or hemostat application to the galea with external reflection will temporarily control most bleeding areas. The wound then should be explored with a gloved finger. Evidence of bone fragments or open or depressed fractures necessitate neurosurgical consultation before closure. A running, locked suture closure can help with hemostasis. Pressure applied directly to the repaired wound also enhances hemostasis.

### Subgaleal Hematoma

Subgaleal and cephalohematomas are blood clots beneath the galea and pericranium, respectively. The latter is limited to suture lines lying over only one skull bone. These injuries occur frequently in children younger than 1 year. The child might have a lump that is not noticed for several days. Children with subgaleal hematomas commonly present with a soft, boggy swelling, occasionally in association with a linear fracture. Because of the fluctuant nature of these lesions, they often are diagnosed as a CSF collection that has leaked through the fracture. However, these swellings usually are liquefied subgaleal blood that can spread circumferentially around the entire skull. These lesions should be followed expectantly because attempts at surgical treatment, including aspiration, can predispose to infection. Sufficient blood leakage can occur into the subgaleal space in an infant to produce anemia.

Guidelines for the management of severe head injury were published in 1995 and revised in 2000 by the Brain Trauma Foundation as a joint initiative of the major national neurosurgical organizations.[16] This large-scale literature meta-analysis examined 14 specific management topics and classified standards, guidelines, or options based on high, moderate, or unclear degrees of clinical certainty, respectively. The topics and recommendations pertinent to this course are summarized in Table 9-11.

## Critical Pathway for the Treatment of Established Intracranial Hypertension

Table 9-12 outlines emergency measures for treatment of intracranial hypertension. Patients with severe TBI (GCS score less than 8) should be admitted to a tertiary care facility and evaluated by a trauma surgeon, neurosurgeon, and/or critical care specialist with pediatric expertise. However, cardiorespiratory stabilization and treatment of ICP should be instituted immediately and are more important than immediate referral. If the child presents to a nontertiary care center, consultation with a trauma surgeon, neurosurgeon, and/or critical care physician at the referral center is advisable before transfer. These patients are best transported expeditiously by an ALS service or by a critical care transport team.

## Spinal Injuries

Spinal injuries are relatively uncommon in children. It should be assumed that all children who have sustained multiple trauma or head or neck trauma (blunt or penetrating), have a high-risk mechanism of injury (e.g., motor vehicle crash, ejection from vehicle, lap belt injury, sports injury, fall, or dive), or have been shaken vigorously have a spinal injury until proved otherwise.[17] Most spinal injuries occur in boys and are secondary to blunt trauma, most often motor vehicle crashes. As many as 20% are secondary to penetrating injury from knives and bullets.

Signs and symptoms suggestive of spine or spinal cord damage include:

- Altered level of consciousness
- Abnormal neuromotor or neurosensory examination
- Report of neurologic abnormality at any time after injury
- Neck or back tenderness
- Crepitus or pain on palpation or movement
- Limitation of neck or back motion
- Unexplained hypotension

Table 9-13 summarizes the signs and symptoms of cervical spine injury. Occasionally, bradycardia also can occur because of unopposed parasympathetic tone in a cervical spine injury. In this situation, accompanying signs are those of neurogenic shock (hypotension with warm, flushed skin) and spinal shock (decreased deep tendon reflexes, decreased sensory level, flaccid sphincters, and hypotonia).

Goals in the care of children with spinal trauma include effective stabilization of the primary spinal injury and prevention of progression to a more severe or significant injury. Patient management involves recognition of the possibility of spinal injury and taking steps to prevent secondary injury by adherence to the ABC (airway, breathing, circulation) approach of resuscitation, along with steps to prevent further movement or displacement of a potentially unstable spine. The devastating nature of a cervical cord injury with attendant paralysis or death makes it imperative that a potentially unstable cervical spine injury not be missed.

Cervical spine and cord injury can present anywhere along the continuum of severity. The cervical column can incur a fracture that

**TABLE 9-11** Summary of Recommendations From *Guidelines for the Management of Severe Head Injury*

| Recommendation | Meta-analysis Results | Consensus Indications | Comment |
|---|---|---|---|
| Intracranial pressure monitoring | Insufficient data to support a treatment standard. | GCS score < 8 after cardiopulmonary resuscitation. Abnormal CT scan as defined by the presence of hematoma, contusion, edema, or compressed basal cisterns. | Ventricular catheters connected to an external drain are the most accurate, low cost, and reliable method of monitoring ICP. ICP monitoring is not routinely indicated in patients with mild or moderate head injury. |
| *Intracranial pressure treatment* | Insufficient data to support a treatment standard. | Treatment should be initiated at an upper threshold of 20–25 mm Hg. | Treatment of ICP based on any threshold should be corroborated by frequent clinical examination and CPP. |
| *Guidelines for cerebral perfusion pressure* | Insufficient data to support a treatment standard. | The optimal CPP in children is currently unknown, but a minimum of 50 mm Hg has been recommended. | The lowest acceptable systolic blood pressure in children is 70 + (2 × age in years) up to 90 mm Hg. |
| *Use of hyperventilation in the acute management of severe traumatic brain injury* | In the absence of raised ICP, chronic prolonged hyperventilation ($Paco_2$ < 25 mm Hg) should be avoided. | Hyperventilation therapy may be necessary for brief periods when there is acute neurologic deterioration. | Prolonged hyperventilation may transiently control intracranial hypertension refractory to sedation, paralysis, CSF drainage, and osmotic diuretics. |
| Use of mannitol in severe head injury | Insufficient data to support a treatment standard. | The guideline suggests that mannitol is effective for control of elevated ICP after severe head injury. | Limited data suggest that intermittent boluses may be more effective than continuous infusion. Effective doses range from 0.25 to 1 g/kg body weight. |
| Use of barbiturates for control of intracranial hypertension | Insufficient data to support a treatment standard. | High-dose barbiturate therapy may be considered in hemodynamically stable, salvageable head injury patients with intracranial hypertension refractory to maximal medical and surgical ICP lowering therapy. | Effective treatment requires scrupulous monitoring of red cell mass, perfusion pressures, and circulating volumes. This usually implies need for central venous pressure and vasopressor therapy. |
| *Use of glucocorticoids in the treatment of severe head injury* | The standard is that the use of glucocorticoids is not recommended. | No definitive evidence of therapeutic efficacy has been demonstrated. | |
| Role of antiseizure prophylaxis following head injury | Prophylactic use of phenytoin, carbamazepine or phenobarbital is not recommended for preventing late post-traumatic seizures. | Anticonvulsants may be used to prevent early posttraumatic seizures in patients at high risk for seizures following head injury. | Available evidence does not indicate that prevention of early post-traumatic seizures improves outcome following head injury. |

Adapted from: *Guidelines for the Management of Severe Head Injury.* New York, NY: Brain Trauma Foundation; 2000.

| TABLE 9-12 | Emergency Therapy for Children Who Have Increased Intracranial Pressure Caused by Head Trauma |
| --- | --- |

- Establish controlled ventilation (Paco$_2$ of 35 to 40 mm Hg).
- Maintain oxygenation.
- Stabilize the cervical spine.
- Keep head and neck in midline position.
- Minimize stimuli (ie, suctioning and movements).
- Institute fluid resuscitation for shock and hypovolemia.
- If not in shock, provide fluids at a maintenance rate.
- Monitor heart rate, respirations, blood pressure, cardiac rhythm, and, if indicated, pulse oximetry.
- Administer mannitol 0.25 to 0.5 g/kg IV in cases of documented deterioration despite above measures.

| TABLE 9-13 | Signs and Symptoms of Cervical Spine Injury |
| --- | --- |

- Abnormal motor examination (paresis, paralysis, flaccidity, ataxia, spasticity, rectal tone)
- Abnormal sensory examination (pain, sensation, temperature, paresthesias, anal wink)
- Altered mental status
- Neck pain
- Torticollis
- Limitation of motion
- Neck muscle spasm
- Neck ecchymosis or swelling
- Abnormal or absent reflexes
- Clonus without rigidity
- Diaphragmatic breathing without retractions
- Neurogenic shock (hypotension with bradycardia)
- Priapism
- Decreased bladder function
- Fecal retention
- Unexplained ileus
- Autonomic hyperreflexia
- Blood pressure variability with flushing and sweating
- Poikilothermia
- Hypothermia or hyperthermia

Adapted from: Woodward G. Neck trauma. In: Fleisher GR, Ludwig S, eds. *Textbook of Pediatric Emergency Medicine,* 3rd ed. Baltimore, Md: Williams & Wilkins; 1993. Adapted with permission.

is stable and not a neurologic threat, or a patient can have no evidence of bony injury with a complete cervical cord transection. There is a subset of children (e.g., those with Down syndrome) whose underlying medical problems make them more susceptible to cervical cord injuries as a result of atlantoaxial instability, even following relatively trivial trauma. It is estimated that 3.8% of pediatric patients with multiple trauma have a spine and/or spinal cord injury.[3] Many, if not most, patients with spinal column injuries present without overt neurologic deficits. In several studies, most patients with spinal injuries had evidence of concurrent head injury.

Neurologic damage from spinal injuries can be caused by many different anatomic problems. The spinal canal might be impinged on by fracture fragments, blood, or a herniated disk. The spinal cord can be compromised directly by edema, hypoperfusion, contusion, laceration, or transection. The effects of a head injury can make diagnosis of concurrent spine injury difficult if not impossible in the early stages of evaluation. Although spinal injury must always be assumed, it is helpful when possible to distinguish between neurologic deficits that result from brain trauma and those that result from spinal cord trauma. Brain-injured patients often have diffuse or regional deficits (one side of the body) and intact bulbocavernosus and anal reflexes, whereas patients with spinal cord injuries often present with neurologic deficits in a myotome distribution, neuromotor disparity between arms and legs, flaccidity, absent reflexes, and loss of sphincter tone (spinal shock).

### Immobilization

If a protective helmet is still in place following a sports-related injury, this should be removed slowly and carefully, with lateral expansion of the helmet, rotation of the helmet to clear the occiput, neck support, and stabilization during the removal process. A second rescuer should be available to maintain immobilization from below during this maneuver, using pressure on the jaw and occiput. Following helmet removal, inline immobilization is reestablished from above.[18]

For acute transfer, soft cervical collars offer no protection for an unstable spine, and semirigid collars alone might still allow flexion, extension, and lateral movement of the cervical spine. Ideal immobilization for transport includes a semi-rigid cervical collar (e.g., Stifneck) in conjunction with a full spine board and soft spacing devices between the head and securing straps. For more information on C-spine immobilization see Chapter 22, Critical Procedures.

The child's head is disproportionately large compared with an adult's head. Fifty percent of the postnatal head circumferential growth occurs by age 18 months, whereas 50% of the postnatal growth of the chest does not occur until age 8 years. The disparate growth of the head and trunk results in neck flexion into a position of relative kyphosis when a child is placed on a hard surface.[19] Recommendations include using a spine board with a recess in the head area to accommodate a child's large occiput, or placing a 1-inch blanket under the torso to allow the neck to rest in a neutral position.[20] Cervical spine alignment can be greatly improved by these techniques, with avoidance of inadvertent flexion and anterior displacement of a potentially unstable spine. These amendments to spinal immobilization can be discontinued for patients 8 years or older, in whom cervical spine and body proportions approximate those of an adult.

Inline manual neck immobilization (performed by a caretaker whose sole responsibility is to ensure there is no neck motion) is used to assist with airway maneuvers. Care should be taken to avoid traction (ie, pulling) on the cervical spine to prevent longitudinal stress and secondary cord injury.

## Management

Orotracheal intubation with manual inline cervical stabilization is the preferred method of airway control in children with suspected or proven spine injury. A surgical airway or fiberoptic-assisted intubation performed by skilled personnel can be considered in patients with unstable spinal injury.

A study by Bracken et al suggests that methylprednisolone in a dose of 30 mg/kg over 15 minutes, followed by infusion of 5 to 6 mg/kg per hour for 23 hours, begun within 8 hours after acute spinal cord injury (ASCI), improves functional outcome in some patients.[21,22] Although these studies specifically excluded children younger than 13 years, the poor functional outcome of patients with documented spinal cord injury has led many experts to recommend use of this still controversial protocol in children and adults. Alternatively, Prendergast et al found that methylprednisolone therapy for penetrating ASCI might impair recovery of neurologic function.[23] Short's evidence evaluation of all clinical studies determined that high-dose methylprednisolone use in ASCI cannot be justified.[24]

## Clinical Features

Many clues can aid in the diagnosis of a spinal cord injury (Table 9-13).[25,26] The signs and symptoms can be obvious or masked by other abnormalities, such as altered level of consciousness resulting from hypovolemic shock, a concurrent head injury, or the ingestion of alcohol, drugs, or toxic substances. Head and spinal cord injuries can present with overlapping abnormal neurologic signs, and differentiation of causation can be difficult. A complete history is imperative to assess whether abnormal neurologic function, such as paresthesias, paralysis, or paresis, was present at any time after injury. These symptoms might have been transient and might not be present at the time of examination or volunteered by the patient during the history taking, but still suggest an underlying spinal cord injury. The physical examination should include assessment of the patient for neck or paraspinal back tenderness, pain, limitation of motion, and muscle spasm, as well as for neurologic signs, particularly those of neurogenic shock (i.e., hypotension, bradycardia, peripheral flush) and spinal shock (i.e., flaccidity, areflexia, loss of anal sphincter control).

A catastrophic cervical spinal cord injury should be strongly suspected in any child who has sustained cardiac arrest shortly after trauma. Following successful CPR, vigorous isotonic crystalloid resuscitation and pressor support might be needed. A careful assessment of the cervical spine will address three issues: fracture identification, determination of subluxation/malalignment, and suspicion of ligamentous laxity. In the acute setting, begin with a lateral cervical spine film and a CT scan of the cervical spine. Spinal cord injury without radiographic abnormality is more common in children, and an MRI of the cervical spine might also be needed.[27] If in doubt, prolonged immobilization is essential until an injury is unequivocally recognized or ruled out, and might be needed for a week or longer.

## Diagnostic Studies

### Pediatric Versus Adult Anatomy

The anatomy and evaluation of the pediatric spine differ in many ways from those of the adult spine. The fulcrum of the cervical spine of an infant is at approximately C2-3. By 5 to 6 years of age it is located at C3-4, and by age 8 it is at the same level as adults at C5-6. This is in part the result of the relatively large head size of a child compared with that of an adult. The higher fulcrum of a child's spine, along with relatively weak neck muscles and poor protective reflexes, accounts for fractures in younger children that involve the upper cervical spine. Older children and adults have fractures that more often involve the lower cervical spine.

The large amount of cartilage in the pediatric spine can cushion forces distributed to the spine and make radiographic evaluation challenging. The radiolucent nature of cartilage mandates the ability to evaluate and appreciate soft tissue abnormalities on the radiograph. The pediatric cervical spine appears to have more anterior and posterior movement than its adult counterpart, due not only to the radiolucent cartilage but also to ligamentous laxity and relatively horizontal facet joints. These differences in part account for the anterior pseudosubluxation (physiologic subluxation) that can be seen between C2-3 and C3-4 up to the age of 16 years. These factors also allow the apparent predental space (between the dens and anterior ring of C1) to

be increased to a maximum of 5 mm (adult maximum is 3 mm). Moreover, cartilaginous growth centers (synchondroses) can look like fractures to the untrained eye.

The pediatric cervical spine also has the ability to revert to a relatively normal appearance after a significant distortion, which can hinder the radiographic search for abnormalities. Neurologic symptoms from spinal cord compression, including compression by epidural hematomas, can be slower to manifest in a young child than in an adult due to increased room around the spinal cord within the spinal column in a young child.

### Plain Radiography, Computed Tomography, and Magnetic Resonance Imaging

Radiographic evaluation of the cervical spine is an essential step in the assessment. Options include plain radiography, computed tomography (CT), and magnetic resonance imaging (MRI). The CT scan demonstrates fractures quite clearly. A CT scan often is used as a secondary screen when adequate plain radiographs cannot be obtained or to confirm suspected fractures. A CT scan provides good soft tissue detail and allows for the possibility of reconstruction images but does not provide the intrathecal, ligamentous, disk, or vascular detail that can be obtained with MRI. MRI scans are more appropriate for evaluation of the subacute or chronic stages of injury or an acute problem with cord impingement by blood or soft tissues. MRI does not image cortical bone as well as other modalities and should not be used to evaluate the cervical spine for fractures.

The plain radiograph remains the initial test of choice in the acutely traumatized patient. Several authors have attempted to devise criteria to limit the number of patients who receive cervical spine radiographs. The perception of unnecessary tests must be balanced against the severity of consequences that can occur with a missed cervical spine injury. The literature suggests that if the patient does not have a high-risk mechanism of injury (e.g., motor vehicle crash, sports injury, fall, dive, or penetrating neck injury), is awake and alert, is not under the influence of drugs or alcohol, is age appropriate, does not complain of cervical spine pain, has no tenderness or muscle spasm on palpation (especially in the midline), has normal neck mobility without limitation of motion, has a completely normal neurologic examination without history of abnormal neurologic signs or symptoms at any time after the injury, and has no painful distracting injuries that can mask neck pain, the cervical spine can be clinically cleared.

In a substudy of the National Emergency X-Radiology Utilization Study (NEXUS), 3,065 children younger than 18 years were evaluated for cervical spine injury. Only 30 (0.98%) patients had a cervical spine injury. These investigators showed that five criteria (midline cervical tenderness, altered level of alertness, evidence of intoxication, neurologic abnormality, tenderness and distracting injury) had a sensitivity of 100% (CI 87.8% to 100%), a specificity of 19.9%, and a negative predictive value of 100% (CI 99.2% to 100%) in identification of children who required spinal radiographs. Only 88 (3%) patients were younger than 2 years, and none had cervical spine injury, so caution must be used in translating these criteria for cervical spine immobilization to this age group.[28]

When radiographs are obtained, a normal lateral radiograph does not clear the cervical spine but allows assessment of gross malalignment or distraction. The sensitivity of a single lateral cervical spine radiograph for fracture has been reported to vary between 82% and 98%.

A lateral cervical spine radiograph should include C1-7 and the C-7/T-1 junction. Additional films, including an anteroposterior (AP) view of C3-7 and an open-mouth view (AP) of C1-2 (odontoid view) in the age-appropriate child, will increase the sensitivity of the initial radiographic evaluation to greater than 95%. If at any point during the radiographic evaluation a fracture is identified, further plain radiographs often are not necessary. CT at that point might be more useful in delineating the extent of the injury. An algorithm for considering radiographic evaluation is presented in Figure 9.18.

The cervical spine has anterior (vertebral bodies, intervertebral disks, ligaments) and posterior (lamina, pedicles, neural foramen,

facet joints, spinous processes, ligaments) elements. The initial three-view series can provide a good evaluation of the anterior cervical spine, but it is not ideal for evaluation of the posterior cervical spine. Oblique (pillar) views are helpful to evaluate the posterior elements. Flexion and extension films for assessment of ligamentous stability can be obtained in an awake patient by having the patient flex and extend the neck as far as able without discomfort. These films can be inadequate because the neck muscles have splinted the cervical column in a position of comfort or stability and subsequent alignment will not change with flexion or extension. If questions remain concerning the integrity of the cervical spine after obtaining these radiographs, CT should be considered. Radiographic tomograms also can be performed but require patient movement, are time-consuming, and are not easily performed on an acutely ill patient.

**Evaluation of Radiographs**

When evaluating radiographs of the cervical spine, use a systematic approach. The ABCs (alignment, bones, cartilage, soft tissues) method of evaluating the lateral cervical radiograph is useful. Alignment is assessed, as demonstrated in Figure 9.19. The spinal cord lies between the posterior spinal line and the spinolaminal line. The usual lordotic curve of these lines might not be present in children younger than 6 years, in those on hard spine boards (the large occiput forces the neck in a flexed direction), with cervical collars, or with cervical neck muscle spasm. As mentioned, pseudo subluxation or physiologic subluxation can be seen in the upper cervical spine until the age of 16. Gross abnormalities should be detectable through assessment of alignment (Figure 9.20).

When evaluating the bones, look for typical abnormalities, which can be subtle. Compression fractures are suggested by differences in the heights of adjacent vertebral bodies. Structures including the skull, teeth, and the cartilage growth centers can simulate fractures (Table 9-14).

Assess cartilage after bone. Cartilage is radiolucent on plain radiographs. Pediatric spinal columns contain a large amount of car-

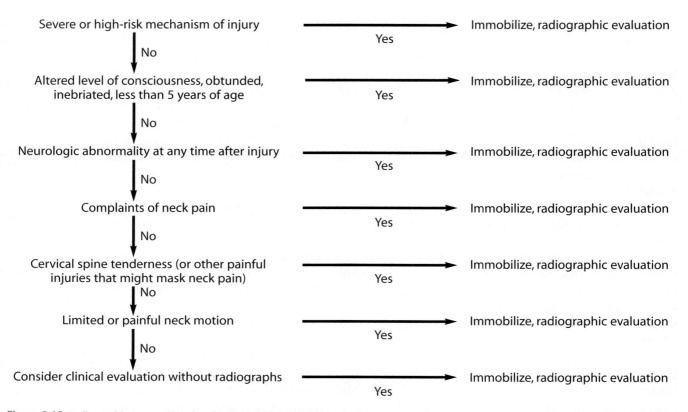

Figure 9.18 Radiographic versus clinical evaluation of the cervical spine in the traumatized patient.
Source: Woodward G. Neck trauma. In: Fleisher GR, Ludwig S, ed. *Textbook of Pediatric Emergency Medicine*. 3rd ed. Baltimore, Md: Williams & Wilkins' 1993. Reprinted with permission.

tilage, which can make radiographic evaluation challenging. Cartilaginous areas include the synchondroses, or growth plates, and intervertebral disk spaces. The growth plates can mimic fractures and be confusing to the uninitiated. Growth plates can be differentiated from fractures by their location and regular, smooth, sharp borders compared with the irregular appearance and often different locations of fractures. Growth centers in the anterior-superior vertebral bodies cause a sloped appearance that can look like anterior compression fractures to the untrained eye. The vertebral disk space also should be evaluated because abnormalities can suggest specific mechanisms of injury. A vertebral disk space that is narrowed anteriorly can indicate disk extrusion from compression, whereas a widened space suggests a hyperextension injury with posterior ligamentous disruption.

Evaluation of soft tissue is extremely important. Abnormal soft tissue spaces might be the only clue to an underlying ligament, cartilage, or subtle bone injury, that is not overt on a plain radiograph. Soft tissue thickening can represent blood or edema, which suggests an underlying injury. A rule of thumb is that the prevertebral (retropharyngeal) space at C3 should be less than two thirds the anteroposterior width of the adjacent vertebral body. This space will approximately double below C4 (the level of the glottis) because the usually nonair-filled esophagus is included in this area. Crying, neck flexion, or the expiratory phase of respiration can produce a pseudothickening in the prevertebral space. Soft tissue abnormality should be reproducible on repeated radiographs if there is an underlying injury.

Multiple types of neck injury can be seen in the child, ranging from minor muscular strains with torticollis to stable bony injuries

**Radiographic Features Suggestive of Cervical Spine Injury/Fractures**

- Loss of normal lordosis
- Vertebral disk space narrowed anteriorly (disk extrusion from compression) or widened (hyperextension injury with posterior ligamentous disruption)
- Prevertebral (retropharyngeal) space at C3, less than two thirds the anteroposterior width of the adjacent vertebral body
- Lateral mass offset by greater than 1 mm (Jefferson's fracture)
- Spondylolisthesis of C2 (Hangman fracture)
- Widened predental space (greater than 5 mm)
- Increased space between the occiput and C1 and/or widened predental space (atlantoaxial dislocation)
- Widening of an intervertebral disk space (distraction injury)
- Odontoid view shows one lateral mass of C1 forward and closer to the midline while the other lateral mass appears narrow and away from the midline (rotatory subluxation)

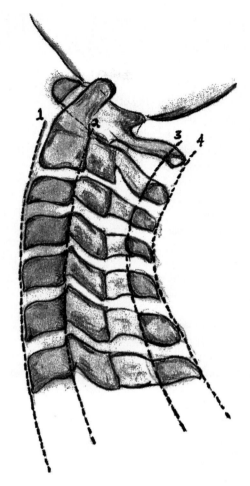

**Figure 9.19** Lordotic curves seen with normal cervical spine alignment 1-4.

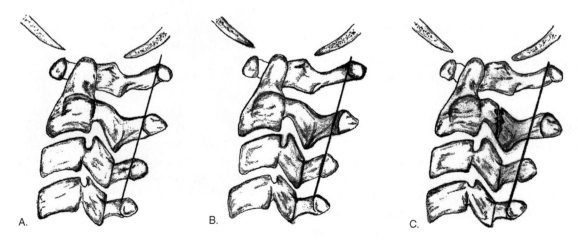

**Figure 9.20** Distinguish true subluxation from pseudosubluxation of the cervical spine. 9.20A Line is drawn from the anterior cortical margin of the spinous process of C1 through the anterior cortical margin of the spinous process of C3; in normal patients without true subluxation the line passes through the anterior cortical margin of the spinous process of C2 or within 1 mm of it. 9-22B Shows psudosubluxation as the line drawn passes through the anterior cortical margin of the spinous process of C2 even though the body of the C2 vertebrae is forward on C3. 9.22 C Shows true subluxation of C2 on C3 and the line drawn does not pass through the aterior cortical margin of C2.

| TABLE 9-14 | Radiographic Characteristics of the Pediatric Cervical Spine |
|---|---|

- Cartilage artifact
  - Tapered anterior vertebrae
  - Apparently absent anterior ring of C1
  - Atlas (C1) body not ossified at birth and might fail to close
  - Axis (C2) four ossification centers
  - Apex of odontoid ossifies between ages of 12 and 15 years
  - Spinous process ossification centers
- Increased mobility
  - Pseudosubluxation
  - C1 override on dens
  - Increased predental space (5 mm maximum)
  - Ligament laxity
  - Facet joints shallow
- Growth plates (synchondrosis)
  - Dens ossifies between ages of 3 and 8 years (can persist into adulthood)
  - Posterior arch of C1 ossifies at age 3 years
  - Anterior arch of C1 ossifies at age 6 to 9 years
- C1 internal diameter reaches adult size at age 3 to 4 years
- C2 through C7 internal diameter reaches adult size at age 5 to 6 years
- Lack of cervical lordosis
- Fulcrum varies with age (see text)
- Soft tissue variability with respiration
- Congenital clefts or other bony abnormalities (os odontoideum), spondylolisthesis, spina bifida, ossiculum terminale
- Rare compression fractures
- Approaches adult characteristics by age 8 years

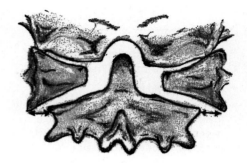

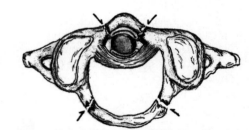

**Figure 9.21A** Jefferson fracture, offset of lateral mass of C1 greater than 1 mm indicating possible fracture.

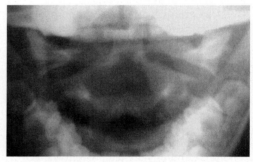

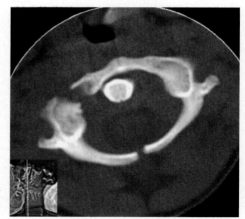

**Figure 9.21B** Jefferson fracture, cross-section demonstrating multiple fracture sites.

to unstable cervical injuries with and without neurologic damage. Five percent or more of patients with a cervical spine injury will have an additional spinal injury at another level, and these injuries should be actively sought.

## Specific Injuries

### Jefferson Fracture

The Jefferson fracture is a bursting fracture of the ring of C1 secondary to an axial load (Figure 9.21A and Figure 9.21B). Although the fracture can be unstable, neurologic impairment often is not present initially since the fracture fragments splay outward and do not physically impinge on the spinal cord. The fracture usually is seen best on the open-mouth odontoid view; the radiographic criterion for diagnosis of a Jefferson fracture is lateral offset of the lateral mass of C1 of greater than 1 mm from the vertebral body of C2. Neck rotation can produce a false-positive result.

Approximately one third of Jefferson fractures are associated with other fractures, most

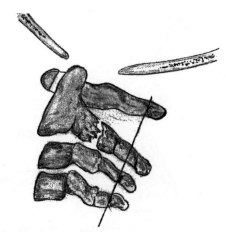

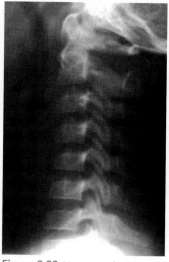

**Figure 9.22** Hangman fracture.

curs as a result of hyperextension that fractures the posterior elements of C2. Hyperflexion after the hyperextension leads to anterior subluxation of C2 on C3 and subsequent cervical cord damage. The subluxation seen with a hangman fracture can sometimes be mistaken for the pseudosubluxation or physiologic subluxation seen in the C2-3 or C3-4 region in approximately 25% of children younger than 8 years, which can occur up to the age of 16 years. Distinguishing between a subtle hangman fracture and pseudosubluxation can be accomplished using the posterior cervical line of Swischuk, depicted in Figure 9.20. A value of greater than 1.5 to 2 mm indicates an occult hangman fracture as the source of the anterior subluxation of C2 on C3. This line should be used only for evaluation of anterior subluxation of C2 on C3.

### Atlantoaxial Subluxation

Atlantoaxial subluxation is the result of movement between C1 and C2 secondary to transverse ligament rupture or a fractured dens (Figure 9.23A, Figure 9.23B, and Figure 9.23C). Ligament instability precipitated by tonsillitis, cervical adenitis, pharyngitis, arthritis, connective tissue disorders, or Down syndrome can allow minor trauma to result in ligamentous damage. Subluxation due to transverse ligament disruption will be evidenced by a widened predental (preodontoid) space on a lateral radiograph. Normal predental measurement in children is less than 5 mm compared with less than 3 mm in adults. Steel's rule of three states that the area within the ring of C1 is composed of one third odontoid, one third spinal cord, and one third connective tissue. Space therefore is available for limited dens movement or predental space widening without neurologic compromise. Neurologic symptoms often are not seen until the predental space exceeds 7 to 10 mm. Dens fractures cause atlantoaxial subluxation more often than ligamentous disruption in a young child because the weakest part of the child's musculoskeletal system is the osseous component. These fractures are seen in young infants secondary to a rapid deceleration while in improperly positioned forward-facing car seats.

often involving C2. The pseudo-Jefferson fracture of childhood is present in 90% of children at the age of 2 and usually normalizes by 4 to 6 years. The pseudo-Jefferson fracture has the radiographic appearance of a Jefferson fracture due to increased growth of the atlas (C1) compared with the axis (C2) and radiolucent cartilage artifact. If a Jefferson fracture is suspected in a child younger than 4 years, a CT scan is usually needed to further elucidate the injury. The CT scan is quite helpful in the evaluation of suspected injuries in the C1-2 area. Odontoid views are difficult to obtain in children younger than 3 years, because they are unable to cooperate with the open-mouth view.

### Hangman Fracture

The hangman fracture is a traumatic spondylolisthesis of C2 (Figure 9.22). This injury oc-

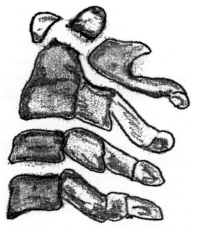

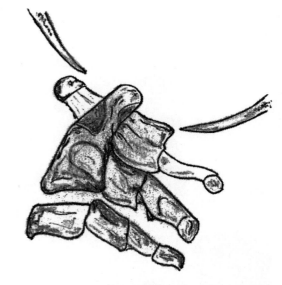

**Figure 9.23B** Widened predental space secondary to transverse ligament rupture.

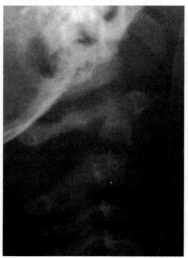

**Figure 9.23A** Dens fracture.

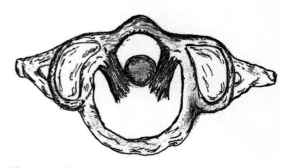

**Figure 9.23C** Transverse ligament rupture.

### Distraction Injury

Distraction injuries result from a longitudinal stress to the cervical column. The most dangerous of these is occipito-atlantal dissociation. These injuries can contribute to a significant percentage of deaths in pediatric acute trauma. Although severe distraction injuries are incompatible with long-term survival, initial CPR might be possible. These injuries can be obvious or subtle on the lateral radiograph. Increased space between the occiput and C1 or widening of an intervertebral disk space without an obvious adjacent compression fracture indicates the possibility of a distraction injury. Distraction injuries also can be seen with difficult newborn deliveries. The spinal cord, however, can distract only one fourth of an inch before there is permanent neurologic damage. An MRI scan is useful in assessing an infant or other stable patient with diminished motor activity who is suspected of having a distraction injury.

### Rotary Subluxation

Rotary subluxation is a cervical spine injury that often is missed or undiagnosed due to difficulty in interpreting the radiographs. Rotary subluxation or displacement can follow minor or major trauma or be spontaneous. These patients rarely present with abnormal neurologic findings. They present in the typical (cock-robin) position, with muscle spasm of the sternocleidomastoid muscle on the same side to which the chin points. In contrast, in patients with muscular torticollis, the chin points to the side opposite that involved. This is logical considering that the action of the sternocleidomastoid is an attempt to reestablish normal neck position.

The CT scan appears to be the most useful diagnostic tool in rotary subluxation. Patients with mild rotary subluxation should be treated with a cervical collar and analgesia for comfort; those with moderate rotary displacement need immobilization and occasionally traction. If there is anterior displacement of C2 on C1, a longer period of immobilization might be necessary to allow injured ligaments to heal.

### Spinal Epidural Hematoma

Spinal epidural hematomas also are seen in the pediatric population. These are venous bleeds that compress the adjacent spinal cord and present with ascending neurologic symptoms hours or days after often apparently minor trauma. An MRI scan is helpful in the evaluation of these patients. Rapid evaluation and surgical decompression are mandatory to prevent further neurologic compromise.

### SCIWORA

SCIWORA occurs mainly in children younger than 8 years who present with or develop symptoms consistent with cervical cord injuries, without radiographic or tomographic evidence of bone abnormality. In children, much of the strength of the spinal column is derived from cartilage and ligaments, although the ligaments are not as strong as in adults. This difference in tensile strength increases the potential for isolated ligamentous injury.[27,29] There is a subset of patients who have initial transient neurologic symptoms, who apparently recover and then return an average of 1 day later with significant neurologic abnormalities. For this reason, many recommend hospitalization and immobilization for young patients who have experienced transient neurologic symptoms.

## Chest Injuries

Blunt thoracic trauma is commonly encountered in children and can cause injuries that require immediate attention to establish adequate ventilation. A child's chest wall is very compliant and allows energy transfer to the intrathoracic structures, frequently without evidence of injury to the external chest wall. The elasticity of the chest wall increases the likelihood of pulmonary contusions and direct intrapulmonary hemorrhage, usually without overlying rib fractures. Significant thoracic injuries rarely occur alone and usually are a component of major multisystem injury. Analysis of the NPTR indicates that mortality from chest injury diagnoses is exceeded only by mortality from CNS injury. In the majority of cases, these two organ systems are both injured, producing an extraordinarily morbid synergy.

### Specific Injuries and Management

Children with pulmonary contusion can initially manifest few physical findings. Early radiographs might show minimal changes that can be confused with evidence of aspiration, which very commonly occurs in children with multisystem injury. A child receiving bag-mask ventilation might accumulate air in the stomach. As the airway is further manipulated, the likelihood of acute gastric dilation associated with vomiting of gastric acid and stomach contents is increasingly likely. Thus, every child with a significant mechanism of injury should be assumed to be at risk of aspiration at the moment of injury and during initial management.

Children with any possibility of pulmonary injury require careful monitoring and serial evaluations of ventilation and oxygenation. For the child on mechanical ventilatory support, this will be manifested by desaturation and increasing peak inspiratory pressures or rising $Pco_2$. Children who are not intubated will develop increasing tachycardia, rales, hemoptysis, and a falling $Sao_2$. Early recognition is critical for effective therapy. Once a child with pulmonary contusion and/or potential aspiration deteriorates to a point that mechanical ventilation is required, a prolonged ventilator course, nosocomial pneumonia, and possibly acute respiratory distress syndrome become increasingly likely. Close attention to detail during initial assessment has a significant role in avoiding what could be a catastrophic synergy of concurrent central nervous system and pulmonary failure.

Pneumothorax can occur with blunt or penetrating trauma and consists of air in the pleural space from lung, tracheobronchial or penetrating injury. Minimal collections of air in the pleural space might be undetected on examination and are seen best on an expiratory chest radiograph or CT scan, although a small air collection can be obscured if a plain radiograph is taken with the patient in the supine position.

Collapse of one lung can produce signs of hypoxia, hyperresonance to percussion, asymmetry of chest wall movement, and decreased breath sounds on the affected side. Treatment involves tube thoracostomy with underwater seal drainage. Bilateral pneumothoraces and tension pneumothorax are life-threatening injuries. With bilateral pneumothoraces, the patient is hypoxic, has minimal or absent breath sounds bilaterally, and is typically hypotensive. A needle or an over-the-needle catheter device placed in the second intercostal space anteriorly or in the fourth to fifth intercostal space laterally in the axillary line (at the level of the nipple) can be lifesaving until chest tubes can be placed. Remember to administer oxygen to all patients who sustain significant blunt chest trauma.

An open pneumothorax can be sucking or not, depending on size and other factors. Fortunately, gunshot and stab wounds are infrequent in childhood, and open pneumothoraces usually occur as the result of extensive animal attack or misadventure with farm or industrial machinery. The presenting injury is usually very dramatic and associated with significant soft tissue loss that can actually mask the presence of the sucking chest wound. These children need immediate sedation and analgesia so that a thorough evaluation of the chest injury can be accomplished. Intrathoracic and atmospheric pressures will rapidly equilibrate; thus, if the opening is larger than the airway, ventilation becomes ineffective. Place an occlusive dressing (gauze impregnated with petroleum jelly) over the wound and tape it on three sides. Insert a chest tube immediately. If the patient exhibits sudden respiratory embarrassment after the closure, suspect tension pneumothorax; remove the dressing briefly to let any air under pressure escape until the chest tube is placed or repositioned.

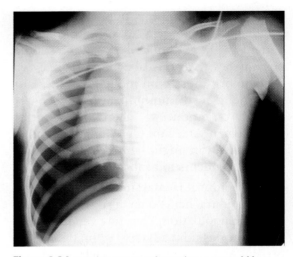

**Figure 9.24** Tension pneumothorax in a 4-year-old boy with blunt chest trauma.

Tension pneumothorax is commonly a lethal chest injury. It frequently develops after the patient's arrival in the hospital and can especially occur in ventilated patients who receive high inspiratory volumes under positive pressure to aerate injured lung parenchyma. The pathophysiology is that of sudden cardiorespiratory failure. The pleural pressure rises and the lung collapses. The mediastinum shifts and the opposite lung compresses. The superior vena cava kinks, leading to decreased venous return. The resulting decreased cardiac output is the immediate threat to life (Figure 9.24).

The diagnosis must be established by physical examination prompted by a high index of suspicion. Classically, the neck veins are distended and the trachea is deviated; however, these findings can not be apparent in a child with a short, fat neck or one who is wearing a cervical collar to immobilize the cervical spine. There are decreased breath sounds with tympany and hypotension. Immediate treatment is required to improve cardiac output, including needle thoracostomy to convert the tension pneumothorax to a simple pneumothorax, followed by placement of a thoracostomy tube. Needle thoracentesis can be performed within seconds and will provide several minutes of stability while a chest tube is inserted.

Traumatic hemothorax is treated with chest tube insertion and concomitant volume

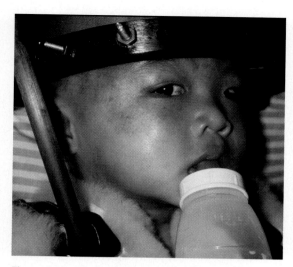

**Figure 9.25** Traumatic asphyxia in a child after being pinned against a garage door by a car. Note the petechiae and subconjunctival hemorrhages in the head and neck area.

replacement. If massive bleeding is noted, the chest tube should be clamped and the patient prepared for immediate thoracotomy. Continued bleeding following chest tube placement (greater than 2 to 4 mL/kg per hour) indicates major vascular injury and the need for open thoracotomy.

Traumatic asphyxia occurs with sudden massive compression of the chest. The pressure is transmitted to the heart, lungs, vena cava, neck, and head. Clinical signs include petechiae of the head and neck, subconjunctival hemorrhages, and occasional depressed level of consciousness (Figure 9.25). Hemoptysis, pulmonary contusion, and great vessel injury can be present. Upper abdominal injuries can also occur. Treatment consists of management of component injuries. Administer oxygen, place chest tubes as needed, limit fluids, and elevate the head of the bed. If PaO$_2$ falls, the use of positive end-expiratory pressure might be indicated.

Cardiac tamponade more commonly occurs as an iatrogenic injury after cardiac catheterization, postoperative open heart surgery, or placement of a central venous catheter. It also can occur with a penetrating or crush injury. Blood accumulates in the pericardial sac so the heart cannot fill during diastole, causing low cardiac output. The diagnostic triad includes shock (associated with narrowed pulse pressure), distended neck veins, and muffled heart sounds. Massive hepatomegaly can be present. Treatment consists of a large fluid bolus and pericardiocentesis. The aspiration of a small volume of fluid from the pericardial space can be lifesaving. If there is time, echocardiography can be helpful in confirming the diagnosis.

## Abdominal Injuries

The onset of symptoms of abdominal injury can be rapid due to massive hemorrhage, or more gradual from an organizing clot, or evolving bacterial or chemical peritonitis. Children with suspected abdominal injuries might need only careful observation, with judicious fluid and blood replacement. The decision to observe injuries of this type should be made only by the surgeon who will be responsible for emergency surgical intervention and perioperative care. If the abdominal injury results in significant blood loss that prevents successful restoration of hemodynamic normality after 40-mL/kg volume restoration, immediate surgical intervention might be necessary.

### Diagnostic Studies

Initially, the abdominal examination might fail to indicate significant pathology, so sequential reexamination is essential to rule out an evolving abdominal problem. Focused Assessment with Sonography for Trauma (FAST) is an excellent method to evaluate for intraperitoneal fluid. New technology has produced small portable devices that are becoming available in every emergency department. The examination in children is not intended to replace detailed studies performed in radiology departments, as up to one third of solid organ injuries in children are intraparenchymal. The FAST exam has one simple mission: the identification of fluid in the pericardium, subhepatic or perisplenic spaces, or the pelvis. The FAST exam can be done quickly and noninvasively on any trauma patient and can often demonstrate significant changes as fluid resuscitation proceeds.

Computed tomography, serial abdominal examination, and monitoring are used in chil-

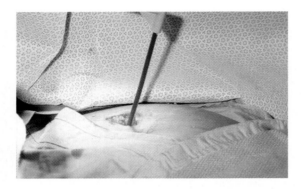

**Figure 9.26** Positive peritoneal lavage in a 16-year-old girl with a ruptured spleen.

dren more often than diagnostic peritoneal lavage (DPL). Even in centers in which radionuclide scanning, CT, and ultrasonography are used to evaluate the intra-abdominal contents, DPL still can occasionally be helpful in the child with a depressed level of consciousness and injuries requiring immediate surgical intervention on another organ system (Figure 9.26). This situation might include a child who requires urgent neurosurgical or orthopedic surgical care. Using DPL to determine abdominal injury is not appropriate in a lucid child who does not require immediate surgery.

## Management

Accurate assessment of abdominal injury remains one of the most challenging aspects of management of the injured child. Although it is rare that a child will require abdominal surgery from trauma, indications for surgery include hemodynamic instability despite maximal resuscitative efforts, a patient who requires transfusion of greater than 50% of total blood volume, radiographic evidence of pneumoperitoneum, intraperitoneal bladder rupture, grade V renovascular injury, gunshot wound to the abdomen, evisceration of intraperitoneal or stomach contents, signs of peritonitis, or evidence of fecal or bowel contamination on diagnostic peritoneal lavage (DPL). A DPL is rarely performed on children because even if frank blood is aspirated, a child would not require surgery unless he

or she becomes hemodynamically unstable after appropriate fluid resuscitation.

Less obvious injuries can emerge gradually as significant threats if not accurately and rapidly identified. These include such things as a small gastrointestinal perforation that stimulates a localized inflammatory process rather than general peritonitis, pancreatic contusion or ductular injury, urinoma, and obstructing duodenal hematoma. As stated earlier, the absence of external injury does not exclude internal derangement. Clinical suspicion and an understanding of the mechanism of injury are critically important. Management of the child with suspected abdominal injury must establish the presence of the injury, the need for surgical intervention, the priority of surgical intervention in relation to other lifesaving maneuvers, the expected natural history of the lesion, and objective findings that will confirm the expected natural history is, in fact, occurring. Only after these questions have been answered can a reasonable plan of management be instituted. The primary tools used to arrive at this therapeutic decision include thorough and repeated physical examinations, FAST examination, and abdominal CT. If time and treatment priority will allow, these should be accomplished in every child at risk within an hour of arrival in the ED.

---

### KEY POINTS

**Management of Abdominal Trauma: Indications for Surgery**

- Hemodynamic instability despite maximal resuscitative efforts
- Requires transfusion of greater than 50% of total blood volume
- Radiographic evidence of pneumoperitoneum
- Intraperitoneal bladder rupture
- Grade V renovascular injury
- Gunshot wound to the abdomen
- Evisceration of intraperitoneal or stomach contents
- Peritonitis—fecal or bowel contamination on DPL

## Liver and Spleen Injuries

The liver and spleen are organs commonly injured from blunt trauma in the child. These injuries can be sufficiently extensive to require immediate exploration, but recent experience indicates that they are frequently self-limited in children. This has stimulated the evolution of protocols in which stable children are managed expectantly with bed rest, frequent exams, serial hemoglobin determinations, monitoring, and surgical supervision. The option of immediate surgical intervention must be available at all times. The decision to treat nonoperatively is solely the responsibility of the surgeon and must be based on physical examination and evaluation.

Essentially, hepatic injuries fall into one of three categories. Those with massive disruption presenting with intractable bleeding are now treated with immediate damage control laparotomy intended to stop bleeding and pack injuries before exsanguination, hypocoagulation, and hypothermia lead to inevitable fatality. These children are then metabolically resuscitated in the PICU and returned to the operating room for further care under more controlled circumstances.

Children with evidence of intraperitoneal hemorrhage documented by CT to be hepatic in origin will usually have spontaneous healing of the organ. These injuries occasionally result in abscesses or hematobilia. As long as the child remains hemodynamically stable, no emergent surgical intervention is necessary. Between these two extremes are those children with significant hepatic disruption that require careful management of fluid volume and red cell mass. These are the patients at risk of sudden exsanguination, and they require scrupulous monitoring in a unit prepared for immediate surgical intervention if so indicated.

## Pancreatic/Duodenal Injuries

High-speed deceleration (such as ejection from a vehicle) or direct blows to the upper abdomen can produce pancreatic or duodenal trauma. The most commonly reported pancreatic lesions are fractures and severe contusions, usually in the midportion of the gland where it overlies the lumbar spine. This can present as relatively acute-onset peritonitis, or it can produce a posttraumatic pseudocyst that develops within days to weeks of injury. Duodenal injury can produce retroperitoneal leak as well as frank duodenal disruption. It should be considered in any child subjected to abuse. Intramural duodenal hematoma is a lesion frequently seen in children who sustain blunt abdominal trauma. It commonly causes signs and symptoms of upper intestinal obstruction. As with pancreatic injuries, a high index of suspicion is the key to expedient and accurate recognition.

## Intestinal Injuries

The intestine can be perforated by deceleration trauma. This is commonly associated with lap belt injuries, and can present with evidence of abdominal wall contusion associated with a lumbar vertebral blowout (Chance) fracture. Intestinal perforation can present immediately with the development of free air, notable on abdominal radiographs, or it can emerge with the evolution of bacterial peritonitis over a period of 12 to 24 hours.

Careful clinical evaluation for at least 24 hours is critical for accurate and timely diagnosis of these injuries in any child considered to be at risk. Because there is no absolutely reliable imaging modality for confirmation of this diagnosis, every child considered at risk for gastrointestinal injury must be monitored for at least 24 hours. Abdominal pain that worsens or persists beyond this period must be explained before the child can be cleared for release. This might require repeat CT with enteric contrast, laparoscopy, or laparotomy based on interpretation of physical findings. Such a progression of clinical evaluation obviously requires that the physician responsible for determination of the need for surgical intervention evaluate the child on arrival to establish the baseline to which subsequent examinations will be compared.

## Genitourinary Injuries

Because torso trauma is a common characteristic of pediatric injury, potential damage to the genitourinary (GU) system must be considered in the evaluation of every injured child.

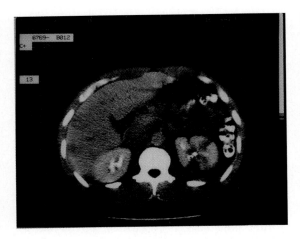

**Figure 9.27** CT scan of the abdomen showing a large left renal laceration with a urinoma. Although large, this laceration healed without surgical intervention.

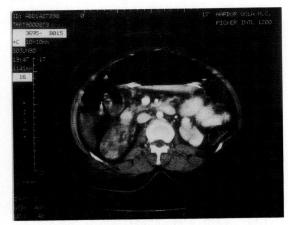

**Figure 9.28** CT scan of the abdomen showing a devascularized right kidney (left side of image) from blunt trauma to the abdomen. Immediate surgical intervention to revascularize the kidney is indicated.

Like hepatic and splenic injuries, most renal lesions will heal without surgical intervention (**Figure 9.27**). Those that require emergent surgery usually involve major renal pedicle disruptions with perinephric hematomas and complete loss of renal function (**Figure 9.28**).

The challenge facing the physician responsible for initial assessment and stabilization is the clinical determination of significant GU injury and the most efficacious method for evaluation of a potential injury. Because most renal injuries involve minor, self-limited contusions, extensive and expensive evaluations can be clinically irrelevant. The combination of significant flank trauma, abdominal injury, and hematuria (even microscopic) in an injured child is an indication for a CT scan with intra-venous contrast to assess bilateral function and absence of extravasation. Lower urinary tract disruption occurs primarily in association with severe pelvic trauma, the prototype of which is the straddle (bicycle) injury. A child who has blood at the urethral meatus requires retrograde urethrography to determine whether a lower urinary tract injury is present. Potential bladder injuries should be assessed with a CT cystogram or formal cystogram following urethrogram.

## Burns

According to the Burn Foundation, an estimated 250,000 children suffer burn-related injuries annually (www.burnfoundation.org/content/view/93/102). Scald injuries are more commonly seen in young children and can be a result of intentional injury. Flame-related injuries more often occur in older children, including those playing with lighters or matches or stoking fires with flammable liquids.

Thermal injuries can be stratified as first, second, third, or fourth degree, or, more preferably, as partial-thickness and full-thickness. First-degree burns (e.g., sunburn) are characterized by erythema and pain with no loss of epidermal integrity. Although first-degree burns generally do not require intravenous fluid replacement, the presence of extensive body surface sunburn in an infant or toddler might require hospitalization for fluid replacement.

## YOUR FIRST CLUE

**Identification of Burn Severity**

- First-degree burn: erythema; pain; no loss of epidermal integrity
- Second-degree or partial-thickness burn: red or mottled appearance; blister formation; moist, weeping appearance
- Third-degree or full-thickness burn: dark, leathery, mottled or white; if surface is red, will not blanch with pressure
- Fourth-degree burn: common with high-voltage electrical injuries; involve destruction of tissues deep to the skin

Second-degree or partial-thickness burns are characterized by a red or mottled appearance. They are recognized by blister formation or a moist, weeping appearance if the epidermis has already sloughed. Because both first-degree and second-degree burns involve partial-thickness destruction, they are painful, especially when exposed to air.

Third-degree or full-thickness burns are dark and leathery, mottled or white and waxy. If the surface is red, it will not blanch with pressure. These full-thickness burns are insensate and dry. Fourth-degree burns are rare and are most common with high-voltage electrical injuries. These burns involve tissues deep into the skin.

Burn depth determines whether epithelialization will occur. Partial-thickness burns are capable of healing, but deep partial-thickness burns can take up to 6 weeks to heal and are more inclined to form hypertrophic scars. Determining burn depth can be difficult, even for experienced burn care providers. Burns that appear shallow immediately following injury can ultimately prove to be deeper. Burns that tend to convert to deeper injuries include scald burns, grease burns, and burns that become infected.[30]

Partial-thickness burns heal through the regeneration of the epidermis by the epidermal appendages (hair follicles, sweat glands). Superficial partial-thickness burns do not require grafting, but might benefit from the placement of biologic dressings (e.g., TransCyte).[31,32] Healing is often complete in 2 weeks or less. Deep partial-thickness burns will take more than 2 weeks to heal and generally benefit from the placement of either biologic dressings or skin grafting. Full-thickness injuries will not regenerate because the epidermal appendages are destroyed. Skin grafting is required unless the injury is minor.

Temperature and duration of contact determine the depth of tissue injury. This is demonstrated best in scald injuries. At 44°C (111°F), cellular destruction will not occur for about 6 hours of contact in adults and older children. A typical setting in the United States for a hot water heater is 140° to 150°F (60° to 65°C), and water at this temperature will pro-

duce a full-thickness burn in as little as 2 to 5 seconds. Lowering the temperature to 130°F (54.4°C) will prolong exposure time to 30 seconds to produce a full-thickness burn, and lowering it further to 120°F (48.8°C) prolongs this time to 5 minutes.[33]

Different types of thermal exposure have different effects. Flash injuries dissipate a large amount of heat for a short duration: they usually are partial-thickness burns. Flame burns can produce high temperature with prolonged contact and are associated with the highest risk of serious full-thickness injury. Contact burns from hot metal including radiators, floor heating grates, oven racks, and irons often produce full-thickness burns with a cutaneous pattern corresponding to the agent of injury.

Smoke inhalation, carbon monoxide poisoning, and airway edema with respiratory compromise are the most common causes of early death after a burn injury. After the first few hours, shock is usually the most common cause of death. Burns involving more than 30% of the body surface area result in a generalized increased capillary permeability. The extravasation of large amounts of fluid into the extravascular space results in hypovolemia, hypoperfusion, and diffuse peripheral edema that affects both burned and unburned tissues. Thermal effects can also result in the destruction of red blood cells. Electrical injuries, burns associated with soft tissue trauma, and those associated with prolonged immobilization of the victim can involve extensive destruction of muscle tissues and threat of myoglobinuria. Gastrointestinal ileus can complicate burns involving a large body surface area.

## Diagnostic Studies

### Laboratory

Children suspected of suffering an inhalation injury should have arterial blood gases and carboxyhemoglobin level measured. A carboxyhemoglobin level in excess of 10 mg % is consistent with a significant inhalation injury. Indications for intubation include persistent or worsening respiratory distress, a $PaO_2$ less than 60 mm Hg or a $PaCO_2$ greater than 50 mm Hg in the face of optimal conservative management.

### Radiology

Children suspected of inhalation injury should have an initial chest radiograph, although this will usually be normal in the first few hours following injury. If the child was also a victim of a car crash, jumped from a burning building, or was involved in an explosion, there is a chance of coexisting multiple injuries; additional screening radiographs might be indicated to rule out specific injuries.

## Management

The upper airway is susceptible to obstruction as a result of exposure to superheated air. Except in severe cases, the subglottic airway is usually protected from direct thermal injury by the larynx. Facial burns, singed nasal hairs and eyebrows, carbonaceous deposits in the oral pharynx and/or carbonaceous sputum, oropharyngeal edema, history of impaired mentation and/or confinement in a closed, burning environment, and voice change, hoarseness, or persistent coughing can indicate inhalation injury or burns.[34]

Initial signs can be subtle. However, progressive airway edema can occur with fluid resuscitation, requiring ongoing evaluation. The small diameter of an infant's and child's airway requires ongoing vigilance and lowers the threshold for intubation. Oxygen should be administered via nonrebreather mask for any suspected inhalation injury and to treat carbon monoxide inhalation.

Estimating burn depth is classified as previously described by degree, or by partial or full thickness. First-degree burns are not included in standard resuscitation formulas. The Lund and Browder chart divides the body surface into areas by percentage. In adults, the "Rule of Nines" is an easy way to determine body surface area. However, this formula is modified in children because of the disproportionate size of the child's head and neck relative to lower extremities. The Lund and Browder chart is typically used for children 10 years old and younger. The palm of the patient's hand (including the fingers) represents approximately 1% of the child's body surface.

The Parkland formula is the most common method of determining fluid resuscitation following a burn. It is intended only as a guide to initiate fluid resuscitation. Continued fluid requirements are dictated by the physiologic status of the patient. Using this formula, the patient receives 2 to 4 mL of lactated Ringer's solution per percentage of burn multiplied by the child's weight in kilograms. The Parkland formula does not include maintenance fluid requirements in a child, so these must be added. Half of the combined resuscitation and maintenance fluid is administered over the first 8 hours, with the remainder given over the next 16 hours. Colloid and blood are not routinely given in the first 24 hours following a burn, but in severe burns the judicious use of albumin might be worthwhile. A dose of 1g/kg can be administered as a bolus over 30 to 90 minutes.

Nasogastric tubes are indicated in patients with burns involving more than 25% of total body surface area. In burns less than 25% total body surface area, a nasogastric tube should be inserted if the child experiences nausea, vomiting, or abdominal distention. If possible, nasogastric or nasojejunal tube feeding should be initiated once the child has stabilized within hours of admission.

Children with burns exceeding 15% of estimated body surface area require intravenous fluid resuscitation. Intravenous lines should be established peripherally, preferably in an unburned upper extremity. If the burns are extensive, the catheter can be placed in any accessible vein. Burn victims are more prone to phlebitis and septic phlebitis in saphenous veins. Fluid replacement is based on an accurate body weight, and the child should be weighed without dressings or clothing as soon as feasible.

Consideration should be given to insertion of a Foley catheter if fluid resuscitation is needed. In thermal, scald, or contact burns, a urine output of 1 to 2 mL/kg per hour is desired, up to a maximum of 30 to 40 mL per hour. If a patient suffers an electrical burn, a urine output of twice that goal is desired because of the increased incidence of myoglobinuria and subsequent renal failure. Resuscitation fluids can be titrated up or down, depending on the ongoing physiologic status of the patient and the adequacy of urine output. If urine output becomes excessive, the rate of fluid infusion should be decreased.

### Initial Burn Wound Care

The first principle in burn wound management is to "stop the fire." All clothing should be removed in the resuscitation area. Some synthetic fabrics can melt into hot plastic residue and continue to burn the patient. Since undue exposure can result in hypothermia, heat lamps should be employed over the patient to maintain optimal temperature. Rings and jewelry should be removed and retained to give to the child's family.

History taking must elicit information and details regarding the circumstances of the injury, specifically where it occurred and whether the victim was using alcohol or drugs at the time. Two historical points that are especially relevant are whether the victim was inside or outside a building, and whether potential additional injury might have occurred as a result of attempts at escape or rescue. Illnesses, medications, allergies, and immunization status are also critical factors that can influence initial care.

The wound should be cleansed with saline. Blisters should be left intact, as they serve as a biologic sterile dressing. Dead skin can be debrided with moist gauze or surgical instruments.

Analgesia and sedation can be administered after resuscitation is begun. Large wounds might require large doses of narcotics to comfort the patient. Initial dosing should be in small increments with careful monitoring of

| TABLE 9-15 | Commonly Used Sedatives and Analgesics for Burn Patients |
|---|---|
| **Drug** | **Dosage** |
| Fentanyl | 1–5 mcg/kg IV |
| Morphine | 0.1–0.2 mg/kg IV/IM |
| Midazolam (Versed) | 0.05–0.2 mg/kg IV/IM |
| Lorazepam (Ativan) | 0.1 mg/kg IV |
| Chloral hydrate | 50–100 mg/kg/dose PO/PR |
| Ketamine | 1–2 mg/kg/dose IV |
| | 3–5 mg/kg IM |

heart rate, respiration, and blood pressure. Guidelines are presented in Table 9-15.

### Circumferential Full-Thickness Burns

Extremities can be burned circumferentially. With fluid resuscitation, edema can increase beneath the unyielding burn eschar, which can lead to decreasing or absent distal vascular perfusion within the first 12 to 24 hours after the injury. Signs include cyanosis, impaired capillary refill, paresthesias, and pain. This usually is a problem only with full-thickness burns, but deep partial-thickness burns can occasionally cause distal ischemia.

After debridement and initial cleansing, further care will be dictated by whether the child is at the final destination. Children who will be transferred to another institution might simply have their wounds dressed with saline, sterile gauze, and bulky dressings. Covering the wounds reduces the pain. Children who are already at a center prepared to care for burn wounds will require a topical antimicrobial agent. Bacitracin ointment can be used on facial burns, while silver sulfadiazine is the topical agent of choice for partial thickness and full thickness wounds elsewhere on the body. Burns to the ears that are partial thickness or full thickness and might involve cartilage are treated with mafenide acetate (Sulfamylon). However, both silver sulfadiazine and mafenide acetate are sulfa-containing and should be avoided in patients with sulfa allergy or glucose-6-phosphate dehydrogenase (G6PD) deficiency. Pillows should be avoided in favor of elevating the head of the bed.

## KEY POINTS

### Initial Management of Moderate to Severe Burns

- Remove clothing
- Assessment of burn size and severity
- Cool burning areas with sterile water
- Keep patient warm to avoid hypothermia
- Early RSI for inhalation injury
- Fluid resuscitation as per Parkland formula
- Assess for need for escharotomies
- Monitor for rhabdomyolysis
- Cover all burned areas with dry, sterile dressings
- Transfer to a specialized burn center for care

The use of systemic antibiotics rarely is indicated in the initial management of the burn wound. Tetanus immunization should be brought up-to-date.

## Pitfalls in Burn Care

Failure to recognize a respiratory or inhalation component of a burn that occurred in an enclosed space, or any associated multiple trauma, can result in a major catastrophe. Avoid underestimation of burn size and depth by approaching the assessment in a disciplined manner. The extent of the burn depth or the possibility of later grafting is not predictable at the time of initial assessment. It is best to be cautious about prognosis.

Nonrecognition of myoglobinuria or hemoglobinuria and of the attendant need for alkalinization of the urine can lead to renal failure. Failure to perform escharotomy and fasciotomy when appropriate can lead to respiratory compromise or loss of an extremity.

## Guidelines for Triage and Disposition

The guidelines in Table 9-16 determine transfer to a burn center. If there is any doubt, admit a burned child to the hospital. Apply these guidelines based on the circumstances of each patient, including age, preexisting medical conditions, extent and nature of thermal injury,

### TABLE 9-16  Criteria for the Transfer of Patients With Burn Injuries

1. Partial-thickness and full-thickness burns greater than 10% of the total body surface area (BSA) in patients under 10 years or over 50 years of age
2. Partial-thickness and full-thickness burns greater than 20% BSA in other age groups
3. Partial-thickness and full-thickness burns involving the face, eyes, ears, hands, feet, genitalia, or perineum, or those that involve skin overlying major joints
4. Full-thickness burns greater than 5% BSA in any age group
5. Significant electrical burns including lightning injury (significant volumes of tissue beneath the surface might be injured and result in acute renal failure and other complications)
6. Significant chemical burn
7. Inhalation injury
8. Burn injury in patients with preexisting illness that could complicate management, prolong recovery, or affect mortality
9. Any burn patient in whom concomitant trauma poses an increased risk of morbidity or mortality can be treated initially in a trauma center until stable before transfer
10. Children with burns seen in hospitals without qualified personnel or equipment for their care should be transferred to a burn center with these capabilities
11. Burn injury in patients who will require special social and emotional or long-term rehabilitative support, including cases involving suspected child abuse and neglect

Adapted from: Committee on Trauma American College of Surgeons. *Resources for optimal care of the injured patient.* Chicago, Il: American College of Surgeons; 1999: pg. 55.

and social circumstances involved.

Transfer to a major burn center can be facilitated through direct telephone communication between the referring and receiving physicians. Preexisting transfer plans are helpful. Maintain adequate records to provide continuity in observation and care. Before a patient leaves the primary facility, prepare him or her for transport with a secure airway, functioning intravenous line, nasogastric tube, urinary catheter, proper burn dressing, and adequate analgesia. All pertinent information regarding tests, temperature, pulse, fluid administration, and urine output should be recorded and sent with the patient. Radiographs taken during assessment should also be sent.

## Electrical Trauma

A number of factors determine the effect of electrical current on the body, including:

- Resistance: Wet skin or water immersion decreases resistance precipitously, thereby increasing current delivered to tissue but resulting in few surface burns. In contrast, in and around tissue with high resistance such as calluses, more heat will evolve, resulting in cellular necrosis and worse surface burns.

- Current type: Alternating current (AC) is much more dangerous at lower voltage than direct current (DC) and can result in ventricular fibrillation at very low voltage. AC also causes tetanic muscle contractions that make many electrical injury victims unable to "let go" after contact with a circuit.

- Current pathway: Current follows the pathway of least resistance from contact point to the ground. Current that crosses the heart or brain is most dangerous.

The most frequent and serious problems involved in electrical injury include third-degree or fourth-degree cutaneous burns, cardiopulmonary arrest or injury, associated physical trauma, infection of burned tissue, myoglobinuria and third-space loss with renal injury, neurologic injury, tympanic membrane rupture, cataracts, and peripheral vessel occlusion.

Four types of electrical burn injury can occur, as follows:

- Direct injury from contact with the electrical source
- Flash burn (similar to a gas flame flash burn)
- Arc burn (measured at 2,500°C)
- Flame injury from ignition of clothing

In addition, blunt injury can occur if a person is thrown by the intense muscle spasm that can be triggered by the electrical current or from falls.

Prolonged hypotension and massive muscle necrosis predispose the electrical burn patient to severe infections, which are the most common causes of death among those who are successfully resuscitated. Although victims of electrical injury can have minimal external manifestations, extensive underlying tissue damage and occult trauma often exist and should be presumed to be present until proved otherwise.[35] In patients injured by generated electrical power sources, care must be taken by rescuers to avoid injury to themselves.

Lightning injuries, which follow the same laws of physics as other electrical injuries, usually present somewhat differently.[35,36] Victims of lightning strike rarely have external or deep internal burn injuries. Cardiac arrest is the main cause of death, although permanent neurologic sequelae often occur in those who survive the initial incident. Lightning injuries rarely have associated myoglobinuria, and fluid resuscitation might not be necessary unless there are massive burns.

### Management

In addition to the standard protocols described in earlier sections of this chapter, there are special characteristics of initial care of the child with an electrical burn. Hypotension is usually secondary to hypovolemia and is treated with a crystalloid fluid challenge of 20 mL/kg, which can be repeated as necessary. If a pressor agent is needed to achieve adequate perfusion, low-dose dopamine is the agent of choice because of its beneficial effect on renal perfusion.

Pay special attention to potential intracranial injury; entrance and exit burn wounds; signs of intra-abdominal hemorrhage, peritonitis, or ileus; evidence of fractures or dislocations; and diminished or absent pulses. Assess the patient for signs of blunt injury that can occur as a result of a fall or being thrown by intense muscle spasm. Traditional burn formulas frequently underestimate crystalloid requirements in patients with electrical injury because of the massive third-space shift that can occur.

Fasciotomies, not just escharotomies, might be necessary because of deep muscle injury.

An indwelling urinary catheter to monitor urine output and a central venous line can be useful. Blood transfusion usually is not required within the first 24 hours of care unless there is ongoing occult hemorrhage. Cardiac dysrhythmias, acidosis secondary to muscle necrosis, renal injury, and gastric dilation might be encountered. If myoglobinuria is present, the goal of fluid resuscitation should be a urine output of 1 to 1.5 mL/kg per hour while the urine is pigmented and 0.5 to 1 mL/kg per hour after the urine clears. Sodium bicarbonate can be added to one-half normal saline (or more dilute crystalloid solutions) to promote alkalinization of the blood to pH 7.35 to 7.40, which will enhance urinary excretion of myoglobin. Mannitol (0.25 to 0.5 g/kg IV bolus followed by continuous infusion at 0.25 to 0.5 g/kg per hour) might be indicated to enhance renal perfusion and avoid myoglobinuric renal failure, one of the main causes of death in the past.

Because lightning injuries seldom involve deep injuries or myoglobinuria, fluid loading, osmotic diuresis, and fasciotomies rarely are needed.

## Disposition

Electrical burns are considered major burns according to the American Burn Association classification system. Transfer to a burn center is appropriate for all seriously injured patients.

Admission to the hospital is recommended for severe electrical burns. However, for the stable patient with relatively isolated burns, including lip burns, studies have shown that the patient can be safely released after 4 hours of observation in the emergency department, provided caretakers are instructed regarding proper methods of controlling late hemorrhage, which can occur from the labial artery.[35]

Cardiac monitoring is controversial. Those with low-voltage electrical injuries probably can be safely discharged if they display no mental status changes or cardiac dysrhythmias. Creatinine phosphokinase level has no relationship to the amount of burn or to the overall prognosis of the electrically injured patient.

Surgical consultation or followup is necessary for victims of electrical injury. For cases of arc burns to the lip, consultation or followup with an experienced oral or plastic surgeon is necessary because severe bleeding can occur when the burn eschar separates from the underlying labial artery (usually 5 to 9 days after the injury) and because long-term splinting, particularly when the burn involves the commissure, might be necessary to avoid microstomia. Growth retardation of the mandible, maxilla, or dentition can occur.

Lightning victims can present more as cardiac or neurologic emergencies than as burn or trauma patients. A baseline ECG is indicated. Changes include nonspecific ST-T wave changes, T-wave changes, axis shift, QT prolongation, and ST-segment elevation. Admission usually is indicated, but children with completely normal examinations, laboratory tests, and ECGs can be discharged if there is adequate home observation and close followup.

## Eschartomy And Fasciotomy

It is important to evaluate the overall status of perfusion serially with Doppler ultrasonography. When signs of decreasing flow are present, longitudinal incisions (escharotomies) should be made on the medial and lateral aspects of the extremity. Incisions must be carried across involved joints. Incise to a depth that allows separation of the cut edges of eschar. This often will decrease the elevated compartment pressure and enhance peripheral circulation. The thorax and abdomen also can sustain extensive full-thickness injury, resulting in respiratory embarrassment. Escharotomies on the chest, back, and abdomen can facilitate more adequate ventilation. Fasciotomy might be necessary with electrical burns to salvage an extremity because of the incidence of deep muscle damage and edema within a fascial compartment. Fasciotomy should be done in an operating room.

## Other Burns

### Abuse

An alarming number of children are subjected to maltreatment.[37] Nonaccidental injury should be suspected and thoroughly investigated if there is evidence of any unusual pattern of the burn wound, or if the history given does not explain the nature of the injury. A clenched fist and "gloved" forearm burn distribution, "stocking" or bilateral lower extremity and buttocks injuries suggest involuntary submersion (Figure 9.29). Cigarette and steam iron pattern burns are suspicious findings that warrant a social services investigation. See Chapter 10, Child Maltreatment.

### Chemical Burns

Early management of most chemical burns, particularly strong acid and alkali burns, must include irrigation with copious amounts of water or saline to dilute any chemical substance. Alkali burns usually are more significant than acid injuries because they penetrate deep into the tissue, and they will require

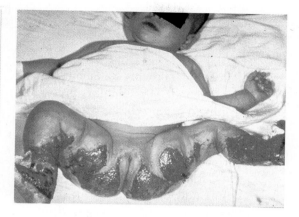

**Figure 9.29** Lower extremity and buttock burn suggesting immersion injury from child abuse.

longer surface irrigation. Avoid self-injury by wearing gloves and protective clothing. After removal of all the chemical substance, the burn wound can be managed with débridement, applications of topical antibiotic creams, and dressings.

## Summary

The continued development of increasingly sophisticated emergency medical systems has improved the quality of care for all pediatric injury victims by establishing evidence-based protocols of care, well-defined primary and definitive care centers, and effective procedures for expeditious transfer. Predetermined referral patterns and transfer agreements facilitate, standardize, and regionalize optimal care for the injured child. The process is complex and relies on accurate clinical assessment, effective initial management, efficient communication, and complete integration of all components. No system will be better than its weakest part. Nor will it be effective if its various components are not applied in an orderly and timely manner. The key to success is a complete understanding of the nature of pediatric injury. Although this will not eliminate the injury, it will significantly enhance the likelihood that its unfortunate victims will not just survive, but will enjoy a quality of life that is the birthright of every child.

# CHAPTER REVIEW

## Check Your Knowledge

1. Which of the following statements regarding secondary brain injury is correct?
   A. Begins to occur 6 hours after a primary traumatic brain insult
   B. Has no long-term consequences once corrected
   C. Most commonly due to respiratory failure and shock
   D. Occurs on the opposite side of the brain following a blow to the head
   E. Occurs rarely in children

2. Proper initial airway management of an agitated 6-year-old who has been struck by a car and who responds to verbal stimulation by flailing all four extremities should be:
   A. Direct oral tracheal intubation
   B. Nasal cannula at 12 L/min oxygen flow
   C. Nasal-tracheal intubation
   D. Rapid sequence intubation using sedation and paralysis after preoxygenation
   E. Sedation and continued bag-valve mask support

3. The target $Pa_{CO_2}$ for initial management of pediatric traumatic brain injury is:
   A. 15 torr
   B. 25 torr
   C. 35 torr
   D. 45 torr
   E. Does not matter

4. Surgical evaluation is necessary for which of the following trauma patients?
   A. Child who has evidence of visceral disruption
   B. Child who is not hemodynamically stable
   C. Child who needs surgical management
   D. One whose injury mechanism or initial clinical findings suggest internal organ system derangement
   E. All of the above

## References

1. Inon AE, Haller JA. Caring for the injured children of our world: a global perspective. *Surg Clin N Am*. 2002;82:435–445.
2. Carrico CJ, Holcomb JB, Chaudry IH. Scientific priorities and strategic planning for resuscitation research and life saving therapy following traumatic injury: report of the PULSE trauma workgroup. *Ann Emerg Med*. 2002; 9:621–626.
3. National Pediatric Trauma Registry. Boston, MA: New England Medical Center; 2000.
4. Rifkinson-Mann S. Head injuries in infants and young children. *Cont Neurosurgery*. 1993;15:1–6.
5. Patel JC, Tepas JJ, Mollitt DL, Pieper P. Pediatric cervical spine injuries: defining the disease. *J Pediatr Surg*. 2001; 36;373–376.
6. Stafford PW, Blinman TA, Nance ML. Practical points in evaluation and resuscitation of the injured child. *Surg Clin N Am*. 2002;82:273–301.
7. Trauma resuscitation and spinal immobilization. In: Hazinski MF, ed. *PALS Provider Manual*. Dallas, Tx: American Heart Association; 2002:258–260.
8. Bruce DA, Alavi A, Bilaniuk L, Dolinskas C, Obrist W, Uzzell B. Diffuse cerebral swelling following head injuries in children: the syndrome of "malignant brain edema." *J Neurosurgery*. 1981;54:170–178.
9. Pigula FA, Wald SL, Shackford SR, Vane DW. The effect of hypotension and hypoxia on children with severe head injuries. *J Ped Surg*. 1993;28: 310–314.
10. Muizelaar JP, Marmarou A, DeSallesa AAF et al. Cerebral blood flow and metabolism in severely head-injured children: Part I. Relationship with GCS, outcome, ICP and PVI. *J Neurosurgery*. 1989;71:63–71.
11. Kitchens J, Groff DB, Nagaraj HS, Fallat ME. Basilar skull fractures in childhood with cranial nerve involvement. *J Ped Surg*. 1991;26(8):992–994.
12. Duhaime AC. Management of pediatric head injury. *Cont Neurosurgery*. 1996;18:1–6.
13. Centers of Disease Control and Prevention. Sports-related recurrent brain injuries - United States. *MMWR Morb Mortal Wkly Rep*. 1997;46: 224–227.
14. Schutzman SA, Greenes DS. Pediatric minor trauma. *Ann Emerg Med*. 2001;37(1):65–74.14.
15. Duhaime AC, Alario AJ, Lewander WJ et al. Head injury in very young children: mechanisms, injury types, and opthalmologic findings in 100 hospitalized patients younger than 2 years of age. *Pediatrics*. 1992;90:179–185.
16. Guidelines for the management of severe head injury. *Brain Trauma Foundation*. 1995.

17. Bonadio WA. Cervical spine trauma in children: Part II. Mechanisms and manifestations of injury, therapeutic considerations. *Am J Emerg Med.* 1993;11:256–278.

18. McSwain ME Jr, Gamelli RL. Helmet removal from injured patients. American College of Surgeons, Committee on Trauma. Poster. 1997.

19. Curran C, Dietrich AM, Bowman MJ et al. Pediatric cervical-spine immobilization: achieving neutral position? *J Trauma.* 1995;39:729–732.

20. Nypaver M, Treloar D. Neutral cervical spine positioning in children. *Ann Emerg Med.* 1994;23: 208–211.

21. Bracken MB, Shepard MJ, Collins WF et al. A randomized, controlled trial of methylprednisalone or naloxone in the treatment of acute spinal-cord injury: results of the Second National Acute Spinal-Cord Injury Study. *N Engl J Med.* 1990;322:1405–1411.

22. Bracken MB, Shepard MJ, Holford T et al. Administration of methylprednisolone for 24 or 48 hours or tirilazad mesylate for 48 hours in the treatment of acute spinal cord injury. *JAMA.* 1997;277:1597–1604.

23. Prendergast MR, Sake JM, Ledgerwood AM, Lucas CE, Lucas WF. Massive steroids do not reduce the zone of injury after penetrating spinal cord injury. *J Trauma.* 1994;37:576–580.

24. Short D. Is the role of steroids in acute spinal cord injury now resolved? *Curr Op in Neurology.* 2001;14:759–763.

25. Bonadio WA. Cervical spine trauma in children. Part I. General concepts, normal anatomy, radiographic evaluation. *Am J Emerg Med.* 1993;11: 158–165.

26. Laham JL, Cotcamp DH, Gibbons PA et al. Isolated head injuries versus multiple trauma in pediatric patients: do the same indications for cervical spine evaluation apply? *Pediatr Neurosurg.* 1994;21:221–226.

27. Pang D, Pollack IF. Spinal cord injury without radiographic abnormality in children—the SCIWORA syndrome. *J Trauma.* 1989;29:654–664.

28. Panacek EA, Mower WR, Holmes JF, Hoffman JR, for the NEXUS Group. Test performance of the individual NEXUS low-risk clinical screening criteria for cervical spine injury. *Ann Emerg Med.* 2001;38:22–25.

29. Ruge J, Sinson GP, McLone DG et al. Pediatric spinal injury: the very young. *J Neurosurg.* 1988;68:25–30.

30. Gibran NS, Heimbach DM. Current status of burn wound pathophysiology. *Clinics in Plastic Surgery.* 2000;27:11–22.

31. Lukish JR, Eichelberger MR, Newman KD et al. The use of a bioactive skin substitute decreases length of stay for pediatric burn patients. *J Pediatr Surg.* 2001;36:1118–1121.

32. Jones I, Currie L, Martin R. A guide to biological skin substitutes. *Br J Plastic Surg.* 2002;55: 185–193.

33. Fallat ME, Rengers SJ. The effect of education and safety devices on scald burn prevention. *J Trauma.* 1993;34:560–564.

34. Monafo WW. Initial management of burns. *NEJM.* 1996;335:1581–1586.

35. Andrews CJ, Cooper MA, ten Duis HJ et al. The pathology of electrical and lightning injuries. In: Wecht CJ, ed. *Forensic Sciences.* New York, Ny: Matthew Bender and Co; 1995.

36. Cooper MA, Andrews CJ. Lightning injuries. In: Auerbach P, ed. *Wilderness Medicine: Management of Wilderness and Environmental Emergencies.* 3rd ed. St. Louis, Mo: Mosby-Year Book; 1995:261–289.

37. Lenoski EF, Hunter KA. Specific problems of inflicted burn injuries. *J Trauma.* 1977;17:842–846.

# CHAPTER REVIEW

A 5-year-old boy is struck by a car while crossing the street. Paramedics find the boy unconscious and lying in the middle of the street about 15 feet from the vehicle. They begin an initial assessment using the Pediatric Assessment Triangle, as follows: appearance is unconscious, not responsive to surroundings; work of breathing is tachypneic, with no retractions; and circulation signs include a pale and diaphoretic color. The paramedics stabilize the cervical spine, administer 100% oxygen by face mask, and attempt intravenous (IV) access en route to the hospital. An IV is placed in the right antecubital fossa, and 50 mL of normal saline is infused prior to arrival.

On arrival in the emergency department the patient's airway is open; increased secretions are noted, and the trachea is midline. There is symmetric chest wall motion and poor tidal volume. No retractions are noted, and breath sounds are equal. The child's color is pale; skin signs show diaphoresis. There is no jugular venous distention, and capillary refill time is 4 seconds. The heart rate is 160, with a thready peripheral pulse quality. Blood pressure is 75/palp. The abdomen is distended and tense on palpation, and the pelvis is stable. The rectal area is normal and negative for occult blood. The patient is still unconscious. There is no spontaneous eye opening. He responds to painful stimuli with flexor posturing. Pupils are at midposition and 4 mm bilaterally sluggish reaction to light. He has a contusion on the forehead, an abrasion on the left arm with swelling at the level of the elbow, an abrasion on the left flank, and deformity on the left femur.

1. *What is the physiologic status of this child?*
2. *What are your initial management priorities?*
3. *Does this patient meet an indication for surgery?*

---

*What is the physiologic status of this child?*

- Hypovolemic shock—decompensated

*What are your initial management priorities?*

- Contact surgeon (nurse or clerk to call with critical information based on primary [initial] survey)
- Suction airway
- Begin rapid sequence induction and endotracheal intubation (indications of decompensated shock and need for neurologic resuscitation, GCS <9)
- Etomidate, lidocaine, succinyl choline, or rocuronium, followed by lorazepam for continued sedation
- Etomidate is the sedative of choice in the hypotensive pediatric trauma patient
- Obtain vascular access in at least two sites (prefer antecubital fossa)
- Fluid resuscitation with normal saline 40 mL/kg, followed by packed red blood cells at 10 mL/kg
- Radiography:
  - Chest: Normal
  - AP Pelvis: Normal
  - C-spine series: Normal
- Obtain blood for type and cross (priority) if able, then send hemoglobin, electrolytes, renal and liver function tests, amylase, glucose, PT, and PTT

CASE SUMMARY 1 CONT

- Initial hemoglobin 10 gm/dL drops to 7 gm/dL after initial resuscitation and up to 9 gm/dL after 200 mL of PRBCs
- LFTs also elevated - alanine aminotransferase (ALT) 100 IU/L and aspartate aminotransferase (AST) 80 IU/L
- Perform trauma exam
- Place urinary catheter - urine 2 +blood, microscopic evaluation with 50 RBCs per hpf
- Nasogastric tube placed - drains gastric contents and air, no blood noted

Additional radiography:

- CT head: normal
- CT abdomen: liver and spleen lacerations (grade II); moderate blood in the peritoneal cavity; renal contusion but bilaterally functioning kidneys
- Reassessment after 2 units of PRBCs and 800 mL of saline; HR = 120; patient is more responsive
- Family informed of patient's condition

*Does this patient meet an indication for surgery?*
Although the patient presented in decompensated shock, initial resuscitation stabilized the patient. This patient now requires further care in a pediatric intensive care unit.

# chapter 10

# Child Maltreatment

Carol D. Berkowitz, MD, FAAP

Meta L. Carroll, MD, FAAP, FACEP

## Objectives

1 Describe common presentations of all forms of child maltreatment, including physical abuse, sexual abuse, child neglect, and Münchausen syndrome by proxy.

2 Describe the diagnostic studies that should be performed in suspected child maltreatment cases.

3 Explain the practitioner's responsibility in notifying authorities of suspected child maltreatment.

## Chapter Outline

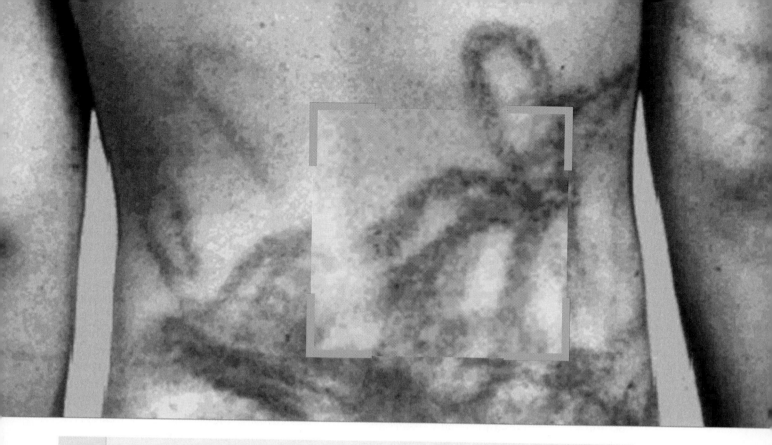

**CASE SCENARIO 1**

A 3-year-old boy is referred to the emergency department from his preschool because he has bruises on his face, left pinna, and lower back. The parents say the child is very active and frequently falls.

1. *What bruises commonly result from accidental injury, and what bruises suggest inflicted trauma?*
2. *What are the appropriate diagnostic studies to evaluate suspected child physical abuse? How does the child's age affect what studies are obtained?*
3. *If inflicted trauma is suspected, what agencies must be notified to assist in the investigation?*

## Introction

According to the US Department of Health and Human Services, approximately 3 million cases of child maltreatment were reported in 2000.[1] Of those, 879,000 cases were confirmed. This represented an increase in confirmed cases, the first such increase in 7 years. In 2000, there were 12.2 cases per 1,000 children.[1] More than 1200 deaths from child abuse were substantiated. For each case of child maltreatment reported, it is projected that there probably are one or two cases that go unrecognized. According to the American Humane Association, maltreatment of children is defined as harm resulting from inappropriate or abnormal child-rearing practices.[1] It includes physical abuse, sexual abuse, emotional abuse, neglect, and Münchausen Syndrome by Proxy.

The most vulnerable populations are infants, preverbal young children, children with chronic disease, and children with disabilities. Factors that increase the risk of physical abuse to a child include social isolation, lack of family supports, chemical dependency, domestic violence, and poverty. It is important to note, however, that physical abuse occurs within families of all cultural backgrounds and socioeconomic strata.

For many children, the emergency department is the point of entry into the health care system. Because some children with minor abuse subsequently might be severely injured or killed, the practitioner working in this area must have a high level of suspicion for signs and symptoms associated with inflicted trauma. A recent report noted that nearly one third of infants diagnosed with abusive head trauma had been evaluated previously in an emergency department for complaints unrecognized as being related to abuse.[2] The possibility of abuse should be considered with every traumatic injury treated. The practitioner should be alert to the possibility of maltreatment by any unexplained or poorly explained injury, evidence of neglect, delay in seeking appropriate medical care, or contradictory histories.

A multidisciplinary approach in which the practitioner works in cooperation with hospital-based nurses and social workers and with community-based child protective service workers, police, and personnel from other agencies has become the model for the evaluation process. In a cooperative multidisciplinary milieu, the child benefits from the knowledge of a broad range of experts, through the elimination of duplication of interviews and examinations, and by the avoidance of many issues that result when agencies work in isolation. Critical decisions affecting the child and the family are more accurately and easily made by a multidisciplinary team.

This section reviews in detail the major categories of child maltreatment: physical abuse, sexual abuse (including acute sexual assault), child neglect, and Münchausen Syndrome by Proxy. In the emergency department, it is difficult to diagnose Münchausen Syndrome by Proxy, a condition frequently associated with multiple hospitalizations and that requires the interaction of a multidisciplinary team for diagnosis.

Psychological/emotional abuse is also difficult to diagnose. Although psychological abuse can occur by itself, it is frequently associated with intentional physical injury and sexual abuse. Psychological injury is often responsible for the most serious long-term morbidity and the cyclic intergenerational pattern of abuse.

# ■ Physical Abuse

## Clinical Features and Assessment

Recognition of physical abuse is important for two reasons: to accurately diagnose and manage the inflicted trauma, and to prevent further injury or death. Abuse occurs in all segments of the population. A careful history and a comprehensive physical examination are needed to detect the signs and symptoms of inflicted injuries.

To adequately evaluate abuse, the physician should follow the guidelines of listen, look, explain, evaluate, record, and report. Obtain a careful, complete history, including the precise details of how the injury occurred from both the caregiver and the child. Conflicting, vague, or evasive answers and changing histories suggest abuse. Was the event witnessed? Does the child accuse the caregiver, or does the caregiver inappropriately blame the child, a sibling, or a third party for causing the injury? Does the caregiver protect his or her companion rather than the child? Is the child unusually fearful or withdrawn, or overly friendly or trusting? Such patterns of behavior often suggest abuse. Does the child engage in pseudomature or seductive behavior, or does he or she voice age-inappropriate sexual verbalizations? This should raise suspicion of sexual abuse. Most importantly, is the history consistent with the injuries?

What are the circumstances surrounding the injury? When did the injury occur? And when did the caregiver seek medical help? Who brought the child to the hospital? Has the child been examined by his or her regular physician? Often, an abused child has been seen by many different physicians to avoid raising suspicion about abuse. Is there a history of previous injuries or ingestions? Multiple prior injuries or a history of being "accident prone" can also be a marker of child abuse.

What is the behavior of the caregiver? Does this person seem under the influence of drugs or alcohol, or bizarre in affect? Does the caregiver show appropriate concern for the condition of the child? Both lack of concern and excessive concern for a minor injury should

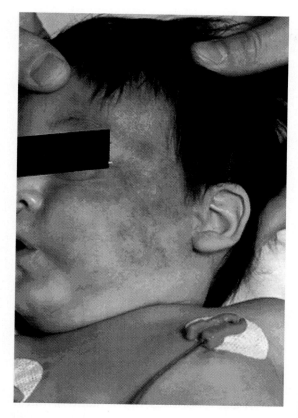

**Figure 10.1** Even minor bruising in an infant should be a red flag.

raise suspicion. Does this person seem overly aggressive, unusually hostile, or excessively critical or demanding of the child or the practitioner? Does this person admit to being abused as a child? Individuals who were abused as children might be caught up in a pattern of intergenerational violence. In summary, key concerns in the medical history are as follows:

- Unusual aspects of the medical history: a history from the child or parent inconsistent with the physical examination, a discrepancy between stories, injuries attributed to a young sibling, or a story that just does not make sense.

- History describing a minor mishap that is inconsistent with a major injury.

- History inconsistent with the developmental capability of the child: infants younger than 6 months rarely injure themselves. Even minor bruising in an infant is a red flag (Figure 10.1).

- Delay in obtaining medical care, or prior sporadic or inconsistent routine health care.

There is an adage, "Those who don't cruise, don't bruise."[3] Common sense and a basic knowledge of motor milestones for infants and children will help in determining the likelihood that the injury occurred in the stated manner.

A complete medical history is essential and should include the following:

- General medical history, including past medical and surgical history, prior injuries and hospitalizations, current medications, allergies, complete review of systems, and current complaints

- Social history, including identifying household members, domestic violence, substance abuse in the household, prior or current involvement with child protective services and/or police, and prior child maltreatment in the household

- Behavioral history, including the description of any change in emotional status, learning problems, school problems, or other behavioral changes

- Developmental history to assess the child's achievement of milestones, current motor skills and dexterity, and to detect significant developmental delay

Finally, for the injured child accompanied by a caregiver who has specific knowledge of the child maltreatment, obtain the name, address, and telephone number of the alleged perpetrator as well as his or her relationship to the child, information that will prove invaluable to the investigation and help ensure the child's future safety.

## YOUR FIRST CLUE

**Signs and Symptoms of Physical Abuse**

- Historical features suggestive of physical abuse
- Inconsistent history
- Delay in seeking medical care
- History of mechanism of injury inconsistent with developmental age

## Physical Examination

When obtaining the history or examining the injured child, note the child's interaction with the parent or caregiver. Is the child comfortable and happy in the caregiver's lap, or does the child avoid the caregiver and seek out each stranger who enters the room? Is the caregiver affectionate, concerned, and warm toward the child, or does he or she demonstrate no bonding or regard for the child?

The complete physical examination includes the child's vital signs; height, weight and head circumference in the infant or child who appears small-for-age, developmentally delayed, or neglected; head and neck exam, noting scalp swelling, fontanel fullness, bruising and petechiae on the face and ears, drainage from ears or nose, hemotympanum, bleeding around the nares, retinal hemorrhages, and abrasions or bruises on the neck; oropharynx exam, noting frenulum tears in the infant, as well as tongue bruising or bite marks, buccal mucosal bruising, and dental trauma; chest exam, identifying chest wall deformities and bruising; abdominal exam, noting distention, tenderness, bowel activity, and skin bruising or marks; genital exam, noting scars, bruises, lesions, abrasions, blood or discharge, and perianal tags, fissures, and bruising; back exam, noting tenderness and bruising; buttocks inspection, noting bruises, scars, patterned marks; exam of the extremities, noting deformity, neurovascular compromise and bruising; and complete neurologic examination.

## Bruises and Bites

The physically abused child might have injuries of the skin, soft tissue, bones, central nervous system, or internal organs. Ninety percent of such children have only superficial injuries such as bruises, bites, lacerations, puncture marks, burns, or signs of strangulation. Common locations for bruises caused by abuse include the buttocks and lower back (from paddling), genitalia and inner thighs (from punishment for masturbation or toilet training accidents), cheeks (from slapping or grabbing), upper lip and frenulum of the

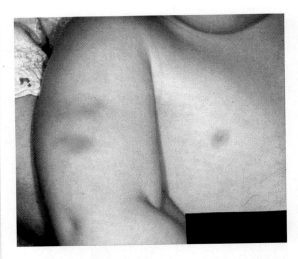

**Figure 10.2** Human hand and fingertip marks can appear as oval bruises.

tongue (from forced feeding or bottle jamming), neck (from strangulation), and ear lobes and pinnae (from boxing, pinching, and slapping). Human hand and fingertip marks can appear as oval bruises, pinch marks as linear marks from the fingers, or actual outlines of handprints (Figure 10.2).

The dating of bruises is at best an inexact science. While traditional teaching has described a predictable progression of bruise coloration (from red to blue, then green, yellow, and brown), the time required for the evolution of the bruise to ultimate healing is dependent on multiple factors. These factors include the depth and location of the injury, the nature of the particular tissue area and its blood supply, the skin complexion, and the presence of repetitively injured tissue. A superficial bruise can appear and heal more quickly, while a deep injury can take days to surface. A blow to an area of loose areolar tissue, around the eyes or genitals, can also bruise and heal more quickly than an area of dense tissue with well-supported blood vessels (e.g., thigh or buttocks). A child whose skin is repetitively injured can also heal more quickly. The dark complexion of some children can hide bruising.[4–6] A study that provided photographic evidence of bruises with known origins and ages provides a succinct summary of what physicians can reliably conclude when

| TABLE 10-1 | Langlois and Gresham: The Color and Age of Bruising* | |
|---|---|---|
| **Color** | **Age** | |
| Blue, purple, or black | From 1 hour to resolution | |
| Yellow | Older than 18 hours | |
| Red | Indeterminate | |

*Bruises inflicted at the same time, on the same person, in the same manner, can appear different and heal at a different rate.

Source: Langlois NEI, Gresham GA. The aging of bruises: A review and study of the color changes with time. *Forensic Science International.* 1991;50:227–238. Reprinted with permission.

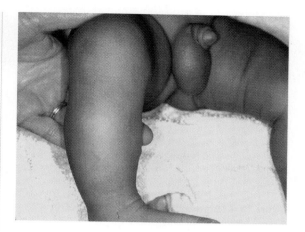

Figure 10.3 Mongolian Spots appear on the buttocks, back, and upper arms of many infants.

evaluating the age of bruising, as summarized in Table 10-1.[7]

While analysis of bruise aging has great limitations, a physician should examine the abused child carefully, note the location, size, shape, and color of each bruise; include a written description of the bruises with an accompanying drawing or body diagram; and consider photography with a ruler and color wheel (for color standardization) in the frame.

It is important to distinguish birthmarks, accidental injuries, and bruises caused by coagulopathies from inflicted trauma. Accidental bruises usually occur over bony prominences, especially the knees, shins, and foreheads of toddlers. Mongolian spots occur on the buttocks, back, and upper arms in many infants, particularly Black, Asian, Native American, and Hispanic infants (Figure 10.3). They are normal birthmarks and not bruises. In addition, people of certain cultures, such as Southeast Asian, might use folk remedies that produce lesions that appear abusive (referred to as Caio gao, they can resemble ecchymoses or hematomas) but are well intentioned and are not fundamentally harmful. Occasionally, excessive bruising might be due to bleeding dyscrasias such as idiopathic thrombocytopenia or von Willebrand disease. Coagulation studies (prothrombin time, partial thromboplastin time, platelet count) must be obtained on all children with extensive bruises.

Bites inflicted by an adult on a child are always abusive and can be identified by the short linear patterned marks of an incomplete bite, and oval or elliptical outlines with central bruising of a complete bite. When evaluating such a bite wound, seek the assistance of a forensic dentist, who will measure and document the bite and provide invaluable assistance in matching the wound with an imprint of the perpetrator's teeth. A quick measurement that can help the emergency physician distinguish a bite inflicted by a child versus an adult is the width of the imprint left by the maxillary canine teeth. A measured width greater than 3 cm corresponds to an adult bite and, as such, constitutes abuse and should prompt reporting and investigation.[8]

## Burns

Burns due to abuse are most commonly immersion burns, patterned contact burns, and cigarette burns. Burns that are deep and involve large areas of skin must be evaluated in the context of the history provided by the caregiver. Most concerning for abuse are immersion burns that characteristically have clearly demarcated edges. They can involve bilateral extremities or buttocks or demonstrate a stocking or glove distribution (Figure 10.4). Such injuries require communication with law enforcement officials, who will investigate the

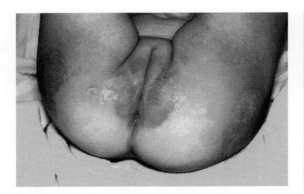

Figure 10.4 Immersion burn of the buttocks.

| TABLE 10-2 | Time and Temperature Required to Produce a Partial-Thickness and/or Full-Thickness Thermal Burn | |
| --- | --- |
| **Temperature °C (°F)** | **Time** |
| 54.4 (130) | 10 seconds |
| 57 (135) | 4 seconds |
| 60 (140) | 1 second |
| 64.9 (149) | 1/2 second |

Adapted from: Jenny C. Cutaneous Manifestations of Child Abuse. In: Reece RM, Ludwig S, eds. *Child Abuse Medical Diagnosis and Management,* 2nd ed. Philadelphia, Pa: Lippincott Williams & Wilkins, 2001: pp 23–45.

home and evaluate the tub, sink, taps, and water temperatures (Table 10-2). The multidisciplinary team then evaluates this information in light of the child's motor skills, the parent's history, and the distribution of burns on the child. The estimation of the severity and involved total body surface area of the burn will determine the need for patient transfer to a burn center for subspecialty care. While uncommon, multisystem injury (i.e., skeletal, head, abdominal) can accompany inflicted burn injury, warranting further trauma workup.

Ambulatory young children might accidentally come in contact with hot objects such as steam irons or curling irons, particularly when left on floors or low tables within easy reach. The resultant burn involves a single site, causes immediate pain and withdrawal of the body part by the child, elicits a rapid response from the caregiver, and usually results in a more superficial injury. More concerning are deep or multiple patterned burns from such household objects—injuries that must be evaluated with caution, as they are more likely to be inflicted by someone else.

Inflicted cigarette burns are usually deep, 8 to 10 mm in diameter, circular, multiple, and found on the hands and feet. When a child accidentally comes into contact with the burning tip of a cigarette, the injury is single, more ovoid in shape (as the child brushes the cigarette tip), and superficial.

The most common burn scenario in children is injury due to the splash or spilling of hot liquids. Typically, young children will attempt to grasp a cup or container from a counter, table or stovetop, splashing the hot liquid down onto the front of themselves, resulting in burns of the face, chest, and upper extremities. The area most severely burned is the site the liquid comes in contact with first. As the liquid runs down and heat dissipates, the resultant burn is less severe and leaves a pattern on the skin that demarcates the flow.[6]

## Head Injuries

The most frequent cause of death in children who are victims of physical abuse is head injury. In a series of patients admitted to the neurosurgical service at Children's Hospital of Philadelphia, at least 80% of the deaths due to head trauma in children younger than 2 years were the result of abuse. The average age of victims of abusive head trauma falls between 5 and 10 months.[9] One retrospective series found one third of all the children younger than 3 years with head injury were abused.[10] The abused infant or child with a head injury might be difficult to recognize, as he or she might be brought into the emergency department for care of respiratory complaints, poor feeding, lethargy, irritability, seizures, vomiting, listlessness, or reports of minor trauma. This absence of accurate history and lack of obvious external signs of injury can result in initial misdiagnosis (e.g., viral syndrome or colic). In an analysis of missed cases of abusive head trauma, 31% of 173 abused children were initially seen by physicians who failed to make the correct diagnosis. More concerning, 15 of the patients were reinjured prior to identification of abusive head trauma.[2] Thus, in all infants and young children with head trauma, careful evaluation of the history, the caregiver, the child's motor development, and the child's exam is critical. Particular care must be taken with the head-injured infant not yet "cruising," or walking. In the absence of a severe nonintentional trauma mechanism (e.g., motor vehicle crash), this young group of patients will rarely sustain severe nonintentional brain injury while under close supervision.

Two mechanisms of injury have been described in abusive head trauma: violent shaking of the infant causing a "whiplash" movement of the head, delivering shearing forces to the brain and intracranial vessels that bridge the subdural space; and a violent impact as the infant's head is slammed against a firm surface (e.g., crib, wall), delivering tremendous force with the abrupt deceleration of the head but providing no external physical evidence of the impact.[9]

The presence of diffuse and multiple retinal hemorrhages in the infant with head injury is highly associated with an abusive mechanism (Figure 10.5). Examination of the retinas using a traditional ophthalmoscope and performed by nonophthalmologists can identify more than 75% of retinal hemorrhages when present. The use of mydriatic drops can greatly facilitate viewing the retina. However, consultation with ophthalmology is essential in obtaining the best possible exam of the retina (through dilated indirect ophthalmoscopy) that allows complete viewing of the retina to its edge (ora serrata) and detailed description of the extent, depth, number, and severity of hemorrhages. The ophthalmologist can also provide essential photographic documentation of retinal findings using a specialized retinal camera. While the term "retinal hemorrhage" is nonspecific and nondiagnostic, an ophthalmologist's description of multiple hemorrhages through-

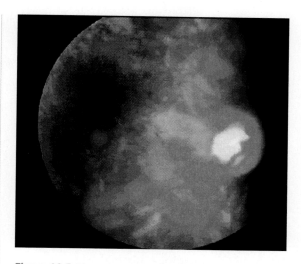

**Figure 10.5** The presence of diffuse and multiple retinal hemorrhages in an infant with head injury is highly associated with an abusive mechanism.

out the retina that extend to the ora serrata in the presence of preretinal, vitreous, or subretinal hemorrhage is virtually pathognomonic of abusive head trauma (in the absence of a severe obvious nonintentional mechanism of injury or life-threatening CNS disease). Without pupillary dilatation, retinal viewing can be difficult and hemorrhages can go undetected. Thus, the emergency physician should remember to document that the exam is "limited" or "preliminary" to prevent confusion about the presence of hemorrhages that are later identified by an ophthalmologist.[11]

For the child who presents with serious head injury and a history of a short fall, the medical literature provides good evidence of the benign nature of injuries that result from minor mechanisms such as rolling off a bed or tumbling down stairs.[12–14] Thus, an alternative explanation is more likely, and further evaluation of the child is essential (i.e., head CT, skeletal survey, retinal examination). Short falls can produce local deformation of the skull or a short linear skull fracture (particularly temporal or parietal areas) with small underlying subdural or epidural blood collections, or contusions. Such mechanisms, however, do not result in complex skull fractures or severe or diffuse brain injury or death.[12–14]

## Diagnostic Studies

The most common CT finding in abusive head trauma is subdural hematoma, particularly along the falx in the parietal and occipital regions. Other findings include mass effect due to subdural hematomas or parenchymal injury, subarachnoid hemorrhage, intraparenchymal hemorrhage, parenchymal tears, loss of gray/white matter differentiation, hemorrhagic contusions, and a "brighter" appearance to the cerebellum relative to the cerebral hemispheres, signaling severe anoxic brain injury and swelling (reversal sign). In some cases, despite the infant's abnormal neurologic exam, the initial head CT can appear normal. Magnetic resonance imaging (MRI) will detect parenchymal injuries missed on CT and is frequently used in dating the abnormal findings, as well as identifying cervical spine injuries that can also result from violent shaking.

---

### THE CLASSICS

**CT Findings in Infants With Intentional Head Injury**

- Subdural hematoma
- Subarachnoid hemorrhage
- Intraparenchymal hemorrhage/ contusion
- Cerebellar injury

---

## Management

In the injured infant with head trauma and suspected abuse, approach management as you would for a child with multisystem trauma. Evaluate the child for occult skeletal and abdominal trauma. Proceed with a skeletal survey, laboratory studies of the blood and urine, and abdominal imaging as appropriate.

## Abdominal Injuries

Injuries due to inflicted abdominal trauma can present in young children with mild symptoms such as poor feeding or listlessness, symptoms specific to the abdomen such as pain and vomiting, or in the child with peritonitis or shock due to bleeding or sepsis. The caregiver might describe a minor accident (e.g., short fall or tumble down stairs), but often no traumatic mechanism is provided. Stairway falls are well documented to result in superficial soft tissue and minor bony injuries, but not abdominal visceral injuries.[14] Most inflicted abdominal injuries are not identified by abdominal bruising. Nonetheless, examine the child carefully for tenderness or bruising of the abdomen, flank, inguinal and perineal areas, and back. Any injury to liver, spleen, pancreas, stomach, or bowel that is unexplained by major accidental trauma must be investigated as an abusive injury. Although these injuries are uncommon, abdominal trauma is the second most common cause of fatal child abuse, with an estimated mortality rate of 40% to 50%.[15] This high rate can be attributed to significant delay in making the diagnosis, requiring that the physician maintain a high index of suspicion in the face of no obvious external injury and an inaccurate history.[16]

Liver injury, including laceration and contusion, can result in bleeding into the peritoneal cavity, or it might be contained by the surrounding liver capsule. Liver enzymes are good markers for injury; AST levels greater than 450 IU/dL and ALT greater than 250 IU/dL are highly sensitive for liver injury seen on abdominal CT.[17] Splenic injury must be suspected in a child with chest or abdominal trauma and can lead to significant blood loss and shock. Suspected splenic injury should also prompt rapid imaging with CT. The most common cause of pancreatitis in the infant and young child is trauma. The young patient with any symptoms referable to the abdomen, or who presents septic or in shock, should have amylase and lipase levels checked—excellent markers of injury to the pancreas. Pancreatic contusion, laceration, or ductal injury is best imaged by CT as well. Ultrasonography is useful in identification of a pancreatic pseudocyst. Stomach or bowel perforation and bowel hematomas without perforation have been reported in cases of physical abuse. The child might present early with peritonitis or hemorrhagic shock, or symptoms can evolve over

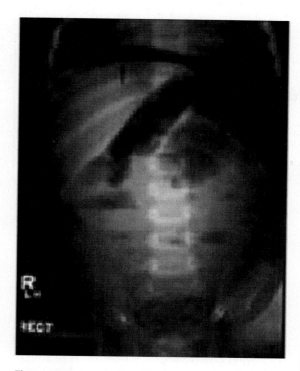

**Figure 10.6** Plain radiograph with free air under the diaphragm from jejunal rupture.

time, with medical attention sought hours to days after the inflicted injury. The most common site of bowel perforation is the duodenum due to its relatively fixed location in the retroperitoneum. Plain radiography of the abdomen can reveal free intraperitoneal air, bedside ultrasonagraphy can detect free fluid, and CT might identify the specific injury (Figure 10.6). However, bowel perforations can be difficult to identify by imaging and should prompt early laparotomy to localize and repair the injury.[16]

For all infants and young children with abdominal injury, optimal management requires early recognition of clinical findings inconsistent with history, rapid assessment and stabilization, early consultation with surgery, detailed abdominal imaging and appropriate laboratory testing, reporting to child protective services and police, and transfer to the appropriate trauma or tertiary care center if necessary. Particular patterns and vital signs are associated with certain types of injuries.[15] Once the abdominal injury is identified and definitive care provided, continued evaluation for evidence of multisystem trauma

is necessary, which can include skeletal survey and head imaging.

## Skeletal Injury

Although young and school-aged children commonly sustain fractures, all skeletal injuries must necessitate a thoughtful assessment in the ED. Nonintentional fractures generally found in active, ambulatory children are isolated fractures and usually involve certain anatomic locations. These locations include the distal radius and ulna, supracondylar area of the humerus, mid to lateral portion of the clavicle, mid or distal tibia, distal fibula, and in older, preschool and school-aged children, the area involving the growth plates near joints (i.e., Salter-Harris fractures).

In contrast, inflicted skeletal trauma found in younger children and infants usually cannot be explained by simple accidents because of their small body mass and early motor skills. In the infant not yet pulling to stand, any fracture should be concerning, and the history and mechanism of injury provided by the caregiver should be evaluated with care. Any concern about abusive fractures in an infant should prompt further radiographic study (i.e., skeletal survey) and protective services investigation.[18,19]

Fractures at sites that are infrequently fractured, in the absence of a major mechanism of injury (e.g., pedestrian hit by a car) should raise an immediate concern about physical abuse. These include the scapulae, ribs, pelvis, and vertebrae. So too, multiple fractures of varying stages of healing in an infant or otherwise healthy child with normal bones are highly suspicious for physical abuse (Figure 10.7). Dating of long-bone fractures can be determined with identification of certain radiographic findings, as summarized in Table 10-3. Certain long-bone fractures, including humerus and femur, while not pathognomonic for abuse, certainly raise serious concern for abuse if no appropriate accidental mechanism is provided. Again, such long-bone injuries in a young infant who is not yet standing or cruising require immediate workup with a skeletal survey and protective services investigation.

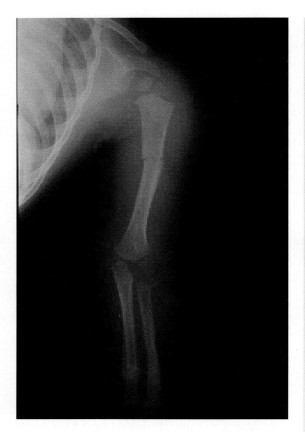

**Figure 10.7** Acute transverse fracture of humerus, healing transverse fracture of distal radius, and nearly healed fracture of the ulna.

| TABLE 10-3 | Dating of Bone Injuries |
| --- | --- |
| **Age of Injury** | **Radiographic Bone Appearance** |
| 0–2 days | Fracture, soft tissue swelling |
| 0–5 days | Visible fragments |
| 10–14 days | Callus, periosteal new bone |
| 8 weeks | Dense callus after fracture |

Fractures highly specific for abuse include the injuries of the metaphyses in infants and young children, described as corner, bucket-handle, or metaphyseal fractures. Forces that twist and shear this immature, weak, and vulnerable area of the infant's bone are the result of two common abuse mechanisms: A violent grasp or twist of the limb, using the arm or leg as a handle, or violent shaking of the infant with resultant flailing limbs.

Rib fractures in infants and toddlers, whether identified incidentally on chest radiograph or in a patient in extremis with serious multisystem injury, are commonly associated with physical abuse. It takes great force to break the ribs of an infant or child; the flexibility and compliance of the young chest wall and ribs make noninflicted mechanisms most unlikely, even secondary to stress such as chest compressions during vigorous resuscitation. One common abuse mechanism of injury is an adult grasping an infant's chest with both hands, and squeezing and compressing the chest while violently shaking the infant. This front-to-back compression of the chest wall fractures the ribs in two areas: near their articulations with vertebrae posteriorly, and along the lateral surfaces. All cases involving rib fractures should be investigated and should prompt careful history-taking, physical exam, skeletal survey, strong consideration for head CT imaging, evaluation for other chest and abdominal trauma, reporting, and hospital admission.

## Diagnostic Studies

### Laboratory

A complete blood cell (CBC) count, including a smear, differential, and platelet count, and coagulation studies (bleeding time, partial thromboplastin time, and prothrombin time) are indicated in patients with multiple bruises to rule out coagulopathy. These studies are also critical evidence in any subsequent trial. Cultures of the base of burns are helpful because bullous impetigo can resemble scald lesions. However, common skin pathogens are frequently cultured from these sites. Liver enzymes, amylase, and lipase levels are indicated in cases of suspected abdominal injuries. Preliminary evidence suggests that the differential rate of rise in the ALT and AST levels might help in the timing of hepatic trauma.[20]

### Radiology

Skeletal trauma in an infant or young child thought to be inflicted warrants at least two radiographic views of the injured extremity, being sure to include the joint above and below the area of suspected fracture. When the child is stable, proceed with a skeletal survey in all infants and toddlers with a fracture that might be from abuse. Also, a skeletal survey is indicated in all patients younger than 2 to 3 years if there is a concern for any abusive injury, including cutaneous, abdominal, or head trauma. The skeletal survey consists of frontal views of the chest, humeri, forearms, hands, pelvis, femurs, legs, and feet, as well as a lateral thoracolumbar view, and frontal and lateral views of the skull. A nuclear medicine bone scan is sometimes used to augment the skeletal survey because of its high sensitivity in identifying acute fractures, particularly those that might not appear on initial skeletal survey (e.g., acute rib fractures), or when the findings on skeletal survey are equivocal. For such equivocal findings, an alternative approach is the use of "coned-down" x-ray views of the skeletal area in question.

When a child's presentation raises concern about head injury due to symptoms, neurologic findings, concerning mechanism, or visible trauma at the head, immediately obtain a noncontrast head CT scan. MRI of the brain is ordered in the inpatient setting in two clinical scenarios: to accurately date the ages of hematomas in infants who have been repetitively injured, and to detect subtle inflicted brain injury not detected by CT. Also, always consider an urgent skeletal survey in the stable infant or young child to identify occult skeletal trauma.

## Management

Part of the appropriate management includes the careful recording of the appearance and lo-cation of all bruises, bites, lacerations, punctures, burns, sores, and signs of choking (e.g., strangulation marks) or restraint (e.g., rope burns) (Table 10-4).[21] Use legible handwriting, and make appropriate diagrams as necessary. Suspicious skin lesions should be photographed using good color-balanced photographic technique. Also record the verbatim statement of the child and parents. Exact record-keeping will become very important if the case comes under scrutiny of the legal system.

Reporting the possible abuse to the appropriate child welfare authorities and law enforcement agencies, as mandated by all states and US territories, should be done immediately on the basis of suspicion. Determining whether abuse actually has occurred is not the responsibility of the physician, but rather of child protection specialists and/or law enforcement officers who are specially trained for this task. However, filing a report of suspected child abuse is required by law. If there is suspicion of child abuse, the child might need to be admitted to the hospital for protection and undergo a complete evaluation.

Manage acute problems such as head, abdominal, and skeletal injuries in an expeditious manner, paying careful attention to the ABCs (airway, breathing, and circulation) of initial assessment and resuscitation. Many infants with such injuries require hospitalization in an intensive care unit. Seek appropriate medical and surgical consultation. Notify the appropriate children's protective services. Law enforcement agencies can also be notified in appropriate cases.

---

### KEY POINTS

**Documenting and Reporting Physical Abuse**

- Document all injuries.
- Obtain photographs of physical findings.
- Record verbatim statement from child/parent.
- Report incident to child protective services.

## TABLE 10-4  Differential Diagnosis of Abuse and Neglect

| Findings | Differential Diagnosis | Diagnostic Assessment |
|---|---|---|
| Bruises | Trauma: nonintentional and intentional<br>Henoch-Schönlein purpura<br>Leukemia<br>Sepsis | PT, PTT, platelet count, bleeding time, CBC<br><br><br>Blood culture, fibrinogen, FSP |
| Burns | Nonintentional/intentional<br>Infection<br>Bullous impetigo | Culture of base of lesion |
| Head injury | Trauma: intentional/nonintentional<br>Aneurysm<br>Tumor<br>Infection | CT scan, ophthalmoscopic exam<br>MRI |
| Abdominal findings<br>　Pain/tenderness<br>　Perforations<br>　Hematomas | Trauma: intentional/nonintentional<br>Tumor<br>Infection | Imaging studies (CT scan)<br>Abdominal ultrasonography urinalysis, liver<br>　enzymes, amylase, cultures |
| Skeletal findings<br>　Fractures<br>Metaphyseal/<br>　epiphyseal | Trauma:birth/intentional/nonintentional<br><br>Osteogenesis imperfecta<br>Rickets<br>Hypophosphatasia<br>Leukemia<br>Tumor: primary and metastatic<br>Scurvy<br>Menke syndrome | X-rays, skeletal survey, bone scan, calcium,<br>　phosphorus, alkaline phosphatase, skin<br>　biopsy, genetic consult, soft tissue swelling,<br>　CBC, VMA, bone marrow, cultures, ESR, bone<br>　biopsy |
| Growth impairment | Organic<br>Nonorganic<br>Mixed type | As suggested by history and physical exam<br>　and PE (e.g., electrolytes,<br>　BUN, organic acids, chromosomes) |

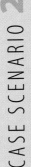

## CASE SCENARIO 2

A 5-year-old girl presents to the emergency department with the complaint of blood on her panties. There is no history of trauma, but the mother states that the daughter often has a yellow stain on her panties. The mother denies any concern about sexual abuse. You are unable to question the girl independently because she is frightened and will not separate from her mother. She will allow an examination if her mother stays with her. The physical examination is normal except for findings in the anogenital area. She is sexual maturity rating 1. The hymen is irregular with fleshy lesions that appear friable on its edge. There is blood on the panties but no frank bleeding. The anal examination is normal.

1. *What are the common causes of anogenital bleeding in children?*
2. *What are the pitfalls in obtaining a history from a child related to sexual abuse?*
3. *What physical findings are associated with acute and prior sexual abuse?*
4. *What is the significance of a sexually transmitted disease in a prepubescent child?*

# Sexual Abuse

## Background and Epidemiology

Child sexual abuse is the involvement of a child in sexual activities that he or she does not understand, for which he or she cannot give informed consent, or that violate social taboos. Such abuse includes oral, vaginal, or rectal contact or penetration; digital contact or penetration; fondling and/or caressing; sexual exploitation; or psychological sexual stress. Although exact prevalence rates are unknown, estimates indicate that 25% of girls and 10% of boys are victims of sexual abuse. And although rates of sexual abuse can be higher for girls, boys are less likely to disclose the abuse. Children are victimized at all ages but are most likely to be abused between the ages of 8 and 12 years. Perpetrators of sexual abuse are most often known and trusted acquaintances, relatives, or household members. The children are befriended, then manipulated or coerced, and can endure long periods of abuse before disclosing it. Sexual abuse must be differentiated from sexual play, which occurs between children of the same age or developmental stage and can represent normal activity in young children. Sexual play involves no coercion, force, or injury to the participants.[22] However, sexual play can occur when there is inappropriate involvement of one of the children in adult sexual activity. For example, it is neither normal nor age-appropriate sexual behavior for a 5-year-old child to put his mouth around the penis of another 5-year-old child.

## Clinical Features

### History

The sexual abuse victim can present for medical evaluation with a clear disclosure of the abuse, or with a variety of behavioral or medical complaints. Behavioral changes might be the only manifestation of abuse and include temper tantrums, clinging to caregivers, sexual acting out, sexual victimization of others, aggression, nightmares, developmental regression, disturbances in appetite, withdrawal, self-injurious behavior, phobias, school problems, and depression. Medical complaints might be quite nonspecific, as in the child with complaints of recurrent abdominal pain or headaches. More specific medical indicators of sexual abuse include genital pain, bleeding, irritation, and itching; sexually transmitted diseases; pregnancy; recurrent urinary tract infections; foreign body in the vagina or rectum; anogenital bruising; and painful defecation or dysuria.

History taking in cases of child sexual abuse must proceed in a manner unlike other pediatric evaluations. The history should be conducted in a quiet, private setting, allowing adequate time for interviewing the parent without interruption. The physician should interview the parent or caregiver alone while the child stays with someone else. Allow the parent to express his or her specific concerns with regard to sexual abuse. If a child's disclosure of abuse prompted the ED visit, obtain information on the circumstances surrounding the disclosure, details of the child's disclosure, and the specifics of the caregiver's questioning of the child. Ask the parent about behavioral changes or any medical complaints or symptoms. For the caregiver who describes genital complaints, feel free to introduce the topic of sexual abuse, proceeding in a gentle and nonjudgmental manner. Alternatively, a parent can present to the ED wanting the doctor to, "Tell me if my child was molested." Explore the parent's specific concerns about behavioral changes, physical symptoms, and household members or other caregivers.

Next, obtain a thorough medical history, including past illnesses, surgeries, chronic conditions, developmental history, medications, and allergies. Ask about current symptoms, including abdominal, urinary, and genital complaints, that will help direct the ensuing medical evaluation. If possible, pinpoint the time and place of the most recent contact between the child and the presumed perpetrator. Also, obtain a detailed social history, including household occupants, child care arrangements, substance abuse and violence within the household, and the mother's history of sexual or physical abuse.

The history provided by a child is the most important aspect of the medical evaluation and diagnosis of child sexual abuse. As such, once the emergency physician has obtained essential information from the parent, he or she must make a determination about the appropriate timing and location of the child interview. For many children, repeated interviewing—by emergency personnel, police, protective services workers, and social workers—might prove deleterious to the child and to the case investigation. With repeated interviewing, a child might feel threatened, intimidated, and doubted. Also, for the physician unaccustomed to asking a young child questions concerning sexual abuse, the interview might include leading questions or suggest answers, and thus contaminate the information subsequently obtained from the child by investigators. Remember that all investigative interviews have civil and criminal ramifications; they can have an impact on custodial arrangements and criminal prosecution. Thus, local protocols that identify children best served by a child advocacy center or sexual abuse specialty clinic should be used, and the complete medical evaluation deferred to the appropriate setting. Such procedures require a multidisciplinary approach that incorporates the expertise of medical, social services, law enforcement, and child advocacy personnel.

Deferral of the complete exam and forensic interview of the child requires that the following criteria are met in the ED:

- Careful screening of the home situation and all caregivers
- Complete medical history
- Child is without medical complaints that suggest genital injury or infection (i.e., no bleeding, discharge, or pain)
- Caregiver compliance with referral plan is ensured
- Child advocacy center or child abuse specialist contacted and followup arrangements made
- Clear safety plan established, ensuring no contact with the presumed perpetrator

- Report made to local child protective services and police
- Child has undergone a medical screening examination in compliance with the federal Emergency Medical Treatment and Labor Act (EMTALA)

However, an emergency medical evaluation should proceed in all cases in which there is reasonable suspicion that a child has been sexually abused within the preceding 72 hours, or the child has medical complaints that raise concern about genital injury or infection, or in all cases in which a child's safety cannot be ensured without a complete medical and psychosocial evaluation.

If indicated and the child is willing to talk about the abuse, the interview of the child should be conducted in privacy, in an unrushed manner, and without the presence of the parent. The physician first establishes rapport with the child by discussing nonthreatening topics, such as birthdays, playmates, pets, or school. Such conversation also helps determine the child's vocabulary and verbal skills. The topic of sexual abuse can be introduced with an open-ended question such as, "Do you know why your mommy brought you to the doctor today?" or "Your mommy told me that someone might have hurt you. Can you talk to me about it?" This allows the child to provide the history in his or her own words, with open-ended prompts such as, "Can you tell me what else happened?" In general, questions that elicit a yes or no answer should be avoided; for example, if a child who acknowledges being touched could be asked to elaborate on the experience with questions such as, "How did it feel?" and "Who have you told about this?" For younger children, a more specific question would be, "Did it hurt you?" or, "Did you tell anyone about it?" Throughout the interview, be sure to reassure the child, offer support, and provide positive statements such as, "You're very brave to talk about this." Such support starts the long process of psychological and emotional healing.

**Historical Features and Symptoms Suggestive of Sexual Abuse**

Historical features:

- Temper tantrums
- Clinging to caregivers
- Sexual acting out or victimization of others
- Aggression
- Nightmares
- Developmental regression
- Disturbances in appetite
- Phobias
- School problems
- Depression

Symptoms:

- Recurrent abdominal pain or headaches
- Genital symptoms
- Sexually transmitted diseases
- Pregnancy
- Recurrent urinary tract infections
- Foreign body in the vagina or rectum
- Anogenital bruising or bleeding
- Painful defecation
- Dysuria

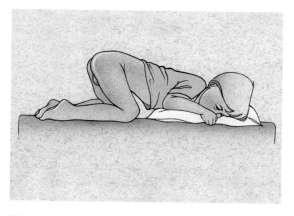

**Figure 10.8** Have the child assume an "up on all fours" position, with the head and chest lowered to the bed and the bottom in the air.

## Physical Examination

Record the stage of development of secondary sexual characteristics (sexual maturity rating) in all children. Perform a general physical examination with special attention to the genital findings. Those findings can differ in acute and chronic molestation. In both instances, note abnormalities in the genital and anal areas. Examine the genital area of the young girl by having her lie supine on the exam table, or sitting in her caregiver's lap, with her legs in a frog-leg position. After initial external inspection, gently hold the labia majora with gloved hands and provide lateral and posterior traction to reveal the labia minora, clitoris, urethra, hymen, hymenal orifice, fossa navicularis, and posterior fourchette. The anus can be viewed with the child in a lateral decubitus position with her knees drawn up to her chest, or lying supine and hugging her knees. In general, all girls should also be examined in the knee-chest position where the full contour of the hymen is more easily evaluated. Contrary to initial concerns that children would find this position anxiety provoking (an attack from the rear), this has not proved to be the case. Have the child assume an "up on all fours" position, with her head and chest lowered to the bed, and her bottom in the air (**Figure 10.8**). Consider demonstrating this position to the patient to help them understand what you'd like them to do. The young boy is best examined lying supine on the bed, with inspection of penis, glans, urethral meatus, scrotum, and perineum and gentle palpation of the testes. Again, the anus can be inspected with the boy lying either supine or on his side, with his knees drawn up, or in the prone knee-chest position. Take note of abrasions, bruises, petechiae, lacerations, scars, sores, ulcers, or other lesions. Carefully document all findings, both normal and abnormal, and use a body diagram with genital detail to draw and describe findings.

## Acute Injury

In general, there is no need to perform an internal pelvic examination on any prepubescent girl unless there is concern about penetrating vaginal or rectal injuries. If there is vaginal bleeding and no external source can be identified, then the child must be referred to a gynecologist or pediatric surgeon for an examination while under anesthesia. Careful external inspection often reveals any acute injury or the abnormal findings of chronic abuse as described below. There might be extragenital bruises and injuries, especially in cases of acute molestation. These can involve grip marks on the forearms where the child was held, or lacerations on the inner lip if the child was struck on the face in an effort to quiet her or him. Look for bruising around the genital and anal areas. There might be abrasions, lacerations, edema, and petechiae. The vagina and rectum might be in spasm after acute trauma. In about 50% of cases, there might be no physical signs after acute anal penetration.

## Chronic or Prior Molestation

Physical findings in a child who is a victim of prior or chronic molestation also might be absent or subtle. Changes in the genital or anal area will depend on the activity engaged in by the child or perpetrator. Exposure, fondling, and oral-genital contact might not produce changes. Chronic or recurrent penile or digital penetration usually will disrupt the hymen. There often are healed tears (transections) that appear as irregularities or scars in the hymen. The hymen itself will lose its thin, fine appearance and will appear thickened. The edge of the hymen will be rounded, and there might be rounded hymenal remnants that resemble the hymenal tags seen in the neonatal period. Scar tissue can form between the hymen and perihymenal tissue. Note the coloring of the genital tissues; blood vessels in areas of previous trauma can appear distorted. An introitus that appears to be gaping, allowing easy visualization of the vaginal rugae, also might be a sign of chronic penetration if the amount of hymenal tissue is reduced. Some investigators have estimated that the average normal transhymenal diameter is 4 mm, but there is great variation depending on the child's age, size, relaxation state and method of examination (e.g., supine with traction or separation, or prone knee chest) and measurement.[23] There might also be findings suggestive of a sexually transmitted infection, such as the presence of a vaginal discharge, ulcers, or polyp-like lesions. Condyloma acuminatum, or venereal warts, can appear as friable, fleshy lesions in the anogenital area. Condyloma latumis, an eruption of flat, broad warts secondary to syphilis.

Chronic anal penetration leads to scarring and observable changes in the anal area in a small percentage of victims. The skin in the perianal area might be thickened, hyperpigmented, and lichenified from chronic frictional irritation. The adiposity in the perianal area can be lost, leading to a funneled appearance, although this finding is very infrequent. Anal fissures can be noted with ongoing abuse. Such fissures can have a characteristic wedge-shaped appearance, being external to the external sphincter and wider distally than proximally. As fissures heal, they can form scars or tags of hypertrophied tissue. The appearance of the rugae in the perianal area can change; rugae become fewer in number, thickened, and more prominent, extending a greater distance from the anus. The anal tone can also change with chronic anal penetration. Observe relaxation and gaping of the external sphincter with separation of the buttocks. In addition, the anal wink, a normal protective reflex, might be lost or diminished. These findings are not significant if there is stool in the rectal ampulla.

Colposcopy is a useful adjunct to the evaluation of a child for chronic sexual abuse. The instrument allows for 5 to 20 times magnification of the area being examined and might reveal evidence of scars or disruptions in the vascular pattern that are not visible to the naked eye. Colposcopy is usually accompanied by video or photo documentation of the examination findings.

Carefully record normal as well as abnormal findings. Diagrams and photographs are helpful in documenting the findings.

## Differential Diagnosis

For children who present with medical symptoms, consideration must be given for other conditions. In the young girl who presents with vaginal or genital bleeding, consider accidental injury, infection (*Shigella*, pinworms, group A β-hemolytic strep), condyloma acuminatum, foreign body, polyps, tumor, precocious puberty, hemangioma, urethral prolapse, and urinary tract infection. In the neonate with vaginal bleeding, maternal estrogen withdrawal is the likely etiology. The differential for vulvovaginal complaints is described in Table 10-5.

## Diagnostic Studies

The laboratory assessment is especially important in cases of acute molestation; collect specimens that will serve as evidence. Details for the proper collection of specimens are usually included in the sexual assault kits kept in emergency departments or supplied by the police who accompany a sexual assault victim to the hospital. In general, collect any loose pubic hairs and, if the victim is post-pubescent, samples of the victim's pubic and scalp hair. A medicine dropper or nonbacteriostatic saline-moistened (not dry), cotton-tipped applicator can be used for specimen collection. Obtain specimens of semen if present; place on a glass slide and air-dry for DNA or other forensic determinations. Place permanent smears in PAP fixative. Semen will fluoresce under a Wood's light, as will urine until it dries, and other substances including some lotions and skin care products.[24] When semen is detected on a non-genital body area, remove dried semen samples with cotton swabs using nonbacteriostatic saline. Perform a pregnancy test on any sexual abuse victim who is at risk.

Obtain specimens to detect sexually transmitted diseases from the body areas listed in Table 10-6 in victims of acute or chronic molestation when signs and symptoms suggest the need. Not all children need to be tested. Obtain serologic testing as listed in Table 10-6. Once a child is out of the newborn period, gonorrhea, *Chlamydia*, and syphilis are presumed evidence of intimate sexual contact. In addition, test any patient with a vaginal discharge for bacterial vaginosis and *Trichomonas vaginalis*.

---

### TABLE 10-5  Vulvovaginal Complaints: Differential Diagnosis

- **Nonspecific vulvovaginitis**
  - Poor hygiene, local irritation, tight-fitting clothing, obesity, lack of estrogenization
- **Infection**
  - Respiratory flora (group A β-hemolytic strep, *Streptococcus pneumoniae*, *N meningitidis*)
  - Enteric flora (*Shigella*, *Yersinia*)
  - Pinworms
  - *Candida*
  - Sexually transmitted infections (*N gonorrhoeae*, *Chlamydia trachomatis*, *Trichomonas*, *Gardnerella vaginalis*, herpes simplex, human papillomavirus)
- **Vaginal foreign bodies (e.g., toilet paper)**
- **Polyps, tumors**
- **Systemic illness**
  - Crohn disease, Kawasaki disease, Scarlet fever
- **Congenital anomalies**
  - Ectopic ureter, double vagina, pelvic fistula
- **Urethral prolapse**
- **Skin diseases**
  - Psoriasis, seborrhea, lichen sclerosus et atrophicus

Adapted from: Vandeven AM, Emans SJ. Vulvovaginitis in the child and adolescent. *Ped in Review*. 1993;14:141–147.

| TABLE 10-6 | STD Testing |
| --- | --- |

**Female Child**

- N *gonorrhoeae* culture: pharynx, vagina, anus
- *Chlamydia* culture: vagina, anus
- Wet prep, Gram stain, culture if vaginal discharge present
- Hepatitis B and C serology, HIV, RPR
- Urinalysis for *Trichomonas*, sperm

  (Note: In the prepubertal girl, cervical cultures are not obtained.)

**Male Child**

- N *gonorrhoeae* culture: pharynx, urethra, anus
- *Chlamydia* culture: urethra, anus
- Wet prep, Gram stain, culture if penile discharge present
- Hepatitis B and C serology, HIV, RPR
- Urinalysis

Adapted from: Hymel KP, Jenny C. Child sexual abuse. *Pediatr Rev.* 1996;17:236–249; and Muram D, Stewart D. Sexual transmitted diseases. In: Heger A, Emans SJ, Muram D, eds. *Evaluation of the Sexually Abused Child,* 2nd ed. New York, Ny: Oxford University Press, Inc; 2000 187–223.

| TABLE 10-7 | Findings and Interpretation: Child Sexual Abuse |
| --- | --- |

- Anogenital Findings
  - Normal anogenital exam
  - Abnormal anogenital exam
  - Indeterminate anogenital exam
- Assessment of Anogenital Findings
  - Consistent with history
  - Inconsistent with history
  - Limited/insufficient history
- Interpretation of Anogenital Findings
  - Normal exam: can neither confirm nor negate sexual abuse
  - Non specific: might be caused by sexual abuse or other mechanisms
  - Sexual abuse highly suspected
  - Definite evidence of sexual abuse and/or sexual contact
- Need further consultation/investigation
- Lab results or photo review pending (can alter assessment)

Source: Findings and Interpretation: Child Sexual Abuse. State of California Office of Criminal Justice Planning. OCJP 925. Revised 07/01/01. pg 6.

With proper consent, try to establish the HIV status of both patient and perpetrator.

For some children, there will be tremendous fear generated by the examination and the collection of laboratory specimens. It is very important that the examiner not produce more fear in the child. Try to gain the child's cooperation by having the child be aware of what is happening and about to happen. The child often can be instructed to obtain his or her own cultures under direct supervision. If the child is uncooperative or out of control, suspend the evaluation.

Avoid the "second sexual assault," when a physical or genital exam in the ED frightens the patient or causes more psychological trauma than the sexual assault itself. It is always better to suspend the evaluation and try again the next day, perhaps in a more quiet setting under more calm circumstances. If the child is bleeding from the site of injury, then the child will have to be examined while under anesthesia. On completion of the evaluation, summarize the findings. Table 10-7 presents a scheme for summarizing

the information and setting a course of action. The California Office of Criminal Justice Planning has many useful forms designed to set a course of action (http://www.ocjp.ca.gov/publications.htm).[25] These forms are used to synthesize the physical findings with the history and are particularly helpful for the forensic assessment of the case.

## Management

Both prepubertal and postpubertal victims of molestation might have sexually transmitted diseases and need appropriate diagnostic evaluations and therapy, unless the patient or family objects (Table 10-8). If an adolescent has a negative pregnancy test in the ED, the possibility of pregnancy still should be discussed, as should the use of an emergency contraceptive drug ("morning-after pill"). Levonorgestrel (Plan B), a totally synthetic progestogen, is associated with less nausea and vomiting and is

**TABLE 10-8  STD Treatment in Child Sexual Abuse (Prepubertal, or Weight Less Than 45 kg)**

| | |
|---|---|
| N gonorrhoeae | Ceftriaxone 50 mg/kg IM/IV × 1 dose |
| | Spectinomycin 40 mg/kg IM × 1 dose |
| C trachomatis | Erythromycin base 50 mg/kg/day po QID × 10–14 days |
| Gardnerella | Metronidazole 5 mg/kg/dose po TID × 7 days<br>or<br>Clindamycin 10 mg/kg/dose po TID × 7 days<br>or<br>Amoxicillin/clavulanic acid 20 mg/kg/dose po BID × 7 days |
| Trichomonas | Metronidazole 10 mg/kg/dose po TID × 7 days |
| Syphilis (incubating) | Ceftriaxone 50 mg/kg IM/IV × 1 dose |
| HSV (first clinical episode) | Acyclovir 400 mg po TID × 7–10 days |
| Hepatitis B* | HBIG 0.06 mg/kg IM + vaccine series |
| HIV (PEP) | Contact infectious disease specialist prior to starting<br>Zidovudine 160 mg/m2 po q6 hours × 28 days<br>and<br>Lamivudine 4 mg/kg po BID × 28 days<br>and<br>Nelfinavir 20–30 mg/kg po TID × 28 days |

*Unimmunized child and perpetrator with acute hepatitis B infection.

Adapted from: Workowski KA, Levine WC. Sexually Transmitted Diseases Treatment Guidelines-2002. MMWR Recommendations and Reports. 2002; 51(RR06): 1–80 and Merchant RC, Keshavarz R. Human immunodeficiency virus postexposure prophylaxis for adolescents and children. *Pediatrics.* 2001; 108:e38.

a currently preferred management strategy. If not available, treatment with Ovral should be offered to patients at risk. The dose is 2 tablets in the ED and 2 additional tablets in 12 hours. An antiemetic before use is recommended. Withdrawal bleeding can occur within the subsequent 21 days.

## Disposition, Reporting, Followup Care

If the child presents with severe symptoms or a serious or life-threatening condition, make immediate arrangements for hospital admission or transfer to a tertiary care facility. In cases in which the perpetrator is unknown but there is significant concern that he or she lives in the child's home, proceed with arrangements for hospital admission or foster care or some other situation with child protective/social service assistance. When the child identifies the presumed perpetrator, discharging the child requires careful formation of a safety plan that ensures the child's protection. The child's parent or primary caregiver must understand that it is mandatory that there be no contact between the child and the presumed perpetrator, and that failure to protect the child will result in removal of the child from the home to safety.

Reassure victims of molestation, both chronic and acute, that they are all right and that their bodies have not been damaged in any way. Some hospitals have victim advocates who support rape victims during the initial emergency department assessment.

Referral to counseling agencies is recommended for all victims of both acute and chronic sexual abuse. Notify law enforcement and children's services of the physical findings of sexual abuse.

The practitioner is obligated by law to report all cases of suspected child abuse.

Although the specifics of reporting differ from state to state, in general, practitioners must make a report by telephone immediately to law enforcement and child protective services. Follow this oral report with a timely written report, preferably immediately but always within 3 days.

Confronting a family about child abuse can be difficult. It is important to keep in mind the vital role of the reporting practitioner as an advocate for the child who is being evaluated. In addition, the abusive parent often is seeking help for himself or herself when bringing in the injured child. The practitioner thus might be able to help not only the child, but also the troubled parent.

Consultation with other professionals (e.g., social workers or psychologists) is helpful in completing the evaluation and disposition planning, especially when evaluating sexually abused children and adolescents.

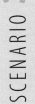

## CASE SCENARIO 3

Police cars bring a 14-year-old girl to the ED. She reports that she was walking home from school when a car pulled up, two men grabbed her, and pulled her into the car. She states that they took her to a house and dragged her up a flight of stairs. One man pointed a gun at her and stood laughing and talking while the second one pulled off her pants and raped her. Then the first man raped her while the second stood holding the gun. She reports no oral or anal penetration, and no condom use. She states that, some time later, the men left the house, allowing her to escape and call the police. When her mother arrives, she states that her daughter is always lying and made up this story to avoid getting into trouble for having sex.

1. *What are the medical treatment priorities for this patient?*
2. *When should HIV prophylaxis be considered?*
3. *The mother refuses to provide consent for the emergency care of her daughter. How should the emergency physician proceed?*

## Acute Sexual Assault

Sexual assault is the sexual contact of one person with another without appropriate legal consent. Legal definitions of rape also include the use of force or threat of force by the perpetrator. An acute assault is one that occurs within 72 hours of presenting for medical evaluation and care. Those most vulnerable to sexual assault include young children, female adolescents, the disabled or developmentally delayed, and those under the influence of drugs or alcohol. In the US, the incidence of rape peaks in female adolescents between 16 and 19 years old; of the 700,000 women that are raped each year, an estimated 61% are younger than 18.[26] An anonymous survey of high school students in the United States revealed that almost 20% reported one episode of forced sexual contact, with approximately half never reporting the assault.[26] Another survey of female adolescents revealed that most knew the perpetrator and that 57% of these assaults occurred during a date.[27] Of the minority of sexual assault victims who seek medical care, more than half might present to the physician with another complaint, further limiting the physician's ability to provide much-needed therapies, and making accurate estimates of disease incidence impossible. In cases of drug-facilitated sexual assault, the substance most commonly identified is alcohol.[26] The reported incidence of male victims of sexual assault in the high school population is 5%.[28]

For the child or adolescent who presents to the ED after a sexual assault, the following should be accomplished: Identify and treat all physical injuries; reduce or eliminate the risk of sequelae of the assault, including genital injury, pregnancy, and sexually transmitted diseases; carefully document the history provided, physical exam findings, and laboratory test results, providing a permanent record of the evaluation; collect forensic evidence and maintain the chain of custody of evidentiary materials; provide referral for followup medical care and psychological counseling; and establish communication with law enforcement for crime investigation and prosecution of the perpetrator. For the minor victim assaulted by a parent or adult in a caregiver role, emergent reporting to local child protective services is critical for the victim's future safety and well-being, as well as the safety of other children in contact with the perpetrator.

## Medical Assessment of Acute Sexual Assault

For the child or adolescent in the ED after a sexual assault, provide a quiet room where the history and physical exam can be conducted in private. The medical assessment can be facilitated by the presence of a victim advocate or hospital social worker who serves to support the victim and ensure that he or she is not left alone. Essential history obtained by the emergency physician includes a general medical history, gynecologic history (including information about menstruation, pregnancies, sexual activity, contraceptive use, and recent surgery or infections), social and developmental history (particularly important in the young child), and a history of the assault.

For the very young child or the victim who is too traumatized to provide detailed information, interview the accompanying caregiver alone, they will provide much-needed medical information and might be able to provide details concerning the child's disclosure of the assault. A child who is unwilling to discuss the assault should not be forced to do so, but might disclose at a later time in a forensic interview or therapeutic setting.

For the adolescent victim who is able to provide details of the assault, obtain a history of the following information: Identifying information about the perpetrator or perpetrators; the date, time, and specific location of the assault; the circumstances and details of the assault; the threats, use of restraints, use of drugs or alcohol, and use of weapons; the physical injuries inflicted before, during, or after the assault; the patient's symptoms; and the patient's activities after the assault (i.e., showering, urinating, douching, changing clothes, eating/drinking, brushing teeth).

For the adolescent victim who is unable to provide such details, focus the history on three main areas: The nature of the sexual contact, the use of force or threats, and the patient's symptoms. Later interviewing by police personnel will likely uncover details of the assault necessary for the investigation and criminal prosecution. In the ED, medical care and psychological support should take top priority.

In the acute sexual assault case involving a young child, take time to establish rapport, assess verbal skills, and determine developmental stage by conversing on nonthreatening topics. Introduce the topic of the assault with a question that is gentle and open-ended. For example, "Do you know why you came to see the doctor today?" or "Your mommy told me that something happened to you that made you feel bad. Can you talk to me about it?" This provides the child an opportunity to explain what happened in his or her own words. Information provided by the child's disclosure leads to more specific questions, which should not be leading or suggest answers. Again, a child who is unwilling or unable to describe details of the assault should not be forced to do so. Reassure the child and turn the focus to physical symptoms, which will assist in the medical evaluation. A forensic interview, also described as a "victim-sensitive interview," can be deferred to a time and place best suited to the young child's needs.

For victims of assault of all ages, be sure to include a therapeutic message throughout the interview. Such statements as, "This was not your fault," "This has happened to other girls and boys," "I'm here to help you get better," and "You are very brave to talk about it" must be said and repeated. Followup counseling for the psychological trauma is essential to recovery, but emotional support and the process of healing should begin in the ED.

## Physical Examination

Physical examination includes careful inspection and documentation of the patient's general physical appearance and demeanor, height and weight, vital signs, and evidence of injury to the head and neck, chest, abdomen, extremities, back, buttocks, and anus. Pay careful attention to skin findings, including bruises, ligature marks, and other injuries, as well as stains, areas of dried secretions, or areas that fluoresce under a Wood's lamp. Examination of the genitalia requires external inspection noting bruising, bleeding, bite marks, petechiae, secretions, stains, or any sign of trauma. For the adolescent female, external inspection, speculum and bimanual exam are needed. In contrast, no speculum exam should be performed on a prepubertal female patient. Rather, assist her in lying supine on the examining table (or sitting in her caregiver's lap) and assuming a frog-leg position for gentle inspection only. Any abnormal or concerning findings on exam should be confirmed by inspecting the child in a second position (i.e., the knee-chest position, in which the child is on all fours on the table with head and chest to the table and bottom in the air). In cases of vaginal bleeding with no visible external trauma, or when there is concern about a foreign body in the anogenital area, prepare the patient for an examination under anesthesia after obtaining the appropriate surgical or gynecologic consultation.

Although physical findings on genital exam of the sexual assault victim can be absent, minimal, or nonspecific, care should be taken to complete a thorough exam under good lighting and with magnification, if available. Most EDs are not equipped for coloposcopy, but such magnification can improve the identification of injuries. A study of female sexual assault victims examined with a colposcope (ages ranged from 11 years to adulthood) identified important genital areas most frequently injured, including the posterior fourchette, labia minora, hymen, and fossa navicularis. The injuries included tears (most often found on the posterior fourchette and fossa), abrasions, and bruising. However, in this series, more than one third of the victims had no visible trauma, which in part demonstrates the rapid healing of highly vascular structures and emphasizes that the history of the assault remains the most important data provided by a patient.[29]

## Diagnostic Testing

While performing the physical exam, be mindful of the requirements of forensic evidence collection. The adolescent or child wearing the same clothing worn at the crime scene, or clothing put on immediately after the assault, should disrobe in the ED on a sheet from the forensic evidence collection kit. This careful collection of debris from the clothing captures material that places the victim and/or perpetrator at the crime scene. Any areas of staining on the skin or stains that fluoresce under a Wood's lamp might be the perpetrator's semen or other secretions and should be swabbed with nonbacteriostatic saline on cotton-tipped swabs. The completed forensic kit includes the patient's clothing, debris collection from clothing, skin swabs, hair combings from the patient's head and pubic area, swabs from the female patient's mouth, vagina and perianal areas, swabs from the male patient's mouth, urethra, and perianal areas, fingernail scrapings, and a sample of blood. Also, collect and package any item that was in or near the vagina during or after the assault (i.e., the speculum, sanitary napkin, tampon, or other foreign body).

Swabs from the mouth, urethra, vagina, perianal areas and skin surface areas should be collected for the forensic kit. Subsequent swabs should be collected for culture testing; these are not placed in the forensic kit, but rather sent to the appropriate hospital lab. For the child who is unable to tolerate evidence collection or culture testing, remember that the first priority during this exam is the patient's comfort and health. Proceed only with those procedures and interventions that are medically necessary. Toxicologic testing should be considered in all cases in which there is reasonable cause to suspect the victim has been drugged. The patient can provide a history of altered mental status or memory deficit, or describe "waking up" in an unfamiliar location. The patient might present to the ED unconscious or with an altered mental status. Obtain urine and blood samples as promptly as possible, and follow the local forensic lab protocols for obtaining consent, specimen collection and labeling, and transfer of specimens to the lab. Table 10-9 summarizes the appropriate diagnostic testing for the sexual assault patient who presents within 72 hours of the attack. Table 10-6 provides the diagnostic testing for the prepubertal female. Table 10-10 summarizes the appropriate 2 week follow-up testing for the sexual assault patient.

## Treatment

Table 10-11 reviews the appropriate dosing of antibiotics used in sexually transmitted disease (STD) prophylaxis for adolescents, while Table 10-8 is for children <45 kg.

Significant controversy exists about the risk of HIV transmission after a sexual assault and the appropriate indications for the use of

| TABLE 10-9 | Diagnostic Testing After Acute Sexual Assault |
|---|---|
| **Adolescent Female** | |
| • Oral | N gonorrhoeae culture |
| • Cervical | N gonorrhoeae and Chlamydia cultures |
| • Vaginal | Wet prep, Gram stain, bacterial culture |
| • Rectal | N gonorrhoeae and Chlamydia cultures |
| • Blood | Hepatitis B and C serology, RPR, HIV |
| • Urine | Urinalysis (and culture as indicated) and urine HCG |
| • Imaging/ labs | As indicated for suspected skeletal, head, chest, abdominal injuries |
| **Male** | |
| • Oral | N gonorrhoeae culture |
| • Urethral | N gonorrhoeae and Chlamydia cultures |
| • Rectal | N gonorrhoeae and Chlamydia cultures |
| • Blood | Hepatitis B and C serology, RPR, HIV |
| • Urine | Urinalysis (and culture as indicated) |
| • Imaging/ labs | As indicated for suspected skeletal, head, chest, abdominal injures (prepubertal female, see Table 10-6) |

Adapted from: Bechtel K, Podrazik M. Evaluation of the adolescent rape victim. *Pediatr Clin North Am.* 1999; 46:809–823.

| TABLE 10-10 | Followup Testing in Sexual Assault |
|---|---|

**Followup Testing at 2 Weeks:**
- If no antibiotics are received at first encounter, consider repeat culture testing.
- If testing and treatment are done at first encounter, review results/discuss current symptoms of patient.

**Followup Testing at 4–6 Weeks:**
- Blood for RPR

**Followup Testing at 12 Weeks:**
- Blood for hepatitis B serology and HIV

**Followup Testing at 6 Months:**
- Blood for HIV

Adapted from: Hymel KP, Jenny C. Child sexual abuse. *Ped in Review.* 1996;17:236–49 and Bechtel K, Podrazik M. Evaluation of the adolescent rape victim. *Pediatr Clin North Am.* 1999; 46:809–823.

| TABLE 10-11 | STD Prophylaxis and Treatment After Sexual Assault (Adolescent, or weight > 45 kg) |
|---|---|
| • *N gonorrhoeae* | Ceftriaxone 250 mg IM |
| • *Chlamydia* | Azithromycin 1 g po or Doxycycline 100 mg po BID × 7 days |
| • *Gardnerella* | Metronidazole 2 g po (or 500 mg po BID × 7 days) or Clindamycin 300 mg po BID × 7 days |
| • *Trichomonas* | Metronidazole 2 g po (or 500 mg po BID × 7 days) |
| • Syphilis | Ceftriaxone 250 mg IM (incubating) |
| • HSV (first clinical episode) | Acyclovir 400 mg po TID × episode) 7–10 days or Famciclovir 250 mg po TID × 7–10 days or Valacyclovir 1g po BID × 7–10 days |
| • Hepatitis B* | HBIG 0.06 mg/kg IM + vaccine series |
| • HIV | Contact local infectious disease specialist before starting Combivir (ziduvidine/lamivudine) 1 tablet po BID × 28 days and Indinavir 800 mg po q8 hours × 28 days |

*Unimmunized teen and perpetrator with acute hepatitis B infection

Adapted from: Workowski KA, Levine WC. Sexually Transmitted Diseases Treatment Guidelines-2002. MMWR Recommendations and Reports. 2002; 51(RR06): 1–80 and Merchant RC, Keshavarz R. Human immunodeficiency virus postexposure prophylaxis for adolescents and children. *Pediatrics*. 2001; 108:e38.

postexposure prophylaxis (PEP) against HIV. The largest body of human and animal data has prompted recommendations for the use of therapy in the occupational setting (e.g., needlestick injuries in health care workers) and perinatal settings. No US guidelines exist for nonoccupational HIV PEP. However, with the presumption of the existence of a brief window after exposure in which the HIV viral load is small and therapy might be efficacious, consideration should be given to offering PEP to the sexual assault victim. Those victims at highest risk should be counseled and offered PEP. Such patients include the victim attacked by a perpetrator with known HIV or at high risk for HIV (e.g., known IV drug user); the victim attacked by multiple perpetrators; and the victim with anal findings consistent with penetration. Provision of the first dose within 1 hour of the assault is ideal but often impossible. Consider providing the medication necessary for the first 72 hours of the PEP regimen, within which time the patient can be seen by a local HIV or infectious disease specialist who will reconsider the risk of HIV and risk/benefit ratio of treatment, provide patient counseling, and establish a followup testing and care plan.[30]

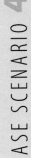

**CASE SCENARIO 4**

A 3-month-old boy with a fever for 1 day is brought to the emergency department by his mother. The mother reports that he is a good eater, taking six to seven 8-ounce bottles of formula a day. The infant is the mother's fourth child. A review of the past medical history reveals that the infant was at the 50th percentile for weight and length at birth and was full term. On physical examination, the infant is now below the 5th percentile for weight and at the 50th percentile for height and head circumference. The temperature is 37.4°C. The infant is apathetic, appears hypertonic, and avoids eye contact. There is mild rhinorrhea, but the throat, ears, and lungs are clear. There is a moderate diaper rash and caked stool in the diaper area. The infant is also dirty and smells like stale milk.

1. *What physical findings are noted with failure to thrive (FTT)?*
2. *What are the interactional characteristics of infants with environmental (nonorganic) FTT?*
3. *What, if any, laboratory studies should be part of the routine evaluation of FTT?*

# Neglect

The most common form of child abuse is neglect; more than 1 million cases of child neglect are reported annually. Neglect can be categorized as physical neglect, which includes medical neglect and failure to provide for common needs such as food, clothing, and shelter; emotional neglect; and educational neglect. Neglect of children is often insidious. It has many profoundly negative consequences and often goes unreported for months or years because of the lack of either positive physical findings or a specific crisis point. The forms of neglect seen most often in the emergency department are abandonment, medical neglect, and nonorganic failure to thrive (FTT).

## Abandonment

Abandonment is leaving a child without proper care or supervision in a situation in which harm can come to the child. There are no specific lengths of time or conditions dictated by society; thus, there must be value judgments made by the health care team in deciding when to initiate a report. Children who are abandoned must be thoroughly examined, assessed for signs of neglect such as malnutrition and dehydration, and reported to child welfare authorities. If there are no provisions for community-based emergency foster care, the child should be admitted to the hospital for protective care.

Some cases of abandonment involve newborn infants whose mothers might not have disclosed their pregnancies. Such infants might be rescued alive from trash receptacles and brought to the emergency department. In recent years, attention has focused on the enactment of safe haven laws, which allow a mother to surrender her newborn infant to hospital personnel or other designated individuals without the risk of criminal prosecution for abandonment.

## Medical Neglect

Medical neglect is a term indicating that, despite appropriate instructions from a health care provider, a parent fails to provide or obtain health services for a child. Because of this parental neglect, the child sustains injury, develops an illness, or has worsening of a medical condition. An example would involve the failure of parents to comply with recommendations for the care of a child's asthma. Such noncompliance can involve failed medical appointments, frequent visits to the emergency department, preventable hospitalizations, and even ICU admissions. Cases of medical neglect can be difficult to document, especially when parents change care providers. When medical neglect is encountered, the physician must file a report with a child protection agency.

## Failure to Thrive

Failure to thrive (FTT) is a disorder characterized by impairment of physical, emotional, and intellectual growth that occurs because of disturbances in the manner in which an infant or child is nourished and nurtured. The hallmark of the disorder is impairment of growth, with height or weight below the fifth percentile or normal height with low weight (low body mass index). Because many chronic medical disorders lead to impairment of physical growth, differentiate the child whose growth is related to environmental factors from the child with a medical problem, although the two conditions are not mutually exclusive.

### Clinical Features

Patients with FTT often present to the emergency department with complaints unrelated to the growth retardation. They also might be victims of physical or sexual abuse. They frequently have concurrent illnesses related to malnutrition, particularly gastroenteritis. An astute practitioner will recognize that a child is malnourished or too small for chronologic age. In all cases, refer to the growth chart, and plot the child's weight, length/height, and head circumference.

### Physical Examination

In an infant the physical examination might reveal findings of malnutrition, such as diminished subcutaneous tissue, thin extremities, and prominent ribs. A child's head might appear disproportionately large because weight and length are more greatly affected than head circumference. The examination might also reveal signs of dehydration. Infants with nonorganic FTT exhibit distinct behavioral characteristics. They often have a watchful, wary, wide-eyed gaze and avoid eye contact. They are hypertonic and dislike close interpersonal interactions, pulling away from the examiner. Observe mother-infant interactions to determine whether these are disturbed. Little vocalization occurs between such a mother and a nonthriving infant. Vocalization that does occur might be negative. A mother frequently will hold an infant at arm's length or leave the child unattended in an infant seat, on the floor, or on the examining table.

## Diagnostic Studies

There are no routine studies in the evaluation of the FTT infant.[31] Obtain studies as suggested by the history and physical findings. Routine health maintenance laboratory studies, such as a hemoglobin or lead level, are appropriate if these have not been obtained.

## Differential Diagnosis

The differential diagnosis of growth impairment is long and includes medical conditions such as genetic, cardiac, gastrointestinal, metabolic, endocrine, and infectious disorders, in addition to growth impairment attributable to a non-nurturing environment. The history and physical examination will suggest whether the condition is related to an in utero insult (maternal infection, drug or alcohol abuse), undernutrition, familial short stature, a specific medical condition, or environmental failure to thrive.

## Management

Infants and children suspected of having FTT might need admission to the hospital. Alternatively, appropriate management and investigative procedures can proceed in an outpatient setting. From 90% to 95% of infants and children with nonorganic FTT gain weight as expected after intervention. Some cases of nonorganic FTT can be reportable under state child abuse reporting laws.

---

**CASE SCENARIO 5**

A 7-year-old girl presents to the emergency department with the complaint of hematuria. The mother, who works as a medical assistant in a physician's office, reports that her daughter has a history of recurrent hematuria and has been worked up extensively in the past at different hospitals in different states. The etiology of the hematuria is unclear, though the daughter is usually treated with antibiotics. The mother has brought in a specimen of urine that appears pink-tinged. She states that if another urine specimen is needed, it should be obtained by catheterization, which the mother volunteers to do, stating she has done it multiple times in the past. The mother voices her concern that the daughter has a rare condition and she hopes that the doctors at your institution will finally be able to determine her problem.

1. *What are the various forms of Münchausen Syndrome by Proxy?*
2. *What approach is necessary to diagnose the condition?*

---

# Münchausen Syndrome By Proxy

Münchausen Syndrome by Proxy (MSBP) is the least common form of child abuse and was initially referred to as the "hinterland of child abuse." The condition was first reported in 1977 by Roy Meadows.[32] Alterative terms have been proposed for the condition, including induced or factitious illness or disorders, factitious disorder by proxy, and pediatric condition falsification.[33] Some evidence suggests that the condition is more common than previously suspected. One report estimated 600 new cases of MSBP involving suffocation and nonaccidental poisoning each year in the United States.[34]

There are, in fact, three different manifestations of MSBP, and these are not mutually exclusive. The types include fabricated, simulated, and induced illness. In the fabricated disorder, the caregiver simply lies about the symptoms. For example, a mother states that her infant has episodes when he stops breathing. In the simulated form, the mother alters laboratory specimens to simulate the findings that would be present if her child had the disease. For example, the mother adds blood (her own or from packaged meat from a butcher) to her child's urine specimen to simulate hematuria. The most dangerous form of MSBP occurs when a parent induces the symptoms in the child. For example, a parent claims that the child has recurrent fevers, and the parent injects the child with a pyrogenic agent such as DaPT. The parent, usually the mother, has access to material because of her job in a medical setting.

## Clinical Features

There are multiple conditions that can present as a manifestation of MSBP. As noted in the case scenario, a bleeding disorder is a common form of presentation. Other symptoms might include apnea, seizures, fever, electrolyte disturbances, allergies, gastrointestinal problems (pain, vomiting, diarrhea, constipation), and educational disabilities.

There are unifying aspects to the history in children with MSBP. Abnormal events such as seizures are usually not witnessed. Physicians have been unable to determine the etiology of the child's problem. The family has moved from one healthcare provider to another in search of answers. The parent is eager for more diagnostic studies, even ones that are invasive. In addition, the parent is a good historian, medically very knowledgeable, and eager to help.

MSBP should be differentiated from cases in which the parent represents the "worried well." These are parents whose children might have had minor illnesses such as ear infections or colds but then appear repeatedly at the physician's office for every minor illness or low-grade fever. Sometimes such parents became concerned during the course of a single illness when the child was subjected to a more extensive diagnostic evaluation such as a lumbar puncture. The parents then became concerned that other febrile illnesses might be indicative of a serious problem. Such parents benefit from an educational approach by an empathetic health care provider.

---

## YOUR FIRST CLUE

**Clinical Features of MSBP**

- Parent might be allied health professional.
- Child with frequent visits to health care often requiring diagnostic procedures.
- Parent medically knowledgeable, eager to help, and shows exaggerated concern.
- Child appears well.
- Multiple physicians cannot determine the etiology of the child's illness.

---

## Physical Examination

Findings on physical examination will vary with the alleged symptomology. Often, the child appears completely well despite the parent's complaints to the contrary. If the child's symptoms have been induced, or if the child has been subjected to invasive procedures such as the insertion of a gastrostomy tube or Broviac catheter, the presence of these devices will be apparent.

## Diagnostic Studies

Diagnostic studies are usually normal. For example, EEGs are normal in the face of MSBP and a history of seizures. Studies can be abnormal when disorders have been induced by the administration of certain agents, such as warfarin to induce a coagulopathy or insulin to induce hypoglycemia.

## Differential Diagnosis

The differential diagnosis includes all medical conditions that present with similar signs and symptoms of the factitious condition.

### Management

Diagnosing MSBP takes a skilled physician and a support team that involves psychologists, social workers, lawyers, law enforcement, and judges. Some institutions have installed covert video surveillance cameras to ensure the safety of the child and intervene if harm is imminent. The use of such cameras has revealed attempts by parents to suffocate infants hospitalized with a history of apnea.[35]

Establishing the diagnosis of MSBP is difficult. In addition, multiple physicians are often involved in the care of the child, including subspecialists and intensivists. Not infrequently, one member of the health care team remains skeptical that the child's problem is simulated, fabricated, or induced. This individual might align with the family and prevent the intervention necessary to ensure the safety of the child and the appropriate psychological services for the parents. The offending parent in a case of MSBP usually does not have a psychosis, but rather a personality disorder. The parent is narcissistic and relishes the attention he or she receives when serving as the historian about the child's illness.

There are multiple risks to the child from MSBP. Symptoms induced by the caregiver can cause permanent damage, disability, or even death. Likewise, invasive diagnostic tests ordered by the healthcare team might be traumatic. In addition, the psychological damage to the child is serious and potentially debilitating. Sometimes these children grow up believing they are invalids, or are unable to trust those closest to them, or both.

## WHAT ELSE?

**Differential Diagnosis of MSBP**
- Bleeding disorder
- Apnea
- Seizures
- Fever
- Electrolyte disturbances
- Metabolic disturbance (hypocalcemia, hyponatremia)
- Allergies
- Gastrointestinal problems (pain, vomiting, diarrhea, constipation)
- Educational disabilities

## Summary

The problems of child abuse and neglect are complex multifactorial issues of individual behavior, family function, and societal stresses. The physician cannot be expected to treat child abuse in the same way as an infectious illness; the management of abuse more closely resembles the treatment of a chronic disease, one that often requires many different therapists from different professional backgrounds and varied hospital-based and community agencies. However, no therapy can begin without recognition and reporting of the problem. In these tasks, the emergency physicians is unique and bears a heavy responsibility for being alert and sensitive and for having the courage to speak up on behalf of the child. Failure to do so unwittingly condones the abuse and positions the child for further injury, both physically and psychologically. The overriding principle to remember is that suspicion equals reporting and reporting equals help.

## THE BOTTOM LINE

- Problems of child maltreatment are complex and multifactorial.
- Management of the child requires multiple disciplines.
- Suspicion for child maltreatment must be reported.
- Reporting prevents further injury or death.

# CHAPTER REVIEW

## Check Your Knowledge

1. When assessing the history of a traumatic injury, which of the following factors should raise concern about inflicted trauma?
   A. History is inconsistent with the development level of the child
   B. Injury is alleged to have been inflicted by a young sibling
   C. Minor mishap has resulted in a major injury
   D. All of the above

2. Which of the following etiologies is the most common cause of death from inflicted trauma?
   A. Abusive head injury
   B. Burns
   C. Inflicted abdominal trauma
   D. Suffocation/strangulation

3. An infant with environmental FTT will manifest any of the following findings except:
   A. Growth impairment
   B. Impaired mother-infant interaction
   C. Skeletal dysplasia
   D. Watchful, wary gaze

4. Which of the following cases would be consistent with MSBP?
   A. Mother who administers Echinacea and goldenseal to her child for upper respiratory symptoms
   B. Mother who administers ipecac to her healthy child and complains about intractable vomiting
   C. Parents who refuse a blood transfusion for their hemorrhaging child because to do so conflicts with their religious beliefs
   D. Parents who refuse to administer insulin to their child with diabetes because to do so conflicts with their religious beliefs

## References

1. Department of Health and Human Services Releases 2000 Child Abuse Report Data. AHA Legislative Activities. American Humane Association. http://www.americanhumane.org/actnoww/2000_abuse_data.htm.
2. Jenny C, Hymel KP, Ritzen A et al. Analysis of missed cases of abusive head trauma. *JAMA.* 1999;281:621–626.
3. Sugar NF, Taylor JA, Feldman KW. Bruises in infants and toddlers: those who don't cruise don't bruise. *Arch Pediatr Adolesc Med.* 1999;153:399–403.
4. Schwartz AJ, Ricci LR. How accurately can bruises be aged in abused children? Literature review and synthesis. *Pediatrics* 1996;97:254–257.
5. Labbe J, Caouette G. Recent skin injuries in normal children. *Pediatrics.* 2001;108:271–276.
6. Jenny C. Cutaneous manifestations of child abuse. In: Reece RM, Ludwig S, eds. Child Abuse Medical Diagnosis and Management. 2nd ed. Philadelphia, Pa: Lippincott Williams & Wilkins; 2001:23–45.
7. Langlois NEI, Gresham GA. The aging of bruises: A review and study of the colour changes with time. *Forensic Science International.* 1991;50:227–238.
8. Hyden PW, Gallagher YA. Child abuse intervention in the emergency room. *Ped Clin of N America.* 1992;39:1053–1081.
9. Bruce DA, Zimmerman RA. Shaken impact syndrome. *Pediatr Annals.* 1989;18:482–494.
10. Reece RM, Sege R. Childhood head injuries–accidental or inflicted? *Arch Pediatr Adolesc Med.* 2000;154:11–15.
11. Levin A. Retinal haemorrhages and child abuse. *Recent Advances in Paediatrics.* 2000;18: 151–219.
12. Tarantino CA, Dowd D, Murdock TC. Short vertical falls in infants. *Pediatr Emerg Care.* 1999;15:5–8.
13. Lyons TJ, Oates RK. Falling out of bed: A relatively benign occurrence. *Pediatrics.* 1993;92: 125–127.
14. Joffe M, Ludwig S. Stairway injuries in children. *Pediatrics.* 1988;82:457–461.
15. Cooper A, Floyd T, Barlow B et al. Fifteen years experience with major blunt abdominal trauma due to child abuse. *J Trauma.* 1988;28:1483.
16. Ludwig S. Visceral injury manifestations of child abuse. In: Reece RM, Ludwig S, eds. Child Abuse Medical Diagnosis and Management. Philadelphia, Pa: Lippincott Williams & Wilkins; 2001:157–172.
17. Hennes HM, Smith DS et al. Elevated liver transaminase levels in children with blunt abdominal trauma: A predictor of liver injury. *Pediatrics.* 1990;86(1):87–90.
18. Thomas SA, Rosenfield NS, Leventhal JM, Markowitz RI. Long-bone fractures in young children: Distinguishing accidental injuries from child abuse. *Pediatrics.* 1991;88: 471–476.

**19.** Bullock B, Schubert CJ, Brophy PD, Johnson N, Reed MH, Shapiro RA. Cause and clinical characteristics of rib fractures in infants. *Pediatrics.* 2000;105:e48.

**20.** Boos S. Personal communication.2002.

**21.** Limbos MA, Berkowitz CD. Documentation of child physical abuse: How far have we come? *Pediatrics.* 1998;102:53–58.

**22.** Hymel KP, Jenny C. Child sexual abuse. *Pediatr in Review.* 1996;17:236–249.

**23.** Heger AH, Ticson L Guerra L et al. Appearance of the genitalia in girls selected for nonabuse: Review of hymenal morphology and nonspecific findings. *J Pediatr Adolesc Gynecol.* 2002;15:27–35.

**24.** Santucci KA, Nelson DG, McQuillen KK et al. Wood's lamp utility in the identification of semen. *Pediatrics.* 1999;104:1342–1344.

**25.** State of California Office of Criminal Justice Planning. Office of Criminal Justice Planning 925, revised 7/1/01, p 6.

**26.** Poirier, MP. CME review article: Care of the female adolescent rape victim. *Pediatr Emerg Care.* 2002;18:53–59.

**27.** Koss, MP, Gidycz CA, Wisinewski N. The scope of rape: Incidence and prevalence of sexual aggression and victimization in a national sample of higher education students. *J Consult Clin Psychol.* 1987;55:162–170.

**28.** Davis TC, Peck GQ, Storment JM. Acquaintance rape and the high school student. *J Adolesc Health.* 1993;14:220–224.

**29.** Slaughter L, Brown CRV, Crowley S, Peck R. Patterns of genital injury in female sexual assault victims. *Am J Obstet Gynecol.* 1997;176:609–616.

**30.** Merchant RC, Keshavarz R. Human immunodeficiency virus postexposure prophylaxis for adolescents and children. *Pediatrics.* 2001;108:e38.

**31.** Berkowitz CD. Failure to thrive, In: Berkowitz, CD, ed. *Pediatrics: A Primary Care Approach.* 2nd ed. Philadelphia, Pa: W.B. Saunders; 2000.

**32.** Meadows R. Münchausen syndrome by proxy: The hinterland of child abuse. *Lancet.* 1977;2:343–345.

**33.** Ayoub CC, Alexander R, Beck D et al. APSAC Taskforce on Münchausen by Proxy, Definitions Working Group. Position paper: definitional issues in Münchausen by proxy. *Child Maltreatment.* 2002;7(2):105–111.

**34.** McClure RJ, Davis PM, Meadows SR et al. Epidemiology of Münchausen Syndrome by Proxy on non-accidental suffocation and non-accidental poisoning. *Arch Dis Child.* 1996;75:57–61.

**35.** Southall DP, Plunkett MCB, Banks MW et al. Covert video recordings of life-threatening child abuse: Lessons for child protection. *Pediatrics.* 1997;100:735–760.

# CHAPTER REVIEW

A 3-year-old boy is referred to the emergency department from his preschool because he has bruises on his face, left pinna, and lower back. The parents say the child is very active and frequently falls.

1. *What bruises commonly result from accidental injury, and what bruises suggest inflicted trauma?*
2. *What are the appropriate diagnostic studies to evaluate suspected child physical abuse? How does the child's age affect what studies are obtained?*
3. *If inflicted trauma is suspected, what agencies must be notified to assist in the investigation?*

On further evaluation, this 3-year-old has a large purple hematoma of his left pinna, four red linear oval marks on his left cheek that appear consistent with a handprint, and a yellow green hematoma measuring 5 × 5 cm on the upper part of the left buttock. There is also a circumferential bruise on the glans of the penis. When questioned by himself, the child states: "Daddy say me bad boy. Me make peepee. Daddy very mad. Me very bad." The CBC, PT, PTT, and platelet counts are all normal. The child also undergoes a skeletal survey, which does not reveal any fractures.

This child's injuries involve the ears and nonbony areas and are all consistent with inflicted trauma. The circumferential injury on the glans of the penis suggests a pinchmark, a not uncommon injury associated with inappropriate punishment for toilet-training accidents. The child's statements would corroborate this conclusion.

Law enforcement and child protective services should be notified about the findings. In addition, the parents need to be advised about the physician's concerns and obligation as a mandated reporter to notify the appropriate agencies.

A 5-year-old girl presents to the emergency department with the complaint of blood on her panties. There is no history of trauma, but the mother states that the daughter often has a yellow stain on her panties. The mother denies any concern about sexual abuse. You are unable to question the girl independently because she is frightened and will not separate from her mother. She will allow an examination if her mother stays with her. The physical examination is normal except for findings in the anogenital area. She is sexual maturity rating 1. The hymen is irregular with fleshy lesions that appear friable on its edge. There is blood on the panties but no frank bleeding. The anal examination is normal.

1. *What are the common causes of anogenital bleeding in children?*
2. *What are the pitfalls in obtaining a history from a child related to sexual abuse?*
3. *What physical findings are associated with acute and prior sexual abuse?*
4. *What is the significance of a sexually transmitted disease in a prepubescent child?*

There are a number of causes of anogenital bleeding in children. In this case the presence of fleshy lesions suggests venereal warts. The lesions in the child's genital area are most consistent with condyloma acuminatum. You obtain additional studies for other sexually transmitted diseases (gonorrhea, *Chlamydia*, syphilis and HIV), which are negative. The case is reported as suspected child sexual abuse to child protective services.

Pitfalls center around the child's age and lack of maturity, and also that the child might not understand that the molestation is wrong. Children also want to please and might answer yes to specific questions; this is why it is best to ask open-ended questions so the child must respond without being prompted. The child subsequently undergoes a forensic interview and discloses that she has been molested by her father for 1 year.

Children have a great capacity to heal injury in the anogenital area. Signs of chronic abuse, depending on the type of abuse, can be subtle and include paucity of hymenal tissue, scarring, and loss of the normal rugal pattern to the anus, or results could be entirely normal.

The presence of a sexually transmitted disease beyond the neonatal period should be presumed secondary to sexual abuse, and a report should be made.

Police cars bring a 14-year-old girl to the ED. She reports that she was walking home from school when a car pulled up, two men grabbed her, and pulled her into the car. She states that they took her to a house and dragged her up a flight of stairs. One man pointed a gun at her and stood laughing and talking while the second one pulled off her pants and raped her. Then the first man raped her while the second stood holding the gun. She reports no oral or anal penetration, and no condom use. She states that, some time later, the men left the house, allowing her to escape and call the police. When her mother arrives, she states that her daughter is always lying and made up this story to avoid getting into trouble for having sex.

1. *What are the medical treatment priorities for this patient?*
2. *When should HIV prophylaxis be considered?*
3. *The mother refuses to provide consent for the emergency care of her daughter. How should the emergency physician proceed?*

The 14-year-old girl was forcibly raped against her will and able to describe genital contact made by two male perpetrators. ED management priorities include reassurance and support for the patient, a complete physical exam, careful inspection of the genital area (which revealed acute abrasions of the fossa and posterior fourchette), thorough documentation of the history provided and exam findings, completion of the forensic kit and transfer of the kit to the crime lab, STD and pregnancy prophylaxis, and reporting to law enforcement. The mother provides no consent for the emergency care, but in the state where this assault occurred, state statutes support the adolescent's desire to seek medical care after sexual assault without parental consent.

# CHAPTER REVIEW

This patient also presents a difficult problem with PEP against HIV. Assaulted by multiple perpetrators, strong consideration is given to starting therapy. The biggest challenge to proceeding with the 30-day PEP regimen however, is a frequent failure of adolescent rape victims to comply with the therapy. Given the mother's lack of support demonstrated in the ED, the patient is unlikely to find the parental support for necessary followup medical care. Careful assessment of the maturity of the patient and her capacity to understand the treatment, its benefits and ill effects, and communication with an alternative supportive adult in the teen's life, will prove invaluable in the care of this patient. Additional consideration is usually given to the background rate of HIV in the community in which the assault occurred.

A 3-month-old boy with a fever for 1 day is brought to the emergency department by his mother. The mother reports that he is a good eater, taking six to seven 8-ounce bottles of formula a day. The infant is the mother's fourth child. A review of the past medical history reveals that the infant was at the 50th percentile for weight and length at birth and was full term. On physical examination, the infant is now below the 5th percentile for weight and at the 50th percentile for height and head circumference. The temperature is 37.4°C. The infant is apathetic, appears hypertonic, and avoids eye contact. There is mild rhinorrhea, but the throat, ears, and lungs are clear. There is a moderate diaper rash and caked stool in the diaper area. The infant is also dirty and smells like stale milk.

1. *What physical findings are noted with failure to thrive (FTT)?*
2. *What are the interactional characteristics of infants with environmental (nonorganic) FTT?*
3. *What, if any, laboratory studies should be part of the routine evaluation of FTT?*

The infant's length and head circumference are normal at the 50th percentile, but the weight is less than 5th percentile. The infant is apathetic and avoids eye contact. Laboratory studies reveal a normal CBC, chemistries, and urinalysis. A home assessment reveals there are limited financial resources and inadequate food. The family is living in an apartment without heat or hot water. The mother feels completely overwhelmed by the situation. Her husband has been unemployed and drinks heavily. She has no one to help her with the children.

Protective services is contacted. They institute a program geared toward family preservation. The family is placed on a waiting list for adequate housing. The three oldest children are enrolled in Head Start. Formula is obtained for the infant, and the family is referred to the food stamp program.

**CASE SUMMARY 5**

7-year-old girl presents to the emergency department with the complaint of hematuria. The mother, who works as a medical assistant in a physician's office, reports that her daughter has a history of recurrent hematuria and has been worked up extensively in the past at different hospitals in different states. The etiology of the hematuria is unclear, though the daughter is usually treated with antibiotics. The mother has brought in a specimen of urine that appears pink-tinged. She states that if another urine specimen is needed, it should be obtained by catheterization, which the mother volunteers to do, stating she has done it multiple times in the past. The mother voices her concern that the daughter has a rare condition and she hopes that the doctors at your institution will finally be able to determine her problem.

1. *What are the various forms of Münchausen Syndrome by Proxy?*
2. *What approach is necessary to diagnose the condition?*

There are three types of Münchausen Syndrome by Proxy, which include fabricated, simulated, and induced illness. In this case, the illness is fabricated by the mother. The urine sample brought in by the mother tests positive for blood. The medical staff requests a fresh specimen. The child is allowed to void into a cup under the direct observation of the nursing staff. The mother is asked to wait outside the restroom. The urine specimen is free of blood. The daughter denies any urine symptoms.

In this case, the approach to establish the diagnosis begins with suspicion of the syndrome. Asking the mother to wait outside the restroom was critical in order to establish that the child indeed has no hematuria. Social service is consulted and prior medical records are requested. The case is referred to child protective services once the records are received and reveal that the child has been seen on 58 different occasions at 32 different hospitals. She has undergone three renal biopsies and multiple different diagnostic studies, all of which have been negative for a cause of hematuria or an underlying medical disorder.

# chapter 11

# Nontraumatic Surgical Emergencies

Pamela J. Okada, MD
Barry A. Hicks, MD

## Objectives

1 Describe the common causes of rectal bleeding in infants with abdominal distention.

2 Recognize that bilious emesis in an infant is a surgical emergency and that malrotation with midgut volvulus must be evaluated and treated immediately.

3 Describe the classic triad of intussusception and recognize that intussusception can present with lethargy.

4 Describe the common causes of testicular pain.

5 Describe the common causes of inguinal or scrotal masses.

6 Establish and discuss the clinical features and emergency management of several important acute surgical disorders in children.

## Chapter Outline

Necrotizing Enterocolitis
Malrotation and Midgut Volvulus
Pyloric Stenosis
Intussusception
Meckel Diverticulum
Testicular Torsion
Pediatric Inguinal Hernia
Appendicitis

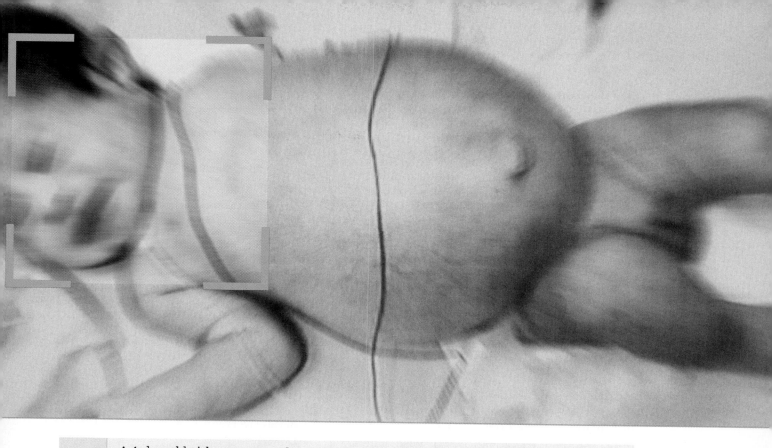

**CASE SCENARIO 1**

A 4-day-old girl presents to the emergency department after an episode of bloody stools and increasing abdominal distention. She has not been feeding well and is sleeping between feedings. She was born at 34 weeks gestation by emergency cesarean delivery because the mother had pregnancy-induced hypertension. The infant did well after delivery and was discharged to home. She had been taking commercial formula every 3 hours, but the past 6 hours has not been feeding at all and has been more lethargic.

On physical examination, the infant is afebrile, with a respiratory rate of 45 breaths per minute and a heart rate of 180 beats per minute (bpm). Head, neck, lung, and heart examinations are normal except for tachycardia. The abdomen is distended; the overlying skin is mildly shiny and erythematous, and bowel sounds are hypoactive. Femoral pulses are present, but capillary refill to the lower extremities is delayed. A stool sample obtained from the diaper is positive for blood.

1. *What could be the cause of rectal bleeding and abdominal distention in this neonate?*
2. *What diagnostic tests could be helpful?*

## Necrotizing Enterocolitis

Necrotizing enterocolitis (NEC) is an acquired neonatal disorder characterized by necrosis of the mucosal and submucosal layers of the gastrointestinal tract. The pathologic hallmarks of NEC are coagulation necrosis, inflammation, and hemorrhage in the involved segment of intestine. NEC is primarily a disease of premature, low birth weight infants and usually presents in the immediate newborn period.

During the 1960s, the incidence of NEC rose dramatically, reflecting the advent of neonatal intensive care units (NICUs). More premature infants were surviving previously fatal pulmonary disease and becoming susceptible to NEC.[1-3]

The origin of NEC is multifactorial. Risk factors of the premature infant include bacterial colonization, intestinal ischemia, hypoxia, and formula feeding with hypertonic formulas or rapid feeding regimens. All of these promote mucosal destruction and stimulate pro-inflammatory mediators that lead to bowel infarction and necrosis. NEC is still recognized as an important cause of morbidity and mortality and continues to be the most common indication for emergency gastrointestinal surgery in the newly born.

Although NEC is considered a disease of the premature, low birth weight infant, it occasionally affects the term newborn infant as well.[4-7] Full-term infants at risk are those with a history of congenital heart disease, perinatal asphyxia, hypoglycemia, polycythemia, respiratory distress, maternal cocaine use, maternal pregnancy-induced hypertension,[4,6–8] or umbilical artery catheters.

In 1978, Bell et al[9] developed a system for the diagnosis of NEC and grading severity of disease. The three-part staging system classified infants as stage I (suspect), stage II (definite), or stage III (advanced) disease. The staging system was later modified to include clinical, gastrointestinal, and radiographic findings and treatment recommendations based on staging of disease.[10]

### Epidemiology

NEC is the most common gastrointestinal emergency seen in the NICU, occurring in 3% to 5% of all admitted infants, or in 1 to 3 per 1,000 live births.[1,11] The more immature the infant at birth, the greater the risk of acquiring NEC. There is no consistent association between sex, race, or socioeconomic status and NEC incidence.

Full-term infants are at low risk for NEC, but between 5% and 25% of all cases of NEC occur in term infants.[4-7] In this group of infants, NEC typically develops within the first few days of life, whereas premature infants are at a prolonged risk and usually develop NEC between the seventh and 14th day of life, and occasionally as late as the third week of life.[4,6]

### Clinical Features

The clinical presentation of a full-term infant with NEC is similar to the preterm neonate and can resemble sepsis. Subtle signs can in-

clude abdominal distention, feeding intolerance, delayed gastric emptying, jaundice, and a change in stooling pattern. More ominous signs and symptoms include abdominal tenderness, bilious emesis, grossly bloody stools, oliguria, hypotension, lethargy, temperature instability, apneic episodes, and respiratory distress.

### Complications

A delay in the diagnosis of NEC can lead to perforation, sepsis, profound metabolic acidosis, disseminated intravascular coagulopathy, respiratory failure, cardiovascular collapse, and death. Unfortunately, with the sudden-onset form of NEC, these complications can occur despite rapid diagnosis and intervention.[12]

The mortality rate from NEC in the full-term infant is 5% compared to 12% to 45% in preterm infants.[4,8,13-16] Long-term complications include intestinal strictures and adhesions (10% to 35%), which can result in bowel

| TABLE 11-1 | Causes of Gastrointestinal Bleeding and Abdominal Distention in the Newborn Infant | | |
|---|---|---|---|
| | | Abdominal Distention | Rectal Bleeding |
| • Swallowed maternal blood | | | + |
| • Hemorrhagic disease of the newborn | | | + |
| • Malrotation with volvulus | | + | + |
| • Intestinal infection | | + | + |
| • Neonatal pseudomembranous colitis | | | + |
| • Necrotizing enterocolitis | | + | + |
| • Hirschsprung disease and associated enterocolitis | | + | + |
| • Cow's milk or soy protein intolerance | | +/− | + |
| • Anal fissure | | | + |
| –Nonaccidental trauma | | | + |
| –Sepsis with intestinal ileus | | + | + |

obstruction, short bowel syndrome (malabsorption syndrome), bacterial overgrowth and life-threatening sepsis, electrolyte and water loss from the ileostomy, or cholestasis secondary to prolonged total parenteral nutrition (TPN) administration.[10,14,17]

## Diagnostic Studies

### Laboratory

Laboratory studies are nonspecific. Stool samples can show occult blood or be grossly bloody. There are numerous causes of gastrointestinal bleeding in the newly born infant.[18-20] However, most of the etiologies are not associated with abdominal distention (Table 11-1).

In more severe illnesses, blood analysis can show respiratory and metabolic acidosis, neutropenia, thrombocytopenia, and evidence of disseminated intravascular coagulopathy. The full-term infant might even show a leukocytosis with a polymorphonuclear predominance. The clinical picture of NEC is similar to the sepsis syndrome, and laboratory studies might help differentiate the two (Table 11-2).

Serum markers, such as plasma intestinal fatty acid binding protein,[21] are currently under investigation to determine their potential for early detection and treatment of NEC. To date there is no consensus on the utility of laboratory markers. Clinical judgment is still the most sensitive and specific indicator of disease.

| TABLE 11-2 | Laboratory Studies to Consider in an Infant with NEC |
|---|---|

- Complete blood cell (CBC) count with differential
- Blood culture
- Electrolytes
- Blood urea nitrogen
- Creatinine
- Glucose
- Cerebrospinal fluid analysis and culture
- Stool for occult blood
- Stool for culture
- Prothrombin time/partial thromboplastin time
- Fibrin split products
- Fibrinogen
- Arterial blood gas
- Urinalysis, urine culture

### Radiography

Plain abdominal radiograph might reveal an ileus, a persistent loop of bowel, pneumatosis intestinalis, portal venous gas, or a gasless abdomen (Figure 11.1 A and B). Two pathognomonic diagnostic radiographic signs are pneumatosis intestinalis (the formation of intramural intestinal gas) and intrahepatic portal venous gas. Portal venous gas (PVG) can be a fleeting radiographic finding, but when

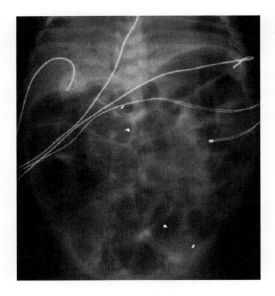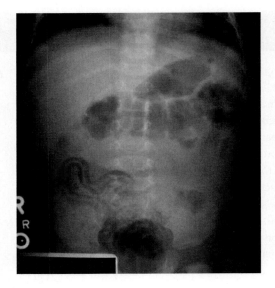

**Figure 11.1 A, B** Examples of pneumatosis intestinalis. In these abdominal radiographs of different patients with NEC, note the gas bubbles located within the bowel wall. This is known as intramural air and is sometimes described as railroad tracks because the inner and outer mucosal walls are separated by the air, giving it an appearance of two parallel lines. The white arrows point this out in 11.1A; 11.1B shows a term infant with impressive pneumatosis intestinalis.

## THE CLASSICS

**Classic Laboratory and Radiographic Findings of NEC**

- Metabolic acidosis
- Neutropenia
- Thrombocytopenia
- Pneumatosis intestinalis
- Intrahepatic portal venous gas
- Pneumoperitoneum

present signifies serious disease (Bell stage II) (**Figure 11.2**). Although PVG can be seen on plain film abdominal radiographs as in Figure 11.2, it can be more easily seen using hepatic ultrasonography.

Pneumoperitoneum is seen in advanced disease (Bell stage III) and signifies bowel perforation (**Figure 11.3**). On a supine radiograph, free air is seen centrally and appears as a vertically aligned ellipse, called the football sign. On a left lateral decubitus radiograph, free air is seen between the liver and the abdominal wall. On a cross-table lateral radiograph, free air is seen anteriorly and is distributed evenly over the entire abdomen. All of these findings occur less frequently in full-term infants.[13,14,22]

**Magnetic Resonance Imaging**

Recently, magnetic resonance imaging (MRI) has come under study as to its use in the diagnosis of intestinal necrosis in the premature infant suspicious for NEC.[23] Areas of intestinal necrosis found at laparotomy corresponded to bubble-like formations in the intestinal segments on MRI. From a logistic standpoint, obtaining an MRI in a premature infant can be prohibitively difficult. Detection of NEC by MRI in the full-term infant might be more feasible but is rarely necessary.

## Differential Diagnosis

The differential diagnosis of NEC includes sepsis with intestinal ileus, intestinal infection, spontaneous bowel perforation (colon, ileum,

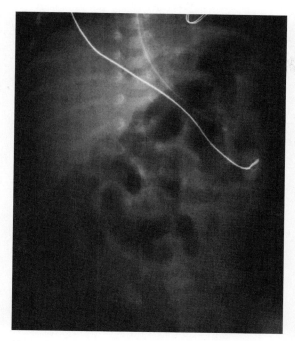

Figure 11.2 Portal venous gas (PVG). Note the tiny air densities superimposed over the liver. These air densities are gas bubbles within the portal venous system or the biliary tree.

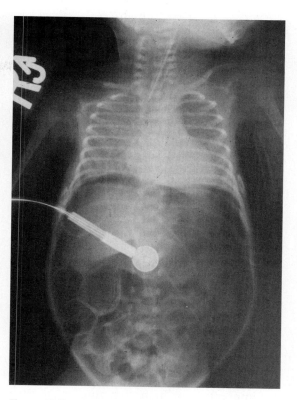

Figure 11.3 Pneumoperitoneum in an infant with NEC. The amount of intraperitoneal air is extensive in this radiograph. Small amounts of free air can be difficult to identify on plain radiographs, especially if taken as a flat plate. Small amounts of free intra-abdominal air can be best seen on an upright, lateral decubitus or a cross-table lateral view.

or stomach), malrotation with volvulus, Hirschsprung disease, neonatal appendicitis, neonatal pseudomembranous colitis, and nonaccidental trauma.

## WHAT ELSE?

**Differential Diagnosis of NEC**
- Sepsis with intestinal ileus
- Intestinal infection
- Spontaneous bowel perforation
- Intestinal obstruction
- Malrotation with volvulus
- Hirschsprung disease
- Neonatal appendicitis
- Neonatal pseudomembranous colitis
- Nonaccidental trauma

## Management

**Emergency Department and Followup Care**
The treatment for uncomplicated NEC (no stricture or perforation) is medical management. Current treatment recommendations are to place an orogastric tube for low intermittent suction, administer broad-spectrum antibiotics (Gram-positive, Gram-negative, and anaerobic coverage is recommended), and stop oral feedings for 10 to 14 days. Hypotension is treated with crystalloid, blood products, and pressors. Ventilation should be assisted if abdominal distention impairs ventilation and oxygenation or for evidence of

sepsis (hypotension, metabolic acidosis). Nutritional support is provided by TPN. This nonsurgical management is successful in 75% of patients.[15] Surgical intervention is indicated if there is evidence of perforation or intestinal necrosis. Relative indications for surgery include clinical deterioration, refractory acidosis, oliguria, hypotension, persistent thrombocytopenia, ventilatory failure, PVG, a fixed dilated loop of bowel, or erythema of the abdominal wall. Surgical interventions include laparotomy with resection and proximal end ostomy, or laparotomy with resection and primary anastomosis, and rarely, peritoneal drainage.[15,24]

### What to Avoid and Why

Failure to recognize that full-term infants can develop NEC is the first problem to avoid. Aggressive early intervention in the term infant has offered a favorable prognosis, with survival rates exceeding 90%.[6]

Avoid relying on systemic findings (such as temperature or hemodynamic instability) or metabolic derangements (such as metabolic acidosis) as determining factors for early surgical intervention. These findings are not reliable early indicators of the extent of disease in the term infant. A number of term infants with pneumoperitoneum or obstruction are otherwise stable but have extensive and advanced disease at laparotomy. It is thought that the term infant has a greater physiologic reserve than the preterm infant, and a low threshold for early laparotomy will improve prognosis.[6]

### Controversies in Management

There are several controversies in the management of NEC, including type and length of intravenous antibiotic coverage, surgical indications (relative versus absolute[9,10]), type of surgical intervention (laparotomy with resection and proximal stoma formation[13] versus laparotomy with resection and primary anastomosis[14]), peritoneal drainage,[15] timing of feeding once the infant is clinically well (10 days versus 14 days of nothing by mouth), and even refeeding formulas (electrolyte solutions versus diluted or full-strength formulas) and regimens (bolus versus continuous feedings).

> ## THE BOTTOM LINE
>
> NEC should be considered as a potential diagnosis in term infants who present with signs of sepsis syndrome. Begin resuscitation with fluids and contact a surgeon early.

**CASE SCENARIO 2**

A 4-week-old boy arrives with a 1-day history of decreased activity and vomiting. The infant is breastfed and has had no difficulty nursing but has vomited intermittently. Over the past 3 hours, the infant has vomited frequently. The last few episodes of vomiting were green in color. The birth history was uncomplicated. The infant was a full-term and born by spontaneous vaginal delivery.

On physical examination, the infant is lethargic, pale, and grunting. His respiratory rate is 60 breaths per minute, heart rate is 190 bpm, blood pressure is 80/60 mmHg, and rectal temperature is 36°C . The anterior fontanel is sunken. The lungs are clear to auscultation, but occasional grunting sounds are noted. Abdominal examination reveals decreased bowel sounds, and the abdomen is distended and tender to palpation. The genital examination is normal. The extremities are mottled with poor perfusion.

1. *What important cause of bilious emesis in an infant must be excluded immediately?*
2. *What is the radiographic study of choice in the evaluation of an infant with bilious emesis?*
3. *Why must the evaluation of an infant with bilious emesis be done emergently?*

# Malrotation and Midgut Volvulus

Malrotation of the midgut occurs when the normal rotational process and fixation of the intestine fail to occur during gestation. Lack of fixation of the small bowel results in obstructing peritoneal adhesive bands (Ladd bands) forming between the cecum and the right abdominal wall. These Ladd bands cause compression of the duodenum and mechanical obstruction (**Figure 11.4**).

A second and far more serious cause of bowel obstruction is malrotation complicated by midgut volvulus (**Figure 11.5**). The small bowel is suspended on a narrow pedicle (containing the superior mesenteric artery), and the small bowel can twist around this narrow axis, resulting in torsion of the entire midgut. This is a surgical emergency because small bowel necrosis can occur in 1 to 2 hours.[25] Midgut volvulus occurs in 70% of infants with malrotation.[26]

The term malrotation focuses attention on the embryology of the defect instead of the anatomic malformation itself. In a normal patient, the small bowel is suspended by mesentery, which is attached to the abdominal wall as a broad fan, and is too broad to twist (**Figure 11.6**). In malrotation, this attachment is a narrow stalk, making it prone to twisting (Figures 11.4 and 11.5). A twist of this stalk results in catastrophic bowel ischemia, which results in infarction unless it is immediately detorsed surgically. This midgut volvulus should be distinguished from sigmoid volvulus, which largely occurs in elderly adults. Malrotation might more accurately be called "guts on a stalk" to stress the anatomy of the malformation and its consequence rather than its embryology.

## Epidemiology

The incidence of malrotation is 1 in 500 live births.[27] Between 25% and 40% of patients with symptomatic malrotation present within the first week of life, an additional 10% (50% total) present within the first month; 75% to 90% present prior to 1 year of age, and the remaining present after 1 year of age. The identification of malrotation after 1 year of age is

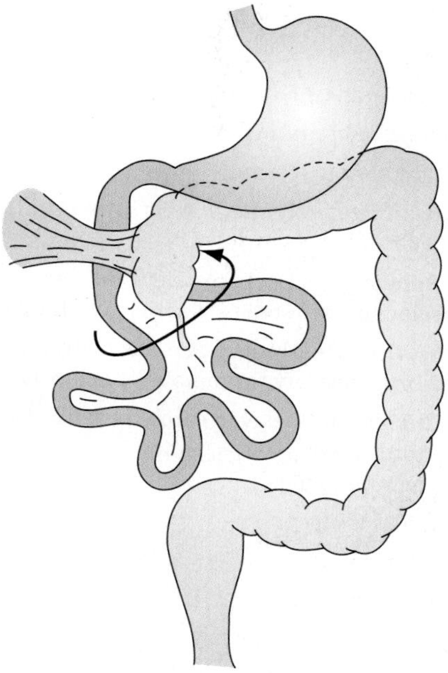

**Figure 11.4** Ladd bands compression of the duodenum. This diagram shows the mesenteric stalk-like attachment of the cecum (Ladd bands) in the malrotation malformation, which can cause a bowel obstruction by compressing the duodenum.

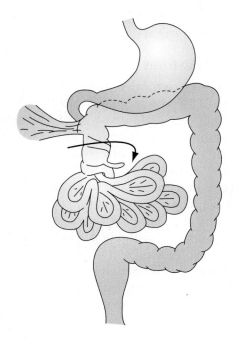

**Figure 11.5** Midgut volvulus. This diagram depicts the catastrophic nature of a midgut volvulus, which results in ischemia and subsequent infarction of most of the small bowel as it twists around its stalk-like mesenteric attachment in the malrotation malformation.

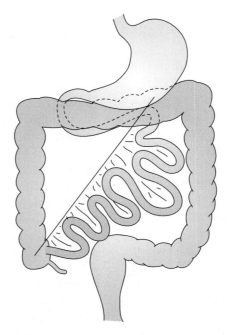

**Figure 11.6** Representation of the normal mesenteric bowel suspension. Note that its attachment is broad, preventing the bowel from twisting on itself.

evenly distributed throughout childhood and is found incidentally in adulthood. There is a 2:1 male predominance in cases presenting in the neonatal period.[27] Mortality from malrotation ranges from 4% to 8%.[28,29]

## Clinical Features

Malrotation typically presents in the first month of life with feeding intolerance, bilious vomiting, and, less consistently, sudden onset of abdominal pain (crying). Bilious emesis is usually the first sign of volvulus and is present in 77% to 100% of cases.[26] Older infants and children can present with vague, nonspecific symptoms such as chronic, intermittent vomiting and cramping abdominal pain, failure to thrive, constipation, bloody diarrhea, and hematemesis.[28,29]

Physical examination might include a normal abdominal examination in 50% to 60% of patients.[26,30] One third of patients present with abdominal distention without tenderness. As intestinal ischemia progresses to necrosis, bowel distention, abdominal pain, and evidence of peritonitis develop. As ischemia progresses to infarction, fever, erythema, and edema of the abdominal wall, peritonitis and abdominal distention worsen, and profound dehydration and vascular collapse occur.

## Complications

In the neonate, volvulus can rapidly result in significant bowel ischemia with abdominal distention, bloody stools, and eventually hypovolemia, shock, and peritonitis. Short of death, intestinal infarction of the entire midgut (nearly all of the small bowel) is the most serious complication of this condition,[28] which is not compatible with survival without lifelong parenteral hyperalimentation or small bowel transplantation.

## Diagnostic Studies

### Laboratory

Laboratory studies are not particularly helpful in the diagnosis of malrotation and midgut volvulus.

### Radiology

Plain films of the abdomen can be normal or can reveal proximal gastric or duodenal distention with or without distal intraluminal air.

On an upright film, triangular gas shadows in the right upper quadrant are produced as the liver edge overlies the air-filled duodenum. This pattern, called the duodenal triangle, has been reported as a plain film sign of midgut volvulus in the neonate.[31]

Malrotation with or without midgut volvulus cannot be excluded by a normal plain radiograph. A limited upper gastrointestinal contrast study, designed to visualize the duodenum and proximal jejunum, is the most reliable method to diagnose malrotation. The malrotated duodenum is often coiled (as in a midgut volvulus) to the right of the midline, giving a corkscrew appearance as seen in Figure 11.7. A cutoff appearance of the contrast ("beak") suggests obstruction from the volvulus.

It is important to identify a malrotation even in the absence of a midgut volvulus. Patients with malrotation are at risk of midgut volvulus later in life. The hallmark radiographic criterion for malrotation is failure of the ligament of Treitz, or the duodenal-jejunal flexure, to cross to the left of the midline.[32] Barium enema and ultrasonography might identify anomalous anatomic findings such as

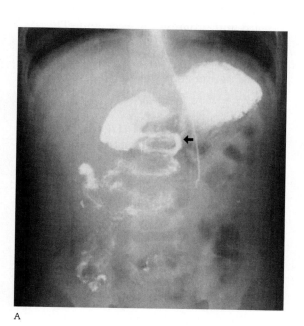

A

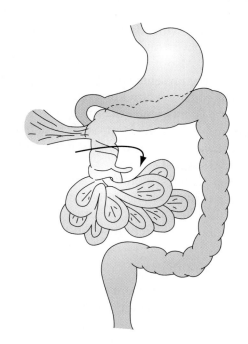

B

**Figure 11.7A, B** Corkscrew appearance of midgut volvulus. The diagram depicts the midgut volvulus. Thin barium permits the coil of the volvulus to be visualized. In other instances, the upper GI contrast will be simply obstructed and the coil will not be visualized.

**Diagnostic Studies for Evaluation of Midgut Volvulus**

Limited upper gastrointestinal (GI) contrast study: The duodenum is coiled (midgut volvulus), or the duodenal-jejunal junction is malpositioned (malrotation).

**Differential Diagnosis of Midgut Volvulus**

- Duodenal web, stenosis, atresia
- Hirschsprung disease
- Meconium ileus
- Imperforate anus
- Intussusception
- Incarcerated inguinal hernia

a nonfixed cecum or an abnormally oriented superior mesenteric artery, but these findings are not as reliable as the abnormally fixed ligament of Treitz on contrast study.

## Differential Diagnosis

The differential diagnosis for the infant with bilious emesis includes duodenal webs, duodenal stenosis, duodenal atresia, and any intestinal obstruction distal to the Ampulla of Vater. Such obstructions include incarcerated inguinal hernia, Hirschsprung disease, meconium ileus, intestinal atresias, and imperforate anus in the young infant, and intussusception in the older infant. However, it is important to remember that an infant with bilious emesis could have a malrotation with midgut volvulus until proved otherwise. Also note that a midgut volvulus infrequently presents with nonbilious emesis.

The phenomenon known as intermittent volvulus occurs when the midgut twists and then untwists on its own. Such patients can present with a history of one or more previous episodes suggestive of an early midgut volvulus, that resolves. Identifying a malrotation in such patients is challenging but beneficial in that it can be corrected before a catastrophic midgut bowel infarction occurs.

## Management

### Emergency Department

Evaluation, resuscitation, surgical consultation, and preoperative preparation proceed simultaneously in patients with suspected malrotation with volvulus. In the emergency department, volume resuscitation, gastric decompression, and broad-spectrum antibiotics are administered.

The surgical procedure for the correction of malrotation, called the Ladd procedure, includes detorsion of the volvulus, division of Ladd bands, separation of the duodenojejunal mesentery from the cecocolic mesentery, and appendectomy. An appendectomy is performed because the colon is positioned on the left side of the abdomen during a Ladd procedure. Subsequent diagnosis of appendicitis could be difficult. A gastrostomy is seldom indicated.

The incidence and type of complications that occur reflect the extent of ischemic bowel and intestinal necrosis found at surgery. With a viable intestine, postoperative care is straightforward and prognosis is excellent. The lifetime risk of adhesive small bowel obstruction is 1% to 10%.[27] Volvulus should not recur once the malrotation is corrected.

With extensive ischemic bowel and intestinal necrosis, the bowel is untwisted and reduced into the abdominal cavity, and 12 to 24 hours later, a "second look" procedure can be performed to assess bowel viability. This allows the surgeon to resect the necrotic bowel and to create an enterostomy at the distal end of the proximal normal bowel. Bowel reconstruction is performed at a later operation. With extensive bowel resection, patients can develop short gut syndrome and might become dependent on TPN.

### What to Avoid and Why

In the management of an otherwise healthy infant with bilious vomiting, a delay in diagnosis must be avoided. Delay can lead to the most serious complication, volvulus with necrosis of the entire midgut. In an acutely ill infant suspected to have malrotation with volvulus, time-consuming studies might be best replaced by laparotomy itself. In an otherwise stable infant, an emergency limited upper GI contrast study should be performed quickly.

### Controversies in Management

Malrotation found incidentally in asymptomatic children should be repaired, but the timing of surgery remains controversial.

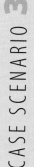

**CASE SCENARIO 3**

A 3-week-old female infant presents with a 4-day history of projectile vomiting. She is a full-term product of a vaginal delivery. There were no complications at birth. For the first 2 weeks of life, the infant would occasionally spit up (normal for age). Currently, the vomiting is very forceful, as if it will "hit the wall." The infant is breastfed, and the vomit appears to be breast milk. There is no history of blood or green-colored emesis, diarrhea, or fever. The mother is frustrated because the infant is losing weight and appears hungry.

On physical examination, the infant is dehydrated, with a sunken fontanel and poor skin turgor. Her respiratory rate is 24 breaths per minute, heart rate is 165 bpm, and temperature is 36.3°C. Cardiac and pulmonary examinations are normal except for tachycardia. Abdominal examination is difficult due to crying and tensing of the abdominal muscles. The infant's genitourinary examination is normal. There is loss of subcutaneous fat of the thighs and buttocks.

1. What maneuver can be done to help facilitate the abdominal examination?
2. What clinical signs can the physician look for during the examination?
3. What ancillary studies could help determine the diagnosis?

## Pyloric Stenosis

Hypertrophic pyloric stenosis (HPS) is the most common surgical cause of vomiting in infants. It is the result of hypertrophy of the circular musculature surrounding the pylorus, leading to compression of the longitudinal folds of mucosa causing obstruction of the gastric outlet.

The hypertrophied pylorus measures the size of an olive and is approximately 2 cm by 1 cm.

Infants with HPS typically present with nonbilious projectile vomiting in the second to fourth weeks of life. Symptoms rarely occur before 2 weeks or later than 4 to 6 months of age.[33]

HPS is primarily a disease of full-term infants. However, cases in the premature infant have been reported. HPS in the premature infant poses a difficult diagnostic challenge. Premature infants, on average, present later (fifth week of life), feed less vigorously, and vomit less forcefully.[34]

The etiology of HPS remains unknown, but both genetic and environmental influences have been implicated. HPS tends to run in families. Siblings of patients with HPS are 15 times more likely to develop the condition than children without a family history of the condition.

Research shows that 5% to 20% of sons and 2.5% to 7% of daughters of affected patients are at risk of developing HPS.[35,36]

Factors that have been implicated in the development of HPS are abnormalities in hormonal control (gastrin, cholecystokinin, secretin, somatostatin, and prostaglandins), abnormalities in pyloric innervation (ganglion cells, peptidergic and nitrergic innervation, nitric oxide synthase deficiency, reduced synapse formation, or reduced nerve-supporting cells), abnormalities of extracellular matrix proteins, abnormalities of smooth-muscle cells, and abnormalities in growth factors.[37-45]

Environmental causes have also been implicated in the development of HPS. These include maternal anxiety, maternal drug use, feeding practices,[46,47] and oral erythromycin use in neonates.[48,49]

### Epidemiology

The incidence of pyloric stenosis is approximately 1.5 to 4.0 per 1,000 live births.[50-59] Male infants are consistently affected more often than female infants, with a 2:1 to 5:1 male to female ratio.[50-54] Although rare, HPS can present in premature infants. The incidence has been reported to be 3.1% of all cases of HPS.[60]

## Clinical Features

The classic history of an infant with HPS is a male infant between 2 and 6 weeks of age with forceful projectile emesis. The emesis is always nonbilious and occurs 10 to 30 minutes after feeding. The infant appears hungry and will usually feed vigorously if given the chance. After 2 to 3 ounces of feeding, the infant will stop eating and play with the nipple, with eyes open wide. Reverse peristaltic waves traveling upward across the abdomen

might be visualized because the gastric contents cannot pass the hypertrophied pyloric sphincter. The ensuing emesis vomit will be expelled with force, as if it is "hitting the wall." Thus it might be more effective to ask parents if the vomitus can hit the wall, rather than asking them if it is projectile (since to a lay person, all vomit projects). The vomitus contains milk and gastric juices; sometimes it may be "coffee ground" in appearance due to gastritis and/or esophagitis.

The overall appearance of the infant presenting with HPS varies. Infants can be generally well appearing [normal pediatric assessment triangle (PAT)], or present with prolonged vomiting, severe dehydration, and lethargy (abnormal PAT). Physical examination findings of dehydration are seen with altered level of consciousness, sunken fontanel, sunken eyes, skin tenting, delayed capillary refill, or mottled and cool extremities. Abdominal findings can include abdominal distention, visible gastric peristaltic waves traveling across the abdomen, and a small mobile mass ("olive") palpable in the midepigastric region. This olive-sized and shaped pylorus is difficult to feel. It is best felt by experienced hands while the child is feed-

---

### YOUR FIRST CLUE

**Signs and Symptoms of Pyloric Stenosis**

Early:

- Normal PAT

Late:

- Appearance: Decreased level of consciousness, decreased activity
- Work of breathing: Effortless tachypnea
- Circulation: Delayed capillary refill, cool, mottled extremities, rapid pulse

Other Findings:

- Male infant
- Nonbilious, projectile emesis
- Appears hungry
- Visible peristaltic waves
- Palpable olive-shaped pylorus in the right upper quadrant

ing (i.e., when the abdominal musculature is most relaxed).

### Complications

If the vomiting is allowed to continue for days, dehydration, weight loss, lethargy, and evidence of shock will occur. Caregivers might give a history of decreased urine output and activity.

## Diagnostic Studies

### Laboratory

Characteristic electrolyte findings are a hypochloremic, hypokalemic metabolic alkalosis. Infants might also exhibit an increased indirect bilirubin, which might be due to increased enterohepatic recirculation, a relative deficiency of hepatic glucuronyltransferase activity, and/or poor caloric intake.[61,62]

### Radiology

Plain films might reveal a large dilated stomach with no air in the small bowel or colon. These findings are consistent with a gastric outlet obstruction.

Until recently, the upper GI was the gold standard for diagnosis of pyloric stenosis. Positive upper GI signs for HPS are the string sign (a single streak of barium in the lumen of the elongated pylorus), the beak sign (the beginning of the elongated pyloric channel), and the double track sign (double streaks of barium passing through the narrow pylorus) (Figure 11.8).[63] More recently, abdominal ul-

trasonography had been used as a noninvasive method to visualize the muscle hypertrophy and measure the pyloric canal length. A muscle thickness of 4 mm or more and a channel length of 15 mm or more confirms the diagnosis of HPS (Figure 11.9 A, B).[64,65] Ultrasonography is advantageous because it is noninvasive, free of ionizing radiation, and is without risk of aspiration of contrast material. Disadvantages of ultrasonography are that it is operator dependent and, in a negative or equivocal study, an upper GI might be necessary.

### THE CLASSICS

**Classic Diagnostic Findings in Pyloric Stenosis**

- Hyponatremic, hypochloremic, hypokalemic metabolic alkalosis
- Sonogram showing thickened and elongated pylorus
- Upper GI contrast study showing the string, beak, or double track signs

## Differential Diagnosis

Although most etiologies are benign and self-limiting, the differential diagnosis of vomiting in an infant is broad. Disorders to consider with HPS include gastroesophageal reflux, overfeeding technique, and cow's milk intolerance. Other primary gastrointestinal conditions include gastric or proximal duodenal web, obstructions, malrotation with midgut volvulus, and gastric volvulus. Vomiting can also be secondary to extraintestinal disorders involving the central nervous system (increased intracranial pressure, intracranial hemorrhage, cerebral edema, space occupying lesions), renal system (obstructive uropathy, renal insufficiency), systemic infection (meningitis, urinary tract infections, or sepsis) or metabolic abnormalities (congenital adrenal hyperplasia or inborn error of metabolism).

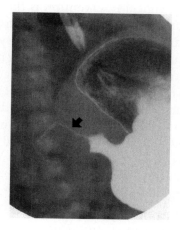

Figure 11.8 String sign of pyloric stenosis seen on barium upper GI series. The "string" represents the thin pyloric lumen.

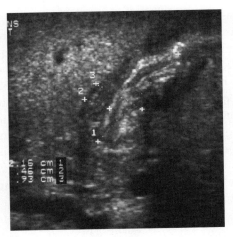

A

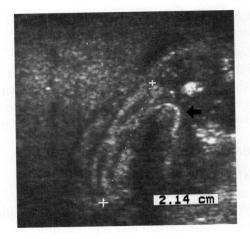

B

**Figure 11.9 A, B** Sonographic imaging in pyloric stenosis. Figure 11.9A shows the measurements of the pylorus. The pyloric length measures 2.16 cm (line #1). The pyloric wall thickness measures 0.46 cm (line #2). The pyloric diameter measures 0.93 cm (line #3). These exceed the measurements of 1.6 cm, 0.4 cm, and 1.4 cm, respectively, which are indicative of pyloric stenosis. Figure 11.9B shows another view of the pylorus. The pyloric length measures 2.14 cm in this view. The black arrow points to a prominent indentation of the pylorus into the stomach, which is also indicative of pyloric stenosis.

## WHAT ELSE?

**Differential Diagnosis of Pyloric Stenosis**

- Gastroesophageal reflux
- Overfeeding
- Cow's milk intolerance
- Malrotation with midgut volvulus
- Necrotizing enterocolitis
- CNS disease (increased intracranial pressure, intracranial hemorrhage, cerebral edema, mass occupying lesions)
- Renal disease (obstructive uropathy, renal insufficiency)
- Infection (meningitis, urinary tract infection, sepsis)
- Metabolic disease (congenital adrenal hyperplasia, inborn error of metabolism)

## Management

### Emergency Department

HPS recognition is important, but surgical correction is not required immediately. Surgical intervention is done after correction of electrolyte abnormalities, normalization of acid base status, and replenishment of fluid deficit. Provide a bolus of 20 mL/kg of normal saline at the time intravenous access is established. Follow the bolus with an infusion of 5% dextrose with 1/2 normal saline at 1.5 times maintenance volume. Correct fluid and electrolyte abnormalities over 24 to 48 hours. Establish good urine output greater than 1mL/kg per hour and then add 20 to 40 mEq/L potassium chloride to the maintenance fluids. Place an orogastric or nasogastric tube to low intermittent suction to decompress the stomach. Provide oxygen and respiratory support as indicated. Surgical intervention is the Fredet-Ramstedt pyloromyotomy, which consists of a longitudinal incision through the hypertrophied muscle down to the underlying mucosa.

Between 6 and 18 hours after surgical correction, infants are allowed to start feedings. Great variability in formula type, feeding regimens, and advancement exists, some advocating ad lib and others standardized feeding regimens. Postoperative emesis is common and occurs in 65% to 90% of patients regardless of the regimen or protocol used.[66-68]

### What to Avoid and Why

Avoid surgical intervention until metabolic alkalosis is resolved. Uncorrected alkalosis can delay recovery from anesthetic agents or cause postanesthetic apnea.

**Controversies in Management**

One area of controversy in management is the approach to repairing the hypertrophied pylorus. Pediatric surgeons might use the traditional abdominal approach, or a laparoscopic technique, or an umbilical fold incision.[50,69] Laparoscopy and the umbilical fold incision provide smaller incisions and better cosmetic results. Laparoscopy requires an increased operative time and causes the potential for respiratory acidosis and hypothermia. The umbilical fold method is not used in infants with a large pylorus and is associated with an increased wound infection rate.

Another area of controversy is the use of nonsurgical approaches to the treatment of HPS. Pyloric stenosis will spontaneously resolve within weeks to months. During this time, the infant can be maintained with parenteral nutrition. Oral atropine sulfate has been shown to reduce the resolution time of pyloric stenosis and reduce the overall costs involved when compared to surgery.[50,70] Because surgical intervention is successful and the complication risk is low, nonsurgical management is not generally accepted in the US, but practices in other countries might differ.

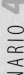

**CASE SCENARIO 4**

A 6-month-old boy presents to a pediatrician's office with 1 day of crying and poor feeding. His mother states that over the past few hours he has had two episodes of vomiting breast milk. There is no fever, diarrhea, or cold symptoms. His mother states that the pain seems so intense that he draws his knees to his chest and "crawls" up her arms and shoulders. Between bouts of pain, he is calm and at times quite sleepy.

On physical examination, the infant is resting in his mother's arms. His respiratory rate is 18 breaths per minute, heart rate is 130 bpm, and rectal temperature is 37.9°C. The anterior fontanel is flat and soft. His lips are pink but dry. His lungs are clear to auscultation without increased work of breathing. The abdominal examination reveals normal bowel sounds, mild tenderness, and a soft mass in the right upper quadrant below the liver border. The genital examination is normal. Soft stool obtained on rectal examination is positive for occult blood. While you discuss further management plans with the mother, the infant begins crying inconsolably.

1. *What could be the cause of this infant's abdominal pain?*

**CASE SCENARIO 5**

The mother of a 9-month-old boy calls you because the baby is sleeping too much. Earlier in the morning he had two episodes of vomiting. The vomit was not green or bloody. The infant passed a stool with mucus and urinated without difficulty.

On physical examination, the infant is lethargic. His respiratory rate is 20 breaths per minute, heart rate is 120 bpm, and rectal temperature is 37.5°C. The anterior fontanel is small and flat. Pupils are 4 mm and reactive. His lungs are clear to auscultation without increased work of breathing, and cardiovascular examination is normal. The abdominal and genital examinations are also normal. The stool is positive for occult blood. The skin examination reveals no evidence of trauma.

1. What surgical emergency could cause lethargy in this infant?
2. What diagnostic test could be performed to diagnose and treat this entity?
3. What is an important complication of an air enema, and how should the physician specifically intervene if respiratory difficulty occurs?

## Intussusception

Intussusception is an invagination of the proximal portion of the bowel into an adjacent distal bowel segment. It is second only to an incarcerated inguinal hernia as the most common cause of intestinal obstruction in infants.

Intussusception is classified according to the site of the inner intussusceptum and the outer intussuscipiens. Approximately 80% to 90% involve invagination of the ileum into the colon (ileo-colic). The remainder are ileo-ileal, ceco-colic, colo-colic, and jejuno-jejunal, in decreasing order of frequency.[71,72]

### Epidemiology

The peak age of occurrence is between 5 and 9 months, with most cases occurring from 3 months to 2 years. Research shows 10% to 25% occur in children older than 2 years. There is a male predominance of 2:1.[71-76] In children younger than 2 years, no pathologic lead point is found in more than 90% of patients.[76] These cases are termed "primary idiopathic" but can be caused by lymphoid hyperplasia of Peyer patches, stimulated by an antecedent viral infection. Pathologic lead points are more commonly found in older children, with Meckel diverticulum being the most common. Other causes of lead points are intestinal duplications, hemorrhagic congestion, and vasculitis of the intestinal mucosa as seen in Henoch-Schonlein purpura, inspissated intestinal secretions as seen in cystic fibrosis, lymphomas, intestinal polyps, foreign bodies, and *Ascaris lumbricoides* infestation.[77–82] There was an association between rotavirus vaccine (Rotashield, Wyeth Lederle Vaccines, Philadelphia, Pa) and intussusception that led to the voluntary withdrawal of the vaccine in 1999.

### Clinical Features

The classic triad of intussusception is intermittent colicky abdominal pain, vomiting, and bloody mucoid ("currant jelly") stools. The majority of infants, however, present with only two symptoms. The most frequent complaint is colicky abdominal pain (85% to 90%) that lasts 2 to 10 minutes followed by a period of relief when the infant appears calm. This pattern usually repeats every 20 to 30 minutes. Classically, the young infant manifests abdominal pain by forcefully drawing up the legs onto the abdomen and crying. The paroxysmal nature of these painful attacks suggests small bowel obstruction. The second most common symptom is vomiting (65% to 80%). Initially, emesis can be nonbilious, but can become bilious or feculent. Stools might initially be negative for blood or positive for occult blood. It is not until significant bowel ischemia occurs that stools become grossly bloody, which is why the presence of "currant jelly" stools is usually a late finding.[71–74] Patients with intussusception can also have fever and can occasionally present without abdominal pain.

Lethargy, hypotonia and pallor are other symptoms seen in intussusception. In a review of patients with lethargy due to intussusception, all had either melena or a palpable abdominal mass on physical examination. The exact mechanism for lethargy in intussusception is unclear. Several mechanisms have been postulated. One hypothesis is that the breakdown of intestinal mucosa and release of endotoxin or other mediators from the bowel enter the bloodstream and then affect the central nervous system. Another mechanism suggests that a release of endogenous opioid from the ischemic bowel contributes to profound lethargy.[83–85] Dehydration can be a contributing factor.

On physical examination, 15% to 30% of infants with intussusception can have a normal examination. Classically, abdominal examination reveals an emptiness in the right lower quadrant; in more than half of the cases, a soft sausage-shaped mass is palpable in the right upper quadrant extending along the transverse colon.[71–73] In patients with extensive involvement of the bowel, the mass might be palpable only on rectal examination. Rarely, protrusion of the intussuscepted intestine occurs through the rectum.[71,73] Differentiating between a simple prolapsed rectum and intussusception is important and is easily accomplished. Ability to insert a finger between the mass (intussusceptum) and the rectal lining indicates an intussusception.

### Complications

With undiagnosed or misdiagnosed intussusception, ischemic bowel will become necrotic and can perforate. Late signs include progressive dehydration, abdominal distention, peritonitis, and hypovolemic shock.

## Diagnostic Studies

### Laboratory

Laboratory tests are nonspecific and generally not helpful. Testing the stool for occult blood can be helpful if positive. Occult blood has been found in 43% of patients with intussusception, and its presence might help increase the index of suspicion for intussusception.[86,87]

### Radiology

Abdominal plain radiographs can be helpful in the diagnosis of intussusception, but if normal, do not exclude the disease. Radiographic findings suggestive of intussusception include a soft tissue mass (Figure 11.10), target sign (Figure 11.11 A, B), absence of cecal gas and stool (Figure 11.12; see also Figure 11.10), meniscus sign (also called

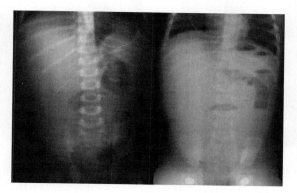

**Figure 11.10** RUQ soft tissue mass in intussusception. There is a fullness in the right upper quadrant with a soft tissue mass (absence of gas). Note that the liver edge (subhepatic angle) is obscured by the mass. This is suspicious for intussusception.

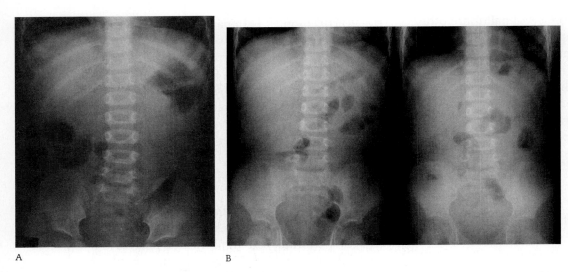

A                                    B

**Figure 11.11 A, B** Target sign in intussusception. This sign is more specific for intussusception. This RUQ soft tissue mass has a target appearance (similar to a faint doughnut). The target signs are not obvious, but they can be clearly identified in these two radiographs. Note that 11.11A demonstrates a crescent sign in the left upper quadrant.

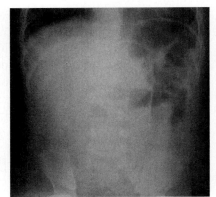

**Figure 11.12** Absence of cecal stool and gas. Note the solid homogeneous nature in the right lower quadrant. The same appearance can be seen in Figure 11.10. This is nonspecific but suspicious for intussusception. Identification of definite gas and stool in the cecum makes it unlikely that an ileo-cecal intussusception is protruding through this area.

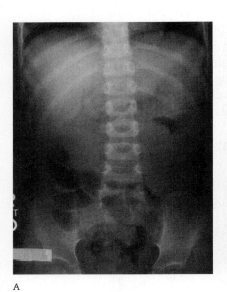

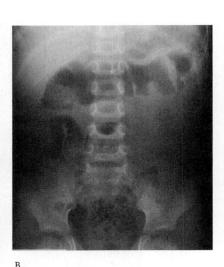

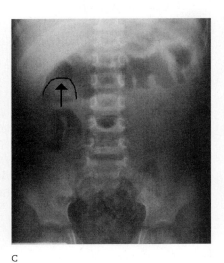

A                              B                              C

**Figure 11.13 A, B, C** Meniscus sign (crescent sign). The crescent sign (LUQ in 11.13A) is formed by the intussusceptum protruding into a gas-filled-pocket. This makes the air pocket resemble a crescent as in the left image. However, in 11.13B, the intussusceptum is traveling superiorly in the right upper quadrant as it approaches the hepatic flexure. Note that the gas-filled pocket is very large, so even though the intussusceptum can be visualized within this gas-filled pocket (pointing superiorly), as in 11.13C, the resultant shape is not a crescent. Thus, the crescent sign is not always crescent shaped. It should be more accurately called "the intussusceptum protruding into a gas-filled pocket sign," but that is too long to say.

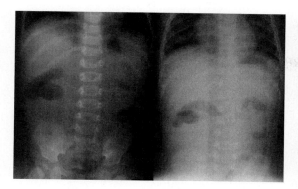

**Figure 11.14** Paucity of bowel gas. This radiograph demonstrates a general paucity of gas. There are only a few bowel loops that are faint on the upright view (right image), and these are actually air-fluid levels, suggesting that this is actually a bowel obstruction that is most likely due to intussusception.

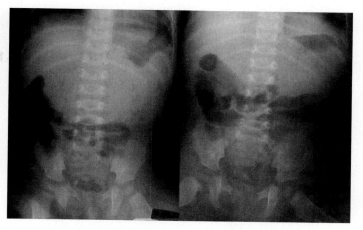

**Figure 11.15** Bowel obstruction. Note the poor distribution of gas on the flat view (left image) and the dilated (smooth) bowel loops on the upright view (right image), which indicate the presence of a bowel obstruction that is most likely due to intussusception. A possible target sign is visible in the right upper quadrant. Figure 11.14 also demonstrates a bowel obstruction due to intussusception.

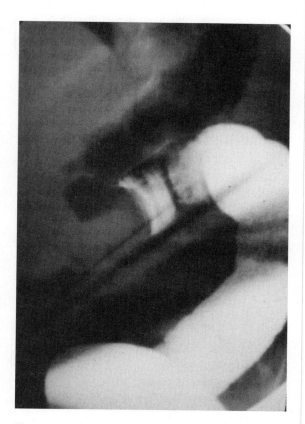

**Figure 11.16** Barium enema diagnosis of intussusception. In this image, barium fills the ascending colon and part of the transverse colon. The barium column encounters a mass within the transverse colon (the intussusceptum).

the crescent sign) (Figure 11.13 A, B, C), paucity of bowel gas (Figure 11.14), and a bowel obstruction (Figure 11.15). Radiographic evidence of small bowel obstruction can be more apparent if the presentation is delayed. A soft tissue mass can be seen in the right upper quadrant in up to 50% of the cases (this includes the target sign). An upright or decubitus plain film is helpful to identify intestinal perforation if present.[88] The barium enema is considered the gold standard study in the diagnosis of intussusception (Figure 11.16). More recently, air contrast enemas have been used and have been shown to be as effective in the diagnosis and treatment of intussusception when used by radiologists skilled in this procedure (Figure 11.17).[89–92] Radiologists who have not been trained in air contrast enemas often prefer barium or water-soluble contrast enemas.

Barium and air contrast enemas are contraindicated in cases involving intestinal perforation, peritonitis, or decompensated shock.

More recently, ultrasonography has been used to diagnose intussusception with up to 100% accuracy when interpreted by a radiologist skilled in the sonographic diagnosis of intussusception. Characteristic sonographic findings are the target sign or doughnut sign on transverse view (Figure 11.18) and the sandwich sign on longitudinal view. The quality of the study and its interpretation are operator dependent. However, when used appropriately,

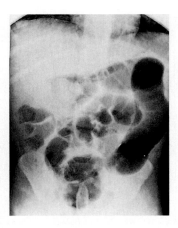

Figure 11.17 Air contrast enema diagnosis of intussusception. In this image, air contrast distends the ascending colon. As the air contrast enters the transverse colon, it encounters a mass (the intussusceptum) just to the right of the midline. This is not as obvious as in the barium enema; because air is normally present in the small bowel as well, the air contrast does not stand out as much.

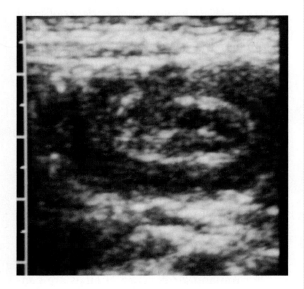

Figure 11.18 Sonographic image of doughnut sign. Similar to the target sign on plain film radiography, this sonographic doughnut sign is indicative of intussusception.

a negative sonogram (that is reliably negative) obviates unnecessary diagnostic enemas. Ultrasonography also can be used to obtain other information, including detection of lead

points.[91–94] If the skill of the available radiologist provides the clinician with only modest certainty, then ultrasonography should not be done, because a negative ultrasound will still require a contrast enema to definitively rule out intussusception, and a positive sonogram will require a contrast enema for confirmation and reduction.

## THE CLASSICS

### Diagnostic Studies for Intussusception

- Soft tissue mass, target sign, crescent sign on plain radiograph
- Target sign by sonography
- Intussusception on air or barium contrast enema

## Differential Diagnosis

The differential diagnosis for intussusception includes conditions that cause intestinal obstruction, abdominal pain, and blood in the stool. These include malrotation with midgut volvulus, Meckel diverticulum, incarcerated inguinal hernia, nonaccidental trauma, and infectious enteritis of the alimentary tract.

## WHAT ELSE?

### Differential Diagnosis of Intussusception

- Meckel diverticulum
- Incarcerated inguinal hernia
- Nonaccidental trauma
- Gastroenteritis
- Cow's milk or soy protein allergy or other benign processes

## Management

### Emergency Department and Followup Care

Once intussusception is suspected, obtain surgical consultation, withhold oral intake, establish intravenous access, and resuscitate the infant with intravenous fluids. Once free peritoneal air is excluded by plain radiography or sonography, nonsurgical reduction by barium or air contrast enema is attempted first. It is successful in 60% to 90% of cases. Contraindications to nonsurgical reduction are signs of peritonitis, hypovolemic shock, or demonstration of a pathologic lead point on a sonogram. Complications of hydrostatic reduction are intestinal perforation and nonreduction. Surgical reduction is necessary when contrast enema reduction is contraindicated or unsuccessful. Laparotomy is performed through a right transverse incision at the level of the umbilicus. The intussusceptum is gently milked out of the intussuscipiens. Nonviable bowel and any lead points are resected. Intussuscepted bowel segments are examined for adequate reperfusion. Appendectomy is also done. Routine use of antibiotics is controversial.

The risk of recurrence of intussusception after surgical reduction is less than 4%. The risk of recurrence of intussusception after contrast enema reduction is 10%. Most first recurrences develop within the first 8 months. Most are not due to pathological lead points and thus can be managed by hydrostatic reduction.[95–97]

### What to Avoid and Why

Complete physical examination and normal plain radiographs are seldom sufficient to eliminate the diagnosis of intussusception with certainty. Consider ultrasonography of the abdomen or an air or barium contrast study to aid in the diagnosis.

Hydrostatic reduction of an intussusception is contraindicated in toxic, ill-appearing patients and patients with evidence of peritonitis. These findings indicate the presence of gangrenous intestine, for which emergency surgery is necessary.

In the patient with profound lethargy, do not forget intussusception as a potential cause. Intussusception is easily treatable, and development of gangrenous bowel can be avoided.

### Controversies in Management

For infants without evidence of peritonitis but with a history of symptoms that exceeds 24 hours and an obstructive pattern on abdominal plain films, management controversies exist. These infants are believed to be at an increased risk of perforation. Some radiologists attempt reduction with gentle hydrostatic pressure while, others recommend surgical correction as first-line therapy.

Postreduction management is also controversial. Patients may be observed in the emergency department for 4 to 6 hours or admitted to the hospital for up to 24 hours after uncomplicated hydrostatic reduction of the intussusception. Patients are observed for evidence of feeding intolerance, peritonitis, and other complications.

---

## KEY POINTS

**Management of Intussusception**
- Fluid resuscitation
- Stop oral intake
- Consult pediatric surgery early
- Obtain appropriate radiographic studies

---

## THE BOTTOM LINE

- Consider intussusception in all infants with abdominal pain and vomiting.
- A normal plain film does not exclude intussusception, so a second study (air/barium enema or ultrasonography) is needed.
- An infant with intussusception can present with profound lethargy.

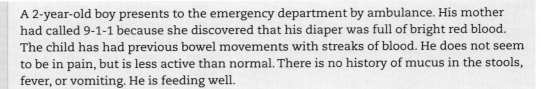

**CASE SCENARIO 6**

A 2-year-old boy presents to the emergency department by ambulance. His mother had called 9-1-1 because she discovered that his diaper was full of bright red blood. The child has had previous bowel movements with streaks of blood. He does not seem to be in pain, but is less active than normal. There is no history of mucus in the stools, fever, or vomiting. He is feeding well.

On physical examination, the child is alert and appropriately fearful. His respiratory rate is 24 breaths per minute and non-labored, heart rate is 140 bpm, blood pressure is 100/60 mmHg, and temperature is 37°C. Head and neck examination reveals pale conjunctivae and mucous membranes. Cardiovascular examination reveals mild tachycardia with a soft 2/6 systolic ejection murmur at the left lower sternal border. Abdominal and genitourinary examinations are normal. Examination of the anus reveals no evidence of trauma, fissures, or tags. Stool is grossly bloody. The skin is without bruising or petechiae.

1. *What are the priorities of management in this child?*
2. *How can the physician differentiate upper gastrointestinal bleeding from lower gastrointestinal bleeding?*
3. *What could be the cause of painless rectal bleeding in this previously healthy child?*
4. *In a child who is actively bleeding from the rectum, would radiographs be helpful or indicated?*

## Meckel Diverticulum

Meckel diverticulum is a congenital true diverticulum of the distal ileum that contains all layers of the intestinal wall. It forms as a result of incomplete obliteration of the omphalomesenteric (vitelline) duct during the ninth gestational week.[98] Normally the omphalomesenteric duct disappears just before the midgut returns to the abdomen. Persistence of some portion of this omphalomesenteric duct results in a constellation of congenital anomalies; Meckel diverticulum is the most common.[99]

Meckel diverticulum is clinically significant because it can contain gastric and pancreatic tissue. Gastric tissue produces acid, which results in ulceration and bleeding. Meckel diverticulum can also remain attached to the body wall by a fibrous cord that forms from incomplete obliteration of the distal portion of the omphalomesenteric duct. This fibrous cord acts as a focus around which the intestines can twist, forming a volvulus and resulting in intestinal obstruction.

Over 60% of children with symptomatic Meckel diverticula are younger than 2 years. Signs and symptoms are typically related to

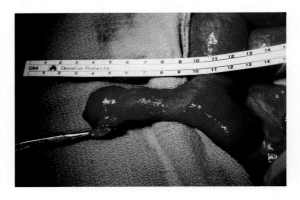

**Figure 11.19** Meckel diverticulum found at laparotomy measuring about 2 inches (5 cm) long.

bleeding, inflammation, or intestinal obstruction.[99]

The "rule of 2s" is often quoted as an easy rule to remember some facts about Meckel diverticulum: 2% incidence, 2 types of heterotopic mucosa (gastric and pancreatic), located within 2 feet of the ileocecal valve, about 2 inches in length and 2 cm in diameter, with symptoms usually occurring before a child is 2 years old (**Figure 11.19**).

### Epidemiology

Meckel diverticulum is the most common congenital anomaly of the gastrointestinal tract and is found in approximately 2% of the population.[100] It occurs in equal frequency between males and females when diverticula are incidentally discovered. However, in symptomatic cases, males are 3 to 4 times more commonly affected than females. An increased incidence of Meckel diverticulum is found in children with esophageal atresia, imperforate anus,[101] small omphaloceles,[102] and Crohn disease.[103]

## Clinical Features

The most common clinical presentations of Meckel diverticulum are lower gastrointestinal bleeding, intestinal obstruction (due to intussusception or volvulus), and inflammatory complications (diverticulitis, similar to appendicitis).[104–106]

Lower gastrointestinal bleeding presents as melena (black, tarry stools) or hematochezia (bright red blood from the rectum). The bleeding from a Meckel diverticulum is generally painless, episodic, and at times, massive. Bowel obstruction can occur due to an intussusception with the diverticulum as the lead point, herniation of the bowel through a patent omphalomesenteric fistula, or volvulus of the distal small bowel. Clinical signs include vomiting, abdominal pain, bloody stools, and a palpable abdominal mass. If symptoms are allowed to progress, signs of dehydration, peritonitis, and shock will develop. Inflammation of a Meckel diverticulum can mimic the clinical picture of appendicitis. The symptoms of Meckel diverticulitis include periumbilical, right lower quadrant, and lower midline pain, vomiting, and diffuse peritoneal irritation.

Complications of unrecognized Meckel diverticulum include massive gastrointestinal hemorrhage, obstruction due to volvulus, intussusception with potential for the development of peritonitis, bowel ischemia, and shock.

Other complications of Meckel diverticulum are rare but have been reported in the literature. These include impaction of foreign bodies (stones, pins, parasites) and future development of primary gastrointestinal cancer such as carcinoid, sarcoma, lymphoma, adenocarcinoma, and leiomyoma.

## YOUR FIRST CLUE

**Signs and Symptoms of Meckel Diverticulum**

Early:

- Appearance: Normal depending on the presentation type
- Work of breathing: Normal
- Circulation: Normal

Late:

- Appearance: Weak
- Work of breathing: Effortless tachypnea (compensatory for metabolic acidosis)
- Circulation: Delayed capillary refill, cool, pallor, poor skin turgor, mottled extremities, rapid pulse

Other Findings:

- Painless, rectal bleeding
- Black, tarry stools

## Diagnostic Studies

### Laboratory

Laboratory studies are nonspecific. Occult bleeding with anemia is an infrequent presentation of Meckel diverticulum. A CBC count, and prothrombin time/partial thromboplastin time (PT/PTT) help differentiate a coagulopathy as the cause of bleeding.

### Radiology

Technetium (TC)-99m pertechnetate scintigraphy, or "Meckel scan," is the diagnostic procedure of choice in children with gastrointestinal bleeding suspicious for Meckel diverticulum. Bleeding Meckel diverticula contain ectopic gastric mucosa in 95% of cases. TC-99m pertechnetate isotope concentrates in the gastric mucosa of the stomach and Meckel diverticulum. As the isotope is excreted, it collects in the urinary bladder. The use of pentagastrin, histamine-2 blockers, and glucagon enhances the accuracy of the scan. Fasting, nasogastric suctioning, and bladder catheterization also increase the diagnostic yield of the scan.[10] A 10-year review of TC-99m scans of Meckel diverticula found 1.7% of scans were false-negative and 0.05% were false-positive. The sensitivity was 85%, the specificity was 95% and accuracy was 90%.[107,108] If bleeding persists after a negative scan and Meckel diverticulum is still suspected, a repeat scan is indicated. If the scan remains negative despite enhancing measures, other studies such as isotope labeled red blood cell scan or angiography can be considered.[109]

cations, hemangiomas, arteriovenous malformations, coagulopathy, and inflammatory bowel disease.

## WHAT ELSE?

**Differential Diagnosis of Meckel Diverticulum**
- Intestinal polyps
- Intestinal hemangiomas
- Intestinal duplications
- Arteriovenous malformations
- Coagulopathy
- Inflammatory bowel disease

## THE CLASSICS

**Diagnostic Findings in Meckel Diverticulum**
Technetium-99m scan shows ectopic gastric mucosa.

## Differential Diagnosis

The differential diagnosis of Meckel diverticulum presenting as lower gastrointestinal bleeding in a child includes gastroenteritis (bacterial), inflammatory bowel disease, polyps, duplications, arteriovenous malformations, intussusception, Henoch-Schönlein purpura, and pseudomembranous colitis. Brisk upper gastrointestinal bleeding caused by peptic ulcer disease and variceal bleeding can also present in a similar manner; however, these usually can be distinguished from Meckel diverticulum by the presence of bloody gastric aspirates, which would indicate an upper GI bleed. In children with massive, painless rectal bleeding, the differential diagnosis is more defined and includes polyps, dupli-

## Management

### Emergency Department

Protect the airway, support respirations, and give oxygen as clinically indicated. Resuscitate with crystalloid fluid (normal saline or Lactated Ringer's solution) in boluses of 20 mL/kg. Transfuse with packed red blood cells (10 mL/kg) for significant hemorrhage. For children with obstructive symptoms, place an orogastric tube for intestinal decompression, give broad-spectrum antibiotics (Gram-positive, Gram-negative, and anaerobic coverage), resuscitate with crystalloid fluid, and consult pediatric surgery emergently for exploratory laparotomy. Rapid relief of the obstruction reduces the risk of ischemic bowel involvement. Patients without obstruction and risk of intestinal ischemia can undergo surgical resection once hemodynamically stable and the hematocrit approaches near normal values.

Surgical resection of the diverticulum is done through a transverse right lower quadrant incision or by laparoscopy. Depending on the extent of involvement, surgical resection will include placement of linear staples at the base of the diverticulum with subsequent amputation, a V-shaped incision at the base of the diverticulum with resection and enteroplasty, or sleeve resection of the involved portion of the ileum with an end-to-end anastomosis of the intestines.[110–112] Appendectomy is also performed.

### What to Avoid and Why

Patients without obstruction should not undergo operation until hemodynamically stable. Bleeding from a Meckel diverticulum is usually episodic and typically stops spontaneously. Surgery can usually be deferred until the patient is stabilized with intravenous fluids and blood products.

### Controversies in Management

Controversy exists over the management of a Meckel diverticulum discovered incidentally at laparotomy. The risk of future complications from an incidentally discovered Meckel diverticulum is estimated to be 4% to 6%.[113,114] Younger age has been associated with an increased risk of complications. Thus, pediatric surgeons will generally remove a Meckel diverticulum found in an infant or young child. Resection is also considered if the diverticulum contains palpable ectopic gastric mucosa, in the presence of omphalomesenteric remnants with abdominal wall attachments, or if there is a history of unexplained abdominal pain. Resection of Meckel diverticulum in an older child and adult without symptoms is controversial. Risks and benefits must be evaluated on an individual basis.[115]

---

## KEY POINTS

**Management of Meckel Diverticulum**
- ABCs
- Gastric decompression
- Fluid resuscitation
- Correct severe anemia

---

## THE BOTTOM LINE

- Determine site of bleeding within the gastrointestinal tract (upper versus lower).
- Emergent surgical consultation for evidence of hemorrhagic obstruction, or peritonitis.
- Correct hypovolemia and anemia before surgery of nonobstructed diverticula.

---

## CASE SCENARIO 7

A 13-year-old boy is brought into the emergency department by his parents at 4:00 AM after he was awakened by a sudden onset of left scrotal pain. The previous day, he was in his usual state of good health and played in his school's football game. He has had several brief, less intense but similar episodes in the past. He now has a tender, swollen left hemiscrotum and the testis appears to ride higher in the scrotum. There is absence of cremasteric reflex on the left. He complains of pain with any movement and is nauseated.

1. *What is your differential diagnosis?*
2. *Are any imaging modalities available or indicated?*
3. *Is there an indication for surgical intervention?*
4. *Is the contralateral testis at risk?*

## Testicular Torsion

Complaints of scrotal pain and swelling in the male pediatric population are a common presenting symptom in the emergency department. The so-called acute scrotum can include several diagnoses that afflict the male population, but distinguishing those boys with acute testicular torsion in a rapid manner is vital for testicular salvage. Tissue loss is directly proportional to the duration of testicular ischemia, and salvage rates drop dramatically when repair is delayed more than 8 hours after the acute event. Even though only some patients with an acute scrotum are found to have acute testicular torsion, it is the working diagnosis until proved otherwise.[116–118]

Testicular torsion has been estimated to occur in 1 out of every 4,000 males before the age of 25.[119] The peak incidence occurs around the age of 13, coinciding with the onset of puberty. Another age peak occurs in the perinatal period and presents as a newborn with a discolored or hard scrotum due to a necrotic testis that is beyond salvage. The occurrence is rare after the age of 30 years.[120]

The cause of testicular torsion in a child appears to be movement of a testis that is abnormally fixed or suspended within its investment by the tunica vaginalis; in the infant, it appears to be lack of fixation of the testicular tunics in the scrotum. If the tunica vaginalis, the portion of the processus vaginalis that normally invests (surrounds) the lower portion of the testis, has an abnormally high attachment to the spermatic cord, the testis is not fixed, and intravaginal torsion can occur. This "bell clapper" deformity allows the testis to lie transversely and to rotate due to poor fixation. Prenatal torsion and torsion of cryptorchid testes are usually due to lack of fixation of the testicular tunics in the scrotum, and hence the entire cord might twist, which is known as extravaginal torsion. Outside of the neonatal period, the bell clapper deformity is the abnormality found in most cases of testicular torsion, and it is commonly bilateral.[117]

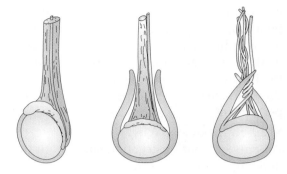

**Figure 11.20** Testicular lie. The diagram on the left shows the normal testicular lie. The middle diagram shows a horizontal lie (the bell clapper deformity), which is prone to torsion. The diagram on the right depicts testicular torsion.

Source: M. Gausche's article: Genitourinary surgical emergencies. *Pediatric Annals.* 1996; 25:458–464. Printed with permission for Gary Strange et al in *Pediatric Emergency Medicine: A Comprehensive Study Guide,* 1996.

### Clinical Features

The typical patient presents with sudden onset of severe pain in the groin or scrotum. Nausea and vomiting are commonly associated symptoms. The patient might have had similar episodes in the past that resolved, suggesting intermittent torsion, or a brief period of torsion that detorsed spontaneously.

Early in the course of testicular torsion, the landmarks and physical findings are most easily examined. As the time of torsion is prolonged, these findings became much less reliable due to pain, inflammation, and swelling. Early signs suggestive of testis torsion include a high-riding testis with a transverse lie, diffuse testicular tenderness, absence of the cremasteric reflex, and a palpable twist of the spermatic cord above the testis (**Figure 11.20**).

### Complications

Delay in reestablishing blood flow to the torsed testis results in the loss of testicular function. Delays can occur both in the patient presenting for evaluation and by the physician recognizing torsion as the etiology of the acute scrotum. Testicular salvage rates of 80% to 96% are possible if surgical intervention is initiated within 8 hours of the acute onset of pain. This salvage rate drops to less than 20% if surgical care is delayed by 12 hours or more.[121,122]

Bilateral testicular loss, though uncommon, can occur both in a synchronous (at the same time) or metachronous (at different times) manner.

## Diagnostic Studies

Laboratory studies are not sufficient for making a definitive diagnosis in the evaluation of the acute scrotum. Imaging studies might, on the other hand, be extremely useful when the diagnosis cannot be made solely based on the history and examination. The two modalities most helpful are testicular scintigraphy and real-time color Doppler sonography.

Testicular scintigraphy uses a radionuclide to analyze testicular perfusion. In most cases, the scan is performed quickly and has a reported positive predictive value of 95%. However, not all centers have immediate access to the technetium-99m pertechnetate at all hours of the day.

Real-time color Doppler sonography allows visualization not only of intratesticular arterial flow, but also of testicular anatomy.

Color Doppler imaging is readily available, noninvasive, and highly accurate. When normal or increased flow to the testis in question is noted, torsion is rapidly excluded. If there is any uncertainty with a technically equivocal study, urgent surgical exploration is indicated.[123] No child with a high clinical index of suspicion for torsion should have a surgical procedure delayed in order to confirm clinical suspicion with a diagnostic study.

## Differential Diagnosis

The three most common causes of the acute scrotum in the pediatric population are testicular torsion, torsion of a testicular appendage, and epididymo-orchitis.[118] Other processes include scrotal trauma, hernias, hydroceles, varicoceles, Henoch-Schonlein purpura, and testicular tumors. Obviously, testicular torsion must be ruled out urgently to prevent testicular loss.

Torsion of a testicular appendage, either an appendix testis or an appendix epididymis, occurs on average at 10 years of age.[124] Sudden onset of pain limited to the scrotum without abdominal or urinary symptoms is most common. Fever is uncommon. Point tenderness at the superior aspect of the testis is sometimes found early in the process, and the "blue dot" sign of a visible tender nodule can be found in one fifth of cases.[118] Most boys with torsion of a testicular appendage have never had a similar episode in the past, and most have a slightly more gradual onset of severity of pain, presenting to a physician more than 12 hours into the illness. Testicular scans and sonograms show increased flow and inflammation in the superior aspect of the testicle. If documented by clinical grounds or confirmed by imaging, treatment is expectant with analgesics alone. However, if there remains any doubt about the diagnosis, emergency scrotal exploration should be performed.

Epididymo-orchitis is the most common cause of the acute scrotum in sexually active males but is actually overestimated in most pediatric centers.[124,125] When a child is found to have documented epididymitis, an underlying anatomic urinary tract anomaly must be sought. The scrotal pain is usually slow in onset, less intense in nature, and associated with pyuria and a leukocytosis. Testicular scintigraphy and sonograms will document normal to increased flow to the affected testis. Treatment is with antibiotics and analgesics following culture. Urine cultures are obtained for antibiotic sensitivity studies, but in many cases, cultures are falsely negative. Positive cultures show that coliforms are usually the cause in prepubertal males; venereal organisms such as *Neisseria gonorrhoeae* and *Chlamydia trachomatis* are often found after puberty. Viral etiologies, including mumps, coxsackievirus, echovirus, and adenovirus have also been implicated.

## WHAT ELSE?

**Differential Diagnosis of Testicular Torsion**

- Torsion of the appendix testis or appendix epididymis
- Epididymitis
- Orchitis
- Incarcerated inguinal hernia
- Scrotal trauma
- Hydrocele
- Varicocele
- Henoch-Schönlein purpura
- Scrotal cellulitis
- Kawasaki disease
- Testicular tumor

## Management

### Emergency Department

Analgesia with an IV narcotic is indicated for patients in significant pain. However, treatment of the pain should not delay evaluation and definitive treatment of the child. If the cause of the acute scrotum has been determined to be testicular torsion or if torsion cannot be excluded in a rapid fashion, emergency scrotal exploration is indicated (**Figure 11.21**). Detorsion of the affected side is performed, and viability is ascertained. If clearly nonviable, the testis is removed. If viable, orchiopexy is performed with 3-point or 4-point fixation with nonabsorbable sutures. The contralateral testis is then explored to be sure the cause of the ipsilateral torsion is the bell clapper deformity, or if the testis is oriented in an abnormal plane due to the high incidence of bilaterality associated with anomalies of testicular fixation.

Manual detorsion can preserve testicular viability and provide time before irreversible necrosis occurs. Administer analgesia first. Because testes usually torse in a medial direction, perform manual detorsion by twisting the affected testis in an outward manner (i.e., such that the anterior surface of the testis is rotated outward, laterally). Twist the patient's right testis to the patient's right, or twist the left testis to the patient's left until the pain is relieved. Successful detorsion can be evident by relief of painful symptoms along with a visible lengthening of the cord structures. More than a 360-degree twist

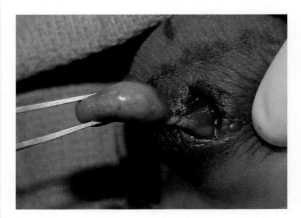

**Figure 11.21** Torsion of the testis.

might be required to fully detorse the affected testis. Manual detorsion is a temporizing procedure only. Definitive surgery to completely relieve the torsion is still indicated. In general, manual detorsion should be performed by the pediatric surgeon or pediatric urologist because it might otherwise confuse the diagnosis and delay needed surgery.

**What to Avoid and Why**
Avoid delay in surgical exploration of an acute scrotum if torsion is suspected. Testicular viability is directly related to the duration of torsion and is affected by patient and physician delay.

**CASE SCENARIO 8**

A 3-month-old boy born at 36 weeks gestation presents to the emergency department with a 12-hour history of agitation, poor feeding, and right scrotal swelling. The parents have never noted this swelling before. The scrotal mass is tense and seems to transilluminate. It is difficult to palpate the testis on the right side. The left hemiscrotum is normal. Initial attempts at reducing the mass are met with a crying child and very anxious parents.

1. *Is this a hydrocele or a hernia?*
2. *Should further attempts be made to reduce the mass?*
3. *When should this lesion be repaired?*

## Pediatric Inguinal Hernia

Inguinal hernias and hydroceles are common findings in the pediatric population. As more premature babies survive, the incidence of hernias and hydroceles is increasing, as are the number of pediatric surgical repairs performed. A hernia is the protrusion of a loop or portion of an organ or tissue through an abnormal opening. Inguinal hernias can be complicated by loss of bowel, testis, and ovary due to incarceration and strangulation.

**Embryology**
During the fifth week of gestation, the gonads develop as retroperitoneal structures. Near the 10th week, through a process of differentiated growth commonly called descent, the gonads can be found close to the groin, and at the internal inguinal ring at 12 weeks. The peritoneum protrudes through the internal ring during the third month to form the processus vaginalis.[126] At 28 weeks gestation, the testes continue their descent, following the gubernaculum through the internal ring toward the scrotum, taking the processus vaginalis (which is attached to the anteromedial portion of the testis) with it.[126] This external phase of descent appears to be dependent on release of testosterone from the fetal testis and from substances produced by the genitofemoral nerve.[127]

Incomplete obliteration of the proximal processus vaginalis, which normally occurs during the ninth month, results in the various types of inguinal hernias and hydroceles encountered in the pediatric population. Fusion of the distal processus with proximal patency results in an inguinal hernia. Complete failure of obliteration leaves a potential space for an inguinoscrotal hernia. Obliteration of the proximal processes with distal patency results in a noncommunicating scrotal hydrocele. If there is a very small proximal opening, a communicating hydrocele can result, with fluid moving between peritoneal and scrotal locations. If a small region along the mid portion of the processus is not obliterated while the distal and proximal portions are obliterated, a hydrocele of the cord, or canal of Nuck in the female, results.

The timing of obliteration of the processus vaginalis is highly variable. Up to 20% of asymptomatic adults have been shown to have a patent processus throughout a normal life.[128] In females, there is no external phase of gonadal descent. However, a peritoneal diverticulum (canal of Nuck) adherent to the round ligament, which corresponds to the processus vaginalis in males, does "descend," and when patent through its attachment to the labia, predisposes to formation of inguinal hernias in females.

## Epidemiology

The anatomic congenital defect that leads to an inguinal hernia in later life occurs in 10 to 20 per 1,000 live births.[129] Prematurity dramatically increases the risk of hernias, with 7% to 10% of infants born at less than 36 weeks gestation having hernias.[130,131] Hernias are more common on the right side in males due to later descent of the right testis.[126] In term infants, hernias are present on the right side in 60%, on the left in 30%, and are bilateral in 10%.[132] The incidence of bilaterality approaches 50% in low birth weight premature infants[133] (Figure 11.22). Males with hernias outnumber females 3:1 to 10:1 in most large series. Many associated conditions have been identified as risk factors for the development of inguinal hernias (Table 11-3).

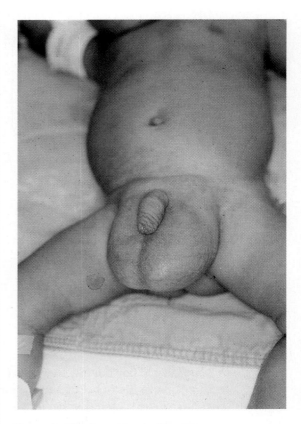

**Figure 11.22** Bilateral inguinal hernias.

### TABLE 11-3 Conditions Associated With Development of Inguinal Hernias

- Positive family history
- Cystic fibrosis
- Undescended testes
- Ambiguous genitalia
- Prematurity
- Exstrophy of bladder
- Low birth weight
- Hypospadias and epispadias
- Hydrops/neonatal ascites
- Peritoneal dialysis
- Ventriculoperitoneal shunt
- Mucopolysaccharidosis
- Connective tissue disorder
- Congenital abdominal wall defects
- Male sex

## Clinical Features

Inguinal hernias and hydroceles in children usually present as an asymptomatic bulge or mass in the groin or scrotum. Most are documented in the first year of life, often when bathing or changing the diaper of a crying or straining child. The groin swelling usually spontaneously resolves when the child relaxes or with gentle manual pressure.

## Complications

If a loop of intestine becomes entrapped (incarcerated) in a hernia, the child soon becomes very uncomfortable and irritable, develops intense pain, and soon has signs of bowel obstruction. If the hernia is not quickly reduced, strangulation occurs with ischemia of the bowel. This can occur in a 4-hour to 6-hour period of time. A tense incarcerated inguinal hernia can also compromise the blood flow to the testis. Prompt reduction of the incarcer-ated hernia is essential to prevent tissue loss and associated complications.

The female with an incarcerated ovary in an inguinal hernia can be relatively asymptomatic until the ovarian blood supply is compromised by torsion or pressure-related ischemia. Although rare, this can occur in a short period of time, and repair of nonreducible hernias in female patients should not be unnecessarily delayed just because there does not appear to be bowel present within the hernia.

## Diagnostic Studies

The physical examination of the child with a suspected inguinal hernia will document the anomaly in the overwhelming majority of cases. Having the child increase intra-abdominal pressure with straining, crying, or in the older child, jumping, will often assist with the demonstration of the inguinal bulge. Additional laboratory or radiographic studies are usually not indicated in the workup for a possible or known inguinal hernia or hydrocele. Although some surgeons will accept the diagnosis based on an accurate history and description by the parents or referring physician, it is not uncommon to require several examinations over a period of time to document the defect definitively.

## Differential Diagnosis

A scrotal hydrocele can often be differentiated from an inguinal hernia by the ability of the examiner to palpate a normal spermatic cord above the mass and feel no continuity of the lesion between the scrotum and the inguinal canal. For abdominal contents to reach the scrotum, they must traverse the inguinal canal. A tense inguinoscrotal hydrocele can be very difficult to differentiate from an incarcerated inguinal hernia by examination alone. However, the hydrocele will typically have caused no symptoms, while the hernia is usually tender and can cause obstructive symptoms. Caution must be used when decisions are made using transillumination of an inguinal or scrotal mass: an incarcerated inguinal hernia might transilluminate as well

---

### YOUR FIRST CLUE

**Signs and Symptoms of Pediatric Inguinal Hernia**

Early, nonincarcerated:

- Appearance: Normal behavior
- Work of breathing: Normal
- Circulation: Normal

Late, incarcerated:

- Appearance: Fussy, irritable, in pain, vomiting; if dehydrated, lethargic
- Work of breathing: If dehydrated, effortless tachypnea (compensatory for metabolic acidosis)
- Circulation: If dehydrated, delayed capillary refill, cool, pallor, poor skin turgor, mottled extremities, rapid pulse

Other findings:

- Poor feeding
- Abdominal distention
- Pain (crying, irritability)
- Lack of bowel movement
- Swelling in groin area that becomes firm and tender

| TABLE 11-4 | Differential Diagnosis of an Inguinal or Scrotal Mass |
| --- | --- |

- Inguinal hernia
- Cryptorchid testis
- Hydrocele
- Varicocele
- Retractile testis
- Torsion of testis
- Torsion of appendix testis
- Trauma
- Lymphadenitis
- Tumor

as a hydrocele! The differential diagnosis of an inguinal or scrotal mass is listed in Table 11-4.

## Management

### Emergency Department

An inguinal hernia will not resolve spontaneously. The patient should be referred to a pediatric surgeon and repair performed shortly following diagnosis. This will reduce the risk of incarceration and its attendant complications, especially in the first year of life.[128] Patients with hydroceles that do not enlarge, are not tense, and are not reducible with manual pressure can be observed because many will resolve in the first year of life.[134]

The child with an incarcerated hernia must be seen as soon as possible by a surgeon. Most incarcerated hernias have not yet strangulated and can be manually reduced. Reduction prevents the need for an emergency surgical procedure, which has significantly increased risks during the repair due to the associated edema and tissue friability.[128,135] However, if the hernia is not reducible without undue pressure, strangulation could be present, and an emergency surgical reduction and repair are indicated. Children who have been vomiting due to incarcerated hernias require intravenous fluid resuscitation. Adjuncts to make the manual reduction easier include Trendelenburg positioning, sedation, and gentle pressure over a period of several minutes.

### What to Avoid and Why

The child with a red, tender inguinal or scrotal mass who appears toxic should not undergo attempts at manual reduction, nor should the child with a bowel obstruction or peritoneal signs. These children should undergo emergent surgical intervention once resuscitated.

### Controversies in Management

The controversies in inguinal hernia management usually center around the indications for contralateral groin exploration and the timing of repair of hernias in the very premature neonate. Surgeons must exercise appropriate judgment based on the age, sex, and comorbid conditions in the child with a hernia.

## KEY POINTS

**Management of Inguinal Hernia**
- ABCs.
- Resuscitate with intravenous fluids.
- Consider orogastric or nasogastric tube.
- Obtain surgical consultation.
- Consider manual reduction with sedation, Trendelenburg position, and gentle upward pressure.

## THE BOTTOM LINE

- Inguinal hernias will not spontaneously resolve.
- Transillumination occurs with both hernias and hydroceles.
- Manual reduction of an incarcerated hernia can be performed.

## CASE SCENARIO 9

An 8-year-old boy presents to the emergency department with a 24-hour history of abdominal pain. Initially the pain was dull, vague, and located in the epigastric and periumbilical regions. This was followed by several hours of nausea and multiple episodes of vomiting. Over the past 6 hours, the pain has become more pronounced in his right lower quadrant. His mother states that several family members have a viral illness. This young boy has a low-grade fever, a normal urinalysis, a white blood cell count at the upper range of normal, and he refuses to ambulate. He has reproducible tenderness in his right lower quadrant despite attempts at distraction.

1. Are other studies indicated prior to disposition?
2. Does the viral illness in the family sway your thinking?
3. Does a normal white blood cell count cloud the picture?

# Appendicitis

Acute appendicitis is the most common condition for which children require emergent abdominal surgery. Prior to 1886, the source of the inflammatory process in the right lower quadrant was thought to be the cecum itself, and descriptions used the term typhlitis, from the Greek typhlon or cecum. Reginald Fitz, in 1886, correctly identified the source of the process as the appendix.[136] As a practicing pathologist, he described the signs and symptoms of both acute and perforated appendicitis and theorized that obstruction of the appendiceal lumen was involved with the process. McBurney, in 1889, described the point of greatest tenderness that bears his name to this day.[137]

## Epidemiology

Complaints of acute abdominal pain account for approximately 4% of office visits in children aged 5 to 14 years.[138] Of these children, acute appendicitis will be the ultimate diagnosis in 1% to 8%.[139–141] The lifetime risk of acute appendicitis is between 7% and 9%.[142] Though uncommon in children younger than 2 years, appendicitis does occur even in the neonatal period. The incidence rises from 1 to 2 cases per 10,000 children per year between birth and 4 years, to approximately 25 cases per 10,000 children per year for children aged 10 to 17 years.[143,144]

A seasonal variation has been documented in the incidence of appendicitis, corresponding somewhat to outbreaks of enteric infections and viral illnesses.[145] A diet high in refined sugars and low in fiber appears to increase the risk of appendicitis. Countries with high dietary fiber intake have less than 10% the incidence of appendicitis compared to Europe and North America.[146,147] It is believed that a high fiber diet speeds stool transit time and decreases the incidence of appendiceal luminal obstruction.

## Clinical Features

The child with acute appendicitis can present with a wide variety of symptoms and complaints. This complex presentation in a child unable to relate a good history contributes to the common misdiagnosis of appendicitis. The classic presentation of periumbilical pain, followed by anorexia, nausea and vomiting, right lower quadrant pain, and then fever is present in less than half of the children with appendicitis.[148,149]

The initial vague periumbilical pain is due to distention of the appendiceal lumen. This referred pain corresponds to the T-10 dermatome shared by the entire midgut. Later, as the appendix becomes inflamed, the adjacent peritoneal irritation causes the pain to localize in the periappendiceal region.

The lack of a classic presentation of appendicitis often results in a delay in the diagnosis. The lack of anorexia is very common in children. Small, frequent, loose stools are also a frequent finding in children with appendicitis, which can mislead clinicians into believing that the child has gastroenteritis. Dysuria with or without mild hematuria and pyuria can be present if an inflamed appendix is lying on the ureter or bladder. Flank or back pain can be the predominant complaint in a child with an inflamed retrocecal appendix.

The child with appendicitis typically appears ill and is hesitant to move. Children writhing in pain or vigorously trying to escape the examiner are unlikely to have appendicitis. A low-grade fever is common. A high fever is more common late in the course with perforated appendicitis. The physical examination in the child with acute appendicitis usually reveals right lower quadrant tenderness with evidence of localized peritoneal irritation. Peritonitis might be suspected if there is sharply increased pain when going over a bump in the road, bumping the stretcher, or on coughing, and is confirmed when there is percussion tenderness or rebound tenderness.[150]

### Complications

Delaying the diagnosis of acute appendicitis can lead to perforation, abscess formation, wound infection, sepsis, bowel obstruction, infertility in females, and death. The risk of appendicitis progressing to perforation is higher in children than in adults. The widely published rates of perforation in large series of children range from 20% to over 70%.[151–154] This is especially common in younger children, because they are not able to communicate as well as older children. Up to 50% of children with perforation can have one of the aforementioned complications following eventual diagnosis.[155]

## Diagnostic Studies

There is no single specific laboratory test that will diagnose appendicitis and rule out other causes for a child's illness. In the child with a very good history and physical examination consistent with acute appendicitis, there is no need for further laboratory or radiographic evaluation. An urgent appendectomy is indicated. But because the classic symptoms are frequently absent, studies are often helpful. An elevated white blood cell count can be present in appendicitis but is not helpful in differentiating perforated from nonperforated appendicitis, and will not exclude other diseases

YOUR FIRST CLUE

**Signs and Symptoms of Appendicitis**
- Appearance: Uncomfortable, abdominal pain, lying still, might be vomiting
- Work of breathing: Normal
- Circulation: Normal

Late:
- Appearance: Severe pain, weak, lethargic, chills
- Work of breathing: Tachypnea (compensatory for metabolic acidosis)
- Circulation: Delayed capillary refill, cool, pallor, poor skin turgor, mottled extremities, rapid pulse

Other Findings:
- Progression of periumbilical to right lower quadrant pain
- Nausea
- Vomiting
- Fever
- Peritoneal irritation
- Percussion tenderness
- Rebound tenderness

associated with an inflammatory process in the abdomen (enteritis, pelvic inflammatory disease, and other infectious diseases).[156] Additionally, a normal white blood cell count in a child with reproducible right lower quadrant tenderness or peritonitis does not exclude the diagnosis of appendicitis.

In those patients with a confusing or unusual presentation, several imaging studies are available. These include plain radiographs, ultrasonography, computed tomography, and barium enema. Plain films can be helpful in cases of a bowel obstruction or perforated viscus, but will usually not be of assistance in uncomplicated appendicitis. A fecalith is visible on plain film radiographs in only 10% of cases (**Figure 11.23 A, B, C, D, E**). Graded compression ultrasonography is particularly useful in the child with equivocal clinical signs and in the female with possible pelvic organ pathology.[157] A focused abdominal CT might be useful in children with an atypical or delayed presentation.

An abscess might be identified that can be drained percutaneously and an interval appendectomy can then be performed several weeks later. Barium enema has been used in the past but adds little to the focused abdominal CT using enteral and intravenous contrast agents.

Imaging and surgical consultation decisions for uncertain cases are evolving and are highly dependent on the expertise available in an institution. The accuracy of ultrasonography is highly dependent on the skill of the clinician interpreting the results. Diagnostic accuracy rates published in studies from tertiary care centers are not necessarily achievable in general hospitals. Ultrasonography is often unable to reveal the appendix, making the study nondiagnostic. CT scanning has a high sensitivity, specificity, and positive predictive value in most studies; however, it requires more time, IV and enteral contrast, and it results in radiation exposure. Surgical consultation is not easily obtainable in many centers. Thus, in many centers, an imaging study (CT or ultrasonography) is performed first, and a surgeon is consulted only if a surgical condition is confirmed, or if the possibility of a surgical condition still cannot be ruled out.

Laparoscopy has gained popularity both as an adjunct in the diagnosis of possible appendicitis and as a therapeutic modality. The postpubertal female with lower abdominal pain is especially well suited for diagnostic laparoscopy and laparoscopic appendectomy if indicated. The pelvic organs are very well visualized, and specific ovarian pathology can be treated with the laparoscope as well.

## THE CLASSICS

**Classic Diagnostic Studies for Appendicitis**

- Leukocytosis, neutrophilia
- Calcified fecalith on abdominal radiograph
- Noncompressible appendix, appendicoliths, or peritoneal fluid/complex mass on sonography

## Differential Disagnosis

The differential diagnosis of abdominal pain is extensive. Most children presenting with abdominal pain do not undergo surgical intervention, so the final diagnosis is often based on presenting signs. The most common diagnoses after excluding appendicitis include gastroenteritis, respiratory infections, urinary tract infections, constipation, gynecologic disorders, and musculoskeletal or abdominal trauma. On initial presentation, children with missed appendicitis are more likely to be younger, have vomiting before pain, complain of dysuria or diarrhea, and have signs of respiratory infections compared to those with documented appendicitis at initial presentation.[149]

## WHAT ELSE?

**Differential Diagnosis of Appendicitis**

- Gastroenteritis
- Mesenteric adenitis
- Constipation
- Ovarian pathology (cyst, teratoma, pelvic inflammatory disease, torsion)
- Meckel diverticulitis
- Lower respiratory infection
- Urinary tract infection
- Musculoskeletal trauma
- Abdominal trauma

## Management

### Emergency Department

Children with suspected appendicitis should be given nothing by mouth, and intravenous fluid resuscitation should be instituted. Prompt surgical therapy will reduce the complications and associated morbidity and mortality in children with appendicitis. Broad-spectrum antibiotics should be considered.

For those who are discharged from the emergency department with a diagnostic impression of a nonsurgical etiology, it should be

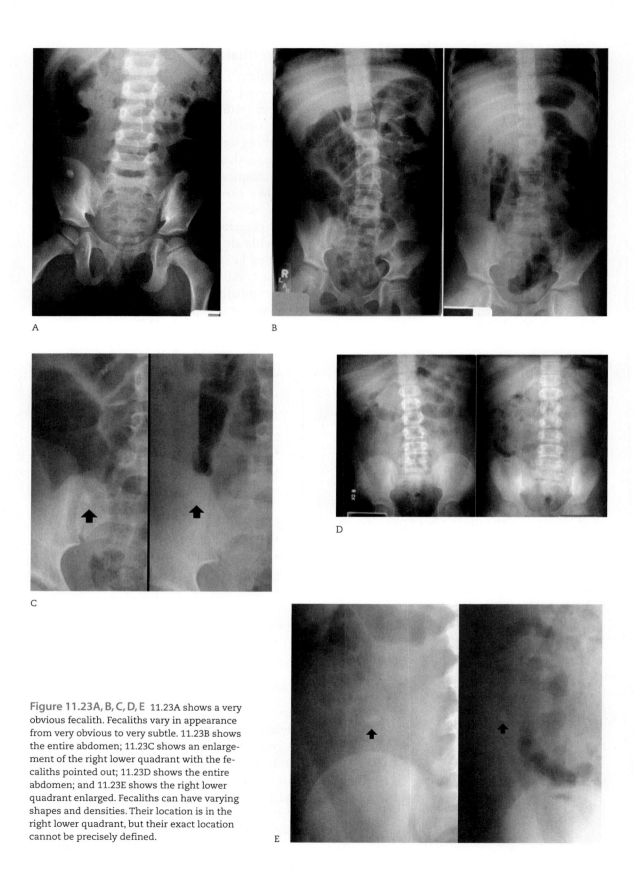

Figure 11.23A, B, C, D, E  11.23A shows a very obvious fecalith. Fecaliths vary in appearance from very obvious to very subtle. 11.23B shows the entire abdomen; 11.23C shows an enlargement of the right lower quadrant with the fecaliths pointed out; 11.23D shows the entire abdomen; and 11.23E shows the right lower quadrant enlarged. Fecaliths can have varying shapes and densities. Their location is in the right lower quadrant, but their exact location cannot be precisely defined.

noted that appendicitis and other serious abdominal conditions can be missed on initial evaluation. This is a high liability risk that can be reduced by providing parents with a standardized set of instructions describing the possibility of a serious condition for which they should return to the emergency department, including the signs and symptoms of appendicitis and other serious conditions.

### Controversies in Management

Controversies exist in several areas in the management of suspected appendicitis. What antibiotic or combination of antibiotics is best suited for the child with simple versus perforated appendicitis? Does the child who presents in the middle of the night require an emergent appendectomy, or is it safe to wait until the next morning? How should the child with a perforated appendix and associated right lower quadrant mass be managed: with emergent appendectomy or with drainage and interval appendectomy? Is laparoscopic appendectomy better than the traditional open approach? The answers to these questions have not been defined, and the emergency physician should consult a surgeon early in the course of management to discuss these issues.

## KEY POINTS

**Management of Appendicitis**
- Stop oral intake (NPO).
- Resuscitate with intravenous fluids.
- Obtain surgical consultation.
- Consider broad-spectrum antibiotics.
- Consider pain medications.

## THE BOTTOM LINE

- Young children are at high risk for perforation.
- Do not delay surgical consultation with ancillary studies if history and physical examinations are classic.
- Children with appendicitis can have a normal white blood cell count.
- Advanced imaging methods might be the only way to definitively diagnose or exclude appendicitis when classic findings are lacking.

# CHAPTER REVIEW

## Check Your Knowledge

1. Which of the following causes of rectal bleeding in a full-term neonate is associated with abdominal distention?
   A. Anal fissure
   B. Hemorrhagic disease of the newborn
   C. Necrotizing enterocolitis
   D. Nodular lymphoid hyperplasia
   E. Swallowed maternal blood

2. Pneumatosis intestinalis and PVG can be viewed on all of the following imaging studies except:
   A. Abdominal CT
   B. Magnetic resonance imaging
   C. Nuclear medicine scan
   D. Plain film radiographs
   E. Ultrasonography

3. Which of the following complications of malrotation is the most serious?
   A. Bowel obstruction from compressing Ladd bands
   B. Hypochloremic metabolic alkalosis
   C. Intermittent volvulus
   D. Midgut volvulus
   E. Sigmoid volvulus

4. Which of the following statements regarding appendicitis in children is correct?
   A. Appendicitis can be definitively ruled out by physical examination
   B. Discharge instruction sheets for patients with benign abdominal pain should not mention signs and symptoms of appendicitis since this would increase liability risk
   C. A normal white blood cell count can be used to confidently rule out appendicitis
   D. Roughly half or more than half of the cases of appendicitis present in a nontypical fashion
   E. The value of ultrasonography in diagnosing appendicitis is not dependent on the skill of the individual performing the procedure

## References

1. Kosloske AM. Epidemiology of necrotizing enterocolitis. *Acta Paediatr Suppl.* 1994;396:2–7.
2. Schwartz RM, Luby AM, Scanlon JW et al. Effect of surfactant on morbidity, mortality, and resource use in newborn infants weighing 500 to 1500 g, *N Engl J Med.* 1994;330:1476–1480.
3. Coit AK. Necrotizing enterocolitis. *J Perinat Neonatal Nurs.* 1999;12:53–68.
4. Wiswell TE, Robertson CF, Jones TA, Tuttle DJ. Necrotizing enterocolitis in full term infants. *Am J Dis Child.* 1988;142:532–535.
5. Polin RA, Pollack PF, Barlow B et al. Necrotizing enterocolitis in term infants. *J Pediatr.* 1976;89:460–462.
6. Andrews DA, Sawin RS, Ledbetter DJ, Schaller RT, Hatach EI. Necrotizing enterocolitis in term neonates. *Am J Surg.* 1990;159:507–509.
7. Martinez-Tallo E, Claure N, Bancalari E. Necrotizing enterocolitis in full-term or near-term infants: risk factors. *Biol Neonate.* 1997;71:292–298.
8. Ng S. Necrotizing enterocolitis in the full-term neonate. *J Paediatr Child Health.* 2001;37:1–4.
9. Bell MJ, Ternberg L et al. Neonatal necrotizing enterocolitis: therapeutic decisions based upon clinical staging. *Ann Surg.* 1978;187:1–7.
10. Walsh MC, Kliegman MD. Necrotizing enterocolitis: treatment based on staging criteria. *Pediatr Clin North Am.* 1986;33:179–201.
11. Stoll BJ. Epidemiology of necrotizing enterocolitis. *Clin Perinatol.* 1994;21:205–218.
12. Kanto WP, Hunter JE, Stoll BJ. Recognition and medical management of necrotizing enterocolitis. *Clin Perinatol.* 1994;21:335–336.
13. Rowe MI, Reblock KK, Kurkchubasche AG et al. Necrotizing enterocolitis in the extremely low birth weight infant. *J Pediatr Surg.* 1994;29:987–990.
14. Kabeer A, Gunnlaugsson S, Coren C. Neonatal necrotizing enterocolitis: a 12-year review at a county hospital. *Dis Colon Rectum.* 1995;38:866–872.
15. Chandler JC, Hebra A. Necrotizing enterocolitis in infants with very low birth weight. *Semin Pediatr Surg.* 2000;9:63–72.
16. Horwitz JR, Lally KP, Chen HW et al. Complications after surgical intervention for necrotizing enterocolitis: a multicenter review. *J Pediatr Surg.* 1995;30:994–998.
17. Simon NP. Follow-up for infants with necrotizing enterocolitis. *Clin Perinatol.* 1994;21:411–424.

18. Stevenson RJ. Gastrointestinal bleeding in children. *Surg Clin North Am.* 1985;16:1455–1480.

19. Vinton NE. Gastrointestinal bleeding in infancy and childhood. *Gastroenterol Clin North Am.* 1994;23:93–122.

20. Caty MG, Azizkhah RG. Acute surgical conditions of the abdomen. *Pediatr Ann.* 1994;23:b192–201.

21. Edelson MB, Sonnino RE, Bagwell CE et al. Plasma intestinal fatty acid binding proteins in neonates with necrotizing enterocolitis: a pilot study. *J Pediatr Surg.* 1999;34:1453–1457.

22. Kliegman RM. Models of pathogenesis of necrotizing enterocolitis. *J Pediatr.* 1990;117: 52–55.

23. Maalouf EF, Fagbemi A, Duggan PJ et al. Magnetic resonance imaging of intestinal necrosis in preterm infants. *Pediatrics.* 2000;105: 510–514.

24. Rescorla FJ. Surgical management of pediatric necrotizing enterocolitis. *Curr Opin Pediatr.* 1995;7(3):335–341.

25. Felter RA. Nontraumatic surgical emergencies in children. *Emerg Med Clin North Am.* 1991;9: 589–610.

26. Torres AM, Ziegler MM. Malrotation of the intestine. *World J Surg.* 1993;17:326–331.

27. Irish MS, Pearl RH, Caty MG et al. The approach to common abdominal diagnoses in infants and children, Part I. *Pediatr Clin North Am.* 1998;45:729–772.

28. Brandt ML, Pokorny WJ, McGill CW et al. Late presentations of midgut malrotation in children. *Am J Surg.* 1985;150:767–771.

29. Messineo A, MacMillan JH, Palder SB, Filler RM et al. Clinical factors affecting mortality in children with malrotation of the intestine. *J Pediatr Surg.* 1992;27:1343–1345.

30. Bonadio WA, Clarkson T, Naus J et al. The clinical features of children with malrotation of the intestine. *Pediatr Emerg Care.* 1991;7: 348–349.

31. Potts SR, Thomas PS, Garstin WIH, McGoldrick J et al. The duodenal triangle: a plain film sign of midgut malrotation and volvulus in the neonate. *Clin Radiol.* 1985;36:47–49.

32. Filston HC, Kirks DR. Malrotation: the ubiquitous anomaly. *J Pediatr Surg.* 1981;16(4 suppl 1):614–620.

33. Zenn MR, Redo SR. Hypertrophic pyloric stenosis in the newborn. *J Pediatr Surg.* 1993;28: 1577–1578.

34. Janik JS, Wayne ER. Pyloric stenosis in premature infants. *Arch Pediatr Adolesc Med.* 1996;150: 223–224.

35. Finsen VR. Infantile pyloric stenosis – unusual family incidence. *Arch Dis Child.* 1979;54: 720–721.

36. Carter CO, Evans KA. Inheritance of congenital pyloric stenosis. *J Med Genet.* 1969;6:233–254.

37. Ohshiro K, Puri P. Pathogenesis of infantile hypertrophic pyloric stenosis: recent progress. *Pediatr Surg Int.* 1988;13:243–252.

38. Dick AC, Ardill J, Potts SR, Dodge JA. Gastrin, somatostatin and infantile hypertrophic pyloric stenosis. *Acta Paediatr.* 2001;90:879–882.

39. Huang PL, Dawson TM, Bredt DS, Snyder SH, Fishman MC. Targeted disruption of the neuronal nitric oxide synthase gene. *Cell.* 1993;75:1273–1286.

40. Vanderwinden J, Mailleux P, Schiffmann SN, Vanderhaeghen J-J, De Laet M-H. Nitric oxide synthase activity in infantile hypertrophic pyloric stenosis. *N Engl J Med.* 1992;327:511–515.

41. Abel RM. The ontogeny of the peptide innervation of the human pylorus, with special reference to understanding the aetiology and pathogenesis of infantile hypertrophic pyloric stenosis. *J Pediatric Surg.* 1996;31:490–497.

42. Subramaniam R, Doig CM, Moore L. Nitric oxide synthase is absent in only a subset of cases of pyloric stenosis. *J Pediatr Surg.* 2001;36:616–619.

43. Shima H, Ohshiro K, Puri P. Increased local synthesis of epidermal growth factors in infantile hypertrophic pyloric stenosis. *Pediatric Res.* 2000;47:201–207.

44. Guarino N, Shimu H, Oue T, Puri P. Glial-derived growth factor signaling pathway in infantile hypertrophic pyloric stenosis. *J Pediatr Surg.* 2000;35:835–839.

45. Guarino N, Yoneda A, Shima H, Puri P. Selective neurotrophin deficiency in infantile hypertrophic pyloric stenosis. *J Pediatr Surg.* 2001; 36:1280–1284.

46. Pisacane A, Luca U, Criscuolo L et al. Breast feeding and hypertrophic pyloric stenosis: population based case-control study. *BMJ.* 1996;312:745–746.

47. Jedd MB, Melton LJ, Griffen MR et al. Factors associated with infantile hypertrophic pyloric stenosis. *Am J Dis Child.* 1986;142:334–337.

48. Honein MA, Paulozzi LJ, Himelright IM et al. Infantile hypertrophic pyloric stenosis after pertussis prophylaxis with erythromycin: a case review and cohort study. *Lancet.* 1999;354: 2101–2105.

49. Hypertrophic pyloric stenosis in infants following pertussis prophylaxis with erythromycin–Knoxville, Tennessee. *Morbidity*

# CHAPTER REVIEW

*and Mortality Weekly Report.* Dec 1999;48: 1117–1120.

50. Letton RW. Pyloric stenosis. *Pediatr Ann.* 2001;30:745–750.

51. Mitchell LE, Risch N. The genetics of infantile hypertrophic pyloric stenosis: a reanalysis. *Am J Dis Child.* 1993;147:1203–1211.

52. Schechter R, Torfs CP, Baleson TF. The epidemiology of infantile hypertrophic pyloric stenosis. *Paediatr Perinat Epedemiol.* 1997;11:407–427.

53. Tam PK, Chan J. Increasing incidence of hypertrophic pyloric stenosis. *Arch Dis Child.* 1991;66:530–531.

54. Applegate MS, Druschel CM. The epidemiology of infantile hypertrophic stenosis in New York state 1983 to 1990. *Arch Pediatr Adolesc Med.* 1995;149:1123–1129.

55. Hedbaack G, Abrahamson K, Husberg B et al. The epidemiology of infantile hypertrophic pyloric stenosis in Sweden 1987–1996. *Arch Dis Child.* 2001;85:379–381.

56. Dodge JA. Infantile hypertrophic pyloric stenosis in Belfast 1957–1969. *Arch Dis Child.* 1975;50: 171–178.

57. Sule ST, Stone DH, Gilmour H. The epidemiology of infantile hypertrophic pyloric stenosis in greater Glasgow area 1980–1996. *Paediat Perinat Epidemiol.* 2001;15:379–380.

58. Spicer RD. Infantile hypertrophic pyloric stenosis: a review. *Br J Surg.* 1982;69:128–135.

59. Shim WK, Campbell A, Wright SW. Pyloric stenosis in the racial groups of Hawaii. *J Pediatr.* 1970;76:89–93.

60. Benson CD, Lloyd JR. Infantile pyloric stenosis: a review of 1120 cases. *Am J Surg.* 1964;107: 429–433.

61. Chaves-Carballo E, Harris LE, Lynn HB. Jaundice associated with pyloric stenosis and neonatal small bowel obstructions. *Clin Pediatr.* 1968;7:198–202.

62. Woolley MM, Bertram FF, Asch MJ, Carpio N, Isaacs H. Jaundice, hypertrophic pyloric stenosis, and hepatic glucuronyl transferase. *J Pediatr Surg.* 1974;9:359–363.

63. Shuman FI, Darling DB, Fisher JH. The radiographic diagnosis of congenital hypertrophic pyloric stenosis. *J Pediatr.* 1967;71:70–74.

64. Blumhagen JD, Noble HG. Muscle thickness in hypertrophic pyloric stenosis: sonographic determination. *Am J Roentgenol.* 1983;140:221–223.

65. Ito S, Tamura K, Nagae I et al. Ultrasonographic diagnosis criteria using scoring for hypertrophic pyloric stenosis. *J Pediatr Surg.* 2000;35:1714–1718.

66. Carpenter RO, Schaffer RL, Maeso CE et al. Postoperative ad lib feeding for hypertrophic pyloric stenosis. *J Pediatr Surg.* 1999;34:959–961.

67. Leinwand MJ, Shaul DB, Anderson FD. A standardized feeding regimen for hypertrophic pyloric stenosis decreases length of hospitalization and hospital costs. *J Pediatr Surg.* 2000;35: 1063–1065.

68. Georgeson KE, Corbin TJ, Griffen JW, Breaux CW. An analysis of feeding regimens after pyloromyotomy for hypertrophic pyloric stenosis. *J Pediatr Surg.* 1993;28:1478–1480.

69. Fujimoto T, Lane GJ, Segawa O et al. Laparoscopic extramucosal pyloromyotomy versus open pyloromyotomy for infantile hypertrophic pyloric stenosis which is better? *J Pediatr Surg.* 1999;34:370–372.

70. Yamataka A, Tsukada K, Yokoyama-Laws Y et al. Pyloromyotomy versus atropine sulfate for infantile hypertrophic pyloric stenosis. *J Pediatr Surg.* 2000;352:338–341.

71. Gross RE, Ware PF. Intussusception in childhood. *N Eng J Med.* 1948;239:645–652.

72. Dennison WM, Shaker M. Intussusception in infancy and childhood. *Br J Surg,* 1970;57: 679–684.

73. Ein SH, Stephens CA. Intussusception: 354 cases in 10 years. *J Pediatr Surg.* 1971;6:16–27.

74. Gierup J, Jorulf H, Livaditis A. Management of intussusception in infants and children: a survey based on 288 consecutive cases. *Pediatrics.* 1972;50:535–546.

75. Hutchison IF, Olayiwola B, Young DG. Intussusception in infancy and childhood. *Br J Surg.* 1980;67:209–212.

76. Stringer MD, Pablot SM, Brereton RJ. Pediatric Intussusception. *Br J Surg.* 1992;79:867–876.

77. Pollack CV, Pender ES. Unusual cases of intussusception. *J Emerg Med.* 1991;9:347–355.

78. Puri P, Buiney EJ. Small bowel tumours causing intussusception in childhood. *Br J Surg.* 1985;72:493–494.

79. Ein SH, Stephens CA, Shandling B et al. Intussusception due to lymphoma. *J Pediatr Surg.* 1986;21:786–788.

80. Navarro O, Dugougeat F, Kornecki A et al. The impact of imaging in the management of intussusception owing to pathologic lead points in children. *Pediatr Radiol.* 2000;30: 594–603.

81. Little KJ, Danzl DF. Intussusception associated with Henoch-Schonlein purpura. *J Emerg Med.* 1991;9:29–32.

82. Choong CK, Kimble RM, Pease P et al. Colocolic intussusception in Henoch-Schonlein purpura. *Pediatr Surg Int.* 1998;14:173–174.

83. Conway EE. Central nervous system findings and intussusception: how are they related? *Pediatr Emerg Care.* 1993;9:15–18.

84. Tenenbein M, Wisemand NE. Early coma in intussusception: endogenous opioid induced? *Pediatr Emerg Care.* 1987;3:22–23.

85. Singer J. Altered consciousness as an early manifestation of intussusception. *Pediatrics.* 1979;64: 93–94.

86. Losek JD. Intussusception: don't miss the diagnosis! *Pediatr Emerg Care.* 1993;9:46–51.

87. Losek JD, Fiete RL. Intussusception and the diagnostic value of testing stool for occult blood. *Am J Emerg Med.* 1991;9:1–3.

88. Teele RL, Vogel SA. Intussusception: the paediatric radiologist's perspective. *Pediatr Surg Int.* 1998;158–162.

89. Bonadio WA. Intussusception reduced by barium enema. *Clin Pediatr.* 1998;27:601–604.

90. Palder SB, Ein SH, Stringer DA et al. Intussusception: barium or air? *J Pediatr Surg.* 1991;26:271–275.

91. Del-Pozo G, Albillos JC, Tejedor D et al. Intussusception in children: current concepts in diagnosis and enema reduction. *Radiographics.* 1999;19:299–319.

92. Kirks DR. Air intussusception reduction: "the winds of change." *Pediatr Radiol.* 1995;25:89–91.

93. Verschelden P, Filiatrault D, Garel L, et al. Intussusception in children: reliability of US in diagnosis – a prospective study. *Radiology.* 1994;191:781–785.

94. Lim HK, Bae SH, Lee KH et al. Assessment of reducibility of ileocolic intussusception in children: usefulness of color Doppler sonography. *Radiology.* 1994;191:781–785.

95. Beasley SW, Auldist AW, Stokes KB. Recurrent intussusception: barium or surgery? *Aust NZ J Surg.* 1987;57:11–14.

96. Ein SH. Recurrent intussusception in children. *J Pediatr Surg.* 1975;10:751–755.

97. Daneman A, Alton DJ. Intussusception: issues and controversies related to diagnosis and reduction. *Radiol Clin North Am.* 1996;34:743–756.

98. Moore KL, Persaud TVN. The developing human. In: Moore KL, Persaud TVN, eds. *Clinically Oriented Embryology.* 6th edition. Philadelphia, Pa: WB Saunders Co.; 1998:292–293.

99. Snyder CL. Meckel's diverticulum. In: Ashcroft KW, Murphy JP, Sharp RJ et al, eds. *Pediatric Surgery.* 3rd edition. Philadelphia, Pa: WB Saunders Co.; 2000:541–544.

100. Matsagas MI, Fatouros M, Koulouras B et al. Incidence, complications, and management of Meckel's diverticulum. *Arch Surg.* 1995;130:143–146.

101. Simms MH, Corkery JJ. Meckel's diverticulum: Its association with congenital malformations and the significance of atypical morphology. *Br J Surg.* 1980;67:216–219.

102. Nicol JW, Mackinlay GA. Meckel's diverticulum in exomphalos minor. *J R Coll Surg Edinb.* 1994;39:6–7.

103. Andreyev HJ. Association between Meckel's diverticulum and Crohn's disease: a retrospective review. *GUT.* 1994;35:788–790.

104. St-Vil D, Brandt ML, Panic S et al. Meckel's diverticulum in children: a 20-year review. *J Pediatr Surg.* 1991;26(11):1289–1292.

105. Brown RL, Azizkhan RG. Gastrointestinal bleeding in infants and children: Meckel's diverticulum and intestinal duplication. *Semin Pediatr Surg.* 1999;8(4):202–209.

106. Yahchouchy EK, Marano AF, Etienne JCF et al. Meckel's diverticulum. *J Am Coll Surg.* 2001;192(5):658–662.

107. Cooney DR, Duszynski DO, Camboa E et al. The abdominal technetium scan (a decade of experience). *J Pediatr Surg.* 1982;17(5):611–619.

108. Sfakianakis GN, Conway JJ. Detection of ectopic gastric mucosa in Meckel's diverticulum and in other aberrations by scintigraphy. *J Nucl Med.* 1981;22:732–737.

109. Ford PV, Bartold SP, Fink-Bennett DM et al. Procedure guideline for gastrointestinal bleeding and Meckel's diverticulum scintigraphy. *J Nuc Med.* 1999;40(7):1226–1232.

110. Teitelbaum DH, Polley TZ, Obeid F. Laparoscopic diagnosis and excision of Meckel's diverticulum. *J Pediatr Surg.* 1994;29(4):495–497.

111. Stylianos S, Stein JE, Flanigan LM. Laparoscopy for diagnosis and treatment of recurrent abdominal pain in children. *J Ped Surg.* 1996;31(8): 1158–1160.

112. Swaniker, F, Soldes O, Hirschl RB. The utility of technatium-99m pertechnetate scintigraphy in the evaluation of patient's with Meckel's diverticulum. *J Pediatr Surg.* 1999;34(5)760–765.

113. Soltero MJ, Bill AH. The natural history of Meckel's diverticulum and its relation to incidental removal. *Am J Surg.* 1976;132:168–171.

114. Cullen JJ, Kelly KA, Moir CR et al. Surgical management of Meckel's diverticulum. *Ann Surg.* 1995; 222(6):770.

115. Arnold JF, Pellicane JV. Meckel's diverticulum: A ten year experience. *Am Surg.* 1997;63:354–355.

116. Lewis AG, Bukowski TP, Jarvis PD et al. Evaluation of acute scrotum in the emergency department. *J Pediatr Surg.* 1995;30:277–282.

117. Kass EJ, Lundak B. The acute scrotum. *Ped Clin North Am.* 1997;44:1251–1266.

118. Knight PJ, Vassy LE. The diagnosis and treatment of the acute scrotum in children and adolescents. *Ann Surg.* 1984;200:664–673.

119. Williamson RCN. Torsion of the testis and other allied conditions. *Br J Surg.* 1976;63:465–476.

120. Melekos MD, Asbach HW, Markou SA. Etiology of acute scrotum in 100 boys with regard to age distribution. *J Urol.* 1988;139:123–125.

121. Fenner MN, Roszhart DA, Texter JH. Testicular scanning: evaluation the acute scrotum in the clinical setting. *Urology.* 1991;38:237–241.

122. Lerner RM, Mevorach RA, Hulbert WC et al. Color Doppler US in the evaluation of acute scrotal disease. *Radiology.* 1990;176:355–358.

123. Kass, EJ Stone KT, Cacciarelli AA et al. Do all children with an acute scrotum require exploration? *J Urol.* 1993;150:667–669.

124. Anderson PAM, Giacomantonio JM, Schwarz RD. Acute scrotal pain in children: prospective study of diagnosis and management. *Can J Surg.* 1989;32:29–32.

125. Caldamone AA, Valvo JR, Altebarmakian VK et al. Acute scrotal swelling in children. *J Pediatr Surg.* 1984;19:581–584.

126. Skandalakis JE, Colborn GL, Androulakis JA et al. Embryologic and anatomic basis of inguinal herniorhaphy. *Surg Clin North Am.* 1993;73:799–836.

127. Davenport M. Inguinal hernia, hydrocele, and the undescended testis. *BMJ.* 1996;312:564–567.

128. Rowe M, Lloyd D. Inguinal hernia. In: Welch K, Randolph J, Ravitch M et al., eds. *Pediatric Surgery.* 4th edition. Chicago, Il: Year Book Medical Publishers; 1986:779–793.

129. Tam P. Inguinal hernia. In: Listen J, Irving JM, eds. *Neonatal Surgery,* 3rd ed. London: Butterworths; 1990:367.

130. Boocock G, Todd P. Inguinal hernias are common in preterm infants. *Arch Dis Child.* 1985;60:669–670.

131. Rajput A, Gauderer MW, Hack M. Inguinal hernias in very low birth weight infants: incidence and timing of repair. *J Pediatr Surg.* 1992;27:1322–1324.

132. Rowe M, Copelson W, Clatworthy H. The patent processus vaginalis and the inguinal hernia. *J Pediatr Surg.* 1969;4:102–107.

133. Rescorla F, Grosfeld J. Inguinal hernia repair in the perinatal period and early infancy: clinical considerations. *J Pediatr Surg.* 1984;19:832–837.

134. Rowe M, Marchildon M. Inguinal hernia and hydrocele in infants and children. *Surg Clin North Am.* 1981;61:1137–1145.

135. Rowe MI, Clatworthy HW. Incarcerated and strangulated hernias in children. *Arch Surg.* 1970;101:136–139.

136. Fitz RH. Perforating inflammation of the vermiform appendix. *Trans Assoc Am Physicians.* 1886;1:107.

137. McBurney C. Experience with early operative interference in cases of disease of the vermiform appendix. *New York Med J.* 1889;50:676.

138. Scholer SJ, Pituch K, Orr DP et al. Clinical outcomes of children with acute abdominal pain. *Pediatrics.* 1996–98;680–685.

139. Reynolds SL, Jaffe DM. Diagnosing abdominal pain in a pediatric emergency department. *Pediatr Emerg Care.* 1992;8:126–128.

140. Reynolds SL, Jaffe DM. Children with abdominal pain: evaluation in the pediatric emergency department. *Pediatr Emerg Care.* 1990;6:8–12.

141. Henderson J, Goldacre MJ, Fairweather JM. Conditions accounting for substantial time spent in hospital in children aged 1–14 years. *Arch Dis Child.* 1992;67:83–86.

142. Addiss DG, Shaffer N, Fowler BS et al. The epidemiology of appendicitis and appendectomy in the United States. *Am J Epidemiol.* 1990;132:910–924.

143. Luckmann R. Incidence and case fatality rates for appendicitis in California. *Am J Epidemiol.* 1989;129:905–918.

144. Brumer M. Appendicitis: seasonal incidence and postoperative wound infections. *Br J Surg.* 1970;57:93–99.

145. Burkitt DP. The aetiology of appendicitis. *Br J Surg.* 1971;58:695–699.

146. Burkitt DP, Walker ARP, Painter NS. Dietary fiber and disease. *JAMA.* 1974;229:1068–1074.

147. Golladay ES, Sarrett JR. Delayed diagnosis in pediatric appendicitis. *South Med J.* 1988;81:38–41.

148. Rothrock SG, Skeoch G, Rush JJ et al. Clinical features of misdiagnosed appendicitis in children. *Ann Emerg Med,* 1991;20:45–50.

149. Golledge J, Toms AP, Franklin IJ et al. Assessment of peritonism in appendicitis. *Ann R Coll Surg Engl.* 1996;78:11–14.

150. Rappaport WD, Peterson M, Stanton C. Factors responsible for the high perforation rate seen in early childhood appendicitis. *Am Surg.* 1989;55:602–605.

151. Savrin RA, Clatworthy HW. Appendiceal rupture: a continuing diagnostic problem. *Pediatrics.* 1979;63:37–43.

152. Marchildon MB, Dudgeon DL. Perforated appendicitis: current experience in a children's hospital. *Ann Surg.* 1977;185:84–87.

153. Adolph VR, Falterman KW. Appendicitis in children in the managed care era. *J Pediatr Surg.* 1996;31:1035–1037.

154. Pieper R, Kager L, Nasman P. Acute appendicitis: a clinical study of 1,018 cases of emergency appendectomy. *Acta Chir Scand.* 1982;148:51–62.

155. Mollitt DL, Mitchum D, Tepas JJ III. Pediatric appendicits: efficacy of laboratory and radiologic evaluation. *South Med J.* 1988;81:1477–1479.

156. Sivit CJ, Siegel MJ, Applegate KE et al. When appendicitis is suspected in children. *Radiographics.* 2001;21:247–262.

157. Barker AP, Davey RB. Appendicitis in the first three years of life. *Aust N Z J Surg.* 1988;58:491–494.

158. Dinkevich E, Ozuah PO. Pyloric stenosis. *Pediatr Rev.* 2000;21:249–250.

159. Gellis SS. Ancient technique of olive detection. *Pediatrics.* 1991;88:655–656.

160. Senquiz AL. Use of decubitus position for finding the "olive" of pyloric stenosis. *Pediatrics.* 1991;87:266 (Comment: Although the title of this citation describes the "decubitus" position, it actually describes a ventral decubitus position which is really a prone position.)

**CASE SUMMARY 1**

A 4-day-old girl presents to the emergency department after an episode of bloody stools and increasing abdominal distention. She has not been feeding well and is sleeping between feedings. She was born at 34 weeks gestation by emergency cesarean delivery because the mother had pregnancy-induced hypertension. The infant did well after delivery and was discharged to home. She had been taking commercial formula every 3 hours, but the past 6 hours, has not been feeding at all and has been more lethargic.

On physical examination, the infant is afebrile, with a respiratory rate of 45 breaths per minute and a heart rate of 180 bpm. The head, neck, lung, and heart examinations are normal except for tachycardia. The abdomen is distended; the overlying skin is mildly shiny and erythematous, and bowel sounds are hypoactive. Femoral pulses are present, but capillary refill to the lower extremities is delayed. A stool sample obtained from the diaper is positive for blood.

1. What could be the cause of rectal bleeding and abdominal distention in this neonate?
2. What studies could help you decide the cause?

The infant is fluid resuscitated, and an orogastric tube at low intermittent suction is placed to decompress the abdomen. Cultures are obtained. Supine and left lateral decubitus plain films of the abdomen reveal pneumatosis intestinalis with PVG.

Ampicillin, gentamicin, and metronidazole are administered by IV. Early surgical consultation is obtained. Enteral feedings are withheld for 10 to 14 days. Parenteral hyperalimentation is given during this time. Once the abdominal radiographs return to normal and 10 to 14 days of bowel rest are completed, feeding using an elemental formula is begun. Formula strength and volume are advanced very slowly. The infant tolerates slow advancement of feedings well without any signs or symptoms of obstruction due to stricture formation.

Laboratory studies are nonspecific. Preterm infants can show neutropenia, thrombocytopenia, or evidence of disseminated intravascular coagulopathy. Full-term infants can exhibit leukocytosis. Plain abdominal films are helpful if positive and characteristically demonstrate an ileus, a persistent loop of bowel, intrahepatic PVG, pneumatosis intestinalis, or a gasless abdomen. Malrotation with midgut volvulus must also be considered and an upper GI series might be warranted.

**CASE SUMMARY 2**

A 4-week-old boy arrives with a 1-day history of decreased activity and vomiting. The infant is breastfed and has had no difficulty nursing, but has vomited intermittently. Over the past 3 hours, the infant has vomited frequently. The last few episodes of vomiting were green in color. The birth history was uncomplicated. The infant was a full-term and born by spontaneous vaginal delivery.

On physical examination, the infant is lethargic, pale, and grunting. His respiratory rate is 60 breaths per minute, heart rate is 190 bpm, blood pressure is 80/60 mmHg, and rectal temperature is 36°C . The anterior fontanel is sunken. The lungs are clear to auscultation, but occasional grunting sounds are noted. Abdominal examination reveals decreased bowel sounds, and the abdomen is distended and tender to palpation. The genital examination is normal. The extremities are mottled with poor perfusion.

1. *What important cause of bilious emesis in an infant must be excluded immediately?*
2. *What is the radiographic study of choice in the evaluation of an infant with bilious emesis?*
3. *Why must the evaluation of an infant with bilious emesis be done emergently?*

Bilious emesis in an infant is considered diagnostic for malrotation with midgut volvulus until proved otherwise. The infant is given oxygen by face mask. Volume resuscitation and gastric decompression improve his circulatory status.

Plain abdominal films reveal absence of free peritoneal air. A limited upper GI contrast study is the study of choice and confirms the presence of malrotation with midgut volvulus. The infant is immediately taken to the operating room to undergo the Ladd procedure with appendectomy.

The evaluation of an infant must be done on an emergency basis because the infant with malrotation and midgut volvulus can infarct the entire midgut in 1 to 2 hours.

**CASE SUMMARY 3**

A 3-week-old female infant presents with a 4-day history of projectile vomiting. She is a full-term product of a vaginal delivery. There were no complications at birth. For the first 2 weeks of life, the infant would occasionally spit up (normal for age). Currently, the vomiting is very forceful, as if it will "hit the wall." The infant is breastfed, and the vomit appears to be breast milk. There is no history of blood or green-colored emesis, diarrhea, or fever. The mother is frustrated because the infant is losing weight and appears hungry.

On physical examination, the infant is dehydrated, with a sunken fontanel and poor skin turgor. Her respiratory rate is 24 breaths per minute, heart rate is 165 bpm, and temperature is 36.3°C. Cardiac and pulmonary examinations are normal except for tachycardia. Abdominal examination is difficult due to crying and tensing of the abdominal muscles. The infant's genitourinary examination is normal. There is loss of subcutaneous fat of the thighs and buttocks.

1. *What maneuver can be done to help facilitate the abdominal examination?*
2. *What clinical signs can the physician look for during the examination?*
3. *What ancillary studies could help determine the diagnosis?*

**CASE SUMMARY 3 CONT.**

The infant is given a bottle of glucose water to facilitate examination of the abdomen. Feeding will allow the abdominal muscles to relax and facilitate palpation of the hypertrophied pyloric muscle in the upper pole of the epigastrium.

Flex the hips and knees to relax the abdominal muscles. Place an orogastric or nasogastric tube to empty the stomach of its contents to facilitate palpation of the hypertrophied pyloric muscle.[158]

The infant should be placed in the prone or lateral decubitus position. This allows the hypertrophied pyloric muscle to fall anteriorly in the abdominal cavity during gentle palpation and examination of the right epigastrium.[159,160] In this case, a small mass is palpated in the midepigastric area. The abdomen is soft and nontender.

Following feeding, look for reverse peristaltic abdominal waves as the intestine moves from the infant's right to left. Peristalsis occurs in the opposite direction as the infant prepares to vomit. After feeding, reverse abdominal peristaltic waves are evident prior to an episode of projectile, nonbilious emesis.

The infant's electrolyte panel shows a hyponatremic, hypokalemic metabolic alkalosis. Intravenous fluids are given, starting with a 20 mL/kg normal saline infusion over 30 minutes followed by 5% dextrose in 1/2 normal saline, with a 20 mEq/L infusion of potassium chloride at 1.5 times maintenance requirement. Fluid and electrolyte losses are calculated and replenished over 48 hours. Once the metabolic abnormalities are corrected, the infant undergoes a pyloromyotomy without complications. She is currently tolerating breast milk and thriving.

**CASE SUMMARY 4**

A 6-month-old boy presents to a pediatrician's office with 1 day of crying and poor feeding. His mother states that over the past few hours he has had two episodes of vomiting breast milk. There is no fever, diarrhea, or cold symptoms. His mother states that the pain seems so intense that he draws his knees to his chest and "crawls" up her arms and shoulders. Between bouts of pain, he is calm and at times quite sleepy.

On physical examination, the infant is resting in his mother's arms. His respiratory rate is 18 breaths per minute, heart rate is 130 bpm, and rectal temperature is 37.9°C. The anterior fontanel is flat and soft. His lips are pink but dry. His lungs are clear to auscultation without increased work of breathing. The abdominal examination reveals normal bowel sounds, mild tenderness, and a soft mass in the right upper quadrant below the liver border. The genital examination is normal. Soft stool obtained on rectal examination is positive for occult blood. While you discuss further management plans with the mother, the infant begins crying inconsolably.

1. *What could be the cause of this infant's abdominal pain?*

The causes of abdominal pain and vomiting in an infant are numerous. These include intussusception, malrotation with midgut volvulus, Meckel diverticulum, incarcerated inguinal hernia, nonaccidental trauma, gastrointestinal tract infections, and cow's milk or soy protein allergy. The infant is sent to the emergency department for fluid resuscitation

# CHAPTER REVIEW

CASE SUMMARY 4 CONT

and surgical consultation. Intravenous normal saline is given, and radiographs of the abdomen are obtained. Laboratory studies are nonspecific. A flat and upright abdominal plain radiograph reveals a paucity of gas in the area below the liver (hepatic flexure) with no free intra-abdominal air. An air contrast enema reveals an ileo-cecal intussusception, which is reduced without difficulty. He is hospitalized for overnight observation. He is discharged home after refeeding the following day without complications.

CASE SUMMARY 5

The mother of a 9-month-old boy calls you because the baby is sleeping too much. Earlier in the morning he had two episodes of vomiting. The vomit was not green or bloody. The infant passed a stool with mucus and urinated without difficulty.

On physical examination, the infant is lethargic. His respiratory rate 20 breaths per minute, heart rate is 120 bpm, and rectal temperature is 37.5°C. The anterior fontanel is small and flat. Pupils are 4 mm and reactive. His lungs are clear to auscultation without increased work of breathing, and cardiovascular examination is normal. The abdominal and genital examinations are also normal. The stool is positive for occult blood. The skin examination reveals no evidence of trauma.

1. *What surgical emergency could cause lethargy in this infant?*
2. *What diagnostic test could be performed to diagnose and treat this entity?*
3. *What is an important complication of an air enema, and how should the physician specifically intervene if respiratory difficulty occurs?*

Intussusception in an infant can present with gastrointestinal symptoms or with profound lethargy. An air contrast enema or a barium contrast enema can be used to diagnose and treat intussusception. An important complication of air contrast enema is perforation of the intestine with accumulation of free intraperitoneal air. An important complication of barium contrast enema is perforation of the intestine with accumulation of barium sulfate suspension, causing barium peritonitis. Management of perforation would include maintaining airway, breathing, and circulation. Emergency paracentesis for peritoneal aspiration of free air might be necessary if respiratory distress occurs. Urgent volume resuscitation with normal saline is mandatory if barium peritonitis occurs. Both would provide temporary relief until immediate surgical correction in the operating room is performed.

The infant is sent to the emergency department for evaluation of altered mental status. Intravenous normal saline is given. Laboratory studies reveal normal electrolyte and glucose levels, normal urinalysis, negative urine toxicology screen, and a normal blood gas analysis. The CBC count shows a leukocytosis without a left shift and a normal hemoglobin and hematocrit. A CT scan of the head is normal. During the evaluation, the infant has three more episodes of vomiting and passes a bloody stool. Surgical consultation is obtained. Abdominal radiographs are normal. An air contrast enema reveals an ileo-colic intussusception, which cannot be reduced by hydrostatic pressure. Surgical reduction is performed without complication and the child does well postoperatively.

A 2-year-old boy presents to the emergency department by ambulance. His mother had called 9-1-1 because she discovered that his diaper was full of bright red blood. The child has had previous bowel movements with streaks of blood. He does not seem to be in pain, but is less active than normal. There is no history of mucus in the stools, fever, or vomiting. He is feeding well.

On physical examination, the child is alert and appropriately fearful. His respiratory rate is 24 breaths per minute and non-labored, heart rate is 140 bpm, blood pressure is 100/60 mmHg, and temperature is 37°C. Head and neck examination reveals pale conjunctivae and mucous membranes. Cardiovascular examination reveals mild tachycardia with a soft 2/6 systolic ejection murmur at the left lower sternal border. Abdominal and genitourinary examinations are normal. Examination of the anus reveals no evidence of trauma, fissures, or tags. Stool is grossly bloody. The skin is without bruising or petechiae.

1. *What are the priorities of management in this child?*
2. *How can the physician differentiate upper gastrointestinal bleeding from lower gastrointestinal bleeding?*
3. *What could be the cause of painless rectal bleeding in this previously healthy child?*
4. *In a child who is actively bleeding from the rectum, would radiographs be helpful or indicated?*

---

First, 100% oxygen by nonrebreathing mask is given. Intravenous access and laboratory tests, including a CBC count with differential, PT/PTT, and type and crossmatch, are obtained. Despite a 20 mL/kg normal saline bolus, tachycardia and pallor continue. A bedside hemoglobin value of 8 mg/dL confirms suspicion of anemia and hypovolemia secondary to blood loss. A 10 mL/kg infusion of type-specific packed red blood cells is started. Technetium-99m pertechnetate scan is inconclusive for a Meckel diverticulum, presumably because of active bleeding and pooling of blood in the intestines. The pediatric surgeon recommends exploratory laparotomy once the patient is hemodynamically stable and hemoglobin normalizes. At laparotomy, a 2-inch diverticulum containing whitish-appearing heterotopic tissue is removed. The child does well postoperatively and has had no further occurrences of rectal bleeding.

To differentiate upper gastrointestinal bleeding from lower gastrointestinal bleeding, place an orogastric or nasogastric tube and lavage with saline. Blood-free aspirates indicate that bleeding is originating from the lower gastrointestinal tract.

Painless rectal bleeding can be due to Meckel diverticulum, intestinal polyps, duplications, hemangiomas, arteriovenous malformations, coagulopathy, peptic ulcer disease, and inflammatory bowel disease. However, the latter two problems are typically associated with abdominal pain and discomfort.

In a child with lower gastrointestinal bleeding, a technetium-99m pertechnetate scan to search for a Meckel diverticulum is frequently obtained. However, if the scan is negative or if the child remains hemodynamically unstable despite volume resuscitation, most pediatric surgeons recommend exploratory laparotomy or laparoscopy for definitive treatment.[112] Some surgeons believe that regardless of scan results, children with brisk, painless lower gastrointestinal bleeding require an exploratory laparotomy and omit the Meckel scan altogether. In a child with a few mild episodes of painless rectal bleeding and a negative Meckel scan, some clinicians will obtain an esophagogastroduodenoscopy (EGD) and a colonoscopy to rule out polyps or other mucosal lesions, but the endoscopy might not be able to directly view a Meckel diverticulum.

A 13-year-old boy is brought into the emergency department by his parents at 4:00 AM after he was awakened by a sudden onset of left scrotal pain. The previous day, he was in his usual state of good health and played in his school's football game. He has had several brief, less intense but similar episodes in the past. He now has a tender, swollen left hemiscrotum and the testis appears to ride higher in the scrotum. There is absence of cremasteric reflex on the left. He complains of pain with any movement and is nauseated.

1. What is your differential diagnosis?
2. Are any imaging modalities available or indicated?
3. Is there an indication for surgical intervention?
4. Is the contralateral testis at risk?

The patient exhibits the classic history and physical findings of testicular torsion. He is given intravenous morphine for analgesia. No laboratory studies or imaging studies are obtained. The patient is taken for emergency scrotal exploration. Detorsion produces a viable-appearing testis. A bell-clapper deformity is noted, and bilateral orchiopexy is performed. The patient does well postoperatively.

The differential diagnosis of testicular torsion includes torsion of the appendix testis or appendix epididymis, epididymitis, orchitis, incarcerated inguinal hernia, trauma to the testis, Henoch-Schönlein purpura, scrotal cellulitis, Kawasaki disease, and testicular tumor.

Imaging modalities are available and include the technetium-99m pertechnetate scan and color Doppler ultrasonography. Imaging studies are helpful in equivocal cases but should not delay surgical consultation. In cases of classic testicular torsion, imaging studies are not indicated. The patient has an acute testicular torsion for which detorsion and orchiopexy are clearly indicated.

The contralateral testis is at risk for future torsion. Testicular torsion in the peri-pubertal male is usually due to abnormal attachments of the tunica vaginalis and usually occurs bilaterally. The testes have a horizontal lie, within the scrotal sac and are likely to become twisted. This abnormality is referred to as the bell-clapper deformity. Bilateral orchiopexy is indicated.

A 3-month-old boy born at 36 weeks gestation presents to the emergency department with a 12-hour history of agitation, poor feeding, and right scrotal swelling. The parents have never noted this swelling before. The scrotal mass is tense and seems to transilluminate. It is difficult to palpate the testis on the right side. The left hemiscrotum is normal. Initial attempts at reducing the mass are met with a crying child and very anxious parents.

1. Is this a hydrocele or a hernia?
2. Should further attempts be made to reduce the mass?
3. When should this lesion be repaired?

Although the scrotal mass transilluminates, there are several clues in the history that support the hypothesis that it is an incarcerated inguinal hernia. The mass is noticed for the first time, is associated with symptoms of agitation, poor feeding, and pain, and is unilateral. Most

CASE SUMMARY 8 CONT

hydroceles are present since birth, asymptomatic, and are more often bilateral. Further attempts at reduction by an experienced surgeon are warranted. Sedation and Trendelenburg positioning might facilitate successful reduction. Manual reduction involves squeezing gently the most dependent portion of the hernia in the direction of the inguinal canal. This is done while holding gentle pressure on the external inguinal ring with the thumb and forefinger of the other hand to "funnel" the incarcerated mass through the inguinal canal.

In this case, surgical consultation is obtained. An intravenous (IV) line and cardiac and pulse oximetry monitors are placed. The infant is given fentanyl (1 mcg/kg IV) and placed in the Trendelenburg position for manual reduction of the incarcerated inguinal hernia. The hernia is not reduced. Maintenance IV fluids are continued, and the infant is taken emergently for intraoperative repair.

In this scenario, the infant requires immediate surgical repair. If manual reduction is successful, elective repair can be performed within the next 12 to 36 hours when swelling has decreased. However, the infant who undergoes successful manual reduction of an incarcerated inguinal hernia should not be discharged, but admitted for observation, due to the small but significant risk of ischemia of the loop of intestine.

CASE SUMMARY 9

An 8-year-old boy presents to the emergency department with a 24-hour history of abdominal pain. Initially the pain was dull, vague, and located in the epigastric and periumbilical regions. This was followed by several hours of nausea and multiple episodes of vomiting. Over the past 6 hours, the pain has become more pronounced in his right lower quadrant. His mother states that several family members have a viral illness. This young boy has a low-grade fever, a normal urinalysis, a white blood cell count at the upper range of normal, and he refuses to ambulate. He has reproducible tenderness in his right lower quadrant despite attempts at distraction.

1. *Are other studies indicated prior to disposition?*
2. *Does the viral illness in the family sway your thinking?*
3. *Does a normal white blood cell count cloud the picture?*

No other studies are indicated for a classic case history as is presented here. A 20 mL/kg normal saline bolus is given by IV route. Surgical consultation is immediately obtained; the diagnosis of appendicitis is made, and morphine sulfate (0.1 mg/kg per dose) is given for pain control. The patient is taken to the operating room and is found to have a ruptured vermiform appendix.

An appendectomy is performed without further complications. IV ampicillin, gentamicin, and clindamycin are given intraoperatively and continued until the child is afebrile, has a normal white blood cell count, and is tolerating a normal diet. This process in otherwise uncomplicated perforated appendicitis takes approximately 5 to 7 days.

The history of viral illness in family members is often present and does not predict the absence or presence of appendicitis.

A normal white blood cell count is seen in approximately 20% of patients with appendicitis; therefore, a normal count does not exclude appendicitis as a diagnosis.

# chapter 12

# Nontraumatic Orthopedic Emergencies

Kemedy K. McQuillen, MD
Ronald I. Paul, MD, FAAP, FACEP

## Objectives

1 Discuss the epidemiology and pathophysiology of nontraumatic pediatric orthopedic conditions.

2 Describe the assessment and management of non-traumatic pediatric orthopedic conditions.

3 Identify the radiographic findings for: developmental dysplasia of the hip, rotational deformities, nursemaid elbow, Legg-Calvé-Perthes disease, slipped capital femoral epiphysis, Osgood-Schlatter disease, and acute septic arthritis.

## Chapter Outline

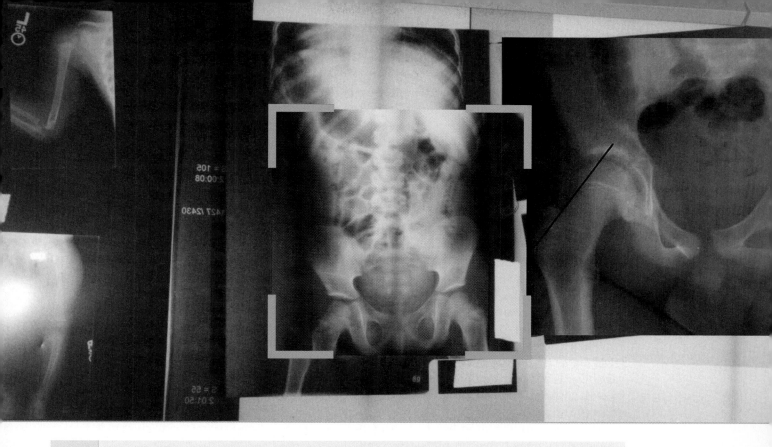

## CASE SCENARIO 1

During your evaluation of a 5-week-old girl, you feel a clunk as you do the Ortolani maneuver on the left hip. You also note asymmetric skin folds and decreased abduction. The rest of the exam, including the right hip, is entirely normal, and the child is in no distress. On questioning, the mother tells you that her daughter was born on time after an uncomplicated antenatal course. Specifically, the mother did not have multiple gestations or oligohydramnios, and the baby was born headfirst. The baby is breastfeeding well and gaining weight. The mother has had no problems with diaper changes, and her daughter does not appear to be in pain. After discussing your findings with the mother, you arrange for further testing and contact a specialist.

1. *What is the diagnosis?*
2. *How do you proceed in your evaluation?*
3. *What is the most likely course of treatment for this child?*

## Developmental Dysplasia of the Hip

As a result of the physiologic and anatomic differences between children and adults, pediatric patients are susceptible to orthopedic problems that do not affect the adult population.

Developmental dysplasia of the hip (DDH), formerly known as congenital dislocation of the hip, is an abnormal formation of the hip joint occurring between organogenesis and fetal maturity.[1] It encompasses a spectrum of disease that ranges from subluxable (loose) hips to frankly dislocated hips. The etiology of DDH is not entirely clear, but it might be related to intrauterine positioning, primary acetabular dysplasia, and/or ligamentous laxity.

In white neonates, the incidence for dysplasia is 1% percent, and the incidence for dislocated hips is 0.1%. It is more common in Native American populations and less common in black, Korean, and Chinese populations. There seems to be a familial predilection. Developmental dysplasia of the hip is more common in girls and most commonly unilateral (80%). With unilateral involvement, there is a slight predilection for the left side.

Associated birth factors include oligohydramnios, breech presentation, torticollis, talipes equinovarus, metatarsus adductus, and being first born.[2] Postnatally, swaddling infants with hips and knees in extension predisposes to dislocation.

## Clinical Features

Developmental dysplasia of the hip might be diagnosed at birth, or, despite frequent and appropriate physical examinations, it might not present until later in life.[3] Conversely, more than 50% of infants found to have unstable hips at birth will go on to develop spontaneous hip stability within 3 to 4 days.[4]

The presentations and physical findings of DDH are as diverse as the disease itself. This variability is due to the differences in the severity of the dysplasia and the progressive changes that occur over time.

In infants up to 6 months of age, the diagnosis of DDH is based on physical examination findings and specific testing. The leg length, skin folds, range of motion, and the Barlow provocative test and the Ortolani reduction maneuver are abnormal (Table 12-1).

Skin fold asymmetry can be noted in the groin, below the buttock, and along the thighs. Skin fold asymmetry is not specific for DDH and can be found in approximately 30% of infants with normal hips. Hip range of motion is also helpful in diagnosing DDH. Asymmetries in hip flexion, abduction, and external rotation should prompt further investigation. The physical diagnostic cornerstones for diagnosing DDH in young infants are the Ortolani reduction maneuver and Barlow provocative test. The Ortolani reduction maneuver is done in an attempt to reduce a dislocated hip back into normal position, and the Barlow provocative test detects the subluxable or dislocatable hip. Abnormal findings include the presence of a "clunk" with the Ortolani test and any abnormal movement between the femoral head and the acetabulum with the Barlow maneuver.

From 4 to 6 months of age, soft tissue contractures develop and the Ortolani and Barlow tests are less helpful in detecting unstable hips, while range of motion abnormalities become more apparent. Limited or asymmetric leg movements or difficulty with diapering might be noticed. On exam there is limited abduction, a relative shortening of the femoral segment (Galeazzi sign), and skin fold asymmetry.

## YOUR FIRST CLUE

**Presentations and Physical Findings of DDH**

- Mother reports difficulty in diapering
- Asymmetric skin folds
- Galeazzi sign present
- Trendelenburg sign present
- Waddling and wide-based gait
- Ortolani reduction maneuver results in "clunk" or "click"
- Barlow provocative test results in "clunk" or "click"
- Reduced range of motion of hip

---

### TABLE 12-1  Ortolani and Barlow Maneuvers

| Ortolani (Reduction) Maneuver | Barlow (Provocative) Test |
|---|---|
| • Stabilize the pelvis with one hand.<br>• With the other hand, slightly abduct the infant's hip.<br>• With the index and long fingers over the greater trochanter, pull the thigh up to gently reduce the hip. | • Stabilize the pelvis with one hand.<br>• Place the thumb on the inner aspect of the thigh near the lesser trochanter.<br>• Adduct the hip.<br>• Exert downward pressure on the thigh with the thumb, pushing it into the table. |

In children with bilateral DDH, the diagnosis is even more difficult beyond the first few months of life because there might be no asymmetry. After contractures develop, physical findings in bilateral DDH include widening of the perineum, abduction less than 4 degrees, and the appearance of abnormally short thigh segments.

With the onset of walking, gait asymmetry or asymmetric intoeing or outtoeing are clues to the presence of DDH. Adduction and flexion contractures, a positive Galeazzi sign, hyperlordosis, and a waddling gait are common findings. Clinical observation will reveal a Trendelenburg sign: While standing, the patient lifts one leg up at a time, and, because the gluteal muscles are weakened on the affected side, the pelvis will drop to the opposite side. With bilateral DDH, the children will present with a wide-based waddling gait.

## Diagnostic Studies

Radiographs of infant hips are extremely difficult to interpret and can provide a false sense of security if they seem normal. At 3 to 6 months of age, the femoral head ossifies. Prior to this time, an abnormal relationship between the upper end of the femur and the acetabulum might not be apparent. Additionally, in infants with unstable but located hips, radiographs show the hip in position and the instability is undetected. A better imaging test

prior to femoral head ossification is ultrasonography.[5] Because a large percentage of infants will have abnormal sonographic evaluation in the first week of life, with many of these abnormalities resolving within a few weeks,[1,6] it is best to delay the ultrasound in children with located but possibly unstable hips until 4 to 6 weeks of age.[3,7] Children with dislocated hips should undergo ultrasonography immediately. After approximately 6 weeks, the ossific nucleus of the femoral head is detectable and radiographs are more likely to reveal abnormalities and asymmetries. A standard anteroposterior pelvis radiograph with both legs extended in neutral abduction is then sufficient for diagnosis.

Findings on radiographic evaluation can be subtle, but two features are typical for DDH: the Shenton line is displaced laterally (Figure 12.1), and the acetabular angle is widened. The Shenton line, an arc running from the inferior border of the femoral neck up and extending to the superior border of the obturator foramen, is used to identify displacement of the hip on an AP pelvis film. The acetabular angle is formed by the angle produced by a line drawn between two points on the acetabulum and the Hilgenreiner line (Figure 12.2). Angles greater than 30 degrees are considered abnormal, and angles greater than 40 degrees indicate dislocation (Figure 12.3).

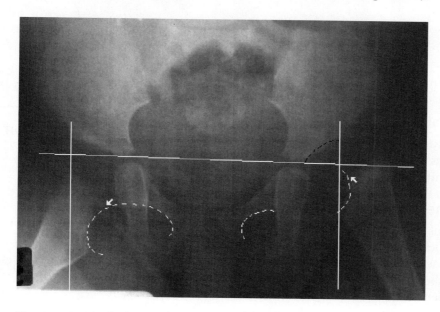

**Figure 12.1** Shenton line displaced laterally in a hip with DDH.

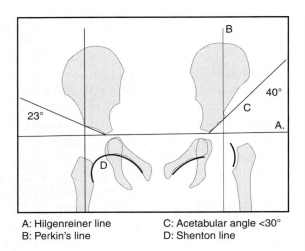

A: Hilgenreiner line
B: Perkin's line
C: Acetabular angle <30°
D: Shenton line

**Figure 12.2** Acetabular angle and Hilgenreiner line.

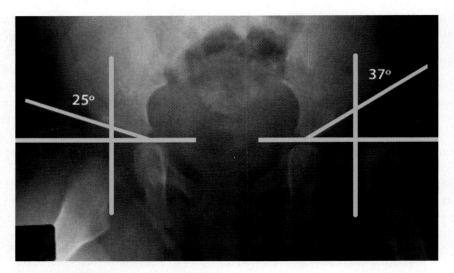

**Figure 12.3** Widened acetabular angle in DDH.

## Differential Diagnosis

The differential diagnosis for DDH is broad and includes trauma, infections, cerebral palsy, and congenital abnormalities.

## Management

Treatment of DDH is most successful when begun early; delays in detection can lead to a significantly worse prognosis. Patients with untreated abnormal hips persisting beyond the newborn period are at risk for osteoarthritis, pain, abnormal gait, leg length discrepancy, and decreased agility. All infants who are seen in the ED should have their hips examined regularly until they are able to walk. Neonates who have a dislocated hip at birth should be referred to an orthopedic surgeon or pediatric orthopedic surgeon if available. When a newborn has a loose but located hip, referral can be made within 2 weeks. Children who present after the newborn period require immediate referral.

The essential goal of treatment is concentric reduction of the hip. After concentric reduction, stability must be obtained so that when the leg is allowed to move, it does not subluxate or dislocate. This position is maintained until all the dysplastic features of the bone and cartilage have resolved. The two most important complications are failure to achieve these goals and aseptic necrosis of the femoral head.

In the first 6 months of life, the Pavlik harness is the mainstay of treatment. It is a dynamic splint that allows movement while preventing hip extension or adduction. If the harness is unsuccessful, a hip spica cast is usually the next choice. Beyond 6 months of age, a hip spica cast or fixed orthosis is required. Surgical release of contracted muscles might be required in older infants and children, with open surgical reduction if complete closed reduction is not achieved. Femoral and/or pelvic osteotomy might be necessary to reduce and stabilize dislocated hips in children older than 2 or 3 years.[8] Beyond 4 years in bilateral cases and 8 years in unilateral cases, reduction should not be attempted. The risk of aseptic necrosis and the potential for a poor result are too high.[2]

---

## KEY POINTS

**Management of Developmental Dysplasia of the Hips**

Birth to 6 months of age

- Infants younger than 6 weeks - Ultrasonography
- Infants older than 6 weeks - Plain radiography
- Orthopedic referral for closed reduction as appropriate and Pavlik harness

6 to 18 months of age

- Plain radiography
- Orthopedic referral for closed reduction and spica cast

Older children

- Plain radiography
- Orthopedic referral for closed reduction or leave unreduced

---

## CASE SCENARIO 2

A woman brings in her 15-month-old daughter because she has noticed that the child's toes point inward when she walks and she often falls when she runs. After falling, the child gets up right away and continues on her way. She does not seem to be in pain and is not bothered by these frequent falls. She is otherwise healthy without any medical problems, takes no medications, and has no allergies.

The patient was a full-term infant delivered vaginally after an uncomplicated antenatal course. She weighed 8 pounds, 5 ounces at birth and had Apgar scores of 9 and 9 at 1 and 5 minutes. She has achieved developmental milestones on schedule and started walking at 12 months. She eats a diverse diet, including meats, fruits, and vegetables, and drinks whole milk. She shows no preference for either hand and uses both well. There is no family history of cerebral palsy, learning disabilities, brain tumors, progressive neurologic diseases, or spina bifida. Of note, when he was a toddler, the child's father's toes pointed in; he wore corrective shoes connected by a bar and currently has a normal gait.

On examination the child is alert and playful and is toddling around the examination room. She is at the 50th percentile for height, weight, and head circumference. Significant physical examination findings include a normal neurologic exam and a normal spine without evidence of a dimple or tuft of hair at the sacrum. Her legs are of equal length. There are no clicks or clunks with Ortolani and Barlow maneuvers, and the hips have a full range of motion. The lateral aspects of the feet are straight; the feet are easily dorsiflexed above the neutral position (90 degrees), and the heel is midline without varus or valgus deformity. When you have the child sit on the examination table with her legs dangling over the edge, you find the lateral malleolus to be aligned with the medial malleolus. As you finish your physical exam, you have the child walk and then run down the corridor while you observe her from the front and back. For best visualization, you do this part of the examination with the child wearing only a diaper. On observation you note that her feet point inward and her patellae point forward as she ambulates. Otherwise she has a normal gait without evidence of spasticity, ataxia, or pain.

1. *What is the diagnosis?*
2. *What is the treatment?*
3. *Does the patient need a referral to an orthopedic surgeon?*

## Rotational Deformities

Parents and grandparents are frequently distressed by their child's intoeing and often seek medical advice. Fortunately, most cases of intoeing are related to age and development and resolve spontaneously as the child grows. Knowledge of the normal musculoskeletal changes that occur through childhood in conjunction with a familiarity of the pathologic causes of intoeing is essential for making the correct diagnosis and appropriate referrals.

Most commonly, the cause of intoeing is related to musculoskeletal development and is considered physiological. Three physiological causes of intoeing include metatarsus adductus, internal tibial torsion, and excessive femoral anteversion.

## Metatarsus Adductus

Metatarsus adductus is an intrinsic curving of the foot that results in intoeing. It is thought to result from compression in utero and occurs in approximately 1 in 1,000 live births. In the past it was associated with DDH, although recent reports have questioned this association.[9] Metatarsus adductus can present in the hospital nursery or can be brought to the attention of a physician at any time during infancy.

### Clinical Features

The diagnosis of metatarsus adductus is made by looking at the sole of the foot. Normally, the lateral border of the foot is straight. In metatarsus adductus, the lateral aspect of the foot has a C-shaped curve. To assess the flexibility of the defect, the heel is held in neutral alignment and the forefoot is abducted. A flexible deformity can be eliminated, and a fixed or rigid defect cannot. Grading of metatarsus adductus is based on the degree of flexibility and the relationship of the toes to a line bisecting the heel. With a normal foot, a line bisects the heel between the second and third toes. The line is at the third toe in a mild deformity, and between the third and fourth toes in a moderate deformity. The line is between the fourth and fifth toes in a severe deformity. The severity of metatarsus adductus is classified as mild/flexible, moderate/fixed, or severe/rigid.

### Management

Mild/flexible and moderate/ fixed metatarsus adductus can initially be treated with stretching exercises; however, despite its commonly prescribed use, the effectiveness of stretching exercises is uncertain.[10] If the deformity does not resolve by 2 to 4 months, a referral for casting is recommended. Every 2 to 3 weeks, two or three casts are applied. Treatment with casting is most effective prior to 6 months of age and ineffective after 2 to 3 years of age. In general, no further intervention is required after the casting is completed. Severe/rigid metatarsus adductus should be referred for serial casting in the first few weeks of life. These patients might require night splinting to maintain correction after the casting is completed. In 85% to 90% of cases, metatarsus adductus resolves spontaneously.[11]

## Internal Tibial Torsion

Internal tibial torsion (ITT) usually presents at walking age with inward pointing of a child's toes during walking or running. Some parents also comment on frequent falling, especially with running. With ITT, intoeing is a reflection of the normal rotational changes of the tibia. At birth, the mean tibial torsion is 5 degrees. Over time, the tibia rotates outward to a mature torsion of 15 to 20 degrees.[10]

### Clinical Features

The diagnosis of ITT is made using the bimalleolar axis (Figure 12.4). With the knee bent to a right angle and the tibial tubercle pointing forward, the examiner places his or her hands on the medial and lateral malleoli. In newborns, the lateral malleolus is 2 to 4 degrees posterior to the medial malleolus; by 5 years old it is 9 degrees posterior, and at maturation it is 15 to 22 degrees posterior. Internal tibial torsion is present if the lateral malleolus is less posterior than this. Tibial rotation is also reflected in the thigh-foot angle (TFA) (Figure 12.5). With the child prone, the foot and the ankle in a neutral position, and the knees flexed to 90 degrees, the TFA is the angle between the axis of the foot and the thigh. An internal TFA is indicative of internal tibial torsion. Observation of the child's gait can also aid in the diagnosis. When the child walks or

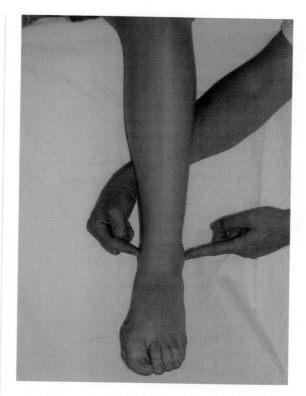

**Figure 12.4** Normal bimalleolar axis due to the posterior position of the lateral malleolus.

runs, the patellae will face forward while the toes point inward. Encircling the patellae with ink will allow for better visualization of its alignment. Varus at the knee often is associated with ITT. Fortunately, by the time 95% of children with ITT reach 7 to 8 years old, the internal tibial torsion has resolved and no intervention is required.

### Management

In the past, severe ITT was treated with a Denis Browne splint (what our patient's father had worn as a child), twister cables that turn the feet out, and various shoe modifications. None of these interventions has been shown to hasten resolution of the malrotation. Additionally, poorly applied Denis Browne splints can be harmful if they cause heel valgus to develop.[11] In severe cases of ITT that do not resolve by 8 years of age, the treatment of choice is a rotational osteotomy of the tibia. However, this procedure is associated with significant complications, including malrotation, angular

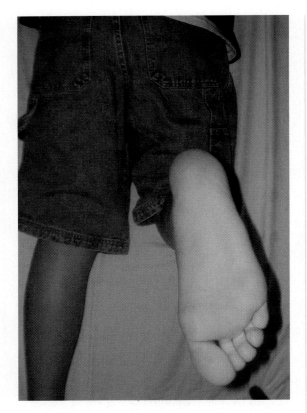

**Figure 12.5** Determination of the thigh-foot angle.

deformity, nonunion, recurrence, and neurovascular complications. Only one study has addressed the arthritic complications of unresolved ITT[12]; however, it was retrospective, unsubstantiated by statistics, and is, thus far, unconfirmed. On the up side, a recent study has suggested that ITT is associated with increased running speed.[13] When sex matched sprinters and nonathletes were compared, sprinters were found to have more internally rotated tibias than did the control group. Without conclusive evidence that ITT can result in long-term disability, it might be preferable to forgo the potentially destructive surgery required to repair the malrotation.

## Excessive Femoral Anteversion

Excessive femoral anteversion is the most common cause of intoeing and, as with metatarsus adductus and ITT, is related to normal rotational changes with skeletal maturation. Intrauterine positioning results in infants being born with externally rotated hips and feet. Over the course of infancy these findings resolve. Additionally, the femur is anteverted relative to the axis of the femoral condyles at the knee. Normal degrees of anteversion are reported; however, there is a wide range of normal, with only 80% of patients' values falling within 10 degrees of the mean.[14] Despite the wide range of values found, all studies document a gradual decrease in anteversion during childhood with an ultimate femoral neck anteversion of 8 to 25 degrees by adulthood. The increased anteversion in newborns can be masked by the external rotation contracture of the soft tissues about the hip. The contracture originates from the externally rotated position of the hips in utero and is perpetuated by the wearing of diapers and positioning of the child postnatally. For this reason, although children with intoeing secondary to excessive femoral anteversion can present as toddlers, they tend to present in early childhood, with maximal average internal rotation in children between 3 and 7 years old.

### Clinical Features

As external rotation contracture of the hip resolves, parents might notice a worsening of the child's intoeing. In addition to intoeing, parents often note that the child sits in the "W" position and is unable to sit cross-legged. Excessive femoral anteversion is often familial, usually bilateral, and tends to affect girls more frequently than boys. The diagnosis is made by internally and externally rotating the hips while the child lies either prone or supine with the hips extended (Figure 12.6).

In children with excess femoral anteversion, most of the arc of rotation will be inward, with internal rotation as much as 90 degrees. External rotation is only 10 to 30 degrees. On observation of the child's gait, note that both the patellae and feet point inward.

### Diagnostic Studies

Although radiography, computed tomography, magnetic resonance imaging (MRI), and ultrasonography can be used to measure the degree of femoral anteversion, the results from these studies show a poor correlation with clinical examination and are not necessary to make

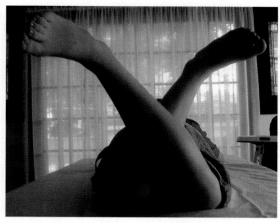

A

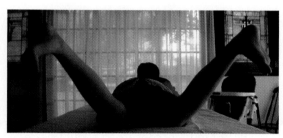

B

Figure 12.6  A. Internal hip rotation. B. External hip rotation.

the diagnosis of excessive femoral anteversion.[9] Additionally, there might not be a radiographic improvement as the degree of intoeing resolves. The absolute precision of clinical measurement of hip rotation has also been called into question; however, the assessment of hip rotation remains the mainstay of diagnosis in the routine clinical setting. Research to evaluate the long-term complications of excessive femoral anteversion is contradictory. Smaller studies suggest that excessive femoral anteversion predisposes patients to osteoarthritis of the hip, while others contradict this claim.[15]

Further workup should be done if the cause of intoeing is thought to be pathologic. This workup might include radiographs of the pelvis, knees, wrists, and spine to confirm or exclude skeletal dysplasia or metabolic bone disease; ultrasonography, radiography or MRI of the hip to exclude DDH; MRI to exclude cerebral palsy, spina bifida, and intracranial abnormality; and blood tests to exclude metabolic bone disease.

## YOUR FIRST CLUE

**Physical Examination Findings in Metatarsus Adductus, Internal Tibial Torsion, and Femoral Anteversion**

Metatarsus adductus:

- Line bisecting the heel lateral to third toe
- C-shaped lateral foot

Internal tibial torsion:

- Bimalleolar axis shows lateral malleolus anterior or less posterior than it should be
- Thigh-foot angle internal

Femoral anteversion:

- Child sits in the "W" position
- Arc of rotation of the hip is inward
- Foot and patella are point inward

## Differential Diagnosis

The differential diagnosis of intoeing is varied; however, the diagnosis can often be made after a thorough history and physical examination with normal growth and neurologic function excluding many of the causes of intoeing.

The physician is able to systematically exclude many of the pathologic causes of intoeing by asking directed questions: a history of hand preference during infancy, spasticity, problems during pregnancy and/or delivery, and unilateral intoeing would suggest cerebral palsy; asymmetric leg length with limited external rotation or abduction of the hip would suggest DDH; a sacral dimple or hair tuft suggests spina bifida; and a diet devoid of vitamin D would suggest rickets.

## WHAT ELSE?

**Differential Diagnosis of Intoeing**

- Cerebral palsy
- Developmental dysplasia of the hip
- Spina bifida
- Rickets
- Metatarsus adductus
- Internal tibial torsion
- Femoral anteversion

## Management

Nonsurgical treatments have included shoe wedges, torque heels, night splints, and twister cables. As with ITT, these interventions have not been shown to be effective. If intoeing persists after 8 to 10 years of age, is cosmetically unacceptable, and causes functional problems with gait, some recommend derotational osteotomy. Complications occur in approximately 15% of patients and include residual intoeing, avascular necrosis of the femoral head, osteomyelitis, and late-developing valgus deformity. Patients and families should carefully consider the risks and benefits of surgery in light of a paucity of evidence for long-term sequelae. Spontaneous resolution of intoeing secondary to femoral anteversion occurs in more than 95% of affected children.[16]

### KEY POINTS

**Management of Metatarsus Adductus, Internal Tibial Torsion, and Femoral Anteversion**

- Metatarsus adductus
  - stretching or casting
- Internal tibial torsion
  - observation or rotational osteotomy
- Femoral anteversion
  - shoe wedges, torque heels, night splints, and twister; or derotational osteotomy

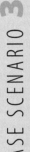

**CASE SCENARIO 3**

A woman brings her 3-year-old son in for evaluation of bowlegs. The boy has had bowlegs since he started walking. The mother was not initially concerned about this because her first son had the same problem and, by 3 years of age, his legs were straight. The child, however, has had progressive worsening and has started to waddle when he walks. He is able to walk and run without difficulty and never complains of pain. He has no history of major trauma to his legs and has never broken a bone. His medical history is remarkable only for the usual childhood viral illnesses. He is on no medications, has no allergies, and has not received any specific therapy for bowlegs. He was born at term after an uncomplicated antenatal course. He was delivered vaginally and was born headfirst. At birth he was 8 pounds, 12 ounces. He eats a well-balanced diet and tends to snack between meals. He drinks at least 24 ounces of whole milk a day. His milestones were achieved on time or early and, although he did not crawl, he walked at 11 months. The mother does not know of anyone else in the family with bowlegs or any other bone problems.

Physical examination reveals a husky boy in no distress. He speaks well and interacts appropriately for age. His height is at the 50th percentile, and his weight is at the 90th percentile. His head, ears, eyes, nose, throat, lung, cardiovascular, abdominal, and neurologic examinations are normal. When he stands with his back to you, with his medial malleoli touching, you measure the intercondylar distance to be 12 cm. As he walks, his gait is even with lateral thrusting of both knees. Supine, his legs are the same length. You are unable to straighten the bowing with the derotational test. In full extension the knees are stable; however, at 10 to 20 degrees of flexion, the medial femoral condyles sublux posteromedially.

1. *What is the next step in the evaluation?*
2. *Do most children outgrow bowleggedness?*
3. *Will this patient?*

## TABLE 12-2 Development of Tibiofemoral Angle During Growth. Note the Normal Physiologic Progression of Bowlegs to Knock-Knees and Then to Normal

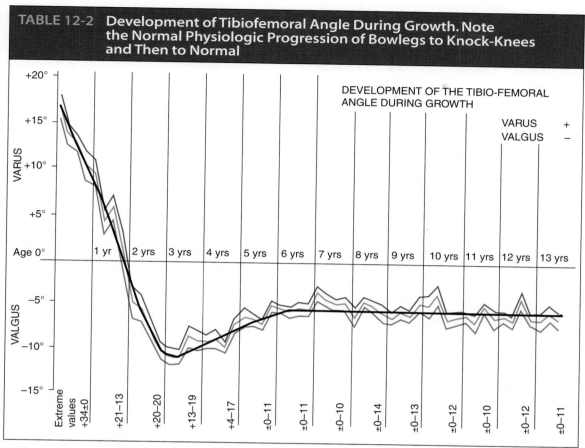

Source: Salenius P, Vankka E. The development of the tibiofemoral angle in children. *J Bone Joint Surg [Am]*. 1975;57A:260. Reprinted with permission.

## Angular Deformities

Bowleggedness or genu varum, is a common physical finding in children younger than 2 years. The bowing tends to become more obvious as the child starts to ambulate and, in the presence of a rotational abnormality such as ITT, is exaggerated.

Secondary to intrauterine positioning, infants are born with a contracture of the medial knee capsule, especially of the posterior oblique ligament. This results in external rotation of the entire lower limb and the genu varum posture of the infant's legs. During the first year of life, this contracture loosens and, depending on the amount that remains, results in children having varying degrees of bowleggedness when they begin to walk. By 18 to 22 months, the contractures stretch and the knees begin to straighten. The varus deformity (bowlegs) becomes a valgus alignment (knock-kneed) during the second and third years of life and then achieves the normal adult alignment of a slight valgus by 7 to 8 years of age. Normals for the tibiofemoral angle during growth are depicted in Table 12-2.

In most cases, bowing is a physiologic abnormality that corrects itself however, any significant bowing beyond 2 years of age tends not to be physiologic.

## Blount Disease

Blount disease, as the most common pathologic condition that results in bowleggedness, deserves special mention. Blount disease is characterized by disordered endochondral ossification of the medial proximal tibial physis. Clinically, it appears as an abrupt varus deformity of the proximal tibia associated with an internal torsion of the tibia. There are two major types of Blount disease: infantile and adolescent. The infantile form is more common and usually found in obese black children younger than 3 years. It is bilateral in up to 75% of cases. This form is more progressive than the adolescent form. Adolescent Blount disease occurs after the age of 6 years and tends to be unilateral. Black children and boys are more commonly affected than white children and girls. Most patients with adolescent Blount disease have a history of childhood bowing that improved but never resolved. When the child has a growth spurt, the varus angle acutely worsens.

The cause of infantile Blount disease is unknown, although it is most likely multifactorial with contributions from hereditary, developmental, and mechanical factors. Environmental and mechanical factors are postulated to have a role in the adolescent form of the disease.[17]

The diagnosis of Blount disease is based on historical features, clinical findings, and radiographs. Clinically, the varus deformity is readily apparent and there is some medial tibial torsion. The beaking of the medial proximal metaphysis is often palpable. Affected children might walk with a waddle (or a limp in unilateral disease) and demonstrate a lateral thrust of the knee during ambulation. The knee tends to be stable in full extension but, at 20-degree flexion, can have posteromedial subluxation of the femoral condyle into the depressed medial tibial plateau. The subluxation, or Siffert-Katz sign, can be present before there are any changes on x-rays. In the later stages of the disease, clinical features can include pain and instability of the knee with ambulation.

## Clinical Features

Adolescent Blount disease is more commonly unilateral, and leg shortening is common. The varus deformity tends to be less than 20 degrees, and medial torsion of the tibia is mild or absent. Locking or popping of the knee and pain are more common than in the infantile form. The patient's gait can be antalgic and show a mild lateral knee thrust; instability of the knee is uncommon, but at 20-degree flexion, there can be mild laxity of the medial collateral ligament. Varus deformity of the knee is common in children; however, pathologic causes should be excluded. The history of present illness should include onset and progression of symptoms, alleviators and exacerbators, and any prior interventions. A comprehensive medical history including birth, growth, and developmental histories, dietary habits, and family history should be elicited. Children with pathologic genu varum frequently have a history of walking at an early age, being overweight, and having pain with ambulation. Physical examination components include the assessment of weight, height, and nutritional status, a comprehensive neurologic examination, skin evaluation for signs of neurofibromatosis, and joint inspection for evidence of inflammatory changes. On examination of the affected extremity, the derotation test and the determination of the intercondylar distance will help differentiate physiologic from pathologic causes of bowing. The derotation test differentiates physiologic bowing secondary to tight knee ligaments from more serious pathology. It is done by flexing the knee to 90 degrees, holding the femur steady in one hand, and attempting to externally rotate the knee. Alternatively, it can be done with the child on his or her back by externally rotating the tibia to match the external rotation of the femur. With physiologic bowing, these maneuvers derotate the contracted medial knee capsule and the deformity disappears. The intercondylar distance is determined by measuring the distance between the femoral condyles while the child is standing with medial malleoli touching; distances greater than 6 cm are abnormal. Other concerning findings on physical examination include small size, excessive weight for height, significant asymmetry, severe deformity, palpable metaphyseal beaking, knee pain, and knee instability or lateral thrust with ambulation.

## Diagnostic Studies

Children with persistent bowing beyond 2 years old and those patients with concerning findings on history or physical examination should have radiographs from hip to ankle, with the focus being on the knees. The child

**Signs and Symptoms of Blount Disease**

- Intercondyle distance greater than 6 cm
- Short stature
- Weight excessive for height
- Severe deformity
- Palpable metaphyseal beaking
- Knee instability
- Knee pain
- Presence of Siffert-Katz sign

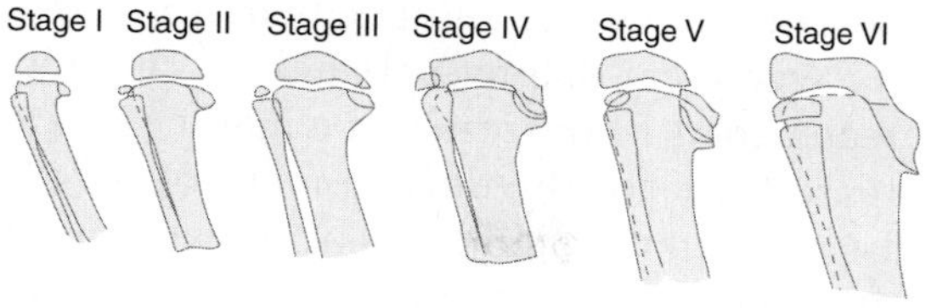

**Figure 12.7** Langenskiold's six stages of Blount disease. Source: Bradway JK, Klassen RA, Peterson HA. Blount Disease: a review of the English literature. *J Pediatr Orthop.* 1987;7:472–480. Reprinted with permission.

should be standing with both kneecaps pointing forward.[19] On plain radiographs, physiologic bowing might show an exaggerated metaphyseal-diaphyseal angle of the proximal tibia, a finding also seen in Blount disease. In physiologic bowing, however, this change also tends to be seen in the distal femur and distal tibia.

Radiographic findings in pathologic causes of bowing can include widened physes at all the joints and bowing of the femur and tibia as is seen in rickets, or overgrowth of the fibula compared with the tibia and asymmetry in the growth of the proximal tibial metaphysis as is seen in achondroplasia, the most common genetic condition that leads to bowing.

Radiographically, infantile Blount disease is a progressive disease classified according to radiographic findings as defined by Langenskiold's six stages of Blount disease (**Figure 12.7**). Radiographic findings include abrupt varus angulation at the metaphysis of the proximal tibia, a widened and irregular physeal line medially, a medially sloped and irregularly ossified epiphysis, and prominent beaking of the medial metaphysis with lucent cartilage island within the beak. Drennan's angle, or the metaphyseal-diaphyseal angle, is measured. If it is greater than 11 degrees in children older than 2 years or greater than 16 degrees in children younger than 2 years, it is abnormal.[18] It is important to remember that, to diagnose Blount disease, there must be other radiographic findings in addition to an excessive Drennan angle. The isolated finding of an increased metaphyseal-diaphyseal angle might represent nothing more than physiologic bowing that will resolve spontaneously. The prognosis for infantile Blount disease is variable, with progression being the norm. Complete regression has been documented in early stages of the disease.

There is not a radiographic classification system for adolescent Blount disease. Radiographic findings include widening of the medial growth plate, a normal or slightly wedge-shaped epiphysis, and a narrow area about midway in the medial physeal line, with sclerosis on the epiphyseal and metaphyseal sides of this area.

In addition to diagnosing pathology, radiographs can also be helpful in alerting the physician to those children who need close

**Radiographic Signs of Blount Disease**

- Metaphyseal beaking
- Varus angulation of proximal tibia
- Irregularly ossified epiphysis
- Excessive Drennan angle

observation. Levine and Drennan noted that a metaphyseal-diaphyseal angle of the tibia greater than 11 degrees was a marker for increased risk for the development of Blount disease.[18] In their study, 29 of 30 extremities with metaphyseal-diaphyseal angles greater than 11 degrees went on to develop Blount disease, while only 3 of 58 extremities with angles less than 11 degrees had subsequent changes consistent with Blount disease. These high-risk children should not be treated until they show definitive signs of Blount disease because some children with significant varus deformities go on to complete spontaneous resolution.

Blood tests in the evaluation of bowlegs are directed by the suspected diagnosis.

## Differential Diagnosis

In most cases, bowing is a physiologic abnormality that corrects itself. However, any significant bowing beyond 2 years of age tends not to be physiologic and can be due to a number of pathologic conditions.

## Management

The management of bowleggedness is based on the underlying cause. Most cases are physiologic and resolve spontaneously. They are treated with observational management and can be followed by the primary care provider. If physiologic genu varum fails to resolve by 7 to 8 years old, orthopedic referral is appropriate. Pathologic conditions should be referred for specialized management. The treatment of Blount disease is determined by patient age, severity of the varus deformity, and

Langenskiold stage. Milder cases of infantile Blount disease in children younger than 3 years are initially treated with braces. More severe or progressive angular deformities are treated surgically with a corrective osteotomy with or without physeal bar resection. Mild, nonprogressive adolescent Blount disease is treated with observation. If the deformity is progressive or causes significant disability, surgical treatment should be considered.

A father brings in his 2-year-old daughter because she will not move her left arm. Earlier that day, as she was walking with her mother, she tripped and her mother grabbed her arm to prevent her from falling. Since that time she has not moved her arm and cries if anyone touches it. The father thinks she has hurt her wrist. The girl is otherwise healthy without any medical problems or allergies. She is not taking any medications. Excluding the left arm, the physical exam is entirely normal. The child is holding her left arm at her side in mild flexion with the forearm pronated. Her wrist, elbow, and shoulder are nontender. She has no tenderness of any of her bones in her left upper extremity.

1. *What is the diagnosis?*
2. *How do you treat it?*
3. *What is the prognosis?*

# Radial Head Subluxation

Radial head subluxation, commonly referred to as nursemaid elbow, is a frequent condition encountered in the emergency department (ED). Classically, it occurs when there is a sudden traction on a child's arm. Simple maneuvers like swinging a child by the wrists or pulling the child up by the hands are associated with radial head subluxation. Other associated histories include taking off or putting on a sweater or coat, falls, and self-induced episodes during temper tantrums. In up to one half of cases, no history of sudden traction of the arm is elicited. However, many of these infants likely had unwitnessed falls or pulls of their arms by other children. Studies have shown a higher frequency of occurrence in the left arm, and a slightly higher incidence in girls compared to boys. Radial head subluxation usually occurs between 1 and 5 years of age, with an average age of approximately 2.5 years.[20–22] There are reported cases in infants younger than 6 months.[23] A recurrence rate has been described of up to 26%.[21]

The proposed mechanism of injury is the entrapment of the annular ligament between the radial head and capitellum.

## Clinical Features

The child usually presents with the affected arm held at the side in mild flexion with the forearm pronated. Frequently, children hold their wrists as they attempt to support their arms and elbows, causing parents to erroneously think the injury is at the wrist instead of the elbow. Patients can have bilateral involvement of both arms.[21,24] Most children have a nontender examination of the extremity unless the forearm is supinated, which causes the child to cry and resist supination.

## YOUR FIRST CLUE

**Nursemaid Elbow**
- History of traction to the arm or swinging of the child by the arms
- Absence of edema or bruising of the upper extremity
- Child holds the arm by the side with forearm flexed and pronated

## WHAT ELSE?

**Differential Diagnosis for Nursemaid Elbow**
- Fractures of the upper extremity
- Osteomyelitis
- Cellulitis
- Tumor

There should be no edema or induration at the elbow. If detected, the physician should consider other diagnoses, including elbow fracture, contusion, or infection.

### Differential Diagnosis

The differential diagnosis for nursemaid elbow includes trauma, infection, and tumor. If the history and physical findings are not classic, then radiographs will help distinguish these conditions from nursemaid elbow.

### Diagnostic Studies

Radiographs, if obtained, can either be normal or reveal an abnormality in a line drawn through the longitudinal axis of the radius and capitellum.[25] In uninjured elbows this line should bisect the capitellum. A patient with a true radial head subluxation might return from the radiology department with a reduced subluxation, as positioning for a lateral elbow radiograph sometimes provides the necessary treatment procedure even before the radiograph is taken. Overall, radiographs are not recommended before attempts at reduction, especially if there is a classic history of a pulled arm and a compatible examination. Even without a classic history, many practitioners will attempt a reduction if the examination is compatible with radial head subluxation and then reevaluate clinically prior to getting a radiograph.[26]

### Management

Treatment of radial head subluxation is fairly straightforward, with two different types of procedures described. The classic method of reduction involves supination of the wrist/forearm followed by flexion at the elbow (**Figure 12.8**). Studies have found this technique to be successful in 80% to 90% of cases.[21,22] An alternative technique is hyperpronation at the wrist; flexion is not required[27] (**Figure 12.9**). Although

> ## KEY POINTS
>
> ### Management of Nursemaid Elbow
> - Management of patients with classic presentation of not moving the arm after traction or swinging should include immediate reduction.
> - Obtain radiographs in children with physical findings suggestive of trauma or when the history includes trauma.
> - Reduction techniques include hyperpronantion or supination followed by flexion of the elbow.

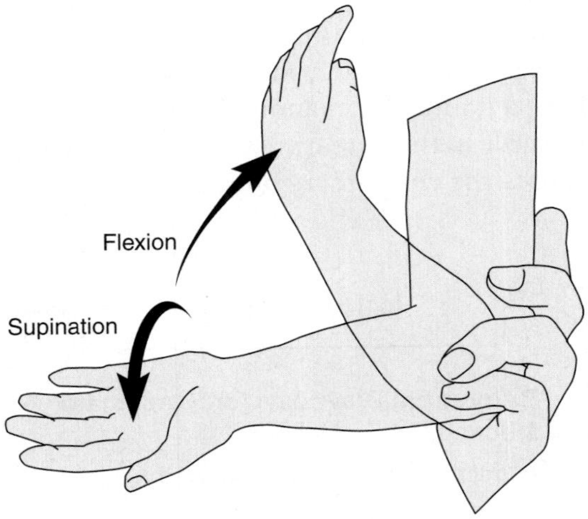

Flexion

Supination

**Figure 12.8** Treatment of radial head subluxation with supination and flexion.
Source: Macias CG, Bothner J, Wiebe R. A Comparison of supination/flexion to hyperpronation in the reduction of radial head subluxations. *Pediatrics*. 1998;102:10. Reprinted with permission.

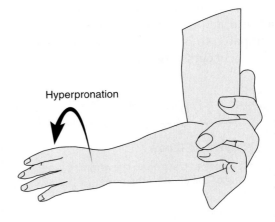

Hyperpronation

**Figure 12.9** Treatment of radial head subluxation with pronation.
Source: Macias CG, Bothner J, Wiebe R. A Comparison of supination/flexion to hyperpronation in the reduction of radial head subluxations. *Pediatrics*. 1998;102:10. Reprinted with permission.

both techniques have been found to be highly successful, hyperpronation might provide a slightly higher success rate, especially in the left arm.[27,28] In addition, one study suggested that it might be less painful to the patient.[28] It is helpful to know both techniques, as some patients who have failed one type of reduction will subsequently reduce when the alternative procedure is applied. In both treatment modalities, a palpable or audible click at the radial head is highly associated with a successful reduction and the child is usually using the arm fully within 10 to 15 minutes. Children younger than 2 years have been associated with a slower return of use of the arm perhaps because it takes the younger child longer to realize that the arm is no longer painful. Occasionally, the subluxed elbow cannot be reduced even after several attempts. In these cases, the elbow should be splinted in 90 degrees and referred for orthopedic followup. Most of these patients will have normal use of the arm at followup.[29]

There are no known complications of either reduction technique in patients with radial head subluxation. If attempts at reduction occur in patients with other injuries, complications can be seen, including displacement of previously nondisplaced fractures and unnecessary pain. In most cases the diagnosis is obvious and the treatment is straightforward. Once reduced, the arm should be painfree and need no specific followup. Guidance should be given, however, to avoid sudden traction on the arm to prevent recurrences.

## CASE SCENARIO 5

A woman presents with her 4-year-old daughter. For the past 3 weeks, the child has been intermittently limping and complaining of right leg pain. She has otherwise been well without fever, chills, or a preceding viral illness. She does not have a history of recent injury to her leg. She has never been hospitalized and is not taking any medications. On physical exam, the girl is in the 10th percentile for height and weight. She has a normal physical exam except for her right leg. Her legs are the same length and she limps on the right leg. She has normal range of movement of her ankle and knee and has no bony tenderness. When you attempt to move her hip, she tenses up and whimpers. She has limited hip range of motion in all directions. There is no redness, swelling, or deformity of her right leg. Anteroposterior and frog-leg lateral radiographs of the pelvis show the right femoral head to be smaller than the left with a relatively widened joint space. Her CBC count and ESR are normal.

1. What is the diagnosis?
2. What is the treatment for this illness?
3. What is the prognosis?

## Legg-Calvé-Perthes Disease

Legg-Calvé-Perthes (LCP) disease is a localized disorder of the hip characterized by ischemic necrosis of the femoral head, subsequent collapse, and fragmentation, followed by reossification. Although the disease was first described in the early 1900s, its causes and methods of treatment remain elusive and controversial.[30] The origin of LCP disease is thought to be a localized manifestation of a generalized disorder of the epiphyseal cartilage.[31] This process is manifested in the femoral head because of its precarious blood supply. The ischemic injury to the femoral head might be due to abnormal viscosity and clotting.[31]

Most cases of LCP disease occur between the ages of 4 and 9 years, although cases have been reported as early as 2 years or as late as 13 years.[32] The disease affects boys more often than girls and is found to be bilateral in 10% of cases.[30] A history of other family members with the disease has been found in about 10% of cases.[30] Low birth weight and growth delay have been associated with LCP disease, with some patients having a bone age that is between 1 and 3 years below chronological age.[30,32]

## Clinical Features

Clinical symptoms in patients with LCP disease typically include pain and/or limp in the affected extremity. Similar to patients with slipped capital femoral epiphysis (SCFE), symptoms can be referred to the groin, thigh, or knee. Therefore, any child presenting with knee pain should have a thorough examination of the hip. A history of minor trauma frequently brings the chronic symptoms to medical attention but is not the cause of the disease. Gait disturbances can be due to pain, limb length discrepancy, or to a limited range of motion at the hip. The examination should include gait, limb length measurement, and range of motion at the hip. Limited internal rotation and abduction at the hip joint is frequently found.

## Diagnostic Studies

The diagnosis of LCP disease is confirmed with anteroposterior and frog-leg lateral pelvis radiographs.[32] Initially, the femoral head appears smaller and the articular cartilage space appears wider than the contralateral normal side. Within several months, a crescent-shaped radiolucent line can be seen on the lateral radiograph (crescent sign). This is caused by subcortical collapse of the trabecular bone. Later, the femoral head develops a fragmented appearance and is less radiopaque (Figure 12.10). Reossification then takes place, but a residual deformity in the femoral epiphysis and acetabulum can persist.

## Differential Diagnosis

The differential diagnosis of Legg-Calvé-Perthes disease includes other entities that present with

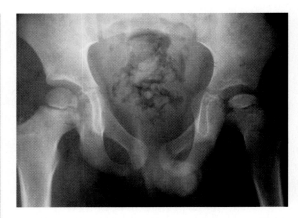

**Figure 12.10** Anteroposterior radiograph of Legg-Calvé-Perthes disease.

knee or hip pain in children, including septic arthritis, transient synovitis, fractures, malignancies, and SCFE.[32] Although SCFE usually presents in older children, there is overlap of age presentations between 10 and 13 years. Radiographs should easily distinguish these two entities. Other diagnoses can be eliminated by either history or radiographic evidence.

## Management

Treatment of LCP disease is controversial.[30,33] Long-term studies of the natural history are rare and multiple classification schemes exist, which makes it more difficult to compare treatment modalities. The disease process is self-limiting but can last for several years. The early goals of treatment are to alleviate pain and hip stiffness. The limp can persist for 2 to 4 years.[32] Nonsteroidal anti-inflammatory medications and reduction of activities will help reduce pain. Occasionally, non–weight-bearing with crutches and/or braces will be necessary. A physical therapy program might improve range of motion and decrease stiffness. Long-term goals of therapy include reducing residual deformities of the femoral head and surrounding acetabulum. One approach to maintaining a spherical femoral head on reossification is femoral head containment, which requires positioning the proximal femur in abduction with braces or doing so during surgical procedures.[32] Prognosis depends primarily on age of healing, with better outcomes found in younger children, especially those whose diagnosis is made before the age of 5 years.[33] Long-term studies reveal a higher incidence of osteoarthritis and total hip replacement as patients approach their sixth and seventh decades of life.[30] These late-term complications might be dependent on the shape of the femoral head and acetabulum at the time of healing.

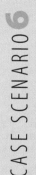

**CASE SCENARIO 6**

A mother and her 12-year-old son present to the emergency department after he collided with another boy while playing baseball. Following the collision, which is described as minor, he started to complain of left knee pain. He tells you he has been having mild, intermittent knee pain for the past 2 months but it is now worse and he cannot walk. He denies hip, ankle, or foot pain. No other injuries were sustained in the collision. On physical exam, he is in the 90th percentile for weight and 25th percentile for height. On examination, he is lying on the stretcher with his leg held in flexion with external rotation and abduction. The knee, ankle, and foot are normal. Any attempt to move his hip elicits extreme pain and he has very limited range of motion, especially with abduction and internal rotation.

1. *What is the diagnosis?*
2. *What should not have been done during the physical exam?*
3. *How do you diagnose this condition?*

## Slipped Capital Femoral Epiphysis

Slipped capital femoral epiphysis (SCFE) occurs when the femoral head (epiphysis) slips posterior and inferior relative to the femoral neck (metaphysis). Although it is the most common orthopedic hip disorder in adolescence, SCFE is frequently misdiagnosed early in its course because of the variety of presenting symptoms. Delays in diagnosis can lead to a more difficult treatment course and a less favorable prognosis. Therefore, SCFE has to be considered whenever a patient presents with a limp, or hip, thigh, or knee pain, or both.

In the past, patients with SCFE were classified by duration of symptoms.[34] Those with symptoms of less than 3 weeks' duration were classified as acute. Patients with symptoms of more than 3 weeks' duration were classified as chronic, and those with a long duration but sudden increase in symptoms were classified as acute or chronic. The problem with this classification scheme is that the duration of symptoms is often vague, making it impossible to accurately classify the disease. In addition, classification based solely on length of symptoms was not found to be prognostic with regard to longer-term outcome. Recently, a different classification system has been used based on the type of symptoms.[34] Patients that can ambulate with or without crutches are classified as having stable SCFE, whereas patients with unstable SCFE are nonambulatory even with crutches. The latter form is treated much more like an acute fracture of the femur across the growth plate and has a poorer prognosis due to an increased incidence of avascular necrosis of the femoral head. Approximately 90% of SCFE cases are stable and therefore have a favorable prognosis.[34]

The overall incidence of SCFE is 1 to 3 per 100,000, with a slightly higher incidence in black children.[35,36] Males are affected almost twice as often as females. In two thirds of cases, children are found to be obese; it is thought that the increased weight during the early adolescent growth spurt years increases the stress across the physeal plate, which is already oriented vertically and posteriorly. The average age for development of SCFE is 12 years (± 1.5) in girls and 13.5 years (± 1.7) in boys. Patients should be carefully observed because bilateral involvement develops in up to 40% of children within 18 months of presentation.[37] Although most cases are considered idiopathic, there are associations described with hypothyroidism, growth hormone administration, renal osteodystrophy, and radiation therapy. The incidence of hypothyroidism is so low in patients with SCFE that routine thyroid function testing is not recommended unless the clinical presentation is atypical or the patient presents with bilateral hip involvement.

## Clinical Features

Patients with SCFE usually present with a history of intermittent limp of several weeks' du-

ration with either hip, thigh, or knee pain. Often a vague history of trauma or a fall brings attention to the limp and is the initial reason for the visit. In one study, 29% of patients were misdiagnosed at the initial visit, mostly because the main symptom was thigh pain instead of hip pain.[36] Diagnoses frequently given at the initial visit include Osgood-Schlatter disease, growing pain, thigh contusion, and muscle strain. Physical examination findings depend on the degree and chronicity of slippage. Patients with early symptoms can have an antalgic gait with discomfort in the groin, thigh, and knee. If chronic slippage has developed, discomfort of the hip is seen when the hip is rotated internally and externally. Range of motion at the hip might be decreased, particularly in abduction and internal rotation. Patients with acute slippage will present with severe pain, similar to those with an acute fracture. Attempts to rotate or flex the hip are not advised as they can cause severe discomfort. The hip is typically held in a position of flexion, external rotation, and abduction. The acute slippage can disrupt circulation to the femoral head, especially the superior retinacular arteries, which supply blood flow to the outer two thirds of the femoral head, thus increasing the risk for avascular necrosis of the femoral head.[38]

## Diagnostic Studies

The diagnosis of SCFE can be confirmed with plain film radiographs. Both anteroposterior and frog-leg pelvic radiographs should be obtained (Figure 12.11). Early in the course, anteroposterior radiographs can appear normal

## YOUR FIRST CLUE

### Signs and Symptoms of Slipped Capital Femoral Epiphysis

- Obese preadolescent or adolescent
- Hip, thigh, groin, or knee pain
- Limp
- Decreased range of motion of the hip

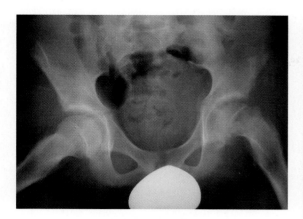

**Figure 12.11** Frog-leg view of a left slipped capital femoral epiphysis.

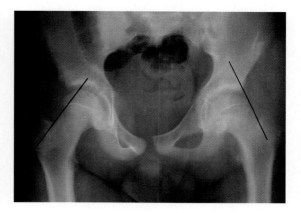

**Figure 12.12** Anteroposterior radiograph of slipped capital femoral epiphysis revealing normal Klein line on right hip, intersecting the edge of the epiphysis, and an abnormal Klein line on the left hip, missing the epiphysis.

because the early slippage is in the posterior direction and will be seen only on a lateral view. The first radiographic sign is physeal widening; obtain an anteroposterior (AP) pelvic view to compare the width of the physis between the right and left sides of the hip. In normal pelvic radiographs, the Klein line can be drawn along the anterior neck of the femur at the base of the greater trochanter and should intersect the epiphysis (**Figure 12.12**). In patients with SCFE, an abnormal Klein line does not intersect the epiphysis as it should.[34] With an unstable slip, radiographs show an abrupt displacement of the femoral head posterior, inferior, and medial relative to the femoral neck. These patients are in such severe pain that only one projection of the hip can be obtained, usually an anteroposterior view.

## Differential Diagnosis

The differential diagnosis includes other causes of hip and knee pain, including toxic synovitis, septic hip, LCP disease, Osgood-Schlatter disease, and other hip and knee conditions.

## Management

Treatment is always surgical, so early orthopedic consultation is advised. Once diagnosed, patients should be non-weight-bearing on the affected extremity to prevent further slippage. Initial ED management consists of bed rest, pain management, and relief of muscle spasms.

### THE CLASSICS

**Radiographic Signs of Slipped Capital Femoral Epiphysis**
- Physeal widening
- Klein line
- Epiphysis inferior and posterior

Treatment of patients with stable SCFE consists of a single screw placed through the femoral neck into the epiphysis, thus eliminating the possibility of further slippage. The treatment of patients with unstable SCFE is more controversial both in the type of surgical procedure recommended and the timing of the procedure.[39]

The most common complications are avascular necrosis of the femoral head and chondrolysis. The risk of either process increases with the severity of the initial slippage.[40,41] Children with avascular necrosis can have a rapidly developing arthritis of the hip, ultimately requiring a hip replacement early in adulthood. Chondrolysis, a loss of articular cartilage, can occur in 5% to 7% of patients with SCFE and can lead to chronic pain and loss of normal hip motion. Barring the development of either complication, the child can resume running and contact sports may resume after closure of the physis.

**CASE SCENARIO 7**

A woman brings her 2-year-old son, to see you because he has a fever and has been crying. He had been well until yesterday, at which time he became quite cranky with frequent crying spells. Later that day he developed a fever of 102°F, which the mother treated with ibuprofen. His fever came down but he continued to cry intermittently, especially with diaper changes. He has been lying around and seems to be favoring his left leg. He has no current cold symptoms, vomiting, diarrhea, or rash. He has not had any recent falls or accidents. Three weeks earlier, he had a cold that got better without any treatment. The child is very healthy, has never been admitted to the hospital, and has never been seriously ill. He takes no medications and has no allergies.

As you start to examine the child, you notice that he is lying still on the bed and looks tired but not toxic; he has no increased work of breathing, and his skin is flushed. His initial assessment is normal except a heart rate of 140 beats/min and a temperature of 39°C. On focused and detailed physical examination, you find no abnormalities on his head, eyes, ears, nose, throat, lung, abdominal, lung, and cardiovascular exams. His cranial nerves are intact. Deep tendon reflexes are normal, but as you lift his left leg to check his left patellar reflex, he winces with pain. The remainder of his neurological exam is normal. On extremity exam, he has full range of movement of both upper extremities and his right lower extremity. His left foot, ankle, and knee are normal. On examination of the left hip, he cries with pain and pushes your hand away. He has limited range of motion of his left hip, especially with flexion, abduction, and external rotation. There is no redness, swelling, or warmth of the left hip.

After your exam, you discuss your concerns with the mother and order blood tests and radiographs. As you wait for results, you treat the child's pain and fever and call a consultant.

1. *What is the diagnosis?*
2. *What tests were ordered, and why?*
3. *Who did you consult, and why?*

## Acute Septic Arthritis

Septic arthritis refers to microbial invasion and infection of the joint space. Bacterial pathogens are common in patients with acute septic arthritis, while fungal and mycobacterial pathogens tend to be associated with chronic septic arthritis. Acute septic arthritis occurs in all age groups but is more common in children. Approximately 70% of cases occur in children younger than 4 years, and the peak incidence is between 6 and 24 months. Boys are affected twice as frequently as girls. Predisposing factors include preceding viral infection, trauma, immunodeficiency, hemoglobinopathy, hemophilia with recurrent hemarthroses, diabetes, intravenous drug abuse, rheumatoid arthritis, and intra-articular injections or surgeries. Seventy-five percent of septic arthritis cases involve the joints of the lower extremity, with the knee being most commonly and the hip second most commonly involved. Other affected joints, in order of involvement, include the ankle, elbow, shoulder, and wrist. Over 90% of cases are monoarticular.

Hematogenic seeding, local spread, or traumatic or surgical infection can cause septic arthritis. In children, it most commonly results from hematogenic spread as bacteria pass into the synovial space through the highly vascular synovial membrane. The synovial membrane lacks a limiting basement membrane, which facilitates bacterial translocation. The bacteria then bind to bone and cartilage and initiate an inflammatory response that breaks down the joint by two mechanisms: directly through the effects of proteolytic enzymes, and indirectly through pressure necrosis caused by accumulation of purulent synovial fluid.

The contiguous spread of infection from osteomyelitis to the joint space occurs in approximately 10% of cases and is more common in newborns and young infants. The most common bacterial causes of septic arthritis are listed in Table 12-3. Additional causative organisms include *Neisseria gonorrhoeae* in neonates and sexually active adolescents, *Pseudomonas aeruginosa* and *Candida* in intravenous drug abusers, *Salmonella* in children with sickle cell disease, and Gram-negative bacteria in children with immunosuppression.

## Clinical Features

The clinical picture of septic arthritis varies with age. Infants tend to have fever, failure to feed, lethargy, pseudoparalysis of the extremity, and pain with diaper changes. Most older children have systemic symptoms of fever, malaise, poor appetite, and irritability as well

## YOUR FIRST CLUE

**Signs and Symptoms
of Septic Arthritis**

- Irritability
- Fever
- Erythema
- Limp or refusal to walk
- Decreased range of motion of the affected limb
- Hip held in abduction and external rotation

| TABLE 12-3 | Septic Arthritis Pathogens and Treatment | |
| --- | --- | --- |
| **Age** | **Organism** | **Treatment** |
| Birth to 2 months | Group B *Streptococcus*<br>S aureus<br>Gram-negative rods | Nafcillin 50 mg/kg and gentamicin 2.5 mg/kg; add vancomycin 10 mg/kg if staph is suspected or known |
| 2 months to 3 yr | S aureus<br>H influenzae<br>S pneumoniae | Nafcillin 50 mg/kg and ceftriaxone 50 mg/kg; add vancomycin 10 mg/kg if staph is suspected or known |
| 3 years to 12 yr | S aureus<br>S pneumoniae<br>S pyogenes | Nafcillin 50 mg/kg and ceftriaxone 50 mg/kg; add vancomycin 10 mg/kg if staph is suspected or known |
| > 12 yr | S aureus<br>S pneumoniae<br>N gonorrhoeae | Nafcillin 50 mg/kg and ceftriaxone 50 mg/kg; add vancomycin 10 mg/kg if staph is suspected or known |

as localized symptoms of pain, with limp or refusal to walk. With septic arthritis, the onset of symptoms is more acute than seen with osteomyelitis. Physical examination reveals local erythema, warmth, and swelling. If the hip is affected, it is often held in flexion, abduction, and external rotation. Range of motion is decreased due to pain and muscle spasm, and passive joint movement is painful. In infants, joint dislocation might be observed.

## Diagnostic Studies

Helpful initial laboratory studies for diagnosis of septic arthritis include a white blood cell count, ESR, C-reactive protein (CRP), and blood cultures. No single blood study is diagnostic of septic arthritis, and no single blood test is consistently elevated in septic arthritis. A combination of history, physical examination, and laboratory test results will suggest the diagnosis and prompt an evaluation of synovial fluid. On the first day of illness, a CRP might be more appropriate than an ESR: CRP levels increase early in infection, while the ESR is slower to rise. Practitioners may order both CRP and ESR, as they might be useful in tracking the course of the infection.

Blood cultures are positive in 29% to 40% of cases of septic arthritis.[42–44] Identification of the causative organism not only helps direct antibiotic treatment but also provides an organism for serum bactericidal testing when the child is switched to oral antibiotics.

Synovial fluid evaluation is the mainstay for diagnosing septic arthritis. If septic arthritis is suspected, joint aspiration should be performed without delay and the sample sent for Gram stain, aerobic and anaerobic cultures, cell count with differential, and glucose. The synovial fluid of septic arthritis tends to be turbid or grossly purulent with a white blood cell count greater than 40,000 cells/mm$^3$ and a predominance of polymorphonuclear cells. Synovial glucose can be low (synovial fluid/blood glucose less than 0.5) and protein and lactate elevated (Table 12-4). Because of the intrinsic immunoglobulins in the synovial fluid, cultures of the fluid will be positive in only half of children with a clinical picture consistent with septic arthritis. Synovial fluid culture can be done using agar plates or blood

### THE CLASSICS

**Diagnostic Studies in Septic Arthritis**

- WBC is elevated >15,000 mm$^3$ (50%)
- ESR is elevated >60 mm/hr (>90% of cases)
- C-reactive protein >20 mg/L (94%)
- Synovial fluid white cell count greater than 40,000 cells/mm$^3$ and a preponderance of polymorphonuclear cells

| TABLE 12-4 | Synovial Fluid Findings in Different Types of Arthritis. | | | | |
|---|---|---|---|---|---|
| | Character | WBC count (cells/mm$^3$) | PMNs (%) | Mucin clot | Other |
| Normal | Clear; yellow | <200 | <10 | Good | |
| Juvenile rheumatoid arthritis | Turbid | 250–50,000 | 50–70 | Fair to poor | 50% with decreased complement |
| Reactive arthritis | Cloudy to turbid; can be clear | 1,000–150,000 | 50–70 | Fair to poor | Increased complement |
| Lyme arthritis | Turbid | 500–100,000 | >50 | Poor | |
| Septic arthritis | Turbid; white-grey | 10,000–250,000 | >75 | Poor | Low glucose High lactate |

culture media. Either way, the specimen requires immediate inoculation.

In septic arthritis, plain radiographs of the hip can be normal or, in the presence of a large joint effusion, can show periarticular soft tissue swelling, widening of the joint space, obliteration or displacement of the gluteal lines, and asymmetric fullness of the iliopsoas and obturator soft tissue planes (**Figure 12.13**). Late in the course of infection, subchondral bone erosions and narrowing of the joint space can be seen.

Ultrasonography is much more sensitive than plain radiography in the detection of hip effusion and provides direct visualization of the fluid and needle during joint aspiration. Scintigraphy can also be useful in diagnosing septic arthritis: during the "blood pool" or delayed images of the joint, symmetric uptake in the periarticular tissues on both sides of the joint is seen. Scintigraphy is diagnostic of septic arthritis earlier than other imaging techniques and is also a useful adjunct in identifying associated osteomyelitis or avascular necrosis of the femoral head. CT and MRI can confirm the presence of an effusion but do not differentiate septic from nonseptic arthritis.

## Management

Septic arthritis requires immediate admission, antibiotics, and surgical intervention. Surgical options range from needle aspiration to open surgical drainage; however, no randomized controlled trials exist that compare these two treatment approaches. Some authors recommend surgical drainage in all infants and young children with septic arthritis because needle aspiration has been shown to be inferior in this population.[43] Indications for surgical drainage in children with septic arthritis include involvement of the hip joint, the presence of large amounts of pus or debris in the joint, loculated fluid, recurrence of joint fluid after four or five aspirations, and lack of clinical improvement within 3 days of the initiation of appropriate therapy.[45–47] In joints other than the hip, the need for surgical drainage is determined on a case-by-case basis.

Empiric antibiotic therapy for septic arthritis is directed against the most likely organisms based on patient age and comorbidities. (See Table 12-3.) Treatment can then be changed after culture results and sensitivities are known. To maximize culture results, antibiotics should not be given until a specimen

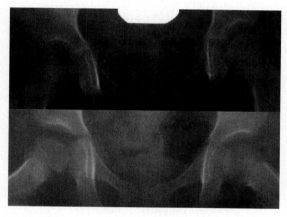

**Figure 12.13** Septic arthritis of the hip with large joint effusion.

## THE CLASSICS

**Joint Effusions/Joint Space Widening in the Hip on Plain Radiographs:**

- Infants—measure from the inner border of the ramus to the top femur at the junction with the physis

- Children—measure from the teardrop on the pelvis to the femoral head; >2 mm difference between the sides with the hips in neutral position is abnormal

## KEY POINTS

**Management of Septic Arthritis**

- Admission
- Parenteral antibiotics
- Surgical intervention: aspiration and/or surgical drainage

of joint fluid is obtained. However, antibiotic therapy should not be delayed if arthrocentesis cannot be performed in a timely manner. Initial treatment is parenteral to ensure adequate serum concentrations of antibiotic. After the patient's clinical condition is stabilized, oral antibiotic therapy can be instituted. In general, doses 2 to 3 times those used for mild infections are sufficient. Response to therapy is measured with clinical improvement and acute phase reactants, including the ESR or CRP.

The mortality rate associated with septic arthritis has fallen to less than 1% but the morbidity remains significant. Sequelae include leg length discrepancy, persistent pain, limited range of motion and ambulation, and aseptic necrosis of the femoral head. Predictors of poor outcome include infection of the hip and shoulder, adjacent osteomyelitis, a delay of 4 days or more before antibiotics and surgical intervention, and prolonged time to sterilization of synovial fluid.

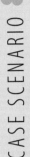

## CASE SCENARIO 8

A 12-year-old and her mother come to see you because the girl has been having right knee pain. It started about 1 month ago and has been getting worse. The pain is worse when she goes up or down stairs and when she plays soccer. It also hurts when she touches it. There is a small amount of swelling of the knee but no redness. She has not fallen on the knee and there are no other complaints. On examination of the right knee, she has point tenderness at the tibial tubercle. There is full range of motion of the knee and on extension against resistance her pain is reproduced. Her ligaments are stable and there is no knee effusion.

1. *What is the diagnosis?*
2. *Does she need an x-ray?*
3. *What is the treatment?*

## Osgood-Schlatter Disease

Osgood-Schlatter disease is generally a benign lesion of the tibial tubercle at the site of the patellar tendon insertion. It affects adolescents during growth spurts and is most commonly seen in boys 12 to 14 years old and in girls 10 to 11 years old.[48] Most cases are unilateral, but bilateral cases are not uncommon. Osgood-Schlatter disease occurs frequently in boys due to greater participation in sports. It is becoming more common in girls as they are increasingly involved in athletic activities. Common sports associated with Osgood-Schlatter disease include basketball, football, soccer, gymnastics, and ballet. During these activities, repetitive quadriceps stress contractions apply through the patellar tendon its insertion at the tibial tuberosity. This can result in a partial avulsion fracture through the ossification center, which subsequently leads to heterotopic bone formation at the tendon insertion

site. Tibial tuberosity fuses with the tibial etaphysic at age 15 years in girls and 17 years in boys. The avulsed segment can fail to unite, leaving a small palpable mass.[48]

### Clinical Features

Patients with Osgood-Schlatter disease present with a painful soft tissue swelling at the tibial tubercle. The area is very tender to palpation

### YOUR FIRST CLUE

**Signs and Symptoms of Osgood-Schlatter Disease**

- History of repetitive running, jumping, or sports activity
- Swelling and pain over the tibial tubercle
- Pain over tibial tubercle with knee extension or squatting

and the pain can be reproduced by having the patient extend the knee against resistance or by squatting with the knee in full flexion. History usually reveals that running, going up and down stairs, and jumping cause increased pain.

### Diagnostic Studies

The diagnosis of Osgood-Schlatter disease is usually clinical. Radiographs are frequently obtained to rule out other conditions, including neoplasm, cysts, infections, stress fractures, and other musculoskeletal diseases involving the knee. Although a lateral knee radiograph might reveal a fracture through the tibial tubercle, frequently only soft tissue swelling is seen. Some patients who present with radiographic fragmentation of the tubercle will develop chronic symptoms. Those with no fragmentation are usually asymptomatic at long-term followup.[49]

### Management

Management of patients with Osgood-Schlatter disease is almost always nonsurgical and depends on the extent of the presenting symptoms.[48] Patients with mild symptoms should be given nonsteroidal anti-inflammatory drugs and be advised to avoid activities that cause repeated quadriceps contraction. For many adolescents, the latter advice is frequently hard to follow. Symptoms usually improve in weeks to months. More advanced cases can be treated with a knee immobilizer (and, rarely, a cylindrical cast). Steroid injections are not indicated. Rarely, patients with unresolved lesions will require surgery directed at excision of all the intratendon ossicles and possible removal of the tibial tubercle.[50] In most patients, the condition is self-limiting and results in no long-term complications.

## Summary

The approach to children with orthopedic complaints should be based on age, history of symptoms, and physical findings. Causes of nontraumatic orthopedic conditions vary significantly with age, and a complete history and physical examination will be necessary to exclude systemic disease.

---

### KEY POINTS

**Management of Osgood-Schlatter Disease**

- Mild to moderate symptoms
  - decrease activity; nonsteroidal anti-inflammatory agents
- Moderate to severe symptoms
  - knee immobilizer or cylindrical cast
- Very severe cases
  - surgical intervention (rare)

---

### THE BOTTOM LINE

- Causes of nontraumatic orthopedic emergencies vary with patient age.
- Obtain a complete history to include character, location, quality, and time course of symptoms.
- Establish if the condition is associated with an acute traumatic event or repetitive activity.
- Always examine the hips in any patient with knee pain.
- Radiographs might be needed to establish the diagnosis.
- Prompt orthopedic or primary care referral is necessary.

# CHAPTER REVIEW

## Check Your Knowledge

1. Which of the following statements regarding Legg-Calvé-Perthe disease is correct?
   A. Can be bilateral
   B. Classically presents in toddlers
   C. Generally seen in large, obese children
   D. Has no findings on x-ray

2. Which of the following statements regarding SCFE is correct?
   A. Most common in the early 20s
   B. Occurs when the femoral head slips anterior and superior relative to the femoral neck
   C. Often presents as knee pain
   D. Treated nonsurgically

3. Which of the following statements regarding septic arthritis is correct?
   A. Always yields bacterial growth from the synovial fluid
   B. Most common in teenagers
   C. Most commonly caused by *N meningitidis*
   D. Treated with joint drainage and intravenous antibiotics

4. Which of the following statements regarding children with Osgood-Schlatter disease is correct?
   A. All have knee effusions
   B. Have increased pain when they squat with the knee in full flexion
   C. Require surgery for a cure
   D. Usually play a lot of video games

## References

1. Marks DS, Clegg J, al-Chalabi AN. Routine ultrasound screening for neonatal hip instability: can it abolish late-presenting congenital dislocation of the hip? *J Bone Joint Surg Br.* 1994;76:534–538.
2. Novacheck TF. Developmental dysplasia of the hip. *Pediatr Clin North Am.* 1996;43(4):829–848.
3. Donaldson JS, Feinstein KA. Imaging of developmental dysplasia of the hip. *Pediatr Clin North Am.* 1997;44:591–614.
4. Barlow TC. Early diagnosis and treatment of congenital dislocation of the hip. *J Bone Joint Surg Br.* 1962;44:292.
5. Boal DK, Schwenkter EP. The infant hip: assessment with real-time ultrasound. *Radiology.* 1985;157(3):667–672.
6. Tionnis D, Storch K, Ulbrich H. Results of newborn screening for congenital dislocation of the hip with and without sonography and correlation of risk factors. *J Pediatr Orthopaed.* 1990;10:145–152.
7. Gull F, Muller D. Results of hip ultrasonographic screening in Austria. *Orthopade.* 1997;26:25–32.
8. French LM, Dietz FR. Screening for developmental dysplasia of the hip. *Am Fam Physician.* 1999;60(1):177–184.
9. Karol LA. Rotational deformities in the lower extremities. *Curr Opinion Pediatr.* 1997;9:77–80.
10. Dietz FR. Intoeing–fact, fiction and opinion. *Am Fam Physician.* 1994;50(6):1249–1259.
11. Pontes IV, Becker JR. Congenital metatarsus adductus: the results of treatment. *J Bone Joint Surg.* 1966;48A:702–711.
12. Turner MS, Smillie IS. The effect of tibial torsion on the pathology of the knee. *J Bone Joint Surg [Br].* 1981;63:396–398.
13. Fuchs R, Staheli LT. Sprinting and intoeing. *J Pediatr Orthop.* 1996;16:489–491.
14. Heinrich SD, Sharps CH. Lower extremity torsional deformities in children: a prospective comparison of two treatment modalities. *Orthopedics.* 1991;14:655–659.
15. Eckhoff DG, Kramer RC, Alongi CA, VanGervon DP. Femoral anteversion and arthritis of the knee. *J Pediatr Orthop.* 1994;14:608–610.
16. Bruce RW. Torsional and angular deformities. *Pediatr Clin North Am.* 1996;43(4):867–881.
17. Salenius P, Vankka E. The development of the tibiofemoral angle in children. *J Bone Joint Surg [Am].* 1975;57A:260.
18. Bradway JK, Klassen RA, Peterson HA. Blount disease: a review of the English literature. *J Pediatr Orthop.* 1987;7:472–480.
19. Levine AM, Drennan JC. Physiological bowing and tibia vara: the metaphyseal-diaphyseal angle in the measurement of bowleg deformities. *J Bone Joint Surg [Am].* 1982;64:1158–1163.
20. Do TT. Clinical and radiographic evaluation of bowlegs. *Curr Opinion Pediatr.* 2001;13:42–46.
21. Choung W, Heinrich SD. Acute annular ligament interposition into the radiocapitellar joint in children (nursemaid's elbow). *J Pediatr Orthop.* 1995;15(4):454–456.
22. Schunk JE. Radial head subluxation: epidemiology and treatment of 87 episodes. *Ann Emerg Med.* 1990;19(9):1019–1023.****
23. Quan L, Marcuse EK. The epidemiology and treatment of radial head subluxation. *Am J Dis Child.* 1985;139:1194–1197.

24. Newman J. "Nursemaid's elbow" in infants six months and under. *J Emerg Med.* 1985;2(6): 403–404.

25. Foster DL. Bilateral nursemaid's elbow. *Pediatr Emerg Care.* 1991;7:128.

26. Frumkin K. Nursemaid's elbow: a radiographic demonstration. *Ann Emerg Med.* 1985;14(7): 690–693.

27. Sacchetti A, Ramoska EE, Glascow C. Nonclassic history in children with radial head subluxations. *J Emerg Med.* 1990;8(2):151–153.

28. Macias CG, Bothner J, Wiebe R. A comparison of supination/flexion to hyperpronation in the reduction of radial head subluxations. *Pediatrics.* 1998;102(1):e10.

29. McDonald J, Whitelaw C, Goldsmith LJ. Radial head subluxation: comparing two methods of reduction. *Acad Emerg Med.* 1999;6(7):715–718.

30. Jones J, Cote B. "Irreducible" nursemaid's elbow. *Am J Emerg Med.* 1995;13(4):491.

31. Wenger DR, Ward WT, Herring JA. Legg-Calvé-Perthes disease. *J Bone Joint Surg.* 1991;73(5):778–788.

32. Weinstein SL. Natural history and treatment outcomes of childhood hip disorders. *Clin Orthop.* 1997;344:227–242.

33. Koop S, Quanbeck D. Three common causes of childhood hip pain. *Pediatr Clin North Am.* 1996;43(5):1053–1066.

34. Herring JA. The treatment of Legg-Calvé-Perthes disease. A critical review of the literature. *J Bone Joint Surg.* 1994;76(3):448–458.

35. Stanitski CL. Acute slipped capital femoral epiphysis: treatment alternatives. *J Am Acad Orthop Surg.* 1994;2(2):96–106.

36. Swiontkowski MF, Gill EA. Slipped capital femoral epiphysis. *Am Fam Physician.* 1986;33(4):167–171.

37. Loder RT. Slipped capital femoral epiphysis. *Am Fam Physician.* 1998;57(9):2135–2142.

38. Ledwith CA, Fleisher GR. Slipped capital femoral epiphysis without hip pain leads to missed diagnosis. *Pediatrics.* 1992;89(4): 660–662.

39. Maeda S, Kita A, Funayama K, Kokubun S. Vascular supply to slipped capital femoral epiphysis. *J Pediatr Orthop.* 2001;21(5):664–667.

40. Loder RT. Unstable slipped capital femoral epiphysis. *J Pediatr Orthop.* 2001;21(5):694–699.

41. Rattey T, Piehl F, Wright JG. Acute slipped capital femoral epiphysis. Review of outcomes and rates of avascular necrosis. *J Bone Joint Surg.* 1996;78(3):398–402.

42. Bennett DM, Mannyak SS. Acute septic arthritis of the hip in infancy and childhood. *Clin Orthop.* 1992;281:123–132.

43. Syriopoulou V, Smith A: Osteomyelitis and septic arthritis. In: Feigin R, Cherry J, eds. *Musculoskeletal Infections: Pediatric Infectious Disease.* 3rd ed. Philadelphia, Pa: WB Saunders; 1992:727–753.

44. Dunkle LM. Toward optimum management of serious focal infections: the model of suppurative arthritis. *Pediatr Infect Dis J.* 1989;8:195–196.

45. Nelson JD, Koontz WC. Septic arthritis in infants and children: a review of 117 cases. *Pediatrics.* 1996;38:966–971.

46. Green NE, Edward K. Bone and joint infections in children. *Orthop Clin North Am.* 1987;18:555–576.

47. Nade S. Acute septic arthritis in infancy and childhood. *J Bone Joint Surg Am.* 1983;65: 234–241.

48. Dunn JF. Osgood-Schlatter Disease. *Am Fam Physician.* 1990;41(1):173–176.

49. Krause BL, Williams, JP, Catterall A, Chir M. Natural history of Osgood-Schlatter disease. *J Pediatr Orthop.* 1990;10(1):65–68.

50. Binazzi R, Felli L, Vaccari V, Borelli P. Surgical treatment of unresolved Osgood-Schlatter lesion. *Clin Orthop.* 1993;(289):202–204.

CASE SUMMARY 1

During your evaluation of a 5-week-old girl, you feel a clunk as you do the Ortolani maneuver on the left hip. You also note asymmetric skin folds and decreased abduction. The rest of the exam, including the right hip, is entirely normal, and the child is in no distress. On questioning, the mother tells you that her daughter was born on time after an uncomplicated antenatal course. Specifically, the mother did not have multiple gestations or oligohydramnios, and the baby was born headfirst. The baby is breastfeeding well and gaining weight. The mother has had no problems with diaper changes, and her daughter does not appear to be in pain. After discussing your findings with the mother, you arrange for further testing and contact a specialist.

# CHAPTER REVIEW

CASE SUMMARY 1 CONT.

1. *What is the diagnosis?*
2. *How do you proceed in your evaluation?*
3. *What is the most likely course of treatment for this child?*

In this case, the infant showed signs of developmental dysplasia of the hip (DDH): asymmetry of skin folds and asymmetrical range of motion of the hip. Because she was only 5 weeks old, routine radiographs may not be helpful and you obtained an immediate ultrasound of both hips. On ultrasound she was found to have a normal right hip with DDH of the left hip. The baby was seen by an orthopedic surgeon within 2 days and placed in a Pavlick harness. He instructed the parents in the use and care of the harness, as well as how to change diapers and handle the infant without disrupting the alignment of the hip. The orthopedist is confident that this infant's hip will respond to this therapy and will continue to follow her closely for the next several months.

CASE SUMMARY 2

A woman brings in her 15-month-old daughter because she has noticed that the child's toes point inward when she walks and she often falls when she runs. After falling, the child gets up right away and continues on her way. She does not seem to be in pain and is not bothered by these frequent falls. She is otherwise healthy without any medical problems, takes no medications, and has no allergies.

The patient was a full-term infant delivered vaginally after an uncomplicated antenatal course. She weighed 8 pounds, 5 ounces at birth and had Apgar scores of 9 and 9 at 1 and 5 minutes. She has achieved developmental milestones on schedule and started walking at 12 months. She eats a diverse diet, including meats, fruits, and vegetables, and drinks whole milk. She shows no preference for either hand and uses both well. There is no family history of cerebral palsy, learning disabilities, brain tumors, progressive neurologic diseases, or spina bifida. Of note, when he was a toddler, the child's father's toes pointed in; he wore corrective shoes connected by a bar and currently has a normal gait.

On examination the child is alert and playful and is toddling around the examination room. She is at the 50th percentile for height, weight, and head circumference. Significant physical examination findings include a normal neurologic exam and a normal spine without evidence of a dimple or tuft of hair at the sacrum. Her legs are of equal length. There are no clicks or clunks with Ortolani and Barlow maneuvers, and the hips have a full range of motion. The lateral aspects of the feet are straight; the feet are easily dorsiflexed above the neutral position (90 degrees), and the heel is midline without varus or valgus deformity. When you have the child sit on the examination table with her legs dangling over the edge, you find the lateral malleolus to be aligned with the medial malleolus. As you finish your physical exam, you have the child walk and then run down the corridor while you observe her from the front and back. For best visualization, you do this part of the examination with the child wearing only a diaper. On observation you note that her feet point inward and her patellae point forward as she ambulates. Otherwise she has a normal gait without evidence of spasticity, ataxia, or pain.

CASE SUMMARY 2 CONT.

1. *What is the diagnosis?*
2. *What is the treatment?*
3. *Does the patient need a referral to an orthopedic surgeon?*

Reassurance is the mainstay of treatment in most cases of rotational deformities. The girl has internal tibial torsion and can be observed for the next several years to ensure that her lower extremity rotational development progresses as expected and her intoeing resolves. If, however, her intoeing persists or worsens as she approaches school age, a referral to an orthopedic surgeon may be indicated. The mother was given a thorough explanation of the abnormality and reassured that this problem should resolve on its own. The other rotational abnormalities can be treated in much the same way with orthopedic referrals made in a timely fashion (by 2 to 4 months of age for a flexible metatarsus adductus and sooner for a rigid metatarsus adductus, and by 8 to 10 years of age for excessive femoral anteversion) to allow for treatment at the optimal time.

CASE SUMMARY 3

A woman brings her 3-year-old son in for evaluation of bowlegs. The boy has had bowlegs since he started walking. The mother was not initially concerned about this because her first son had the same problem and, by 3 years of age, his legs were straight. This child, however, has had progressive worsening and has started to waddle when he walks. He is able to walk and run without difficulty and never complains of pain. He has no history of major trauma to his legs and has never a broken a bone. His medical history is remarkable only for the usual childhood viral illnesses. He is on no medications, has no allergies, and has not received any specific therapy for bowlegs. He was born at term after an uncomplicated antenatal course. He was delivered vaginally and was born headfirst. At birth he was 8 pounds, 12 ounces. He eats a well-balanced diet and tends to snack between meals. He drinks at least 24 ounces of whole milk a day. His milestones were achieved on time or early and, although he did not crawl, he walked at 11 months. The mother does not know of anyone else in the family with bowlegs or any other bone problems.

Physical examination reveals a husky boy in no distress. He speaks well and interacts appropriately for age. His height is at the 50th percentile, and his weight is at the 90th percentile. His head, ears, eyes, nose, throat, lung, cardiovascular, abdominal, and neurologic examinations are normal. When he stands with his back to you, with his medial malleoli touching, you measure the intercondylar distance to be 12 cm. As he walks, his gait is even with lateral thrusting of both knees. Supine, his legs are the same length. You are unable to straighten the bowing with the derotational test. In full extension the knees are stable; however, at 10 to 20 degrees of flexion, the medial femoral condyles sublux posteromedially.

1. *What is the next step in the evaluation?*
2. *Do most children outgrow bowleggedness?*
3. *Will this patient?*

# CHAPTER REVIEW

In this case, the boy had multiple red flags in his history and physical exam. He is an obese child whose deformity is worsening. While walking he had lateral thrusting of the knees; a finding that is never seen with physiologic bowing. His intercondylar distance was excessive and the derotational maneuver was ineffective. Findings on the boy's x-rays were consistent with stage II infantile Blount disease. He was referred to an orthopedic surgeon who treated him with braces and will follow his progress closely.

A father brings in his 2-year-old daughter because she will not move her left arm. Earlier that day, as she was walking with her mother, she tripped and her mother grabbed her arm to prevent her from falling. Since that time she has not moved her arm and cries if anyone touches it. The father thinks she has hurt her wrist. The girl is otherwise healthy without any medical problems or allergies. She is not taking any medications. Excluding the left arm, the physical exam is entirely normal. The child is holding her left arm at her side in mild flexion with the forearm pronated. Her wrist, elbow, and shoulder are non-tender. She has no tenderness of any of her bones in her left upper extremity.

1. *What is the diagnosis?*
2. *How do you treat it?*
3. *What is the prognosis?*

The girl has radial head subluxation of her left arm. You explain the injury to the father and the girl. After explaining the hyperpronation reduction technique, you proceed with the maneuver and feel a clunk under your thumb. Within five minutes the girl is playing and using her left arm normally. The father is told that this is a common problem in young children and it may recur but should not cause any long-term problems. You also instruct him to avoid maneuvers that put traction on the arm in order to minimize the risk of recurrence.

A woman presents with her 4-year-old daughter. For the past 3 weeks, the child has been intermittently limping and complaining of right leg pain. She has otherwise been well without fever, chills, or a preceding viral illness. She does not have a history of recent injury to her leg. She has never been hospitalized and is not taking any medications. On physical exam, the girl is in the 10th percentile for height and weight. She has a normal physical exam except for her right leg. Her legs are the same length and she limps on the right leg. She has normal range of movement of her ankle and knee and has no bony tenderness. When you attempt to move her hip, she tenses up and whimpers. She has limited hip range of motion in all directions. There is no redness, swelling, or deformity of her right leg. Anteroposterior and frog-leg lateral radiographs of the pelvis show the right

CASE SUMMARY 4 CONT.

femoral head to be smaller than the left with a relatively widened joint space. Her CBC count and ESR are normal.

1. *What is the diagnosis?*
2. *What is the treatment for this illness?*
3. *What is the prognosis?*

The girl has LCP disease. The mother is informed that LCP is a progressive disease with a variable prognosis. The girl is under five years of age, so her prognosis is better than if she had presented later in childhood. You also let the mother know that treatment modalities are quite variable. She needs to see an orthopedic surgeon who will consider her age and degree of femoral head deformity and formulate a treatment plan. The girl is sent home with an appointment to see an orthopedist in 3 days.

CASE SUMMARY 6

A mother and her 12-year-old son, present to the emergency department after he collided with another boy while playing baseball. Following the collision, which is described as minor, he started to complain of left knee pain. He tells you he has been having mild, intermittent knee pain for the past 2 months but it is now worse and he cannot walk. He denies hip, ankle, or foot pain. No other injuries were sustained in the collision. On physical exam, he is in the 90th percentile for weight and 25th percentile for height. On examination, he is lying on the stretcher with his leg held in flexion with external rotation and abduction. The knee, ankle, and foot are normal. Any attempt to move his hip elicits extreme pain and he has very limited range of motion, especially with abduction and internal rotation.

1. *What is the diagnosis?*
2. *What should not have been done during the physical exam?*
3. *How do you diagnose this condition?*

The boy has (acute on chronic) unstable SCFE. Because of the instability of the hip, manipulation during initial evaluation should be minimized. He had AP and frog leg pelvic radiographs done that showed the slippage, and an orthopedic surgeon was consulted. He is admitted to the hospital for pain control and complete bed rest, and is scheduled for surgical stabilization.

CASE SUMMARY 7

A woman brings her 2-year-old son, to see you because he has a fever and has been crying. He had been well until yesterday, at which time he became quite cranky with frequent crying spells. Later that day he developed a fever of 102°F, which the mother treated with ibuprofen. His fever came down but he continued to cry intermittently, especially with diaper changes. He has been lying around and seems to be favoring his left leg. He has no current cold symptoms, vomiting, diarrhea, or rash. He has not had any recent falls or accidents. Three weeks earlier, he had a cold that got better without any treatment. The child is very healthy, has never been admitted to the hospital, and has never been seriously ill. He takes no medications and has no allergies.

As you start to examine the child, you notice that he is lying still on the bed and looks tired but not toxic; he has no increased work of breathing, and his skin is flushed. His initial assessment is normal except a heart rate of 140 beats/min and a temperature of 39°C. On focused and detailed physical examination, you find no abnormalities on his head, eyes, ears, nose, throat, lung, abdominal, lung, and cardiovascular exams. His cranial nerves are intact. Deep tendon reflexes are normal, but as you lift his left leg to check his left patellar reflex, he winces with pain. The remainder of his neurological exam is normal. On extremity exam, he has full range of movement of both upper extremities and his right lower extremity. His left foot, ankle, and knee are normal. On examination of the left hip, he cries with pain and pushes your hand away. He has limited range of motion of his left hip, especially with flexion, abduction, and external rotation. There is no redness, swelling, or warmth of the left hip.

After your exam, you discuss your concerns with the mother and order blood tests and radiographs. As you wait for results, you treat the child's pain and fever and call a consultant.

1. *What is the diagnosis?*
2. *What tests were ordered, and why?*
3. *Who did you consult, and why?*

The boy's white blood cell count is elevated with a left shift and his CRP is 19. The radiograph of his left hip shows slight widening of the joint space with no bony abnormality. These findings in a child with his clinical picture are highly suggestive of septic arthritis of the hip. The consultant, an orthopedic surgeon, agrees with clinical assessment and takes the boy to the operating room to tap his hip. The boy's synovial fluid is purulent, has a white count of 90,000 mm$^3$ with a preponderance of polymorphonuclear cells. On gram stain, the synovial fluid shows white blood cells and gram positive cocci in clusters. Intravenous antibiotics were started intraoperatively. His hip was surgically drained and intravenous antibiotics were continued until he became afebrile and his hip pain resolved. He was then switched to oral antibiotics and discharged home. He continues on oral antibiotics and has remained afebrile and pain free.

A 12-year-old and her mother come to see you because the girl has been having right knee pain. It started about 1 month ago and has been getting worse. The pain is worse when she goes up or down stairs and when she plays soccer. It also hurts when she touches it. There is a small amount of swelling of the knee but no redness. She has not fallen on the knee and there are no other complaints. On examination of the right knee, she has point tenderness at the tibial tubercle. There is full range of motion of the knee and on extension against resistance her pain is reproduced. Her ligaments are stable and there is no knee effusion.

1. *What is the diagnosis?*
2. *Does she need an x-ray?*
3. *What is the treatment?*

The girl has Osgood-Schlatter disease. It was exacerbated with daily playing during soccer season. She does not need a radiograph for this diagnosis. She was treated with nonsteroidal anti-inflammatory medications and rest (avoidance of activities causing repeated quadriceps contraction) and her symptoms resolved completely. She is advised that her symptoms may recur until her tibial tuberocity fuses at approximately 15 years of age.

# chapter 13

# Medical Emergencies

Jeffrey R. Avner, MD, FAAP
Ghazala Q. Sharieff, MD, FAAP, FACEP, FAAEM

## Objectives

1 Formulate a diagnostic evaluation of a child with a fever.

2 Describe emergencies encountered with children with sickle cell disease.

3 Identify rashes that indicate serious illnesses.

4 Recognize signs and symptoms of genitourinary emergencies in male patients.

5 Plan management of hypertensive urgencies and emergencies.

6 Classify etiologies of syncope.

## Chapter Outline

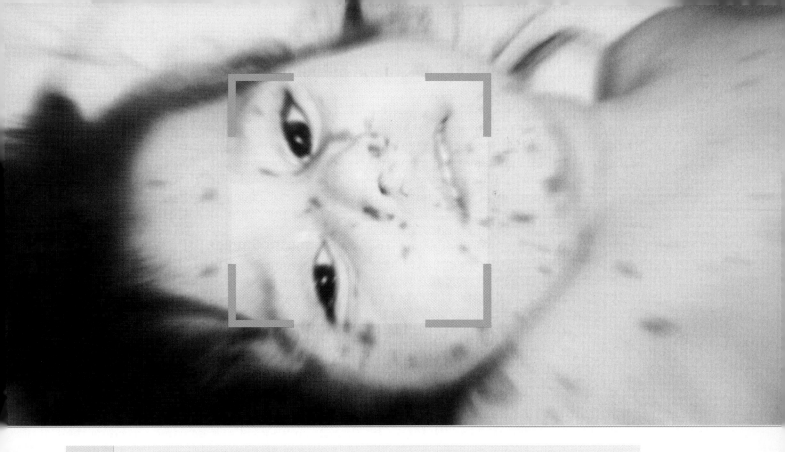

A previously healthy 15-month-old boy is brought to the emergency department with a 1-day history of fever and "not acting like himself." He was well until 3 days ago when he had symptoms of an upper respiratory tract infection. Yesterday he developed a low-grade fever that his mother treated with ibuprofen. Today he has continued fever and decreased oral intake, urine output, and activity level. He has no history of vomiting, diarrhea, cough, or rash. He is not taking any prescription medication.

On physical examination he appears tired and cranky when stimulated. His breathing is not labored, and he is pink. His respirations are 40/min, pulse is 162/min, blood pressure is 92/70 mmHg, and temperature is 38.9°C (102°F). He has dry lips but moist mucous membranes without oral lesions. His neck is supple. An examination of lungs, heart, abdomen, and extremities is unremarkable. There are a few scattered petechiae on his abdomen and lower extremities. His peripheral pulses are normal, and capillary refill time is 3 seconds.

1. *What is your general impression of this child?*
2. *What are the most likely diagnoses?*
3. *What would be your initial management strategy?*

## Introduction

A myriad of conditions presents to the emergency department as medical emergencies. Fortunately, most emergencies have recognizable presenting signs and symptoms, allowing the clinician to formulate an appropriate management plan. At the same time, the clinician must be aware of those conditions that can be life-threatening so that immediate care and treatment are not delayed. This chapter will address both common and life-threatening medical emergencies.

## Sepsis

The body's host defense system responds to an infectious agent with a complex cascade of cytokines and other proinflammatory mediators that repair existing damage caused by the microorganism and limit new damage. This inflammatory response is regulated through the cellular and humoral immune systems, as well as the reticuloendothelial system. In certain situations, this regulation is lost, leading to a massive systemic reaction that results in damage ranging from tissue and capillary injury to organ dysfunction. The term sepsis is often used to refer to a process of systemic inflammation accompanied by systemic signs such as alteration in body temperature, tachypnea and tachycardia, leukocytosis, or leukopenia. It is also helpful to categorize sepsis in the following clinical categories: bacteremia, systemic inflammatory response, sepsis, severe sepsis (failure of an organ system), septic shock, and multiorgan dysfunction syndrome. Infection is the most common cause of sepsis; however, there can be other etiologies such as trauma, burns, and neoplasms.

## Clinical Features

The pathophysiology of bacteremia is essentially a battle between the infecting organism and the host defense. The organism tries to multiply and invade various organ systems while the host tries to contain and then eliminate the organism. If the host wins, there is complete resolution; if the organism wins, there is focal infection. The effects of this battle are the signs of inflammation, which produce characteristic clinical manifestations. Fever is usually apparent, especially early in the course of bacteremia. Hypothermia, while less common, portends a worse prognosis. As the severity of sepsis increases, so do the clinical features. In response to vascular and tissue injury, the body generates lactic acid. Initially, there is tachycardia and an increase in cardiac output in order to preserve systemic blood pressure and organ perfusion. Tachypnea results from increased oxygen demands as well as a response to metabolic acidosis. Hypoxemia can affect other organ systems, including the central nervous system (confusion, lethargy, irritability) and the kidneys (decreased urinary output). Increased capillary leak and vascular permeability cause volume depletion, increased systemic vascular resistance, and the clinical signs of decreased peripheral perfusion. After volume resuscitation, there is usually a decrease in systemic vascular resistance. Vasodilation and warm extremities, despite the presence of inadequate organ perfusion, characterize the "warm shock" of sepsis.

## Diagnostic Studies

The peripheral white blood cell count in children with sepsis typically shows a leukocytosis with a left shift of the differential (increased band forms). In overwhelming sepsis, the white blood cell count can be low, with or without neutropenia. Hypoglycemia is common, especially in young infants, due to limits in their glycogen stores, but conversely can be elevated due to stress.[1] Serum bicarbonate is usually low, consistent with metabolic acidosis resulting from cellular demand exceeding the supply of necessary substrates. Depending on the degree of metabolic acidosis and the child's respiratory reserve, there can be a partial respiratory compensation. Thus, arterial blood gas analysis can show a low pH (less than 7.25), a base deficit, and, if there is respiratory compensation, a low $P_{CO_2}$ (less than 35). In severe sepsis, respiratory failure can exacerbate metabolic acidosis. If capillary leak is present, the serum albumin, total protein, and total calcium will be low; therefore, it is also important to measure the ionized calcium, which is independent of the albumin level.[1] Disseminated intravascular coagulation can cause abnormalities in coagulation studies and thrombocytopenia. Cultures of the blood, urine, spinal fluid, and/or stool are necessary for determining a bacterial etiology. It must be emphasized that antibiotics and other supportive therapy should not be delayed while attempting to obtain laboratory tests.

Infants who appear ill and those with respiratory findings should have a chest radiograph to evaluate the presence of pneumonia, pulmonary edema, and atelectasis. Cardiac size on a chest radiograph might identify hypovolemia (small heart), cardiac failure (large heart), or congenital heart disease (characteristic findings). If cardiac disease or dysfunction is considered, an ECG should be obtained. An abdominal radiograph might show evidence of intestinal perforation (free air), small bowel obstruction (dilated small bowel loops with air-fluid levels), or intussusception (paucity of air in the right lower quadrant). Additional imaging studies may include ultrasonography and computed tomography (CT) scanning.

## Differential Diagnosis

Many diagnoses may present as sepsis. Infection is the most common cause of sepsis in children. Common bacterial causes are shown in Table 13-1.[1] Children with congenital cardiac lesions, especially those that have left-sided outflow tract obstruction (coarctation of the aorta, hypoplastic left heart syndrome) present with tachycardia, tachypnea, poor peripheral perfusion, and cold, mottled extremities. Depending on the type of congenital heart lesion and the duration of illness, a heart murmur or signs of congestive heart failure (hepatomegaly, rales) might or might not be present. Diagnosis is supported by findings characteristic of a heart defect on chest radiograph and ECG and then is usually confirmed by echocardiography. Supraventricular tachycardia (SVT) is a common dysrhythmia in childhood. SVT might be well tolerated in infants for as long as 24 to 48 hours; however, prolonged tachycardia will cause signs and symptoms of heart failure. Similarly, myo-

carditis presents with fever, ill appearance, and congestive heart failure.

Infections of the gastrointestinal (GI) tract can lead to an intra-abdominal abscess with peritonitis, bowel ischemia, or perforation of the intestinal wall. Necrotizing enterocolitis (NEC) usually presents with the sudden onset of bilious vomiting, abdominal distention, lethargy, and lower GI bleeding. Although most common in premature infants, NEC can occasionally occur in stressed, full-term infants. Diagnosis is confirmed by the presence of pneumatosis intestinalis on abdominal radiograph, but this finding is variable. A volvulus or malrotation of the GI tract presents with abdominal pain, bilious vomiting, and melena. Abdominal x-ray might show loops of small bowel overriding the liver shadow with paucity of air in the GI tract distal to the volvulus. Children with intussusception classically present with intermittent, severe, crampy abdominal pain and vomiting. As the intussusception progresses, lethargy or paradoxical irritability develops. As the bowel becomes ischemic, guaiac-positive stools are seen and often there is passage of red, bloody mucus, referred to as "currant jelly stools," which is a late finding in intussusception.

Congenital adrenal hyperplasia, usually caused by deficiency of the enzyme 21-hydroxylase, presents in the first few weeks of life with vomiting, diarrhea, lethargy, and

| TABLE 13-1 | Common Bacterial Causes of Sepsis and Empiric Therapy | |
|---|---|---|
| Age | Etiology | Empiric Therapy |
| Infant < 4–6 weeks | Group B *Streptococcus* <br> Gram-negative bacilli | Ampicillin and cefotaxime <br> OR ampicillin and gentamicin |
| Infants > 4–6 weeks | *Pneumococcus* <br> *Meningococcus* | Cefotaxime or ceftriaxone; <br> add vancomycin if suspected gram-positive |
| Children | *Pneumococcus* <br> *Meningococcus* <br> *Staphylococcus aureus* | Cefotaxime or ceftriaxone; <br> add vancomycin if suspected gram-positive <br> or high staphylococcal or pneumococcal resistance |
| | Group A *Streptococcus* | Penicillin and clindamycin |
| For presumed pseudomonal infection, add ceftazidime or cefepime. | | |

Source: Schexnayder SM. Pediatric septic shock. *Pediatrics in Review.* 1999;20:301–308. Reprinted with permission.

shock. Female patients might have virilization of the external genitalia; male patients might have hyperpigmentation of the nipples and scrotum. Hyponatremia, hyperkalemia, and metabolic acidosis are typically noted.

Many inborn errors of metabolism can present as sepsis. Following a minor stress, such as a viral illness, the infant becomes tachycardic, tachypneic, acidotic, and frequently hypoglycemic. Treatment is aimed at reducing the catabolism by administering intravenous fluids and glucose.

## Management

Management of any child with suspected sepsis begins with rapid assessment of the airway, breathing, and circulation (ABCs). High-flow oxygen should be given and intravenous access obtained. Early antibiotic therapy is essential and must not be delayed while attempting other procedures. Begin empiric therapy based on possible etiology of the sepsis as outlined in Table 13-1.[1] It is important to note that in some cases of bacterial sepsis, antibiotics can worsen the clinical findings through the release of endotoxins from lysed organisms. Cardiovascular support usually begins with intravenous isotonic fluids (normal saline or Lactated Ringer's solution). If perfusion does not improve after repletion of the intravascular space, inotropic drugs (dopamine, dobutamine, or epinephrine) might be needed. All ill-appearing children should have a rapid bedside glucose determination and, if hypoglycemic, be given intravenous glucose. Other electrolyte abnormalities should also be addressed.

# Fever in Children at Risk for Sepsis

## Fever in the Immunosuppressed Child

Advances in care and treatment have led to high survival rates for children with cancer, human immunodeficiency virus (HIV), sickle cell disease, and other immunosuppressive disorders. In many cases, management of these children has moved from the inpatient to the ambulatory setting. Thus, presentation of immunocompromised children to the emergency department is common. Although fever in these children often represents benign illness (upper respiratory infection, otitis media, viral syndrome), the risk of serious bacterial illness can be as high as 20%.[2] Therefore, fever in children who are immunosuppressed requires immediate attention.

The degree of immunosuppression varies with the child's underlying disease and can often be estimated by specific laboratory tests. In general, children are considered severely neutropenic if their absolute neutrophil count (ANC) is less than 500. In addition to a low ANC, a low total lymphocyte count, and in particular a low CD4 lymphocyte count, is a risk factor for serious bacterial illness in children with HIV.

## Clinical Features

General appearance is an important clinical feature in children who are immunosuppressed. However, fever might be the only sign of serious illness. Although a child may appear well at presentation, the potential for acute deterioration mandates immediate evaluation. Some children with sepsis present with alteration in mental status (lethargy, irritability), signs of increased work of breathing (tachypnea, retractions), and decreased peripheral perfusion (prolonged capillary refill, mottled extremities, weak pulse). Particular attention should be given to potential sites of bacterial invasion to the bloodstream. Many children who are immunosuppressed have indwelling intravascular catheters. Repeated use of these catheters for blood drawing and intravenous medications, as well as irritation of the catheter insertion site, increase the likelihood of colonization and eventual invasion of bacteria. Catheter infections are often indolent; presenting with low-grade fever over several days. Other sources of bacteria are the respiratory tract, GI tract, genitourinary tract, perineum, and skin. Although bacterial infections are a common cause of morbidity, certain viral infections can disseminate, causing cardiovascular collapse and death. In particular, vesicles on the skin can be a sign of herpes simplex or varicella zoster infections.

## Diagnostic Studies

All children with fever who are potentially immunosuppressed should have a complete blood cell (CBC) count with attention to the degree of leukopenia or leukocytosis. Comparison with recent white blood cell counts is particularly helpful for children undergoing chemotherapy and those children with HIV. Blood and urine cultures should be obtained. Children with indwelling intravascular catheters need both a blood culture from the catheter as well as from a peripheral site in order to determine whether the catheter is the source of infection. These blood cultures should be of sufficient volume to allow detection of fungi as well as aerobic and anaerobic bacteria. Children in respiratory distress should have continuous pulse oximetry measurements. If respiratory failure is suspected, arterial blood gas analysis should be performed to determine the level of respiratory compromise. Specific areas of potential focal infection might require further investigation with radiography, ultrasonagraphy, or CT of the chest, abdomen, or sinuses.

## Differential Diagnosis

Gram-positive bacteria account for most cases of sepsis. Children with indwelling intravenous catheters are at risk for line sepsis by coagulase-negative *Staphylococcus* or *Staphylococcus aureus* (*S aureus*). Pus and erythema are often found at the catheter insertion site, or erythema and tenderness can be found along the catheter tract. Signs of cellulitis, skin irritation, and abrasions can also be a source of invasion by *Staphylococcus*. Mucosal tenderness, sores, or ulcers suggest infection with *Streptococcus viridans*. Gram-negative infections with *Escherichia coli* (*E coli*), *Klebsiella*, and *Pseudomonas aeruginosa* are less common but potentially more virulent. Typhlitis, a bowel injury of the terminal ileum and cecum associated with chemotherapy, should be suspected in any child with neutropenia and abdominal tenderness.

In addition to these considerations, children with HIV are at high risk for sepsis due to infection with *Pneumococcus* and *Salmonella,* which can present without antecedent illness or focus of infection on physical examination. *Pneumocystis carinii* pneumonia usually occurs in young children and is accompanied by tachypnea, cough, and hypoxemia.

### Management

Rapid assessment and immediate management of suspected sepsis in immunocompromised children is often lifesaving. Regardless of the clinical appearance or the height of fever, all children need a complete examination, CBC count with a manual differential, and, if neutropenic, empiric antibiotic therapy. Often empiric therapy can be based on a combination of factors including likely pathogens, previous history of sepsis, and local antibiotic resistance patterns. Usual therapy includes an antipseudomonal antibiotic (e.g., ceftazidime). If high rates of Gram-negative resistance are known, an aminoglycoside can be added to the empiric treatment. Due to concerns of increasing Gram-positive resistance, vancomycin should be reserved for suspected catheter-related infections, children with severe mucosal damage, or those who present in shock. Regardless of the antibiotic choice, close monitoring is essential. If the bacterial load is high, the massive lysis of cells after antibiotic administration can cause cardiovascular instability within hours.

The management of children with HIV is controversial. Children who are febrile but appear well and have an ANC above 500 can usually be managed as outpatients with oral or parenteral antibiotics and close followup. Ill-appearance or a low ANC requires admission and empiric parenteral antibiotics.

## Fever in Very Young Infants

Infants younger than 2 months have immature immune responses and might not be able to contain certain infections. Although most well-

appearing febrile infants have benign, self-limited illness, those with serious bacterial illness are often difficult to diagnose and have high morbidity. In fact, up to 10% of febrile infants in this age group have SBI, including almost 3% with bacteremia or bacterial meningitis.[3–8] Therefore, fever is an important symptom for identifying infants who need immediate evaluation and treatment.

### Clinical Features

Although most febrile infants who have serious bacterial illness appear ill, fever might be the first and only presenting sign. Useful clinical clues from observation include quality of the infant's cry, general activity and alertness, skin color, hydration status, and reaction to stimulation. However, clinical impression alone is an unreliable predictor of serious infection. At this age, the ability of the infant to interact in a clear, social manner, such as with a social smile, is inconsistent. Thus, a febrile infant can present with signs of sepsis—irritability, lethargy, bulging fontanel, tachypnea, grunting, poor peripheral perfusion—or the infant can appear well.

### Diagnostic Studies

Although some differences in practice patterns exist, most agree that febrile infants younger than 1 month should have a sepsis (or SBI) work-up consisting of a CBC count with a manual differential of the white blood cells, urinalysis, lumbar puncture, and cultures of blood, urine, and spinal fluid. A chest radiograph is needed for evaluation of respiratory symptoms, and a stool culture should be obtained if there is diarrhea. Evaluation of the febrile infant 1 to 2 months old is controversial. Conservative management requires the same diagnostic testing as for the infant younger than 1 month. However, some clinicians withhold the lumbar puncture if the infant appears well and the other test results are unremarkable. Regardless of age, if the infant is in shock or has episodes of apnea, the lumbar puncture should be deferred until the infant is stable, and antibiotics should be administered prior to diagnostic study results.

## Differential Diagnosis

Life-threatening illness in febrile infants is usually the result of bacteremia, sepsis, or bacterial meningitis. In infants younger than 1 month, infection is usually due to organisms acquired perinatally—group B streptococci, Gram-negative enteric organisms, and *Listeria*. Infants older than 6 weeks have infections with community-acquired organisms such as *Pneumococcus*, *Neisseria meningitidis* and, with declining incidence, *Haemophilus influenzae* type B. Infants 4 to 6 weeks old can be infected with organisms common in either age group. Other areas of focal bacterial infection that occur include urinary tract infection, bacterial gastroenteritis, cellulitis (including omphalitis and mastitis), pneumonia, and otitis media.

Although bacterial infection is the primary concern because of the high morbidity, benign viral illness is the most common cause of fever in the well-appearing infant. During the winter months, respiratory syncytial virus (RSV) may present with tachypnea, wheezing, and respiratory distress. Apnea and cyanosis can be presenting signs of RSV in infants younger than 6 weeks, especially if they were born prematurely. Aseptic meningitis is common in the summer months and presents with mild irritability and fever. Although most cases of aseptic meningitis are self-limited, herpes encephalitis can be life threatening.

## Management

Febrile infants with ill-appearance or other signs of serious bacterial infection mandate a sepsis workup and empiric treatment with antibiotics. As noted earlier, because of concerns of apnea and/or bradycardia, the lumbar puncture should be deferred if the infant is in shock or apneic; however, do not delay treatment with antibiotics. There are several approaches to the management of well-appearing febrile infants. In an effort to avoid routine hospitalization, investigators have devised low-risk criteria to identify febrile infants unlikely to have serious illness (Table 13-2). Most experts agree that infants younger than 1 month should have a sepsis workup and routine hospitalization. Well-appearing febrile infants 1 to 2 months old judged to be at low risk who have no focal findings on physical examination, are not chronically ill, and have close followup can be managed as outpatients. All high-risk infants, regardless of age, should be treated with empiric antibiotics (one combination option includes ampicillin and cefotaxime). The use of empiric antibiotics as part of outpatient management for well-appearing, low-risk, 1- to 2-month-old infants is controversial.[3, 4, 6–8] Options are close followup alone, or treatment with parenteral ceftriaxone once daily until cultures are negative.

## Fever With Petechiae

Although most etiologies of petechiae in children are benign, the combination of fever and petechiae raises the concern of invasive bacterial illness, especially due to meningococcus (*Neisseria meningitidis*). Meningococcus was found to be present in only about 2% of children with petechiae who were well enough to be managed as outpatients, but in up to 20% of those managed as inpatients.[9] Furthermore, the mortality rate associated with meningococcus is as high as 20%.

### Clinical Features

There is a continuum of clinical features of meningococcemia, ranging from asymptomatic to mild infection to sepsis and shock. The prodrome can include an upper respiratory illness with early symptoms of fever, headache, fatigue, myalgias, and arthralgias. Within hours,

## TABLE 13-2 Low-Risk Criteria for Febrile Infants

|  | Boston (Baskin, J Peds, 1992) | Philadelphia (Baker NEJM, 1993) | Rochester (Jaskiewicz, Ped 1994) |
|---|---|---|---|
| Age (days) | 28–89 | 29–56 | 0–60 |
| Temp (°C) | >38 | >38.2 | >38 |
| WBC | <20,000 | <15,000 | 5,000–15,000 |
| Differential WBC count | Not specified | Band total neutrophils < 0.2 | Absolute band count < 1,500 |
| Urinalysis | <10 WBC/hpf | <10 WBC/hpf, no bacteria | <10 WBC/hpf |
| CXR | No infiltrate | No infiltrate | Not required |
| CSF (WBC/mm$^3$) | <10 | <8 | Not required |

Adapted from: Avner JR, Baker MD. Management of fever in infants and children. *Emerg Med Clin North Am.* 2002;20(1):49–67

Baker MD, Avner JR. Management of fever in young infants. *Clin Pediatr Emerg Med.* 2000;1:102–108.

Baker MD, Bell LM, Avner JR. Outpatient management without antibiotics of fever in selected infants. *N Engl J Med.* 1993;329:1437–1441.

Jaskiewicz JA, McCarthy CA, Richardson AC, et al. Febrile infants at low risk for serious bacterial infection—an appraisal of the Rochester criteria and implications for management. *Pediatrics.* 1994;94:390–396.

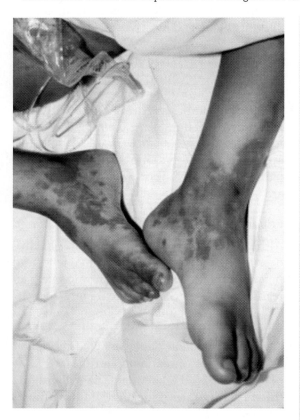

Figure 13.1 Purpura in a patient with meningococcemia.

the child may become lethargic, tachypneic, and tachycardic, with poor peripheral perfusion. Petechiae can be present at any stage of the illness. In the more fulminant cases, petechiae progress to purpura (Figure 13.1).

## YOUR FIRST CLUE

**Signs and Symptoms of Meningococcemia**

- Fever
- Headache
- Fatigue
- Myalgias
- Arthralgias
- Lethargy
- Rigors
- Tachypnea
- Tachycardia
- Skin signs of shock
- Petechiae/purpura

### Diagnostic Testing

All children with fever and unexplained petechiae should have a CBC count, with attention to the platelet count and white blood cell differential, coagulation studies (PT and PTT), as well as a blood culture. Because streptococcal pharyngitis can present with petechiae, a throat culture and rapid antigen should be considered. A lumbar puncture should be performed if the child appears ill or has signs of meningitis, assuming the child is clinically stable and has normal coagulation and platelet counts. Many physicians also recommend a lumbar puncture for children younger than 12 months because they have a higher incidence of meningococcemia and are often difficult to evaluate clinically.

### Differential Diagnosis

Most diagnoses in children with fever and petechiae are viral. In particular, influenza, enterovirus, infectious mononucleosis, adenovirus, atypical measles, and other viral illnesses can present with petechiae. In addition to meningococcemia, bacterial etiologies include *Pneumococcus, H influenzae* type b, group A *Streptococcus, S aureus, E coli,* and *Neisseria gonorrhoeoe.*[10] Rocky Mountain spotted fever presents with petechiae over the wrists and ankles accompanied by headache and myalgias. Children with leukemia often have associated bone pain and organomegaly. Signs of heart failure or a history of acute rheumatic fever or congenital heart disease accompanies bacterial endocarditis.

One important caveat in the evaluation of the child with fever is the presence of petechiae above the nipple line (upper chest and face). Increases in intrathoracic pressure that can accompany cough and emesis can cause petechiae in the distribution of the superior vena cava. If petechiae are restricted to this distribution with a clear etiology and the child appears well, the risk of serious bacterial illness is unlikely.

### Management

Children who are ill appearing or immunocompromised need an immediate evaluation for sepsis, empiric parenteral antibiotics, and hospitalization. The management of the well-appearing child with fever and no clear source of the petechiae is somewhat controversial.[9] Children younger than 12 months have a higher risk of invasive bacterial illness and therefore should be hospitalized and treated with empiric antibiotic therapy. Older children with a white blood cell count between 5,000 and 15,000, a band count less than 500, normal ANC, normal prothrombin time, and normal cerebrospinal fluid studies (if obtained) can be observed in the emergency department for several hours and then managed as outpatients if they remain well and no new petechiae develop. Use of empiric antibiotics in the outpatient management of these children is varied. Children who are well appearing and have pharyngitis with a positive streptococcal antigen test can be treated as outpatients with an antistreptococcal antibiotic.

## Sickle Cell Disease

A single amino acid substitution of valine for glutamate in the β chain of the hemoglobin molecule is responsible for sickle cell disease. This disorder is most commonly seen in African, Indian, Middle Eastern, and Mediterranean populations. In the United States, approximately 0.15% of the black population carries the homozygous form of sickle cell disease, and 8% carry the hemoglobin (HbS) gene.

### Clinical Features

Although symptoms of sickle cell disease can present in infancy, most patients present after 6 months of age. The sickle cells are more readily deformed than normal red blood cells, and this leads to hemolysis and thrombosis within the small blood vessels, with resultant tissue ischemia and end-organ damage. There are four classic presentations of sickle cell disease: vaso-occlusive crises, splenic sequestration, aplastic crises, and infectious crises.

#### Vaso-occlusive Crises

These painful crises typically involve the chest, abdomen, extremities (usually the long bones such as the tibia, femur, and humerus), and back. Infants can present with dactylitis (swelling of the hands and feet) due to occlusion of the nutrient arteries supplying the metacarpals and metatarsals (Figure 13.2). Triggers for all vaso-occlusive crises include infections, dehydration, high altitudes, hypoxia, stress, and cold water immersion. Priapism, a result of vaso-occlusion of the corpus cavernosum, is a true emergency because sustained priapism can result in impotence. Acute chest syndrome presents with cough, chest pain, tachypnea, and dyspnea. Although initial chest radiographs can be negative, an infiltrate might develop 2 to 3 days after symptom onset (Figure 13.3). Between 5% and

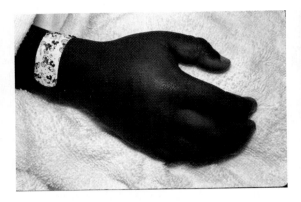

Figure 13.2 Child with dactylitis.

10% of children will develop cerebral disease such as seizures, coma, thrombotic strokes, subarachnoid hemorrhage, and cranial nerve palsies (Figure 13.4).

### Splenic Sequestration Crises

This crisis typically occurs in children younger than 5 years and presents with hypotension, pallor, and splenomegaly. Preceding infections with parvovirus B19, echovirus, and rhinovirus have been implicated. Reticulocyte counts are elevated and hemoglobin levels are markedly decreased. Rapid treatment with blood transfusions (initial rate of 10 mL/kg of packed RBCs) is imperative. Exchange transfusion and splenectomy might also be warranted.

### Aplastic Crises

This crisis occurs when erythropoiesis is inhibited, resulting in hemoglobin levels less than 1 to 3 g/dL and low reticulocyte count (less than 3%). Possible etiologies include parvovirus B19, bone marrow toxic drugs, and folic acid deficiency. Treatment includes blood transfusions and supportive therapy.

### Infectious Crises

Splenic infarction due to multiple episodes of splenic thrombosis usually results in splenic autoinfarction (and functional asplenia) by the age of 5 years. Therefore, in these children, infections with the encapsulated organisms (such as *Streptococcus pneumoniae*, *H influenzae* type b, *E coli*, and *S aureus*) can lead to overwhelming sepsis and death. Patients with sickle cell disease are also at increased risk for meningitis, bacteremia/septicemia, urinary tract infections, bacterial pneumonia, and osteomyelitis. The

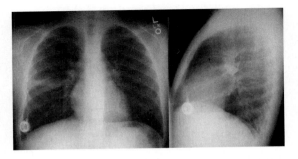

Figure 13.3 Acute chest syndrome. This 13-year-old with sickle cell disease developed cough, chest pain, and tachypnea. This chest radiograph demonstrates streaky infiltrates in his right lung.

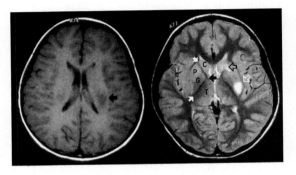

Figure 13.4 Patients with sickle cell disease are at increased risk for thrombotic strokes. This MRI image of a 7-year-old shows a T1 (left) and a T2 (right) image taken at different levels. On the T1 image, the ventricles appear to be dark and the infarct visible in the posterior left putamen is also dark (black arrow). The T2 image is a lower cut through the center of the infarct. The T2 image shows the CSF within the ventricles to be white. Normal anatomic structures are identified in the right brain (left side of T2 image) (C=caudate nucleus, P=putamen, G=globus pallidus, T=thalamus, white arrows=anterior and posterior limbs of internal capsule, black arrow=genu of internal capsule). The infarct appears as a white lesion in the left caudate nucleus (black outlined arrow) and the left putamen (white outlined arrow). Note the obvious distortion of the anterior limb of the left internal capsule, compared to the right. The posterior limb of the left internal capsule is also slightly distorted (compared to the right) adjacent to the infarct in the putamen. This study is read as an infarct in the left basal ganglia, the posterior limb of internal capsule, and the head of the caudate.

most common causes of pneumonia are *S pneumoniae* and *Mycoplasma*. Fifty percent of osteomyelitis cases are caused by *Salmonella typhimurium*, with *S aureus* and *E coli* also being contributing organisms. Prophylactic oral penicillin for children younger than 6 years has

**Signs and Symptoms of Sickle Cell Crisis in Infants and Children**

- Vaso-occlusive crisis: Bone pain, dactylitis, priapism, chest pain, shortness of breath, seizures, coma, stroke, subarachnoid hemorrhage, and cranial nerve palsies
- Splenic sequestration: Hypotension, pallor, and splenomegaly
- Aplastic crisis: Pallor, tachycardia
- Infectious crisis: Fever, meningismus, tachypnea, cough

decreased the incidence of sepsis. In addition, vaccination against *S pneumoniae* and *H influenzae* type b are crucial for patients with sickle cell disease because these two organisms are the most common bacterial pathogens.

## Diagnostic Studies

Patients who present with a sickle cell crisis should have a CBC count and reticulocyte count performed. Typical hemoglobin levels in patients with sickle cell disease range from 6 to 9 g/dL; baseline platelet counts and white blood cell counts are often elevated. Typical baseline reticulocyte counts range from 5% to 15%; counts less than 3% should raise the suspicion of an aplastic crisis. Blood cultures should be obtained in patients with a fever (temperature >38°C). A lumbar puncture should be performed if meningitis is suspected. Urinalysis and urine culture are indicated in patients with fever, dysuria, or hematuria. Liver enzyme studies might be warranted in the evaluation of right upper quadrant pain or if cholecystitis is suspected. Chest radiographs should be obtained in patients with dyspnea, fever, cough, or hypoxia. Other testing might include a bone scan or MRI (osteomyelitis), extremity radiographs (avascular necrosis of the femoral or humeral head), or a head CT or MRI (transient ischemic attack or cerebral infarct).

## Management

Patients who present with a sickle cell crisis are typically dehydrated and therefore might require a fluid bolus with 20 mL/kg of normal saline solution. Ongoing fluid therapy should be 1.5 times the maintenance rate. Pain control is imperative; many patients have tried oral analgesics prior to presenting to the emergency department and will require parenteral therapy. Morphine, hydromorphone, and ketorolac are good analgesic agents. Meperidine should be used with extreme caution because high doses can lead to seizures. Supplemental oxygen can be beneficial. Patients with splenic sequestration, aplastic crises, CNS syndromes, priapism, and acute chest syndrome often require a blood transfusion to decrease the concentration of circulating sickled red blood cells. Severe cases can ultimately require exchange transfusion. Patients with priapism require prompt urologic consultation; surgical intervention might be necessary if the priapism is not relieved. Patients who fail outpatient pain management and require multiple doses of parenteral medications should be managed as inpatients with patient-controlled analgesia.[11]

**Management of Sickle Cell Crisis in Infants and Children**

- Assess and treat for signs of respiratory distress, failure, and shock.
- Obtain vascular access and begin fluid resuscitation.
- Provide pain control.
- Obtain blood for CBC and reticulocyte count.
- Send other laboratory studies as indicated.
- Begin antibiotic therapy for documented infections.
- Transfuse as indicated.
- Prompt urologic consultation is indicated for cases of priapism.

# Dermatologic Emergencies

Almost any infectious illness can present with skin manifestations, as do many systemic inflammatory conditions. In most cases, rashes are part of a benign illness. However, certain rashes can be a warning sign of a more serious disease.

## Clinical Features

A thorough history and physical examination often lead to a diagnosis. Information about the child's general health, immune status, medication use, and history of chronic illness can identify risk factors for associated illness. Related symptoms might include a viral prodrome, fever, mucous membrane involvement, myalgias, arthralgias, or arthritis. Progression of the rash—how the rash started, inciting agents, spread, duration, presence of pruritis—is also important.

On physical exam, identify the type of primary lesion. A macule is a small, flat lesion with a different skin color. A papule is a small, elevated lesion. A vesicle is a blister containing clear fluid; a pustule contains purulent fluid. A bulla is a large blister. The rash can be generalized, suggesting a diffuse exposure or a systemic illness, or confined to specific areas. There can be characteristic patterns such as linear (poison ivy) or dermatomal (herpes zoster), or a characteristic appearance such as purpura or target lesions.

## Diagnostic Studies

Laboratory evaluation is based on the nature of the rash, appearance of the child, and likely etiologies. If the child is febrile and ill appearing, obtain a CBC count, ESR, and blood culture. In addition to evaluation for possible sepsis, children with purpura and/or petechiae should have platelet count and coagulation studies (PT, PTT, bleeding time) to investigate for bleeding disorder. The presence of multinucleated giant cells on a Tzanck smear (obtained by unroofing an intact blister) is consistent with herpes simplex, varicella, and herpes zoster. Gram stain of fluid from a lesion might be consistent with bacterial etiologies but is often indeterminate.

## Differential Diagnosis

The differential diagnosis of dermatologic lesions is extensive. Although many rashes are self-limited, it is important to identify those rashes that are potentially life threatening.

### Maculopapular Rashes

Erythema multiforme is a hypersensitivity reaction characterized by diffuse erythematous macules with central clearing called target or iris lesions (Figure 13.5). Drug exposure (especially penicillins, sulfonamides, and anticonvulsants) and herpes infection are common etiologies when a cause is identified. Most cases of erythema multiforme are self-limited, but the presence of mucus membrane involvement can be a sign of progression to Stevens-Johnson syndrome, which has a mortality rate of up to 25%. Children with Stevens-Johnson syndrome have areas of extensive mucosal necrosis accompanied by severe systemic symptoms, including ill-appearance, fever, cough, vomiting, and diarrhea. Rocky Mountain spotted fever presents with a maculopapular or petechial rash, usually beginning on the wrists and ankles. Systemic symptoms include fever, headache, and lethargy. Kawasaki disease is an illness characterized by fever for at least 5 days and four of the following five features: rash, conjunctivitis, mucositis (red lips, strawberry tongue), erythema, swelling of the hands and feet, and adenopathy (usually a single, nontender cervical node). Coronary artery aneurysms develop in about 20% of untreated children. See Chapter 4, Cardiovascular System.

Many viral illnesses have characteristic maculopapular rashes. In measles, the rash begins on the face and then progresses to the torso and extremities over a 3-day period. Cough, coryza, and conjunctivitis accompany the rash. Erythema infectiosum (fifth disease), caused by parvovirus B19, presents with a slapped cheek erythema or a lacy erythematous rash on

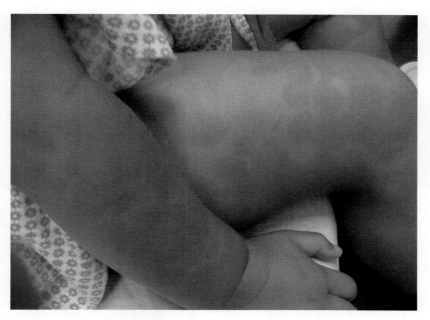

**Figure 13.5** Erythema multiforme.

the torso and extremities (**Figure 13.6**). The appearance of young children is usually asymptomatic, but adolescents can have mild fever and arthralgias. Transmission of this virus to pregnant women is a concern. Roseola associated with human herpes-virus 6 infection presents with 3 days of high fever followed by defervescence and appearance of a diffuse, rose-colored papular rash.

Toxic shock syndrome (TSS) is an acute systemic illness characterized by fever and a diffuse macular erythematous rash with rapid onset of hypotension, renal failure, and multisystem organ involvement. TSS is caused by toxin-producing strains of either *S aureus* or *Streptococcus pyogenes* (group A *Streptococcus*). Although public awareness increased in the early 1980s when TSS was associated with tampon use in menstruating women, currently menstrual cases account for less than 50% of reported cases.[12] Risk factors for *S aureus*-mediated TSS include primary *S aureus* infection (e.g., cellulitis, carbuncle, osteomyelitis, sinusitis), postoperative wound infection, skin or mucus membrane disruption (e.g., burns, influenza, varicella), and surgical/nonsurgical foreign body placement (e.g., catheters, tampons, sutures).[12] *S pyogenes*-mediated TSS in children is usually associated with varicella or some other viral infection.

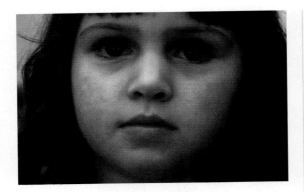

Figure 13.6 "Slapped cheek" rash of erythema infectiosum.

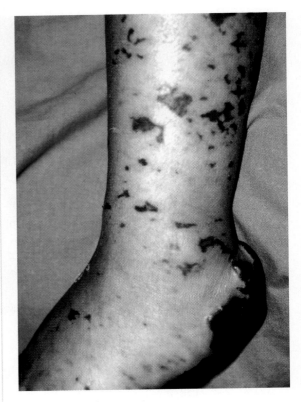

Figure 13.7 Child with meningococcemia and purpura fulminans.

## Purpuric Rashes

Purpura results from bleeding into the skin and, unlike most other rashes, does not blanch when pressure is applied across the skin surface. The most common causes of purpura in children are local trauma, sepsis, vasculitis, and bleeding disorder. When accompanied by fever or ill-appearance, purpura, like petechiae, can be a sign of invasive bacterial illness or disseminated viral illness. In particular, sepsis caused by meningococcemia can lead to disseminated intravascular coagulation resulting in diffuse areas of purpura, some evolving with central necrosis (Figure 13.7). Henoch-Schönlein purpura (HSP) is the most common vasculitis in children, usually occuring between the ages of 3 and 9 years. This leukocytoclastic vasculitis of the small blood vessels involves primarily the skin, gastrointestinal tract, joints, and kidneys. The characteristic rash of HSP is palpable purpura located predominant on the buttocks and lower extremities (Figure 13.8). Associated symptoms include colicky abdominal pain, gastrointestinal bleeding, arthritis, and hematuria. Although some children with HSP develop intussusception or glomerulonephritis, most recover uneventfully. Purpura can be a presenting sign of a bleeding disorder such as hemophilia or von Willebrand disease. Idiopathic thrombocytopenic purpura, an immune disorder causing increased platelet destruction, is the most common cause of thrombocytopenia in children, usually occuring in children 2 to 4 years old. The child appears well but has bruising, purpura, petechiae, or mucosal bleeding. The remainder of the blood count in idiopathic thrombocytopenic purpura is normal, whereas children with leukemia often have significant anemia and thrombocytopenia.

## Vesiculobullous and Vesiculopustular Rashes

Herpes-virus is a common cause of vesicular eruptions in children. Herpes simplex virus causes gingivostomatitis, usually accompanied by fever and irritability. In varicella (chicken pox), the cutaneous lesions follow a mild prodrome of fever, sore throat, and malaise. The rash begins with scattered pruritic papules that progess to vesicles on a red base, central umbilication, and then crusting. Smallpox has been eradicated for more than 20 years but remains a bioterrorism threat. The vesicles of smallpox are similar to varicella. However, there are key differences in their presentations. Varicella lesions occur in crops that appear at different stages through the course of the illness, whereas

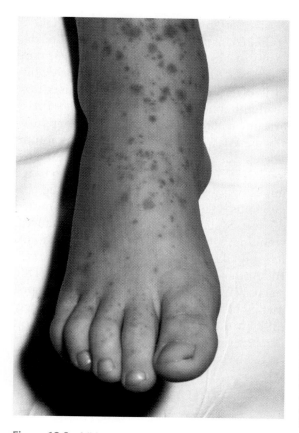

**Figure 13.8** Child with Henoch-Schönlein purpura.

smallpox lesions are all in the same stage. Varicella usually begins on the torso and spreads to the extremities; smallpox begins on the arms, face, and legs and progresses to the torso over about 7 days. Scab formation occurs in 4 to 7 days after the rash begins in varicella and in 10 to 14 days in smallpox. Herpes zoster is a reactivation of dormant varicella that presents with pain, itching, and then grouped papular vesicles in a dermatomal distribution (Figure 13.9). Any herpes infection can disseminate in an immunosuppressed child and is life threatening.

Staphylococcal scalded skin syndrome (SSSS) is a severe systemic reaction to a staphylococcal toxin and occurs primarily in young children and infants. After a prodrome of fever, malaise, and crusting around the mouth or nose, a fine erythematous rash erupts on the face and neck. Over the next 1 to 2 days, the rash spreads over the entire body and the skin becomes very tender. At this stage, slight skin pressure causes sloughing of the upper epidermis or blister formation (Nikolsky sign). Desquamation occurs 1 to 2 weeks after the initial infection. Toxic epidermal necrolysis

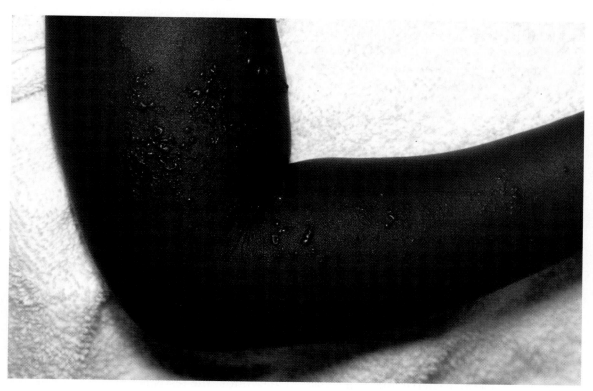

**Figure 13.9** Girl with shingles (herpes zoster).

(TEN), a hypersensitivity reaction to medications, presents with similar clinical findings as SSSS. However, TEN has higher morbidity and mortality due in part to the fact that the skin sloughing in TEN is at the dermal-epidermal junction, unlike the superficial epidermal sloughing of SSSS.

## Management

Management of dermatologic emergencies is based on the underlying etiology. Most viral illnesses require supportive care and maintenance of the child's hydration status. Antiviral agents such as acyclovir can provide a small amount of benefit in healthy children. However, herpesvirus infection in neonates or children who are immunocompromised warrants hospital admission, monitoring, and parenteral antiviral therapy. Rashes typical of bacterial infection or sepsis should be treated with the appropriate antibiotics. Severe, diffuse skin reactions such as TSS, SSSS, TEN, or Stevens-Johnson syndrome call for intensive monitoring, fluid therapy, and burn care. Early treatment of Kawasaki disease with intravenous immunoglobulin and aspirin might prevent the development of coronary artery aneurysms. Children with bleeding disorders may require transfusion of blood or coagulation factors. Many cases of idiopathic thrombocytopenic purpura require no therapy; however, a very low platelet count or persistent symptoms might respond to intravenous immunoglobulin or steroids. $Rh_0(D)$ immune globulin is the preferred treatment for children with idiopathic thrombocytopenic purpura with an intact spleen who are Rh positive. Children with suspected HSP should have a urinalysis to check for hematuria and if positive, measurement of BUN and creatinine.

## Epididymitis

### Clinical Features

Epididymitis results from inflammation of the epididymis, which is located along the posterior aspect of the testis and serves as the storage center for sperm. Bacterial infection is the most common etiology, with the causative organism varying by age. Adolescents should be evaluated for possible sexually transmitted diseases, such as *Neisseria gonorrhoeoe* and *Chlamydia trachomatis*. Patients can have a history of previous urinary tract infections, anatomic abnormalities, or prior genitourinary instrumentation. Patients with epididymitis usually present with a tender, edematous scrotum. The epididymis is in its normal location, posterolateral to the testes. A urethral discharge might be present, particularly when the epididymitis is secondary to a sexually transmitted disease. Systemic symptoms such as nausea, vomiting, low grade fever, and lower abdominal, scrotal, and testicular pain can also be present. As the swelling increases, obliteration of the sulcus between the testis and epididymis occurs, making differentiation from torsion extremely difficult. Relief of pain with scrotal elevation (Prehn's sign) can be present but is unreliable. A reactive hydrocele might also be noted.

### YOUR FIRST CLUE

**Signs and Symptoms of Epididymitis**
- Scrotal swelling and pain
- Nausea, vomiting, low grade fever
- Tender epididymis and scrotum
- Urethral discharge might be present.
- Prehn sign might be present.
- Reactive hydrocele

### Diagnostic Studies

A urinalysis and urine culture should be obtained. However, a lack of pyuria does not rule out epididymitis because between 20% to 50% of patients can have a normal urinalysis. A leukocytosis can be present on a peripheral blood smear. Any urethral discharge should be cultured and sent for Gram stain, including studies for *N gonorrhoeoe* and *C trachomatis*. Color-flow duplex Doppler sonography or radionuclide scintigraphy can be used to exclude testicular torsion. In epididymitis, the testis is normal and vascular flow is preserved or increased.[13]

## Differential Diagnosis

Although acute scrotal, testicular, or penile pain can be caused by a benign underlying diagnosis, the emergency physician is always concerned about the diagnoses that can cause irreversible genitourinary injury with resultant testicular loss, atrophy, or infertility. Patients who present with acute pain should be evaluated for testicular torsion, paraphimosis, strangulated or incarcerated inguinal hernia, foreign body tourniquet, testicular rupture, or hemorrhage into a testicular mass. Other diagnoses to consider include torsion of the testicular appendages, epididymitis, phimosis, balanitis, priapism, orchitis, Henoch-Schönlein purpura, idiopathic scrotal edema, varicocele, and hydrocele. The diagnosis that must be excluded is testicular torsion because misdiagnosis can result in testicular infarction (Table 13-3).[14]

## Management

If there is urethral discharge, the patient should be treated for both *N gonorrhoeoe* and *C trachomatis*. The treatment for sexually acquired epididymitis is ceftriaxone 125 mg IM, or cefixime 400 mg PO as a single dose, followed by either doxycycline 100 mg PO twice a day, tetracycline 500 mg PO 4 times a day, or azithromycin 1 g PO as a single dose. Patients younger than 9 years should be treated with erythromycin (50 mg/kg per day divided 4 times a day) instead of doxycycline. Nonsexually acquired epididymitis can be treated with cephalexin orally for 10 days. Other treatment options for nongonococcal epididymitis include ampicillin, erythromycin, and cephalexin. Bacterial resistance patterns vary geographically, so all emergency staff should know local resistance patterns. Patients with systemic symptoms and toxicity should be admitted for intravenous antibiotics with either ceftriaxone or cefotaxime. In addition to antibiotic administration, pain control is imperative. Scrotal elevation, placement of ice packs on the swollen area, nonsteroidal anti-inflammatory agents, as well as narcotic medications might be necessary. Children will need close urologic followup to ensure that there are no contributing urologic abnormalities,

| TABLE 13-3 | Painful Causes of Scrotal/Testicular Swelling |
|---|---|

- Epididymitis
- Testicular torsion
- Torsion of the appendix testis
- Incarcerated strangulated hernia
- Paraphimosis
- Priapism
- Penile tourniquet syndrome
- Testicular rupture
- Hemorrhage into a testicular tumor

Source: Herman MI. Scrotal pain and swelling. In: Barkin RM ed. *Pediatric Emergency Medicine Concepts and Clinical Practice*, 2nd ed. St Louis, Mo: Mosby;1140, Reprinted with permission.

and might require voiding cystourethrography and renal ultrasonography. If epididymitis is found to be sexually transmitted in a young child, the appropriate child protective agency should be contacted immediately and a report filed by the emergency department provider.

## KEY POINTS

**Management of Epididymitis**
- Analgesics
- Obtain diagnostic studies (urinalysis, urine culture, color Doppler ultrasonography)
- Begin antibiotic therapy
  - Child—treat as urinary source
  - Adolescent—treat for sexually transmitted disease

## Balanitis/Balanoposthitis

### Clinical Features

Balanitis (inflammation of the glans) and balanoposthitis (inflammation of the glans and the foreskin) occur in up to 3% of uncircumcised males. The primary cause of balanoposthitis is infection; however, chemical irritation, trauma, fixed drug eruption, or contact dermatitis can also be contributory. The typical organisms involved in infection-related balanoposthitis are Gram-positive and Gram-negative organisms that are normal flora. Group A β-hemolytic streptococci have been reported to cause balanitis.[15] *Candida albicans* can also be contributory in prepubertal males and recurrent cases should raise the suspicion of diabetes mellitus. In adolescents, sexually transmitted diseases can lead to inflammation and subsequent balanoposthitis. Physical examination can reveal penile erythema, edema, and occasionally a discharge. Systemic symptoms are unusual.

### Differential Diagnosis

Other causes of scrotal and testicular swelling, both painful and nonpainful, are listed in Tables 13-3 and 13-4.[14]

### Diagnostic Studies

The diagnosis of both balanitis and balanoposthitis is clinical. Culturing any discharge for streptococcal antigens can sometimes identify the causative organism. Adolescent males should also be cultured for *N gonorrhoeoe* and *C trachomatis* if the clinical presentation is suspicious for sexually transmitted diseases.

### Management

The mainstay of management is emphasis on adequate hygiene with gentle retraction and cleaning of the foreskin and sitz baths to reduce inflammation. In patients with cellulitis, a 5- to 7-day course of a first-generation cephalosporin might be required. If group A β-hemolytic *Streptococcus* is identified, aggressive management with antistreptococcal antibiotics is required. Those patients with *Candida* infections should be treated with topical or oral antifungals depending on the presentation of the patient. Inflammation can also be treated with 0.5% hydrocortisone cream applied sparingly to the area; however, this is not usually necessary in routine cases. Circumcision might be required for recurrent disease.

| TABLE 13-4 | Painless Causes of Scrotal/Testicular Swelling |
|---|---|

- Phimosis without uropathy
- Henoch-Schönlein purpura
- Varicocele
- Hydrocele
- Inguinal hernia
- Idiopathic scrotal edema
- Testicular tumor

Source: Herman MI. Scrotal Pain and Swelling. In: Barkin RM, ed. *Pediatric Emergency Medicine Concepts and Clinical Practice*, 2nd ed. St Louis, Mo: Mosby;1140. Reprinted with permission.

## KEY POINTS

**Management of Balanoposthitis**

- Sitz baths
- Topical antibacterial ointment—mild cases
- Oral antibiotic therapy (cephalexin)—cellulitis
- Antifungal therapy as indicated

## Urinary Tract Infections – Cystitis and Pyelonephritis

Diagnosing urinary tract infections (UTIs) in infants and young children can be challenging because the clinical signs are often nonspecific (fussiness, fever, lethargy). Early diagnosis is imperative to avoid the potential complications of sepsis and renal scarring. The risk of developing UTIs before age 12 is approximately 3% for girls and 1% for boys. Seven percent of children younger than 2 years with a temperature greater than 39°C and presenting without a source have an occult UTI. Newborn males are more likely to develop a UTI than newborn females. Beyond the newborn period, UTIs are more common in females. Girls younger than 2 years and uncircumcised boys younger than 6 to 12 months are especially at risk. Up to 4% of children with a fever and upper respiratory tract infection or acute otitis media have an associated UTI.[16]

*E coli* is the predominant cause of UTIs in children, although *Klebsiella* is more common in newborn children. *Enterobacter, Proteus, Morganella, Serratia,* and *Salmonella* are also important pathogens. In neonates and young infants, bacteremia is considered the route of infection to the urinary tract. A common cause of UTIs in toilet-trained females is improper wiping after urination. In older children, infection from the lower tract is often the cause of upper tract infection. Vesicoureteral reflux from the bladder into the ureter is a common cause of pyelonephritis and can lead to renal scarring. Renal scarring can occur in 27% to 64% of children after pyelonephritis and can cause renal failure and hypertension.[16]

## Clinical Features

In infants, the signs and symptoms of UTIs or pyelonephritis are usually nonspecific and include decreased oral intake, lethargy, jaundice, and irritability. Children 3 months to 2 years of age can present with nonspecific complaints and/or abdominal pain, vomiting, and fever. Young children might not be able to verbalize when urination is painful. Children older than 2 years might present with abdominal pain, dysuria, or hematuria. New bedwetting might be a sign of a UTI. Cystitis is usually associated with local symptoms such as suprapubic tenderness and dysuria, whereas patients with pyelonephritis typically have more systemic complaints such as fever, costovertebral angle tenderness, and vomiting.

Underlying renal disease or urinary tract abnormality should be considered in a child with hypertension, elevated BUN, elevated creatinine, abnormal electrolytes or acidosis, significant hematuria, or difficulty with urination.

## Diagnostic Studies

There are several methods for collecting urine samples from children. Because of the difficulty in cleaning the perineal area, the bag-collection method poses an increased risk of contamination, with false-positive results ranging from

---

### YOUR FIRST CLUE

**Signs and Symptoms of Urinary Tract Infection**

- Infancy:
  - Poor oral intake
  - Jaundice
  - Irritability
  - Fever
- Child:
  - Abdominal pain
  - Vomiting
  - Fever
  - Abdominal tenderness
  - Dysuria
  - Flank pain/tenderness

---

12% to 83%.[16] While a negative urine culture from a bag specimen can be helpful, a positive culture, especially one with multiflora organisms, must be confirmed by urethral catheterization or suprapubic bladder aspiration.

For a clean-catch urine sample from a toilet-trained child, the parent can clean the child with soap and water prior to urination. A urine sample with greater than 10 WBC/hpf and a significant number of epithelial cells should be considered contaminated, and either an improved clean-catch method or catheterization must be tried. Females with a vaginal discharge or vaginal bleeding should be catheterized.

Suprapubic bladder aspiration or bladder catheterization is less prone to contamination and is the method of choice for obtaining urine samples in ill- or septic-appearing infants.[17] Urethral catheterization is relatively simple and poses little risk, although it might be more difficult in uncircumcised boys or in young infants. There is a slight risk of both trauma to the urethra and the introduction of bacteria into the urinary tract with this technique. A Number 5 feeding tube can be used in young infants. In children younger than 2 years, urinalysis alone is not considered adequate for ruling out UTIs. As many as 10% to 50% of patients with UTIs can have a false-negative urinalysis (bacteria without pyuria).[18] Nitrite and leukocyte esterase urinalysis markers have the highest combined sensitivity and specificity for infection.

### Differential Diagnosis

There are several other causes of dysuria in children. Irritants such as bubble bath or soaps can cause a local irritation and dysuria. A retained foreign body in the vagina (such as toilet paper) can cause irritation or a bacterial growth with associated dysuria and vaginal discharge. Pinworms in the genitourinary area can cause itching and scratching. Balanitis in uncircumcised males can also cause dysuria and pyuria. Accidental injuries to the genital area can cause abrasions, lacerations, and subsequent dysuria. Sexual or physical abuse must always be considered in any young child with a history of multiple UTIs.

### Management

Because of the risk of associated sepsis and pyelonephritis, infants younger than 3 months with a UTI are typically admitted to the hospital for empiric intravenous antibiotic therapy.[19] Recent studies suggest that well-appearing children between 3 months and 2 years of age without signs of toxicity can be managed as outpatients with good followup.[20] Followup is essential to ensure resolution of the infection and to obtain imaging studies to determine the presence of renal scarring, posterior urethral valves, and vesicoureteral reflux. Oral antibiotic therapy might need to be adjusted based on local patterns of resistance, but choices include cephalosporins (cephalexin [1st generation], cefprozil [2nd generation], loracarbef [2nd generation], cefdinir [3rd generation], cefpodoxime [3rd generation]), amoxicillin clavulanate, or trimethoprim/sulfamethoxazole (TMP/SMZ), all of which should be administered for 10 days for UTI and 14 days for pyelonephritis.

In older children (older than 5 years) with a simple cystitis, a short 3- to 5-day course of antibiotics such as amoxicillin, amoxicillin clavulanate, any of the cephalosporins listed earlier, TMP/SMZ, or for those older than 18 years, ciprofloxacin. In older children with pyelonephritis, a longer course of antibiotics (generally 14 days) is recommended.

## KEY POINTS

**Management of Urinary Tract Infection**

- Obtain clean urine sample for urinalysis and culture.
  - Infant or toddler: Urethral catheterization or, rarely, suprapubic aspiration
  - Child: Clean catch, midstream sample
- Begin oral antibiotic therapy based on local patterns of resistance.
- Admit infants younger than 3 months or children with toxic signs and symptoms.

## Hypertension

Hypertension is defined as a systolic or diastolic blood pressure higher than 2 standard deviations above the mean for the age and sex of the patient. This diagnosis requires accurately measured blood pressures over the course of several weeks. A correct-sized cuff should be chosen (80% to 100% of the circumference and two thirds of the length of the upper arm). A child who is in pain or is agitated can have falsely elevated blood pressure readings, so repeat measurements should be obtained when the patient is more comfortable.

Hypertension occurs throughout childhood in both males and females. Predisposing factors include obesity, physical inactivity, and strong family histories. Primary, or essential, hypertension is unrelated to a second systemic disease. Secondary hypertension results from endocrinologic, cardiac, neurologic, or other factors like certain drugs or poisons. Children with significant hypertension usually have an underlying renal (e.g., glomerulonephritis) or renovascular cause.

## Clinical Features

Hypertension in children can occur from various clinical presentations. Asymptomatic or mildly symptomatic hypertension can be discovered during routine vital signs tests performed on children evaluated in the emergency department for an unrelated illness. On questioning, these children might complain of headaches, abdominal pain, irritability, or nose bleeds. Sometimes personality changes and difficulties in school are noted.

Hypertensive urgencies are considered severe elevations in systolic and/or diastolic blood pressures (patients younger than 10 years—systolic blood pressure of 160 mm Hg or higher, diastolic blood pressure of 105 mm Hg or higher; patients older than 10 years—systolic blood pressure of 170 mm Hg or higher, diastolic blood pressure of 110 mm Hg or higher) but without signs of end-organ damage.

Patients with hypertensive emergencies have clinical signs of end-organ damage such that severe elevation in blood pressure is associated with acute neurologic changes or encephalopathy, pulmonary edema, myocardial ischemia, or severe proteinuria. An ECG might show signs of ischemia or ventricular hypertrophy. Chest radiographs might reveal cardiomegaly or pulmonary edema. Rapid treatment of a hypertensive emergency is crucial. However, overly aggressive treatment of the long-standing hypertension can produce relative hypotension and lead to worsening neurologic sequelae.

Symptoms of hypertensive encephalopathy include headache, vomiting, altered mental status, vision disturbances (including blurred vision and diplopia), and seizures or stroke. Papilledema, decreased retinal venous pulsations, and cranial nerve palsies might be found on exam. The diagnosis is confirmed when the symptoms and signs improve rapidly after the blood pressure is lowered. The differential diagnosis of hypertensive encephalopathy includes meningitis, brain tumor, intracerebral hemorrhage, stroke, or uremia.

## YOUR FIRST CLUE

**Signs and Symptoms of Hypertensive Emergencies in Children**

- Encephalopathy
  - Headache
  - Vomiting
  - Altered mental status
  - Vision disturbance
  - Seizure
  - Stroke
  - Papilledema
  - Cranial nerve palsies
- Pulmonary edema
- Myocardial ischemia
- Severe proteinuria

## Diagnostic Studies

In addition to a thorough history and physical examination, laboratory and radiographic studies can help determine both the cause of the hypertension and whether a hypertensive emergency exists.

## THE CLASSICS

**Definition of Hypertension in Children**
Systolic or diastolic blood pressure greater than 2 standard deviations above the mean for the age and sex of the patient on repeat measurements with correct-sized cuff.

## Management

Initial management of severe hypertension begins with an evaluation of the ABCs of resuscitation. Pertinent historical questions include a previous history of hypertension, UTIs, hematuria, or edema or umbilical artery catheterization. A history of joint pain or swelling, palpitations, weight loss, flushing of the skin, drug ingestion, or family history of hypertension is important.

Physical examination should focus on the central nervous system and cardiovascular system. Examination of the optic fundus might show papilledema or hemorrhages. Signs of congestive heart failure or a difference in the upper and lower extremity blood pressures should be noted. A renal cause for the hypertension is suggested by the presence of peripheral edema or palpable kidneys. An abdominal bruit suggests renovascular hypertension. Initial laboratory tests include a CBC, electrolytes, BUN, creatinine, urinalysis, urine culture, chest x-ray, and ECG.

Any child with findings consistent with a hypertensive emergency (e.g., end-organ damage by physical exam, laboratory, or radiographic results) should have an intravenous line placed. Continuous blood pressure readings must be provided; an arterial catheter is preferable. The goal of therapy is to reduce the mean arterial blood pressure by 10% to 20% over several minutes to hours, depending on the nature of the emergency. Headache and vomiting require blood pressure control over several hours, whereas intracranial bleeding or herniation would require reduction over several minutes. To avoid overly aggressive treatment and resultant relative hypotension, medications that can be titrated by intravenous infusions are preferred.[18] Nitroprusside (0.3 to 0.5 mcg/kg per minute), hydralazine (0.1 to 0.2 mg/kg), esmolol (load of 100 to 500 mcg/kg followed by a maintenance drip of 25 to 100 mcg/kg per minute), labetalol (0.2 to 1 mg/kg bolus, followed by 0.4 to 1 mg/kg per hour) or phentolamine (0.1 mg/kg) are good choices. Admission to a pediatric intensive care unit bed should be arranged.

β-blockers are contraindicated in patients with decreased cardiac output and clinical signs of congestive heart failure. Oral nifedipine is contraindicated in patients with signs of end-organ damage (such as an intracerebral bleed) because of the inability to accurately control the blood pressure reduction.[18]

Patients with hypertensive urgency should be started on an oral antihypertensive agent in order to prevent end-organ sequelae. Angiotensin-converting enzyme inhibitors (captopril 0.3 to 6 mg/kg/24 hours divided every 6 to 12 hours) or calcium channel blockers (nifedipine 0.25 to 0.5 mg/kg) are useful first-line agents. The child should be observed for a few hours after administration of the medication to evaluate effectiveness. The child can then be discharged home on the agent used to lower the blood pressure with close followup. However, if these medications are unsuccessful in lowering the blood pressure or reducing the symptoms, the patient should be admitted to a monitored bed for further evaluation and therapy.

Children with mildly elevated blood pressures (5 to 10 mmHg above normal) unrelated to their emergency department visits require repeated blood pressure measurements before treatment for hypertension is begun. If the blood pressure is moderately elevated and the patient is asymptomatic, the patient can be discharged home for outpatient workup of the hypertension.

## KEY POINTS

**Management of Hypertensive Emergencies**

- Lower arterial blood pressure by 10% to 20% over minutes to hours, depending on symptoms.
- Avoid overly aggressive treatment and hypotension.
- Admit patient to a pediatric intensive care unit.

## Acute Glomerulonephritis

The most common type of glomerulonephritis seen in the United States in children between the ages of 3 and 7 years is poststreptococcal glomerulonephritis (PSGN). PSGN is a nonsuppurative complication of infection with strains of nephritogenic *Streptococcus*, which is not generally preventable by antibiotics. There is typically a delay in the onset of nephritis of approximately 8 to 14 days following pharyngitis and 14 to 21 days following a streptococcal skin infection.

## Clinical Features

Up to 70% of patients present with gross hematuria or tea-colored urine. Dependent edema is also present. Other signs and symptoms include mild to moderate hypertension, pallor, oliguria, nausea, fever, abdominal pain, vomiting, and headache. Less frequent but more severe presentations include UTIs, congestive heart failure, and hypertensive encephalopathy.

## Diagnostic Studies

The hallmark of glomerulonephritis is red blood cell casts in freshly spun urine. Hematuria, pyuria, and proteinuria can also be present. Blood chemistry evaluation might show an elevated BUN, creatinine, potassium, and chloride, with low sodium, bicarbonate, and albumin. Hemoglobin and platelet counts are typically normal, although there can be a dilutional anemia. Cultures of the throat and skin lesions should be obtained. Other lab tests to obtain include antistreptolysin O titers (elevated with pharyngitis), anti-DNase B (elevated with pyoderma), antihyaluronidase (elevated), and C3 complement (decreased).

## THE CLASSICS

### Diagnostic Findings in Glomerulonephritis

- Urinalysis reveals red cell casts.
- Blood chemistry can show elevated BUN, creatinine, potassium, and chloride and decreased sodium, bicarbonate, albumin, and complement.

## Differential Diagnosis

Other causes of glomerulonephritis include hereditary nephritis, lupus nephritis, IgA nephropathy, Henoch-Schonlein purpura nephritis, toxin-mediated nephritis (lead, hydrocarbons, and mercury), and membranoproliferative glomerulonephritis.

## Management

Patients with acute renal insufficiency should be placed on fluid restriction and a low sodium/low protein diet. Patients with congestive heart failure should be placed on fluid restriction and given diuretics (furosemide), morphine (0.1 mg/kg), and oxygen. Hypertension and hypertensive encephalopathy should be treated as outlined in the prior hypertension section. Hyperkalemia can be treated with kayexalate (1 g/kg), bicarbonate (1 mEq/kg), calcium gluconate (100 mg/kg), or glucose and insulin (2 to 4 mL/kg D25 solution and 0.1 units/kg of insulin). Patients with PSGN should be managed as inpatients with a nephrology consultation.

# Nephrotic Syndrome

Hypoproteinemia, proteinuria, and edema characterize nephrotic syndrome. Primary nephrotic syndrome applies to diseases limited to the kidney; renal biopsy is used to categorize patients and will determine therapeutic and prognostic decisions. Secondary nephrotic syndrome results from systemic illnesses such as PSGN.

Between 2 and 7 cases of nephrotic syndrome per 100,000 children are diagnosed each year. Boys are affected twice as often as girls, but this ratio equalizes by adulthood. Primary nephrotic syndrome occurs more commonly in children younger than 5 years and secondary occurs more often in older children. Of children with nephrotic syndrome, 90% have the primary disease, with 85% having minimal change nephrotic syndrome, 10% focal sclerosis, and 5% mesangial proliferation. The etiology of primary nephrotic syndrome is thought to be idiopathic, but various theories involving bacterial or viral infections, allergic reactions (pollens, poison ivy), or drug ingestion (heroin, mercury) have been implicated.

## Clinical Features

Characteristic findings include edema, hypoalbuminemia, proteinuria, and hyperlipidemia. The onset of edema can be insidious, often beginning with periorbital edema. As a child's weight increases from the retained fluid, parents might report that the child's pants and shoes are tight. The edema continues to progress but the child usually does not appear ill unless pulmonary edema or ascites are present. Anorexia, nausea, and vomiting can be present as a result of edema of the intestinal wall. Hypertension, hematuria, or oliguria might also occur. Acute renal failure is rare in primary nephrotic syndrome.

Children with nephrotic syndrome are at risk for thrombosis, with up to 2% of nephrotic children having thromboembolic complications. Renal vein thrombosis can cause flank pain, hematuria, and worsening renal function. Children with nephrosis should not undergo punctures to deep vessels because of this risk of thrombosis. Most cases of nephrosis are treated with corticosteroids. Side effects of corticosteroid use include acute mood changes (from depression to mania), irritability, excessive crying, and sleeping difficulties. Because of steroid therapy and decreased levels of immunoglobulins, children with nephrosis are at risk for bacterial infections, such as E coli and S pneumoniae.

### Diagnostic Studies

Proteinuria in nephrotic syndrome is defined as >3.5 gram protein $1.73m^2/24$ hrs, or greater than 50 mg/kg/24 hours. This corresponds to 3+ or 4+ on the "dipstick" reading. Specific gravity may be high due to the proteinuria. Microscopic hematuria may also be present. Total serum protein usually is low at 4.5 to 5.5 g/dL and serum albumin is less than 2 g/dL.

Hyperlipidemia can occur due to the increased serum cholesterol. Hyponatremia can be present, but other electrolytes are usually normal. BUN and creatinine are also usually normal, and hemoglobin and hematocrit levels can be elevated due to hemoconcentration.

A chest radiograph might reveal a pleural effusion or pulmonary edema. The heart appears normal or small on chest radiograph due to intravascular hypovolemia. An abdominal radiograph might reveal ascites, and renal ultrasonography can help rule out renal abnormalities. A renal biopsy is important for diagnostic and therapeutic decisions and should

be obtained in children older than 6 years, or if there is evidence of hematuria, elevated BUN, persistent hypertension, or failure to respond to steroids.

### Differential Diagnosis

Other renal diseases that cause edema include glomerulonephritis and renal failure. A vasculitis or acute thrombosis of the renal vessels must also be considered. Gastrointestinal causes that produce hypoproteinemia include cirrhosis, cystic fibrosis, and protein-losing enteritis.

### Management

Despite the edema, children with signs of hypovolemia or shock should be resuscitated in the usual manner with a crystalloid solution. However, if the patient is hypertensive, treatment should be initiated.

After consultation with a pediatric nephrologist, patients between 12 months and 5 years old with no gross hematuria and no large loss of protein or complement are treated with corticosteroids (prednisone 2 mg/kg/24 hour orally divided either 2 or 3 times a day). Relapses or steroid resistance might necessitate a second course of steroids. Diuretics such as furosemide might be necessary if respiratory distress or significant ascites are present. Salt restriction is usually required. Fluid intake should be restricted only if edema is present despite salt restriction or if the child exhibits hyponatremia due to an impaired ability to excrete excess water. The relative immunocompromised state of nephrotic children increases their risk of infection. A fever or signs of peritonitis must be evaluated thoroughly. A paracentesis should be performed and fluid sent for Gram stain and culture. These children should be admitted and antibiotic therapy initiated.[21]

## Syncope

Syncope is a sudden brief loss of consciousness associated with a decrease in muscle tone that usually results from a transient decrease in cerebral blood flow. Most cases of syncope are self-limited and are of benign etiology.[22]

The incidence is more common in adolescence, but syncope can be seen at any age.

## Clinical Features

By the time the child arrives in the emergency department, the episode of syncope is usually resolved. Therefore, information on most of the clinical features must be obtained from a careful history. Helpful clues are obtained from the circumstances immediately preceding the event (specific activities, environmental factors, and physical complaints), the duration of the syncope, and the physical signs during the event (tonic-clonic movements, cyanosis).

## Diagnostic Studies

Because the differential diagnosis of syncope can range from benign to life-threatening etiologies, the initial workup is varied and based on probable diagnoses.

## Differential Diagnosis

The most important aspect in the evaluation of a child with syncope is differentiating life-threatening causes from those of relatively benign etiologies. It is helpful to divide the etiologies of syncope into three clinical categories: vasovagal (neurocardiogenic), cardiac, and noncardiac.

## WHAT ELSE?

**Differential Diagnosis of Syncope**
- Breath-holding spell
- Cardiac disorders
- Hyperventilation
- Hypoglycemia
- Hypovolemia
- Migraine
- Pregnancy
- Psychiatric disorder
- Seizure disorder
- Subarachnoid hemorrhage

### Vasovagal

Vasovagal syncope is the most common etiology. Often there is a clearly identifiable precipitating event such as fear, pain, exhaustion, or prolonged standing. The child might feel faint, lightheaded, sweaty, and/or short of breath. The child then loses consciousness and falls slightly forward. During the event, there is usually bradycardia associated with the transient hypotension. After a short time, the child awakens but might complain of mild headache, nausea, and/or fatigue. Physical examination is unremarkable.

### Noncardiac

Most noncardiac etiologies are not episodes of true syncope but rather loss of consciousness as an associated symptom. Seizure is usually associated with tonic-clonic movements and incontinence. In contrast to vasovagal syncope, children with seizures usually have a postictal state and do not remember the events immediately preceding the loss of consciousness. Orthostatic syncope can be the result of dehydration, anemia, or associated medication use. Breath-holding spells occur in young children, typically 6 months to 4 years old. The child becomes upset or angry (as when a favorite toy is taken away), begins to cry, holds his breath, and then passes out, occasionally with a twitch or jerk of the extremities. These breath-holding spells can be pallid (the child's face turns pale) or cyanotic (perioral or facial cyanosis). Although very concerning to the parents and other caregivers, breath-holding spells are benign. Situational syncope follows specific events such as micturation, giggling, cough, or venipuncture. Psychiatric (hysterical) syncope usually occurs in front of an audience when children faint and fall gently backward, rarely hurting themselves. Other than hypoglycemia, metabolic causes of syncope are rare. Other noncardiac causes of syncope include pregnancy, hyperventilation, migraine, and subarachnoid hemorrhage.

### Cardiac

Although uncommon, cardiac causes of syncope are potentially life threatening. Therefore, every evaluation for syncope must involve careful history, physical examination, and laboratory testing, if necessary, for cardiac causes. Warning signs include palpitations, tachycardia, chest pain, or syncope associated with exercise. There is then a controlled fall followed by the loss of consciousness. Cardiac etiologies can be grouped into outflow obstruction (myxoma, critical aortic stenosis), myocardial dysfunction (hypertrophic cardiomyopathy), and dysrhythmias (ventricular tachycardia, prolonged QT syndrome, sick sinus syndrome).

## Management

Initial management is based on the likely diagnoses. Emergency evaluation should include a serum hemoglobin, serum glucose, ECG, and urine pregnancy test (as appropriate). Other studies will be based on history and physical exam findings. If cardiac syncope is suspected, ECG, chest radiograph, serum creatinine phosphokinase (with isoenzymes if elevated), and cardiology consultation should be obtained.

Further monitoring as an inpatient as well as an echocardiogram and a Holter monitor might be needed. Evaluation for noncardiac causes might include serum hemoglobin, serum glucose, electroencephalogram, and urine pregnancy test and toxicology screen.

## KEY POINTS

**Management of Syncope**
- Complete a thorough history and physical examination.
- Obtain blood for serum hemoglobin, serum glucose.
- ECG
- Urine pregnancy test (as appropriate)
- Cardiology consultation for all children with suspected cardiac syncope

# CHAPTER REVIEW

## Check Your Knowledge

1. Which of the following pathogens has been associated with aplastic crises in sickle cell disease?
   A. *E coli*
   B. *Klebsiella*
   C. Parvovirus B19
   D. *Salmonella typhimurium*

2. All of the following statements are true except:
   A. If there is significant scrotal swelling, it can be difficult to differentiate between acute testicular torsion and epididymitis
   B. If there is urethral discharge, a sexually transmitted disease is most likely responsible for the epididymitis, and the patient should be treated for both gonorrhea and chlamydial infection
   C. Many patients with epididymitis may have a normal urinalysis
   D. Relief of pain with scrotal elevation (Prehn sign) is reliable in differentiating between testicular torsion and epididymitis

3. An 8-month-old child is brought to the ED for evaluation of fever, vomiting, and listlessness. On examination, the infant is lethargic with a temperature of 103°F, a weak pulse of 160/min, a respiratory rate of 44/min, and cool, mottled extremities with a capillary refill of 6 seconds. After evaluation of the ABCs, which of the following is the next step in management?
   A. Attempt oral fluids with a rehydration solution
   B. Give an intravenous normal saline bolus; if the white blood cell count is elevated, give parenteral antibiotics
   C. Obtain a blood culture, attempt a lumbar puncture, and then give parenteral antibiotics
   D. Obtain a blood culture, give an intravenous normal saline bolus and intravenous antibiotics

4. A 13-year-old girl is brought to the ED on hot summer morning after she passed out in church. According to bystanders, she was standing when she fainted. By the time the ambulance arrived, she was awake. She has no significant past medical history, and her physical exam is normal. Which of the following is the most likely etiology of her syncope?
   A. Breath-holding spell
   B. Dysrhythmia
   C. Seizure
   D. Vasovagal

## References

1. Schexnayder SM. Pediatric septic shock. *Pediatr Rev.* 1999;20:301–308.
2. Dayan PS, Pan SS, Chamberlain JM. Fever in the immunocompromised host. *Clin Pediatr Emerg Med.* 2000;1:138–149.
3. Avner JR, Baker MD. Management of fever in infants and children. *Emerg Med Clin North Am.* 2002;20(1):49–67.
4. Baker MD, Avner JR. Management of fever in young infants. *Clin Pediatr Emerg Med.* 2000;1:102–108.
5. Baker MD, Avner JR, Bell LM. Failure of infant observation scales in detecting serious illness in febrile 4–8-week-old infants. *Pediatrics.* 1990;85:1040–1043.
6. Baker MD, Bell LM, Avner JR. Outpatient management without antibiotics of fever in selected infants. *N Engl J Med.* 1993;329:1437–1441.
7. Baskin MN, O'Rourke EJ, Fleisher GR. Outpatient treatment of febrile infants 28 to 89 days of age with intramuscular administration of ceftriaxone. *J Pediatr.* 1992;120:22–27.
8. Jaskiewicz JA, McCarthy CA, Richardson AC et al. Febrile infants at low risk for serious bacterial infection—an appraisal of the Rochester Criteria and implications for management. *Pediatrics.* 1994;94:390–396.
9. DiGiulio GA. Fever and petechiae: No time for a rash decision. *Clin Pediatr Emerg Med.* 2000;1:132–137.
10. Mandl KD, Stack AM, Fleisher GR. Incidence of bacteremia in infants and children with fever and petechiae. *J Pediatr.* 1997;131:398–404.
11. Steinberg M. Management of sickle cell disease. *N Engl J Med.* 1999;340:1021–1030.

12. American Academy of Pediatrics. Toxic shock syndrome. In: Pickering LK, ed. *2000 Red Book: Report of the Committee on Infectious Diseases.* 25th ed. Elk Grove Village, Il: American Academy of Pediatrics;2000:576–581.

13. Mufti RA, Ogedegbe AK, Laftery K. The use of Doppler ultrasound in the clinical management of acute testicular pain. *Br J Urol* 1995;76:625–627.

14. Herman, MI. Scrotal pain and swelling. In: Barkin RM, ed. *Pediatric Emergency Medicine Concepts and Clinical Practice.* 2nd ed. St Louis, Mo: Mosby;1140–1142.

15. Orden B, Martinez R, Lopez de los Mozos A, Franco A. Balanitis caused by group A beta-hemolytic streptococci. *Pediatr Infect Dis J.* 1996;15:920–921.

16. Shaw KN, Gorelick MH. Urinary tract infection in the pediatric patient. *Pediatr Clin North Am.* 1999;46(6):1111–1124.

17. American Academy of Pediatrics, Committee on Quality Improvement Subcommittee on Urinary Tract Infection. Practice parameter: the diagnosis, treatment, and evaluation of the initial urinary tract infection in febrile infants and young children. *Pediatrics.* 1999;103:843–852.

18. McCollough M, Sharieff G. Renal and genitourinary tract disorders. In: Marx J, Hockberger R, Walls R, eds, *Rosen's Emergency Medicine Concepts and Clinical Practice.* 5th ed. St Louis, Mo: Mosby, 2002 2326–2343.

19. Crain EF, Gershel J. Urinary tract infections in febrile infants younger than 8 weeks of age. *Pediatrics.* 1990;83(3):363–367.

20. Hoberman A et al. Oral versus intravenous therapy for urinary tract infections in young febrile children. *Pediatrics.* 1999;104:79–86.

21. Mahan, JD, Turman MA, Mentser MI. Evaluation of hematuria, proteinuria, and hypertension in adolescents. *Pediatr Clin North Am.* 1997;44(6):1573–1589.

22. Willis J. Syncope. *Pediat Rev.* 2000;21:1–8.

## Additional Reading

Halsam DB. Managing the child with fever and neutropenia in an era of increasing microbial resistance. *J Pediatr.* 2002;140:5–7.

Leung AKC, Chan KW. Evaluating the child with purpura. *Am Fam Physician.* 2001;64:1–12.

Narchi H. The child who passes out. *Pediatr Rev.* 2000;21:1–9.

Satish RR, Sheldon RS. At the bedside: syncope. *Evidence-based Cardiovascular Med.* 2001;5:1–4.

Wheeler AP, Bernard GR. Treating patients with severe sepsis. *N Engl J Med.* 1999;340:207–213.

CASE SUMMARY 1

A previously healthy 15-month-old boy is brought to the emergency department with a 1-day history of fever and "not acting like himself." He was well until 3 days ago when he had symptoms of an upper respiratory tract infection. Yesterday he developed a low-grade fever that his mother treated with ibuprofen. Today he has continued fever and decreased oral intake, urine output, and activity level. He has no history of vomiting, diarrhea, cough, or rash. He is not taking any prescription medication.

On physical examination he appears tired and cranky when stimulated. His breathing is not labored, and he is pink. His respirations are 40/min, pulse is 162/min, blood pressure is 92/70 mmHg, and temperature is 38.9°C (102°F). He has dry lips but moist mucous membranes without oral lesions. His neck is supple. An examination of lungs, heart, abdomen, and extremities is unremarkable. There are a few scattered petechiae on his abdomen and lower extremities. His peripheral pulses are normal, and capillary refill time is 3 seconds.

# CHAPTER REVIEW

**CASE SUMMARY 1 CONT.**

1. *What is your general impression of this child?*
2. *What are the most likely diagnoses?*
3. *What would be your initial management strategy?*

---

On presentation, the child is ill-appearing, febrile, tachycardic, and tachypneic with a physical exam remarkable for scattered petechiae on the abdomen and lower extremities. The primary concern is whether this child is in shock. The tachycardia and slightly delayed capillary refill with a normal peripheral pulse and blood pressure are consistent with compensated shock. Since the child is febrile, has a history of an upper respiratory tract illness with no history of excessive fluid loss, the most likely etiology of the shock is sepsis. Any ill-appearing child with fever and petechiae should be assumed to have a serious bacterial illness, most likely meningococcemia. While many other conditions such as viral infection (influenza, enterovirus, infectious mononucleosis, and adenovirus), group A streptococcae infection, and Rocky Mountain spotted fever can present with fever and petechiae, meningococcal infection is rapidly progressive and life-threatening. Initial management begins with 100% oxygen by a nonrebreather mask. Continous pulse oximetry showed an oxygen saturation of 98% with the oxygen therapy. An intravenous line was placed and blood was sent for CBC count, serum electrolytes, coagulation studies, and culture. Rapid bedside glucose determination was 120. Since the child was tachypneic and had signs of shock, the lumbar puncture was deferred and intravenous antibiotics were administered immediately. An intravenous bolus of normal saline was given because of poor oral intake and decreased urine output with no signs of cardiac or pulmonary disease. The child was admitted to a monitored inpatient unit.

His initial lab tests showed a white blood cell count of 21,000 with 25% band forms. Serum bicarbonate was 11, prothrombin time 15, and partial prothrombin time 28. Over the next several hours he became more obtunded, developed purpura, had increasing respiratory distress, and labile blood pressure. He was intubated, ventilated, and intravenous pressors were initiated. His blood culture grew *N meningitidis*.

# chapter 14

# Neonatal Emergencies

David J. Burchfield, MD, FAAP
Rodney Brian Boychuk, MD

## Objectives

1. Relate the history of resuscitation.

2. Outline the sequence of care in the resuscitation of the newly born.

3. Describe the difference between the newly born and newborn and the common reasons they require or seek emergency care.

4. Describe the diagnosis, management, and disposition of specific diseases of the newly born and newborn presenting to the emergency department.

## Chapter Outline

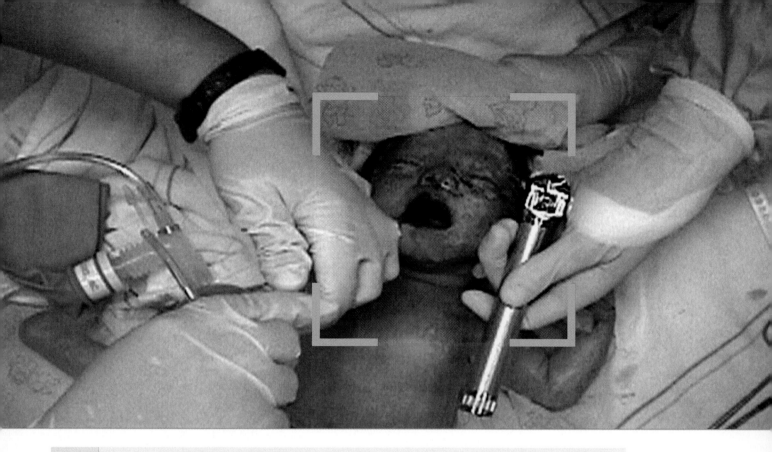

**CASE SCENARIO 1**

A 16-year-old girl arrives in your emergency department with abdominal pain. She states she is pregnant. The patient states she is having abdominal pains about every 1 to 2 minutes. Her appearance is anxious but alert; she breathes rapidly with the pain but then slows her rate in between episodes of pain. There are no retractions, and her skin color is normal. Vital signs reveal a respiration rate of 22, a heart rate of 120, a blood pressure of 100/70 mmHg, and a temperature of 38°C.

1. *What three questions should the patient be asked to predict the need for resuscitation of the newly born?*
2. *What priorities of care should be initiated to resuscitate the newly born?*

## Introduction

In medicine, few patients present a challenge as daunting as the neonate. Historically, the neonatal age group extends from the time of delivery (birth) to 28 days. Because specific high-risk emergency conditions are recognizable immediately at birth or during the transitional period (birth to extrauterine life, or when the fetus is physiologically converting newborn life), it is appropriate to discuss them as a special group, termed newly born.[1] This chapter focuses on problems likely to be encountered by the emergency physician or office-based practitioner. Diseases usually encountered in the neonatal intensive care unit,

such as respiratory distress syndrome, are beyond the scope of this discussion. The chapter will begin with a review of resuscitation principles, highlighting the differences in neonatal physiology that can make resuscitation procedures unique. In the second part of the chapter, other non–resuscitation emergencies will be discussed using a symptom-based approach to help the clinician develop a differential diagnosis and ultimate treatment plan.

## Resuscitation of the Newly Born

The probability of death or lifelong neurological injury is higher when a baby is born in the non–delivery room setting.[2] The treatment received in the first few minutes of life can carry lifelong consequences. Knowing and applying resuscitation techniques in newborns can have a positive impact on the long-term quality of life.

## Preparation for Delivery

### Resuscitation-Oriented History

If time permits before the baby is born, a brief resuscitation-oriented history should be obtained to help facilitate a possible resuscitation. Although much of the maternal history will be important after the baby is born, the only critical data needed just prior to delivery can be limited to three questions (Table 14-1). These questions are:

1. Do you have twins? If multiple newborns are expected, preparation for each infant must be made, including setting up multiple resuscitation areas, stocked with appropriate equipment for each, and establishing a resuscitation team for each baby.

2. When is your due date? A significant number of unplanned deliveries will be preterm (less than 36 weeks), which can require different sizes of equipment and will increase the chances of the baby(ies) being depressed at birth, requiring medical resuscitation.

3. What color is the amniotic fluid? Greenish color of the amniotic fluid signifies the passage of meconium in utero. Meconium passage is a sign of two

possible problems: a distressed newborn and/or airway obstruction in the newborn. In some instances, endotracheal intubation and clearing the airway of meconium are indicated,[3] so preparation of appropriate equipment including endotracheal intubation and suction equipment will be necessary.

### Preparation of Equipment

Assume that the infant will be depressed, and locate all necessary equipment in advance. Equipment should include, as a minimum, a neonatal manual resuscitator (less than 750 mL capacity), newborn and premature-sized masks, intubation equipment including appropriate-sized endotracheal tubes and laryngoscope blades, an oxygen source, and suction (Table 14-2).

The steps for preparation of equipment should include providing a warm environment for the newborn. A preheated radiant warmer works best for this purpose, but other provisions can be made. A supply of towels, preferably warmed, will be necessary to adequately dry the infant. The baby's oxygen utilization increases exponentially with decreasing body surface temperature, so limiting this requirement is important in the stressed newborn.

## Immediate Care of the Newborn

Most full-term newborns are healthy and require no specific treatment, but the initial steps in caring for the newly born can prevent secondary, avoidable complications in an otherwise healthy baby, as well as provide important precursors for any resuscitation.[4]

| TABLE 14-1 | Brief Resuscitation History |
|---|---|
| Question | Implication |
| Do you have twins? | More than one newborn will require additional equipment and staff. |
| When is your due date? | <36 weeks gestation increases need for resuscitation. |
| What color is your amniotic fluid? | If green, then meconium is present, and your management will depend on how vigorous the baby is at delivery. |

**TABLE 14-2  Equipment for Neonatal Resuscitation**

- Manual resuscitator (500–750 mL)
- Masks (two sizes, term and premature)
- Dry towels/blankets
- Suction equipment
- Endotracheal tubes (sizes 2.5, 3.0, 3.5)
- Laryngoscope and blades (sizes 0, 1)

### Dry and Warm the Baby

Unless immediately dried, the baby can lose tremendous amounts of heat through evaporation and radiation.[5] Drying the infant thoroughly, even if depressed, should take minimal time but can have an important role in reducing heat loss and tissue oxygen requirements.

### Clear the Airway

The newborn's head is disproportionately large compared to the older child or adult, which leads to flexion of the neck in the supine position. Positioning the baby on its back with the head slightly extended will increase the patency of the airway. In addition, neonates are born with copious upper airway fluid[6-8] (amniotic fluid) that can secondarily occlude the airway, even in a vigorous baby. Take time to ensure a clear airway by routinely suctioning the mouth and nose.

### Assess Breathing

Most babies will be crying, and this is proof of breathing. If the baby has no respiratory effort, it could be in either primary or secondary apnea. In primary apnea, the baby will recommence breathing with stimulation. Drying and clearing of the airway should be adequate stimulation to initiate breathing in the patient with primary apnea. With secondary apnea, the baby will not initiate spontaneous ventilation with simple stimulation and will require artificial ventilation. For these reasons, when apnea is discovered following the initial steps of drying and positioning the baby, assume that the patient is in secondary apnea and proceed to bag-mask ventilation.

### Assess Heart Rate

In the newly born, low heart rate is a sign of hypoxia, not intrinsic heart disease. The crying, active newborn has an adequate heart rate. Assess heart rate carefully in the baby who is not active or who requires ventilation. This can be done through auscultation or through palpating the pulse in the umbilical cord. Even if it appears that the baby is making respiratory efforts, if the heart rate is low it usually means that the respiratory effort is not adequate and should be assisted. Treat heart rates less than 100/min with positive pressure ventilation and 100% oxygen.

### Assess Color

In utero, the fetus thrives with an arterial oxygen concentration of 25–28 torr.[9] At birth, the baby begins to breathe oxygen and the arterial oxygen concentration quickly rises to 50 to 70 torr. Until the baby has established regular ventilation, the physician should expect cyanosis. If the baby is breathing regularly and maintains central cyanosis, then administration of passive oxygen (blow-by oxygen) is indicated. This can be administered through oxygen tubing held next to the patient's face, or preferably, through a flow-controlled resuscitation bag-mask, with the mask held lightly on the face. Peripheral cyanosis, or cyanosis limited to the distal extremities, is common and does not require treatment.

### Meconium Presence in Amniotic Fluid

If meconium is present in the amniotic fluid, routine intrapartum oropharyngeal and nasopharyngeal suctioning is no longer recommended.[10] The mouth and trachea should be suctioned (**Figures 14.1 and 14.2**) if any of the following is present: the baby is not vigorous; respiratory effort is weak; muscle tone is poor; or heart rate is less than 100/min.[3]

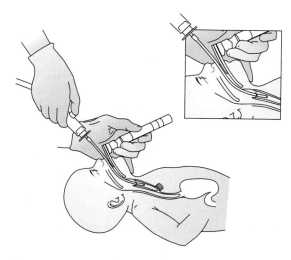

**Figure 14.1** Suctioning the trachea when meconium is present and the baby is not vigorous.
(Source: Kattwinkel J, ed. *Textbook of Neonatal Resuscitation.* 4th ed. Elk Grove, Il: American Academy of Pediatrics and American Heart Association; 2000:2–8.)

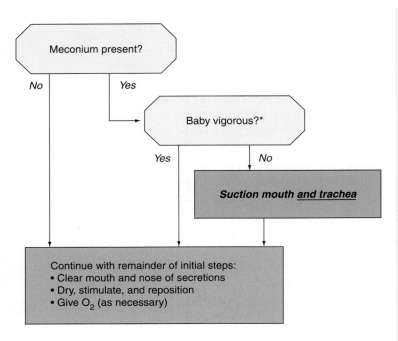

* "Vigorous" is defined as strong respiratory efforts, good muscle tone, and a heart rate greater than 100/min.

Figure 14.2 Management algorithm if meconium is present in amniotic fluid.

### Depressed Newly Born

The infant who is not breathing when born is a serious challenge to the practitioner. Coordinating and administering emergency care will have profound influences on the long-term quality of life for that patient.

Most infants who require resuscitation have arrived in that state due to hypoxia and acidosis, and treatment is directed at reversal of these two states. This is accomplished best with bag-mask ventilation and oxygen. Figure 14.3 summarizes the steps of newborn resuscitation.

### Bag-Mask Ventilation of the Newly Born

Artificial ventilation should be used in all babies with apnea or with heart rates less than 100/min.[11] After positioning the infant supine with slight head extension, place the mask firmly over the mouth and nose without putting pressure on the eyes. Too much pressure can stimulate the trigeminal reflex, a parasympathetic reflex that causes bradycardia. Apply enough pressure to see chest rise. If the depressed newborn has made no spontaneous respiratory effort, the pressure required for the initial breaths can be as high as 60 mmHg due to retained lung liquid. Deliver 40 to 60 breaths per minute, assessing the heart rate approximately every 30 seconds (Figure 14.4).

### Chest Compression

Most infants with bradycardia will improve their heart rate with adequate ventilation and not require chest compressions. Administer chest compressions when the heart rate is less than 60/min despite a 30-second trial of positive pressure ventilation. It is important to coordinate ventilations and chest compressions, because ventilation will be compromised if it is being delivered simultaneously with chest compressions. Deliver 3 compressions, then pause for a positive pressure breath. There should be approximately 120 events per minute of CPR: 90 compressions plus 30 breaths. Continue this sequence until the heart rate has risen above 60/min. Continue positive pressure ventilation until the heart rate is above 100/min and the patient is breathing spontaneously.

### Medications

When beginning chest compressions, also prepare for administration of epinephrine. Epinephrine is indicated when the heart rate remains below 60/min after 30 seconds of assisted ventilation plus 30 seconds of chest compressions. A logistical problem is establishing an administration route. Although intravenous administration is the preferred route, it is difficult to establish access in an acidotic/hypoxic baby. Therefore, emergency intubation might be necessary for epinephrine administration.[12] Umbilical vein catherization can provide a route for medications as well as for fluids (see Chapter 22, Critical Procedures).

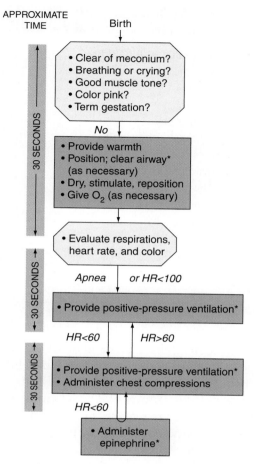

APPROXIMATE TIME

Birth

30 SECONDS

- Clear of meconium?
- Breathing or crying?
- Good muscle tone?
- Color pink?
- Term gestation?

*No*

- Provide warmth
- Position; clear airway* (as necessary)
- Dry, stimulate, reposition
- Give O₂ (as necessary)

- Evaluate respirations, heart rate, and color

30 SECONDS

*Apnea*   or *HR<100*

- Provide positive-pressure ventilation*

*HR<60*      *HR>60*

30 SECONDS

- Provide positive-pressure ventilation*
- Administer chest compressions

*HR<60*

- Administer epinephrine*

*Endotracheal intubation may be considered at several steps.

**Figure 14.3** Steps of newborn resuscitation. (Source: Kattwinkel J, ed. *Textbook of Neonatal Resuscitation* 4th ed. Elk Grove, Il: American Academy of Pediatrics and American Heart Association; 2000:2–5.)

## Conditions That Make Resuscitation of the Newly Born Challenging

If the baby is still not responding to resuscitation, then other causes that challenge standard resuscitation techniques must be sought. Generally, difficulty in achieving stability in an infant during resuscitation falls into five major categories: 1) technical problems, 2) unrecognized pulmonary problems, 3) severe metabolic problems, 4) developmental (congenital) anomalies of the organ systems involved, and 5) severe anemia (Table 14-3).

**Postresuscitation Care**

Following resuscitation, the infant is at high risk for postresuscitation complications. Monitoring the patient for further apnea is very important. Intravenous access should be established and an intravenous glucose solution (10% in water, 4 mL/kg per hour) should be initiated to prevent hypoglycemia. Hypocalcemia can also be a problem but typically does not appear for several hours.

The patient should be placed in a thermoneutral environment. Cold stress can increase oxygen utilization, while overheating can have a negative impact on cerebral injury.[13]

## Fever

In the first few days of life, elevated temperature (greater than 38°C, or 100.4°F) can be due to environmental factors, but in neonates beyond the first few days of life, fever virtually

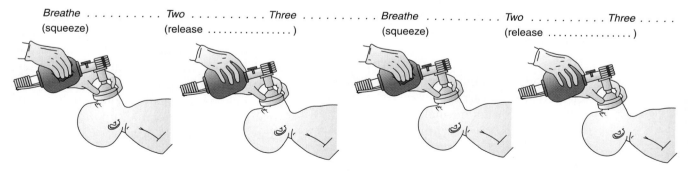

*Breathe* . . . . . . . . . . *Two* . . . . . . . . . . *Three* . . . . . . . . . . *Breathe* . . . . . . . . . . *Two* . . . . . . . . . . *Three* . . . . .
(squeeze)           (release . . . . . . . . . . . . . . . )              (squeeze)           (release . . . . . . . . . . . . . . . )

**Figure 14.4** Bag-mask ventilation in a neonate. (Source: Kattwinkel J, ed. *Textbook of Neonatal Resuscitation* 4th ed. Elk Grove, Il: American Academy of Pediatrics and American Heart Association; 2000:3–26.)

| TABLE 14-3 | Conditions That Make Resuscitation of the Newly Born Challenging |
|---|---|

**TECHNICAL PROBLEMS**
- Esophageal intubation
- Mainstem intubation
- Hyopoxia
- Hypoventilation secondary to low assisted ventilation rate
- Hypoventilation secondary to low ventilatory pressure

**UNRECOGNIZED PULMONARY PROBLEMS**
- Pneumothorax, pneumopericardium
- Meconium aspiration syndrome
- Diaphragmatic hernia
- Hypoplastic lungs
- Bacterial pneumonia
- Other restrictive intrathoracic problems

**SEVERE METABOLIC PROBLEMS**
- Acidosis
- Hypoglycemia
- Hypothermia

**OTHER PROBLEMS**
- Developmental (congenital)
- Anomalies of:
  – Cardiovascular system
  – Respiratory system
  – Central nervous system
  – Severe anemia, hypovolemia

always signals an acute infectious disease. Most of these infections are caused by viruses and are self-limited illnesses. However, a significant number of febrile neonates have bacterial infections. It is axiomatic that any bacterial infection in a neonate is a serious illness. Neonates have immature immune systems that cannot localize and eliminate a bacterial focus, thus making them vulnerable to hematogenous dissemination and the development of devastating illness such as meningitis or sepsis. These problems can originate from sites of infection, such as the middle ear, that in older infants and children would be unlikely sources for the development of systemic infection. Even neonates with an obvious focus of infection such as cellulitis, can have positive blood cultures.

## Clinical Features

The general appearance of the febrile neonate is of paramount importance. If the baby is neither lethargic nor irritable, is eating well, and otherwise appears normal, consideration of environmental overwarming can be considered, especially if the fever is not documented in the emergency department (ED). Inquire about the baby's home environment. How was the baby dressed? Do the parents tend to keep the house warm? Perform a complete physical examination, looking for a potential infectious focus. Observe the neonate eating. Repeat the temperature measurement while the baby is appropriately dressed. If all of these are normal, environmental conditions are likely. Irritability is a cause for concern, and lethargy is ominous. Any febrile neonate with apnea or cyanosis is gravely ill. The patient should be assessed for signs of cardiovascular instability such as mottled extremities, diminished peripheral pulses, or delayed capillary refill. These patients require aggressive fluid resuscitation and might require intubation and artificial ventilation (see Chapter 13, Medical Emergencies).

## Management

In the truly febrile neonate, complete blood cell count should be determined,[14] and cultures should be done of the blood, urine, and cerebrospinal fluid.[15] Because a viral illness presumes exclusion of a bacterial etiology, febrile neonates usually are hospitalized and treated with parenteral antibiotics until cultures are definitively negative.

## Bacterial Sepsis

Newly born and newborn infants whose maternal antepartum or partum events include pro-

## YOUR FIRST CLUE

**Signs and Symptoms of Serious Illness in the Neonate**

Cardiorespiratory Symptoms

- Rapid breathing
  - Pneumonia
  - Bronchiolitis
  - Congenital diseases
- Cough
- Nasal congestion
- Noisy breathing/stridor
- Apnea/periodic breathing
- Blue spells/cyanosis
- Cardiopulmonary failure

Crying/Irritability/Lethargy

- Testicular torsion
- Traumatic conditions
  - Battered child syndrome (fractures, burns, etc.)
  - Falls (skull and extremity fractures)
  - Open diaper pin
  - Strangulation of digit or penis
  - Corneal abrasion or foreign body
- Infections
  - Meningitis
  - Generalized sepsis
  - Otitis media
  - Urinary tract infection
  - Gastroenteritis

Eye Symptoms

- Discharge
- Redness

Fever

Gastrointestinal Symptoms

- Feeding difficulties
- Regurgitation
- Vomiting
- Diarrhea
- Abdominal distention
- Constipation
- Intestinal colic
- Incarcerated hernia
- Anal fissure

Skin Symptoms

- Jaundice
  - ABO/Rh incompatibility
  - Sepsis
  - Congenital infections
  - Bruising
  - Physiological
  - Bile duct atresia
  - Hepatitis
  - Hemolytic anemias
  - Hypothyroidism
  - Breast milk jaundice
- Diaper rash/oral thrush

---

longed rupture of membranes (PROM) (greater than 24 hours), maternal chorioamnionitis, fever,[16] foul lochia, urinary tract infections, fetal monitoring, or asphyxia are all predisposed to bacterial sepsis. Infections can occur early (0 to 4 days of age) from Group B streptococci and *Escherichia coli* (60% to 70%) and *Listeria, Klebsiella, Enterococcus, Streptococcus pneumoniae,* Group A streptococci, and *Staphylococcus aureus.* Late infection (greater than 5 days age) usually is from Group B streptococci, *E coli, Klebsiella, S aureus,* or *Staphylococcus epidermidis, Pseudomonas, Serratia,* or *Haemophilus influenzae.*

Presentation is usually subtle with signs and symptoms that can include jaundice, irritability, sleepiness, poor feeding, fever, or hypothermia. More obvious serious signs include abdominal distention or vomiting, poor perfusion or shock, respiratory distress, cyanosis or apnea, petechiae or bleeding, lethargy, irritability, or seizures.

Newborns initially might or might not look ill[16] and do not exhibit the typical meningeal signs with meningitis. The history must be focused on associated signs or symptoms such as poor feeding, lethargy, irritability, vomiting, apnea, and so on, while physical findings must focus on the appearance of the assessment triangle as well as the work of breathing and circulation. Early signs and symptoms in a febrile newborn do not correlate well with the subsequent severity of the disease.

Associated metabolic disorders such as hypoglycemia, metabolic acidosis, hypocalcemia, or hyponatremia can also be present. Fever or hypothermia can be absent! Other laboratory findings can include thrombocytopenia, neutropenia, and DIC. The most important issue when considering neonatal sepsis/meningitis is to not delay antibiotic administration.

### Management

Any febrile neonate without an identifiable focus of infection should have a complete sepsis workup, including complete blood cell (CBC) count, blood culture, lumbar puncture (LP) with cerebrospinal fluid (CSF) analysis and culture, catheterized urinalysis and culture, and chest radiograph if any respiratory symptoms are present. If the newborn is too unstable to undergo an LP, or if CT imaging is preferred prior to an LP (i.e., concern of increased intracranial pressure), administer the antibiotics immediately and do the LP later. Management includes stabilization of the ABCs (airway, breathing, circulation) and empiric broad-spectrum antibiotic treatment (e.g., ampicillin plus cefotaxime or gentamicin).[17] These patients can also present as gravely ill, requiring intubation, ventilation, fluid resuscitation, inotropic infusion, and other support.

Infections occurring after 5 days of life are termed late onset, occurring secondary to infectious exposure from the postnatal environment or, less likely, from the mother's genital tract (e.g., late onset GBS sepsis).

Gram negative organisms (e.g., *E coli*, *Klebsiella*, *Enterobacter*) often are hematogenously spread from the urinary tract, while *S aureus* can result in septic arthritis, breast abscess, or cellulitis. *Salmonella* infection (infectious gastroenteritis) can result in bacteremia with seeding of the joints or meninges.

Herpes simplex virus infection, usually acquired during delivery, generally presents in the first 2 weeks of life. This can present with signs of sepsis, or with localized skin vesicles and mouth ulceration, or meningitis (CNS involvement). If considered, intravenous (IV) acyclovir must be started in the ED.

## Lethargy

When awake, most neonates are alert and interact with their environment. They can fix and follow with their eyes, move their extremities spontaneously, and will suck a bottle. Be concerned about any neonate who is lethargic or listless, is difficult to awaken, will not fixate, has poor tone, or will not suck. The observations of the primary caregiver are important and should be considered. A chief complaint of "she just isn't herself" should be heeded. In the absence of other signs and symptoms, lethargy usually implies an acute metabolic disorder, infectious disease, or neurologic abnormality.

A complete physical examination should ensue, with particular focus on assessment of oxygenation, ventilation, and cardiovascular stability (Table 14-4). A fontanel that is full or loses vascular pulsations suggests increased intracranial pressure. Pupils should be assessed for symmetry and response to light. An appropriate evaluation can be tailored to findings from the physical examination and might include evaluation of neonatal reflexes.

Newborns with an inborn error of metabolism present with a number of nonspecific symptoms (similar to hypoglycemia) after a period of normal behavior, activity, and feeding.[18] The symptoms are in part dependent on the type of inborn error but might include: 1) lethargy; 2) seizures or hypotonia; 3) vomiting; 4) respiratory distress or apnea; 5) jaundice, with or without hepatomegaly; 6) failure to thrive; and 7) unusual odor.

### Management

Acute management includes cardiorespiratory and oxygen saturation monitoring. Compromise of either of these requires immediate intubation. Intravenous access should be established and glucose administration started. After

| TABLE 14-4 | Lab Evaluation of Lethargic Neonate |
| --- | --- |
| **Test** | **Abnormal in . . .** |
| CBC with differential and platelet count | Sepsis, severe anemia |
| Serum glucose | Sepsis, metabolic abnormalities |
| Electrolytes, blood urea nitrogen, creatine, calcium | Metabolic abnormalities, renal conditions |
| Serum ammonia | Metabolic abnormalities (urea cycle defects) |
| Arterial pH, lactate | Metabolic abnormalities, shock, CNS disturbances |
| Blood, urine, CSF cultures | Sepsis |
| Brain imaging | Intracranial trauma, hemorrhage, anomaly |

obtaining appropriate cultures, empiric therapy with broad-spectrum antibiotics, such as ampicillin and gentamicin or cefotaxime should be initiated for possible sepsis unless another etiology is obvious. If an inborn error of metabolism is suspected, initial rapid laboratory evaluation should include glucose, electrolytes, arterial blood gases (ABG), CBC, liver function tests, ammonia, and urine for ketones, reducing substances, and glucose. Initial treatment in the ED includes stopping formula feedings and starting an IV fluid containing glucose. Sodium bicarbonate might be required to treat metabolic acidosis, which is frequently severe. Transfer to an appropriate intensive care unit (ICU) setting should be expedited.

## Irritability

It is essential to distinguish the truly irritable neonate from one who simply cries more than usual. Irritability implies that the baby is in pain. Rocking or cuddling might not console the neonate because it is in pain. The irritable baby should be undressed completely and examined from head to toe. Abdominal tenderness can indicate peritonitis. The fingers, toes, and genitalia should be inspected carefully to exclude strangulation by a hair or piece of thread. Scrotal examination should be conducted and include an evaluation for incarcerated hernia.

### WHAT ELSE?

Differential Diagnosis of:

**Infection**
- Septic arthritis
- Urinary tract infection
- Meningitis
- Septic shock

**Trauma**
- Occult fractures
- Shaken baby syndrome

**Other**
- Metabolic disease
- Corneal abrasions
- Hair tourniquet

### Differential Diagnosis

The differential diagnosis is wide and includes meningitis, shaken baby syndrome, urinary tract infection, septic arthritis, and abuse. Traumatic lesions such as occult fractures or corneal abrasions are possible. Early shock can cause irritability or alternating lethargy and irritability due to decreased brain perfusion.

### Management

In the absence of another explanation, the irritable neonate requires a full evaluation for sepsis, trauma, and meningitis. Admission is prudent until a diagnosis is reached.

## Apnea

Many neonates present to the ED with the complaint from parents that they stopped breathing. Many normal infants have episodes during which normal breathing is interrupted by short pauses; however, they remain asymptomatic. Apnea episodes accompanied by symptoms are always a concern. Apnea accompanied by changes in skin color (cyanosis or mottling) that lasts more than 10 seconds, is recurrent, or appears later than 2 weeks of age, warrants further evaluation.

### Differential Diagnosis

The differential diagnosis for apnea is broad and includes infectious, metabolic, and neurologic causes. A complete history, physical examination, and laboratory evaluation will help distinguish these causes.

### Management

In cases of pathologic apnea, admission to a pediatric intensive care unit is desirable. Admission to a general pediatric floor is acceptable when careful monitoring can be ensured. In the ED, it is essential that the patient be on a cardiac monitor. Neonates with recurrent apnea might require intubation and ventilatory support. Any metabolic abnormality should be corrected, and empiric antibiotic therapy should be considered.

### WHAT ELSE?

**Differential Diagnosis of Neonatal Apnea**

- **Infections:** Sepsis, pneumonia, meningitis, encephalitis, pertussis, respiratory syncytial virus.
- **Metabolic:** Hypoglycemia, electrolyte abnormalities, inborn errors of metabolism.
- **Neuromuscular:** Seizures, infant botulism, child abuse (shaken baby syndrome), intracranial hemorrhage.
- **Gastrointestinal:** Gastroesophageal reflux.
- **Cardiac:** Dysrhythmias.
- **Hematologic:** Anemia.

## Cyanosis

Cyanosis can be peripheral or central. Peripheral cyanosis, also termed acrocyanosis, involves cyanosis limited to the hands and feet. It is common in the immediate newborn period and, as an isolated finding, is of no consequence. It is also common in newborn infants with polycythemia who are cold stressed, but it is also seen in healthy newborns. Outside of the immediate newborn period (1 to 2 days), acrocyanosis is less common and more concerning. Central cyanosis involves the body as well as the extremities.

### Differential Diagnosis

The differential diagnosis of central cyanosis includes pulmonary and cardiac diseases as well as central nervous system and metabolic problems.

### Management

Care of these infants should include a careful evaluation of the cardiovascular system (blood pressure, heart murmurs, pulses, and perfusion) as well as a CBC. Distinguishing between primary heart and lung disease in a newborn with respiratory distress can be

### WHAT ELSE?

**Differential Diagnosis of Cyanosis in Neonates**

**Pulmonary/Lung Disease**
- Upper airway obstruction
- Space-occupying lesion in the thoracic cavity (hypoplastic lungs)
- Persisting pulmonary hypertension (PPHN)

**Cardiac**
- Congenital heart disease
- Hypoxemia
- Polycythemia
- Methemoglobinemia

**Hematologic Symptoms**
- Severe anemia (hemoglobinopathy or blood loss)

difficult. Clues helpful in defining whether the problem is primarily cardiac or pulmonary include evaluation of clinical features, chest x-ray, blood gases, and the "hyperoxia test."

## Clinical Features

Usually a newborn with heart disease shows more tachypnea than retractions, while both are common with lung disease. Abnormal findings related to the cardiovascular system, such as heart murmur, poor pulses, or enlarged liver, point to cardiac rather than pulmonary disease. If the infant is being ventilated, a poorly compliant (stiff) lung favors the diagnosis of lung disease.

Neonates with central cyanosis should be admitted to an ICU setting where continuous monitoring can occur. Initial workup should include chest radiograph, arterial blood gas while breathing 100% oxygen, and CBC and differential. A baby that does not increase its $Po_2$ above 100 mmHg when breathing 100% oxygen is likely to have congenital heart disease. Arrangements for transfer to a pediatric ICU with pediatric cardiology support should follow. If congenital heart disease is expected, infusion of $PGE_2$ 0.1 mcg/kg per minute can be life-saving. The side effects of $PGE_2$ are minimal compared with the potential benefits. Approximately 10% of patients will show a side effect of apnea.

## Congenital Heart Disease

Congenital heart disease (CHD) is a common problem for the neonate, most often presenting either immediately after birth or in the first week of life. CHD is covered in greater detail in Chapter 4, Cardiovascular System.

Although congenital heart disease is typically divided into cyanotic or acyanotic, the appearance of other signs and symptoms must be recognized for appropriate diagnosis and treatment to occur (Table 14-5). After birth, the ductus arteriosus normally closes, at first functionally (at about 10 to 15 hours of life),[19] then anatomically (by about 2 to 3 weeks of life). However, the ductus can remain open in the presence of hypoxia, acidosis, and with ductal-dependent lesions such as hypoplastic left heart, coarctation of the aorta, interrupted aortic arch, or pulmonic or aortic stenosis. When the patent ductus arteriosus (PDA) does close, these newborns develop acute severe signs and symptoms of cardiogenic shock and congestive heart failure. Although many patients with CHD will present with tachypnea, tachycardia, sudden onset of cyanosis, or pallor, others typically present with vague and nonspecific signs and symptoms of congestive heart failure. These include lethargy, poor feeding or sweating while feeding, cyanosis that worsens with crying, and failure to thrive. In these infants, initiation of $PGE_2$ 0.1 mcg/kg per minute can be lifesaving.

## Grunting

Grunting is a short, low-pitched sound heard during expiration. During grunting respiration, the neonate is exhaling while simultaneously closing the glottis. Physiologically, this mechanism conserves lung volume by not allowing for full expiration.[20] It typically signifies parenchymal pulmonary disease leading to poor pulmonary compliance. Chest radiographs are indicated to diagnose potential pulmonary disease, and the neonate should be admitted for close observation and treatment.

## Vomiting

Vomiting is a common complaint in the neonate, and a difficult one to gauge because all babies spit up. Regurgitation of milk is very common, and physicians should ask questions that will differentiate between spitting up and vomiting. Regurgitation is typically nonforceful, with no retching, and is effortless. In the otherwise asymptomatic neonate, better burping and smaller, more frequent feedings can improve this symptom.

Vomiting must be distinguished as bilious or nonbilious. Bilious vomiting in a newborn signifies an upper gastrointestinal obstruction and is a medical emergency requiring immediate attention.[21] The most dangerous problem this indicates is a malrotation with subsequent

## TABLE 14-5 Presenting Symptoms and Other Findings of Cardiac Disease in the Newly Born and Neonate

### Newly Born (immediately after birth)

| Symptoms | Differential Diagnosis |
|---|---|
| Hydrops | • AV malformation<br>• Arrhythmias<br>　– Heart block<br>　– Supraventricular tachycardia (SVT)<br>• Myocarditis<br>• Severe chronic fetal anemia |
| Shock (cardiac muscle dysfunction) | • Hypoxemic-ischemic injury<br>• Myocarditis<br>• Sepsis<br>• Metabolic<br>　– Hypoglycemia<br>　– Hypocalcemia |
| Heart murmur | • Closing PDA<br>• Pulmonic or aortic stenosis<br>• Mitral or tricuspid valvular insufficiency |
| Cyanosis | Fixed right to left shunts<br>• Transposition of the great arteries<br>• Truncus arteriosus<br>• Tricuspid atresia<br>• Total anomalous pulmonary venous return (TAPVR)<br>• Pulmonary atresia or stenosis<br>• Double outlet right ventricle<br>• Single ventricle |

### Neonate (after the transitional period)

| Symptoms | Differential Diagnosis |
|---|---|
| Shock (first week of life) | • Newly born defects (above)<br>• Hypoplastic left heart (when PDA closes)<br>• Pulmonic or aortic stenosis<br>• Interrupted aortic arch<br>• Critical coarctation of the aorta<br>• TAPVR<br>• Arrhythmias<br>　– Heart block<br>　– SVT |
| Heart murmur (first month of life)<br>A. (dependent on ↓ PVR or ↑ SVR)<br><br>B. (not dependent on PVR or SVR) | • Ventricular septal defect (VSD)<br>• AV canal defects<br>• Patent ductus arteriosus (PDA)<br>• Newly born defects (above) |

*(continues)*

| TABLE 14-5 | Presenting Symptoms and Other Findings of Cardiac Disease in the Newly Born and Neonate (*Continued*) |
|---|---|
| Cyanosis | • Newly born defects (p. 488)<br>• Tetralogy of Fallot |
| Congestive heart failure<br>(Tachycardia, Tachypnea, Hepatomegaly,<br>    Large heart on x-ray) | • Coarctation of the aorta<br>• VSD<br>• Truncus arteriosus<br>• Endocardial cushion defect<br>• PDA<br>• Arteriovenous malformation |
| Cardiomegaly on x-ray | • Congestive heart failure<br>• Myocarditis<br>• Overhydration<br>• Pericardial effusion<br>• Metabolic disturbances<br>  – Acidosis<br>  – Hypoglycemia |

volvulus, which has a high mortality rate due to intestinal infarction.

Persistent nonbile-stained vomiting also signifies a possible bowel obstruction. Sometimes a history of polyhydramnios can be elicited. Although it can present earlier, pyloric stenosis most commonly comes to medical attention in the third to fourth week of life.

Vomiting is sometimes seen with increased intracranial pressure as well as sepsis/meningitis, which should be considered in the lethargic or febrile infant.

## Management

Bilious vomiting should be managed aggressively and rapidly. Resuscitation and evaluation for malrotation and midgut volvulus must proceed. Because this condition causes compromise to the blood supply (superior mesenteric artery) of the gastrointestinal tract, begin fluid resuscitation and contact a pediatric surgeon quickly. The diagnostic test of choice is an upper gastrointestinal (GI) series.

## Constipation

More than 90% of newborns will pass their first stool in the first 24 hours of life.[22] However,

### KEY POINTS

**Management of Bilious Vomiting in the Neonate**

- Continuous OG/NG suction with large bore, soft tube (10 Fr)
- Place IV, give fluid bolus 10 mL/kg saline or Ringer's lactate solution
- Continuous fluids at 1.5 maintenance
- CBC, serum electrolytes
- Urgent surgical referral (transfer as appropriate)
- Urgent upper GI

because infants are often discharged from the hospital within the first 24 hours of life, emergency physicians are often called on to evaluate the complaint of constipation. A history of meconium-stained amniotic fluid should be sought and is reassuring. Failure to pass the first stool by 36 hours of life warrants an evaluation. Causes for this include meconium plug syndrome, Hirschsprung disease, hypothyroidism, and hypoplastic left colon.

## Diarrhea

Diarrhea is present when there is an increase in the frequency and water content of the stools. In many neonates, especially breast-fed babies, frequent stools are normal, and it is a change in the pattern that is significant. Diarrhea can result from overfeeding, using a formula with a high osmotic content, or one of the carbohydrate malabsorption syndromes.

For the neonate, infectious etiologies cause the most concern, especially when the pathogen is bacterial. *Salmonella* gastroenteritis can be associated with bacteremia. Rotavirus is a common cause of profuse, watery diarrhea and can rapidly result in significant dehydration. Diarrhea can be a nonspecific manifestation of systemic illness, such as a urinary tract infection. It is important to try to determine the frequency of bowel movements and character of the stools. Blood in the stools can be due to structural abnormalities such as intussusception or anal fissure, but also can result from a bacterial infection.

### Management

The physical examination focuses on the general appearance of the neonate and state of hydration. In the febrile neonate with diarrhea, stool microscopy is indicated to assess the presence of fecal leukocytes or red blood cells (both are common in *Salmonella* gastroenteritis). If bacterial enteritis is suspected, stool cultures are indicated. In the febrile patient, cultures of blood, urine, and cerebrospinal fluid also should be considered. Hospital admission and empiric antibiotic therapy are prudent. An enzyme-linked immunosorbent assay for rotavirus is indicated during periods of expected epidemics.

## Seizures

Neonatal seizures are fairly common. The immaturity of the nervous system is such that seizures result in a wide variety of nonspecific symptoms. Focal convulsions are common and can be limited to one extremity or to the muscles of the face, especially the eyes.

### TABLE 14-6 Differentiation of Seizures from Jitteriness

| Variable | Seizure | Jitteriness |
|---|---|---|
| Rate | 1–3/sec | Fast |
| Amplitude | May be unequal | Equal |
| Stimulus sensitive | No | Very |
| Suppressed by passive restraint | No | Yes |

They can be accompanied by spells of apnea or bradycardia, often associated with cyanosis. Occasionally, it is extremely difficult to distinguish seizure activity from the normal tremulousness (jitteriness) many neonates exhibit. To help differentiate the two, evaluate the rate and amplitude of the jerking, and see if the movement can be precipitated by a stimulus such as gentle shaking or a loud noise, or suppressed by passive restraint (holding the arm or leg) (Table 14-6).

Seizures occurring within the first 24 hours after delivery most often are secondary to perinatal hypoxic ischemic disease, birth trauma, metabolic disease, or congenital malformations of the central nervous system. The baby is likely to be extremely ill. Seizures occurring after the second postnatal day are more commonly due to central nervous system infection and, in the preterm infant, intracranial hemorrhage. Herpes simplex should always be considered when seizures occur in the first 4 weeks of life. Rarely, neonatal seizures are due to inborn errors of metabolism. An extremely rare but treatable metabolic cause of neonatal seizures is pyridoxine dependency. In cases of intractable seizures, pyridoxine (50 to 100 mg IV) is administered while the infant undergoes continuous EEG monitoring (Table 14-7).

### Management

The evaluation of neonatal seizures includes serum glucose, electrolytes, calcium, phosphate, and magnesium; CBC; and cultures of the blood, CSF, and urine. Spinal fluid should

## TABLE 14-7 Etiology of Newborn Seizure Versus Age

**Less Than 24 Hours Old**
- Hypoxic-ischemic encephalopathy
- Birth trauma
- Intracranial hemorrhage
- Congenital malformations of CNS
- Hypoglycemia/hypocalcemia
- Infection
- Pyridoxine deficiency

**24 to 72 Hours Old**
- Sepsis/CNS infection
- Trauma/intracranial hemorrhage
- Metabolic (hypoglycemia, hypocalcemia, hypomagnesemia, hyponatremia/hypernatremia, hyperphosphatemia)
- Inborn errors of metabolism
- Drug withdrawal
- Congenital anomalies or developmental brain disorders
- Hypertension

**More Than 72 Hours Old**
- Infection (consider herpes simplex)
- Congenital anomalies or developmental brain disorders
- Metabolic or inborn error of metabolism
- Drug withdrawal
- Hypertension

be sent for polymerase chain reaction (PCR) and culture for herpes simplex. If no metabolic or infectious etiology of the seizures is discovered, computed tomography is indicated.

Acutely, seizures usually can be controlled with benzodiazepines (see Chapter 5, Central Nervous System). Phenobarbital is useful for chronic control. The prognosis of neonatal seizures depends on the etiology.

## Withdrawal

Neonates born of narcotic-addicted mothers often experience narcotic withdrawal syndrome. Common signs include tremulousness, tachypnea, vomiting, diarrhea, and irritability. Convulsions are uncommon but more likely when the mother is addicted to methadone than to heroin. Symptoms usually appear within 24 to 48 hours of birth but can be delayed.

### Management

The diagnosis most often is made by obtaining a history of maternal drug abuse. Hypoglycemia, hypocalcemia, and central nervous system infection must be excluded. Hospitalization for parenteral fluids and controlled withdrawal with the use of sedatives or narcotics might be necessary.

## Gastrointestinal Bleeding

Gastrointestinal bleeding can be the result of swallowed maternal blood either during delivery or from cracked, bleeding nipples during breastfeeding, causing hematochezia or hematemesis. Neonatal (fetal) blood can be differentiated from maternal blood by the Apt test, which is useful in differentiating swallowed maternal from neonatal blood.

Upper GI bleeding can result from stress ulcers, hemorrhagic gastritis, esophagitis, varices from portal hypertension, vascular malformations, and bleeding diathesis such as hemorrhagic disease of the newborn.

### Management

Whenever bleeding is noted from either the upper or lower gastrointestinal tract in the first 24 to 48 hours of life, an attempt should be made to determine whether it is maternal or fetal blood (Apt test).

Diagnosis and treatment consist of placing a nasogastric (NG) tube in all patients with melena or hematemesis while baseline laboratory data (coagulation studies, CBC, liver enzymes, type and match, x-ray) are obtained. Hospital admission is prudent if any of these conditions is being considered. A prolonged prothrombin time (PT) is treated with vitamin K, while a coagulopathy requires fresh frozen plasma.

## Umbilical Problems

Umbilical concerns that result in ED presentations frequently involve umbilical discharge or "bleeding" after the dried umbilical cord falls off (usually about 10 to 14 days). Delayed separation (beyond the third week) can be normal or secondary to problems such as immune deficiency[23] or sepsis. "Bleeding" is frequently exacerbated by constant irritation from the diaper rubbing the cord stump. Other concerns include granulation tissue (pink-red raw tissue mass requiring silver nitrate cauterization); omphalitis (periumbilical cellulitis with erythema, induration, and purulent discharge); umbilical hernia (of no immediate concern); or umbilical discharge. Brown discharge can be from an omphalomesenteric duct, while yellow discharge is from a patent urachus; both require surgical evaluation. Omphalitis requires blood cultures, IV antibiotic treatment, and hospitalization. Consider *Streptococcus*, *Staphylococcus*, and *Clostridium* species and coliform bacteria.

## Hyperbilirubinemia

Jaundice is caused by elevated bilirubin, which is the end product of heme degradation. It is ultimately dependent on liver function. Bilirubin can exist in one of two forms, either unconjugated (indirect-reacting) bilirubin, which is fat soluble and can cross the blood-brain barrier, or conjugated (direct-reacting) bilirubin, which is water soluble and does not cross the blood-brain barrier. The type of elevated bilirubin is dependent on the cause.

There are three fundamental causes of hyperbilirubinemia, which include: increased heme degradation (hemolysis), resulting in an indirect hyperbilirubinemia; delay in maturation or inhibition of conjugation mechanism (within the liver), also resulting in an indirect hyperbilirubinemia; or interference with excretion of bilirubin (from the liver), resulting in a direct hyperbilirubinemia. The type of bilirubin is helpful in classifying the cause of hyperbilirubinemia and the presence or absence of liver disease.

Unconjugated (indirect acting) hyperbilirubinemia is very common during the newborn period, usually peaking at 3 days of age in term newborns, with a rise up to 12 mg/dL considered normal.[24] The term "physiologic jaundice" is used to describe this condition, which is multifactorial but thought to be primarily due to a normal delay in maturation of the conjugation mechanism of the liver. There are a number of additional causes affecting the liver's conjugation mechanism, resulting in an "indirect hyperbilirubinemia" (greater than 12 mg/dL at 3 days of age in term newborn). Some of these include prematurity, hypoxia and acidosis, metabolic causes (dehydration, hypoglycemia), endocrine causes (hypothyroidism), breast milk inhibitors, GI obstruction, maternal diabetes, Down's syndrome, and inadequate fluid and caloric intake. Certain factors are associated with an exaggerated physiologic jaundice, such as breastfeeding and Asian race.

The second fundamental cause of unconjugated (indirect) hyperbilirubinemia is secondary to hemolysis or extravasation of blood, both of which result in increased bilirubin production. Intrinsic hemolysis is secondary to congenital defects of either the red blood cell (RBC) membrane (hereditary spherocytosis),

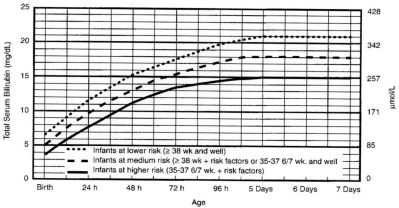

Legend within chart:
- •••• Infants at lower risk (≥ 38 wk and well)
- – – – Infants at medium risk (≥ 38 wk + risk factors or 35-37 6/7 wk. and well)
- —— Infants at higher risk (35-37 6/7 wk. + risk factors)

Y-axis (left): Total Serum Bilirubin (mg/dL) — 0, 5, 10, 15, 20, 25
Y-axis (right): µmol/L — 0, 85, 171, 257, 342, 428
X-axis: Age — Birth, 24 h, 48 h, 72 h, 96 h, 5 Days, 6 Days, 7 Days

- Use total bilirubin. Do not subtract direct reacting or conjugated bilirubin.
- Risk factors: isoimmune hemolytic disease, G6PD deficiency, asphyxia, significant lethargy, temperature instability, sepsis, acidosis, or albumin <3 g/dL (if measured).
- For well infants 35-37 6/7 wk, can adjust TSB levels for intervention around the medium risk line. It is an option to intervene at lower TSB levels for infants closer to 35 wks and at higher TSB levels for those closer to 37 6/7 wk.
- It is an option to provide conventional phototherapy in the hospital or at home at TSB levels 2-3 mg/dL (35-50 mmol/L) below those shown, but home phototherapy should not be used in any infant with risk factors.

**Figure 14.5** Management of hyperbilirubinemia in the newborn. (Source: American Academy of Pediatrics, Subcommittee on Hyperbilirubinemia. Management of hyperbilirubinemia in the newborn infant 35 or more weeks of gestation. *Pediatrics.* 2004;114:297-316.)

or RBC hemoglobin (thalassemia, sickle cell disease, both of which are very uncommon in the early newborn period), or RBC enzyme deficiency (G6PD, pyruvate kinase). Extrinsic hemolysis is common and occurs secondary to isoimmunization (e.g., ABO incompatibility, Rh disease), bacterial sepsis, or drugs. Extravasation of blood can be secondary to a cephalohematoma, vacuum extractor hematoma, bruising with breech presentation, traumatic or premature delivery, or IVH.

Conjugated (direct) hyperbilirubinemia is said to occur when more than 20% of the total bilirubin is conjugated (direct acting) and is always abnormal. This occurs when there is interference with the excretion of bilirubin from the liver, and it can be secondary to either intrahepatic or extrahepatic obstruction. Although both types of bilirubin are elevated, the terms "conjugated" or "direct-acting" is used.

Intrahepatic obstruction may be secondary to hepatitis from intrauterine infections, postdelivery infections (bacterial sepsis, herpes simplex), or neonatal viral hepatitis B. Congenital metabolic deficiencies (galactosemia, alpha-1 antitrypsin deficiency) will have similar findings. Extrahepatic causes include biliary atresia or extrinsic obstruction of the bile ducts (choledochal cyst).

## Management

The ED evaluation of a neonate presenting with jaundice should include measurement of the total and direct bilirubin; hemoglobin, blood smear and reticulocyte count; ABO; Rh grouping; and direct Coombs test. G6PD screening and other study work ups can be guided as indicated by clinical findings (cultures, viral studies). The level and type of bilirubin will immediately define the need and direction of further tests. Direct hyperbilirubinemia always needs further work up, while an elevated unconjugated bilirubin level might not need any further studies if otherwise normal. However, if the unconjugated bilirubin exceeds normal values for age (see standard texts) or is rising faster than expected, further testing is indicated.

A low hemoglobin with an elevated reticulocyte count suggests hemolysis, which can be secondary to isoimmunization or RBC membrane or enzyme defects. Blood grouping and a positive Coombs test diagnoses isoimmunization, while a blood smear can give clues to RBC structural problems that lead to hemolysis. G6PD deficiency is an X-linked recessive disorder mainly affecting black males.[25] The initial treatment for unconjugated hyperbilirubinemia is age dependent and starts with phototherapy (Figure 14-5).

# CHAPTER REVIEW

## Check Your Knowledge

1. An EMS crew arrives with a newly born infant that is mottled, limp, and has a heart rate of 80/min. Your first step should be:
   A. Bag-mask ventilation
   B. Chest compressions
   C. Dry the infant while suctioning the airway
   D. Intravenous access
   E. Narcan administration IM

2. An 8-day-old infant is brought to the ED for evaluation of fever and lethargy. The baby had a temperature of 38°C at home, refused to feed, and is difficult to awaken. Physical examination reveals the baby to be listless. The neck is supple. Appropriate steps by the emergency physician include:
   A. A full sepsis evaluation and admit
   B. IV fluid resuscitation with 20 mL/kg normal saline and discharge if the baby can take a bottle
   C. Observe in ED for 1 hour
   D. Take a further history as to the baby's environment
   E. Take a urine culture and close followup

3. All of the following questions are part of the resuscitation-oriented history for a woman in labor except:
   A. Do you abuse alcohol?
   B. Do you have twins?
   C. What color was the amniotic fluid?
   D. What is your due date?

4. An obese 17-year-old girl presents with abdominal pain. She is having severe back pain as well, which seems to be colicky in nature. On physical exam, you feel an abdominal mass; on pelvic exam, you find a baby's head crowning. She promptly delivers what appears to be a full-term newborn. The amniotic fluid is clear. The baby is cyanotic and limp. The cord is clamped and cut. The baby has been dried and warmed but remains limp and cyanotic. What is the next step in your resuscitation?
   A. Begin bag-mask ventilation
   B. Begin chest compressions
   C. Continue to dry and warm the baby
   D. Perform endotracheal intubation
   E. Place an umbilical vein catheter

## References

1. Kattwinkel J, Niermeyer S, Nadkarni V, et al. Resuscitation of the newly born infant: an advisory statement from the Pediatric Working Group of the International Liaison Committee on Resuscitation. *Resuscitation.* 1999;40:71–88.

2. World Health Organization. *World Health Report.* Geneva, Switzerland: World Health Organization; 1995.

3. Wiswell TE, Gannon CM, Jacob J, et al. Delivery room management of the apparently vigorous meconium-stained neonate: results of the multicenter, international collaborative trial. *Pediatrics.* 2000;105:1–7.

4. Niermeyer S, Kattwinkel J, Van Reempts P, et al. International guidelines for neonatal resuscitation: an excerpt from the Guidelines 2000 for Cardiopulmonary Resuscitation and Emergency Cardiovascular Care: International Consensus on Science. Contributors and Reviewers for the Neonatal Resuscitation Guidelines. *Pediatrics.* 2000;106:E29.

5. Dahm LS, James LS. Newborn temperature and calculated heat loss in the delivery room. *Pediatrics.* 1972;49:504–513.

6. Kattwinkel J, ed 4th ed *Textbook of Neonatal Resuscitation.* Elk Grove, Il: American Academy of Pediatrics and American Heart Association; 2000:2–8.

7. Bland RD, Hansen TN, Haberkern CM, et al. Lung fluid balance in lambs before and after birth. *J Appl Physiol.* 1982;53:992–1004.

8. Bland R. Formation of fetal lung liquid and its removal near birth. In: Polin RA, Fox WW, eds. *Fetal and Neonatal Physiology.* Vol. 1. Philadelphia, Pa: WB Saunders Co; 1992:782–789.

9. Teitel DF, Iwamoto HS, Rudolph AM. Effects of birth-related events on central blood flow patterns. *Pediatr Res.* 1987;22:557–566.

10. ECC Committee, Subcommittees, and Task Forces of the American Heart Association. 2005 American Heart Association guidelines for cardiopulmonary resuscitation and emergency cardiovascular care: part 13: neonatal resuscitation guidelines. *Circulation*. 2005;112(Suppl I):IV-190.

11. Saugstad OD. New guidelines for resuscitation of the newly born infant. *J Matern Fetal Neonatal Med*. 2002;11:2–3.

12. Roberts JR, Greenburg MI, Knaub M, Baskin SI. Comparison of the pharmacological effects of epinephrine administered by the intravenous and endotracheal routes. *JACEP*. 1978;7:260–264.

13. Perlman JM. Maternal fever and neonatal depression: preliminary observations. *Clin Pediatr (Phila)*. 1999;38:287–291.

14. Procop GW, Hartman JS, Sedor F. Laboratory tests in evaluation of acute febrile illness in pediatric emergency room patients. *Am J Clin Pathol*. 1997;107:114–121.

15. Kumar P, Sarkar S, Narang A. Role of routine lumbar puncture in neonatal sepsis. *J Paediatr Child Health*. 1995;31:8–10.

16. Escobar GJ, Li DK, Armstrong MA, et al. Neonatal sepsis workups in infants >/=2000 grams at birth: a population-based study. *Pediatrics*. 2000;106:256–263.

17. Odio CM. Cefotaxime for treatment of neonatal sepsis and meningitis. *Diagn Microbiol Infect Dis*. 1995;22:111–117.

18. Ellaway CJ, Wilcken B, Christodoulou J. Clinical approach to inborn errors of metabolism presenting in the newborn period. *J Paediatr Child Health*. 2002;38:511–517.

19. Clyman RI, Chan CY, Mauray F, et al. Permanent anatomic closure of the ductus arteriosus in newborn baboons: the roles of postnatal constriction, hypoxia, and gestation. *Pediatr Res*. 1999;45:19–29.

20. Lindroth M, Johnson B, Ahlstrom H, Svenningsen NW. Pulmonary mechanics in early infancy: subclinical grunting in low-birth-weight infants. *Pediatr Res*. 1981;15:979–984.

21. Godbole P, Stringer MD. Bilious vomiting in the newborn: how often is it pathologic? *J Pediatr Surg*. 2002;37:909–911.

22. Sherry S, Kramer I. The time of passage of the first stool and first urine by the newborn infant. *J Pediatr*. 1955;46:158.

23. Bissenden JG, Haeney MR, Tarlow MJ, Thompson RA. Delayed separation of the umbilical cord, severe widespread infections, and immunodeficiency. *Arch Dis Child*. 1981;56:397–399.

24. Maisels MJ, Newman TB. Jaundice in full-term and near-term babies who leave the hospital within 36 hours: the pediatrician's nemesis. *Clin Perinatol*. 1998;25:295–302.

25. Southgate WM, Wagner CL, Wagstaff P, Purohit DM. Hyperbilirubinemia in the newborn infant born at term. *J S C Med Assoc*. 2002;98:92–98.

**CASE SUMMARY 1**

A 16-year-old girl arrives in your emergency department with abdominal pain. She states she is pregnant. The patient states she is having abdominal pains about every 1 to 2 minutes. Her appearance is anxious but alert; she breathes rapidly with the pain but then slows her rate in between episodes of pain. There are no retractions, and her skin color is normal. Vital signs reveal a respiration rate of 22, a heart rate of 120, a blood pressure of 100/70 mmHg, and a temperature of 38°C.

1. *What three questions should the patient be asked to predict the need for resuscitation of the newly born?*
2. *What priorities of care should be initiated to resuscitate the newly born?*

What three questions should patient be asked to predict the need for resuscitation of the newly born?

1. Do you have twins? If yes, then prepare appropriate equipment and staff to handle two resuscitations.
2. When is your due date? If less than 36 weeks, then the need for a resuscitation of the newborn is more likely.
3. What color is your amniotic fluid? If green, then meconium is present, and you should suction the nose and mouth of the baby when the head delivers. After complete delivery of the newborn, tracheal suctioning should begin if the newborn is not vigorous or lacks muscle tone, has a heart rate is less than 100/min, or lacks respiratory effort.

What priorities of care should be initiated to resuscitate the newly born?
- Clear meconium as needed when head delivers.
- Deliver baby.
- Assess breathing, tone, and color. If not normal, then warm, dry, position, stimulate, and give oxygen.
- Begin bag-mask ventilation if apneic or heart rate is less than 100/min.
- Assess heart rate. If less than 60 bpm after 30 seconds of bag-mask ventilation, begin chest compressions and prepare medications.

# chapter 15

# Procedural Sedation and Analgesia

Alfred Sacchetti, MD, FACEP

## Objectives

1 Identify clinical circumstances in which procedural sedation or analgesia is indicated in the care of children.

2 Provide a pharmacologic basis for pediatric procedural sedation and analgesia.

3 Describe the basis for the development of safe and effective procedural sedation and analgesia practices.

4 Discuss alternative nonpharmacologic approaches to the care of children who require analgesia or sedation.

## Chapter Outline

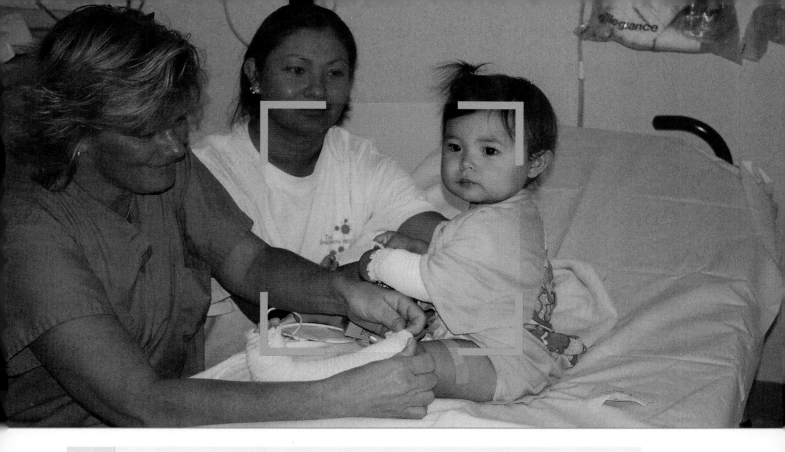

**CASE SCENARIO 1**

An 18-month-old boy is brought to the emergency department after his 3-year-old sibling knocked him down three stairs. He sustained a closed-head injury and a 4-cm forehead laceration when he struck a low coffee table. His mother, who witnessed the event, noted that the child was unresponsive for a few minutes following the initial injury. On awakening, he cried briefly but has been abnormally quiet and withdrawn since the event. He has vomited three times and is irritable in his mother's arms, but has no other signs of injuries. The physician plans to order a computed tomography (CT) scan to evaluate the child's head injury and repair his forehead laceration.

1. *What are the procedural sedation options for this child for CT scanning and laceration repair?*
2. *Can a single agent be used for both procedures?*

## Introduction

Traditionally, the pain management requirements of children have largely been ignored, with multiple studies documenting inadequate analgesia in the pediatric age group. Control for painless and painful procedures consisted of verbal reprimands and reassurances of, "It's okay," while sedation was limited to a single oral agent or intramuscular (IM) combination that produced significant oversedation for extended periods of time.

Fortunately, this field has evolved dramatically in the past decade. The introduction of new pharmacologic agents, as well as monitoring modalities and protocols, presents pediatric care providers with multiple sedation and analgesia options, with improved safety and efficacy to address the various clinical scenarios. Despite these advances, some clinicians are still reluctant to use sedation and analgesia in pediatric patients, even for painful conditions or procedures. This section will describe the different approaches for the delivery of procedural sedation and analgesia in children.

Procedural sedation and analgesia (PSA) overlaps many fields, including anesthesiology, critical care, emergency medicine, and pediatrics. As a result, various definitions have been put forth to describe similar management

## TABLE 15-1  JCAHO Sedation Level Definitions

| | |
|---|---|
| Minimal Sedation (Anxiolysis) | A drug-induced state during which patients respond normally to verbal commands. Although cognitive function might be impaired, ventilatory and cardiovascular functions are unaffected. |
| Moderate Sedation/Analgesia ("Conscious Sedation") | A drug-induced depression of consciousness during which patients respond purposefully to verbal commands, either alone or accompanied by light tactile stimulation. No interventions are required to maintain a patient's airway, and spontaneous ventilation is adequate. Cardiovascular function is usually maintained. |
| Deep Sedation/Analgesia | A drug-induced depression of consciousness during which patients cannot be easily aroused but respond purposefully following repeated or painful stimulation. The ability to independently maintain ventilatory function might be impaired. Patients might require assistance in maintaining a patent airway, and spontaneous ventilation may be inadequate. Cardiovascular function is usually maintained. |

Source: Joint Commission Resources. *Comprehensive Accreditation Manual for Hospitals (CAMH)*. Oakbrook Terrace, Il: Joint Commission on Accreditation of Healthcare Organizations; 2002:TX-15, definitions 1–3. Reprinted with permission.

protocols or strategies used in these different venues for the care of children.[1–5] Table 15-1 lists the most recent definitions proposed by the Joint Commission on Accreditation of Healthcare Organizations (JCAHO).[6]

Because of the extreme variability in children's responses to medications and tolerance of procedures, it is not always possible to predict the degree of sedation required, or achieved, in a given case.[7] A procedure expected to be completed with only moderate sedation can evolve to require deep sedation and analgesia. Alternatively, only moderate sedation/analgesia might be required and targeted, but deep sedation/analgesia is actually attained. As a result, operational definitions describing the intended purpose of PSA are more useful in helping clinicians approach the treatment of any given child. From a practice perspective, sedation and analgesia requirements can be defined by five clinical scenarios: simple analgesia, anxiolysis, procedural sedation for painless intervention, procedural sedation for painful intervention, and extended sedation. These scenarios are specifically defined in Table 15-2. Procedural sedation can be described by a single definition; however, from the patient care perspective, the selection of agents to use is determined by whether a procedure is painful or painless.[8]

## Clinical Features

### Preparation and Monitoring

Preparation for analgesia, anxiolysis, or PSA begins with patient assessment. Although some variation is expected, all pediatric pain management or sedation needs must be examined in the context of their clinical scenario. A focused history and physical examination are part of the initial evaluation and should include specific questions concerning past medical history, medication allergies or reactions, previous sedation or analgesia experiences,

**TABLE 15-2   Procedural Sedation and Analgesia Clinical Scenarios**

| Clinical Scenario | Definition | Examples |
|---|---|---|
| Simple Analgesia | Relief of pain without production of an altered mental state. Sedation might be a secondary effect of medications administered for this purpose. | Administration of an opioid to a patient with an undisplaced extremity fracture or abdominal pain. |
| Anxiolysis | A state of decreased apprehension concerning a particular situation; there is no change in patient's level of awareness. | Benzodiazepine administration to an adolescent following severe emotional traumatic event. |
| Procedural Sedation for Painless Intervention<br><br>Procedural Sedation for Painful Intervention | A technique of administering sedatives, analgesics, and/or dissociative agents to induce a state that allows the patient to tolerate unpleasant procedures while maintaining function. Intended to result in a depressed level of consciousness but allow the patient to maintain airway control independently and continuously. | Barbiturate use to permit a CT scan in a toddler following seizure.<br><br>Ketamine administration to a child for debridement of burns. |
| Extended Sedation | Intentional depression of a patient's sense of awareness of surroundings to permit cooperation with ongoing care. Loss of protective airway reflexes and respiratory drive might be an intended consequence of such care in patients in whom ventilatory management has been assumed. | Barbiturate or benzodiazepine infusion to facilitate ventilator management in a head injury victim. |

## THE CLASSICS

**Important Principles in Emergency Sedation and Analgesia for Children**

- Children are undertreated for pain and anxiety.
- Appropriate monitoring of children undergoing PSA includes bedside monitoring by an experienced clinician with the training and competence to provide airway support and rescue from respiratory or cardiovascular sequelae of deep levels of sedation.
- Monitoring should in most cases include continuous pulse oximetry

and family medication histories. Questions concerning last meals and recent activities are appropriate for ED patients but might not be needed in intensive care unit (ICU) patients. Unless there is reliable evidence to the contrary, it is probably safest to proceed as if a child has eaten recently. A good mnemonic that covers all the salient historical points in a child undergoing procedural sedation is AMPLE:

- Allergies
- Medications
- Previous procedures and past medical history
- Last meal
- Events prior to procedure

The classification system developed by the American Society of Anesthesiologists (ASA) can help guide the management of PSA candidates. (Table 15-3). As a general rule, ASA class I and II patients can be safely managed by nonanesthesiologists, while ASA class IV and V patients are best managed in conjunction with an anesthesiologist or subspecialty consultant when possible. ASA class III patients can be managed by emergency physicians, intensivists, and other providers, although input from an anesthesiologist can be useful depending on the clinical scenario. In emergent circumstances, it might be necessary to begin treatment immediately while consultant input is sought for higher risk patients.[8]

An example of a class II patient is one with well-controlled asthma: a patient with poorly controlled asthma would fall into class III. Patients with diseases of two systems (e.g., diabetes and asthma) might be considered to be in Class III even if each were relatively well controlled. Some practitioners believe that patients with certain congenital problems such as Down's syndrome and some skeletal dysplasias should be in class III because of multiple anomalies associated with these conditions.

Additional preparation includes determination of medications and routes of administration as well as initiation of appropriate patient monitoring. If intravenous medications are to be used, some form of vascular access must be established. Supplemental oxygen and suction capabilities along with respiratory and cardiovascular monitoring equipment should be readily available in every area in which PSA will be performed.

Explanation of the planned sedation or analgesia to the child and parent or other caregiver should not be overlooked during medical preparations. Assurance that a child's pain will be addressed or anxiety managed is extremely comforting to both patient and family. Written consent might be required in some institutions.

The degree to which a child's respiratory or cardiovascular status is continuously monitored is scenario specific. Children receiving

| TABLE 15-3 | American Society of Anesthesiologists Physical Status Classification |
|---|---|
| Class I | Normal healthy patient |
| Class II | Patient with mild systemic disease |
| Class III | Patient with severe systemic disease |
| Class IV | Patient with severe systemic disease that is a constant life threat |
| Class V | Moribund patient who is not expected to survive without the procedure |
| E | Emergency procedure |

simple analgesics or anxiolytics will generally not require any ongoing monitoring beyond initial, and possibly repeated vital signs. Those undergoing procedural sedation will require more intensive monitoring. At the least, continuous pulse oximetry should be maintained on any child with an intentionally depressed level of awareness. Cardiac and blood pressure monitoring is strongly recommended for ASA class III patients and is mandatory for class IV and V patients.[9] Pulse oximetry will detect arterial hypoxia, but this is not necessarily an early indicator of hypoventilation or airway obstruction. Elevation of end-tidal carbon dioxide levels has been reported in children managed with respiratory depressant medications.[10,11] Whether clinically significant hypoventilation actually occurs in these patients is unclear, and the role of routine capnometry in ASA I or II patients has not been established. An absent capnography waveform can be the earliest warning sign of airway obstruction. The use of capnography, especially in situations such as CT or MRI where patients cannot be directly observed, can allow early detection and relief of airway obstruction (absent waveform) before desaturation and its consequences occur. Alternatively, careful patient observation by an experienced clinician will also detect hypoventilation or airway obstruction prior to the development of hypoxia. Continuous cap-nometry should be considered in patients sensitive to both carbon dioxide tension as well as oxygen saturation, including those with elevated intracranial pressure or certain cardiac lesions.[8]

Any monitoring initiated on a child must be continued beyond the time required to perform the procedure. For painful activities such as fracture reductions or burn debridement, the level of sedation can increase dramatically after the stimulus of the procedure is removed.

Specified disposition criteria should be established for children undergoing procedural sedation. As a general rule, a child must return to baseline respiratory status prior to consideration for discharge. Airway reflexes must also be present unless altered by some preexisting condition. Both level of consciousness and voluntary motor control should be observed to be spontaneously improving, although both of these might not return completely to baseline for some time if certain longer-acting agents are used.[12] Parents should be warned of this possibility and instructed not to allow children to engage in unsupervised play or activities that require coordination until all residuals of the treatment medications have dissipated.

## Pain Assessment

The ability to provide pain relief to any patient requires an effective means of assessing that patient's degree of discomfort. Simple, subjective assessment by parents and practitioners correlate poorly with children's pain.[13,14] Objective and visual analog tools have been designed to better facilitate pain-related communication between patients and practitioners. The problem of pain assessment is compounded further in children because of the variable communication skills present in different age groups. Purely observational scoring systems have been developed for neonates and infants, while progressively more interactive scales have been used for older children.[15–17] Figure 15.1 A, B, and C contain examples of three age-related scoring systems.

The selection of any single pain scoring system is not as important as the consistent application of some form of repeated patient assessment. Toddlers and small children in particular might be hesitant to verbalize their discomfort, and mechanisms should be in place to specifically offer these patients pain medication. In communicative children, the regular presentation of the option for analgesia can be even more effective than using clinical judgment based on a scoring system to determine when pain medications are needed.

For children with altered mental status, communicative handicaps, or central nervous system (CNS) injuries, it can be difficult to determine if appropriate procedural sedation is being provided during a painful procedure (although the FLACC scale described in Figure 15.1A does not rely on patient self-reporting). In these children, the use of a bispectral index monitor might be helpful. This device uses head electrodes to create a quantifiable modified electroencephalogram that can reflect the level of consciousness of any sedated patient. Use of the bispectral index monitor can ensure appropriate sedation (but not pain assessment) for children who otherwise cannot be assessed clinically.[18]

## Management

### Principles of Analgesia and Sedation and Routes of Administration

The determination of the need for some form of analgesia or sedation is made by the clinicians immediately caring for a child. Regardless of the potential etiology of a patient's pain, there is never an indication to withhold analgesics while awaiting an examination by a consultant or the results of a diagnostic study. Published studies contradict the notion that the appropriate use of opioid analgesics masks the important physical findings in any symptom complex, including those in children with abdominal pain, head injuries, hernias, extremity

FLACC Observation Scale for Infants and Small Children

| Category | Scoring | | |
|---|---|---|---|
| | 0 | 1 | 2 |
| Face | No particular expression or smile | Occasional grimace or frown, withdrawn disinterested | Frequent to constant quivering chin, clenched jaw |
| Legs | Normal position or relaxed | Uneasy, restless, tense | Kicking, or legs drawn up |
| Activity | Lying quietly, normal position, moves easily | Squirming, shifting back and forth, tense | Arched, rigid or jerking |
| Cry | No cry (awake or asleep) | Moans or whimpers; occasional complaint | Crying steadily, screams or sobs, frequent complaints |
| Consolability | Content, relaxed | Reassured by occasional touching, hugging or being talked to, distracted | Difficult to console or comfort |
| FLACC: F-Face, L-Legs, A-Activity, C-Cry, C-Consolability | | | |

**Figure 15.1A** Pain assessment scale.
Source: Merkel SI, Voepel-Lewis T, Shayevitz JR, Malviya S. The FLACC: a behavioral scale for scoring postoperative pain in young children. *Pediatr Nurs.* 1997;23:293–297. Reprinted with permission.

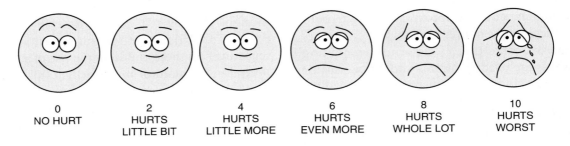

| 0 NO HURT | 2 HURTS LITTLE BIT | 4 HURTS LITTLE MORE | 6 HURTS EVEN MORE | 8 HURTS WHOLE LOT | 10 HURTS WORST |

**Figure 15.1B** Faces scale for children older than 3 years.
Source: Wong DL, Hockenberry-Eaton M, Wilson D, Winkelstein ML, Schwartz P. *Wong's Essentials of Pediatric Nursing*, 6th ed. St Louis, Mo: Mosby, Inc.; 2001:1301. Copyrighted by Mosby, Inc. Reprinted with permission.

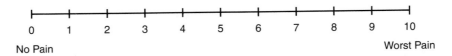

0   1   2   3   4   5   6   7   8   9   10
No Pain                                  Worst Pain

**Figure 15.1C** Linear scale for older children and adolescents.

injuries, or headaches.[19] In older or emancipated adolescents, the administration of opioid analgesics does not interfere with their ability to provide consent for any surgical procedures.

Not every child undergoing a procedure or study requires some form of sedation. Cooperation can sometimes be elicited by imaginative cajoling or distraction for brief diagnostic studies such as simple head CT scans. Even briefly painful procedures such as reduction of a subluxed radial head can be performed without sedation if completed quickly and efficiently. The decision to proceed without pharmacologic assistance is determined by clinical experience and anticipated duration of the procedure.

If the need for some form of analgesia or sedation is established, then a determination must be made as to the optimal approach for that particular child. Available options on the best technique, route of administration, medications, monitoring, followup, and personal preferences must all be considered. Every procedural sedation case should be approached with the realization that any given child might require substantially more sedation than expected, and that the personnel and equipment required for any degree of sedation should be present at the bedside or immediately accessible.

If a pharmacologic approach is selected for a child, the route of administration of the medication must be determined. The potential options for route of administration, along with their advantages and disadvantages, are presented in Table 15-4. In selecting a route of administration, the clinician must balance ease of administration with reliability of onset, duration of action, ability to titrate, and patient tolerance.

Oral administration of medications is convenient and well tolerated in patients of all ages. Medications given in this manner can be liquids, pills, and even gelatin cubes.

Transmucosal delivery routes include intranasal, transbuccal, and rectal. All of these have been described for use in infants and small children. Intranasal medications are delivered as either drops or as a spray. Transbuccal medications are generally delivered in a lollipop-like hard candy that the child sucks on; this permits medication absorption through the mucosal surfaces of the cheeks and beneath the tongue. Rectal medications are administered either as a suppository or as a liquid. Liquid medications are generally injected into the rectum with a soft catheter attached to a syringe. The child's gluteals are then held together to allow time for absorption.

Both the oral and transmucosal routes have the advantage of ease of administration regardless of the vehicle for the medications. The primary disadvantage of these routes is the difficulty in titrating doses to a specific effect. Because of variabilities in the absorption of medications given in these ways, the time to onset can never be determined exactly. Medications must be absorbed first, producing a delay between administration of a drug and onset of action. Physicians managing such patients might be uncertain whether a lack of effect in the patient is the result of a delay in absorption or an inadequate dose. This might not be an issue for children receiving simple analgesia or anxiolysis, but can be a major obstacle for those undergoing procedural sedation. If the transmucosal route is selected, it should only be used with medications demonstrating a predictable response with a single dose.

Transdermal medications can also be given, although they are generally used for provision of local anesthesia or long-term analgesia.[20]

Parenteral administration of drugs provides a more rapid onset with more predictable outcomes. Intravenous, IM, and subcutaneous injections all bypass the problems associated with absorption of a drug across a mucosal barrier. The major disadvantage of these approaches is that they require some form of painful injection.

| TABLE 15-4 | Routes of Pharmacologic Administration | | | |
|---|---|---|---|---|
| Route | Comfort | Reliability | Titratable | Efficacy |
| Oral | ++++ | ++ | + | +++ |
| Transmucosal | | | | |
|   Rectal | + | ++ | + | ++ |
|   Nasal | + | ++ | + | ++ |
|   Buccal | +++ | ++ | ++ | ++ |
| Parenteral | | | | |
|   Intramuscular | + | +++ | ++ | +++ |
|   Subcutaneous | ++ | +++ | ++ | +++ |
|   Intravenous* | + | +++ | ++++ | ++++ |

*Consider PCA device

For intramuscular and subcutaneous medications, a separate injection is required for each administration, making these routes less desirable for procedures requiring multiple doses or titration.[21] Intravenously administered medications require an initial needlestick, but all subsequent doses are delivered painlessly. The minimal time delays between administration of a drug and observation of an effect allows for much easier titration to effect with this route.

Patient-controlled analgesia (PCA) is an option for most children older than 3 years.[22] Most of these systems use intravenously administered opioid analgesics delivered through an infusion pump. The pumps are programmed to allow the children to self-administer pain medications as needed while using lockout features to prevent accidental delivery of excessive amounts. These devices have been used in acute care settings and are ideal for children with exacerbations of recurrent painful conditions.

Inhaled nitrous oxide has also been used successfully in children. The onset time is virtually immediate with this delivery route, making titration to response exceptionally sensitive. Delivery mechanisms are the primary limiting factor to this route of administration. Older children can use self-delivery systems that utilize demand valves to shut off flow when the appropriate level of sedation is achieved. Younger children receive inhaled nitrous oxide through a fixed delivery system that must be controlled externally.[23,24]

Because of their imaginative and curious natures, children are also good candidates for nonpharmacologic analgesia and sedation techniques. Distraction techniques using visual or audio cues have proved effective in diverting children's attention from brief painful procedures or extended nonpainful diagnostic studies.[25,26] Hypnosis of toddlers and young children has also been shown to be effective for brief injections, laceration repairs, and even fracture management.[23] In newborns, nonnutritive sucking or pacifier use can reduce the distress associated with heel blood sampling and circumcision.[27,28] Sleep deprivation prior to a scheduled nonpainful diagnostic study is also very useful when planned in advance.

# Medications Used in Analgesia and Sedation

There is no single ideal agent for pediatric pain control, anxiety management, or procedural sedation. As in all other areas of medicine, the best medication for a given patient will be determined by the clinical scenario, the child's age, history and physical exam, and the personal preferences and experience of the clinician providing the care. What is universal is that a sound knowledge of the pharmacology of sedation or analgesia agent is essential to its safe and effective use. Table 15-5 summarizes medications used in pediatric sedation and analgesia.

Classification systems have been proposed based on the sedative or analgesic properties of medications. However, many of the newer agents have actions common to more than one class, making definitive groupings difficult. A more practical approach is to examine individual medications within their pharmacologic classes but apply them clinically based on their individual properties.

## Acetaminophen

Acetaminophen is a pure analgesic with both antipyretic and analgesic actions. It has an excellent safety profile and is frequently combined with opioid analgesics for management of mild to moderate pain.

## Nonsteroidal Anti-Inflammatory Drugs

This class of drugs also possesses both antipyretic and analgesic actions. The NSAIDs,

**TABLE 15-5  Medications**

| Medication | Dose (mg/kg) | Route | Max Unit Dose (mg) | Duration | Precautions | Comments |
|---|---|---|---|---|---|---|
| Acetaminophen | 10–20 | Oral/Rectal | 1,000 | 4 hr | | |
| Ibuprofen | 5–10 | Oral | 800 | 6 hr | | |
| Ketorolac | 0.5 | IM/IV | 30 mg IV or 60 mg IM | 4–6 hr | | |
| Morphine | 0.1 | IM/IV | 10 | 3–4 hr | Histamine release, respiratory depression | |
| Fentanyl | 0.001–0.005 | IM/IV | 0.05 | 0.5–1 hr | Rigid chest | Decrease dose in infants |
| | 0.005–0.015 | Transmucosal | 400 mcg | 0.5–1 hr | Vomiting | |
| Meperidine | 1–2 | IM/IV | 100 | 3–4 hr | Toxic metabolites | Seizure, irritability |
| Hydromorphone | 0.01 | IM/IV | | 3–4 hr | | |
| Hydrocodone | 0.2 | Oral | 10 | 4–6 hr | | Combine with acetaminophen |
| Codeine | 1–2 | Oral | 60 | 4–6 hr | GI upset, vomiting | Combine with acetaminophen |
| Pentobarbital | 2–5<br>4 | IV<br>IM | 200 | 0.5–1.5 hr | Titrate IV | Avoid all barbiturates in children with porphyria |
| Methohexital | 0.5–1 | IV | 100 | 20–60 min | Respiratory depression | |
| | 18–25 | Rectal | | | Respiratory depression | |
| Thiopental | 2.5–5 | IV | 300 | 20–60 min | Respiratory depression | |
| | 25 | Rectal | | | | |
| Midazolam | 0.05–0.2 | IV/IM | | 1–2 hr | Respiratory depression | Agitation with low dose |
| | 0.3–0.7 | Oral | | | | |
| Chloral Hydrate | 50–100 | Oral/Rectal | 1,000 | 6–24 hr | Liver disease | |
| Propofol | 0.5–1 | IV bolus | 100 | 6–10 min | Respiratory depression | |
| | 1–3 mg/kg/h | Drip | | | | |
| Etomidate | 0.1–0.3 | IV bolus | 20 | 15–20 min | Myoclonic jerks | |
| Ketamine | 3–5 | IM | | 1–2 hr | Airway secretions | |
| | 1–2 | IV | | 0.5–1 hr | | |
| | 6–10 | PO | | 2–3 hr | | |

*(continues)*

TABLE 15-5    Medications (*Continued*)

| Medication | Dose (mg/kg) | Route | Max Unit Dose (mg) | Duration | Precautions | Comments |
|---|---|---|---|---|---|---|
| Naloxone | 0.005–0.01 (partial reversal), 0.1 (total reversal) | IV/IM | 2 | 20 min | | Opiate antagonist |
| Nalmefene | 0.00025–0.00050 | IV | 0.0040 | | | Long-acting opiate antagonist |
| Flumazenil | 0.01 | IV | 0.2 | 30 min | | Benzodiazepine antagonist |
| Lidocaine | | Infiltrated | 4.5 mg/kg | 30–120 min | | |
| Lidocaine with epinephrine | | Infiltrated | 7 mg/kg | 1 hr | | |
| Bupivacaine | | Infiltrated | 2.5 mg/kg | 2–8 hr | | |

All drugs should be titrated to effect and administered at intervals consistent with their onset and interactions with other drugs being administered.

as this group is known, produce their effect through enzyme inhibition in the prostaglandin synthesis pathways. As a result, these drugs are most effective for prostaglandin-mediated pain such as that produced by biliary or renal colic, dysmenorrhea, and inflammatory arthritis. They have also proved effective in the treatment of mild to moderate pain associated with musculoskeletal injuries and surgery. The NSAIDs also decrease blood flow to the gastric mucosa, which can produce gastritis or ulcers with chronic use. These issues are generally not a concern with short-term use in children with no underlying gastrointestinal problems. NSAIDs have an antiplatelet effect, which can aggravate bleeding and bruising in some types of injuries, especially trauma.

Ibuprofen is the prototypical NSAID. It is effective alone for relief of mild pain but can be combined with opioid analgesics for management of more severe pain.[29]

Ketorolac is no more potent than ibuprofen or other orally administered NSAIDs but has the option for parenteral administration. Because the mechanism involves decreased production of a prostaglandin precursor, there is a delay in onset of its analgesic effect even with IM or intravenous use. In addition to the typical NSAID indications mentioned, ketorolac has also been used successfully for sickle cell crisis and postoperative pain.[30–32]

## Opioid Analgesics

Medications in this group vary from mild to potent analgesics applicable to an entire spectrum of painful conditions, from minor extremity trauma to general anesthesia. All of the opioids produce pain relief through stimulation of opioid receptors in the CNS.

All of the clinically used opioid analgesics stimulate each of the receptors to some degree, although preferential activity of different receptor types does exist between various drugs. Most of the variability in the observed actions of different drugs results from their receptor binding behavior as well as their metabolism and ability to enter the CNS. Some synthetic opioids possess both agonist and antagonist opioid receptor actions. Opioid analgesics also produce some degree of sedation, and, although not a primary action, this effect can be used to some advantage in patients with both pain and anxiety. All of the opioids can produce dose-related respiratory depression, which is more prominent in infants and young children. Hypoxia and hypercarbia can both result from depressed ventilation, and in sensitive children these changes can result in elevation of intracranial pressure. Hypotension as a result of both peripheral vasodilation and myocardial depression is another potential systemic physiologic effect of this group of agents. Many of the opioids also release histamine, and transient urticaria or flushing can occur. All of the drugs in this class have the potential to induce nausea. Concomitant administration of a phenothiazine or other antiemetics has not been shown to prevent this effect in controlled trials, although many clinicians find that the use of these agents does help in some patients in whom nausea occurs.

Morphine sulfate is the classic opioid analgesic. It is a potent pure agonist with excellent analgesic properties. Morphine can be administered orally, intramuscularly, subcutaneously, intravenously, intra-articularly, epidurally, and intrathecally. When delivered intravenously its actions can be easily titrated. Morphine is unusual in that it is better absorbed subcutaneously than intramuscularly, which allows for use of a much smaller and less painful needle for delivery.

Meperidine is a semisynthetic opioid agonist with analgesic properties similar to morphine. Meperidine is frequently described as producing more euphoria than morphine, although the clinical significance of this in children is unclear. One of the major disadvantages of meperidine is that one of its principal metabolites, normeperidine, can accumulate with repeated dosing. Normeperidine has a longer half-life than its parent meperidine and is associated with CNS stimulation, dysphoria, and seizures. Normeperidine can interact adversely with certain monoamine oxidase (MAO) inhibitors and should be avoided in any patients taking this class of drugs.

Hydromorphone is a more potent semisynthetic opioid with excellent analgesic properties. Its pharmacology is similar to that of other opioid agents, and it is frequently preferred for PCA programs.

Fentanyl is an extremely potent synthetic opioid analgesic. Unlike other agents that are dosed as milligrams per kilogram, fentanyl is dosed in micrograms per kilogram. It has very little histamine-releasing effect and a very flat cardiovascular response curve, making it suitable for patients with cardiac pathology, asthma, or hypotension. The increased potency of fentanyl extends to its sedative and respiratory depressant actions as well, with a much greater apnea risk than either morphine or meperidine. Fentanyl also tends to induce more nausea and vomiting in children, particularly when administered as a transbuccal lollipop. Reports differ on the effects of fentanyl on intracranial pressure (ICP). Some case studies have demonstrated increases in ICP, while others indicate a decrease with fentanyl administration. The onset of action of this drug is very rapid, with a correspondingly short duration of action of only about 30 to 60 minutes. The clinical characteristics of fentanyl make it more appropriate for procedural sedation rather than simple analgesia. When used in this manner, it is commonly combined with a pure sedative. One characteristic unique to high-potency opioids such as fentanyl is chest wall rigidity, which occurs if it is administered too rapidly.[33]

Two relatives of fentanyl, alfentanil and sufentanil, have also been used for pediatric PSA. Sufentanil is 10 times more potent than fentanyl. Alfentanil is 5 to 10 times less potent than fentanyl and has a shorter half-life (15 to 30 minutes compared to 60 to 75 minutes for sufentanil and fentanyl).[34] Remifentanil is a relatively new synthetic opioid that demonstrates equal potency to sufentanil but with a much shorter duration of action. Remifentanil has an almost immediate onset of action when administered intravenously but a half life of only 5 minutes. It has a significant potential for respiratory depression; apnea has been reported in up to 50% of children treated with remifentanil for procedural sedation.[35–39]

Codeine is a low-potency opioid agent. Although it can be administered parenterally, codeine is most commonly given orally in combination with acetaminophen for mild to moderate pain. Gastrointestinal discomfort and nausea are recognized side effects of this drug.

Hydrocodone is an opioid agonist used primarily in combination with acetaminophen or ibuprofen as an oral preparation to treat moderate to severe pain. It is similar in action to codeine but more potent with fewer gastrointestinal side effects.

## Opioid Antagonists

Because all opioid medications act through a specific receptor site, their actions can be reversed through blockade of the opioid receptors. Naloxone is the traditional opioid antagonist and rapidly reverses the respiratory and cardiovascular depressant effects of any opioid agent. The half-life of naloxone is approximately 60 minutes, which is shorter than the duration of action of many opioid drugs. Because of this, any patient administered this agent must be observed beyond this time frame to be certain a relapse does not occur. An alternative agent, nalmefene, has a 10- to 12-hour duration of action and might be more appropriate if extended observation is not possible. Analgesic effects are also reversed with administration of naloxone and nalmefene. Nalmefene has not been approved for use in children younger than 12 years, although anecdotal reports have documented its use in younger children.

## Barbiturates

As a class, the barbiturates are the model sedative-hypnotic agents. They produce their effects through binding to the γ- aminobutyric acid receptor site (GABA) within neuronal membranes. This is the primary neuroinhibitor of the CNS. The site itself is a five-protein complex surrounding a chloride ion pore. When activated, the pore opens, allowing chloride to enter the cell, thus hyperpolarizing the cell membrane and making it more difficult to stimulate.

The barbiturates bind to two of the pore's proteins and activate the chloride channel. All of the barbiturates operate through this same mechanism, and the differences in clinical characteristics reflect chemical differences in lipid solubility, CNS penetration, and metabolism. Their neuroinhibitory actions are the source of the barbiturate's sedative, hypnotic, and anxiolytic properties. Because their CNS actions are relatively nonspecific, the barbiturates also depress respirations and, like the opioids, can produce hypoxia and hypercarbia. Also like the opioids, the barbiturates can induce hypotension through both myocardial and peripheral vascular effects. The neuroinhibitory actions of these drugs have additional applications in that they can interrupt seizure activity, reduce cerebral metabolism, and lower elevated ICP. Barbiturates are also metabolically very active compounds that induce liver enzymes and affect the pharmacokinetics of many other drugs. The barbiturates are also unique in that they can induce hemolysis in patients with porphyria. The barbiturates are not analgesics and possess no inherent pain relief properties. However, if a deep enough state of sedation is induced, brief painful procedures can be performed.

Pentobarbital is a short-acting sedative hypnotic agent typically used for painless diagnostic procedures. The recommended protocol for pentobarbital use involves titrated intravenous doses. Once a patient is appropriately monitored, a loading dose of 2.5 mg/kg is administered by IV. If the child is not sleeping within 1 to 2 minutes, a dose of 1.25 mg/kg is administered, followed another 2 minutes later by a final dose of 1.25 mg/kg if needed. In general, the second or third dose is rarely required. Children older than 12 years are more difficult to sedate with this protocol, although this might only represent the fact that children of this age who require sedation are more likely to have significant underlying neurodevelopmental problems that require additional agents. In direct comparisons with other pure sedatives, pentobarbital is consistently shown to be equipotent or superior for painless diagnostic studies.[40,41]

Methohexital is a very rapid-acting, short duration, potent barbiturate. Administered intravenously, it is generally used as an induction agent for general anesthesia, although its use has been described for emergency department procedural sedation. In children, methohexital is commonly used as a rectal preparation for sedation in painless diagnostic studies. Administered in this manner, it acts rapidly and consistently with a reasonable safety profile with proper monitoring for respiratory depression, which can occur in 3% to 10% of patients.[42,43]

Thiopental is almost identical to methohexital in both action and use.[44]

## Benzodiazepines

As a family of drugs, the benzodiazepines parallel the barbiturates. The benzodiazepines also activate the GABA receptor, although they bind to the two other proteins not used by either the barbiturates or GABA. As would be expected, the clinical actions of this class of drugs include sedation, hypnosis, respiratory depression, and antiseizure activity. The cardiovascular depression is not as prominent as with the barbiturates, and they tend to show more diversity in action because of differences in CNS distribution. The benzodiazepines also appear to be more variable in their dose-response relationships in children than both opioids and barbiturates. As a result, it is possible to produce disinhibition and agitation even with recommended doses.

Midazolam is a short-acting, rapid-onset benzodiazepine sedative used for painless diagnostic studies or in combination with opioids for painful procedures. This drug can be administered orally, intranasally, intravenously, and, rarely, intramuscularly. The recommended dose range for midazolam can be broad, and paradoxical reactions are well documented. The treatment of a child who becomes agitated after receiving this medication is additional medication until sedation is achieved.[41,45,46] Midazolam is also a potent amnestic agent, useful for sexual assault examinations.

Diazepam is very similar to midazolam in its actions, with a slightly longer time to onset but a very similar duration of action. Diazepam should not be given IM (poor absorption); it must be given slowly by IV (because of pain). Lorazepam is a long-acting benzodiazepine sedative-hypnotic used primarily for seizure control and anxiolysis.

## Benzodiazepine Antagonists

As with the opioids, the action of the benzodiazepines can be reversed with an antagonist. Flumazenil competitively inhibits all of the actions of the benzodiazepines and will effec-tively reverse sedation, respiratory depression, and hypotension. Flumazenil will also antagonize the antiseizure properties of the benzodiazepines and should be used with extreme caution in children with underlying seizure disorders treated with benzodiazepines.

## Other Sedative/Hypnotic Agents

Propofol is an ultra–short-acting sedative hypnotic agent with an extremely rapid onset. It is a modified phenol; the exact mechanism of action of this agent is unclear, although some suspect both a direct membrane effect as well as a GABA receptor action. Used for both rapid sequence intubation and procedural sedation, propofol has an immediate onset with duration of action of 6 to 8 minutes. The speed of onset is related to its high lipid solubility, which allows it to easily penetrate the highly lipophilic CNS. For procedural sedation, propofol is generally titrated beginning with a 0.5 mg/kg bolus. For more prolonged sedation, such as for ventilator management, a continuous infusion is required. Like the barbiturate induction agents, propofol will induce apnea if injected rapidly or in too large a dose. It will also produce hypotension secondary to peripheral vasodilation. Reports of a fatal propofol infusion syndrome have been described in patients on high doses of propofol for extended periods of time. Propofol infusion syndrome is most likely caused by an interference by propofol with electron transport in the mitochondria. Cases of propofol infusion syndrome have been noted in patients receiving greater than 4 mg/kg per hour for more than 48 hours. Propofol is a potent skeletal muscle relaxant, which makes it particularly valuable for reduction of large joint dislocations. Propofol also possesses antiemetic properties. The lipid-like nature of propofol requires that it be suspended as an emulsion. The lipid formulation is an extremely good medium for bacterial growth, and extreme care must be taken to prevent infection when administering propofol. Propofol should be drawn up under aseptic conditions just prior to administration. The syringe should be kept capped. Opened propofol should be discarded after 6 hours. Some of the generic preparations of propofol have a high sulfite concentration in their suspensions, which can induce bronchospasm in susceptible asthmatic patients. The sedative effects of propofol make it useful for both painful and painless procedures, while its short duration of action reduces postprocedure monitoring times.[39,47–50]

Etomidate is another anesthesia induction agent used in procedural sedation in children. Etomidate does have the potential to induce myoclonic jerks, making it unsuitable for use in conjunction with diagnostic procedures that require a motionless patient. Etomidate also produces nausea and vomiting in some patients. Use of etomidate has been documented to produce adrenal suppression. This depression is clinically insignificant when a single dose is administered, although long-term infusions have been fatal in some instances.[51]

Chloral hydrate is a pure oral sedative hypnotic agent. Chloral hydrate produces a very consistent sedation with 50 to 75 mg/kg and is used commonly for painless diagnostic studies. The major disadvantage of this medication is its prolonged duration of action, which can be 2 to 24 hours. Chloral hydrate should not be used in children with underlying liver pathology.[12]

Ketamine is the only dissociative procedural sedation agent. By disrupting communication between the cortical and limbic systems, ketamine induces a trance-like state. The dissociative state has been described as, "Someone is doing something painful to my body, but I'm separated from my body right now, so I don't notice it." Patients are not asleep in the traditional sense but tolerate both painful procedures and painless diagnostic studies. Unlike any of the other agents, ketamine is a mild sympathomimetic that produces increases in both heart rate and systolic blood pressure. It also increases intracranial and intraocular pressure and should not be used in patients with open globe injuries or those who have preexisting intracranial hypertension. These actions are mediated by endogenous release of epinephrine, which is also responsible for the bronchodilatory effects. Ketamine can have an anticholinergic effect and inhibit norepinephrine reuptake (potentiating β effects), adding to its bronchodilatory effects. Even though its effect on the lower airway muscles is relaxation, ketamine causes an exaggeration of upper airway reflexes, leading to an increased incidence of coughing and risk of laryngospasm, especially if large boluses (greater than 1 mg/kg) are given rapidly. Ketamine also differs from other sedative-hypnotics or opioids in that it does not blunt the ventilatory response to carbon dioxide; therefore, it is less likely to produce respiratory depression, but apnea can occur if large doses are given. Ketamine does produce excessive salivation, which can contribute to the incidence of coughing and risk of laryngospasm. Some practitioners pretreat their patients with either atropine or glycopyrrolate prior to administration. Because of these effects, ketamine should be used with caution in patients with oral pathology or upper respiratory infections in whom the risk of laryngospasm is greatest.[52,53]

Ketamine produces very vivid dreams in children and can produce agitated emergence reactions in 2% to 17% of patients. Emergence reactions appear to be related most closely to the state of agitation of the child prior to the administration of ketamine and the noise and activity of the area where the child recovers. The concomitant administration of benzodiazepines with ketamine has been recommended to reduce the incidence of emergence agitation. However, recent small, well-controlled ED studies have shown no significant reduction in agitation with benzodiazepine use,[54–56] although midazolam can reduce the incidence of vomiting.[56] Vomiting also occurs in a small proportion of patients given ketamine and is usually brief and self-limited. Ketamine might have the greatest margin of dosing safety of all procedural sedation medications. Patients administered 10 times the intended dose suffered no significant adverse outcomes.[57] Despite the large therapeutic index, patients given ketamine require preparation and vigilance equal to that afforded patients given other sedative-hypnotics.

Droperidol is a butyrophenone used in the pharmacologic control of acutely psychiatrically agitated patients. Useful for both psychotic conditions and alcohol-induced delirium in older adolescents, droperidol has also been combined with fentanyl to produce general anesthesia. Droperidol produces rapid somnolence, although patients are easily aroused and exhibit no significant respiratory depression. Recently, the Food and Drug Administration (FDA) issued what is termed a black box warning for cases of arrhythmias thought to be due to prolongation of QT interval produced by droperidol administered as an antiemetic following general anesthesia. The emergency medicine and pediatric implications of this warning are unclear, and the significance of the warning itself has been questioned. At present, there is no effective alternative sedative agent that exhibits the agitation control of droperidol without significant respiratory compromise. When droperidol is used, it is mandatory to also provide cardiac monitoring in light of the liability risk engendered by the FDA warning.[58]

Diphenhydramine is a common antihistamine with sedative-hypnotic effects. Available as an over-the-counter sleep aid and antihistamine, it can also be administered to children to provide cooperation for control during painless diagnostic studies. Diphenhydramine is particularly effective in children who are already exhausted from extensive crying. Hydroxyzine, another H1 receptor antagonist, has been used effectively in combination with chloral hydrate for sedation for dental procedures in children.

Nitrous oxide is an inhalation agent available for acute use as a fixed nitrous oxide-oxygen mixture. It has a rapid onset and offset of action and is excreted unmetabolized from the lungs. Nitrous oxide produces a dose-related sedative-hypnotic effect that can induce general anesthesia at higher concentrations. The minimum recognized effective mixture is 30% nitrous oxide and 70% oxygen, although to be truly effective, a 50/50 mixture is probably required. Nitrous oxide is best used for short, painful procedures. Because the gas readily diffuses into any body cavity, it should not be used in patients with bowel obstruction or pneumothorax.[23,24,59]

High concentrations of sucrose appear to provide good analgesia as measured by less crying or fewer actions suggestive of pain in neonates when administered 1 to 3 minutes or more prior to a procedure. Generally 1 mL to 2 mL of a 30% sucrose solution is used and supplemented with nonnutritive sucking. The proposed mechanism of effect of sucrose is thought to be through enkephalin release.[27,28]

## Local Anesthetics

Two local anesthetics commonly used in the management of acute painful conditions in children are lidocaine and bupivacaine. Both of these agents inhibit nerve conduction through blockade of sodium channels in the axons of sensory nerves. These agents are infiltrated directly into a wound or injected around a peripheral nerve to produce a nerve block. In all instances, care must be taken to avoid excessive dosing of either lidocaine or bupivacaine. Agitation is the mildest toxic effect noted, while seizures and even death can result from severe overdoses.

A Bier block provides regional anesthesia distal to the elbow or the knee. It is performed by administering dilute lidocaine IV into a distal vein after a tourniquet has been applied. A detailed description of how to perform a Bier block is beyond the scope of this chapter. When performing a Bier block, it is essential that the limb first be exsanguinated and a double tourniquet used to prevent inadvertent release of drug into the circulation. Only dilute lidocaine is used for a Bier block because bupivacaine is much more cardiotoxic, with a higher risk for morbidity if the drug enters the circulation in large amounts (e.g., tourniquet failure).

The pain of injection of local anesthetics can be reduced through buffering. Adjusting the pH closer to 7.4 allows more rapid absorption of the anesthetic into the myelinated axon fibers and decreases the pain on injection. Buffering can be accomplished by creation of an approximate 9:1 lidocaine to bicarbonate (8.4%) ratio solution. For a fresh 30-mL bottle of lidocaine, this would require removing 3 mL of solution and replacing it with 3 mL of sodium bicarbonate solution. Other procedures shown to reduce the pain of injection include warming of solutions, use of small-gauge needles (27g or 30g), and slow infiltration (as opposed to rapid infiltration).

Lidocaine is an amide anesthetic with a rapid onset of action and a duration of 30 to 120 minutes. A more prolonged effect results when the drug is combined with epinephrine to produce localized vasoconstriction. The maximum recommended dose of this drug is 4.5 mg/kg when used alone and 7 mg/kg when combined with epinephrine for subcutaneous infiltration. A 1% solution of lidocaine contains 10 mg of lidocaine for every 1 mL of solution. Lidocaine solutions containing epinephrine should not be injected for nerve blocks near end arteries (fingers, toes, penis). In these locations, plain lidocaine or bupivacaine should be used.

Bupivacaine is another amide anesthetic with a slightly slower onset of action but a duration of action of 2 to 8 hours. The safe dose of bupivacaine is up to 2.5 mg/kg (1 mL/kg of a 0.25% solution) for subcutaneous infiltration or nerve block.

Tetracaine is generally used either in drops for ophthalmic anesthesia or in combination with lidocaine and epinephrine as a topical wound anesthetic preparation. Commonly referred to as LET (lidocaine, epinephrine, tetracaine) or LAT, this solution produces good wound anesthesia without the need for infiltration with a needle. To correctly use topical anesthetics for local lacerations, a cotton ball is saturated with the LET solution. The edges of the laceration are pulled apart, and the cotton ball is placed directly into the wound and loosely taped in place with a single piece of tape. If the solution is not dripping out of the wound, an inadequate amount of solution is being applied. Older preparations of such solutions used cocaine in place of lidocaine, but these have been replaced with the safer LET solutions. LET can be prepared as a combination of lidocaine (4%), epinephrine (0.1%), and tetracaine (0.5%). Some institutions add a thickening agent to produce a gel instead of a solution.

Another alternative to painful percutaneous procedures in children is the use of topical anesthetic agents. The thinner stratum corneum in children permits greater penetration of topical anesthetic agents to the underlying nerve endings, producing very effective elimination of pain sensation in the skin for intravenous insertions or lumbar punctures. Most topical preparations contain some eutectic mixture of local anesthetics such as lidocaine, prilocaine, tetracaine, or amethocaine and are available in ready-to-apply creams such as EMLA and ELA-Max. Topical agents are best applied 60 minutes prior to the percutaneous procedure, although some anesthesia can be present at 30 minutes. Attempts to shorten the time to anesthesia by heating the area, stripping with tape, or adding nitroglycerin preparations have had limited success.[60–62]

## Medication Selections

The decision regarding which agent to use must be made, again, based on the child's medical history, the clinical scenario, and physician preference. Providing clinicians with the widest possible selection of agents permits the greatest opportunity to select the medication or medication combination most appropriate for any given child.

For simple analgesia, the use of acetaminophen, ibuprofen, or a combination of either with an oral opioid is appropriate. For more severe painful conditions, a parenteral opioid analgesic is commonly used.

Anxiety can be managed with an oral sedative, a parenteral benzodiazepine, or a barbiturate.

Painful procedures can be managed with a high-potency opioid analgesic, ketamine, etomidate, propofol, or an opioid-sedative combination. Fentanyl has been combined successfully with midazolam or propofol for such procedures. When combining opioid analgesics and sedatives, their effects are enhanced, but the risk of respiratory depression is enhanced as well. Because of this, the doses of both agents should be decreased to start, and they should be titrated more carefully. As a general rule with such combinations, the opioid is administered first and followed after a few minutes by the sedative. Nitrous oxide has also been used for many of these procedures. Procedural pain associated with angiography or the repair of complex lacerations frequently can be managed with a pure sedative and a local or topical anesthetic agent.

For painless diagnostic studies, pure sedatives, potent opioids, ketamine, and etomidate have all been used.

The specifics of the particular case help to determine which agent within a group of agents should be used. Drugs such as the barbiturates or propofol, which lower cerebral metabolism and ICP, might be selected for a child with possibly elevated ICP, while hypovolemic children should be treated with a drug that will help support blood pressure, such as ketamine or etomidate. In addition, sedation regimens that might result in hypercarbia due to hypoventilation should be used cautiously in patients who might have intracranial hypertension, because these patients might lack normal autoregulation of cerebral blood flow, and they might experience great increases in ICP, which can worsen cerebral perfusion.

Some possible medication options for different clinical scenarios are presented in Table 15-6.

The presence of so many different options for pediatric procedural sedation indicates that no single drug or drug combination is clearly superior. In a study of sedation preferences for posttraumatic head CT scans, more than 20 different regimens were described.[63] Multiple comparisons of different medications or combinations have been performed and some trends have been noted, but no single agent has emerged as a consensus choice by anesthesiologists, emergency physicians, pediatricians, or intensivists. Depending on the study examined, virtually all of the agents listed in Table 15-6 have been reported to be the most effective agent for a given condition. For this reason, it is important for all clinicians to be as knowledgeable as possible about the analgesic and sedation options available.

Children with special health care needs require analgesia and sedation for problems common to all children, as well as for conditions related to their underlying diagnoses. Regardless of the indications, the approach is the same as for any other child. The fact that many of these children are already taking medications sometimes simplifies or complicates the selection of a sedation or analgesia agent. Use of a drug within a class of agents already taken by a child can reduce the risk of unexpected responses or drug interactions. For example, a child taking phenobarbital along with other medications is probably best sedated with pentobarbital or methohexital for a CT scan or MRI. If an analgesic or sedative class of agents is not among the medications a child is taking, then one must be selected taking into account the child's unique physiology.

In children with cardiac problems, a palliative procedure might have been performed using a shunt or some form of mixing communication between the pulmonary and systemic circulations. In these children, a balance must be maintained between the resistance in the two circulations. Analgesic or sedative agents that decrease peripheral vascular resistance can direct blood flow from the pulmonary to the systemic circulation, resulting in cyanosis. In these instances, a relatively neutral agent such as fentanyl or ketamine might be the best choice. Although carefully titrated, propofol use has been reported in these instances.[64]

Children with intracranial lesions might receive any number of agents, although care should be taken to prevent cerebral vasodilation secondary to either hypoxia or hypercarbia. Agents such as ketamine that increase ICP should also be used with caution. When sedated, children who are developmentally delayed can develop a greater narrowing of their upper airways compared to other children.[65]

Children with underlying respiratory problems also require careful monitoring during procedural sedation. Generic preparations of propofol are known to be formulated with sulfites, which can trigger bronchospasm in susceptible patients.

Children with endocrine problems, particularly those with adrenal problems and those

## TABLE 15-6   Sedation Options

| Scenario | Options |
|---|---|
| Extremity Injury (Minor) | Oral opioid |
| | Acetaminophen or ibuprofen with or without an opioid |
| Extremity Injury (Major) | Parenteral or oral opioid |
| | PCA |
| | Regional anesthesia |
| | Ketamine |
| | Propofol |
| | Etomidate |
| | Nitrous oxide |
| Small Area Burn | Oral opioid |
| | Acetaminophen or ibuprofen with or without an opioid |
| | IM opioid |
| | Local anesthetic infiltration |
| | Topical anesthetic (LET) |
| Large Area Burn | IV opioid |
| | Regional anesthesia |
| | PCA |
| | Ketamine |
| Multiple Minor Injuries | Parenteral opioid |
| | Acetaminophen or ibuprofen with or without an opioid |
| | Distraction |
| | Hypnosis |
| | Oral opioid |
| Multiple Trauma | IV opioid |
| | Ketamine |
| | Etomidate |
| | PCA |
| | Fentanyl |
| | Remifentanil |
| Joint Dislocation | Propofol |
| | Nitrous oxide |
| | IV opioid/sedative |
| | Diazepam |
| | Etomidate |
| | Intra-articular lidocaine |
| Abdominal Pain (*if Biliary/Renal Colic) | Parenteral opioids |
| | Ketorolac* |
| | PCA |
| Pelvic Pain (Nonpregnant) | Parenteral opioids |
| | Oral NSAIDS |
| | Ketorolac |

*(continues)*

## TABLE 15-6    Sedation Options (Continued)

| Scenario | Options |
|---|---|
| Pregnant Non-OB Painful Condition | Oral opioid<br>Acetaminophen and opioid<br>IM/SQ opioid<br>Distraction<br>Regional anesthesia |
| Toothache | Oral opioid<br>Acetaminophen or ibuprofen with or without an opioid<br>Hypnosis<br>Local anesthesia |
| Laceration in Cooperative Child | Lidocaine<br>Bupivacaine<br>LET |
| Laceration in Uncooperative Child<br>(Many sedative analgesic combinations are possible. A few are listed here.) | Oral midazolam and local anesthetic or LET<br>Fentanyl and midazolam<br>Propofol and local anesthetic<br>Ketamine and local anesthetic |
| Lumbar Puncture<br>(Many sedative and analgesic options are possible. Only a few are listed here.) | Propofol<br>Ketamine<br>Fentanyl and midazolam<br>Pentobarbital<br>Local anesthesia |
| CT/ MRI<br>    (*If no risk elevated ICP) | Pentobarbital<br>Propofol<br>Fentanyl* or remifentanil*<br>Methohexital IV/PR<br>Midazolam<br>Diphenhydramine<br>Chloral hydrate<br>Ketamine* |
| Outpatient Painless Diagnostic Study Hospital Sedation Unit | Midazolam PO<br>Chloral hydrate<br>Pentobarbital PO<br>Diphenhydramine<br>Sleep deprivation |

with alterations in cellular immunity, should probably not be treated with etomidate because of its adrenal suppression effects. Barbiturates should be avoided in children with porphyria, while chloral hydrate should not be used in patients with liver failure.

Complications can and do occur with pediatric analgesia and sedation.[66] Overwhelmingly, most of these complications are related to patient monitoring or airway difficulties. Both multiple medications with synergistic effects on ventilation and airway patency and procedural sedation conducted in inappropriately equipped facilities have been noted to increase the risk of an adverse outcome in sedated children. Problems are uncommon in children sedated in emergency departments, intensive care units, properly attended radiology suites, or correctly staffed endoscopy units.[67–70]

Hypoxia is not a problem in a sedated child when it is recognized and treated promptly. In most instances, repositioning of the head, lifting of the jaw, or administration of supplemental oxygen is all that is required to treat this problem. Brief bag-mask ventilation might be required in more severe cases. Reversal agents are rarely indicated, as much of the apnea produced with procedural sedation is short-lived and related to rapid injection of a medication.

Hypoxia can be fatal if it is unrecognized and/or uncorrected. Continuous pulse oximetry during procedural sedation by personnel trained to recognize and react to airway obstruction and/or hypoxia will minimize this problem. Immediate access to physicians adept at pediatric airway management is also important in any facility contemplating pediatric procedural sedation.

Because hypoxia can be a sign (albeit late) of hypoventilation, some authors have suggested that administration of prophylactic supplemental oxygen to a sedated child could delay the early detection of this problem. In these cases, the fear is that more extreme hypoventilation, carbon dioxide retention, and respiratory acidosis will occur before hypoxia appears if a child is routinely given oxygen during procedural sedation. To date there is no evidence supporting or refuting this concept. Observation of the patient should allow detection of airway obstruction and/or significant hypoventilation before a decrease in oxygenation occurs. Oxygen supplementation provides a margin of safety and a longer time to correct the problem. In addition, combining capnography with pulse oximetry serves to detect airway obstruction through loss of carbon dioxide waveform at an earlier time, often prior to desaturation, and can provide an additional margin of safety.

In outpatient facilities, a sedative should not be administered until the child is present in the facility and under the observation of competent staff. By the same token, children should not be discharged until respiratory status and protective airway reflexes have returned to baseline. Deaths have occurred in sedated children in car seats during transport home from outpatient diagnostic sites. Physicians asked to arrange outpatient procedures that require sedation should only allow them to be performed in sites with the capabilities to monitor and react to sedated children.

## Summary

The successful delivery of procedural sedation or analgesia to a child is more than simply the knowledge of pharmacology and a working pulse oximeter. The entire treatment team including nurses, technicians, aids, and physicians must all have an understanding of the entire clinical scenario and how the PSA fits into the care of this particular patient. A formal presentation of all potential procedural sedation and analgesia protocols for all combinations of different agents and clinical scenarios is beyond the scope of this text. Even Table 15-6 barely touches the multitude of options used in clinical practice. Table 15-7 is an example of how a PSA agent such as propofol might be applied in a clinical setting. The safe application of such a protocol will hinge on the unit's education, pretreatment, monitoring, and credentialing practices.

## THE BOTTOM LINE

Administration of sedation and analgesic agents by appropriately trained and credentialed clinicians is safe and effective and offers optimal care to pediatric patients.

## TABLE 15-7   Sample Protocol for the Use of Propofol for Procedural Sedation

| | |
|---|---|
| Clinical indication: | • Extended sedation for painless diagnostic procedure. |
| Intended sedation level: | • Moderate sedation to deep sedation. |
| Anticipated agent and route: | • Propofol intravenous |
| Specific precautions: | • Hypotension |
| | • Egg allergies |
| | • Asthma |
| Supervising physician: | • Credentialed for use of propofol. |
| Location: | • Approved unit for use of propofol sedation. |
| Preparation: | • History and physical exam to be performed in compliance with the hospital's pre-procedure assessment protocols and to include at the least: |
| |   – Direct inspection of mouth and posterior pharynx |
| |   – Assessment of lungs and respiratory capabilities |
| |   – Recent vital signs |
| |   – Cardiac monitoring, continuous pulse oximetry, intermittent BP monitoring |
| |   – Immediate access to suction, airway supplies, oxygen |
| |   – Normal saline infusion |
| |   – Nasal prongs (optional)* |
| |   – Pretreatment of vein with lidocaine (optional to reduce infusion pain)† |
| Medication delivery: | • Propofol bolus 0.5–1 mg/kg over 2–3 minutes |
| | • Propofol infusion 1–3 mg/kg/hr |
| | • Inadequate sedation: Rebolus 0.5 mg/kg, infusion increase 1 mg/kg/hr |
| Postprocedure care: | • Terminate infusion |
| | • Continue monitoring until return to baseline physical exam (6–10 min) |

\* Some practitioners routinely begin low-dose nasal oxygen for all patients sedated with propofol; others administer oxygen only if hypoxia is detected. Regardless of the use of oxygen, placement of the nasal prongs prior to performance of the procedure allows oxygen administration, if needed, without removal and repositioning of the child within a diagnostic device such as an MRI or CT scanner.

† Intravenous infusion is stopped and vein is occluded with a finger 1–2 cm proximal to catheter tip. Slow infusion of 0.5–1 mL of 1% lidocaine, without epinephrine, not to exceed 1 mg/kg. (1% lidocaine contains 10mg/1 mL). Hold finger occlusion in place for 2 minutes.

# CHAPTER REVIEW

## Check Your Knowledge

1. What is the ASA classification for a 7-year-old child with occasional asthma relieved with PRN albuterol MDI puffs?
   A. Class I
   B. Class II
   C. Class III
   D. Class IV

2. Which of the following agents would be a good choice for sedation of an alert and normally acting obese 9-month-old who rolled off a changing table and requires a CT scan for a possible head injury?
   A. Chloral hydrate PO
   B. Ketamine IM
   C. Oral midazolam
   D. Rectal methohexital
   E. All of the above

3. Discharge criteria following procedural sedation include:
   A. 2 hours of observation after conclusion of procedure
   B. Return to baseline ambulation status
   C. Return to baseline level of alertness
   D. Return to baseline respiratory status

4. What is the maximum volume of 1% lidocaine with epinephrine that can be safely given as a subcutaneous infiltration in a 20-kg child?
   A. 14 mL
   B. 20 mL
   C. 27 mL
   D. 38 mL

## References

1. ACEP. Clinical policy for procedural sedation and analgesia in the emergency department. *Ann Emerg Med*. 1998;31:663–677.
2. Green SM, Krauss B. Procedural sedation terminology: moving beyond "conscious sedation." *Ann Emerg Med*. 2002;39(4):433–435.
3. Krauss B. Management of acute pain and anxiety in children undergoing procedures in the emergency department. *Pediatr Emerg Care*. 2001;17:115–122.
4. Sacchetti AD, Schafermeyer R, Gerardi M et. al. Pediatric analgesia and sedation. *Ann Emerg Med*. 1994;23:237–250.
5. American Academy of Pediatrics. The assessment and management of acute pain in infants, children and adolescents. *Pediatrics*. 2001;108:793–797.
6. JCAHO. *Standards intent statement and examples for sedation and anesthesia care of patients*. In: *Comprehensive Accreditations Manual for Hospitals*. Oakbrook Terrace, Il: Joint Commission on Accreditation of Healthcare Organizations; 2000;Tx-15.
7. Dial S, Silver P, Bock K, Sagy M. Pediatric sedation for procedures titrated to a desired degree of immobility results in unpredictable depth of sedation. *Pediatr Emerg Care*. 2001;17:414–420.
8. Sacchetti AD, Turco T, Carraccio C et. al. Procedural sedation for children with special health care needs. *Pediatr Emerg Care*. 2003; 155: 496–500.
9. Sacchetti AD, Gerardi M. Procedural sedation for patients with special health needs. In, Krauss B, Brustowicz RB, eds. *Pediatric Procedural Sedation and Analgesia*. Baltimore, Md: Lippincott Williams & Wilkin; 1999:189–199.
10. McQuillen KK, Steele DW. Capnography during sedation/analgesia in a pediatric emergency department. *Pediatr Emerg Care*. 2000;16:401–404.
11. Miner JR, Heegaard W, Plummer D. End-tidal carbon dioxide monitoring during procedural sedation. *Acad Emerg Med*. 2002;9:275–280.
12. D'Agostino J, Terndrup TE. Chloral Hydrate versus Midazolam for sedation of children for neuroimaging: a randomized clinical trial. *Pediatr Emerg Care*. 2000;16:1–4.
13. Singer AJ, Gulla J, Thode HC. Parents and practitioners are poor judges of young children's pain severity. *Acad Emerg Med*. 2002;9:609–612.
14. Kelly AM, Powell CV, Williams A. Parent visual analogue scale ratings of children's pain reported by child. *Pediatr Emerg Care*. 2002;18:159–162.
15. Merkel SI, Voepel-Lewis T, Shayevitz JR, Malviya S. The FLACC: a behavioral scale for scoring postoperative pain in young children. *Pediatr Nurs*. 1997;23:293–297.
16. Buchholz M, Karl HW, Pomietto M, Lynn A. Pain socres in infants: a modified infant pain scale versus visual analogue. *J Pain Symptom Manag*. 1998;15:117–124.
17. Hicks CL, von Baeyer CL, Spafford PA, van Korlaar I, Goodenough B. The Faces pain scale—revised: toward a common metric in pediatric pain measurement. *Pain*. 2001;93:173–183.
18. Berkenbosch JW, Fichter CR, Tobias JD. The correlation of the bispectral index monitor with

clinical sedation scores during mechanical ventilation in the pediatric intensive care unit. *Anesth Analg.* 2002;94:506–511.

19. Kim MK, Strait RT, Sato TT, Hennes HM. A randomized clinical trial of analgesia in children with acute abdominal pain. *Acad Emerg Med.* 2002;9:281–287.

20. Collins JJ, Dunkel L, Gupta SK et. al. Transdermal fentanyl in children with cancer pain: feasibility, tolerability & pain. *J Pediatr.* 1999;134:319–323.

21. McGlone RG, Ranasinghe S, Durham S. An alternative to "Brutacaine": a comparison of low dose intramuscular ketamine with intranasal midazolam in children before suturing. *J Accid Emerg Med.* 1998;15:231–236.

22. Shin D, Kim S, Kim CS, Kim HS. Postoperative pain management using intravenous patient-controlled analgesia for pediatric patients. *J Craniofac Surg.* 2001;12:129–133.

23. Luhmann JD, Kennedy RM, Jaffe DM, McAllister JD. Continuous-flow delivery of nitrous oxide and oxygen: a safe and cost-effective technique for inhalation analgesia and sedation of pediatric patients. *Pediatr Emerg Care.* 1999;15:388–392.

24. Annequin D, Carbajal R, Chauvin P, Gall O, Tourniaire B, Murat I. Fixed 50% nitrous oxide oxygen mixture for painful procedures: a French survey. *Pediatrics.* 2000;105:E47.

25. Baghdadi ZD. Evaluation of audio analgesia for restorative care in children treated using electronic dental anesthesia. *J Clin Pediatr Dent.* 2000;25:9–12.

26. Rusy LM, Weisman SJ. Complementary therapies for acute pediatric pain management. *Pediatr Clin North Am.* 2000;47:589–599.

27. Stevens B, Ohlsson A. Sucrose for analgesia in newborn infants undergoing painful procedures. *Cochrane Database Syst Rev.* 2001;4:CD001069.

28. Carbajal R, Chauvet X, Couderc S, Olivier-Martin M. Randomised trial of analgesic effects of sucrose, glucose and pacifiers in term neonates. *BMJ.* 1999;319:1393–1397.

29. Tobias JD. Weak analgesics and nonsteroidal anti-inflammatory agents in the management of children with acute pain. *Pediatr Clin North Am.* 2000;47:527–543.

30. Beiter JL Jr, Simon HK, Chambliss CR et. al. Intravenous ketorolac in the emergency department management of sickle cell pain and predictors of its effectiveness. *Arch Pediatr Adolesc Med.* 2001; 155:496–500.

31. Lieh-Lai MW, Kauffman RE, Uy HG, Danjin M, Simpson PM. A randomized comparison of ketorolac tromethamine and morphine for postoperative analgesia in critically ill children. *Crit Care Med.* 1999;27:2786–2791.

32. Harwick WE, Givens TG, Monroe KW, King WD, Lawley D. Effect of ketorolac in pediatric sickle cell vaso-occlusive pain crisis. *Pediatr Emerg Care.* 1999;15:179–182.

33. Sharar SR, Carrougher GJ, Selzer K, O'Donnell F, Vavilala MS, Lee LA. A comparison of oral transmucosal fentanyl citrate and oral oxycodone for pediatric outpatient wound care. *J Burn Care Rehabil.* 2002;23:27–31.

34. Bates BA, Schutzman SA, Fleisher GR. A comparison of intranasal sufentanil and midazolam to intramuscular meperidine, promethazine and chlorpromazine for conscious sedation in children. *Ann Emerg Med.* 1994;24:646–651.

35. Keidan I, Berkenstadt H, Sidi A, Perel A. Propofol/remifentanil versus propofol alone for bone marrow aspiration in paediatric haemato-oncological patients. *Paediatr Anaesth.* 2001; 11:297–301.

36. Litman RS. Conscious sedation with remifentanil and midazolam during brief painful procedures in children. *Arch Pediatr Adolesc Med.* 1999;153: 1085–1088.

37. Litman RS. Conscious sedation with remifentanil during painful medical procedures. *J Pain Symptom Manage.* 2000;19:468–471.

38. Donmez A, Kizilkan A, Berksun H, Varan B, Tokel K. One center's experience with remifentanil infusions for pediatric cardiac catherization. *J Cadiothorac Vasc Anesth.* 2001;15:736–739.

39. Duce D, Glaisyer H, Sury M. An evaluation of propofol combined with remifentanil: a new intravenous anaesthetic technique for short painful procedures in children. *Paediatr Anaesth.* 2000;10:689–690.

40. Greenberg SB, Adams RC, Aspinall CL. Initial experience with intravenous pentobarbital sedation for children undergoing MRI at a tertiary care pediatric hospital: the learning curve. *Pediatr Radiol.* 2000;30:689–691.

41. Moro-Sutherland D, Algern JT, Penelope TL, Kozinetz A, Shook, J. Comparison of intravenous midazolam with pentobarbital for sedation for heat computed tomography imaging. *Acad Emerg Med.* 2000;7:1370–1375.

42. Pomeranz ES, Chudnofsky CR, Deegan TJ, Lozon MM, Mitchiner JC, Weber J. Rectal methohexital sedation for computed tomography imaging of stable pediatric emergency deparment patients. *Pediatrics.* 2000;105:1110–1114.

43. Sedik H. Use of intravenous methohexital as a sedative in pediatric emergency departments. *Arch Pediatr Adolesc Med.* 2001;155:665–668.

44. Beekman RP, Hoorntje TM, Beek FJ, Kuijten RH. Sedation for children undergoing magnetic resonance imaging: eficacy and safety of rectal thiopental. *Eur J Pediatr.* 1996;155:820–822.

45. Karian VE, Burrows PE, Zurakowski D, Connor L, Mason KP. Sedation for pediatric radiological procedures: analysis of potential causes of sedation failure and paradoxical reactions. *Pediatr Radiol.* 1999;29:869–873.

46. Havel CJ, Strati RT, Hennes H. A clinical trial of propofol vs. midazolam for procedural sedation in a pediatric emergency department. *Acad Emerg Med.* 1999;6:989–997.

47. Golden S. Combination propofol-ketamine anaesthesia in sick neonates. *Paediatr Anaesth.* 2001;11:119–122.

48. Jayabose S, Levendoglu-Tugal O, Giamelli J et. al. Intravenous anesthesia with propofol for painful procedures in children with cancer. *Am J Pediatr Hematol Oncol.* 2001;23:290–293.

49. Skokan EG, Pribble C, Bassett KE, Nelson DS. Use of propofol sedation in a pediatric emergency department: prospective study. *Clin Pediatr.* 2001;40:663–671.

50. Cannon ML, Glazier SS, Bauman LA. Metabolic acidosis, rhabdomyolysis and cardiovascular collapse after prolonged propofol infusion. *J Neurosurg.* 2001;95:925–926.

51. Dickinson R, Singer A, Carrion W. Etomidate for pediatric sedation prior to fracture reduction. *Acad Emerg Med.* 2001;8:74–77.

52. Green SM, Rothrock SG, Harris T, Hopkins GA, Garrett W et. al. Intravenous ketamine for pediatric sedation in the emergency department: safety profile with 156 cases. *Acad Emerg Med.* 1998;5:971–976.

53. Green SM, Denmark TK, Cline J et. al. Ketamine sedation for pediatric critical care procedures. *Pediatr Emerg Care.* 2001;17:244–248.

54. Green SM, Kupperman N, Rothrock SG, Hummel CB, Ho M. Predictors of adverse events with intramuscular ketamine sedation in children. *Ann Emerg Med.* 2000;35:35–42.

55. Sherwin TS, Green SM, Khan A, Chapman DS, Dannenberg B. Does adjunctive midazolam reduce recovery agitation after ketamine sedation for pediatric procedures? A randomized double-blind placebo controlled trial. *Ann Emerg Med.* 2000;35:229–238.

56. Wathen JE, Roback MG, Mackenzie T, Bothner JP. Does midazolam alter the clinical effects of intravenous ketamine sedation in children? A double-blind, randomized, controlled, emergency department trial. *Ann Emerg Med.* 2000;36:579–588.

57. Green SM, Clark R, Hostetler MA et. al. Inadvertent ketamine overdose in children: clini-cal manifestations and outcome. *Ann Emerg Med.* 1999;34:492–497.

58. Horowitz BZ, Bizovi K, Moreno R. Droperidol— behind the black box warning. *Acad Emerg Med.* 2002;9:615–617.

59. Luhmann JD, Kennedy RM, Porter FL, Miller JP, Jaffe DM. A randomized clinical trial of continuous flow nitrous oxide and midazolam for sedation of young children during laceration repair. *Ann Emerg Med.* 2001;37(1):20–27.

60. Kleiber C, Sorenson M, Whiteside K, Gronstal BA, Tannous R. Topical anesthetics for intravenous insertion in children: a randomized equivalency study. *Pediatrics.* 2002;110(4):758–761.

61. Chen BK, Cunningham BB. Topical anesthetics in children: agents and techniques that equally comfort patients, parents, and clinicians. *Curr Opin Pediatr.* 2001;13(4):324–330.

62. Liu DR, Kirchner HL, Petrack EM. Does using heat with eutectic mixture of local anesthetic cream shorten analgesic onset time? A randomized, placebo-controlled trial. *Ann Emerg Med.* 2003;42(1):27–33.

63. Conners GP, Sacks WK, Leahey NF. Variations in sedating uncooperative, stable children for post-traumatic head CT. *Pediatr Emerg Care.* 1999;15:241–244.

64. Gozal D, Rein AJ, Nir A, Gozal Y. Propofol does not modify the hemodynamic status of children with intracardiac shunts undergoing cardiac catherization. *Pediatr Cardiol.* 2001;22:488–490.

65. Elwood T, Hansen LD, Seely JM. Oropharyngeal airway diameter during sedation in children with and without developmental delay. *J Clin Anesth.* 2001;13:482–485.

66. Pena BM, Krauss B. Adverse events of procedural sedation and analgesia in a pediatric emergency department. *Ann Emerg Med.* 1999;34:483–491.

67. Cote CJ, Karl HW, Notterman DA, Weinberg JA, McCloskey C. Adverse sedation events in pediatrics: analysis of medications used for sedation. *Pediatrics.* 2000;106:633–644.

68. Hoffman GM, Nowakowski R, Troshynski TJ, Berens RJ, Weisman SJ. Risk reduction in pediatric procedural sedation by application of an American Academy of Pediatrics/American Society of Anesthesiologists process model. *Pediatrics.* 2002;109:236–243.

69. Blike G, Cvravero J, Nelson E. Same patients, same critical events—different systems of care, different outcomes: description of a human factors approach aimed at improving the efficacy and safety of sedation/analgesia care. *Qual Manag Health Care.* 2001;10:17–36.

70. Cote CJ, Notterman DA, Karl HW, Weinberg JA, McCloskey C. Adverse sedation events in pediatrics: a critical incident analysis of contributing factors. *Pediatrics.* 2000;105:805–814.

**CASE SUMMARY 1**

An 18-month-old boy is brought to the emergency department (ED) after his 3-year-old sibling knocked him down three stairs. He sustained a closed-head injury and a 4-cm forehead laceration when he struck a low coffee table. His mother, who witnessed the event, noted that the child was unresponsive for a few minutes following the initial injury. On awakening, he cried briefly but has been abnormally quiet and withdrawn since the event. He has vomited three times and is irritable in his mother's arms, but has no other signs of injuries. The physician plans to order a computed tomography (CT) scan to evaluate the child's head injury and repair his forehead laceration.

1. *What are the procedural sedation options for this child for CT scanning and laceration repair?*
2. *Can a single agent be used for both procedures?*

---

This case presents a unique challenge because both a painless procedure and a painful procedure must be addressed. Multiple options can be considered for procedural sedation. The possibility of increased ICP makes ketamine or fentanyl lower priority choices. A pure sedative with ICP-lowering characteristics would be appropriate for CT scanning cooperation but would not permit repair of the laceration alone. Combining such a sedative with local anesthesia of the wound might help, although the injection process itself might produce excessive agitation that would require additional doses of the sedative, and this might result in a relative overdose once the stimulus of the injection is removed and the child is placed in the CT scanner. One alternative would be to use an IV pentobarbital or rectal methohexital sedation protocol in combination with LET anesthesia of the laceration. This approach would permit the LET to take effect during the CT scan procedure, while enough residual sedation would remain after the CT scan to permit cooperation for repair of the laceration without need for an injection.

# chapter 16

# Interface With EMS

Michael G. Tunik, MD, FAAP
George L. Foltin, MD, FAAP, FACEP

## Objectives

1 Describe the components of the EMSC continuum of care.

2 Explain the differences in levels of care (BLS and ALS) and providers (EMT, EMT-P).

3 Discuss the physician's role in EMS and EMSC.

## Chapter Outline

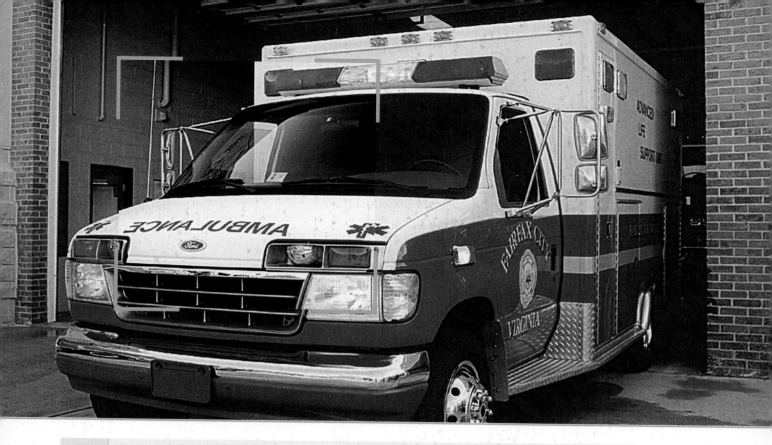

## CASE SCENARIO 1

A 2-year-old girl wanders outside to the pool in her back yard. Her mother, distracted by a telephone call, rushes outside and finds her daughter floating face down in the water. She pulls her out of the pool, performs CPR, and calls 9-1-1.

1. *What process and resources provide support for pediatric-specific training, equipment, assessment, treatment, triage, and transport in an EMS system?*
2. *What is the role of the physician in the EMS system's ability to care for individuals?*

## Introduction

Health care professionals should have an understanding of their emergency medical services (EMS) systems, as they have a critical role in the care of acutely ill and injured children.

### Definitions

- EMS system—a group of emergency health care delivery organizations that, together, allow for the appropriate delivery of out-of-hospital care and transport of persons who suffer sudden illnesses or injuries.

- Emergency medical services for children (EMSC)—those components within the EMS system that address the needs of children. A program and philosophy that supports the seamless integration of pediatric care capability.

- The EMSC continuum of care—encompasses all aspects of the care provided to an acutely ill or injured child. Begins with prevention, followed by EMS access: the recognition of an emergency, access to a telephone-activated emergency 9-1-1 system where available, and ambulance dispatch; prehospital care, including triage and transport; stabilization care in an emergency department; interhospital care/interfacility transport; definitive care, including inpatient care, trauma centers, pediatric critical care networks; and rehabilitation. The continuum goes full circle when the child returns to the community and has access to a primary care physician for immunizations and illness and injury prevention.[1]

- Medical home/family-centered care—the combination of family and primary care physician responsible for day-to-day care of a child, and integration of the services involved in the EMSC continuum of care such as injury prevention, recognition of an emergency, and access to EMS.

- Medical oversight, direct and indirect—direct (online) medical oversight (formerly direction or control) refers to medical personnel authorized to assist out-of-hospital personnel with medical and procedural decisions via telephone or radio. Medical oversight personnel are based at a receiving facility, a central medical facility, or an EMS agency. Indirect (off-line) medical oversight refers to physicians who provide input and collaborate on writing and modifying treatment protocols, triage criteria, and equipment lists, as well as assume responsibility for quality improvement. A committee of physicians who work with the EMS medical director usually provides this input. This is an excellent forum for physicians to become involved as advocates for the special needs of children.[2]

- Medical oversight physician—a physician who participates in the EMS system by developing guidelines for prehospital provider training, ambulance equipment, prehospital care protocols, and online (direct) medical oversight.

- Primary transport—transport from the scene of an injury or illness to a hospital emergency department (ED).

- Secondary transport—transport from an ED or community hospital to a specialty or definitive care center.

## Epidemiology

Children account for 25% to 30% of ED visits nationally. Seriously ill children are frequently transported by their caregivers for medical evaluation. Many children, however, are assessed, treated, and transported by EMS personnel. Approximately 6% to 10% of all EMS calls are for patients younger than 19 years.[3-5] Most children require transport between the hours of 12 noon and 12 midnight. Although a majority of pediatric calls receive only basic life support (BLS) interventions, about one-third require advanced life support (ALS) responses. Children transported to emergency departments by EMS personnel are at least 5 times more likely to require admission than are those who arrive by other methods.[6]

In EMS transported patients, the most common mechanisms of injury are vehicular trauma (including as a vehicle occupant or pedestrian and bicycle collisions), falls, and burns. Traumatic complaints predominate in children older than 2 years, with a peak in vehicular trauma among adolescents.[3-5] The most common medical complaints are seizures, respiratory distress, submersion, and poisonings. For children younger than 2 years, the majority of calls are for medical problems. Types of illness and patterns of injury in children differ from that of adults, requiring education and treatment protocols specific to children's needs.

## Origin of EMS Systems

Trauma surgeons working in the Korea and Vietnam conflicts recognized that rapid transport and surgical repair of traumatic injuries improved survival. They applied these principles to victims of motor vehicle trauma in the United States in the 1960s; previously, these patients had high mortality rates because of poor access to rapid transport to surgical care.[7] In 1966, Pantridge and colleagues, who brought health care to chest pain patients at home in Ireland, demonstrated that early defibrillation of adults with ventricular dysrhythmias, prior to arrival at a hospital, improved survival.[8] EMS systems were thus developed to provide stabilization and rapid transport for trauma victims and early defibrillation for adult ventricular dysrhythmias. Specific pediatric needs were not initially recognized or addressed.

## Models of Prehospital Care

### The Trauma and Medical (Cardiac) Models

Two models, the trauma model and the medical model, have influenced the approaches to prehospital care. Both are based on data collected on adult patients. A primary goal in providing medical (cardiac) care of the adult, both in the prehospital and hospital setting, is the rapid delivery of advanced life support to prevent or reverse sudden cardiac death (e.g., defibrillation of ventricular dysrhythmias). The approach to trauma care is to maintain the airway and ventilation, provide hemorrhage control, and transport the patient rapidly to a regional trauma center for definitive care by an awaiting surgical team. Prehospital interventions for trauma patients should not lengthen transport time.[9]

### The Pediatric Prehospital Care Model

Cardiac disease and cardiac arrest are uncommon prehospital problems in children, whereas respiratory distress and seizures are more common in children cared for by EMS systems. Children suffering out-of-hospital respiratory arrest appear to have improved survival rates in an urban short transport system if airway and ventilation are provided by bag-mask ventilation.[10] Clearly, skills in airway management and ventilation are critical for prehospital providers caring for children. The pediatric prehospital care model should be conservative (i.e., providing BLS care, focusing on airway and ventilation, and transport to pediatric-capable hospital EDs) yet permissive (i. e., providing ALS care) when clear life saving benefits are apparent (e.g., defibrillation for ventricular dysrhythmias, bronchodilators for reactive airway disease, anticonvulsants for status epilepticus).[11]

Certain realities affect pediatric prehospital care: many prehospital providers had primary training that did not incorporate the pediatric educational courses and resources developed by the EMSC program, and most prehospital providers will get infrequent exposure to critically ill and injured children.[12] Therefore, there is a need for pediatric continuing medical education and frequent refreshing of critical pediatric skills, such as bag-mask ventilation.[13]

## Federal EMSC Program

### Origin of EMSC

The federal EMSC program was established in 1985 to help reduce childhood disability and death due to severe illness or injury. Recognition that the trauma mortality rate for children was double that of adults, and that most EMS systems lacked pediatric equipment, protocols for the care of children and provider training in pediatrics were incentives for EMSC program development.[14,15] Calvin Sia, MD and Sen Daniel Inouye (D, Hawaii) set the EMS for Children program in motion. Sen Orrin Hatch (R, Utah) and Sen Lowell Weicker (R, Conn) joined Sen Inouye in authoring the first EMSC legislation (Public Law 98-555), which established a national EMSC Program.[14-16] The EMSC program is currently federally funded by the Health Resources and Services Administration (HRSA) Maternal and Child Health Bureau (MCHB) and the Department of Transportation (DOT) National Highway Traffic Safety Administration (NHTSA).

### Phases of Care in EMS-EMSC Systems

The phases of care in the EMS-EMSC systems are as follows:

1. Entry Phase—includes recognition of an emergency and activation of the EMS system (through a 9-1-1 call if available).
2. Response Phase—immediate care by bystanders, police, appropriate prearrival instructions by EMS dispatch, dispatch priority for BLS or paramedic (ALS) ambulance.

3. Treatment and Triage—care by EMS providers (first responder, emergency medical technician [EMT], paramedic [EMT-P]), including scene assessment; patient assessment (using a standard assessment approach, e.g., the Pediatric Assessment Triangle); a focus on initial stabilization of airway, ventilation, and circulation; maintenance of temperature; making triage decisions (based on severity of illness or injury); and primary transport to a hospital ED, a pediatric critical care center, or trauma center. Focus on rapid transport, identification of appropriate destination and method of transport based on severity of condition and distance from the ED.

4. Hospital Phase—stabilization in a hospital ED, transfer (secondary transport) to a pediatric-capable trauma center or critical care center, and definitive care (operating room [OR], pediatric intensive care unit [PICU], and inpatient ward).

5. Rehabilitation Phase—appropriate physical or mental rehabilitation needed to allow discharge to ongoing family-centered care, preferably at home.

6. Ongoing Care—prevention and care of chronic medical problems; focus on child, family, and primary care provider (Table 16-1).

### Entry Phase

The entry phase requires that a problem be identified as an emergency by the patient, parent, other caregiver, or observer. Education of parents, teachers, and other caregivers is important, to ensure that initial first aid/CPR can be administered when needed, and that true emergencies are correctly identified. Patient education materials reviewing what defines an emergency and when to activate the EMS 9-1-1 system, are available (Table 16-2).[17] After an emergency is identified, the EMS system should then be activated. In many areas of the United States, this is done via "9-1-1" telephone systems. Systems with enhanced 9-1-1 capabilities (i.e., "9-1-1-e") can automatically trace caller locations, thereby enabling medical assistance to be dispatched even if the caller is un-

| TABLE 16-1   EMS-EMSC System |
| :--- |
| • Prevention phase (illness and injury prevention) |
| • Entry phase (recognition of an emergency at home/scene/professional office, 9-1-1 system access) |
| • Response phase (ambulance dispatch, prehospital assessment) |
| • Treatment and triage phase (patient assessment, care by EMS responders, primary transport) |
| • Hospital phase (ED care, interfacility transport/definitive inpatient care, or, PICU care) |
| • Rehabilitation phase (physical rehabilitation, home care) |
| • Ongoing care (medical home/family-centered care) |

Adapted from: Dieckmann RA. *Pediatric Emergency Care Systems: Planning and Management.* Baltimore, Md: Williams & Wilkins; 1992.

able to provide that information. In areas without 9-1-1 telephone access, contact usually is provided through an emergency telephone number for the local law enforcement agency, fire department, ambulance service, or hospital. If medical assistance is required, the call is routed to a medical dispatcher. Using only the limited amount of information available by telephone, the medical dispatcher must be able to recognize and appropriately triage both adult and pediatric emergencies.[18]

Based on the complaint and additional information, the dispatcher determines the required level of EMS response and activates the appropriate ambulance/response units. If indicated, the dispatcher should instruct the caller in first aid and immediate BLS measures necessary for patient support until the EMS unit arrives. The dispatcher's actions and instructions usually are dictated by protocols.[18] The development of specific pediatric dispatch protocols and dispatcher training, as well as assessment of the accuracy and efficacy of the protocols, are goals of EMSC.

EMS provider agencies have many organizational structures (volunteer, municipal, part of fire department, or separate EMS agency) but are functionally divided into those providing First Responder, BLS services, ALS services, or

## TABLE 16-2   Parent/Patient Education: What Is an Emergency, When to Call 9-1-1

### What Is an Emergency?

- An emergency is when you believe a severe injury or illness is threatening your child's health or might cause permanent harm.
- A child needs emergency medical treatment right away.
- Emergencies can result from medical (or psychiatric) illnesses or injuries.
- Your child could show any of the following signs:
  - Acting strangely or becoming more withdrawn and less alert
  - Less of or lack of a response when talking to the child
  - Unconsciousness or lack of response
  - Rhythmic jerking and loss of consciousness (a seizure)
  - Increasing trouble with breathing
  - Skin or lips that look blue, purple, or gray
  - Neck stiffness or rash with fever
  - Increasing or severe persistent pain
  - A cut or burn that is large, deep, or involves the head, chest, or abdomen
  - Bleeding that does not stop after applying pressure for 5 minutes
  - A burn that is large or involves the hands, groin, or face
  - Any loss of consciousness, confusion, headache, or vomiting after a head injury
- Ask your child's pediatrician in advance what you should do in case of an emergency.
- Call your child's pediatrician if you think your child is ill.
- Take a BLS course at your local hospital or school.
- Call the Poison Center at once if your child has swallowed a suspected poison or another person's medication, even if your child has no signs or symptoms.
- Call 9-1-1 (or your local emergency number) for help if you believe your child's life might be in danger or that your child is seriously ill or injured.

### In Case of an Emergency:

- Stay calm.
- Start rescue breathing or CPR if your child is not breathing.
- Call 9-1-1 if you need immediate help.
- If you do not have 9-1-1 service in your area, call your local emergency ambulance service or county emergency medical service.
- Apply continuous pressure to the site of bleeding with a clean cloth.
- Place your child on the floor with his or her head turned to the side if he or she is having a seizure. Do not put anything in his or her mouth.
- Do not move your injured child unless there is immediate danger.
- Stay with your child until help arrives.
- Bring any medication your child is taking with you to the hospital.
- Bring any suspected poisons or other medications your child might have taken.
- After you arrive at the ED, make sure you tell the emergency staff the name of your child's pediatrician. Your pediatrician can work closely with the emergency physicians and nurses and can provide them with more information about your child.

Adapted from: American Academy of Pediatrics, "When Your Child Has a Medical Emergency."

a combination. First responders provide first aid, basic airway management such as airway clearance, CPR, newborn deliveries, basic wound care, and hemorrhage control. An Emergency Medical Technician-Basic (EMT-B) can provide all first responder skills plus patient assessment, oxygen administration, assisted ventilation (via bag-mask), splinting, spinal immobilization, patient transport, and in some systems, assistance in administering auto-injected epinephrine, and inhaled bronchodilators. An EMT-Intermediate (EMT-I) is considered to be at an intermediate level of training between BLS and ALS providers. Depending on the state and the EMS system, the EMT-I is allowed to perform intubation, intravenous (IV) access, and manual defibrillation and may be able to administer some medications. EMT-Paramedic (EMT-P) can obtain vascular access; deliver inhaled, IV, intraosseous (IO), intramuscular (IM), and tracheal medications; perform endotracheal or nasotracheal intubation, needle or surgical cricothyrotomy, and 12-lead ECG analysis.[2,19] Although a majority (two thirds) of pediatric patients receive only BLS support, many have the potential to deteriorate and require constant reassessment by an ALS team. A major goal of the EMSC program is to identify methods to correctly match the severity of illness or injury, as assessed by EMS dispatchers, to the level of EMS care dispatched.[6]

## Response Phase

First responders and EMT-B providers sometimes perform initial life saving interventions, including airway clearing maneuvers, hemorrhage control, mouth-to-mask ventilations, compressions, and defibrillation using an automated external defibrillator (AED). On patient contact, EMS providers first perform a scene assessment for safety hazards and environmental/visual information that might affect patient assessment and care (Figure 16.1). Observation of a trauma scene can clarify the mechanism of injury by noting details such as the condition of a car or bicycle or the presence of other victims and the nature of their injuries. Other scene details can help to assess the possibility of neglect or abuse or assist in the identification of a poison. Bystanders might be able to provide historical information, such as initial level of consciousness or seizure activity, as well

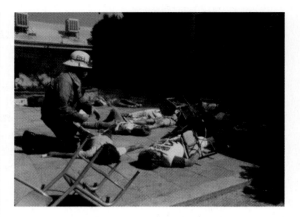

**Figure 16.1** Scene assessment for safety hazards.

as treatments provided before the arrival of EMS. Family members might not know these details. Discussion between emergency physicians and EMS personnel provides critical details frequently unavailable from any other source.

The EMS provider then performs a rapid patient assessment. Emphasis is placed on early recognition of abnormalities in the airway and breathing because most critically ill pediatric patients, including victims of serious blunt trauma, have associated respiratory distress or failure. Determination of vital signs in the field is performed. Due to the wide range of variability of normal pediatric vital signs and the difficulty of accurate measurement in the field (especially blood pressure in younger children), a goal of EMSC is to teach EMS providers to look for abnormalities in mental status, respiratory effort, and peripheral perfusion in assessing for respiratory failure and shock. Having a readily available reference list for normal pediatric vital signs by age is also recommended.

## Treatment and Triage Phase

Patient assessment and treatment often occur simultaneously. Assessment follows an approach that has become an integral part of many pediatric resuscitation and prehospital education courses and resources. This approach is based on the pediatric assessment triangle (PAT). The PAT focuses assessment on appearance, work of breathing, circulation to the skin, and continuous reevaluation (Figure 16.2). Treatment is protocol driven, with each EMS system having written treatment protocols for children. Model pediatric protocols have been developed

(Table16-3).[20] Treatment focuses on airway management, assisted ventilation, oxygen administration, prevention of hypothermia, and rapid transport to definitive care. ALS should be provided when necessary and appropriate providers are available on scene. Initial treatment on the scene should be focused on airway maintenance, assisted ventilation, spinal immobilization, and treatment for severe respiratory impairment (e.g., epinephrine for anaphylaxis, bronchodilators for reactive airway disease) (Figure 16.3). Other treatments are frequently provided on scene or en route if there is unavoidable transport delay due to an extrication problem or anticipated prolonged transport time.

The patient should be triaged to an appropriate destination based on age, mechanism of injury or illness, and measures of acuity. Triage and treatment decisions will be dictated by protocol or made with the assistance of direct (on-line) medical oversight. (Figure 16.4) Thus, another goal of EMSC is to ensure that the physicians and nurses providing direct medical control are trained in special issues pertaining to the care of children in the field, including all pediatric treatment protocols, medication dosing, and triage decisions. There are validated pediatric trauma triage tools (e.g., Pediatric Trauma Score);

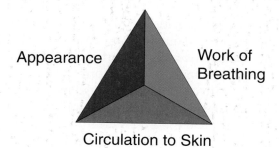

Figure 16.2 The pediatric assessment triangle (PAT).

| TABLE 16-3 | Model Pediatric Protocols by Medical Condition |
| --- | --- |

- General patient care
- Trauma
- Burns
- Foreign body obstruction
- Respiratory distress, failure, or arrest
- Bronchospasm
- Newborn resuscitation
- Bradycardia
- Tachycardia
- Nontraumatic cardiac arrest
- Ventricular fibrillation or pulseless ventricular tachycardia
- Asystole
- Pulseless electrical activity
- Altered mental status
- Seizures
- Nontraumatic hypoperfusion (shock)
- Anaphylactic shock/allergic reaction
- Toxic exposure
- Near-drowning
- Pain management
- Sudden infant death syndrome (SIDS)

Source: Mulligan-Smith D, O'Connor RE, Markenson D. EMSC Partnership for Children: NAEMSP Model Pediatric Protocols. *Prehospital Emergency Care.* 2000; 4:111–130. Reprinted with permission.

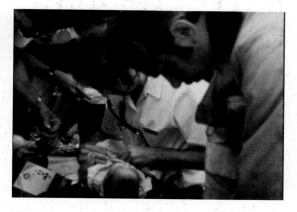

Figure 16.3 Initial treatment should focus on airway maintenance, assisted ventilation, and spinal immobilization.

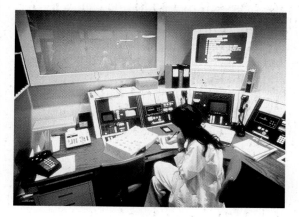

Figure 16.4 Specially trained nurse at a base hospital providing medical oversight for paramedics in the field.

however, no triage tool for medical illness has been developed and validated for the out-of-hospital setting. A goal of EMSC is to develop and validate a simple and functional medical triage score.

Once treatment and triage have been initiated, providers must make transport decisions. They must decide how (e.g., ground vehicle or air ambulance, ALS or BLS) and when to transport the patient. Traumatized children should be transported as soon as the airway has been stabilized and hemorrhage controlled, with other interventions performed en route. The definitive treatment for ongoing internal hemorrhage from trauma is surgical, so expeditious transport to a hospital is critical. Some patients with medical conditions receive emergency treatment in an effort to stabilize before and during transport (e.g., anticonvulsants for status epilepticus, epinephrine for anaphylaxis).

Frequent reassessment and ongoing treatment are continued during transport. Requirements for radio or telephone contact with the receiving facility vary, but continuous availability of direct medical oversight is optimal. A good example is contact with a poison center for directions on management of a pediatric ingestion or poisoning during transport. At the receiving hospital, the EMS providers should report the patient's status, pertinent information from the scene, interventions performed en route, and clinical course during transport. Responsibility for patient care is then transferred to the hospital staff, which initiates the next phase in the EMSC continuum.

### Safety of Children During Transport

Guidelines to make ambulance transport safe for children are being developed. A list of do's and don'ts is available from the EMSC program and includes the following:

- Drive cautiously at safe speeds and observe traffic laws.
- Tightly secure all monitoring devices and other equipment.
- Ensure available restraint systems are used by EMTs and other occupants, including the patient.
- Transport children who are not patients in a different (passenger) vehicle, and be sure that they are properly restrained whenever possible.
- Encourage use of the DOT NHTSA Emergency Vehicle Operating Course (EVOC), National Standard Curriculum.[21]

## Hospital Phase

### Triage and Transport to Hospitals With Pediatric Capabilities

Hospitals prepared to care for critically ill or injured children should be identified and be part of a written protocol or online medical oversight-driven triage process. Hospitals within an EMS system have varying pediatric capabilities and resources. Some EMS systems have regionalized pediatric care, while others have chosen to improve the pediatric capability of all hospitals in the system. Guidelines for pediatric preparedness of emergency departments have been developed.[22-25] Not all hospitals have used available guidelines at this time.[27,28] Ideally, children should be transported to the closest facility with pediatric emergency capabilities.

Although the rehabilitation phase is the last in the EMS-EMSC phases of care, an additional phase in the continuum of care is a child's ongoing care in the community. This is actually the end as well as the beginning, as it involves returning the child to the community and medical home or physician. Physicians can help educate local EMS agencies about the most prevalent injuries in the community, and then involve them in prevention activities. This can include bike helmet giveaways/bicycle rodeos, fire safety/smoke detector checks, or water safety/pool fencing campaigns.

## Medical Home

At the center of the EMSC system, there is a primary care physician who can coordinate care for the pediatric patient (Figure 16.5). Every child should have a medical home[1] (parent and primary physician) responsible for:

- Educating the family on prevention so there will be less need to use the system for the child
- Appropriately recognizing acute illness or severe injury requiring the use of EMSC

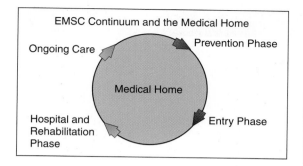

**Figure 16.5** The EMSC continuum of care and the medical home.

- Activating the EMS system and instructing the family on how and when to access EMS

## EMSC Landmarks

### Institute of Medicine Report

The Institute of Medicine (IOM) published a report on EMSC in 1993 that, while recogniz-ing significant advances in EMSC, suggested improvements in several areas. These included communication, access to care, data collection, physician involvement, equipment, education of providers, research, and EMS system infrastructure.[29] This has led to the numerous advances that follow.

### Prehospital Provider Education in Pediatrics

The EMSC program has sponsored initiatives to provide education in pediatric emergency care for prehospital professionals. The EMSC Program National Education of Out-of-Hospital Providers Task Force evaluated curricula and made recommendations for future EMS educational curriculum design and topic areas. Recommended topic areas to be covered in the paramedic curriculum are listed in Table 16-4. The task force also outlined essential pediatric skills for para-medic providers (Table 16-5).[30]

| TABLE 16-4 Paramedic Pediatric Curriculum Content |
|---|

- Patient assessment
- Growth and development
- EMS for children
- Illness and injury prevention
- Respiratory emergencies (airway and breathing problems)
  - Respiratory distress, respiratory failure, respiratory arrest
  - Possible causes of respiratory emergencies:
    - Airway obstruction (upper airway and lower airway obstruction)
    - Fluid in the lungs
- Cardiovascular/circulatory emergencies
  - Shock (compensated and decompensated shock)
  - Rate and rhythm disturbances, cardiopulmonary arrest
- Altered mental status
  - Possible causes:
    - Airway/breathing problems, shock, seizures, poisoning, metabolic, occult trauma, serious infection
- Trauma
  - Burns
- Child abuse and neglect

- Behavioral emergencies
  - Suicide, aggressive behavior
- Child-family communications
- Critical incident stress management
- Fever
- Medical-legal issues
  - DNR, consent, guardianship, refusal of care
- Newborn emergencies
- Near-drowning
- Pain management
- Poisoning
- SIDS and death in the field
- Transport considerations
  - Destination issues, methods for transport (safety seats and parental transport)
- Infants and children with special needs
  - Technologically assisted children
    - Tracheostomy care, apnea monitors, central lines, chronic illness, gastrostomy tubes, home artificial ventilators, and shunts

Adapted from: Gausche M, Henderson DP, Brownstein D, Foltin G. The education of out-of-hospital medical personnel in pediatrics: Report of a national task force. *Ann Emerg Med.* 1998;31:1:58–63, and *Prehosp Emerg Care.* 1998;2:56–61; and American Academy of Pediatrics. Out-of-hospital care of pediatric patients. In: Seidel JS, Knapp J, eds. *Childhood Emergencies in the Office, Hospital, and Community: Organizing Systems of Care.* 2nd ed. Elk Grove, Il: American Academy of Pediatrics; 2000:187–201.

## TABLE 16-5    Critical Skills for Paramedics

### Assessment of Infants and Children

Use of a Length-Based Resuscitation Tape
- Airway management
  - Mouth-to-mouth barrier devices
  - Oropharyngeal airway
  - Nasopharyngeal airway
  - Oxygen delivery system
  - Bag-mask ventilation
  - Tracheal placement confirmation devices ($CO_2$ detection)
  - Optional: Rapid sequence intubation
  - Foreign body removal with Magill forceps
  - Needle thoracostomy
  - Nasogastric or orogastric tubes
  - Suctioning
  - Endotracheal intubation
  - Tracheostomy management
- Monitoring
  - Cardiorespiratory monitoring
  - Pulse oximetry
  - End-tidal $CO_2$ monitoring and/or $CO_2$ detection

- Vascular access
  - Intravenous line placement
  - Intraosseous line placement
- Fluid/medication administration
  - Tracheal
  - Intramuscular
  - Intravenous
  - Nasogastric
  - Nebulized
  - Oral
  - Rectal
  - Subcutaneous
- Cardioversion
- Defibrillation
- Drug dosing in infants and children
- Stabilization/extrication
  - Car seat extrication
  - Spinal stabilization

Adapted from: Gausche M, Henderson DP, Brownstein D, Foltin G. The education of out-of-hospital medical personnel in pediatrics: Report of a national task force. *Ann Emerg Med.* 1998;31:1:58–63, and *Prehosp Emerg Care.* 1998;2:56–61; and American Academy of Pediatrics. Out-of-hospital care of pediatric patients. In: Seidel JS, Knapp J eds. *Childhood Emergencies in the Office, Hospital, and Community: Organizing Systems of Care.* 2nd ed. Elk Grove Village, Il: American Academy of Pediatrics; 2000:187–201.

Several pioneering programs in pediatric prehospital education have been developed. These include:

- The Center for Pediatric Emergency Medicine's Teaching Resource for Instructors in Prehospital Pediatrics (TRIPP). The TRIPP resource is now available in BLS and paramedic versions (www.cpem.org).[31,32]
- The Pediatric Education for Prehospital Professionals (PEPP) Course (www.PEPPsite.com). The first national course for pediatric education for out-of-hospital providers, PEPP was established by the American Academy of Pediatrics (AAP) in collaboration with Jones and Bartlett Publishers in 2000.[33]
- The National Association of EMTs (NAEMT) Pediatric Prehospital Care Course (PPC) is designed to provide education at the EMT-I and paramedic levels (www.naemt.org).[34]

## Pediatric Protocols for Prehospital Care

The National Association of EMS Physicians (NAEMSP), as part of the Partnership for Children program (supported by EMSC), developed model protocols for out-of-hospital care of children.[20] In order to develop these new pediatric protocols, the medical literature was evaluated to identify those out-of-hospital interventions that are evidence based, and existing protocols from many EMS systems in the United States were reviewed and collated. The topics covered by the pediatric prehospital emergency protocols that were developed are listed in Table 16-3; the protocols are available from NAEMSP at www.naemsp.org or the EMSC Web site at www.ems-c.org.

## Care of Children in the Emergency Department: Guidelines for Preparedness

Initial efforts to develop guidelines for emergency departments that care for children originated in California.[22-26] Data suggest that many EDs are not fully prepared to care for pediatric patients; despite this finding, few of the guidelines for ED care of children have been widely adopted.[27,28] The EMSC program, through the Partnership for Children, therefore established a task force led by the American College of Emergency Physicians (ACEP) and AAP to develop guidelines for ED pediatric preparedness to be used nationally.[26] These guidelines developed by ACEP and AAP have been supported in concept by 17 professional organizations, and efforts are ongoing to evaluate the impact of these guidelines on ED pediatric preparedness.[26] The guidelines are available on the ACEP (www.acep.org) and AAP (www.aap.org) Web sites.

## EMSC Support of National Resource Centers and a National Research Network

The EMSC program currently supports two national resource centers. The EMSC National Resource Center (NRC), based in Washington, DC (www.ems-c.org), provides technical support, information dissemination, and topic-specific expertise. The National EMS Data Analysis Resource Center (NEDARC) based in Salt Lake City, Utah (www.nedarc.org), provides resources on data collection, analysis, and linkages. In 2001, the EMSC program funded the Network Development Demonstration Project (NDDP). The goal of the NDDP is to develop an infrastructure for collaborative research in EMSC. Four regional research node centers, with more than 20 affiliated hospital EDs, make up this Pediatric Emergency Care Applied Research Network (PECARN).

## Other EMSC-Supported Programs

Over the years, numerous programs have been funded by EMSC for state EMSC system development, regional EMSC conferences, national organizations, and research initiatives. Some of these are listed in Table 16-6.

| TABLE 16-6 EMSC Supported Programs |
|---|
| • National Resource Centers: NRC and NEDARC |
| • EMSC Development Demonstration Grants (formerly state planning and implementation grants) |
| • Network Development Demonstration Project (NDDP) |
| • Pediatric Emergency Care Research Network (PECARN) |
| • EMSC Partnership Demonstration Grants |
| • Interagency Committee on EMSC Research (ICER) |
| • EMSC Regional Symposium Supplementation Grants |
| • EMSC Targeted Issue Grants |
| • Trauma/EMS Systems |
| • Partnership for Children |
| • Clinical Practice Guidelines |
| • Enhancing Patient Safety |

## Other EMSC Initiatives

### Priorities in EMSC Research—Research Task Force

A consensus group reviewed priorities for research in EMSC. Fifteen topic areas were given a high priority, and these are listed in Table 16-7.[35]

### Emergency Information Form

Children with special health care needs (CSHCN) bring unique problems to providers of prehospital and emergency care. The Emergency Information Form (EIF) was created to delineate in a clear and concise manner the complicated medical conditions, baseline abnormalities in mental, respiratory, and circulatory status, and baseline vital signs of a CSHCN. It helps a caregiver know what is normal for the individual child, and it helps that provider determine the severity of anatomic or physiologic change due to illness or injury. CSHCN are frequently managed by several specialists, making it difficult for emergency care providers to readily access complete information on their medical care from one source. In a collaborative effort of the EMSC program, ACEP and the AAP produced policy statements that outline the contents and format of an EIF.

| TABLE 16-7 | Priorities for Research in EMSC |
|---|---|

1. Major clinical entities including, shock, respiratory distress, asthma, brain injury, multiple organ trauma, seizures, poisoning, behavioral disorders, burns, fever
2. Development and validation of outcome measures
3. Injury prevention
4. Medical informatics
5. Effective ways to measure, improve, and upgrade the quality of EMS care and systems
6. Prevention and relief of physical and emotional pain
7. Effectiveness and cost of out-of-hospital interventions
8. Pediatric resuscitation
9. Costs of EMSC—direct, indirect, and marginal
10. Access to EMS for children
11. Development and validation of injury and illness scores
12. Educational issues, such as training, retraining, and skill retention
13. Public education in injury prevention, basic emergency care skills, and the use of EMS systems
14. Triage in the out-of-hospital and emergency department settings
15. Children with special health care needs

Source: Seidel JS, Henderson D, Tittle S et al.: Priorities for research in emergency medical services for children: Results of a consensus conference. *Ann Emerg Med.* 1999;33:206–210. Reprinted with permission.

This form would be completed by a child's physician and provided to prehospital providers and emergency physicians.[36,37]

## Physician's Role in EMSC

Physicians have an important role in supporting and advancing EMSC. They must be well informed about their regional EMS systems, as well as the resources, collaborative efforts, and products developed by the EMSC program. The educational programs and resources developed to educate prehospital providers in the care of children should be incorporated into prehospital provider training and continuing medical education (CME). Model pediatric prehospital care protocols and recommended ambulance equipment lists are available to guide regional EMS systems in providing appropriate prehospital care for children. Individual physicians should be involved on EMS and hospital committees to ensure incorporation of these pediatric-focused resources. Guidelines for preparedness of EDs in the care of children also exist. Emergency physicians and pediatricians must take leadership roles in their EMS systems and hospital EDs to make sure that

these innovative products and resources are used effectively.[2,38] Some of these are listed in Table 16-8.

| TABLE 16-8 | Physician's Role in EMSC |
|---|---|

- Emphasize safety and injury prevention.
- Encourage parents to become certified in BLS/CPR.
- Advocate for injury prevention and safety campaigns.
- Support/develop legislation supporting injury prevention and safety.
- Ensure that children are up-to-date on immunizations.
- Maintain office emergency preparedness and ED preparedness for children.
- Frequently practice pediatric resuscitation.
- Maintain skills in emergency pediatrics, especially airway management.
- Become familiar with local prehospital care providers, EDs, and transport services.
- Be available for consultation to local EDs.
- Serve as medical advisors to the local EMS system.
- Stay informed on issues pertaining to EMSC.

## Future of EMSC

Aspects of EMSC have been integrated into the EMS systems of all 50 states. The EMSC program has accomplished much to improve the care of ill and injured children. Products associated with EMSC programs can be found by contacting the EMSC National Resource Center (www.ems-c.org). Nevertheless, there are still challenges ahead. These include a need for all children cared for in all EMS systems to benefit from the education, training, and information developed by the EMSC program. Research studies must evaluate the national impact of many EMSC programs and initiatives. With continued collaboration of national, public, and government organizations and programs focused on improving the emergency care of children, the future of children cared for in our EMS systems is very encouraging.

# CHAPTER REVIEW

## Check Your Knowledge

1. Which of the following illnesses is the most common across all age groups to be cared for by EMS?
   A. Poisoning
   B. Rashes
   C. Respiratory distress
   D. Seizures
   E. Submersion

2. Which of the following statements regarding prehospital providers' care of children is correct?
   A. They are comfortable managing critically ill children
   B. They frequently provide assisted ventilation for a child
   C. They infrequently (1% to 5%) transport seriously ill or injured children
   D. They require frequent refreshing of pediatric knowledge and skills

3. All of the following treatments or services can be provided by an EMT-B except:
   A. Assisted ventilation
   B. Cardiac compressions
   C. Immobilization
   D. Manual defibrillation
   E. Patient transport

4. The role of the physician in EMS includes all of the following except:
   A. Becoming familiar with local prehospital care providers, EDs, and transport services
   B. Emphasizing safety and injury prevention
   C. Maintaining office emergency preparedness and ED preparedness for children
   D. Providing funding for issues pertaining to EMSC
   E. Serving as medical advisors to local EMS systems

## References

1. Dieckmann, RA. The EMS-EMSC continuum. In: Dieckmann, RA. *Pediatric Emergency Care Systems: Planning and Management.* Baltimore, Md: Williams & Wilkins; 1992: 3–17.
2. American Academy of Pediatrics. Out of hospital care of pediatric patients. In: Seidel JS, Knapp J, eds. *Childhood Emergencies in the Office, Hospital, and Community: Organizing Systems of Care.* 2nd ed. Elk Grove Village, Il: American Academy of Pediatrics; 2000:187–201.
3. Seidel JS, Hornbein M, Yoshiyama K, Kuznets D, Finkelstein JZ, St. Geme JW. Emergency medical services and the pediatric patient: Are the needs being met? *Pediatrics.* 1984;73:769–772.
4. Tsai A, Kallsen G. Epidemiology of pediatric prehospital care. *Ann Emerg Med.* 1987;16:284–292.
5. Babl FE, Vinci RJ, Bauchner H, Mottley L. Pediatric pre-hospital advanced life support care in an urban setting. *Pediatr Emerg Care,* 2001;17:5–9.
6. Foltin G, Pon S, Tunik M, et al. Pediatric ambulance utilization in a large American city: A systems analysis approach. *Pediatr Emerg Care.* 1998;14:254–258.
7. Boyd DR. The history of emergency medical services (EMS) systems in the United States of America. In: Boyd DR, Edlich RF, Micik S, eds. *Systems Approach to Emergency Medical Care,* Norwalk, Ct: Appleton; 1983:1–82.
8. Pantridge JF, Geddes JS. Cardiac arrest after myocardial infarction. *Lancet.* 1966;1:807–808.
9. Foltin GL, Tunik MG. Emergency medical services for children, In: Barkin RM, ed. *Pediatric Emergency Medicine: Concepts and Clinical Practice.* 2nd ed. St Louis, Mo: Mosby–Year Book, Inc; 1997:23–41.
10. Gausche M, Lewis RJ, Stratton SJ, et al. Effect of out-of-hospital pediatric endotracheal intubation on survival and neurological outcome: A controlled clinical trial. *JAMA.* 2000;283:783–790.
11. Foltin GL, Salomon M, Tunik M, Schneiderman W, Treiber M. Developing advanced life support for children in the prehospital setting: The New York City experience. *Pediatr Emerg Care.* 1990;6:141–144.
12. Gausche-Hill M, Lewis RJ, Gunter CS, Henderson DP, Haynes BE, Stratton SJ. Design and implementation of a controlled trial of pediatric endotracheal intubation in the out-of-hospital setting. *Ann Emerg Med.* 2000;36: 356–365.

13. Glaeser PW, Linzer J, Tunik MG, Henderson DP, Ball J. Survey of nationally registered emergency medical services providers: pediatric education. *Ann Emerg Med.* 2000;36:33–38.

14. Seidel JS, Henderson DP, eds. *EMSC—Emergency Medical Services for Children: A Report to the Nation.* Washington, DC: National Center for Education in Maternal and Child Health; 1991.

15. Seidel JS. History of EMS for children. In: Dieckmann RA, ed. *Pediatric Emergency Care Systems: Planning and Management.* Baltimore, Md: Williams & Wilkins; 1992:18–23.

16. Post C, Treiber M. History. In: Kuehl AE, ed. *Prehospital Systems and Medical Oversight.* 3rd ed. Dubuque, IA: National Association of EMS Physicians, Kendall/Hunt Publishing Company; 2002:3–19.

17. American Academy of Pediatrics. TIPP sheet: When your child needs emergency medical services. Available at: http://www.aap.org/family/tipp%2Dems.htm.

18. Foltin GL, Schneiderman WJ, Dieckmann RA. 911 and ambulance dispatch. In: Dieckmann RA, ed. *Pediatric Emergency Care and Systems: Planning and Management.* Baltimore, Md Williams & Wilkins; 1992:109–116.

19. Pointer JE, McGuire TL. Levels of providers. In: Kuehl AE, ed. *Prehospital Systems and Medical Oversight.* 3rd ed. Dubuque, Ia: National Association of EMS Physicians, Kendall/Hunt Publishing Company; 2002:106–113.

20. Mulligan-Smith D, O'Connor RE, Markenson D. EMSC Partnership for Children: NAEMSP Model Pediatric Protocols. *Prehosp Emerg Care.* 2000;4:111–130.

21. EMS for Children National Resource Center. The do's and don'ts of transporting children in an ambulance. Available at: http://www.ems-c.org/products/frameproducts.htm.

22. Seidel JS, Tittle S, Henderson DP, et al. Guidelines for pediatric equipment and supplies for emergency departments. *Ann Emerg Med.* 1998;31:54–57.

23. American Medical Association, Commission on Emergency Medical Services. Pediatric emergencies. An excerpt from "Guidelines for Categorization of Hospital Emergency Capabilities." *Pediatrics.* 1990;85:879–887.

24. American College of Emergency Physicians. Emergency care guidelines. *Ann Emerg Med.* 1997;29:564–571.

25. American Academy of Pediatrics, Committee on Pediatric Emergency Medicine. Guidelines for pediatric emergency care facilities. *Pediatrics.* 1995;96:526–537.

26. American Academy of Pediatrics, Committee on Pediatric Emergency Medicine; and American College of Emergency Physicians, Pediatric Committee. Care of children in the emergency department: Guidelines for preparedness. *Pediatrics.* 2001;107:777–781, and *Ann Emerg Med.* 2001;37:423–427.

27. Athey J, Dean JM, Ball J, et al. Ability of hospitals to care for pediatric emergency patients. *Pediatr Emerg Care.* 2001;17:170–174.

28. McGillivray D, Nijssen-Jordan C, Kramer MS, Yang H, Platt R. Critical pediatric equipment availability in Canadian hospital emergency departments. *Ann Emerg Med.* 2001;37: 371–376.

29. Durch JS, Lohr KN, eds. *Emergency Medical Services for Children.* Washington, DC: National Academy Press; 1993.

30. Gausche M, Henderson DP, Brownstein D, Foltin G. The education of out-of-hospital medical personnel in pediatrics: Report of a national task force. *Ann Emerg Med.* 1998;31:1:58–63, and *Prehosp Emerg Care.* 1998;2:56–61.

31. Foltin GL, Tunik MG, Cooper A, Markenson D, Treiber M, Phillips R, et al, eds. *Teaching Resource for Instructors in Prehospital Pediatrics (EMT-Basic).* New York, Ny: Maternal and Child Health Bureau; 1998.

32. Foltin GL, Tunik MG, Cooper A, et al. *Paramedic Teaching Resource for Instructors in Prehospital Pediatrics.* New York, Ny: Center for Pediatric Emergency Medicine, 2002.

33. Dieckmann RA, Brownstein D, Gausche-Hill M, eds. *Pediatric Education for Prehospital Professionals.* Sudbury, Ma: Jones and Bartlett Publishers, Inc; 2000.

34. Markenson D, ed, *Pediatric Prehospital Care.* Upper Saddle River, Nj: Prentice Hall; 2002.

35. Seidel JS, Henderson D, Tittle S, et al. Priorities for research in emergency medical services for children: Results of a consensus conference. *Ann Emerg Med.* 1999;33:206–210.

36. Sacchetti A, Gerardi MJ, Barkin R, et al. Emergency data set for children with special needs. *Ann Emerg Med.* 1996;28:324–327.

37. American College of Emergency Physicians. Emergency information form for children with special health care needs. *Ann Emerg Med.* 1999;34:577–582.

38. Wheeler DS. Emergency medical services for children: A general pediatrician's perspective. *Curr Probl Pediatr.* 1999;29:221–241.

# CHAPTER REVIEW

A 2-year-old girl wanders outside to the pool in her back yard. Her mother, distracted by a telephone call, rushes outside and finds her daughter floating face down in the water. She pulls her out of the pool, performs CPR, and calls 9-1-1.

1. *What processes and resources provide support for pediatric-specific training, equipment, assessment, treatment, triage, and transport in an EMS system?*
2. *What is the role of the physician in the EMS the system's ability to care for children?*

The EMS system responds by dispatching EMT and paramedic units. The mother's CPR efforts combined with assisted ventilation with appropriate pediatric equipment by EMTs and paramedics resuscitate the toddler. The child is transported to a hospital with pediatric emergency and critical care staff. She is stabilized in the ED and transferred to the pediatric intensive care unit. After 2 days, she is transferred to the pediatric floor with no apparent neurologic deficits and is discharged to home after 1 week of hospitalization. Her pediatrician provides her family with information on four-sided pool fencing on her next followup visit. The physicians and nurses at the hospital are actively lobbying their state legislators to create a law requiring 4-sided fencing around all in-ground pools.

# chapter 17

# Disaster Management

Lou E. Romig, MD, FAAP, FACEP

## Objectives

1 Describe the special vulnerabilities of children during and after a disaster.

2 Design an evacuation plan for home, office, and hospital.

3 Compare the roles of local EMS and federal agencies in their response to a disaster.

## Chapter Outline

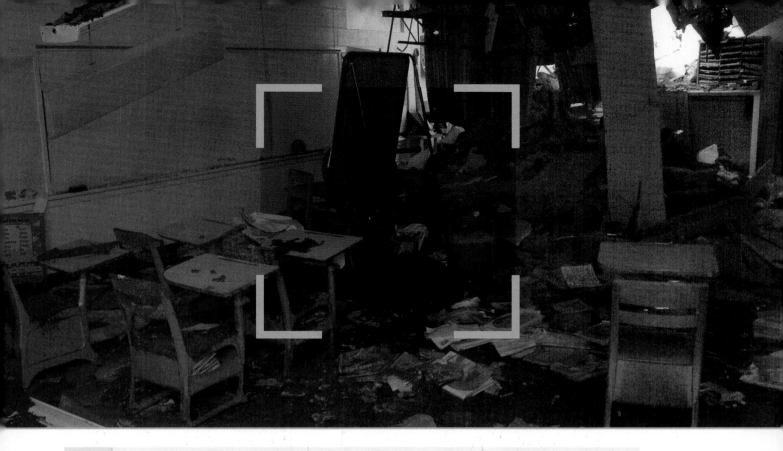

## CASE SCENARIO 1

A disaster shelter with 130 evacuees is struck and heavily damaged by a tornado during the storm. Per local protocol, emergency medical services units are unable to respond due to the intensity of the weather. Adult and pediatric victims of the tornado start arriving by the carload at the nearby emergency department, stating that other victims will be following them, as it is impossible to travel further to other facilities.

1. Does your hospital disaster plan consider self-referred victims instead of just those arriving by emergency medical services? Is your emergency department staff prepared to perform primary disaster triage?
2. Does your hospital disaster plan consider adequate staffing and resources to allow emergency medical services to function at high demand levels with minimal outside assistance?

## Introduction

A disaster can be defined as any occurrence that taxes or overwhelms local response resources. For example, in a nonmedical setting, a disaster could be an irreversible crash of a company's computer network. Some disasters do not generate unusual numbers of medical patients but can tax resources for shelters, nutrition, safety/law enforcement, or transportation. In the medical setting, disasters usually entail the presence or potential presence of a number of victims that overwhelms agency-specific or local resources. A vehicle collision with six critical victims could con-stitute a disaster for a small emergency medical services (EMS) system and/or the local hospitals that a larger EMS and hospital system would be able to handle easily with the available resources.

Table 17-1 lists types of disasters, with examples of each. Note that some disasters occur suddenly, with little to no warning. Risk-specific planning and preparation are especially critical in these types of disasters, as response resources must be ready to be marshaled and dispatched immediately. Other disasters, such as floods and hurricanes, usually provide advance warning or have a gradual onset that allows for additional preparations before the

## TABLE 17-1  Types of Disasters

**Natural**
- Hurricanes or cyclones
- Tornadoes
- Floods
- Mudslides
- Tsunamis
- Ice or hail storms
- Droughts
- Wildfires
- Earthquakes
- Infestations or disease epidemics

**Technological**
- Hazardous materials releases or spills
- Nonintentional explosions or collapses
- Transportation crashes or derailments
- Power outages

**Terrorism/International Violence**
- Bombings or explosions
- Chemical agent releases
- Biological agent releases
- Nuclear agent releases
- Multiple or mass shootings
- Cult-related violence
- Riots
- Arson

**Humanitarian Disasters/Complex Emergencies**
- War or violent political conflict
- Genocidal acts
- Droughts
- Famine
- Shelter or feeding or medical care of displaced populations

critical stage ensues. Most often, natural disasters are thought of as geological or weather related; however, many disasters arise from the use or misuse of technology. Others are intentional, triggered by political or ideological motives. Humanitarian disasters (also sometimes called "complex emergencies") usually involve multiple resource shortages for large populations over long periods. Those affected are often a displaced, or refugee, population. Many disasters have some degree of physical, mental, or emotional effect on significant numbers of people, without regard to sex, age, ethnicity, or any factor other than proximity to the event. Indeed, terrorist attacks have demonstrated that disasters can have marked psychological effects on people who had no physical connection to the attack itself. It is this widespread impact that makes terrorist attacks so effective. To think that children are infrequent victims, directly or indirectly, of disaster is to ignore reality. To fail to consider the needs of children in disaster planning and response at all levels is to potentially jeopardize one of our most precious resources.

# Emergency Management Process

Emergency management in the context of disasters is traditionally divided into four phases: planning, response, recovery, and mitigation. Although it is usually the emergency managers working for government and public safety agencies who adopt this structure for action, this approach can help guide preparedness activities for hospitals, private offices, and organizations, as well as individuals and families.

Planning comprises all activities and actions taken in advance of a disaster. Planning should be based on analysis of a community's or organization's risks for exposure to specific types of disasters. Plans should take into account the frequency of occurrence of each type of disaster, the anticipated magnitude of effect, the degree of advance warning or suddenness of onset and offset, characteristics of the populations most likely to be affected, the amount and types of resources available within the community or organizational structure, and the ability to function independently without additional outside resources for periods of time.

Planning should not completely ignore low-probability disasters. Some incidents have relatively small chances of occurring but, if they do occur, are likely to have a disproportionately profound effect. An example of this is hospital preparedness for patients potentially contaminated with nuclear, biological, or chemical agents. One unrecognized or inadequately decontaminated or isolated patient can close an entire emergency department (ED) or hospital for hours, days, or weeks. Even though the probability of such an event at any given hospital remains relatively low, our new global awareness of the increasing possibility of such incidents has triggered a widespread demand for hospital-based training and planning, as well as federal funding in the United States to encourage such preparation within our medical systems (See Chapter 18, Preparedness for Acts of Nuclear, Biological, and Chemical Terrorism).

Response comprises all activities and actions taken during and immediately after a disaster. This includes initial search and rescue, damage assessment, evacuation, sheltering, and many other activities. Disaster response in the United States is usually coordinated by local agencies but can be augmented by state and federal response resources. The response phase lasts until the initial casualties have either been rescued or acknowledged as lost and sufficient resources have been made available to allow the population to assess damages and begin plans for restoration and recovery. This phase can last hours to weeks.

The recovery phase is the period in which the affected organization or community works toward re-establishing self-sufficiency. This is the period of new community planning, rebuilding, and the re-establishment of government and public service infrastructure. It is also the period in which outside support services are gradually withdrawn.

The response and recovery phases can represent a challenge from the medical standpoint because injuries can increase during damage assessment and physical rebuilding. Emotional and mental health problems often become evident in this time period as well; as reality sinks in, future challenges become much more overwhelming. Some victims feel abandoned as immediate response resources withdraw and attention and assistance from other communities wane.

Mitigation is the phase in which all other aspects of emergency management are scrutinized for "lessons learned"; the lessons are then applied in an effort to prevent the recurrence of the disaster itself or to lessen the effects of subsequent incidents. Mitigation and planning are continuous operations, as lessons learned from a previous disaster are rolled into planning for the next one. Mitigation includes preventive and precautionary actions such as changing building codes and practices, redesigning public utilities and services, revising mandatory evacuation practices and warning policies, and educating members of the community.

## Children and Disaster Planning

Families and individuals should have their own disaster plans that are aimed at allowing them to remain self-sufficient for the first 3 days following a disaster. Local and federal response resources take time to mobilize, even with good organizational planning. A family plan should consider the risks the family is most likely to encounter, key decisions they might have to make on very short notice, and additional needs by those with special health care requirements.

### Risk Analysis

In the same way that community emergency managers must devise risk-specific plans, families also should plan for specific disasters. Table 17-2 lists some of the questions families must answer to assess their own risks in case of disaster. The American Academy of Pediatrics (AAP), the American College of Emergency Physicians (ACEP), and 27 other state and national organizations developed the "Family Readiness Kit" to help families learn to deal with children in various disaster scenarios (Figure 17.1).

Disasters with advance warning allow for last-minute preparations, but those occurring

| TABLE 17-2 | Risk Analysis for Family Disaster Planning |
| --- | --- |

**Analyzing Your Family's Risks in Disasters**

- What natural disasters are most likely to strike your community?
  - Will you have adequate advance notification to finish preparations, or must you maintain constant preparedness?
  - Is there a seasonal nature to your most likely disasters?
  - Will you be able to ensure the safety and location of all family members before the disaster strikes, or will you need to make plans for reunification?
  - Are your residence, schools, and places of business in special risk zones such as flood or storm surge zones?
  - Is your residence as well constructed, reinforced, and prepared for the specific types of disasters as possible?
- Are your home, places of business, and schools and childcare facilities located in an area at risk as targets for terrorist attacks or technological incidents?
- Is any family member obligated to be away from the family, especially in an at-risk service position, during or immediately after a disaster strikes?
- Does any member of your family have special health care needs that would affect the resources you need during and after a disaster?

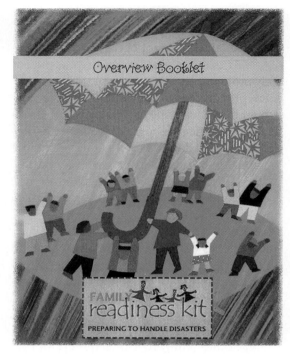

**Figure 17.1** Family readiness kit.

suddenly demand a constant state of readiness. Seasonal disasters such as hurricanes or winter storms are amenable to preparation updates and stock inventory/rotation at the beginning of the season. Sudden disasters sometimes find family members in scattered locations, in which case plans should be made for those who will try to pick up specific family members. A physical or telephone rendezvous point should be designated to aid in reunification. Families with residences in storm surge or flood zones or those in remote areas should consider evacuation. Likewise, families living in at-risk housing such as mobile or waterfront homes should consider early evacuation.

Some residences, businesses, schools, and childcare centers are located in or near areas that are potential terrorist targets or sites at risk for technological disasters. Childcare centers were located in both the Alfred P. Murrah Building in Oklahoma City and one of the World Trade Center towers. Some industrial plants have childcare centers located on site or nearby for the convenience of their work-

ers. Schools and hospitals (especially pediatric hospitals) could be at risk as terrorist targets specifically because an intentional attack on innocent children would inspire high levels of terror and insecurity. Military, research, and public utility facilities could also become terrorist targets. As hard as it is to face these realities, families must recognize these kinds of risks and come to grips with them.

Many healthcare providers have professional and ethical obligations to respond before, during, and after disasters. They and their family members must acknowledge how their professional duties will affect their families, especially when those duties place them at unusual personal risk. Family members should recognize and respect the duty, training, and skills, but healthcare providers also must recognize and respect the wishes and fears of their loved ones. Whenever possible, conflicts should be settled before an incident actually occurs.

Family members with special healthcare needs require specific planning to ensure that their needs are met during a disaster. Such family members might need special sheltering arrangements, or even to be sent out of the anticipated impact zone before a disaster strikes. Incidents such as a power outage can constitute a disaster for a person with special health care needs yet not seriously affect others without those needs.

## Key Decisions

Disasters with a slow onset or advance warning, such as a hurricane or flood, allow time for families to make decisions for action before the event actively affects them. Some of the questions that must be answered are as follows:

1. If the family's residence is in a known evacuation zone, will the family evacuate early, at the last minute, or not at all? Early evacuation helps ensure a more orderly process, with less chance of leaving critical items and supplies behind, less chance of being caught in evacuation gridlock, and a better chance of securing space at a formal shelter or an out-of-area location. Others choose to evacuate at the last possible minute, hoping that a change in circumstances will allow them to remain safely in their own homes. This alternative increases the danger of being caught in deteriorating and possibly dangerous weather or being trapped in or close to their homes by impassable or closed roads and bridges. Some residents refuse to obey even mandatory evacuation orders, often based on past experience in which their homes remained safe when threatened by similar events. Families making this decision must understand that emergency rescue services may be unavailable when they are most needed, and that they are taking full responsibility for the safety and welfare of their family members. Evacuating families must also remember to make advance plans for their pets. Most community shelters will not allow pets to accompany families. Some veterinarians' practices and boarding facilities offer disaster sheltering. Pets and livestock sometimes have a key role in an individual's or family's refusal to evacuate because of concern for their animals.[1]

2. If the family is evacuating, where will they go? Families who anticipate evacuation must identify community shelters in advance so that there will be no question where they will go and how they will get there. Some families choose to leave the target area entirely, driving to stay with out-of-town family or friends or even just heading in a certain direction and counting on being able to find hotel rooms along the way. Those evacuating should consider doing so at the first warning stages to avoid heavy evacuation traffic and deteriorating travel conditions, and to secure hotel rooms before they are sold out to other evacuees. In addition, storms such as hurricanes can be unpredictable in their movement. A small change in a storm's path can send it directly over the most heavily used evacuation routes and destinations. Long-distance evacuees must carefully monitor weather conditions and forecasts before and during travel.

3. Is there a need to evacuate only part of the family? Disaster mechanisms carry with them some very specific risks. Many weather emergencies trigger power outages, some of which last for days to weeks. A family member who needs technological health care assistance such as a ventilator, oxygen compressor, monitor, or renal dialysis might be better off being evacuated early. Children with chronic illnesses such as asthma or diabetes can be at additional risk for exacerbations of their diseases due to stress, an unusual diet, lack of refrigeration for medications, lack of electricity for nebulizer treatments, or a heavy allergen load due to molds, pollens, generator fumes, and burning debris. Children with behavioral or psychiatric disorders might not tolerate the stress and changes in routine that often accompany a significant disaster. It is never easy to send a family member, especially a child, away from home, but it might be in the child's best interest to leave early to stay with other family or friends until the situation at home stabilizes.

**4.** What comes first: family or duty? Family members with public safety and service positions (including hospital employees and staff) often have duties that place them in unusual danger or prevent them from being with their families at a critical time. Conflicts between family and professional obligations must be discussed during disaster planning. All family members, including children, must understand why a parent is not be able to be with them, as well as why that parent is knowingly placing himself or herself in potential danger. Care should be taken to ensure that everything possible has been done to keep all family members safe. Emergency personnel away from their families must have the confidence that their families are well taken care of in order to be able to fully concentrate on their duties. Likewise, family members need to know that their loved ones will not take unnecessary risks and will be protected in every way possible. Some hospital-based personnel have the choice to be with their families during a disaster such as a hurricane or ice storm, and then respond for duty shortly after the crisis has passed, or to be at the hospital during the event and return to their families soon afterward. This decision should be made by the whole family after advantages and disadvantages have been identified. Emergency personnel who choose to neglect their professional obligations in favor of their families should know in advance about their employers' policies for employees who are absent without leave during an emergency.

### Special Needs Considerations

Families with children or other loved ones who have special health care needs must plan very carefully to meet those needs, either with the assistance of a hospital or shelter or on their own. Extra equipment and supplies should be stocked and inventoried regularly, especially at the beginning of a disaster "season." If the family is planning to stay home during an anticipated event, arrangements should be made to have extra oxygen, batteries, replacement parts, medications, consumables, biohazard disposal equipment, generators, and fuel delivered well in advance, with plans for automatic restocking as soon as possible after the event. Plans should include "bug out" criteria, sets of circumstances under which the family absolutely must evacuate to ensure their own safety and adequate medical care.

Families evacuating from their homes must identify in advance where they will go. Some hospitals open their doors to shelter special needs patients under the care of a few family members but cannot shelter entire families. Likewise, some designated public special needs shelters can accommodate only the special needs patient and one or two caregivers. Some shelters depend on families to provide all equipment, supplies, and patient care; others provide some level of skilled medical assistance and supplies. Some third-party payers have protocols providing for special needs patients in disasters. Hospitals and emergency management agencies might have registries not only for special needs patients but also for those who are frail or might need assistance with evacuation. Families with special health care needs should take advantage of these registries, which also often provide additional educational materials and preparedness checklists. Some home health care agencies and durable medical equipment suppliers furnish disaster planning checklists and assistance.

### Resources for Family Disaster Planning

There are numerous resources for risk-specific family disaster education and planning in print and on the Internet (Figure 17.2). Particularly notable resources are: the American Red Cross, which has numerous pamphlets available in multiple languages; the Federal Emergency Management Agency (FEMA), which has a Web site designed specifically for children; and various medical professional associations such as the AAP and ACEP, which have resources for both medical personnel and the public. Local and state emergency management offices and divisions also have Internet sites and printed educational materials available to the public. See Table 17-3 for a partial list of Internet

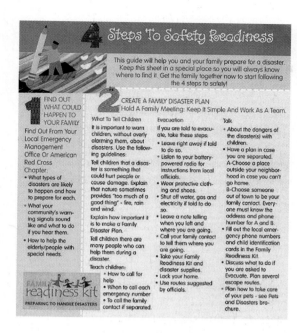

**Figure 17.2** Disaster preparedness for families.

<table>
<tr><td>

**TABLE 17-3** Internet Resources for Family Disaster Education and Planning

- Federal Emergency Management Agency (FEMA)
  FEMA Publications Library
  http://www.fema.gov/library/prepandprev.shtm
  FEMA for Kids
  http://www.fema.gov/kids/index.htm
- American Academy of Pediatrics (AAP)
  Family Readiness Kit: Preparing to Handle Disasters
  http://www.aap.org/family/frk/frkit.htm
- American College of Emergency Physicians (ACEP)
  Family Disaster Preparedness
  http://www.acep.org/1,2892,0.html
- American Red Cross Community Disaster Education Materials
  http://www.redcross.org/pubs/dspubs/cde.html
  US Search and Rescue Taskforce
  Family Disaster Planning
  http://www.ussartf.org/family_disaster_planning.htm
- National Disaster Education Coalition
  Talking About Disaster: Family Disaster Planning
  http://www.nfpa.org/Education

</td></tr>
</table>

resources for family disaster education and planning.

## Planning by Community Medical Practitioners

Medical practitioners in the community should have disaster plans for their offices and staff. If a disaster strikes suddenly during working hours, office staff members must know what to do immediately to ensure their own safety, assist others in the office, and secure and protect the physical property of the practice, especially patient records. Similar protective measures should be taken in the warning period before a disaster of slower onset, especially if the office is in an evacuation zone. The physician must have plans for dealing with hospitalized patients during a disaster, which special needs patients to direct to special shelters, how to handle calls from patients, how to notify patients of practice status, and how to continue to serve patient needs if the office is significantly damaged or disabled.[2–4]

Primary care practitioners can have a key role in encouraging and educating patients and their families to make home disaster plans. Anticipatory guidance sessions and materials can provide families with information about their community's specific disaster risks and provide preparedness checklists for the home. Practice Web sites can include links to resources such as those listed in Table 17-3 and feature targeted disaster planning tips at appropriate times of the year, similar to targeted safety and injury prevention tips. After a disaster occurs, primary care offices can act as distribution centers for information about local and federal recovery resources, medical problems to anticipate in the aftermath, and critical incident stress reactions and interventions.[4]

A school bus full of elementary students and their chaperones on a field trip skids on a patch of ice and overturns. Several children are thrown free of the bus. Some children and adults have left the bus under their own power; others are trapped inside the badly damaged bus. The air is full of the screams and cries of children.

1. *Are your local emergency medical services agencies prepared to appropriately rescue, triage, treat, and transport this number of patients, especially the seriously injured children?*
2. *Which of your local hospitals would be able to handle critically ill children? Will the closest trauma center be able to handle all of these patients? Some local emergency departments have low pediatric volumes. Will they be able to assist with some of the less critical victims?*

## Planning by EMS Agencies

EMS agencies (including fire/EMS departments) are crucial resources in disaster preparedness and response. They could be called on before a disaster to assist with evacuations of hospitals, nursing homes, and other skilled care facilities and provide medical staffing for shelters. Many fire departments and EMS agencies in the United States offer their stations as community disaster shelters. After a disaster, EMS providers perform search and rescue, provide medical care, and distribute information to the public.

Planning and preparation are the keys to the successful functioning of EMS providers before, during, and after a disaster. The most effective plans are often those that most closely match an agency's daily activities. Unfortunately, because children are an infrequent part of most EMS providers' daily encounters, they and their needs are often allotted only small consideration in EMS disaster plans.

EMS agencies customarily have a plan for dealing with all aspects of multiple and mass casualty incidents. There is no universally acknowledged definition or patient count that distinguishes a multicasualty incident from a mass casualty incident. Such definitions are often agency-specific and depend on the available resources of the agency and its mutual aid partners. In general, multiple casualty incidents usually are those that can be handled by local resources, and those requiring aid from multiple agencies or from outside the community are deemed mass casualty incidents.

For the purposes of this discussion, the abbreviation "MCI" will be used to denote both mass and multiple casualty incidents.

### Triage

Triage is commonly used in both the field and ED settings, sometimes based on objective guidelines, sometimes on instinct and experience. Triage in the MCI setting, however, demands a more restricted, objective approach than daily triage with a much more limited number of patients per call. MCI primary triage is focused on a very rapid limited patient assessment with the goal of getting to every victim in a short time and making initial judgments of patient salvageability and resource requirements. In a true MCI, designated triage personnel do not render treatment, including CPR or continuing ventilation/airway management, to any victim until primary triage has been completed for all victims on scene. In primary triage, each patient is assumed to be as "important" as any other, without regard for age, sex, occupation, or other factors; the triage category is determined solely by the victim's medical status.

Until recently, the triage of children in MCIs has not been guided by MCI-specific, pediatric-specific objective guidelines. Instead, EMS agencies have used adult MCI triage guidelines, such as the START (Simple Triage and Rapid Treatment) system, their daily trauma triage criteria, or no objective triage system at all.[5,6] It is not uncommon for a field

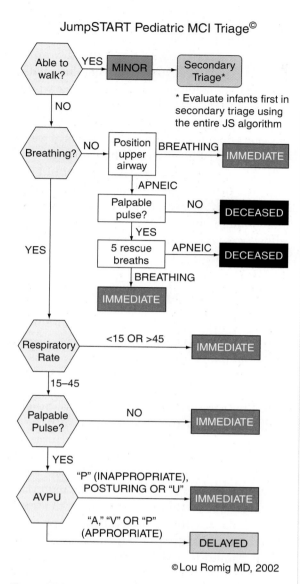

JumpSTART Pediatric MCI Triage©

* Evaluate infants first in secondary triage using the entire JS algorithm

©Lou Romig MD, 2002

**Figure 17.3** JumpSTART© pediatric MCI triage tool.

tional assessment elements designed to detect a child who might be apneic but still have some circulation prior to irreversible heart damage from anoxia. These children, potentially salvageable if respiratory function can be supported or restored, would not be recognized by the START system, in which no pulse check is performed on apneic patients who remain apneic after the upper airway is opened.

Regardless of what system is used for MCI primary triage in the field, every patient must receive at least one detailed secondary assessment either on scene (if transport to an ED is delayed for any reason) or in the ED, at which time the triage category can be upgraded or down graded. Triage is a dynamic process and continues until the patient reaches a facility where definitive assessment and care can be rendered. Note that no MCI triage system has been validated by research, although some elements used by these tools have been found to have more predictive value than others.[9,10]

In large-scale MCIs, victims sometimes arrive at area EDs without being assessed, treated, or transported by EMS. This is particularly true for pediatric victims, who can be easily transported by private vehicle or police car. ED personnel might need to perform initial MCI-style triage instead of using their ordinary triage procedures if large numbers of victims arrive in an uncontrolled manner. In these cases, EMS-based objective tools such as START and JumpSTART© can be helpful for initial patient categorization and assignment of ED resources.

## Treatment

EMS agencies must also plan to be able to provide at least basic treatment to an unusual number of pediatric patients. This requires not only adequate knowledge and training of the providers, but also sufficient supplies and pediatric equipment. Although field interventions are usually limited in an MCI, pediatric-specific disaster supplies should include appropriate equipment for spinal immobilization, including pediatric-sized cervical collars, appropriate oxygen masks and airway management equipment, small intravenous (IV) catheters, intraosseous needles, and methods to prevent hypothermia.

EMS provider to confess that he or she would likely classify most pediatric MCI victims in the most urgent triage categories simply to ensure they got the most rapid care. Until recently, there was no published objective pediatric MCI triage system in the United States; however, the JumpSTART© pediatric MCI triage tool is now being adopted by EMS agencies around the country.[7,8] JumpSTART© parallels the previously mentioned START system's algorithm, using physiologic decision points adapted for ranges of pediatric normals (**Figure 17.3**). In addition, it incorporates addi-

In addition, personnel should be able to recognize when minimal intervention is needed for a pediatric patient. Time and personnel spent trying to establish an IV on a very stable child might be better used for interventions on another patient who needs fluid resuscitation or airway management.

### Transport

EMS agencies must have knowledge of the pediatric capabilities of their area hospitals. Large MCIs might require hospitals that usually do not receive seriously injured or even stable pediatric patients to care for such patients in an effort to avoid overloading other facilities. The sickest children should be transported to facilities best equipped to treat them, and children with minor injuries can go to other EDs with lesser capabilities. It might be necessary to transport family members to different facilities. Good documentation by EMS transport supervisors can facilitate family reunification.

### Extraordinary Care After Disasters

EMS providers customarily act as a bridge between the patient and more traditional medical care. Patients treated by EMS providers or those not transported ("walking wounded"), are encouraged to seek further evaluation and treatment in an ED or by their primary care physicians. When a community's medical infrastructure has been damaged, however, those resources might not be readily accessible due to closure of facilities or because victims have little to no egress from their locations. In such circumstances, EMS is often the only form of medical attention that can physically reach patients until additional resources have been established. Emergency planning might call for EMS vehicles and crews to go from neighborhood to neighborhood to assess damage and care for the ill and injured. After Hurricane Andrew in 1992, EMS crews entering neighborhoods for the first time frequently encountered multiple victims with minor injuries asking for first aid or medical advice. Under normal circumstances, each patient encounter would have been documented with a run report and a signed release if the patient refused to seek further medical care. Instead, EMS and fire rescue crews cleaned and dressed wounds and gave basic medical advice, sometimes without full documentation. To do otherwise would have slowed service to the community in need. EMS agencies should anticipate that large-scale disasters might generate large numbers of walking wounded who need only first aid and those who require simple advice. They should determine what degree of documentation is needed for such patient encounters and how much judgment outside of protocols they will allow personnel under these extraordinary circumstances.

## Planning by Hospitals

Hospitals are required by various accrediting agencies to have hospital disaster plans. Hospital plans commonly cover two types of disasters: those occurring inside the hospital (internal disasters) and those occurring outside the hospital (external disasters), potentially leading to an acute increase in patient load.

Internal disasters include utility failures, fires, explosions, structural collapses, construction incidents, and hazardous materials releases. They also include violent incidents taking place within the facility and apparent or attempted kidnappings. Internal disaster plans should be risk-specific and detail how to protect the staff, visitors, and patients, secure property, and contain hazards (Figure 17.4). They should also detail how and where each type of staff member should respond, as well as provide for methods to organize and maintain control over the staff's response. Internal disasters can be particularly hazardous to staff members who attempt rescues for which they are not trained. As a part of their disaster training, hospital staff members should be educated about the most common hazards in the hospital setting (especially hazardous materials), the training and equipment needed to respond safely in different types of hazardous environments, basic safety precautions, and when they should wait for trained rescuers.

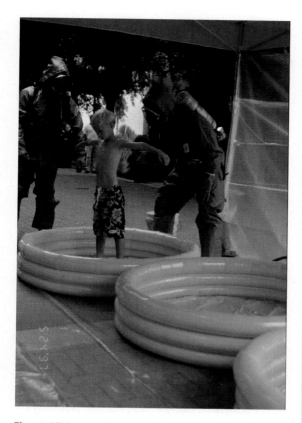

**Figure 17.4** Hazardous materials drill at a hospital.

Most hospital disaster planning and preparation centers on external disasters. External disaster plans commonly detail how immediately available equipment, services, and personnel are deployed in anticipation of an acute increase in patient load. The plan might require that additional personnel be called into the hospital for a major incident. The tendency is to place emphasis on the potential acute patient load, but the continuing care and welfare of patients already in the hospital must be maintained as well. External disaster plans should also detail when and how hospital personnel and resources might respond to the scene of a disaster. As with staff responses to internal disasters, any such plans should focus on maintaining the safety of the responding personnel. Ideally, any response outside hospital property should be planned with and integrated into the community's established emergency response plans, as untrained re-

sponders, however well-meaning, can become victims themselves.

Some external disaster plans, such as those for hurricanes, prepare for disasters of delayed onset, with the goal of ensuring that adequate personnel and resources are in the hospital before and during the disaster to handle an increased load after the disaster passes; that adequate safety precautions have been taken; and that preparations for anticipated utility outages and supply shortages have been completed. Some hospitals open their facilities as disaster shelters for staff and patient families, special needs patients, and the public. Sheltering has its own unique logistic challenges that must be covered in disaster plans.

Hospitals are more commonly adopting a modified incident command system, better allowing them to integrate into the plans of responding outside agencies and maintain a consistent structure despite turnover of personnel. The Hospital Emergency Incident Command System (HEICS),[11] developed at the direction of the California Emergency Medical Services Authority, has become a common platform for hospital disaster planning throughout the United States.

In large-scale federally declared disasters, hospitals must be able to interface with disaster response agencies. Federal Disaster Medical Assistance Teams (DMATs) might set up field emergency care facilities that transfer patients to local EDs. They can also be of assistance with patient followup in their field units or during shelter sick calls. DMAT members also might be used as hospital relief staffing. Hospitals might be asked to provide personnel for public health missions, set-up vaccination programs, assist with public health surveillance and data collection, provide telephone consultation for shelter personnel, or assist with organization and distribution of medical supplies. Hospital and ED administrators should have a basic understanding of the Federal Disaster Response Plan and response resources as well as the local emergency management plans and command structure.[12] Hospitals might choose to designate and train one or more staff members to act as liaisons with local, state, and federal response agencies.

Hospitals might also plan to support community physicians who have lost their practice locations by allowing them to use hospital facilities to see their patients. These physicians might also be used as additional personnel to see patients presenting to the ED or clinic with simple primary care needs, allowing emergency medical staff to focus on the more urgent patients. Community physicians can also be very useful in staffing telephone hotlines for medical questions from shelters and the public, although liability might be a concern, even in postdisaster setting.

Hospital disaster plans should include critical incident stress management services and interventions for staff members who suffer survivor guilt, guilt for leaving their families, stress from personal losses, and other expected psychological consequences. Posttraumatic stress disorder and other stress-related syndromes are not uncommon after disasters. They can affect individual staff members and compromise staff morale, attendance, and work efficiency.

## Planning by Community Agencies

Most accredited public schools are required to have disaster plans. Many private schools have plans as well. School disaster plans should cover a diversity of disasters as well as unusual occurrences such as fire, school violence, student abduction, terrorist attack, and community violence (riots) (Figure 17.5). Many schools act as community shelters; this aspect must also be addressed in school disaster plans and integrated with those of the agency responsible for sheltering (Red Cross, local EMS, or local emergency management).

Plans should include continuous oversight of student medical and emergency contact records and methods to reunite children with their family members. Procedures for seeking emergency medical care for students in the absence of a guardian should be clearly delineated. Ideally, school staff members should be

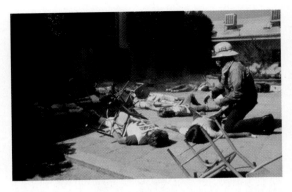

**Figure 17.5** School-based disaster response involving EMS resources.

trained in basic life support and first aid and perhaps even in basic safety precautions, rescue techniques, and triage procedures.

The National Association of School Nurses has prepared position statements on "School Nurse Role in Emergency Preparedness"[13] and "Emergency Care Plans for Students with Special Health Care Needs,"[14] and has developed a course on managing school emergencies[15] that covers much of the training needed not only by nurses but potentially by other school staff members. School disaster plans should also consider post-incident stress management for both students and staff, as well as more formal psychological monitoring and intervention for events involving violence, loss of a student or staff member, and those having community-wide impact.

Any facility that supervises children, such as childcare centers and community youth centers, should also have a disaster plan that focuses on ensuring the children's safety, accessing and interacting effectively with community emergency responders, guardian notification, and family reunification. As with hospitals, schools, and public safety agencies, these facilities should not only have disaster plans on paper, but should also educate staff members and exercise their plans.

Facilities providing supervision and/or medical care on a residential or periodic basis for special needs children should not only have basic disaster plans but also plans for medical record maintenance and access by emergency care personnel to pertinent records. Some EMS agencies keep registries of special needs children in their jurisdictions, with information on facility locations and building plans, usual patient census, hospital preferences, staff medical capabilities, and critical individual medical information. Agencies that routinely transport special needs children are increasingly keeping emergency medical information on board transport vehicles in case of crashes, sudden illness, or other incidents on the road.

AAP and ACEP have jointly developed the Emergency Information Form (EIF) for children with special health care needs, which can provide a child's critical medical information to any emergency medical care provider. In some areas, this EIF has been incorporated into EMS dispatch systems so that responding EMS crews can get information while responding to the call.[16]

## Planning by Community Emergency Management

To ensure a well-rounded emergency plan that addresses the needs of all interest groups, community emergency managers often enlist the assistance of nongovernment organizations that represent and advocate for the welfare of population groups such as the elderly, the disabled, children, and families. Hospital and professional medical associations, school boards, parent-teacher organizations, and social service agencies can act as advocates for the interests and welfare of these potential victims. Although children and families must be considered in all aspects of planning, disaster sheltering typically raises the most challenges.

Table 17-4 lists a number of issues that must be considered in community shelter planning. Although families are expected to provide their own basic supplies for the first few days, long-term sheltering demands that supplies be made available to displaced families. Diapers and other disposable wastes (such as biomedical waste) present potential problems because they can create hazardous and nonhygienic conditions if they are not properly managed pending final disposal. Younger children and those with special dietary requirements might not

| TABLE 17-4 | Pediatric Issues in Disaster Shelter Planning |
|---|---|

**Supplies and Services**
- Access to telephone consultation for medical questions
- Basic pediatric first aid equipment and guidelines
- Child-appropriate snacks and foods
- Diapers and other supplies for infant hygiene
- Games and other distractions for children
- Infant formula and rehydration solutions

**Staffing**
- Prepare staff members to help supervise children when parents start recovery efforts.
- Set contingencies so that the entire family of a child with special health care needs can be together.
- Train staff members in basic pediatric emergency care.
- Use family volunteers to help supervise children.

**Safety**
- Childproof the shelter to promote safety for children and the elderly.
- Sequester sick children and their families to reduce the spread of illness.
- Set ground rules for a healthy environment (limit or forbid smoking, drinking, weapons).
- Supervise interactions between children and frail (often elderly) shelter occupants.

be able to tolerate shelter food, especially MREs (Meals Ready to Eat), which are typically high in salt content and increase free water requirements. Families with infants on elemental or other special formulas might not have access to additional supplies in the initial post-disaster phase, although part of their family plans should be to bring a significant supply with them to the shelter. Hospitals and stores with these special stocks might be the best suppliers of special formulas; advance planning might include arranging with these organizations to supply special nutrition to shelters as needed. Children in shelters must be supervised and kept constructively occupied as much as possible. Supervised activities are a good opportunity to provide children with the information and reassurance they need, while allowing them to participate in familiar activities and routines. Drawing and other creative activities can help children express their feelings and deal with their stress.

Although shelters are not staffed by medically trained personnel, each shelter and shelter staff must be prepared for emergencies among the evacuees, including the children. Basic first aid supplies and guidelines should be available. If possible, shelter staff should have direct access to EMS (perhaps by radio if telephone lines are not operable), and possibly have a designated resource to advise on medical issues. Charts with pictures of infectious diseases with rashes (e.g., chickenpox, measles) can help identify shelter families that should be isolated to minimize contagion. Ideally, shelter plans should include isolation protocols. Long-term sheltering might incorporate plans for shelter sick calls, provided by community medical staff (public health staff or volunteer community practitioners). The National Disaster Medical System (NDMS) might also be activated, allowing DMAT personnel to conduct shelter sick calls.

Safety must be as much of a concern in a shelter as in any home. Both children and the elderly must be considered in creating a safe shelter. Shelter residents must be warned to try to secure their medications and medical supplies such as lancets for blood glucose testing, as well as other personal supplies (e.g., soaps, perfumes) that might cause injury to a child. Cords, oxygen tubing, and other trip hazards must be secured and watched carefully. Bathrooms and floors should be monitored for slip hazards. Rooms not actively in use for sheltering should be locked, and exits should be monitored. Shelter residents must be informed about emergency exits and procedures. Children should be monitored when they are around frail persons to prevent nonintentional injury. Finally, shelter rules about smoking, alcohol and other drug use, and weapons should be explicit and enforced as strictly as possible. If weapons are to be allowed in a shelter, all possible precautions must be taken to keep them out of the hands of children.

Children with special needs might include those with chronic or acute illnesses not usually considered in typical special needs definitions. Children with asthma might need aerosol treatments; families will likely bring their own aerosol machines but need access to power to use them. Families not in shelter but in homes without power might come to a shelter or hospital just to find power to give aerosol treatments. Families of children with diabetes might seek refrigerator or cooler space for their insulin. Families with infants and frail children might seek temporary shelter from heat, cold, sun, wind, or rain.

Officially designated special needs shelters must be prepared to accept pediatric evacuees, preferably with their entire families. If entire families are not allowed, some families might choose to take a special needs child to a regular shelter so the family can stay together. This might not be in the child's best interest from a medical standpoint. Special needs shelters must be as prepared to address children's needs as well as they do adults', including supplementing pediatric supplies and having access to pediatric-specific resources for assistance.

## Response and Recovery Phases

Response comprises all activities and actions taken during and immediately after a disaster. This includes initial search and rescue, damage assessment, evacuation, sheltering, and many other activities. Disaster response in the United States is usually coordinated by local agencies but can be augmented by state and federal response resources. The response phase lasts until the initial casualties have either been rescued or acknowledged as lost and sufficient resources have been made available to allow the population to assess damages and begin plans for restoration and recovery. This phase can last hours to weeks.

The recovery phase is the period in which the affected organization or community works toward re-establishing self-sufficiency. This is the period of new community planning, rebuilding, and the re-establishment of government and public service infrastructure. It is also the period in which outside support services are gradually withdrawn.

The response and recovery phases can represent a challenge from the medical standpoint because injuries can increase during damage assessment and physical rebuilding. Emotional and mental health problems often become evident in this time period as well; as reality sinks in, future challenges become much more overwhelming. Victims sometimes feel abandoned as immediate response resources withdraw and attention and assistance from other communities wane.

## Emergency Medical Services

EMS and other public safety agencies are the first official line of response during and after disasters. Response duties for EMS providers might include search and rescue, multicasualty triage, initial treatment and transport, establishment of casualty collection points, damage assessment, and hazard mitigation in addition to their usual EMS responsibilities. Non–disaster-related EMS and public safety demands continue and might even increase in a disaster. In community-wide disasters, mutual aid agreements allow outside EMS agencies to respond to assist local resources, both inside the damage zone and throughout the community. In large-scale disasters, especially those affecting the EMS system itself (as in the World Trade Center incident, or when stations and equipment are damaged), outside EMS, fire, and law enforcement agencies from around the country send personnel and apparatus to operate in the affected area under guidance by local authorities. Good emergency planning will ensure that the mutual aid effort is controlled under a unified command structure and monitored to ensure that the entire community's EMS requirements are met.

The FEMA Community Emergency Response Team (CERT) program is receiving increasing attention around the United States. The CERT concept was developed and implemented by the Los Angeles Fire Department in 1985, as a way to train and prepare volunteer civilian teams to augment emergency response resources after an earthquake. FEMA recognized the concept and now assists with the development of local CERTs using an all-hazards curriculum developed by the Emergency Management Institute and the National Fire Academy. CERTs have been established by neighborhood associations, church groups, community service organiza-

tions, special interest clubs, and many other types of organizations. Team members are trained in disaster preparedness, emergency medical assessment and basic triage and treatment, light search and rescue, basic fire suppression, disaster psychology, and volunteer management. Additional information about the CERT program is available on the FEMA Web site.[17]

## Hospitals

In disasters with large numbers of casualties or disruption of the community's medical infrastructure, functional hospitals will be challenged to deal with increased patient loads not only immediately after the disaster, but also for weeks or months to follow as the infrastructure is restored. Staffing requirements might increase at a time when staff members themselves have been affected by the disaster and require time off to care for their families, secure their property, and begin the rebuilding process. Additional staffing needs can be met by using temporary agency personnel or pulling staffing from other hospitals in a network. In a federally declared disaster, personnel from DMATs, the US Public Health Service, and the Veterans Administration might be assigned to assist with hospital staffing. Current federal initiatives include the development of a volunteer Medical Reserve Corps (MRC). MRC members would most likely be used to augment local medical resources, possibly to include supplementing clinic and hospital staffing.[18]

Some hospitals and medical professional associations choose to send response resources into an affected area to set up independent patient care sites or to augment existing medical facility capabilities. This kind of response should be preplanned to ensure adequate credentialing and validation of staff, provision of adequate supplies and support services, and coordination with local emergency management to prevent duplication of services and ensure that resources are sent where they are needed most. Hospitals must consider the financial implications of such response services, as expenses might not be reimbursed through FEMA or other agencies.

## Federal Agencies

The Federal Disaster Response Plan details the roles and coordination of various federal agencies and resources expected to respond to a federally declared disaster; Emergency Support Function Eight (ESF 8) is the portion of the plan dealing with health and medical issues.[11] The National Disaster Medical System (NDMS) is a consortium of government, public, and private agencies responsible for providing medical assistance under ESF 8. The NDMS was initially established to organize a domestic response to the evacuation of large numbers of casualties into the United States from a war zone. Its role now has expanded to include responses to all types of disasters, including terrorist events. NDMS resources include US Public Health Service teams, Veterans Administration personnel, DMATs, Veterinary Medical Assistance Teams (VMATs), and Disaster Mortuary Teams (DMORTs). More information is available about these teams on the NDMS Web site.[19]

DMATs are volunteer teams made up of physicians, nurses, EMS providers, logisticians, and other administrative and support personnel. The original concept of a DMAT was to act as the civilian equivalent of a Mobile Army Surgical Hospital (MASH) unit, with the capability of acting as a fully equipped emergency care unit with self-sufficiency for 3 days without resupply or other support. A fully deployed DMAT should have the capability to at least stabilize critically ill and injured children and provide basic inpatient-type care for stable children until other resources are available. Currently, not every DMAT has a pediatrician on call, but several do.

The first large-scale deployment of DMATs in the MASH-type role was after Hurricane Andrew in Dade County, Florida, in 1992. DMAT missions since then have evolved to include replacement of hospital and EMS personnel, special medical coverage for mass gatherings such as the Olympics, shelter sick-call and outpatient clinic services (New York State ice storms, several flood deployments), and medical support for responders (World Trade Center and Pentagon bombings, and wildfires). In some of these missions, the US Public Health Service requisitions the services of specific types of team members rather than entire teams. DMATs sometimes function as local and state resources and respond to state-declared disasters or provide medical coverage for local mass gathering events. There are also several specialty DMATs, including two pediatric DMATs, based in Boston and Atlanta. Other specialty units address burn care and mental health.

VMATs and DMORTs are other NDMS resources. VMATs have been deployed to care for displaced and injured animals after disasters and to support search and rescue canines. They provided an invaluable service at the World Trade Center site, with hundreds of patient contacts for the care of injured search canines, and prevention of injuries to the animals and their partners. DMORTs comprise mortuary and forensic specialists. These teams have been deployed even more often than DMATs, as their specialty in handling, identifying, and preserving human remains has proved invaluable, especially after terrorist attacks and aircraft crashes.

Urban Search and Rescue taskforces (USARs) are teams of personnel trained in heavy rescue and special search operations; they are usually based in fire departments. Federally coordinated by FEMA, USARs also include medical specialists, communications specialists, and engineers. Although most USAR physicians are emergency physicians and surgeons, several are pediatricians. USAR medical capabilities for dealing with children should be at or above the level of a well-trained and equipped advanced life support EMS service in the United States. The USAR medical team members are primarily responsible for the health and welfare of human and canine team members, who often work in very hazardous environments. A medical team's secondary and tertiary duties are to care for entrapped victims and other disaster victims. In a large-scale disaster, USARs perform search and rescue, provide initial treatment for entrapped victims, and then turn the patients over to local hospitals or on-site DMATs. Most USARs respond domestically; however, several have been designated for international response as well. USARs have responded to numerous earthquakes in the United States and around the world, as well as major terrorist events in the United States. More information about USARs is available on the FEMA Web site.[20]

### Individual Volunteerism

Numerous opportunities exist for individuals with medical training who want to volunteer for disaster response. CERTs train and work within their own communities. Some medical professional associations maintain registries of members available to respond after disasters. The Red Cross and Salvation Army are critical response resources and always need volunteers, especially to work in shelters. The previously mentioned federal disaster teams are made up of volunteers and always need more personnel.

Volunteering with an organization integrated into disaster planning is more productive and much safer than going into a disaster zone alone. Volunteer organizations provide training and ensure that safety measures are taken for the protection of personnel. They will ensure that supplies and support services are available and will work within the emergency management command structure to put volunteers where they will be of most use. For an individual to pack his or her car with supplies and head into a chaotic disaster scene is potentially foolish and dangerous, regardless of any altruistic motivation. Just as individual physicians should carefully plan and prepare in advance in case they become disaster victims, they should also plan and prepare to be disaster response volunteers.

### Mitigation Phase

Mitigation is the phase in which all other aspects of emergency management are scrutinized for "lessons learned." The lessons are then applied in an effort to prevent the recurrence of the disaster itself or to lessen the effects of subsequent incidents. Mitigation and planning are continuous operations, as lessons learned from previous disasters are rolled into planning for the next one. Mitigation includes preventive and precautionary actions such as changing building codes and practices, redesigning public utilities and services, revising mandatory evacuation practices and warning policies, and educating members of the community.

### Pediatric Medical Issues After Community-wide Disasters

Small-scale multiple casualty incidents occur daily in the United States. Few present unusual challenges to the local medical systems other than in the number of patients that must be managed at one time. Except in earthquakes, explosions, building collapses, and some types of terrorist attacks, the same holds true for large-scale disasters. Sudden, violent disaster mechanisms can produce major trauma cases, including

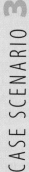

**CASE SCENARIO 3**

A major earthquake severely damages large portions of a major city, including several major hospitals and many private health care offices and facilities. Thousands of people are left homeless, and many have been injured. Hospitals have already been overloaded due to a very active influenza season.

1. *Does your hospital or office have a realistic evacuation plan?*
2. *Is your hospital or office prepared to take on extra loads for potentially long periods of time when the local medical infrastructure is damaged?*
3. *How can your hospital and community medical practitioners benefit from, interact with, and assist response teams from the National Disaster Medical System?*

patients needing field amputations or management of crush syndrome.[21–23] For the most part, medicine after a disaster is much the same as it was before the disaster, with more minor injuries, more people with exacerbations of their chronic illnesses, and a number of patients seeking what is ordinarily considered primary care. This is true for children as well as adults.

## Predisposition of Children to Illness and Injury After a Disaster

Children can be unusually predisposed to injury after a disaster. Adults who normally supervise them might be preoccupied with recovery tasks. They also can be at risk from increased environmental hazards such as collapsed or exposed construction elements, the availability of dangerous tools such as chainsaws, exposure to the elements, animals, and insects, and the availability of hazardous chemicals and objects such as kerosene, gasoline, candles, and generators. Children often want to assist with repairs and might wind up on rooftops or climbing around building or tree wreckage. Disruption of traffic control devices such as traffic lights and signs can lead to an increase in vehicle-related trauma. Families and business owners protecting their property from looters might have weapons that are not secured against curious children. Increased stress levels among adults might even lead to an increase in domestic violence and child abuse.[24] The world can be a much more dangerous place after a disaster; supervision of children is even more important than usual, and even more difficult if the normal supervisory resources of school and childcare are not available.

Acute infectious illnesses generally conform to the patterns existing in the community at the time of the disaster. An epidemic of bronchiolitis or chickenpox will continue to cause problems, possibly to greater degrees because of group sheltering or lesser degrees because children are not crowded together in classrooms. An acute change in diet can lead to food intolerances and gastroenteritis. Exposure to the sun and heat or a shortage of potable water can cause dehydration. Cold environments might lead to hypothermia. Generator and kerosene heater use can lead to carbon monoxide poisoning. Children with allergy-based diseases might have acute exacerbations due to increased and unavoidable allergens in the environment. Any child on medications for a chronic condition can have an acute exacerbation if he or she can not get, or forgets to take, medications. Children with behavioral or psychiatric disorders might get acutely worse because of stress and disruption of their daily routines. Finally, stress itself can produce a variety of symptoms in children, including headache, abdominal pain, chest pain, vomiting, diarrhea, constipation, changes in sleeping patterns, and changes in appetite.

After a community-wide disaster, public health officials commonly monitor for water- and food-borne diseases, such as cholera and other enteric diseases; however, such epidemics have not yet proved to be a problem in the United States. Likewise, although patients frequently request tetanus boosters after a disaster, children who are up-to-date with vaccines do not need them.

## Constraints on Family Access to Care

After disasters, families might not have the ability to seek care for their ill or injured family members as quickly as they ordinarily would. Geographically close medical facilities might not be operational. Families might have lost their means of transportation, or the transportation and road system might be disrupted so badly by damage or disaster relief traffic that a trip outside of the area for medical care could take an entire day. Standing in line for hours for basic survival needs such as food, water, ice, and other supplies might take precedence over seeking medical attention for a seemingly minor complaint. Once a family makes it to medical care, they might not be able to comply well with followup instructions. Good home wound care becomes difficult when water for bathing is in short supply, and every-other-day wound checks can be impossible in the face of other challenges. A child with asthma who needs frequent aerosol treatments might have to be taken from the home every few hours to a place with a generator.

Pharmacies might not be open in the affected area; families might need to take one or two trips out of the area to drop off and pick up prescriptions. These kinds of access to care limitations require changes in decision-making patterns on the part of emergency care providers.

## Constraints on Normal Emergency Department Decision Making

Table 17-5 lists some of the constraints of practicing emergency medicine in a postdisaster setting. Emergency and primary care practitioners might need to change their usual prescribing

---

### TABLE 17-5 Changing Emergency Department Decision Patterns

**Constraint: Lack of Electricity at Home**

**Altered Decision Patterns:**

- Prescribe metered-dose inhalers with spacer chambers for inhaled medications.
- Provide a few power outlets or pressurized oxygen/room air tanks or outlets for use by families for aerosol treatments with their own medications.
- For younger children, prescribe chewable tablets and liquid medication preparations that do not require refrigeration. Consider nonchewable tablets and use of a pill cutter.
- Lower admission threshold for children who require treatment with hardwired electrical equipment.

**Constraint: Unavoidable Environmental Exposure**

**Altered Decision Patterns:**

- Distribute sunscreen, sunburn care products, insect repellant, umbrellas, hats, disposable fans, chemical cold or hot packs.
- Advise family of ongoing risks and possible need to send the child away from the area.
- Distribute safety literature about preventive measures and what to look for in cases of environmental illness.

**Constraint: Infectious Diseases**

**Altered Decision Patterns:**

- Consider parenteral antibiotic treatment as starter dose.
- Consider acceptable shorter course of antibiotics and increased dosing interval to improve compliance.
- Consider need for isolation. Decrease admission threshold if child and family are living in a shelter environment and can not make alternative arrangements.
- Demonstrate a child's ability to take and keep down fluids before discharge with gastroenteritis. Liberalize IV and/or formal oral rehydration practices and antiemetic administration.
- Distribute oral rehydration solution, diapers, diaper wipes, alcohol-based hand cleansing solutions.
- Distribute educational literature regarding measures to prevent spread of disease.

**Constraint: Poor Followup/Decreased Access to Care**

**Altered Decision Patterns:**

- Learn what temporary medical facilities have been set up in the affected area, and ask patients to follow up there if possible. Send a note with patient describing what care is needed.
- Specifically instruct families as to what complications absolutely require further medical evaluation.
- Distribute wound care supplies.
- Instruct families in suture removal procedures.
- Confirm alternative contact methods (e.g., leaving message with relative) for children discharged with pending test results, especially cultures.
- Confirm actual current address (e.g., shelter, relative's house) as well as usual address.
- Decrease admission decision thresholds for any condition that might require frequent followup or pose a risk of sudden deterioration.

patterns to accommodate family needs, and they might have to admit children who would ordinarily be discharged with close outpatient followup. Supplies for injury and illness prevention and health maintenance can be distributed by hospitals to patient families and visitors. Targeted patient and family education efforts should be increased in an environment in which access to care is restricted. The media can be very helpful in printing and airing safety and health tips, as well as the locations of temporary medical facilities and pharmacies.

## Pediatric Mental Health Issues After Disasters

In many ways, children are better suited to deal with the psychological aftermath of a disaster than adults are. Most children have enough mental and emotional flexibility to adapt; they benefit from their ability to express their feelings freely, and they have fewer worries than adults who are trying to put their lives back together do.

Children can and do, however, suffer from acute and chronic emotional distress and mental illness after disasters. Many studies have shown that children experience a variety of psychological sequelae, including posttraumatic stress disorder, even if they were not directly involved in the disaster themselves.[25–34] In the immediate postdisaster stage, it is important to reestablish a sense of order and routine and to ensure children that they are safe. Expect regressive behavior; children might wet the bed or cling to their parents instead of showing their usual independent spirit. They can experience rapid mood changes, interrupted sleep, and nightmares.

It is important to explain a disaster to children in words they can understand, not to lie about loved ones or acquaintances who might have been injured or killed, and to encourage children to express their feelings in talk, play, or art. Adults should express their own concerns and feelings in front of their children but should not subject children to extreme emotional displays. Children should be shown im-

ages of the disaster so they have an authentic picture of what happened, but this should be done in an environment that permits guided discussion. Do not allow children to watch television news clips that repeatedly display disturbing images or footage that graphically portrays injury and death. Children who exhibit signs of ongoing stress and depression, such as headaches, chronic abdominal pain, recurrent nightmares, changes in sleep patterns, deterioration in behavior or school performance, personality changes, drug abuse,[35] or suicidal ideation should undergo full medical and psychological evaluation. Monitoring children for signs of mental illness after a disaster should be a part of recovery planning by families, school systems, social service agencies, primary care providers, and mental health professionals.[36–38]

## Summary

Disasters of all types and sizes occur daily, striking without regard for the ages of their victims. Children can and will be directly and indirectly affected by many kinds of disasters. The issues of children and families must be included in disaster planning at all levels, from family preparedness, to office and hospital preparedness, to community emergency management.

The United States is fortunate to be rich in disaster response resources on local, state, regional, and national levels. All responders must be trained and equipped at their appropriate levels to address the unique physical, medical, and emotional needs of children and their families in a disaster setting. Many more responders are needed to ensure that all possible resources can be made available to disaster victims. Medical professionals can find many opportunities to help. Some opportunities demand little time and energy; others require a significant commitment to training, team management, and response. All volunteer efforts can be both personally and professionally rewarding.

Children are at increased risk for injury and illness both during and after disasters;

however, with the exception of the more sudden, violent types of disasters, most injuries and illnesses are in keeping with typical childhood patterns. Emergency and primary care providers in the post-disaster setting must be prepared to adjust their normal practices to conform to the constraints placed on patients and their families. Mental health issues have been frequently identified in pediatric disaster victims and can affect children and their families far beyond the time when physical injuries have healed. All child advocates must be aware of these potential problems and learn how to incorporate childhood mental health surveillance and interventions into their ongoing disaster plans.

# CHAPTER REVIEW

## Check Your Knowledge

1. After a disaster, families should plan to be self-sufficient for:
   A. 12 hours
   B. 24 hours
   C. 48 hours
   D. 72 hours

2. Which of the following factors can precipitate problems for children with special health care needs after a disaster?
   A. Inability to avoid allergens
   B. Lack of electricity
   C. Lack of refrigeration/cooling capabilities
   D. Stress and disruption in daily routines
   E. All of the above

3. Which of the following statements about multicasualty triage is correct?
   A. An objective triage system helps to optimize patient classification and resource allocation
   B. Children should automatically be given the highest triage priorities
   C. Responders should attempt to resuscitate all children in full cardiopulmonary arrest in a mass casualty incident setting
   D. Triage personnel should go to the most critical patients first
   E. All of the above

4. Which of the following issues should be included in hospital disaster planning?
   A. A command structure, such as HEICS
   B. Critical incident stress monitoring and services
   C. External disasters
   D. Internal disasters
   E. All of the above

## References

1. Heath SE, Kass PH, Beck AM, Glickman LT. Human and pet-related factors for household evacuation failure during a natural disaster. *Am J Epidemiol.* 2001;153(7):659–665.
2. Jacob J. Disaster plan can safeguard your practice, records. American Medical Association Web site. Available at: http://www.ama-assn.org/sci-pubs/amnews/pick_01/bica1022.htm. Accessed June 23, 2001.
3. Klinzing G, McClure C. Could your office cope with disaster? American Academy of Family Physicians Web site. Available at: http://www.aafp.org/fpm/990900fm/26.html. Accessed June 23, 2001.
4. Committee on Pediatric Emergency Medicine. The pediatrician's role in disaster preparedness. *Pediatrics.* 1997;99(1):130–133.
5. Benson M, Koenig KL, Schultz CH. Disaster triage: START then SAVE—a new method of dynamic triage for victims of a catastrophic earthquake. *Prehospital Disaster Med.* 1996;11(2):117–124.
6. Van Amerongen RH, Fine JS, Tunik MG, et al. The Avianca plane crash: an emergency medical system's response to pediatric survivors of the disaster. *Pediatrics.* 1993;92(1):105–110.
7. Smith M. Get smart: JumpSTART! *Emerg Med Serv.* 2001;30(5):46–48, 50.
8. Romig LE. Pediatric triage: a system to JumpSTART your triage of young patients at MCIs. *JEMS.* 2002;27(7):52–63.
9. Garner A, Lee A, Harrison K, Schultz CH. Comparative analysis of multiple-casualty incident triage algorithms. *Ann Emerg Med.* 2001;38(5)541–548.
10. Meredith W, Rutledge R, Hansen AR, et al. Field triage of trauma patients based upon the ability to follow commands: a study in 29,573 injured patients. *J Trauma.* 1995;38:129–135.
11. Hospital Emergency Incident Command System Update Project. California Emergency Medical Services Authority Web site. Available at: http://www.emsa.cahwnet.gov/dms2/heics3.htm. Accessed June 24, 2002.
12. Introduction to the Basic Plan of the Federal Response Plan, April 1999. FEMA Web site. Available at: http://www.fema.gov/rrr/frp/frpintro.shtm. Accessed July 17, 2002.
13. Position Statement: School Nurse Role in Emergency Preparedness. National Association of School Nurses (NASN) Web site. Available at: http://www.nasn.org/positions/emergencyprep.htm. Accessed June 24, 2002.
14. Position Statement: Emergency Care Plans for Students with Special Health Care Needs. NASN Web site. Available at: http://www.nasn.org/positions/emer_care.htm. Accessed June 24, 2002.
15. Managing School Emergencies. NASN Web site. Available at: http://www.nasn.org/continuinged/mse.htm. Accessed June 24, 2002.
16. Emergency Preparedness for Children with Special Health Care Needs. AAP Web site.

Available at: http://www.aap.org/advocacy/epquesansw.htm. Accessed June 24, 2002.

17. Community Emergency Response Teams. FEMA Web site. Available at: http://training.fema.gov/EMIWeb/cert. Accessed July 17, 2002.

18. Medical Reserve Corps. Citizen Corps Web site. Available at http://www.citizencorps.gov/medical.html. Accessed September 30, 2002.

19. About Teams. NDMS Web site. Available at: http://www.ndms.dhhs.gov/NDMS/About_Teams/about_teams.html. Accessed July 17, 2002.

20. National Urban Search and Rescue Response System. FEMA Web site. Available at: http://www.fema.gov/usr/. Accessed July 17, 2002.

21. Donmez O, Meral A, Yavuz M, Durmaz O. Crush syndrome in the Maramara earthquake, Turkey. *Pediatr Int.* 2001;43(6):678–682.

22. Iskit SH, Alpay H, Tugtepe H, et al. Analysis of 33 pediatric victims in the 1999 Marmara, Turkey earthquake. *J Pediatr Surg.* 2001;36(2):368–372.

23. Quintana DA, Parker JR, Jordan FB, et al. The spectrum of pediatric injuries after a bomb blast. *J Pediatr Surg.* 1997;32(2):307–310.

24. Curtis T, Miller BC, Berry EH. Changes in reports and incidence of child abuse following natural disasters. *Child Abuse Negl.* 2000;24(9):1151–1162.

25. Shaw JA, Applegate B, Tanner S, et al. Psychological effects of Hurricane Andrew on an elementary school population. *J Am Acad Child Adolesc Psychiatry.* 1995;34(9):1185–1192.

26. Shaw JA, Applegate B, Schorr C. Twenty-one month follow-up study of school-age children exposed to Hurricane Andrew. *J Am Acad Child Adolesc Psychiatry.* 1996;35(3):359–364.

27. La Greca A, Silverman WK, Vernberg EM, Prinstein MJ. Symptoms of posttraumatic stress in children after Hurricane Andrew: a prospective study. *J Consult Clin Psychol.* 1996;64(4):712–723.

28. Pfefferbaum B, Nixon SJ, Tucker PM, et al. Posttraumatic stress responses in bereaved children after the Oklahoma City bombing. *J Am Acad Child Adolesc Psychiatry.* 1999;38(11):1372–1379.

29. Yule W, Bolton D, Udwin O, et al. The long-term psychological effects of a disaster experienced in adolescence: I: The incidence and course of PTSD. *J Child Psychol Psychiatry.* 2000;41(4):503–511.

30. Yule W, Bolton D, Udwin O, et al. The long-term psychological effects of a disaster experienced in adolescence: II: General psychopathology. *J Child Psychol Psychiatry.* 2000;41(4):513–523.

31. Pfefferbaum B, Seale TW, McDonald NB, et al. Posttraumatic stress two years after the Oklahoma City bombing in youths geographically distant from the explosion. *Psychiatry.* 2000;63(4):358–370.

32. Goenjian AK, Molina L, Steinberg AM, et al. Posttraumatic stress and depressive reactions among Nicaraguan adolescents after hurricane Mitch. *Am J Psychiatry.* 2001;158(5):788–794.

33. Kitayama S, Okada Y, Takumi T, et al. Psychological and physical reactions on children after the Hanshin-Awaji earthquake disaster. *Kobe J Med Sci.* 2000;46(5):189–200.

34. Jones RT, Ribbe DP, Cunningham PB, et al. Psychological impact of fire disaster on children and their parents. *Behav Modif.* 2002;26(2):163–186.

35. Vlahov D, Galea S, Resnick H, et al. Increased use of cigarettes, alcohol, and marijuana among Manhattan, New York, residents after the September 11th terrorist attacks. *Am J Epidemiol.* 2002;155(11):988–996.

36. Dyregrove A. Family recovery from terror, grief and trauma. International Critical Incident Stress Foundation (ICISF) Web site. Available at: http://www.icisf.org/articles/Acrobat%20Documents/TerrorismIncident/Terrorovertime.htm. Accessed July 18, 2002.

37. Raundalen M, and Dyregrov A. Terror: How to Talk to Children. ICISF Web site. Available at: http://www.icisf.org/articles/Acrobat%20Documents/TerrorismIncident/Dyregrov_terrorism.htm. Accessed July 18, 2002.

38. Children's Reactions and Needs after Disaster. ICISF Web site. Available at: http://www.icisf.org/articles/Acrobat%20Documents/TerrorismIncident/Children_and_terroristattack.htm. Accessed July 18, 2002.

A disaster shelter with 130 evacuees is struck and heavily damaged by a tornado during the storm. Per local protocol, emergency medical services units are unable to respond due to the intensity of the weather. Adult and pediatric victims of the tornado start arriving by the carload at the nearby emergency department, stating that other victims will be following them, as it is impossible to travel further to other facilities.

1. *Does your hospital disaster plan consider self-referred victims instead of just those arriving by emergency medical services? Is your emergency department staff prepared to perform primary disaster triage?*
2. *Does your hospital disaster plan consider adequate staffing and resources to allow emergency medical services to function at high demand levels with minimal outside assistance?*

The hospital activates its disaster plan and sets up a triage area in the parking lot, where all patients are sent initially. Emergency department nurses and a physician begin the process of patient triage, and critically ill or injured patients are then taken directly into the emergency department. Those with serious problems are triaged and treated in the urgent care/fast-track clinic area, and the less urgent patients are cared for in the parking lot, or await space in the emergency department. The hospital disaster plan includes calling in additional physicians, nurses, social work, administrative, and other support staff from all areas of the hospital.

A school bus full of elementary students and their chaperones on a field trip skids on a patch of ice and overturns. Several children are thrown free of the bus. Some children and adults have left the bus under their own power; others are trapped inside the badly damaged bus. The air is full of the screams and cries of children.

1. *Are your local emergency medical services agencies prepared to appropriately rescue, triage, treat, and transport this number of patients, especially the seriously injured children?*
2. *Which of your local hospitals would be able to handle critically ill children? Will the closest trauma center be able to handle all of these patients? Some local emergency departments have low pediatric volumes. Will they be able to assist with some of the less critical victims?*

The emergency medical services system calls a mass casualty incident, activates its disaster plan, and calls for mutual aid ambulances. Children and adults are appropriately triaged, and contact is made with local hospitals regarding patient capabilities. The nearby pediatric trauma center receives all of the seriously and moderately injured children, while seriously and moderately injured adults are transported to the adult trauma center. The "walking wounded" (minor injuries), are transported to another (nontrauma center) local hospital.

**CASE SUMMARY 3**

A major earthquake severely damages large portions of a major city, including several major hospitals and many private health care offices and facilities. Thousands of people are left homeless and many have been injured. Hospitals have already been overloaded due to a very active influenza season.

1. *Does your hospital or office have a realistic evacuation plan?*
2. *Is your hospital or office prepared to take on extra loads for potentially long periods of time when the local medical infrastructure is damaged?*
3. *How can your hospital and community medical practitioners benefit from, interact with, and assist response teams from the National Disaster Medical System?*

---

One of your offices has been slightly damaged by the earthquake, but the other is still functioning. The medical records are secure in the damaged office, and duplicates exist at the other office. Due to the magnitude of the earthquake, you realize that your injured patients are likely to go to the local emergency department, so you go to the hospital to lend assistance, as you are on staff there. It is important to realize that federal aid often is not available within the first 24 hours of the disaster—this is why local resources are critical in the first 24 to 48 hours of a disaster.

# chapter 18

# Preparedness for Acts of Nuclear, Biological, and Chemical Terrorism

Fred M. Henretig, MD
Michele R. McKee, MD, FAAP

## Objectives

1 Distinguish signs and symptoms of common childhood illnesses from those caused by biological agents.

2 Formulate a treatment plan for children exposed to chemical agents.

3 Discuss short-term and long-term effects of radiation exposure in children.

## Chapter Outline

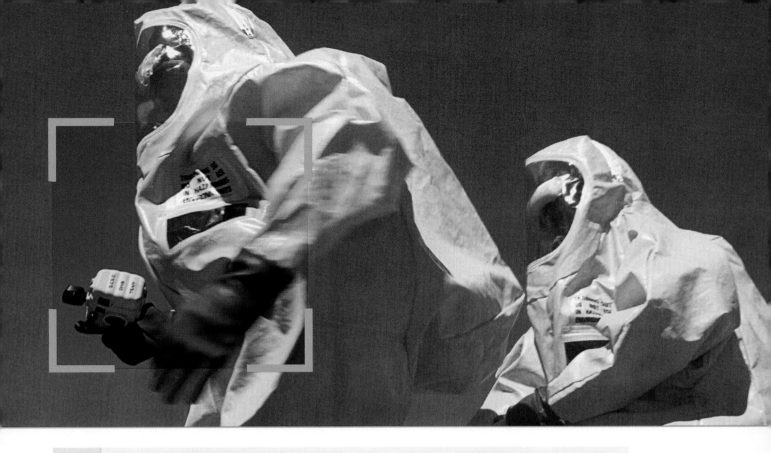

## CASE SCENARIO 1

You receive a call from paramedics who are bringing in many students from a nearby school. The students are complaining of burning eyes and throat pain.

1. *What agents are most likely to cause these symptoms?*
2. *What type of decontamination is needed?*
3. *What do you tell parents?*

## Introduction

The tragic events of September 11, 2001, and the subsequent outbreak of mail-borne anthrax cases have escalated concern among pediatricians and related child health professionals regarding possible acts of terrorism directed against children. An emerging threat is terrorism using weapons of mass destruction (WMD), or "unconventional threats," including those due to biological, chemical, and radiation exposures. Numerous reviews and consensus guidelines for biological agents,[1–6] an article focusing on pediatric issues in biological and chemical terrorism,[7] and a summary of nuclear and radiological exposures[8] have been published. In addition, several relevant Internet Web sites have been developed to provide a more detailed description of individual agents and up-to-date management advice (Table 18-1).

## Epidemiology of WMD Terrorism

Most authorities expect that a terrorist attack with biological or chemical agents would utilize an aerosol route of exposure. A radiological attack might include explosions at a nuclear reactor, a "dirty bomb" utilizing conventional explosives to disperse radioactive

| TABLE 18-1 | Resources/contacts |
|---|---|

**In-House**
- Epidemiology
- Hospital administrator
- Infection control
- Nuclear medicine/radiology staff consultation
- Public affairs
- Radiation safety office

**Off-Site**
- Center for Civilian Biodefense Strategies (www.hopkins-biodefense.org)
- Centers for Disease Control (at request of state/territory agency, clinical resource, www.bt.cdc.gov)
- Emergency Response Hotline
- Federal Bureau of Investigation (crisis management, www.fbi.gov)
- Federal Emergency Management Agency (consequence management, www.fema.gov)
- Federal Emergency Management Association
- Local/state health departments (www.statepublichealth.org/index.php and www.cdc.gov/other.htm#states)
- Nuclear, biological, chemical resources (www.nbc-med.org)
- Poison Control Center
- The Radiation Emergency Assistance Center/Training Site (REAC/TS, www.orau.gov/reacts)
- US Armed Forces Radiobiology Research Institute (www.afrri.usuhs.mil)
- US Army Medical Research Institute of Chemical Defense
- US Army Medical Research Institute of Infectious Disease (www.usamriid.army.mil)
- US Military Agency Resources (educational and practical resources)

material, or conceivably a nuclear weapon. A chemical or radiological attack would likely combine elements of the traditional mass casualty disaster and a hazardous materials incident. Most victims would be recognized early on, and many would receive field care and decontamination by emergency medical services (EMS) personnel. Still, many patients will self-transport to hospitals without prior care; hospitals have to be vigilant and prepared to provide some decontamination and

triage capacity as well as definitive care. Every hospital emergency department should have some preparation for such an incident, including familiarity of these agents by health care providers, some stocking of appropriate antidotes, a quickly deployable decontamination unit, and personal protective equipment (PPE) for those emergency department staff who will be expected to assist with decontamination and provide emergent resuscitative care, prior to or coincident with decontamination.

In contrast, a biological event would likely present similarly to a natural infectious disease epidemic, with numerous patients becoming ill at points remote in time and place from the exposure. However, such an intentional epidemic would likely be more compressed in time due to the synchronous exposure, involve relatively exotic diseases uncommon in a given geographic area, and might exhibit particularly high rates of morbidity and mortality. Pediatricians and emergency physicians would likely be the first responders for pediatric victims in this context. Early recognition of such an epidemic would be very advantageous in mitigating the number of casualties, and would likely provide some protection for physicians themselves. Education regarding these agents and heightened anticipation on the part of emergency, pediatric, and primary-care physicians can facilitate such early recognition.

## Specific Vulnerabilities in Children

Several physiologic, developmental, and psychological considerations unique to children can increase their vulnerability to a WMD attack.[9] Children have higher minute ventilation and "live closer to the ground," potentially enhancing exposure to airborne toxins, infectious particles, or radioactive fallout. Infants and toddlers would be limited in their ability to escape danger, particularly if adult caregivers were critically injured or dead. The witnessed loss of parents or siblings might lead to extraordinary posttraumatic stress reactions. In addition, our national EMS system might be less capable of handling a large surge in pediatric patients than it would be for adults, given the less frequent EMS experience with critical pediatric patients and diminished capacity for rapid expansion of pediatric hospital beds. EMS staff garbed in bulky PPE would be particularly handicapped when challenged by the need to perform emergency procedures on infants and small children.

## Major Biological Agents

Though numerous infectious pathogens or biological toxins might be utilized to cause intentional harm, the Centers for Disease Control and Prevention (CDC) has classified six biological agents as those posing the greatest terrorist threat: anthrax, smallpox, plague, botulinum, tularemia and viral hemorrhagic fevers (VHFs). The United States has been inflicted by only two documented large-scale attacks. The first occurred in 1984 in Oregon when a religious cult infected over 750 persons with Salmonella.[10] The second one was the October 2001 outbreak related to anthrax-contaminated mail.[6]

### Clinical Features

The natural diseases caused by these agents have characteristic incubation periods from time of exposure, ranging from 1 to 5 days for anthrax, plague, and botulism (though low-dose exposure to weaponized anthrax spores can result in very prolonged incubation, up to 6 to 8 weeks), 2 to 10 days for tularemia, 7 to 17 days for smallpox, and 4 to 21 days for VHFs. Anthrax, plague, tularemia, smallpox, and VHFs are infectious diseases, and all begin with a nonspecific flu-like prodrome of fever, fatigue, malaise, and headache that can last 1 to 3 days before more characteristic signs and symptoms evolve. Diagnosis of the first patients to present would therefore be very difficult in this context. Unfortunately, antibiotic treatment for inhalational anthrax and pneumonic plague is most effective in preventing mortality when begun within the first day or two. Even so, the recognition of subsequent characteristic clinical syndromes of these diseases might allow earlier treatment for those affected individuals who follow. Botulism, a syndrome caused by the systemic absorption of a bacterial toxin, is actually more familiar to pediatricians than to most other US physicians because of the occurrence of infantile botulism. Patients poisoned by inhaling weaponized botulinum toxin are likely to present very similarly to those with natural disease. Smallpox causes a unique exanthem that is unfamiliar to most practicing pediatricians today and might be confused with severe varicella. The clinical features, appropriate laboratory tests, and antibiotic therapy for these diseases are described below and summarized in Table 18-2.

## Anthrax

Anthrax is caused by *Bacillus anthracis,* a Gram-positive, sporulating, rod-shaped bacterium.[1] Natural anthrax is a rare bacterial disease in the United States, but has now become infamous after the October 2001 outbreak. In nature it manifests as cutaneous, gastrointestinal, or inhalational forms, contracted by human contact with infected animals or animal products such as unprocessed wool or animal hides, or by eating contaminated meat. In the recent mail-borne attack, there were 22 cases, characterized as either cutaneous or inhalational,[11] with five deaths, all in the inhalational group.[6] The only pediatric victim was a 7-month-old boy with cutaneous anthrax on his arm, initially suspected of having a brown recluse spider bite. He also developed microangiopathic hemolytic anemia and renal insufficiency, but survived.[11]

### Clinical Features

Cutaneous anthrax begins as a papular lesion and progresses rapidly over 7 to 10 days through several stages of vesicle to ulcer to deep, black eschar, with marked surrounding edema. The lesions remain relatively painless, an important distinguishing feature

**TABLE 18-2    Critical Biological Agents of Terrorism**

| Disease | Etiology | Clinical Findings[1] | Incubation Period | Diagnostic Samples | Diagnostic Assay | Isolation Precautions[2] | Initial Treatment | Prophylaxis |
|---|---|---|---|---|---|---|---|---|
| Anthrax | Bacillus anthracis | Inhalational: febrile prodrome with rapid progression to mediastinal lymphadenitis, mediastinitis (chest x-ray: +/− infiltrates, widened mediastinum, pleural effusions); sepsis; shock; meningitis | 1–5 days | Blood CSF Pleural fluid | Culture Gram stain ELISA PCR | Standard | Ciprofloxacin: 10–15 mg/kg (max 500 mg) IV q12h, or Doxycycline: 2.2 mg/kg (max 100 mg) IV q12h[3] | Ciprofloxacin: 10–15 mg/kg (max 500 mg) PO q12h × 60d, or Doxycycline: 2.5 mg/kg (max 100 mg) PO q12h × 60d[4] |
| | | Cutaneous: papule progressing to vesicle, to ulcer, then to depressed black eschar, with marked edema | | Skin biopsy | Immunohisto-chemical assay | | | |
| Plague | Yersinia pestis | Febrile prodrome with rapid progression to fulminant pneumonia with bloody sputum, sepsis, DIC | 2–4 days | Blood Sputum Lymph node aspirate | Culture Gram or Wright-Giemsa stain ELISA, IFA Ag-ELISA | Pneumonic: droplet until patient treated for 3 days | Gentamicin: 2.5 mg/kg IV q8h[5] or Doxycycline: 2.2 mg/kg (max 100 mg) IV q12h, or Ciprofloxacin 15 mg/kg (max 500 mg) IV q12h, or Chloramphenicol 25 mg/kg (max 1 g) IV q6h | Doxycycline 2.2 mg/kg (max 100 mg) 10d PO q12h × 10d, or Ciprofloxacin 20 mg/kg (max 500 mg) PO q12h × 10d, or Chloramphenicol 25 mg/kg (max 1 g) PO q6h × 7d |
| Smallpox | Variola virus | Febrile prodrome Synchronous vesicopustular eruption, predominant on face and extremities | 7–17 days | Pharyngeal swab Scab material | ELISA, PCR Virus isolation | Airborne, droplet, contact | Supportive care | Vaccination within 4 days (consider Vaccinia immunoglobulin: 0.6 mL/kg IM within 3 days of exposure for vaccine complications, immunocompro-mised persons) |

*(continues)*

**TABLE 18-2  Critical Biological Agents of Terrorism (Continued)**

| Disease | Etiology | Clinical Findings[1] | Incubation Period | Diagnostic Samples | Diagnostic Assay | Isolation Precautions[2] | Initial Treatment | Prophylaxis |
|---------|----------|---------------------|-------------------|-------------------|-----------------|-------------------------|-------------------|-------------|
| Tularemia | *Francisella tularensis* | Pneumonic: abrupt onset fever, fulminant pneumonia (chest x-ray: prominent hilar adenopathy) Typhoidal: fever, malaise, abdominal pain | 2–10 days | Blood Sputum Serum Tissue | Culture[6] Serology: agglutination EM | Standard | Gentamicin 2.5 mg/kg IV q8h[5], or Doxycycline 2.2 mg/kg (max 100 mg) IV q12h, or Ciprofloxacin 15 mg/kg (max 500 mg) IV q12h, or Chloramphenicol 15 mg/kg (max 1 g) IV q6h | Doxycycline 2.2 mg/kg (max 100 mg) PO q12h×14d, or Ciprofloxacin 15 mg/kg (max 500 mg) PO q12h×14d |
| Botulism | *Clostridium botulinum* toxin | Afebrile Descending flaccid paralysis Cranial nerve palsies Sensation and mentation intact | 1–5 days | Nasal swab | Mouse bioassay, Ag-ELISA | Standard | CDC trivalent antitoxin (serotypes A, B, E), 1 vial (10 mL) IV DOD heptavalent antitoxin (serotypes A–G) (IND) California Dept of Health immunoglobulin (IND) | None |
| Viral hemorrhagic fevers | Arenaviridae (Lassa fever) Filoviridae (Ebola, Marburg) | Febrile prodrome; rapid progression to shock, purpura, bleeding diathesis | 4–21 days | Serum Blood | Viral isolation Ag-ELISA RT-PCR Serology: Ab-ELISA | Contact, droplet; consider airborne if massive hemorrhage | Supportive care Ribavirin (arenaviruses) 30 mg/kg IV initially 15 mg/kg IV q6h × 4d 7.5 mg/kg IV q8h × 6d | None |

[1]Syndrome expected after aerosol exposure.

[2]Brief definition of isolation precautions:

Standard—hand-washing; gloves, masks, eye protection , face shields, and nonsterile, fluid-resistant gowns for blood, body fluid exposure; appropriate handling of patient care equipment, linens, etc; avoidance of needle-stick, sharps injury.

Airborne—standard, + private, negative-pressure room with external exhaust or HEPA filtered recirculated air; special "fitted" and " sealing" respirator masks, e.g., N95.

Droplet—standard, + private room, "routine" mask within 3 feet of patient.

Contact—standard, + private room; gloves at all times; hand-washing after glove removal; gowns at all times, removed prior to leaving patient's room.

Adapted from: American Academy of Pediatrics. Infection control for hospitalized children. In: Pickering LK, ed. 2000 *Redbook: Report of the Committee on Infectious Diseases*. 25th ed. Elk Grove Village, IL. American Academy of Pediatrics; 2000: 127–137.

[3]CDC recommended one or two additional antibiotics for inhalational anthrax in Fall 2001 outbreak: rifampin, vancomycin, penicillin or ampicillin, clindamycin, imipenem, or clarithromycin. Recommendations in future outbreaks might evolve rapidly, and frequent consultation with local health departments and CDC (1-770-488-7100; www.bt.cdc.gov) is encouraged.

[4]Amoxicillin 80 mg/kg/day divided q8h can be substituted if strain proves susceptible.

[5]Streptomycin 15 mg/kg IM q12h may be substituted if available.

[6]Laboratory must be notified that tularemia is suspected.

Key: CSF= cerebrospinal fluid; ELISA= enzyme-linked immunosorbent assay; Ag=antigen; PCR= polymerase chain reaction; max=maximum dose; DIC= disseminated intravascular coagulation; IFA=immunofluorescent assay; EM= electron microscopy; DOD= Department of Defense; IND=investigational new drug; RT= reverse transcriptase; Ab=antibody

Reprinted with permission from Henretig et al., 2002.[7]

Reprinted from *Journal of Pediatrics*, Vol. 141, No. 3, Tables 3 and 4 from Henretig FM et al., "Biological and Chemical Agents of Terrorism" pg 311–326 ©2002, with permission from Elsevier Science.

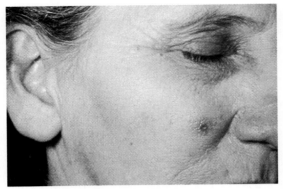

A. Lesion as seen on fourth day.

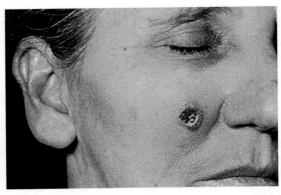

B. Lesion as seen on sixth day.

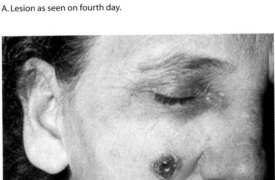

C. Lesion as seen on eleventh day.

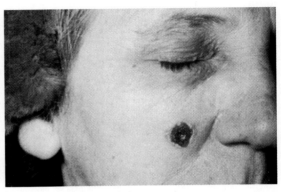

D. Lesion as seen on thirteenth day.

**Figure 18.1** Stages of development of cutaneous anthrax.

from ordinary cellulitis (**Figures 18.1 A, B, C, D**). Inhalational anthrax begins with a 1-day to 2-day febrile prodrome. In contrast to viral flu-like syndromes, patients have a paucity of upper respiratory findings. This prodromal phase is followed by abrupt onset of a severe respiratory syndrome with dyspnea, cyanosis, and shock due to fulminant hemorrhagic, necrotizing mediastinitis.

## Diagnostic Studies and Management

Chest radiographs might reveal mediastinal widening, infiltrates, and pleural effusion (**Figure 18.2**). This phase can progress to sepsis and meningitis, and mortality is very high in patients who present with fulminant disease prior to the onset of antibiotic therapy. Patients with inhalational anthrax are not contagious to health care providers, though

### YOUR FIRST CLUE

**Signs and Symptoms of Anthrax Infections**

- Cutaneous: Relatively painless papule that progresses over 7 to 10 days to form a black eschar
- Inhalational: Nonspecific febrile illness followed by abrupt onset of severe respiratory distress and shock

### THE CLASSICS

**Radiographic Findings of Inhalational Anthrax**

- Mediastinal widening
- Infiltrates
- Pleural effusion

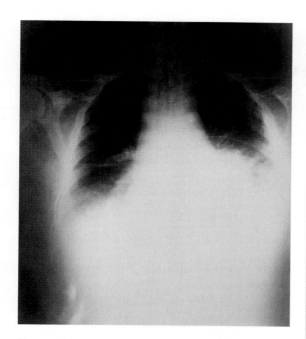

Figure 18.2 Chest radiograph demonstrating mediastinal widening and pleural affusion association with inhalational anthrax.

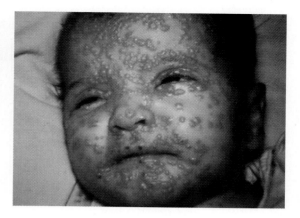

Figure 18.3 Smallpox lesions in a child.

contact precautions are recommended for patients with cutaneous disease. Antibiotic therapy for inhalational or severe cutaneous anthrax includes ciprofloxacin or doxycycline and two or three additional antibiotics (see Table 18-2). Although ciprofloxacin and doxycycline are traditionally used sparingly in children, they are the drugs of choice for inhalational anthrax.

## Smallpox

Smallpox is a viral infection considered eradicated world-wide since the late 1970s.[2] Bioterrorism experts fear that some virus could have fallen into terrorist hands, especially during the collapse of the former Soviet Union, which had large stockpiles of a weaponized form of this agent.

### Clinical Features

Smallpox presents with a febrile prodrome followed by a characteristic vesiculopustular exanthem, with individual lesions similar to

those of varicella. In contrast, however, smallpox lesions appear synchronously; they begin and concentrate on the face and extremities, then extend toward the trunk (Figure 18.3). Smallpox is also typically accompanied by high fever and prostration, uncommon in ordinary varicella. Historically, mortality rates approached 30%, with death thought to be due to hypotension and immune-complex-associated toxemia. The disease is highly contagious. Airborne, droplet, and contact precautions are recommended for unvaccinated caregivers. There are currently no proven antiviral therapies, but vaccination within 3 to 4 days of exposure might prevent or mitigate infection. This

## YOUR FIRST CLUE

**Distinguishing Smallpox From Chickenpox Infections**

**Features of Smallpox**

- Vesicular lesions in similar stage of development that begin on the face and extremities and spread to trunk and abdomen
- Concentration of lesions on face and extremities
- High fever
- Prostration

is a live virus vaccine, so immunocompromised individuals should not be vaccinated or come into close contact with recent vaccinees.

## Plague

Plague is caused by *Yersinia pestis,* a Gram-negative bacterium, and occurs infrequently in the southwest United States, where it might present in bubonic, septic, or pneumonic forms.[3] Airborne exposure would likely present as pneumonic plague, a severe, hemorrhagic bacterial pneumonia with the potential to progress to sepsis, disseminated intravascular coagulation, and meningitis. Patients with pneumonic plague typically manifest significant hemoptysis and rapid progression to respiratory failure.

### Diagnostic Studies and Management

Chest radiographs might reveal patchy or consolidated pneumonia. As in inhalational anthrax, mortality is nearly universal in patients presenting with advanced pneumonic plague. Plague is highly contagious; droplet precautions are required. Streptomycin or gentamicin are considered antibiotics of choice.

## Botulism

Botulism is the syndrome caused by intoxication with botulinum toxin, one of the most potent toxins known.[4] It can occur naturally after ingestion of preformed toxin in contaminated food (food-poisoning form) or intestinal production of toxin (infantile form), or,

rarely, when *Clostridium botulinum* infects a wound and toxin is elaborated at the infected site. Botulinum toxin impairs release of synaptic acetylcholine, particularly at the neuromuscular junction.

Affected patients are afebrile and present with a symmetric, descending flaccid paralysis with marked bulbar findings, although sensation and mental status remain intact. Infants demonstrate poor tone and decreased suck. Differential diagnosis includes meningitis, polio, Guillain-Barré syndrome, myasthenia gravis, and transverse myelitis. Being toxin mediated, it is not contagious, and special infection control precautions are unnecessary. A botulinum antitoxin is available that might mitigate progression, but it does not typically reverse the disease. Supportive care with mechanical ventilation might be required for months in severe cases.

## Tularemia

Tularemia is caused by *Francisella tularensis,* a Gram-negative coccobacillus.[5] Inhalational exposure following a terrorist attack would likely result in pneumonic or typhoidal forms, the latter a syndrome including fever, malaise, abdominal pain, and diarrhea. The disease is not contagious, though the organism is highly infectious and poses a risk to laboratory staff. Streptomycin and gentamicin are preferred antibiotics, while doxycycline, ciprofloxacin, and chloramphenicol are acceptable alternatives.

## Viral Hemorrhagic Fevers

Viral hemorrhagic fevers (VHFs), particularly those due to Filoviridae (e.g., Ebola, Marburg disease) and Arenaviridae (e.g., Lassa fever) are feared because of their contagion potential and high lethality.[11] They typically begin with a febrile prodrome but can also cause early facial flushing and conjunctival infection, reflecting early vascular involvement. These evolve rapidly to shock and widespread mucous membrane hemorrhage. The VHFs require contact and droplet precautions, possibly expanding to include airborne precautions as well for patients with massive hemoptysis and/or hematemesis. Treatment is primarily supportive, though ribavirin might have some benefit for arenaviral disease.

## Chemical Agents

The major chemical weapons of concern are nerve agents such as sarin, used by the Japanese Aum Shinrikyo cult in the infamous Tokyo subway attack in 1995.[12] Other potential chemical agents of terror include vesicants (e.g., mustard), cyanide, pulmonary agents such as chlorine or phosgene, and riot-control or lacrimating (tear-gas) agents. The nerve agents and cyanide have specific antidotes, and both nerve agents and vesicants pose a significant contamination hazard to ED personnel.[7,13] The other agents are outlined in Table 18-3. Chemical agents would cause relatively rapid onset of clinical effects, ranging from seconds or minutes (potent nerve agents) to several hours (e.g., skin blistering and eye inflammation after vesicant contact, pulmonary edema after phosgene exposure).

## Nerve Agents

These agents are organophosphate compounds acting as acetylcholinesterase inhibitors, with toxic effects due to excessive accumulation of acetylcholine at cholinergic synapses. They cause a clinical syndrome very similar to that caused by organophosphate pesticide poisoning, though typically of much greater lethality and with greater immediate central nervous system (CNS) toxicity, in addition to the expected cholinergic effects. Significant vapor exposure would cause rapid onset of rhinorrhea, miosis, and dyspnea due to excessive respiratory secretions and bronchospasm; with high concentrations of vapor,

---

## YOUR FIRST CLUE

**Mnemonics for Signs and Symptoms of Nerve Agent Poisoning**

**DUMBELS**
- Diarrhea, dyspnea, diaphoresis
- Urination
- Miosis
- Bronchospasm, bronchorrhea
- Emesis
- Lacrimation
- Salivation

**SLUDGE**
- Salivation
- Lacrimation
- Urination
- Defecation
- Gastric cramping
- Emesis

TABLE 18-3  Primary Chemical Agents of Terrorism

| Agent | Toxicity | Clinical Findings | Onset | Decontamination[1] | Management |
|-------|----------|-------------------|-------|--------------------|------------|
| Nerve agents: Tabun, Sarin, Soman, VX | Anticholinesterase: muscarinic, nicotinic and CNS effects | Vapor: miosis, rhinorrhea, dyspnea<br>Liquid: diaphoresis, vomiting<br>Both: coma, paralysis, seizures, apnea | Seconds: vapor<br>Minutes-hours: liquid | Vapor: fresh air, remove clothes, wash hair<br>Liquid: remove clothes, copious washing skin, hair with soap and water, ocular irrigation | ABCs<br>**Atropine:** 0.05 mg/kg IV[2], IM[3] (min 0.1 mg, max 5 mg), repeat q2–5min prn for marked secretions, bronchospasm<br>**Pralidoxime:** 25 mg/kg IV, IM[4] (max 1 g IV; 2 g IM), may repeat within 30–60 min prn, then again q1h for 1 or 2 doses prn for persistent weakness, high atropine requirement<br>**Diazepam:** 0.3 mg/kg (max 10 mg) IV; Lorazepam: 0.1 mg/kg IV, IM (max 4 mg); Midazolam: 0.2 mg/kg (max 10 mg) IM prn seizures, or severe exposure |
| Vesicants: Mustard | Alkylation | Skin: erythema, vesicles<br>Eye: inflammation<br>Respiratory tract: inflammation | Hours | Skin: soap and water<br>Eyes: water (only effective if done within minutes of exposure) | Symptomatic care |
| Lewisite | Arsenical | | (immediate pain with Lewisite) | | (possibly BAL 3 mg/kg IM q4–6h for systemic effects of Lewisite in severe cases) |
| Pulmonary agents: Chlorine Phosgene | Liberate HCL, alkylation | Eyes, nose, throat irritation (especially chlorine)<br>Respiratory: bronchospasm, pulmonary edema (especially phosgene) | Minutes: eyes, nose, throat irritation, bronchospasm;<br>Hours: pulmonary edema | Fresh air<br>Skin: water | Symptomatic care |
| Cyanide | Cytochrome oxidase inhibition: cellular anoxia, lactic acidosis | Tachypnea, coma, seizures, apnea | Seconds | Fresh air<br>Skin: soap and water | ABCs, 100% oxygen<br>Na bicarbonate prn metabolic acidosis<br>Na nitrite (3%):<br>Dose (mL/kg)  Estimated Hgb (g/dL)<br>0.27    10<br>0.33    12 (est. for average child)<br>0.39    14<br>(max 10 mL)<br>Na thiosulfate (25%): 1.65 mL/kg (max 50 mL) |

TABLE 18-3  Primary Chemical Agents of Terrorism (Continued)

| Agent | Toxicity | Clinical Findings | Onset | Decontamination[1] | Management |
|---|---|---|---|---|---|
| Riot Control agents: CS (Tear Gas) CN (Mace™) Capsaicin (pepper spray) | Neuropeptide substance P release; alkylation | Eye: tearing, pain, blepharospasm Nose and throat irritation Pulmonary failure (rare) | Seconds | Fresh air Eyes: lavage | Ophthalmics topically, symptomatic care |

[1]Decontamination, especially for patients with significant nerve agent or vesicant exposure, should be performed by health care providers garbed in adequate personal protective equipment. For ED staff, this consists of non-encapsulated, chemically-resistant body suit, boots and gloves with a full face air purifier mask/hood.[15]

[2]Intraosseous route is likely equivalent to intravenous.

[3]Atropine might have some benefit via endotracheal tube or inhalation, as might aerosolized ipratropium.

[4]Pralidoxime is reconstituted to 50 mg/mL (1 g in 20 mL water) for IV administration, and the total dose infused over 30 min, or may be given by continuous infusion (loading dose 25 mg/kg over 30 min, then 10 mg/kg/hr). For IM use, it might be diluted to a concentration of 300 mg/mL (1 g added to 3 mL water - by analogy to the US Army's Mark 1 autoinjector concentration), in order to effect a reasonable volume for injection. Each Mark 1 kit holds 2 auto injectors, one each of atropine 2 mg ( 0.7 mL), and pralidoxime 600 mg (2 mL); while not approved for pediatric use, they might be considered as initial treatment in dire (especially prehospital) circumstances, for children with severe, life-threatening nerve agent toxicity who lack intravenous access, and for whom more precise, mg/kg IM dosing would be logistically impossible. Suggested dosing guidelines are offered; note potential excess of initial atropine and pralidoxime dose for age/weight, though within general guidelines for recommended total over first 60-90 min of therapy of severe exposures:

| Approximate Age | Approximate Weight | Number of Autoinjectors (each type) | Atropine dose range (mg/kg) | Pralidoxime dose range (mg/kg) |
|---|---|---|---|---|
| 3-7 yrs | 13-25 kg | 1 | 0.08-0.13 | 24-46 |
| 8-14 yrs | 26-50 kg | 2 | 0.08-0.13 | 24-46 |
| >14 yrs | >51 kg | 3 | 0.11 or less | 35 or less |

Key: CNS = central nervous system; ABCs = airway, breathing and circulatory support; Hgb = hemoglobin concentration; min = minimum; max = maximum; prn = as needed; BAL = British Anti-Lewisite

Reprinted from Journal of Pediatrics, Vol. 141, No. 3, Tables 3 and 4 from Henretig FM et al., '"Biological and Chemical Agents of Terrorism" pg. 311-326 ©2002, with permission from Elsevier Science.

symptoms would progress rapidly to include coma, seizures, paralysis, apnea, and death unless immediate antidotal therapy was provided. Patients exposed to nerve agent vapor represent a modest contamination hazard to health care providers, since slight off-gassing can occur from contaminated hair or clothing. Disrobement and a brief soap and water shower should suffice for decontamination. For patients exposed to a liquid nerve agent, more scrupulous decontamination with thorough scrubbing is warranted; contaminated skin and clothes would be highly toxic to unprotected caregivers, so appropriate PPE must be worn by involved ED staff.[14]

Mainstays of therapy include cardiopulmonary resuscitation and adequate provision of oxygen, as well as antidotal therapy and supportive care. Atropine is used to counter muscarinic effects, particularly excess secretions and bronchospasm compromising respiratory function. Pralidoxime (2-PAM) restores intact cholinesterase if used prior to induction of irreversible enzyme changes ("aging") and is particularly effective in reversing muscle weakness. Benzodiazepines should be used aggressively to control seizures, and consideration of their use in severe cases even prior to seizure onset is warranted.

## Vesicant Agents

The vesicants mustard and Lewisite have been military chemical weapons and are now feared as potential terrorist agents. There was considerable clinical experience with mus-

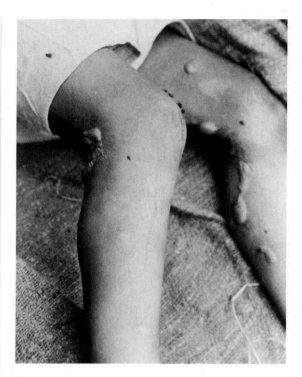

**Figure 18.4** Skin damage caused by mustard gas.

tard in World War I. This agent typically caused skin blistering, eye injury (conjunctivitis, keratitis), and, with heavier exposures, pulmonary tract inflammation (runny nose, sneezing, hoarseness, bloody nose, cough, sinus pain, and dyspnea) several hours after exposure (Figure 18.4). In very severe cases, bone marrow suppression and gastrointestinal mucosal injury (diarrhea, nausea, and vomiting) were also observed. Therapy consists of decontamination as soon as possible after exposure and supportive care. Mustard-contaminated patients or clothing would also pose considerable cross-contamination risk to caregivers and would require precautions similar to those used in managing liquid nerve-agent victims.

## Cyanide

Cyanide inhibits mitochondrial oxidative metabolism by interfering with cytochrome oxidase function in the electron transport chain. Thus, highly metabolically active tissues, especially the brain and heart, are most

### YOUR FIRST CLUE

**Signs and Symptoms of Vesicant Agent Exposure**
- Skin blistering
- Eye irritation and inflammation
- Respiratory symptoms
- Gastrointestinal symptoms

affected. Use by terrorists would likely involve a vapor release within an enclosed space. Victims with low vapor exposure would experience the following symptoms within minutes of exposure: tachypnea, restlessness, dizziness, weakness, headache, nausea and vomiting, and tachycardia. Victims with high vapor exposure would rapidly lose consciousness, develop seizures, and become apneic, though without the typical muscarinic signs of the comparably poisoned nerve agent victim.

## Management

Management begins with cardiopulmonary resuscitation and provision of 100% oxygen. In severe cases antidotal therapy might offer additional benefit. Methemoglobin-forming agents, such as sodium nitrite will allow methemoglobin to disassociate some cyanide from heme-containing enzymes. However, the formation of excess methemoglobin can compromise oxygen delivery in a patient with already inhibited cellular oxidation and must be avoided by careful dosing based on weight and estimated hemoglobin concentration in pediatric patients (Table 18-3).[7] This should be followed by a sulfate donor, sodium thiosulfate, that converts cyanide to the less toxic thiocyanate, which is then renally excreted. In mild to moderate cases, sodium thiosulfate alone can be beneficial and safer.

## Radiation Exposure

The third of the three unconventional threats discussed in this chapter is that of major radiation exposure. Terrorist incidents involving the use of radiation would likely involve four potential scenarios: the nonexplosive dispersal of radioactive substances, dispersal via a conventional explosive device ("dirty bomb"), conventional attacks on nuclear power plants resulting in radiation release and contamination, and finally, of course, the unimaginable detonation of a nuclear weapon.[15–17]

The first three of these scenarios would likely result in a relatively manageable disaster from the perspective of EMS preparedness. While panic and psychological stress might be rampant, most victims would not be exposed to life-threatening doses of radiation, and the health effects of small-dose radiation are delayed by years. Further, the risk of clinically significant exposure to health care workers from contaminated patients is far less than that posed by victims of a chemical attack.[15] In contrast, a nuclear detonation in any populated area would have horrific effects and most likely overwhelm all attempts at adequate preparedness. In brief, even a small nuclear weapon

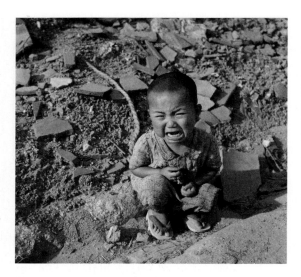

**Figure 18.5** Victim of Hiroshima.

of about 12.5-kiloton energy (comparable to the 13-kiloton bomb dropped on Hiroshima) would devastate a city such as New York. If detonated at ground level in the city's port area, the blast and thermal effects would kill an estimated 52,000 people immediately and cause 44,000 cases of radiation sickness (with an additional 10,000 fatalities) (**Figure 18.5**). Radiation fallout would kill an additional 200,000 people and further result in several hundred thousand with radiation sickness.[15,16]

Numerous sources of radioactive material exist that could be potentially accessed by those with terrorist intentions. Since 1970 there has been a six-fold increase in nuclear material in peaceful programs. The International Atomic Energy Agency (IAEA) currently notes 438 nuclear power reactors, 651 research reactors (284 operational), and 250 fuel cycle plants in operation worldwide.[17] These data do not include the numerous radiation sources used in medicine, industry, agriculture, and research. Fortunately, to date there have been no large-scale intentional attacks with radioactive material. The 1986 nuclear reactor accident in Chernobyl and the 1987 accidental exposure to radioactive cesium from a scrapped medical source in Goiânia, Brazil, represent two notable unintentional radiation exposures that affected large populations.

Evidence of terrorist groups attempting to obtain nuclear materials, in particular from the former Soviet Union, has surfaced. In October 2001, Turkish police arrested two men with weapons-grade plutonium, and the Russian Defense Ministry reported averting terrorist attempts to break into two Russian nuclear storage sites.[16] The IAEA reports 175 cases of nuclear trafficking since 1983, of which 18 cases involved enriched uranium or plutonium.[17]

## Physics

Ionizing radiation is characterized by its associated mass and penetration ability. Alpha particles (two protons, two neutrons) are fully stopped by dead layers of skin or clothing and generally do not pose a significant external exposure hazard, but they can produce internal damage. Beta particles (electrons) are primarily found in fallout radiation and can damage the basal striatum of the skin. These dermal "beta burns" can appear similar to thermal burns. Gamma rays are nonparticulate, have high penetrability, and are emitted during nuclear detonation and fallout. They are uncharged and similar to x-rays. Neutrons are uncharged particles that penetrate similarly to gamma and x-irradiation but are not present in fallout. However, their energy deposition is more concentrated, and they can cause 20 times more damage than gamma rays.[15,18]

Radiation is usually expressed in units of rads or Grays. A radiation-absorbed dose (rad) is a measure of the energy deposited in matter by ionizing radiation. A Gray (Gy) is an international measure of the absorbed dose, where 1 Gy = 1 J/kg = 100 rad. Radiation doses that people receive are measured in units called rem (radiation equivalent, man) or the international measure Sv (Sievert). One Sv is equal to 100 rem.[18] Essentially, one can consider a Gray and a Sievert equal when considering beta and gamma rays. (Also, 1 Gy = 100 cGy, 1 Gy = 1000 mGy, and 1 cGy = 1 rad.) Scientists estimate that the average person in the United States receives a dose of about one-third of 1 rem per year. Eighty percent of typical human exposure comes from natural sources, and the remaining 20% comes from artificial radiation sources, primarily medical x-rays.

A routine pediatric radiologic study such as a chest x-ray exposes a patient to 0.1 to 0.2 mGy, angiocardiography to 0.55 to 1.6 2 mGy, and computed tomography of the head (head CT) to 15 mGy.[19] It is recommended that emergency personnel may enter an area to perform critical, time-sensitive tasks at radiation exposures of up to 0.1 Gy per hour.[15] With acute, whole body radiation exposures, symptoms begin at about 1 Gy. Persons with 4 to 6 Gy of such exposure are at risk of 50% to 100% mortality without medical treatment, and similar exposures above 10 Gy are almost always fatal even with optimal medical care.[15]

## Types of Exposure and Clinical Features

Radiation injury can result from localized or whole body external radiation, or from contamination (deposition) of radioactive materials that can be external (cutaneous) or internal via inhalation, ingestion, wound contamination, or skin absorption. Generally, rapidly dividing cells, such as those of the bone marrow and intestinal mucosa, are most readily injured by a given exposure. With higher doses, there is concomitant injury to the microvasculature with marked fluid and electrolyte loss contributing to hypovolemic shock, and neurologic effects due to cerebral vascular leak and edema.

At doses less than 1 Gy, acute injury is usually modest; most cells survive but can still be susceptible to subsequent malignant changes. There is an increased risk of leukemia at doses as low as 0.4 Gy.[19] The onset of cancer is typically as early as 2 years postexposure for leukemia, and 5 to 10 years or more for radiation-induced solid malignancies.[15]

Localized radiation injury (or radiation burn) is typically associated with the handling of radioactive sources. Most often the hands or buttocks and upper thighs are affected (these latter two from carrying the radioactive source in a pants pocket). Radiation burns are similar to those caused by thermal injury (Figure 18.6). However, they develop af-

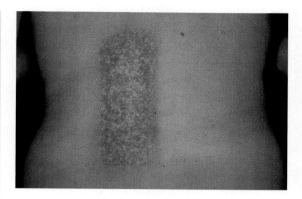

**Figure 18.6** Radiation burn to the skin.

ter a latent interval of several days and are typically less painful, presenting with erythema, followed by blistering, and ultimately ulceration and/or tissue necrosis due to vascular insufficiency.

Whole body exposure to penetrating radiation or internal absorption will result in the acute radiation syndrome. The symptoms vary with individual radiation sensitivity, type of radiation, and dose absorbed (Table 18-4). Within 6 to 12 hours of a significant exposure, the syndrome typically begins with a prodromal phase. This is manifested by rapid onset of nausea, vomiting, diarrhea, fatigue, weakness, fever, and headache. The gastrointestinal manifestations last 24 to 48 hours. However, the fatigue and weakness can persist for an indefinite period of time. This is followed by a latent phase, during which the patient is relatively asymptomatic. The latent phase typically lasts up to 2 or more weeks, though it can be absent in very severe exposures. Radiation lesions, or beta burns, often with hair loss of the scalp, begin approximately 2 weeks after exposure. The most common sites affected include the head, neck, axilla, antecubital fossa, and dorsum of the feet.[20] The manifest illness phase follows, and the form it takes is dose dependent. At doses exceeding 2 Gy (200 cGy), the bone marrow is injured, with the resulting hematopoietic syndrome. Many patients will have lymphopenia within 48 hours of exposure, which can predict the occurrence of this syndrome. The absolute lymphocyte count (ALC) obtained soon after exposure can serve as a marker for the degree of exposure (ALC

**TABLE 18-4   Acute Radiation Syndrome**

Whole body radiation from external radiation or internal absorption

| Phase of Syndrome | Feature | Subclinical Range | | Sublethal Range | | Lethal Range | |
|---|---|---|---|---|---|---|---|
| | | 0–100 rad (cGy) | 100–200 rad (cGy) | 200–600 rad (cGy) | 600–800 rad (cGy) | 600–3000 rad (cGy) | >3000 rad (cGy) |
| Initial or Prodromal | Nausea, vomiting | none | 5–50% | 50–100% | 75–100% | 90–100% | 100% |
| | Time of onset | | 3–6 hrs | 2–4 hrs | 1–2 hrs | <1 hr | <1 hr |
| | Duration Lymphocyte count | | <24 hrs | <24 hrs <1000 at 24 h | <48 hrs < 500 at 24h | <48 hrs | <48 hrs |
| | CNS function | No impairment | No impairment | Routine task performance Cognitive impairment for 6–20 hrs | Simple and routine task performance Cognitive impairment for >24 hrs | Progressive incapacitation | |
| Latent | Duration | > 2 wks | 7–15 days | 0–7 days | 0–2 days | None | |
| "Manifest Illness" (obvious illness) | Signs and symptoms | None | Moderate leukopenia | Severe leukopenia, purpura, hemorrhage Pneumonia Hair loss after 300 rad (cGy) | | Diarrhea Fever Electrolyte disturbance | Convulsions, ataxia, tremor, lethargy |
| | Time of onset | | > 2 wks | 2 days–2 wks | | 2–3 days | 1–48 hrs |
| | Critical period | None | None | 4–6 wks | | 5–14 days | 1–48 hrs |
| | Organ system | None | | Hematopoietic and respiratory (mucosal) systems | | GI tract Mucosal systems | CNS |
| Hospitali-zation | % Duration | 0 | <5% 45–60 days | 90% 60–90 days | 100% 90+ days | 100% 2 weeks | 100% 2 days |
| Fatality | % | 0% | 0% | 0–80% | 90–100% | 90–100% | 100% |
| Time to Death | | | | 3 wks–3 months | | 1–2 wks | 1–2 days |

Source: *Terrorism with Ionizing Radiation General Guidance: Pocket Guide*, US Department of Defense and Veterans Affairs, 2001.

$<1000/mm^3$ moderate, $<500/mm^3$ severe). These patients usually have maximal neutropenia and thrombocytopenia at 3 to 4 weeks, when infection and hemorrhage are the primary challenges to medical care. With doses from 6 to 30 Gy, the manifest illness phase can also encompass a gastrointestinal syndrome, with recurrence of nausea, vomiting, and diarrhea about 1 week or less after the prodromal phase. This is quickly followed by sepsis, metabolic disturbances, and usually death, even with optimal medical care. Finally, a neurovascular syndrome is described in victims exposed to doses above 30 Gy. The patient usually develops almost immediate nausea, vomiting, and prostration, followed shortly by shock, ataxia, and convulsions. The pathology is believed to be diffuse vascular injury leading to hypotension and cerebral edema. Death typically ensues within several days. Of note, a 25-year followup of children and adults exposed to radioactive fallout in the Marshall Islands has demonstrated an increased risk of thyroid nodules and hypothyroidism.[21]

Contamination with radioactive materials represents the third major type of radiation injury. This occurs when radioactive dirt or liquid remains on a body surface (external) or is inhaled, ingested, or absorbed through skin or open wounds (internal). This form of radiation exposure is the only type to involve any risk to health care workers, though the danger is minimal in treating patients during transport to hospital. External contamination is rarely a significant medical risk even to the patient. Internal contamination may be more serious. Many radioisotopes are potentially harmful. However, experience at Chernobyl and the threat related to terrorist attacks on domestic nuclear reactors have focused attention particularly on the risk of inhaled and ingested radioactive iodine exposure, since radioactive iodine is a normal fission product found in reactor fuel rods. This form of contamination is highly associated with increased risk for thyroid cancer. While this represents a chronic exposure outcome, it is predominant in children, and an effective antidote (potassium iodide) exists that must be given emergently.

The data from the 1986 Chernobyl accident estimated exposure based on the following items: direct thyroid measurements in a segment of the exposed population, measurement of $I^{131}$ in milk consumed and quantity of milk consumed, inference from ground deposition of long-lived radioisotopes, and reconstruction of the nature and extent of the actual radiation release. Clinical data show a marked increase in childhood thyroid cancer beginning 4 years after the exposure for the inhabitants of Belarus and the Ukraine. Depending on the degree of radioactive contamination, incidence rates have increased from 30-fold to 100-fold. The most marked increase in thyroid cancer exhibited a dose-response at exposures above 5 cGy. Iodine deficiency might also have had a crucial role.[22]

## Management

The optimal management of a radiation exposure incident would properly require considerable community and EMS planning, and these needs have been recently reviewed elsewhere.[15,16,18] The following refers to the emergency department approach to exposed victims.

Treatment of local radiation burns is primarily supportive. Plastic surgical management will usually be required for severe cases. While overly aggressive debridement should be avoided, these burns might require grafting, or even amputation, in some cases.

Acute radiation syndrome treatment is also primarily supportive. These patients are very prone to hemorrhage and infection due to their severe bone marrow depression, and their management is often further complicated by denuded intestinal mucosa as a portal of entry for enteric organisms. However, most of the significant medical management challenges will not arise for days to weeks after initial presentation.

Victims with evidence of external contamination require decontamination, which is usually provided prior to further medical care. A radiation counter (for alpha, beta, and gamma radiation) is used to ascertain degree of contamination and subsequent adequacy of decontamination. However, if life-threatening conditions are present, these may be attended to by personnel garbed in traditional protective masks, gloves, gowns, and booties as per universal precautions, even prior to decontamination, or in conjunction with disrobement. Patients may be transported wrapped in cloth sheets to minimize facility contamination. The treatment area should be one with controlled access. As soon as feasible, thorough decontamination should be effected by clothing removal (about 90% effective in and of itself) and washing with soap and water. Washing should be gentle and should avoid abrading skin. Special attention is afforded to hair, face, and hands, especially skin folds, ears, and the area under the fingernails, which can hide residual particles. Open wounds should be covered to avoid inadvertent internal contamination. If wounds are already contaminated, they should be irrigated and treated conventionally. If possible, wound closure should be performed as soon as possible after whole body radiation exposure exceeds 1 Gy in order to mitigate potential infection as bone marrow suppression evolves.

Internal contamination raises many of the most challenging issues for the emergency management of patients with radiation injury. In general, the sooner specific therapy is initiated, the better. Unfortunately, optimal treatment requires a precise knowledge of the specific type of contamination, which is rarely known immediately. There are several generic principles that can be applied, such as reducing absorption, enhancing elimination, chelation therapy, and blockage and/or displacement by nonradioactive materials. The most important of these, particularly after a nuclear weapon detonation or attack on a nuclear reactor, is the use of potassium iodide (KI) to prevent accumulation of radioactive iodine in the thyroid. Again, the experience from Chernobyl has been very instructive and prompted the revision of guidelines for treatment.[23,24] Previous guidelines were tempered by limited data from the exposures of Hiroshima and Nagasaki, the Nevada and Hampton domestic test sites, and the Bikini Island detonation, which exposed inhabitants of the Marshall Islands of Rongelap, Ailinginae, Rongerik, and Utirik. Acute treatment with KI as soon as possible within 24 hours postexposure is indicated as an adjunct to evacuation, sheltering, and containment of contaminated foodstuffs.

The recently revised guidelines for KI dosing can be found in Table 18-5. These revised recommendations adhere to the principle of minimum effective dose and suggest a decreased dose compared to older standards. The protective effects of KI last approximately 24 hours, and most individuals could be redosed daily until a significant risk of exposure no longer exists.[23] How-

**TABLE 18-5** Threshold Thyroid Radioactive Exposures and Recommended Doses of KI for Different Risk Groups

| Patient Age | Predicted Thyroid Exposure (cGy) | KI Dose (mg) | #130 mg Tablets | #65 mg Tablets |
|---|---|---|---|---|
| >40 yrs* | ≥500 | 130 | 1 | 2 |
| >18–40 yrs | ≥10 | 130 | 1 | 2 |
| Pregnant/Lactating | ≥5 | 130 | 1 | 2 |
| >12–18 yrs** | ≥5 | 65 | ½ | 1 |
| >3–12 yrs | ≥5 | 65 | ½ | 1 |
| >1 month–3 yrs*** | ≥5 | 32 | ¼ | ½ |
| Birth–1 mo***,† | ≥5 | 16 | ⅛ | ¼ |

*Comments*

\* Older patients are more likely to suffer side effects from KI including iodine-induced thyrotoxicosis, goiter, and hypothyroidism in iodide deficient areas.

\*\* Adolescents approaching ≥70 kg should be given the full adult dose (130 mg).

\*\*\* Infants may be given KI as a fresh saturated solution diluted in milk, formula or water.

†Neonates should have TSH and free $T_4$ monitored with free $T_4$ (levothyroxine) replacement therapy as needed.

Side effects may also include GI distress, rash, and sialadenitis.

Adapted from: *Potassium Iodide as a Thyroid Blocking Agent in Radiation Emergencies*, November 2001, FDA- CDER.

ever, fetal and neonatal exposure to iodine, both stable and radioactive, can result in hypothyroidism. Thus, special attention should be paid to newborns and to pregnant or lactating women. Redosing of KI in these groups is usually not recommended and would be reserved for cases involving severe contamination, with close monitoring of the infant's thyroid function postpartum.[23] Iodine is one of many radioactive substances that might have internal radiation effects. Other substances include americium, cesium, cobalt, plutonium, radium, strontium, tritium, uranium, and phosphorus. De-

pleted uranium is not considered a radiological or chemical threat. Treatment for internal contamination with these radioactive substances is outlined in Table 18-6,[18] though decisions about such exotic therapeutic approaches for specific patients would warrant expert consultation. Evidence-based recommendations for pediatric patients are particularly scanty.

## Early Recognition

Unfortunately, in our current era, physicians facing an unusual increased volume or presentation of patients should at least ask themselves if the situation they are facing is conceivably due to a terrorist attack. They might consider three critical questions: are there epidemic numbers of patients? Are there common exposure sources? Could symptoms be exotic disease presentations?

A large number of patients, out of proportion to the time of year and expected clinical syndromes, might trigger suspicion of an emerging natural infectious disease, but could also represent a terrorist incident. A

## YOUR FIRST CLUE

**Three Critical Questions in the Recognition of a Potential Terrorist Attack**

- Are there epidemic numbers of patients?
- Are there common exposure sources?
- Are there exotic disease presentations?

## TABLE 18-6 Radioactive Elements and Treatment Modalities

| Radioactive Element | Absorption | Therapeutic Approach | Treatment |
|---|---|---|---|
| Americium-241 | Wounds, ±GI | Chelation | DTPA or EDTA if in first 24–48 hours |
| Cesium-137 | Inhalation, GI, wound | Reduction of GI absorption | Prussian blue (IND) |
| Cobalt-60 | Inhalation, <5%GI | Reduction of GI absorption chelation if severe | Gastric lavage, purgatives; severe cases use penicillamine |
| Iodine-131,132,134,135 | Primarily thyroid | Blockage mobilization | Potassium iodide; alternatives are propylthiouracil or methimazole |
| Phosphorus-32 | All sites | | Lavage, aluminum hydroxide, oral phosphates |
| Plutonium-239,238 | Inhalation, ±GI wounds variable | Reduction of GI absorption chelation | CaDTPA within 24 hours followed by ZnDTPA (IND) |
| Radium-226 | GI | Reduction of GI absorption Mobilization | 10% magnesium sulfate lavage followed by saline and magnesium purgatives, ammonium chloride can increase stool elimination |
| Strontium-90 | Inhalation, GI | Reduction of GI absorption blockage, displacement, mobilization | Aluminum phosphate PO, stable strontium can competitively inhibit metabolism; increase urinary excretion by acidification with ammonium chloride and large doses of calcium |
| Tritium (hydrogen-3) | Inhalation, GI | Dilution | Hydration with caution to avoid iatrogenic water intoxication |
| Uranium-238,235,239 | Inhalation | Mobilization | Sodium bicarbonate and tubular diuretics to decrease renal toxicity |

*Uranium included for completeness, not considered to be a serious radiation threat.
DTPA: diethylenetriaminepentaacetic acid; IND: investigational new drug; EDTA: calcium edentate.
Source: Data for this table derived from references 8, 18.

history of geographical relatedness among patients, or some observation of an unusual source of exposure, such as an explosion, discovery of a suspected aerosol delivery device, cloud of vapor, unusual odor, or visible powder, would reinforce such suspicion. An exotic disease presentation, such as several of the syndromes caused by major biological, chemical, or radiological weapons, is relatively unusual and might be characteristic. If a physician believes he or she is seeing the crest of such a wave of patients, immediate reporting to public health authorities and law enforcement agencies is appropriate, even without a specific diagnostic impression.

## THE BOTTOM LINE

- In these turbulent times, physicians caring for childhood emergencies may face patients who are victims of terrorism. Familiarity with clinical syndromes associated with biological, chemical, and radiological weapons may enable practitioners to recognize such an outbreak early in its evolution.

- Recognition of a terrorism incident can lead to lifesaving treatment, protection of the physician and other patients, and early public health interventions that might mitigate the potential catastrophe.

## Check Your Knowledge

1. A biological weapons attack would most likely resemble which of the following mass casualty emergencies?
   A. Earthquake
   B. Large bomb blast
   C. Release of chlorine from a train wreck
   D. Severe influenza epidemic
   E. Tornado

2. Which of the following syndromes is common to most of the high threat biological agents?
   A. Characteristic rash
   B. Encephalopathy
   C. Febrile prodrome
   D. Pneumonia
   E. Renal failure

3. Distinguishing features of botulism from other causes of paralysis include which of the following?
   A. Hallucinations
   B. High fever
   C. Intact sensation
   D. Normal bulbar function
   E. Severe paresthesias

4. Which of the following patients poses the least potential hazard to health care providers?
   A. An adolescent with untreated pneumonic plague
   B. An asymptomatic adolescent with mustard agent on skin
   C. Children exposed to high doses of ionizing radiation
   D. A child with fever and extensive lesions of smallpox
   E. An infant with nerve agent on clothing

## References

1. Inglesby TV, Henderson DA, Bartlett JG, et al. Anthrax as a biological weapon: medical and public health management [consensus statement]. *JAMA.* 1999;281:1735–1745.

2. Henderson DA, Inglesby TV, Bartlett JG, et al. Smallpox as a biological weapon: medical and public health management [consensus statement]. *JAMA.* 1999;281:2127–2137.

3. Inglesby TV, Dennis DT, Henderson DA, et al. Plague as a biological weapon: medical and public health management [consensus statement]. *JAMA.* 2000;283:2281–2290.

4. Arnon SS, Schechter R, Inglesby TV, et al. Botulinum toxin as a biological weapon: medical and public health management [consensus statement]. *JAMA.* 2001;285:1059–1070.

5. Dennis DT, Inglesby TV, Henderson DA, et al. Tularemia as a biological weapon: medical and public health management [consensus statement]. *JAMA.* 2001;285:2763–2773.

6. Inglesby TV, O'Toole T, Henderson DA, et al. Anthrax as a biological weapon, 2002: updated recommendations for management. *JAMA.* 2002;287:2236–2252.

7. Henretig FM, Cieslak TJ, Eitzen EM Jr. Medical Progress: biological and chemical terrorism. *J Pediatr.* 2002; 141:311–326. Corrections *J Pediatr.* 2002; 141:743–746.

8. Mettler FA, Voelz GL. Major radiation exposure: what to expect and how to respond. *N Engl J Med.* 2002;346:1554–1561.

9. White S, Henretig F, Dukes R. Vulnerable populations in the setting of bioterrorism. *Emerg Med Clin North Am.* 2002;20:365–392.

10. Torok TJ, Tauxe RF, Wise RP, et al. A large community outbreak of salmonellosis caused by intentional contamination of restaurant salad bars. *JAMA.* 1997;278:389–395.

11. US Army Medical Research Institute of Infectious Diseases. *Medical Management of Biological Casualties Handbook.* Ft Detrick, MD: US Army Medical Research Institute of Infectious Diseases; 1998.

12. Okumura T, Takasu N, Ishimatasu S K, et al. Report on 640 victims of the Tokyo subway sarin attack. *Ann Emerg Med.* 1996;28:129–135.

13. US Army Medical Research Institute of Chemical Defense. *Medical Management of Chemical Casualties,* 3rd ed. Aberdeen Proving Ground, Md: US Army Medical Research Institute of Chemical Defense; 1999.

14. Macintyre AG, Christopher GW, Eitzen E Jr, et al. Weapons of mass destruction events with contaminated casualties: effective planning for health care facilities. *JAMA.* 2000;283:242–249.

15. Mettler FA, Voelz GL. Major radiation exposure: what to expect and how to respond. *N Engl J Med.* 2002;346:1554–1561.

16. Helfand I, Forrow L, Tiwari J. Nuclear terrorism. *BMJ.* 2002;324:356–359.

17. IAEA News. Calculating the new global nuclear terrorism threat. *Sci Total Env.* 2002;284:269–272.

18. Jarrett DG. *Medical Management of Radiation Casualties Handbook.* Bethesda, Md: Armed Forces Radiobiology Research Institute; 1999.

# CHAPTER REVIEW

19. AAP Committee on Environmental Health. Risk of ionizing radiation exposure to children: a subject review. *Pediatrics.* 1998;101:717–719.

20. Conrad RA, Rall JE, Sutow WW. Thyroid nodules as a late sequela of radioactive fallout. *N Engl J Med.* 1966;274:1391–1399.

21. Larsen PR, Conard RA, Knudesen KD, et al. Thyroid hypofunction after exposure to fallout from a hydrogen bomb explosion. *JAMA.* 1982;247:1571–1575.

22. Schwenn MR, Brill AB. Childhood cancer 10 years after the Chernobyl accident. *Curr Opin Pediatr.* 1997:9:51–54.

23. US FDA Center for Drug Evaluation and Research Guidance. *Potassium Iodide as a Thyroid Blocking Agent in Radiation Emergencies.* Rockville, Md: US FDA Center for Drug Evaluation and Research Guidance; November 2001. (http://www.fda.gov/cder/guidance/index.htm).

24. World Health Organization. WHO guidelines for iodine prophylaxis following nuclear accidents: update, Geneva, Switzerland: World Health Organization; 1999.

You receive a call from paramedics who are bringing many students from a nearby school. The students are complaining of burning eyes and throat pain.

1. *What agents are most likely to cause these symptoms?*
2. *What type of decontamination is needed?*
3. *What do you tell parents?*

---

A quick look at the list of signs and symptoms of chemical agents reveals that riot control agents (tear gas, Mace™, pepper spray) are the most likely, although pulmonary agents such as chlorine and phosgene, and even vesicants such as mustard and Lewisite, must also be considered. Because of the possibility of the latter two agents, full decontamination procedures should apply. However, if prearrival information can be obtained such as how fast symptoms occurred, whether anyone saw anything sprayed, or school location (e.g., near a chemical plant), you might be able to determine that vesicants are less likely (vesicant symptoms take hours to occur, while pulmonary agents take minutes, and riot control agents seconds).

Decontamination for vesicants includes disrobing patients, then washing the skin with soap and water, and water only for the eyes. For pulmonary agents and riot control agents, fresh air and water to skin or eyes are required.

Depending on EMS, hazardous materials evaluation, and even police reports, it is key to reassure parents that the main treatment for mild cases of exposure to these agents is symptomatic care, and that they are not contagious.

# chapter 19

# Children With Special Health Care Needs: The Technologically Dependent Child

Terry A. Adirim, MD, MPH

## Objectives

1 Explain how children with special health care needs differ from healthy children with regard to vital signs, size, and developmental level.

2 Describe the types of emergencies that medical personnel might encounter in children with special health care needs.

3 Discuss the management of various technologies used for children with special health care needs, including tracheostomy tubes, home mechanical ventilators, central venous lines, feeding tubes, and ventriculoperitoneal shunts.

## Chapter Outline

Introduction
Tracheostomies and Home Ventilation
Feeding Tubes and Gastrostomy Tubes
Central Venous Catheters
Dialysis Shunts and Peritoneal Dialysis Catheters
Ventriculoperitoneal Shunts

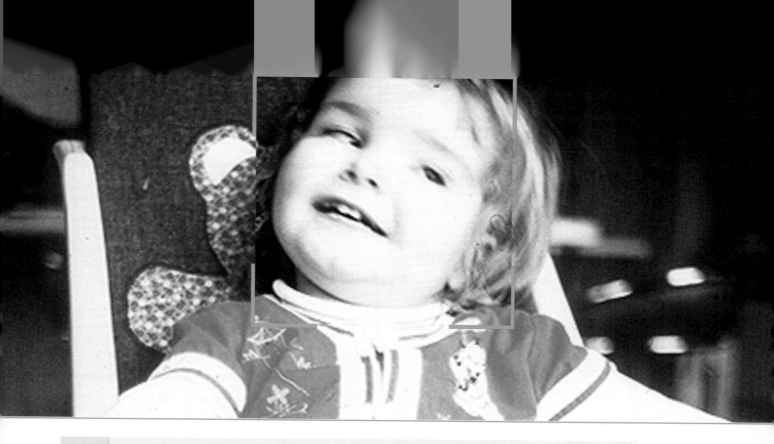

**CASE SCENARIO 1**

A 6-month-old girl with a tracheostomy tube, ventriculoperitoneal shunt, and gastrostomy tube is brought to your emergency department because she has been having difficulty breathing. She was born prematurely and was only recently discharged from the neonatal intensive care unit. The mother states that the child has had a fever since the night before, and that today she needed to increase her oxygen flow. At baseline, this child is ventilated only at night and is currently being weaned from mechanical ventilation. The tracheostomy was performed for mechanical ventilation and tracheal stenosis. During the day, the child usually receives 0.25 L $F_{IO_2}$. The mother states that the child's secretions have increased and she is suctioning more frequently. On examination, the child is awake but fussy, with subcostal and intercostal retractions, and her color is normal. Her respiratory rate is 60 breaths/min, heart rate is 180 beats per minute (bpm), blood pressure is 90/60 mmHg, and her temperature is 38.6°C. Oxygen saturation as measured by pulse oximetry is 90% on her baseline supplemental oxygen. The lung examination is notable for diffuse crackles and wheezes. Capillary refill is less than 2 seconds, and the extremities are well perfused.

1. *What is your initial assessment of this child's presentation?*
2. *How do you manage this presentation? Where do you start?*
3. *What issues do you need to consider?*

## Introduction

An estimated 34% of all emergency department (ED) visits involve children and adolescents. More than half of these visits are medically related, and a subset of these patients comprises children with special health care needs (CSHCN).[1,2] CSHCN are children who have a variety of chronic health and behavioral conditions that are potentially disabling. A subset of these children are technology assisted. They are children who depend on medical devices to support bodily functions.[3] In 1998 a national consensus group created an official definition of special needs children. This definition is: "Children with special health care

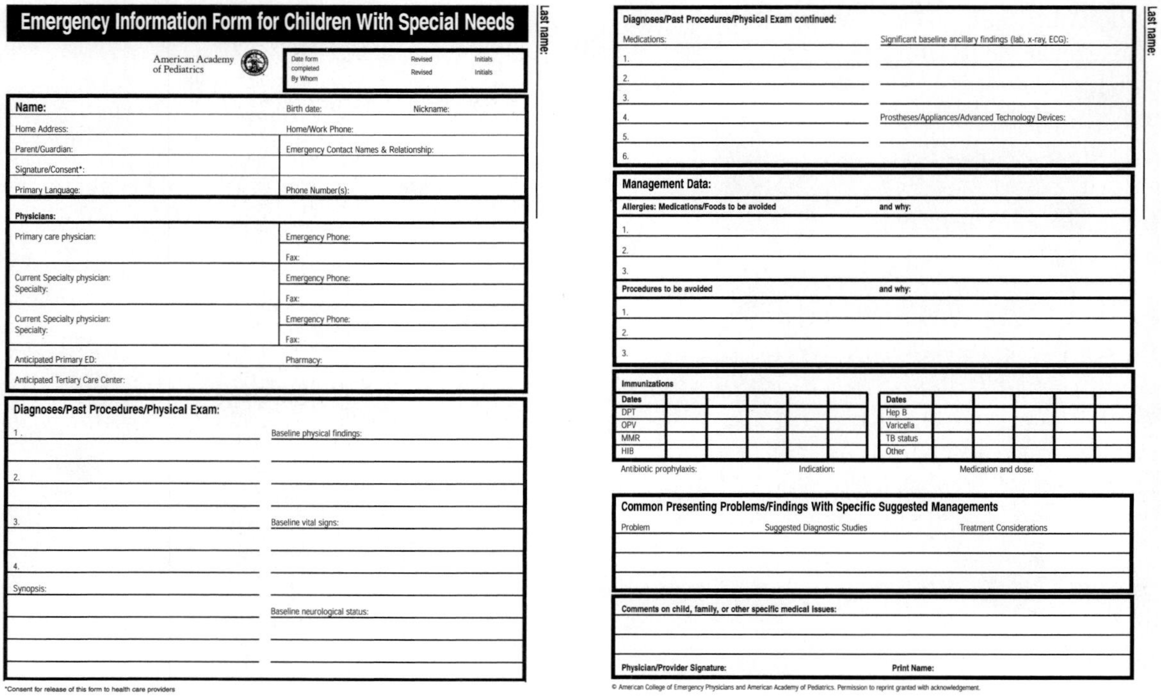

Emergency Information Form for Children With Special Needs

Last name:

American Academy of Pediatrics

Date form completed By Whom | Revised | Initials | Revised | Initials

Name: | Birth date: | Nickname:

Home Address: | Home/Work Phone:

Parent/Guardian: | Emergency Contact Names & Relationship:

Signature/Consent*:

Primary Language: | Phone Number(s):

Physicians:

Primary care physician: | Emergency Phone: | Fax:

Current Specialty physician: Specialty: | Emergency Phone: | Fax:

Current Specialty physician: Specialty: | Emergency Phone: | Fax:

Anticipated Primary ED: | Pharmacy:

Anticipated Tertiary Care Center:

Diagnoses/Past Procedures/Physical Exam:

1. | Baseline physical findings:

2.

3. | Baseline vital signs:

4.

Synopsis: | Baseline neurological status:

*Consent for release of this form to health care providers

Diagnoses/Past Procedures/Physical Exam continued:

Medications: 1. 2. 3. 4. 5. 6.

Significant baseline ancillary findings (lab, x-ray, ECG):

Prostheses/Appliances/Advanced Technology Devices:

Management Data:

Allergies: Medications/Foods to be avoided | and why: 1. 2. 3.

Procedures to be avoided | and why: 1. 2. 3.

Immunizations

| Dates | | | | | | Dates | | | | | |
|---|---|---|---|---|---|---|---|---|---|---|---|
| DPT | | | | | | Hep B | | | | | |
| OPV | | | | | | Varicella | | | | | |
| MMR | | | | | | TB status | | | | | |
| HIB | | | | | | Other | | | | | |

Antibiotic prophylaxis: | Indication: | Medication and dose:

Common Presenting Problems/Findings With Specific Suggested Managements

Problem | Suggested Diagnostic Studies | Treatment Considerations

Comments on child, family, or other specific medical issues:

Physician/Provider Signature: | Print Name:



Figure 19.1 Emergency information form for children with special needs.

needs are those who have or are at increased risk for a chronic physical, developmental, behavioral, or emotional condition and who also require health and related services of a type or amount beyond that required by children generally."[4] Based on this definition, it is estimated that more than 12 million, or 18%, of children in the United States have special health care needs.[5] One study at a tertiary care pediatric ED found that almost a quarter of their visits were by CSHCN. Not unexpectedly, they found that these children tended to be sicker, were 33 times more likely to need intensive care unit (ICU) admission, and that more than half of these children needed the consultation of a subspecialty service.[1]

The driving forces behind the large numbers of special needs children presenting to EDs for care are multifaceted. Advances in medical science and technology have enabled children with complex medical problems to live longer lives. Also, economic pressures from health care payers and the advent of family-centered care have increased the numbers of these children cared for at home as opposed to in institutional settings.

Most parents and caregivers of CSHCN have specialized training in the care of their children. They are very well versed in the care of their children's technology and medical conditions. They often carry detailed care plans that are developed with teams of specialists. One example of a program that provides information to medical care providers is the American Academy of Pediatrics and American College of Emergency Physicians "Emergency Preparedness for Children with Special Health Care Needs Program." This is an emergency notification program designed to provide specific information to medical caregivers about the special needs child. An Emergency Information Form (EIF), downloadable at www.aap.org and www.acep.org, is completed by the child's primary care physician and/or family and is carried with the child, or the child is enrolled in the MedicAlert program (Figure 19.1). MedicAlert personnel enter the information from the EIF into a database accessible to health care providers in an emergency.

Other programs, like "EMS Outreach" from Children's National Medical Center in Washington, DC, serve a similar function but are aimed at the prehospital professional. Enrollees in this program complete a medical information form that caregivers carry with them. This information is kept in a database and is updated every 6 months.

Although most caregivers are adept at handling many of their children's emergencies, they still seek help for a variety of reasons, including: the need for respite, equipment malfunction, an overwhelming medical problem, and the need for help with transport to the child's home hospital

Medical personnel should to be aware that CSHCN differ from well children in a variety of ways. They can be neurologically impaired and therefore developmentally delayed. Their growth might be impaired, so they might be smaller than other children of the same age. Also, depending on a child's condition, vital signs might also be different, and thus change management strategies. Medical personnel cannot rely on ages and weight-based norms and should either ask caregivers for this information or use length-based tapes when estimating weight and determining fluid and medication management. Developmentally delayed children might not be able to respond in the manner expected for age. Baseline vital signs can be altered, especially in children with cardiac conditions or on mechanical ventilators. For example, a child with complex congenital heart disease might have a baseline pulse oximetry reading of 85%. Also, some children have sensorineural deficits such as blindness and deafness. Medical care providers caring for special children should be sensitive to these situations. In addition, many of these children have latex allergies, so latex-free equipment should be used when caring for CSHCN.

This chapter will focus on technology-dependent children. The more common technologies used in CSHCN will be discussed. These include tracheostomy care and home mechanical ventilation, feeding tubes, central venous lines, and ventriculoperitoneal shunts.

## Tracheostomies and Home Ventilation

### Tracheostomy Tubes

A tracheostomy is a surgical opening in the anterior aspect of the neck (stoma) through the trachea that is meant to bypass the upper airway. A tracheostomy tube is placed in the stoma to either facilitate mechanical ventilation, provide a bypass of the upper airway, or to improve pulmonary toilet. Tracheostomy tubes allow for long-term management of the airway and for respiratory support of breathing. There are several conditions for which a child might need a tracheostomy. The more common conditions include but are not limited to tracheal stenosis, tracheomalacia, certain craniofacial anomalies, bronchopulmonary dysplasia, muscular dystrophy, spinal cord injury, and traumatic brain injury.

Tracheostomy tubes are used by most children and adolescents with tracheostomies. The tube keeps the stoma patent and can be attached to a mechanical ventilator (**Figure 19.2**).

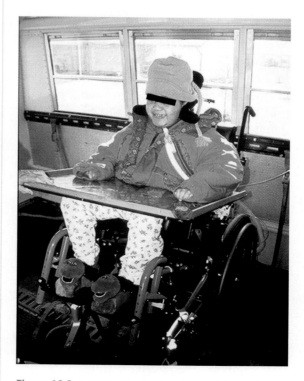

**Figure 19.2** A child with a tracheostomy might require continuous support of ventilation with a portable ventilator.

Tracheostomy tubes come in various sizes. There are several manufacturers, so there are variations in the way that they are sized and marked. Brands include Shiley, Bivona, Holinger, Portex, and Berdeen. Typically, the sizes are marked on the packaging and on the flange, or wings, of each tube (Figure 19.3). They range in size from 00 for newborns to 7.0 for older adolescents.[6] The inner and outer diameter ranges are provided so that comparisons between brands can be made. They range from 2.5 mm for infants to 10.0 mm for adolescents and adults. This information is also provided on the packaging or on the flange of the tube. This information is also important for emergency personnel when replacing a tracheostomy tube or when choosing a tracheal tube for oral intubation or use through the stoma. The inner diameter of a tracheostomy tube is the size to choose for tracheal tube insertion. Tracheostomy tubes also come in various lengths. Neonatal tubes are shorter than pediatric tubes, although the inner diameters might be the same.

There are several types of tracheostomy tubes and attachments. Types include single cannula tubes, double cannula tubes, cuffed tubes, and fenestrated tubes (Figure 19.4).[3] Neonates, infants, and young children use single cannula tracheostomy tubes (Figure 19.5). As a child's trachea gets larger, a double cannula tube should be used. It contains an outer tube that stays in the stoma and an inner tube that is removable for cleaning and pulmonary

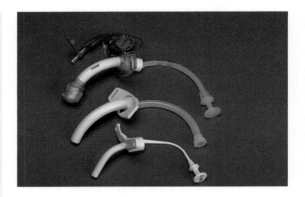

Figure 19.4 Fenestrated, double lumen, and single lumen tracheostomy tubes (top to bottom).

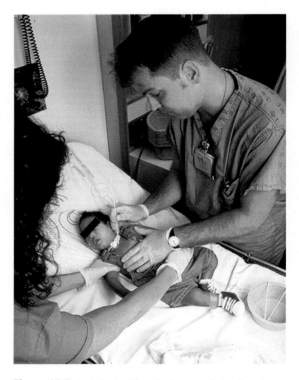

Figure 19.5 An infant with a single cannula tracheostomy tube in place.

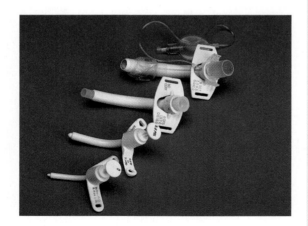

Figure 19.3 Tracheostomy tube sizes are marked on the flange, or wings.

toilet. Tracheostomy tubes for older children and adolescents often have an inflatable cuff to keep the tube in place and to prevent air leaks. Fenestrated tubes have a hole in the cephalic portion of the tube that redirects air into the upper airway, allowing the child to speak and breathe through the nose and mouth. This is facilitated by a decannulation plug attached to the opening of the tube.

Attachments to the tracheostomy tube include a tracheostomy nose, a tracheostomy collar, and a speaker valve. A tracheostomy nose is placed over the external opening of the tracheostomy tube of a nonmechanically ventilated child to provide air filtration and humidification. A tracheostomy collar is used to provide humidified air or supplemental oxygen to the nonmechanically ventilated patient. A speaker valve is an attachment that redirects airflow through the upper airway to facilitate speech.

## Tracheostomy Emergencies

There are many reasons a child with a tracheostomy tube can become sick, including an exacerbation of an underlying pulmonary disease. Signs and symptoms of respiratory distress include nasal flaring, retractions, increased respiratory rate, decreased breath sounds, decreased oxygen saturation, cyanosis, wheezing, rales, and increased secretions. Other causes can include a mucus plug of the tracheostomy tube or equipment failure.

The management approach to the child with a tracheostomy should begin as with any other child, with a history and attention to the ABCs (airway, breathing, circulation). Sudden onset of respiratory distress can lead one to predict a mucous plug or equipment failure as opposed to a pulmonary infection, in which fever and a more progressive onset of deterioration of respiratory status would be expected. Assessment of the airway should include inspection of the tracheostomy tube for patency. Next, breathing is assessed by observation and auscultation of the chest. Finally, circulation is assessed by assessing color, perfusion, pulses, and auscultation of the heart sounds.

For the child with a tracheostomy tube and a pulmonary exacerbation, infection and reactive airway disease are the most likely causes. Acute treatment would include administration of a bronchodilator nebulizer treatment through the tracheostomy or in-line with the ventilator in a mechanically ventilated child. If the child has a fever, infection should be considered and proper tracheostomy cultures and antibiotic coverage provided. Chest radiography should also be considered. Hospital admission is determined by a combination of factors, including age, medical history, severity of illness, and diagnosis. Medical personnel should consider transporting a medically complex child, if appropriate, to his or her home hospital under the advice of the physicians who know the child best.

For the child with sudden onset of respiratory distress, suctioning the tracheostomy tube can be helpful. If suctioning 2 to 3 times does not relieve the obstruction or respiratory distress, then the medical provider should consider changing the tracheostomy tube because a thick mucus plug might be obstructing airflow through the tube. See Table 19-1 for the steps for emergency tracheostomy tube change. As with any procedure, the practitioner should be prepared and have the appropriate supplies available (Table 19-2). If the ED or ambulance service does not have all of the supplies needed, parents and other caregivers often have them.

## Home Mechanical Ventilation

Many children with tracheostomies are also mechanically ventilated. Indications for mechanical ventilation include severe lung disease and abnormal respiratory drive either from central causes or secondary to paralysis. Some children are dependent on ventilators 24 hours a day, some while asleep, and some part of the day.

Two types of ventilators are used: pressure-cycled ventilators and volume ventilators. Pressure-cycled ventilators tend to be used in infants. They are set to deliver a given pressure with each breath. Volume ventilators give a tidal volume with each breath. There are two common modes of ventilations: intermittent mandatory ventilation (IMV) and continuous mechanical ventilation (CMV). IMV mode delivers a mechanical breath between the patient's own respirations to ensure that the patient achieves a certain number of breaths per minute. The ventilator synchronizes its breaths with the patient's breaths. The CMV ventilator, on the other hand, is set to deliver a certain number of breaths per minute regardless of whether the patient can breathe without assistance.

Some ventilators have an assist control mode during which the ventilator gives an augmented

| TABLE 19-1 | Steps for an Emergency Tracheostomy Tube Change |
| --- | --- |

1. **Prepare a replacement tracheostomy tube** of the same size. Ask parents for one if you do not have one.
2. For cuffed tracheostomy tubes, **deflate the balloon** by connecting a syringe to the valve on the pilot balloon. Draw air out until the pilot balloon collapses. Cutting the pilot balloon will not deflate the cuff.
3. If the child has a double cannula tracheostomy tube, **remove the inner cannula.** If removal of the inner cannula fails to clear the airway, the outer cannula should then be removed.
4. **Cut the cloth or Velcro ties** that hold the tracheostomy tube in place.
5. **Remove the tube** using a slow outward motion.
6. Gently **insert the same size tracheostomy tube** with the obturator in place. Point the curve of the tube downward. *Never force the tube.* The tube may be lubricated with a water-soluble gel or by dipping it into normal saline prior to insertion.
7. Securely hold the flange (wings) while removing the obturator, ventilate, assess tube placement, and ensure proper placement. **Then secure tube with tracheostomy ties** (or Velcro strap).
8. If the tube cannot be inserted easily, withdraw it and **attempt to pass a smaller sized tracheostomy tube** if available.
9. If insertion of a smaller tracheostomy tube fails or a smaller size is not available, then attempt to **insert an endotracheal tube (ETT)** into the stoma no more than one to two inches into opening. Select an ETT with an inner diameter that is equal to or smaller than the inner diameter of the last tracheostomy tube attempted. Aim downward when inserting an ETT into the stoma. If the ETT has a cuff, inflate it after checking proper placement. Note that this is only a temporizing measure until definitive treatment can be sought. An ETT in the stoma is not stable.
10. **If there is no improvement in the child's clinical condition, attempt oral endotracheal intubation** if this child does not have a preexisting upper airway obstruction. Bag-mask ventilation can also be attempted if there is no preexisting upper airway obstruction. If this is not possible, then attempt to ventilate the child by placing a manual resuscitator (bag-mask) directly over the stoma while covering the mouth and nose.

Source: Adirim TA, Smith EL, Singh T. In: *Special Children's Outreach and Prehospital Education.* Sudbury Ma: Jones and Bartlett, 2006. Reprinted with permission.

| TABLE 19-2 | Supplies Needed for Tracheostomy Tube Change |
| --- | --- |

- Same size tracheostomy tube that is "ready to go" (with ties in place)
- One size smaller tracheostomy tube
- Various sized endotracheal tubes
- Laryngoscope
- Suction catheters (6.0F, 8.0F, 10.0F)
- Normal saline for suctioning (premeasured ampules, "bullets," or vials, if available)
- Towel for shoulder roll
- Sterile gloves and face mask
- Scissors
- Oxygen and suction
- Bag-mask resuscitator with appropriately sized face masks
- Water-soluble lubricating gel
- Nebulizer setup

Source: Adirim TA, Smith EL, Singh T. In: *Special Children's Outreach and Prehospital Education.* Sudbury, Ma: Jones and Bartlett, 2006. Reprinted with permission.

## YOUR FIRST CLUE

**Recognizing Illness in a Child With Special Health Care Needs**

- Parent or caregiver says "something is different."
- Increased work of breathing
- Need for increased oxygen
- Fever
- Change in level of functioning
- Altered level of consciousness

volume of air at the same time the patient takes a breath. There are five types of ventilator alarms. They include: low pressure/apnea, low power, high pressure, setting error, and power switchover.

The causes of a low pressure alarm include a loose or disconnected circuit, a leak in the circuit, and a leak around the tracheostomy site. Check that all circuits are connected; if so, check the tracheostomy for leaks. The low power alarm means that the internal battery is nearly spent and the ventilator should be plugged into an electrical outlet. A high pressure alarm indicates an obstructed circuit or that the patient is having bronchospasm. Clear the obstruction or administer a bronchodilator or both. A setting error signifies that a setting might have been improperly adjusted. Under these circumstances the patient should be manually ventilated until the ventilator can be set properly. Any time the ventilator switches from AC power to battery, an alarm will sound. Check to make sure the battery is powering the unit and press the "alarm silent" button.[7]

A ventilator-dependent child is at risk for airway and breathing emergencies. Possible causes of respiratory distress in a ventilator-dependent child include airway obstruction (obstructed tracheostomy tube), an obstruction or leak in the ventilator tubing, problems with the oxygen supply, equipment failure involving the ventilator, and an acute medical condition. If a ventilator-dependent child is found to be in respiratory distress and the cause is not easily determined, then the child should be taken off the ventilator and manually ventilated with a bag-mask ventilator. Manually ventilating the child can help determine if the problem is equipment failure or a medical condition.

## Feeding Tubes and Gastrostomy Tubes

Feeding tubes and gastrostomy tubes are placed in children who need long-term nutritional supplementation or who cannot consume food by mouth. There are many conditions that necessitate placement of an artificial feeding tube. Some of these include severe developmental delay and/or cerebral palsy, coma, short bowel syndrome, swallowing difficulties, burns to mouth and esophagus, failure to thrive, and chronic diseases that affect nutrition such as cystic fibrosis.

A feeding tube is a long catheter usually inserted through the nose or mouth of the child into the stomach or jejunum. The terminology used for these tubes includes nasogastric (NG tube), orogastric (OG tube), nasojejunal (NJ tube) and orojejunal (OJ tube).

Gastrostomy tubes (G-tubes) go directly into the stomach from a site on the abdomen (**Figure 19.6**). Most G-tubes are inserted surgically or endoscopically by gastroenterologists,

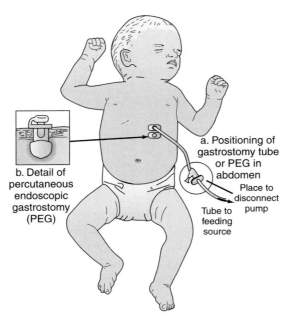

b. Detail of
percutaneous
endoscopic
gastrostomy
(PEG)

a. Positioning of
gastrostomy tube
or PEG in
abdomen

Place to
disconnect
pump

Tube to
feeding
source

**Figure 19.6** Gastrostomy tube.

surgeons, or radiologists, either at the bedside or in an outpatient procedure area, by using a procedure called percutaneous endoscopic gastrostomy (PEG). There are several types of low profile gastrostomy tubes in use, including the Button and Mic-Key.

A jejunostomy tube (J-tube) is often placed in children with gastroesophageal reflux. The tube is placed in the stomach and then passed through the duodenum into the jejunum.

## Feeding and Gastrostomy Tube Emergencies

There are many potential feeding and gastrostomy tube emergencies. The main complication with a feeding tube is displacement, which can lead to aspiration of fluid. A G-tube can become completely displaced or leak gastric contents, or the tube can become obstructed. When presented with a child who has one or more of these problems with a feeding or G-tube, assessment of respiratory and hydration status is important, especially in those children who are totally dependent on their feeding tubes for hydration and nutrition. Also, ask about medications and if any doses were missed.

## Management

If the child has a feeding tube that has been displaced, ask if it ends in the stomach or jejunum. An NG or OG tube can be replaced with a tube of the same size and length of the old catheter. The depth of insertion is estimated by measuring the catheter along its intended path: from the nose or mouth, down the esophagus, and into the stomach. The cm marking at this length should be noted. Then lubricate the tube and gently insert to this mark. Confirm tube location by instilling 10 to 30 cc of air into the tube while listening over the stomach for any sound of air. If air is heard, the tube is in the proper position and should be taped in place. If air is not heard, or the child is not crying, remove the tube and repeat the procedure.

An NJ or OJ tube is often a specially weighted tube that requires insertion under fluoroscopic guidance, so the appropriate specialist must be called for its insertion.

If a child has leaking around the G-tube or J-tube, attempt to determine the cause. Some possible causes of leakage include balloon deflation, coughing, constipation, bowel obstruction, and seizures. Addressing the cause might solve the problem, or consultation with the subspecialty service that manages the child's tube might be necessary.

An obstructed tube can be cleared with either a proteolytic enzyme solution or Coca-Cola, but if these methods are unsuccessful, it should be replaced. G-tubes that have been displaced should be replaced as soon as possible so that the stoma does not constrict and make replacement much more difficult. J-tube placement is more problematic because, after placing a tube in the stomach, passing the tube to the jejunum is usually done under fluoroscopy by a radiologist familiar with this procedure. When replacing a G-tube, the medical practitioner should determine when the tube was first inserted. For tubes in use for less than 3 months, consultation with the person or institution that performed the procedure is necessary, because the track might not be fully formed and insertion by a practitioner not adept at replacing these tubes might create a false track.

When performing the reinsertion procedure, the practitioner should use a similar size and type of G-tube. The different types of tubes include Mic-Key tubes or Buttons. Parents often have an extra tube with them, but if not, and the ED does not have G-tubes, a Foley catheter can be used to temporarily keep the stoma open until definitive placement can occur. Patients should not be discharged home without a definitive G-tube placed. Discussion with the subspecialty service managing the tube is important for further advice. See Table 19-3 for a description of the G-tube insertion procedure. If there is a delay in G-tube replacement, assessment of hydration is important. For the child who cannot take fluids orally, intravenous hydration should be considered.

---

**TABLE 19-3  Steps for Gastrostomy Tube Insertion**

1. Have same size G-tube and one size smaller available.
2. Check the balloon for leaks by placing in 3 to 5 cc water. Deflate balloon prior to insertion.
3. Lubricate tip with water-soluble gel.
4. Insert G-tube into stoma.
5. If the tube will not pass through the stoma after 2 to 3 attempts, the procedure should be attempted with one size smaller tube. Repeat balloon check and lubrication.
6. If the smaller tube will not pass, then attempt to dilate the stoma as follows:
   1) Have three sizes smaller Foley or other catheters available.
   2) Insert the smallest size, lubricated catheter into the stoma. Repeat with larger catheters in a stepwise fashion until the appropriate size catheter is able to pass through the stoma.
   3) Pass the appropriate size G-tube into the stoma.
7. Instruct patient and family to follow up with the medical practitioner who regularly manages the tube. If insertion of tube is not successful, the child needs to be transferred for definitive care.

Source: Adirim TA, Smith EL, Singh T. In: *Special Children's Outreach and Prehospital Education.* Sudbury, Ma: Jones and Bartlett; 2006. Reprinted with permission.

---

## CASE SCENARIO 2

A 6-year-old boy with acute lymphocytic leukemia presents to your emergency department with history of fever. His mother states that he last had chemotherapy 3 days prior to this emergency department visit. He was fine until this morning when he began to complain that he was not feeling well. His mother took his temperature orally and found that it was 38.2°C. She called the pediatric oncologist who advised that she take the child to the emergency department. The mother denies history of sore throat, vomiting, diarrhea, and contact with anyone who was ill. His mother states that he has a Broviac venous catheter.

On exam, the child is alert, has no labored breathing, but is somewhat pale. His vital signs are respirations 22 breaths/min, pulse 120 bpm, blood pressure 90/50 mmHg, and temperature is 38.6°C orally. His mucous membranes appear moist but pale. He has alopecia and is anicteric. His head and neck exam is otherwise normal. His lungs are clear to auscultation and his heart exam is notable for a soft systolic ejection murmur at the left sternal border. His Broviac catheter site appears clean and dry and the catheter is intact. His abdomen is soft and there are no masses or hepatosplenomegaly. His extremities are warm and well perfused.

1. What is your initial assessment of this child's presentation?
2. What historical factors impact on your diagnostic work-up and management?
3. How do you manage this child?

## Central Venous Catheters

Central venous catheters, or central lines, are used to deliver medications, blood products, and nutrition directly into a central vein. Blood samples can also be drawn from these lines. There are many circumstances under which a child would need a central venous line. These include cancer and the need for chemotherapy, sickle cell disease and the need for frequent transfusions, infections and the need for long-term antibiotic therapy, and various conditions in which nutritional supplementation is needed, such as in short bowel syndrome.

There are three types of catheters. Peripherally inserted central venous catheters (PICC) are long catheters inserted into the cephalic vein via the antecubital fossa. The catheter is advanced into the subclavian vein. These tubes are placed in children who need temporary venous access for antibiotic therapy. Some potential complications include easy dislodgement because they are not sutured in place, infection (but less of a risk than with other central lines), and obstruction.

Tunneled central venous catheters are placed surgically. They are inserted directly into a central vein, most commonly the subclavian, cephalic, or jugular. There are three common types: Broviac, Hickman, and Groshong. The first two are most common in children. The distal ends rest outside the chest and can have one to three ports. Implanted vascular access ports (Port-A-Cath, PAS Port, and Med-A-Ports) are also common in children. The insertion sites and method are the same as for the tunneled central venous catheters. The distal end of the catheter consists of a reservoir that is covered with a self-healing rubber septum. This reservoir rests subcutaneously, and a special needle is needed to access this line.[8]

### Management

The advantages of the implanted vascular ports are that they only need to be flushed with heparin once a month and after each access as opposed to daily heparin flushes. Another benefit is that they are hidden and might be more acceptable to older children when body image is more of an issue. See Table 19-4 for how to access Broviac and Hickman catheters and Table 19-5 for how to access Port-A-Caths.[9]

### Central Venous Catheter Emergencies

There are several circumstances under which a child with a central line will present for emergency treatment. These include damage to the catheter, air embolus, catheter dislodgement, and fever. Damaged catheters should be clamped proximal to the break with a hemostat. If the catheter is dislodged, apply direct pressure at the entry site to prevent or stop bleeding. This is a potentially life-threatening emergency. The child should be brought to a facility that can repair or replace the catheter. Air emboli or blood clot in the tubing can cause sudden onset of respiratory distress, chest pain, and altered mental status. If an embolus is suspected in a child with a central line, the medical practitioner should first manage the patient, with attention to airway, breathing, and circulation. The line should be clamped; the child should be placed on the left side and given oxygen. Peripheral intravenous placement should be considered. Hyperbaric therapy should be considered for a significant air embolus.

Fever is a common problem in children with central lines and should be considered an emergency. The central line is a foreign body that can act as a direct conduit for microorganisms from the outside world into the child's system. This is especially problematic in immunocompromised children, such as those undergoing treatment for cancer, as these children can easily develop sepsis.

### Management

Management of children with central lines and fever should include evaluation of ABCs, obtaining blood samples for CBC count and cultures from the central line and a peripheral vein, and starting broad-spectrum antibiotics until culture results are known. Obtain other cultures of urine, joint fluid, or cerebrospinal fluid as indicated. If the child with a central line and fever is not immune suppressed and appears well, then the practitioner can consider discharging the child home. However, if the child with a central

## TABLE 19-4   How to Access Broviac, Hickman Catheters

1. Prepare equipment.
2. Use sterile technique.
3. Clamp catheter at least 3 inches from cap. Either use the patient's clamp or a clamp without teeth.
4. Put sterile towel under catheter.
5. Remove cap at end of catheter and attach 10 mL syringe filled with sterile normal saline.
6. Unclamp catheter and slowly inject 3 to 5 mL of saline into catheter.
7. Aspirate back into syringe to check for blood return.
8. If resistance is met to instillation of saline or no blood returns, reclamp catheter and either reposition the catheter or the patient and try procedure again.
9. If blood return is achieved, inject the remaining sterile saline into the catheter and reclamp and remove syringe. Intravenous tubing can then be attached to the catheter. Be sure to purge the line of any air bubbles prior to infusing fluid.
10. If the practitioner needs to draw blood prior to infusing fluids, withdraw 8 to 9 mL of blood, reclamp the catheter, and discard the syringe. Attach an empty 10 mL syringe and remove needed blood for diagnostic tests, then return to Step 9.
11. After completion of procedure, inject 3 to 5 mL of heparin into catheter, replace cap and apply dressing.

Source: Fuchs SM. Accessing indwelling central lines. In: Henretig FM, King C, eds. *Textbook of Pediatric Emergency Procedures.* Baltimore, Md: Williams & Wilkins Co.; 1997:811–820. Reprinted with permission.

## TABLE 19-5   Accessing Totally Implanted Catheters (Port-A-Caths)

1. In a non-emergency, an anesthetic cream (EMLA) should be placed over the site 30 to 60 minutes prior to skin puncture.
2. Prepare equipment.
3. If EMLA is on-site, remove dressing and wipe cream away.
4. Perform procedure under sterile conditions; wearing sterile gloves.
5. Palpate reservoir. Wash overlying area with povidone-iodine or other sterile cleanser, then alcohol.
6. Attach a 10 mL syringe filled with sterile saline to T-connector tubing and flush saline through tubing.
7. Attach extension tubing to Huber needle and flush needle with saline to remove air. Clamp the extension tubing.
8. Put on new pair of sterile gloves.
9. Locate center of septum and stabilize reservoir between thumb and index finger. Slowly but firmly insert needle through septum to back of reservoir.
10. Unclamp extension tubing and slowly instill 2 mL saline.
11. If resistance is met, do not force. Reclamp.
12. If resistance is not met, infuse 3 mL more saline into port.
13. Aspirate fluid back into syringe and check for blood return. If blood is needed for diagnostic purposes, then attach an empty 10 mL syringe to extension tubing and withdraw 8 to 9 mL of blood, reclamp catheter, and discard syringe.
14. Attach 10 mL syringe with saline and slowly inject into reservoir and reclamp extension tubing. Tape needle in place, maintaining it at a right angle to septum.

Source: Fuchs SM. Accessing indwelling central lines. In: Henretig FM, King C, eds. *Textbook of Pediatric Emergency Procedures.* Baltimore, Md: Williams & Wilkins, Co.; 1997:811–820. Reprinted with permission.

line and fever is neutropenic (absolute neutrophil count less than 500), the child should be admitted to the hospital for intravenous antibiotics pending blood culture results.

## Dialysis Shunts and Peritoneal Dialysis Catheters

Approximately 150 cases of chronic renal failure per million persons are diagnosed in the United States each year. Most of these cases are in the adult population,[10] as end-stage renal disease is not a common pediatric problem. Less than 15 per million children develop chronic renal failure. In fact, less than 1% of all hemodialysis patients are children. Children tend to be treated more often with transplantation and therefore might need hemodialysis or peritoneal dialysis only temporarily.

### Dialysis Shunts

Hemodialysis is performed several times a week, because permanent vascular access is important. A child might have a synthetic graft or arteriovenous fistulae created by a surgeon. These sites should not be accessed outside of the dialysis laboratory except in extreme emergency situations. These grafts and fistulae are susceptible to multiple complications. Some of these include graft degeneration, stenosis of the graft or fistulae, vascular aneurysm, fistula rupture, thrombosis, and infection. All of these complications should be managed by the child's nephrologist and surgeon. Until definitive care can be undertaken by appropriate specialists, management of the symptoms resulting from complications is important. Some of these children manifest signs and symptoms of volume overload and metabolic derangements, and these should be addressed in the emergency setting. Hyperkalemia is the most immediately life-threatening and should be promptly diagnosed and treated.[10] Children with dialysis shunts and fever should have blood samples drawn and empiric antibiotics started pending culture results.

### Peritoneal Dialysis Catheters

Peritoneal dialysis catheters tend to be more common in children than dialysis vascular shunts, because peritoneal dialysis is a temporary form of managing end-stage renal disease that can be accomplished at home. A peritoneal dialysis catheter is a foreign body that provides a portal of entry for microorganisms from the external environment and therefore subjects patients to the risks of infection, most notably peritonitis.[10] This is considered a life-threatening emergency. The signs and symptoms of peritonitis include fever, abdominal pain, distended abdomen, and rebound tenderness.

## Management

The dialysate (fluid from the peritoneal cavity) should be sent for culture, and antibiotics should be infused into the peritoneal cavity by personnel comfortable with this procedure.[11] The decision regarding systemic antibiotic treatment should be made after assessing the child's appearance and looking for signs and symptoms of sepsis. Treatment should be undertaken with consultation from the child's nephrologist.

## Ventriculoperitoneal Shunts

Ventriculoperitoneal (VP) shunts are catheters inserted into the ventricles within the brain then threaded under the skin from the skull to the peritoneum, where excess cerebrospinal fluid (CSF) is drained (Figure 19.7).[12] (For more information on VP shunts, see Chapter 5, Central Nervous System). In some cases, the distal end of the shunt is placed in the pleural space between the chest wall and the lung (also called a VP shunt), or in the right atrium of the heart (VA shunt). Both of these locations allow CSF to drain, but each can result in unique complications. There are many medical conditions in which a VP or VA shunt is necessary. The most common is hydrocephalus, where there is a blockage in the CSF circulation system. The lateral ventricles enlarge with nonabsorbed CSF, causing an increase in intracranial pressure. Hydrocephalus is found in formerly premature babies who sustain an intraventricular bleed in the neonatal period, and also in children with brain tumors, spina bifida, myelomeningocele, and post-traumatic injury. These children should be assumed to have latex allergies and the necessary precautions taken.

## Shunt Emergencies

A child with a VP shunt is at higher risk of developing an infection of the shunt within the first 3 months postoperatively. Symptoms include fever, ill appearance, erythema over the shunt site and/or tubing, tenderness over the tubing, abdominal pain and tenderness,

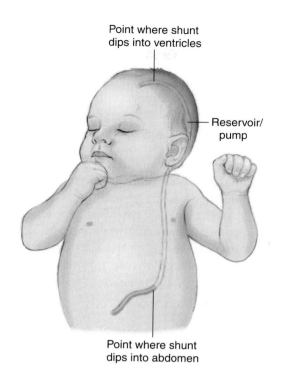

**Figure 19.7** A VP shunt directs CSF from the ventricles to the abdomen or, more rarely, the heart.

vomiting, and altered mental status. If a VP shunt infection is suspected, management should include assessment of the airway, breathing, and circulation and obtaining diagnostic lab work. CSF should be drawn from the shunt by a neurosurgeon and sent for a cell count and culture. Broad-spectrum antibiotics should be administered pending cell count and culture. Neurosurgeons should manage all shunt infections.

Peritonitis is another complication of VP shunts. The tip of the shunt empties into the peritoneal cavity, and a foreign body can serve as a nidus for infection. Signs and symptoms include fever, vomiting, abdominal pain and tenderness, and abdominal distention. A pseudocyst can cause symptoms similar to peritonitis, except a fever is not usually present. Management should be similar to that for VP shunt infections and should include diagnostic lab work, broad-spectrum antibiotics, and consultation with the neurosurgeon. Although infections of VP and VA shunts will not result in peritonitis, infection of the CSF can lead to pleural effusions and bacteremia, respectively.

The most common complication of a VP shunt is obstruction or malfunction. These can occur if there is an increase in protein in the CSF, causing a blockage in the tubing, or if there is a mechanical disruption in the shunt tubing, which can cause a buildup of CSF in the ventricles, and therefore an increase in intracranial pressure. Signs and symptoms include headache, nausea, vomiting, irritability, altered mental status, ataxia, change in vital signs, and in infants, a bulging fontanel. Late signs include those of the Cushing triad: bradycardia, irregular respirations, and hypertension. Initial management should include assessment and management of the airway, breathing, and circulation; oxygen supplementation; raising the child's head to 30°; if there are signs of increased intracranial pressure, providing bag-mask ventilation and preparing for intubation; obtaining intravenous access; and contacting a neurosurgeon as soon as possible. If the patient is stable, obtain a head CT and shunt series radiographs (head, chest, and abdomen) as needed. The definitive treatment for VP shunt malfunction is surgical shunt revision.

## THE CLASSICS

**Radiographic Findings of Shunt Obstruction/Malfunction**
- Enlarged ventricles (CT)
- Disconnected shunt (shunt series)
- Pseudocyst (ultrasonography)

## THE BOTTOM LINE

- The initial priorities are the same; follow the ABCs.
- Ask parents/caregivers about the child's baseline, or look for an EIF form.
- Use parents/caregivers assistance.
- Obtain an accurate weight; do not depend on age-appropriate norms.
- Learn about the technology devices used by dependent children.

## Check Your Knowledge

1. What should be your first step in managing a child with a tracheostomy tube and respiratory distress?
   A. Assess color
   B. Auscultate chest
   C. Remove tracheosotomy tube
   D. Suction tracheostomy

2. If a gastrostomy tube is clogged, which of the following can be used to clear it?
   A. Coca-Cola
   B. Ginger ale
   C. Hydrogen peroxide
   D. Pancrease
   E. Using more pressure

3. All of the following statements regarding a central line are correct except:
   A. Commonly used tunneled central venous catheters in children include Broviac and Hickman; the distal ends rests outside the chest and can have 1 to 3 ports
   B. Implanted central vascular access ports have a distal end of the catheter, which consists of a reservoir covered with a self-healing rubber septum
   C. Tunneled central venous catheters are inserted surgically into a central vein, most commonly the subclavian, cephalic, or jugular
   D. A regular needle can be used to access an implanted port

4. Which of the following would be the most critical and worrisome sign or symptom of a shunt obstruction?
   A. Bulging fontanel
   B. Cushing's triad
   C. Headache
   D. Nausea
   E. Vomiting

## References

1. Reynolds S, Desguin B, Uyeda A et al. Children with chronic conditions in a pediatric emergency department. *Pediatric Emergency Care.* 1996;12: 166–168.
2. Weiss HB, Mathers LJ, Forjuoh SN, and Kinnane JM. *Children and Adolescent Emergency Department Visit Databook.* Pittsburgh, Pa: Center for Violence and Injury Control, Allegheny University of the Health Sciences; 1997.
3. Foltin GL, Tunik MG, Cooper A, Markenson D, et al (eds). *Teaching Resource for Instructors in Prehospital Pediatrics, Version 2.0.* New York, Ny: Center for Pediatric Emergency Medicine; 1998.
4. Commentaries: a new definition of children with special health care needs. *Pediatrics.* 1998; 102(1):137–140.
5. Newacheck, PW, Strickland B, Shonkoff JP et al. An epidemiologic profile of children with special health care needs. *Pediatrics.* 1998;102(1):117–121.
6. Kallis JM. Replacement of a tracheostomy cannula. In: Henretig F. and King, C. eds. *Textbook of Pediatric Emergency Procedure.*, Baltimore, Md: Williams & Wilkins Co.; 1997: 82:873.
7. Adirim TA, Smith EL, and Singh T. In: *Special Children's Outreach and Prehospital Education* Sudbury,. Ma: Jones and Bartlett; 2004 (in press).
8. Foltin GL, Tunik MG, Cooper A, Markensson D et al (eds). *Paramedic TRIPP.* Version 1.0. New York, Ny: Center for Pediatric Emergency Medicine; 2002.
9. Fuchs, SM. Accessing indwelling central lines. In: Henretig FM and King C, eds. *Textbook of Pediatric Emergency Procedures.* Baltimore, Md: Williams & Wilkins Co.; 1997:811–820.
10. Krause RS. Renal failure, chronic and dialysis complications. In: Howes DS, Talavera F, Sinert R, Halamka J and Plantz S. eds. *emedicine.* Available at: http://www.emedicine.com/ emerg/topic501.htm. Accessed June 28, 2002.
11. National Kidney Foundation. K/DOQI clinical practice guidelines for vascular access, 2000. *Am J Kidney Dis.* 2001:37;S137–S181 (suppl 1).
12. Dieckmann R, Brownstein, D, Gausche-Hill M, eds. *Pediatric Education for Prehospital Professionals.* Sudbury, Ma: American Academy of Pediatrics/Jones & Bartlett Publishers: 2000:187.

A 6-month-old girl with a tracheostomy tube, ventriculoperitoneal shunt, and gastrostomy tube is brought to your emergency department because she has been having difficulty breathing. She was born prematurely and was only recently discharged from the neonatal intensive care unit. The mother states that the child has had a fever since the night before, and that today she needed to increase her oxygen flow. At baseline, this child is ventilated only at night and is currently being weaned from mechanical ventilation. The tracheostomy was performed for mechanical ventilation and tracheal stenosis. During the day, the child usually receives 0.25 L $FIO_2$. The mother states that the child's secretions have increased and she is suctioning more frequently. On examination, the child is awake but fussy, with subcostal and intercostal retractions, and her color is normal. Her respiratory rate is 60 breaths/min, heart rate is 180 beats per minute (bpm), blood pressure is 90/60 mmHg, and her temperature is 38.6°C. Oxygen saturation as measured by pulse oximetry is 90% on her baseline supplemental oxygen. The lung examination is notable for diffuse crackles and wheezes. Capillary refill is less than 2 seconds, and the extremities are well perfused.

1. What is your initial assessment of this child's presentation?
2. How do you manage this presentation? Where do you start?
3. What issues do you need to consider?

---

The initial assessment of this child reveals that she is in respiratory distress. She has an increased $O_2$ requirement and on lung examination is noted to have retractions, diffuse crackles and wheezes, and a slightly elevated respiratory rate. By history and examination, this child has a fever and increased tracheal secretions. The most likely diagnosis is infection.

The initial management priorities should mirror those of any other child. First, the airway should be assessed and cleared of obstruction. The medical practitioner should suction the tracheostomy tube both for therapeutic and diagnostic reasons. Sending a tracheal aspiration culture for Gram stain and culture and virus respiratory panel could be useful diagnostically and direct antibiotic management. Next, the practitioner should initiate treatment to improve this child's breathing. Suggested therapies could include assisting ventilation via bag-mask ventilation, administration of additional oxygen to maintain saturations above 95%, and bronchodilator nebulizer treatment. If this child's condition deteriorates on oxygen, then consideration of mechanical ventilation is necessary. Serial clinical examinations are invaluable, and arterial blood gas measurements can provide useful information. This child is at risk of ventilatory fatigue and apnea if her respiratory system is stressed beyond her capacity. The practitioner should next prescribe antibiotics for this child. The practitioner should choose a broad-spectrum antibiotic until the tracheal Gram stain and culture results are available.

The following issues should be considered. This child is a young baby who was born prematurely and recently discharged from the neonatal intensive care unit. This baby has chronic lung disease because of her premature lungs and damage from mechanical ventilation, known as bronchopulmonary dysplasia. Children with bronchopulmonary dysplasia are susceptible to pulmonary exacerbations of their lungs and pulmonary infections. They have a low respiratory reserve and even seemingly simple viral infections can be very serious. This child is dependent on an artificial airway that can become obstructed, so careful attention to pulmonary toilet is important. As is the case with this child, premature babies often have multiple medical problems and multiple technologies. In this child, fever and respiratory distress could also be caused by other infections such as sepsis, meningitis, VP shunt infection, and peritonitis from the shunt. A careful history and examination can help the practitioner determine the precise cause of her distress.

There are other issues to consider in the management of special needs children. These children's clinical status can deteriorate much quicker than in healthy children. Communication with the home hospital early in the child's course can be very helpful to practitioners in community hospitals.

A 6-year-old boy with acute lymphocytic leukemia presents to your emergency department with history of fever. His mother states that he last had chemotherapy 3 days prior to this emergency department visit. He was fine until this morning when he began to complain that he was not feeling well. His mother took his temperature orally and found that it was 38.2°C. She called the pediatric oncologist who advised that she take the child to the emergency department. The mother denies history of sore throat, vomiting, diarrhea, and contact with anyone who was ill. His mother states that he has a Broviac venous catheter.

On exam, the child is alert, has no labored breathing, but is somewhat pale. His vital signs are respirations 22 breaths/min, pulse 120 bpm, blood pressure 90/50 mmHg, and temperature is 38.6°C orally. His mucous membranes appear moist but pale. He has alopecia and is anicteric. His head and neck exam is otherwise normal. His lungs are clear to auscultation and his heart exam is notable for a soft systolic ejection murmur at the left sternal border. His Broviac catheter site appears clean and dry and the catheter is intact. His abdomen is soft and there are no masses or hepatosplenomegaly. His extremities are warm and well perfused.

1. *What is your initial assessment of this child's presentation?*
2. *What historical factors impact on your diagnostic work-up and management?*
3. *How do you manage this child?*

This is a well-appearing child with fever. His airway, breathing, and circulation are stable. However, this is a child who is at risk for developing serious infections such as sepsis and so this child's respiratory and circulatory status can change rapidly.

It is important to consider that this child is undergoing treatment for leukemia. Depending on the phase of treatment, this child is at risk for neutropenia (absolute neutrophil count less than 500). Children with neutropenia are at risk for serious infections. In addition, this child has a central line, which also places him at risk for serious infection. Therefore, any child with a central venous line and/or neutropenia who presents with fever needs to be evaluated for serious infection and treated with broad-spectrum antibiotics until culture results are known. This child's appearance should not deter the work-up.

Obtain blood drawn from his Broviac and send to the laboratory for complete blood count and for bacterial cultures. The practitioner should consider sending fungal cultures in the severely immune-compromised child. If this child appears well and is not neutropenic, then the practitioner can consider giving a dose of antibiotics through the Broviac and discharging the child home with close follow-up by the oncologist. If this child is found to be neutropenic, then the child should be admitted for an inpatient stay for antibiotic therapy until culture results are known.

# chapter 20

# Medical-Legal Considerations

Steven M. Selbst, MD, FAAP, FACEP
Andrew O. De Piero, MD

## Objectives

1 Discuss the importance of good communication and proper documentation when caring for pediatric patients and their families in the emergency department.

2 List common diagnoses that lead to malpractice lawsuits and identify methods to reduce malpractice actions in emergency care.

3 Describe issues of confidentiality and consent related to children in the emergency department.

4 Explain the requirements of the Emergency Medical Treatment and Labor Act with regard to evaluating and transferring patients.

5 Outline the pros and cons of having family members present for emergency procedures.

6 Develop an approach to a family whose child has died in the emergency department.

## Chapter Outline

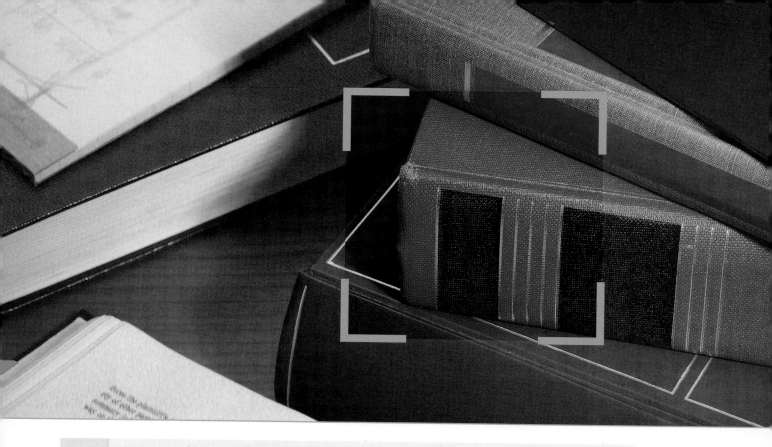

CASE SCENARIO 1

A 12-year-old boy is hit by a car while bicycling. He is brought to the emergency department and found to be hypotensive with abdominal distention and a swollen left thigh. The staff begins fluid resuscitation, and blood is ordered for possible transfusion. The child's condition worsens, and perfusion cannot be maintained with saline alone. His parents are told about his serious condition and the need for surgery and blood transfusion. The parents reply that they cannot consent to a blood transfusion because of their religious beliefs.

1.  *What should you do now?*

CASE SCENARIO 2

Paramedics bring in a 4-year-old boy who was rescued from a house fire, along with his uninjured mother. The child is awake and responds to questions but is mildly tachypneic despite receiving supplemental oxygen. Other vital signs are stable. The physical exam is notable for scattered first- and second-degree burns to less than 5% of the body surface area but involving regions on the face and lips. Carbon deposits are noted in the oropharynx. Concern for inhalational injury prompts the decision to perform endotracheal intubation. The child's mother asks to stay with her son as the intubation is performed.

1.  *How should you respond to the mother's request?*

# Introduction

Legal issues are especially important in the ED. There are guidelines, rules, and laws that govern the relationships among the pediatrician or emergency physician, the patient, the child's family, other medical staff, and community agencies. Children have unique and sometimes complicated medical conditions. They might present with problems such as child abuse or neglect, which pose difficult medical and legal questions. Issues of consent for minors add further legal burdens. The rights of the patient, the physician, the hospital, and the public are intertwined in complex relationships. Physicians and other health care providers must be aware of these relationships and legal guidelines if they are to safeguard the patient, the hospital, the community, and themselves.[1]

Pediatricians, emergency physicians, and others who care for acutely ill and injured children must be aware of relevant laws in order to fulfill their medical responsibilities. They must also be trained to recognize the pediatric diagnoses that pose the highest risk for litigation. They also should be adequately prepared for court when legal proceedings are forthcoming.[1]

# Medical Malpractice and the ED

Providing emergency care to children is a challenging endeavor. Medical malpractice cases disproportionately involve the ED. In one pediatric study, the ED accounted for 45% of 262 hospital-related cases alleging malpractice.[2] There are several reasons that lawsuits seem to originate in the emergency department. The ED can be crowded and lack the warm atmosphere of a pediatrician's private office. Privacy is often limited, and overworked staff might be impatient at times. Perhaps most importantly, patients can become frustrated when they endure long waiting times before they get to see the emergency physician. Sometimes the encounter with the physician can seem impersonal if the overwhelmed physician hurries off to see another patient. Understandably, it is difficult to establish rapport with a patient during a brief emergency encounter, and this puts the emergency physician at a disadvantage.[3]

Most malpractice lawsuits result in out-of-court settlements, or they are dropped altogether. Only about 10% reach a jury verdict. Still, these legal actions can be burdensome and emotionally draining.[1] They are also quite expensive. The median medical malpractice award (verdict by a jury) was $750,000 in 1998 and $800,000 in 1999. Settlements also rose from a median of $500,000 in 1998 to $650,000 in 1999.[4] About 45% of jury awards in 1998–1999 were $1 million or more, compared to 39% in 1997–1998.[5]

A bad outcome might trigger a lawsuit. The bad occurrence might be compounded by poor communication on the part of the physician, or unrealistic expectations on the part of the patient or family. Some families sue to seek revenge against physicians with whom they are unhappy. Others sue to obtain resources they will need to care for a handicapped child. Others sue to relieve their own guilt, and some to "save another patient from the physician" (Table 20-1). Often the lawsuits are instigated by a relative (perhaps a physician) who implies that the treatment given to a child fell below the standard of care.[6] ED staff members can unintentionally precipitate a malpractice lawsuit. Raising the eyebrows, shaking the head, or making comments such as, "I wish you had brought the child here first" might convey to the parents that initial treatment fell below the standard of care.[3,6] The standard of care is defined as that which a reasonable physician in a particular specialty would have

| TABLE 20-1 | Why People Initiate Medical-Legal Action |
|---|---|

- Child has a poor outcome
- Parents want more information
- Breakdown in communication (family and physician)
- Revenge against medical staff
- To obtain financial resources
- Attempt to relieve parental guilt
- Greed

Source: Selbst SM, Korin JB. *Preventing Malpractice Lawsuits in Pediatric Emergency Medicine.* Dallas, Tx: American College of Emergency Physicians; 1998. Reprinted with permission.

given to a similar patient under similar circumstances. Because most clinicians have similar access to information and knowledge, they often are held to a national standard of care no matter where they practice.[1]

Poor care might not necessarily result in a bad outcome, and a bad outcome might not always be the result of poor care. The attorney for the plaintiff must show that there is a relationship between bad practice and bad outcome. The attorney must prove that the physician had a duty to the patient, that this duty was breached, and that this resulted in an injury to the patient.

Some malpractice lawsuits are unavoidable. Children present with unusual or atypical findings, and the diagnosis might be difficult initially. However, pediatricians and emergency physicians should have a high index of suspicion when a child "just doesn't look right" to the parent or the physician. If there is a worrisome history or a suspicious physical exam, it is prudent to observe the child for a period of time in the ED. Persistent vomiting, irritability, lethargy, or inability to drink fluids in the ED can be signs of serious illness. Finally, followup care should be arranged for the very near future after an ED visit. The physician should be particularly concerned if a child does not improve despite the initial recommendations and treatment.[1]

## Statute of Limitations

If there is a poor outcome, parents (or the patient) might find fault with the care delivered many years later. Each state has its own statute of limitations that sets standards for the length of time in which a person may bring a lawsuit for an alleged injury. For most states, the statute of limitations for adult patients is 2 or 3 years from the time an injury that resulted from alleged negligence is discovered, or should have been discovered. When this time has passed, a lawsuit can no longer be brought, regardless of its merits. With children, the time period is extended because they cannot initiate legal action on their own behalf. In many jurisdictions, the time period does not begin for an injured child until he or she has reached the age of majority (18 to 21 years old). Thus, a pediatric patient may bring a lawsuit against a physician for events that took place 20 years earlier.[1,3]

For example, suppose an infant, only a few months old, presents with meningitis that is not promptly diagnosed and results in complications, including delayed development. The family is not obligated to initiate a lawsuit within 2 years of the illness, but rather within 2 or 3 years after the injury (delayed development) is discovered. This could be when the child begins school 5 years later. Some states limit this time period, but it usually extends 7 to 8 years or more after the injury should have been discovered. If the parents do not file a lawsuit, the patient may still decide to sue when he or she becomes an adult, at age 21.[1,3]

## High-Risk Cases in Pediatric Emergency Medicine

Consider the following case: a 15-year-old girl is taken to an ED with complaints of severe abdominal pain.[7] She is evaluated and discharged to home with medication. She returns 3 days later with persistent symptoms. At the second visit, a perforated appendix and peritonitis are found.

The patient sues the hospital and the physicians who treated her initially. She contends that her condition had worsened, and that complications developed because the hospital failed to make the correct diagnosis on the first visit. The hospital claims that the patient was sent home with instructions to see a private doctor the same day. She allegedly ignored those instructions, and thus her condition worsened. A jury returns a verdict in favor of the physicians and the hospital.[8]

Consider a second case: a 7-month-old boy is brought to the ED because of lethargy, irritability, decreased appetite, uncontrollable crying, and stiffening of his extremities.[9] The physician who examines the infant diagnoses an upper respiratory infection and discharges him with a prescription for amoxicillin. Two days later, the baby is taken to another hospital and is given cough syrup. The next day, the baby develops seizures and is rushed to the first ED. He is found to be in a coma and is transferred to a local children's hospital 4 hours later. Bacterial meningitis is diagnosed. The baby suffers brain damage and now has a chronic seizure disorder. It is believed that the infant will not be able to live independently. The family sues the physicians and hospitals that treated the infant initially, claiming that they should have performed a spinal tap when he first presented, before he had the seizure.[10]

The physician at the first hospital claims the baby did not have meningitis at the time of the visit, that a complete examination was performed but negative findings were just not noted in the record.

A jury finds in favor of the first physician and hospital that provided treatment. The other physicians and hospital settle with the family for more than $900,000.

Specific diagnoses are particularly troublesome and are often the subject of malpractice lawsuits in acute pediatric care. For example, febrile children and those with abdominal pain pose high-risk situations. Failure to diagnose meningitis and appendicitis are the leading pitfalls for those treating children. This is not surprising because these conditions can result in serious morbidity or death if not diagnosed and treated promptly. In addition, both of these conditions can have subtle presentations. Many infections progress rapidly, and the diagnosis might not be obvious when the patient first presents to the clinician.[1,3,10] Other errors, such as missed fractures or failure to find a foreign body in a wound, might

| TABLE 20-2 | Common Pediatric Diagnoses Involved in ED Malpractice Claims |
|---|---|

- Appendicitis
- Child abuse
- Dehydration
- Fractures
- Medication errors
- Meningitis
- Meningococcemia
- Myocarditis
- Slipped capital femoral epiphysis
- Testicular torsion
- Wounds and lacerations (foreign bodies and other complications)

Source: Selbst SM, Korin JB. *Preventing Malpractice Lawsuits in Pediatric Emergency Medicine*. Dallas, Tx: American College of Emergency Physicians; 1998. Reprinted with permission.

not result in serious morbidity but are common triggers for malpractice lawsuits. In these cases, the public simply expects the physician to make the diagnoses. The public is aware of great advances in medicine. They expect a good outcome when they seek medical care. Anything less must be someone's fault.[10]

Other pediatric conditions that often result in litigation include failure to diagnose testicular torsion, medication errors, and complications of lacerations.[1,3] A careful approach to these conditions is warranted. Juries are generally sympathetic to children and award large sums when a physician is found negligent. Table 20-2 summarizes the pediatric diagnoses commonly involved in ED malpractice actions.

## Documentation

The importance of careful documentation cannot be overemphasized. Good documentation prevents lawsuits. The patient's chart is generally the first document reviewed by parents, attorneys, and expert witnesses. Its content and appearance could be the difference between being sued or not in those cases where there is a perception of incorrect treatment. A record that demonstrates a thorough examination and testing can suggest to the plaintiff's

| TABLE 20-3 | Crucial Elements of ED Chart Documentation |
|---|---|

- Address chief complaint
- Include pertinent positive, negative findings
- Carefully describe general appearance, state of hydration
- Record allergies, immunizations, medications, past medical history
- Record neatly; note should reflect professional approach
- Include progress or discharge note
- Document your thought process
- Avoid derogatory statements
- Avoid self-serving statements
- Establish agreement with notes of others (EMT, RN)

Source: Selbst SM, Korin JB. *Preventing Malpractice Lawsuits in Pediatric Emergency Medicine*. Dallas, Tx: American College of Emergency Physicians; 1998. Reprinted with permission.

attorney not to proceed further. A record that does not clearly demonstrate an important test or portion of the examination can lead counsel to assume it was not done. The record will often sway the consulting physician who advises an attorney of whether the case has merit and should be pursued. Because it is difficult to predict which patient will have a bad outcome and pursue litigation, each chart should be prepared as if it were to serve as the basis for defense in a lawsuit.[1,3,10] Table 20-3 reviews the important items of the ED medical record.

Because of the extended statute of limitations for children, many years can pass before a physician is advised of malpractice action. Recall of the case can be limited. The physician might be totally dependent on the record for recollection of facts of the case. The document will prove to be the doctor's friend or foe depending on how well it was prepared at the time of treatment. Many malpractice cases have been settled despite appropriate medical care because the care was not substantiated in the medical records.[1,3,10,11]

The history of present illness must be described in the record completely but con-

cisely.[1,3,10] Any information relevant to the chief complaint should be included. It is especially wise to record details about the child's diet, level of activity at home, and medications received. The physical examination should be described in detail, including vital signs. Abnormal vital signs deserve careful attention.[1,3,10] It is particularly important to note the child's general appearance, state of hydration, and level of activity or playfulness in the ED.[1,3,10] A second note or progress note is essential if the child remains in the ED for a significant amount of time. Procedures must be documented in a detailed note. The medical record, of course, must include the diagnostic impression of the physician, and this should be consistent with the treatment rendered.

The medical record should provide meaningful information to another physician if further care is required. The record should display a concerned and professional attitude toward the patient. Only comments that a physician would be comfortable reading in front of a jury should be included. The content and neatness of such a record can greatly affect the way a jury feels about a physician. It should not contain insensitive terms. Avoid derogatory statements or descriptions of the patient's parents.[1,3,10]

The notes of other professionals caring for the child in the emergency setting are also important. Physicians should carefully read the notes of nursing staff, consultants, and prehospital care providers. Emergency medical technicians (EMTs) who transport the child can provide pertinent information such as the patient's name, the condition in which he or she was found, vital signs, and a description of services rendered, such as the administration of oxygen or attempts to establish vascular access. This information can be very helpful in caring for the patient. For example, if a child is involved in a motor vehicle crash, a description of how the patient was found can help the physician determine the most likely type of injury and the appropriate diagnostic studies to obtain. An EMT's description of the crashed vehicle can help determine the magnitude of the injuries sustained. A patient might have related important information to the EMTs, such as drug allergies or medications taken. Copies of the EMT's medical records should be presented to the ED staff, and important information should be shared verbally and entered into the patient's hospital record. The physician's notes should be consistent with those of other professionals who record in the chart.[1,3,10]

In a noisy ED environment with numerous sick and injured patients, physicians understandably make mistakes while charting. Errors should be corrected appropriately. There should be no attempt to cover up mistakes by blacking out words or phrases, as this tends to arouse suspicion. A single line drawn through the error, which is then initialed and dated, is more appropriate. Do not attempt to alter the record later![1,3]

## Communication

Good communication among the medical staff, patient, and family is also extremely important in the ED. There is a direct relationship between good communication skills of the physician and fewer malpractice lawsuits.[6,12] Physicians who generate patient complaints are more likely to be sued.[13] The patient and family must perceive a caring attitude, openness, professional integrity, and standards of excellence. Patients are not always aware of a physician's competence, but they are keenly aware of his or her manner. In other words, when treating children in the ED, accuracy helps. Professional appearance, honesty, and a kind, compassionate attitude are vital.[1]

Good communication is especially important at the time of discharge from the ED. The physician should give written, detailed discharge instructions and go over these carefully with the parent or other caregiver, and with the patient if he or she is old enough to understand. Nonspecific instructions to "give fluids" or return "as needed" are not helpful. Abbreviations should be avoided. The instructions should always include a few examples of worrisome signs to look for at home. Although it is not feasible to list every possible complication, the parents must have a clear notion of when to see their personal pediatrician and what warrants an immediate return to the ED. The parent should be asked to sign the record to indicate that he or she has received and understands the discharge instructions.[1,3,10]

It is important to explain the thought process to a parent at the time of discharge and why followup care is crucial, especially if the child's symptoms change. Write the diagnosis down for other caregivers at home and ask the parents if they have any questions before they leave.[1,3,10]

It is also essential to acknowledge uncertainty. Patients often think highly of physicians and believe that a clinical evaluation provides absolute certainty that the child's condition is benign. However, symptoms of serious illness can develop later (e.g., appendicitis, meningitis), and parents might be reluctant to return to the ED because they were told that the child's condition is benign. Acknowledging that the diagnosis is never totally certain permits patients or parents (in fact, they should be encouraged) to call the ED or return if the child's condition worsens or fails to improve as expected. Additionally, parents might perceive the physician to be arrogant when they are told emphatically that the child's condition is benign, and if it turns out to be serious, they are more likely to sue. Physicians and patients together must be able to accept some degree of uncertainty. If any party is uncomfortable with this, the risk of litigation and dissatisfaction is higher. Direct discussions and communication with the family can improve this situation. Optional diagnostic studies can reduce the level of uncertainty.

## Consultants

Consider the following case: a teenaged boy is stabbed with an ice pick during an altercation and is brought to an ED.[14,15] The physician diagnoses a superficial wound and discharges the patient with instructions to return if his condition changes. The patient returns to the ED 3 hours later with vomiting and abdominal pain. At this time, the chief of surgery is called and the patient is taken to the operating room. An exploratory laparotomy reveals that the patient has a perforated duodenum, which is repaired. However, a second perforation is not noted or repaired, and neither is a laceration to the right kidney and renal vein. Four hours after surgery, the patient suffers cardiac arrest and dies, due to blood loss from the vascular injury that was not found.

The surgeon is sued for deviating from the standard of care. However, the family also sues the first physician for failing to call the surgeon earlier and for releasing the patient from the ED, which caused a delay in surgical intervention. They argue that the surgery was more difficult because of the delay, and that this might have led to the misdiagnosis. The hospital settles with the family for $100,000 before trial. A jury returns a verdict in favor of the physicians.[15]

In a second case, a 14-year-old boy is injured in a motor vehicle crash.[16] He is trapped in a vehicle with his legs under the dash for 30 minutes before he is extricated and brought to an ED. The child complains of bilateral hip pain and cannot stand or bear weight. An emergency physician evaluates the child, obtains radiographs of the hips, and reads them as normal. The boy is admitted to the hospital for pain management. The next day, the hospital radiologist reviews the radiographs and diagnoses bilateral posterior hip dislocations. The report is not placed into the child's chart for 2 days, and no action is taken. The patient undergoes "therapy" in the hospital, and his pain worsens. Orthopedics is consulted when the radiology report is discovered, and the dislocations are reduced. Additional radiographs taken at this time reveal fractures of the femoral heads.

He subsequently develops bilateral hip necrosis. He requires multiple surgical procedures, and 1 year later, he requires bilateral hip replacements. He is expected to have more hip replacements as he ages. The family sues the hospital, the emergency physician, the radiologist, and the primary care physician who managed the hospital admission. They claim that poor communication among the physicians led to a delay in diagnosis and treatment. The case is settled for $1.6 million.[17]

No physician works in isolation in the ED. Frequently there is a need to consult other physicians and specialists while caring for ill and injured children. Emergency physicians should call for help whenever they believe that the care required is beyond their expertise, or when it appears that another opinion will be helpful. Pediatricians, emergency physicians, critical care specialists, trauma surgeons, radiologists, and other experts must work together to manage illnesses and injuries appropriately. Usually these interactions proceed smoothly and consultation leads to improved patient care.[1]

Consultation in a timely manner is expected.[18,19] The more unstable the patient, the more urgent the need for rapid consultation. If there is a true surgical abdomen, for example, it is unwise to delay consultation by waiting for a urinalysis or other study. Likewise, if a child has a clinical picture of testicular torsion, it is appropriate to call for consultation promptly rather than ordering Doppler studies or other tests that might delay definitive care.[18] If the consultant does not arrive in a timely manner, other options should be pursued, including calling the consultant's supervisor, specialty attending, or other sources for help.[19] It is important to document the time the specialist was called, the time he or she arrived, and if applicable, the time he or she assumed care of the patient.

If a family insists on consultation (e.g., a plastic surgeon to suture a facial laceration) it might be wise to comply whenever the request is reasonable. A request for a second opinion should also be honored if at all possible.[20]

Often the emergency physician calls a patient's primary care physician to discuss the need for admission, to obtain special studies, or to get approval for specialty consultation. The opinion of an outside attending physician should be considered advisory only.[20] If the physician providing the care believes admission to the hospital is warranted and the consultant, including the primary care physician, disagrees, then the consultant must come to the ED to evaluate the child. Responsibility for the disposition often rests with the emergency physician, but this responsibility would probably be shared if both have evaluated the child.

If simple, limited information is needed from a consultant, it can be appropriate to obtain this by telephone without direct examination by the consultant. In those cases, it should be made clear that the consultant is being asked solely for advice and there is no request for the consultant to see the patient directly.[1,18] The essence of the telephone conversation should be recorded in the patient's chart. Both the consultant and the emergency physician accept some risk with this type of consultation, as miscommunication on the telephone is possible.[1]

Radiology consultation is common in the ED. The emergency physician should seek radiology consultation if it is available and if there is doubt about the interpretation of a radiograph. In the event of a trial, the emergency physician might be found liable for misreading a child's x-ray. The emergency physician might not be held to the same standard as a radiologist, but a jury will have to determine the level of expertise that the physician should possess.[1] If a radiologist is not available in the ED, the family should be told that the interpretation by the ordering physician is preliminary and that they will be contacted if there is a discordant reading.[1] Because this procedure is not always followed perfectly, it might be preferable to recommend that the parent followup through the primary care physician's office. A preprinted instruction sheet could provide a standardized set of instructions on how parents can do this.

Good communication with consultants is essential (Figure 20.1). Understandably, there are sporadic disagreements about patient management. Consultants are not always correct,

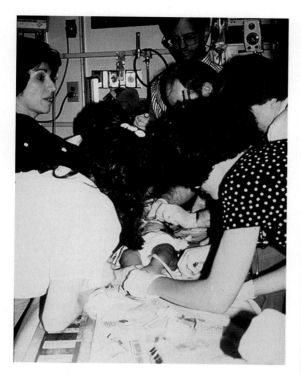

Figure 20.1 Good communication with the consultant is essential.

Source: Selbst SM, Korin JB. *Preventing Malpractice Lawsuits in Pediatric Emergency Medicine.* Dallas, Tx: American College of Emergency Physicians; 1998. Reprinted with permission.

| TABLE 20-4 | Emergency Physician-Consultant Relationship |
| --- | --- |

**Emergency Physician's Role**
- Request consultation when appropriate
- Consult in a timely manner
- Document time of call
- Consult a competent physician
- Communicate important information succinctly
- Request specific advice or ask management questions of the consultant
- Attempt to resolve disagreements

**Consultant's Role**
- Provide timely consultation
- Document time of arrival
- Address specific questions
- Communicate well with emergency physician
- Document findings
- Attempt to resolve disagreements

## THE BOTTOM LINE

- Medical malpractice risk in the ED is disproportionately higher than in other patient care areas.
- Good communication and proper documentation reduce the likelihood of medical malpractice litigation.
- Pay special attention to the diagnoses that most commonly lead to medical malpractice litigation.

and their actions, or inaction, can sometimes result in harm to the pediatric patient. The emergency physician can be sued with a specialist when a patient is harmed by the improper actions of another physician, as illustrated in the case.[21]

Emergency physicians are not legally bound to accept the advice of consultants. Blind acceptance of a consultant's advice can leave the emergency physician liable if a child suffers.[20] However, it is not advisable to reject the advice of a specialist without careful consideration of the consequences. If there are questions about care, it is best to discuss the case personally with the consultant. If recommendations are not followed, the emergency physician should document why suggested studies were not obtained.[1,19] Disputes about care should not be discussed in front of the patient or family. Instead, it is best to try to resolve these amicably, away from the patient, before discharge.[1] Table 20-4 reviews the physician-consultant relationship in the ED.

## Issues of Consent

Consider the following case: an 11-month-old girl is brought to an ED by her aunt because of difficulty in breathing. Her mother is at work. The family claims that an ED clerk told the aunt that the baby could not be treated without the mother's consent. The hospital denies this and says another patient or visitor in the waiting area misled the aunt. The woman leaves the ED with the child and goes to find the mother. The three return to the ED, but the baby is then in cardiac arrest and dies soon after.[1]

Federal law (EMTALA) requires a medical screening examination for all patients presenting to the ED regardless of consent or who brings the child in.

When a child is not in the care of the parents, consent and determination of guardianship should not delay the medical screening examination. Most states have laws that permit treatment of minors (children younger than 18 years) in an emergency and other selected cases. Treatment without parental consent is required to prevent death or serious injury. The greater the risk of serious harm to a child, the more justified it is to act without delay in the absence of the legal guardian. The hospital staff should attempt to locate the legal guardian and obtain consent for treatment, but treatment should not be delayed so as to risk the child's life or health. If a physician is not sure if a patient's medical condition justifies immediate yet unauthorized treatment, it is best to err on the side of treatment rather than to withhold care.[1] A good general principle to follow is to act as a reasonable person would expect a reasonable physician to do.

Adolescents who present for care pose additional dilemmas. Courts in almost all states have agreed that there are some situations in which a minor can be treated in the ED without parental consent or knowledge. Most states recognize an emancipated minor as one who has been married, pregnant, graduated high school, served in the armed forces, or is otherwise independent of parental care or control (Table 20-5). State laws vary; clinicians are advised to become familiar with local statutes. Furthermore, some specific medical conditions allow an adolescent to seek medical care without his or her parents. All states have recognized that many teenagers would avoid treatment of venereal disease if involvement of their parents were required. This could put the patient at risk and lead to increased public health problems as well. Thus, all states allow a minor to receive treatment for venereal disease without parental consent. Some states allow minors to consent to treatment and testing for pregnancy and HIV.[1]

Furthermore, several states allow "mature minors" to give consent for treatment. The mature

| TABLE 20-5 | Criteria for Emancipated Minor (Apply in Most States, But Not All) |
|---|---|

- Married
- Pregnant
- High school graduate
- Self-employed
- Living independently
- Served in armed forces

Source: Selbst SM, Korin JB. *Preventing Malpractice Lawsuits in Pediatric Emergency Medicine.* Dallas, Tx: American College of Emergency Physicians; 1998. Reprinted with permission.

minor doctrine allows minors older than 14 or 15 years to consent for care if they are "sufficiently mature to understand the nature of the procedure and its consequences." The treatment must not involve serious risks. For example, in some jurisdictions, a 15-year-old boy who is assessed to be mature enough to understand can give his own consent to have a finger laceration sutured. The physician must determine that the minor is competent to understand and give consent.[1,22]

Physicians should be aware of problems in treating adolescents who present for care without their parent (Figure 20.2). Their medical histories might be incomplete, and knowledge of important facts such as immunizations or allergies can be lacking. Also, their ability to understand directions might be limited and compliance with treatment poor. Consequently, medical care can be compromised, and the physician faces additional liability risks. The right of confidentiality is extended to a minor who consents to his or her own care. If a minor adolescent is treated in the ED without parents (under a state's mature minor statute) and insists on privacy, this must be respected unless it is believed that failure to inform the parents will harm the patient.[1,23]

It is wise to discuss confidentiality as it applies to billing issues with the adolescent patient in the ED. Most hospitals send the bill to the legal guardian (a confidentiality breach), and the parents would then be likely to ask questions about the visit. In general, parents are not responsible for contracts made by their children, so the adolescent who consented for his or her own care is legally responsible for

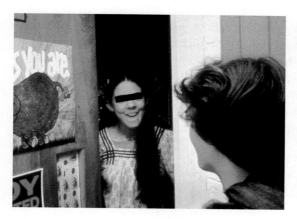

Figure 20.2 Physicians should be aware of problems in treating adolescents who present for care without their parents.

the bill. Ideally, hospital billing and medical record-keeping should be done in a manner that protects the adolescent's right to privacy. Unfortunately, this is not always easy to do.

## Informed Consent

Parents, legal guardians, or emancipated minors have the right to know and make an informed decision about the care to be delivered. They must give informed consent for treatment and significant procedures unless an emergency exists such that there is no time to involve the patient or guardian. In order to make an informed decision, the patient or parent must be autonomous, that is, free of coercion or manipulation by the physician, family, or other forces. Next, the patient or

| TABLE 20-6 | Important Elements of Informed Consent |
| --- | --- |

- Child's diagnosis
- Purpose and nature of planned procedure or treatment
- Risks, side effects (significant or common)
- Reasonable alternatives and their risks
- Prognosis with and without treatment

Source: Selbst SM, Korin JB. *Preventing Malpractice Lawsuits in Pediatric Emergency Medicine.* Dallas, Tx: American College of Emergency Physicians; 1998. Reprinted with permission.

parent must be capable of making the decision. The physician must determine that pain, medications, or hypotension are not impairing his or her ability to decide. Third, there must be adequate disclosure. Physicians are obligated to reveal the significant risks of treatment and of withholding treatment. It is expected that the physician will tell parents whatever information a reasonable person would need to make an informed decision. Alternatives must be disclosed. Many patients and parents want to know the physician's opinion and will follow his or her recommendations if the physician seems trustworthy. Finally, the patient or parent must comprehend the information. The physician must determine if the teenager or parent understands the information presented and is making a reasonable objection or an irrational choice. It is wise to ask the patient or parent to repeat the information given in his or her own words.[24] Table 20-6 summarizes the important features of informed consent to be reviewed with patients or parents.

**CASE SCENARIO 3**

A 4-year-old girl is brought to the emergency department with a history of choking on a peanut. Her past medical history is unremarkable. On examination, she is in mild respiratory distress. Her respiratory rate is 44/minute. She has slight retractions with decreased breath sounds on the right. Chest radiograph is consistent with foreign body aspiration. There is difficulty starting an IV, and the mother has "words" with the nursing staff. When bronchoscopy is suggested, the mother is visibly upset and shouts harshly at the house officer. The mother wants to sign out against medical advice.

1. *How could this situation have been avoided?*
2. *What steps can be taken now to ensure that the child receives the best care possible?*

## Refusal of Care

In general, parents have the right to make decisions about their child's care, and it is presumed they will act in their child's best interests. Some patients or parents refuse treatment or leave the ED against medical advice. This usually occurs when the patient or parent is angry, afraid, feels guilty, is disoriented, or has certain religious beliefs. In some situations, a hostile patient or parent is actually invited or encouraged to leave by an angry or frustrated staff member. When a patient or family leaves the ED without evaluation and treatment, everyone involved can suffer. The child, of course, might have persistent or worsening symptoms from a medical problem that has not been addressed. Likewise, the staff usually feels a sense of failure and frustration when their advice and recommendations are not heeded. Worse yet, the hospital and physicians can be exposed to a lawsuit if the patient suffers serious morbidity or dies after leaving against medical advice, even voluntarily.[1]

The physician should try to understand why the patient or family wants to leave. If the patient or parent seems angry, allow him or her to express concerns without interruption. If a staff member made the family angry, that individual should apologize or avoid contact with the patient. It is never a good idea to challenge a patient to sign out against medical advice, and they should not be threatened with a call to the security officers. Further agitation will accomplish little. Security should be called

| TABLE 20-7 | Required Documentation When Patients Leave Against Medical Advice |
| --- | --- |

- History, examination—parts completed
- Clinical impression
- Treatment risks, benefits explained
- Alternative treatments explained
- Reasons family wanted to leave
- Offer of help to transfer the child
- Invitation to return to ED later
- Signatures of parents (if possible), physicians, witness

Source: Selbst SM, Korin JB. *Preventing Malpractice Lawsuits in Pediatric Emergency Medicine.* Dallas, Tx: American College of Emergency Physicians; 1998. Reprinted with permission.

in only if needed to maintain order. Instead, the staff should remain courteous and flexible in the treatment plan. If the situation reaches an impasse, offer the parents an opportunity to speak to another physician. The primary care physician can often be helpful in such situations. If all attempts to convince the family to stay for treatment are unsuccessful and the family leaves the ED against medical advice, the encounter must be carefully documented (Table 20-7).[1]

In some cases, the patient might not be permitted to leave under any circumstances. A disoriented or impaired teenager or parent may not be permitted to leave the ED. A patient or parent who cannot understand the risks and benefits of treatment or the risks of leaving the ED should not be permitted to make a decision to refuse care. Likewise, any medical problem that presents a life-threatening problem for the child justifies immediate medical care. It should be noted that most courts in the United States will not allow a parent to impose his or her religious beliefs on a minor, especially in a life-threatening situation. If a blood transfusion is considered essential for treatment, it should be given.[25] A court order will be necessary and should be sought simultaneously as treatment is begun. In most cases of leaving against medical advice or refusal of care, it is best to win the cooperation of the parents, but if they refuse, the staff is justified in treating the child. They should report the case as medical neglect and attempt to obtain a court order while emergency care is delivered. If it is unclear whether a life-threatening situation is present, err on the side of treatment. Similarly, in the case of suspected child abuse, when the perpetrator is unknown, the child should not be released despite the parents' wishes or protests.[1]

---

**CASE SCENARIO 4**

A 3-year-old child presents to a small, rural emergency department with a 24-hour history of abdominal pain. The patient also has fever and vomiting but is clinically stable. The child has a past medical history of developmental delay, cerebral palsy, and epilepsy. The emergency department physician establishes a diagnosis of appendicitis and consults a general surgeon. The surgeon agrees with the diagnosis of appendicitis but recommends transfer to a tertiary care center given the patient's complex medical issues. Citing a lack of bed availability within the hospital, the physician at the tertiary care center refuses to accept the patient. The emergency physician disregards the refusal and sends the patient by ambulance to the tertiary care center.

1. Should the patient have been transferred under these circumstances?
2. Is such a refusal justified?

---

## Transfer of Care

Interfacility transfer of patients involves a number of medical and legal considerations. The ability to transfer patients represents a vital component of the health care system. Transfer of patients can occur to provide care not available at the sending facility (both emergent and nonemergent) or as a result of the patient's or primary care provider's request. Discussion of the medical responsibilities involved in transferring patients should be coupled with a discussion of the federal statute governing this process.

The Emergency Medical Treatment and Labor Act (EMTALA) is a section of the Consolidated Omnibus Budget Reconciliation Act (COBRA) passed in 1986 to address the care of emergency patients. While originally designed to prevent the "dumping" of uninsured patients from private to public EDs, its scope has broadened considerably. EMTALA applies to all US hospitals that receive Medicare funds. Failure to comply with EMTALA can result in fines to the physician, which are not covered by malpractice insurance, and the hospital can be terminated from the Medicare program.

EMTALA imposes three essential duties on hospitals. A medical screening examination is required for all individuals who present for evaluation of a medical condition to determine if an emergency medical condition exists. Triage assessment is not considered a medical screening examination. An emergency medical condition is defined as a condition of "acute symptoms of sufficient severity (including severe pain) such that the absence of immediate medical attention could reasonably be expected to result in placing the health of the individual (or, with respect to the pregnant woman, the health of the woman or her unborn child) in serious jeopardy, serious impairment to bodily functions, or serious dysfunction of any bodily organ or part."[26] The medical screening examination must be of similar thoroughness for all patients presenting to the ED with the same complaint. This can involve diagnostic testing and the use of consultants.[27] In the event that an emergency medical condition is discovered, EMTALA requires that the patient be stabilized within the capabilities of the hospital. Under EMTALA, stabilization has occurred when "no material deterioration of the emergency medical condition is likely, within reasonable medical probability, to result from or occur during the transfer of the individual from the facility or . . . ."[26] If the hospital is unable to stabilize the patient with its resources, EMTALA requires that the patient be transferred to a facility able to provide the necessary services. A patient's (or parent's) written informed consent is required to initiate a transfer. The medical benefits must outweigh the risks of transfer, and an appropriate transfer method must be selected. Copies of the medical record should accompany the patient to the receiving facility. Under EMTALA, accepting hospitals are required to accept patients with emergency medical conditions if they possess resources not available at the sending hospital. However, the receiving hospital must have the available bed and personnel to care for the patient. If these requirements cannot be met, the transfer should not occur. Table 20-8 summarizes EMTALA rules.

Emergency physicians are also routinely faced with issues regarding transfer of care within their own institutions. Transfer of care can occur within the ED itself or to inpatient care units. With a transfer of any nature, there is potential for lapses in patient care as well as legal ramifications. Special attention should be awarded to these issues despite the fact that they might represent routine and seemingly benign events in ED care.

The patients in the ED are the primary responsibility of the emergency department attending physician. This may only change when medical orders are written that identify another physician willing to oversee the care of the patient. However, there can be cases in which the patient's primary physician and the emergency physician disagree with the disposition of the patient. The emergency physician is ultimately responsible for arranging the appropriate level of

| TABLE 20-8 | Requirements of EMTALA (Emergency Medical Treatment and Labor Act) |
| --- |
| • Medical screening examination to determine if an emergency medical condition exists |
| • Stabilization within the capacity of the hospital if a emergency medical condition is identified |
| • Transfer (with copies of the entire medical record) to hospital with specialized capabilities if further stabilization is required |
| • Receiving facility must accept the patient if it has appropriate personnel and bed availability |

care for admitted patients.[28] In accepting a lower level of care, the emergency physician implies that the patient's condition is such that more intensive or specialized care is not indicated. Other potential conflicts can arise with the decision to admit or discharge a patient. This is particularly troublesome if the discussion occurs over the telephone. Again, it is important to note that while in the ED, the patient is the responsibility of the emergency physician. If the conflict cannot be resolved, the primary physician must come to the ED and assume responsibility for the care of the patient. However, this approach might not completely absolve the emergency physician and the hospital if the patient deteriorates after discharge. All parties might ultimately share responsibility to varying degrees in the event of a poor outcome. A more cooperative attitude will certainly reduce legal exposure and might ultimately benefit the patient.

In some cases, emergency physicians are asked to write holding or admission orders. These situations often occur at night, and writing these orders is performed as a service to the admitting physician. This creates some responsibility for emergency physicians, as they are continuing to direct a patient's care while being unavailable for further consultation.[29] The American College of Emergency Physicians policy regarding admission orders states that emergency physicians should not be compelled to write any orders beyond treatment in the ED. It also adds that hospitals and

EDs should establish policies clearly delineating responsibility for writing admission orders that guarantee patients are seen in a timely manner.[30] When an emergency physician elects to write admission orders, the orders should be time-limited and clearly identify the attending physician. An attending physician must be available for consultation or questions should the patient's condition change.

Despite a lack of published data, change of shift is accepted as a high-risk situation for patients. These patients are often transferred to the incoming emergency physician with a diagnosis and plan of care. As a result, there is the tendency not to reevaluate these patients. Physicians should be aware of the potential for medical errors associated with change of shift. A formal transfer of care with supporting documentation and complete reassessment by the incoming physician will improve patient care during this high-risk situation. The physician of record is the physician who discharges the patient, but all involved in the child's care will likely be held accountable in the event of a poor outcome.[29]

## THE BOTTOM LINE

- All patients who present to the ED requesting evaluation of a medical condition must receive a medical screening examination.
- Transferring (sending and accepting) patients must be done according to clinical necessity and EMTALA regulations.

## Family Presence

The concept of family member presence during invasive medical procedures continues to develop. Less than 15 years ago, the literature began to identify parental preference for presence during routine procedures such as venipuncture. In the time since, focus has expanded to include parental presence during more invasive procedures and even resuscitations. This change has stimulated significant discussion regarding potential benefits and problems associated with family presence.

The majority of parents want to remain with their children during medical procedures.[31–34] The reasons for this preference vary and are unique to each individual. However, most parents believe that their presence reduces their own anxiety and allows them to comfort their children. In most cases, parents believe that their presence will assist the individuals performing the procedures. As procedures become more invasive, parental desire to be present decreases. Despite this "hierarchy of invasiveness," most parents want to be present during even highly invasive procedures such as lumbar puncture and endotracheal intubation.[35] The majority of families feel that the physician should not make the decision regarding their presence.

Medical personnel have traditionally displayed reluctance toward family member presence. The reasons against parental presence include increased patient and parent anxiety, lack of parental understanding of the procedure, anticipated parental interference, and increased nervousness of the medical staff member performing the procedure. Although a decrease in pain has not been demonstrated in cases of parental presence, similarly no differences have been noted in the number of attempts or time to complete the procedure.[34] Medical personnel experienced with family presence for procedures are known to be more supportive of this concept.

The issue of family presence during resuscitation deserves special consideration, because it often generates the most intense emotions and is the setting in which the request for parental presence is most likely to be denied. Data suggest that a large proportion of parents want to be present during resuscitations[33,35] and this number might increase if the child is likely to die during the resuscitation.[35] The family's presence might help in the acceptance of the child's death. The presence of family members during resuscitations prompts consideration toward medical-legal issues, self-confidence of the medical personnel in their abilities, effects on education, as well as concern regarding the emotional effects of witnessing the death of a child. As with other procedures, the experience of medical personnel with family presence during resuscitation correlates with their support for the process.[36] The effect of family presence with respect to medical-legal issues has yet to be described. Many institutions have policies to facilitate family presence. These policies vary but include the identification of appropriate personnel to stay alongside the family and serve as a liaison. Other policies are related to the safety of family members. This can include simple steps such as requesting that family members remain seated during their child's procedures.

Family presence might not be appropriate in all circumstances. In some cases, the family members are too emotionally distraught to remain with their child or might interfere with the procedure. Others have different reasons for not remaining with their child.

Although there is considerable variation with regard to acceptance and appropriateness of family presence among medical personnel, family members show a strong preference for this model. Medical personnel should be mindful of these preferences with even critically ill patients. Table 20-9 summarizes the pros and cons of having family members present for procedures and resuscitation.

### TABLE 20-9 Family Presence During Invasive Procedures and Resuscitations

| Pros | Cons |
| --- | --- |
| • Most families prefer to be present. | • Can increase patient anxiety |
| • Can reduce parent anxiety | • Can increase parent anxiety |
| • Allows parents the opportunity to comfort child | • Potential for parental interference with procedure |
| • Can assist individual performing the procedure | • Can increase nervousness of individual performing the procedure |
| • Can help in acceptance of child's death | • Can limit teaching opportunities |
| | • Emotional effects of witnessing a child's death |
| | • Medical-legal concerns |

## KEY POINTS

**Presence of Family During the Delivery of Care in the ED**

- Family members often prefer to be present during procedures on their children.
- The family's presence can help in the acceptance of the child's death.

## THE BOTTOM LINE

- If reasonable, permit parents to be present during procedures if they want to be.

## CASE SCENARIO 5

A 3-month-old baby is brought to the emergency department with no pulse and no respirations. The mother had fed the infant at 6:00, and put her back in her crib. She found the infant lifeless at 9:00 and called EMS. The mother attempted CPR before the paramedics arrived, and the paramedics intubated the baby's trachea and continued resuscitation en route to the hospital. In the ED, the baby is noted to have an asystolic rhythm. The temperature is 36°C. Pupils are fixed and dilated.

The ED staff confirm correct placement of the endotracheal tube, place an intraosseous line, and give the infant epinephrine, 3 doses over 15 minutes. The baby has no spontaneous respirations and remains asystolic.

1. *Does the literature support termination of CPR in this case?*
2. *In what clinical situations can prolonged resuscitation be justified?*

# Death and Dying

## Termination of CPR

All patients in cardiac arrest in the ED should undergo cardiopulmonary resuscitation (CPR) unless the patient has signs of irreversible death such as rigor mortis, dependent lividity, or decapitation. Also, CPR should not be initiated if an attempt to resuscitate would put the rescuer at risk (this is unlikely in the ED setting but can apply to prehospital care providers).[37–39] Finally, CPR may be withheld if there is a valid do not resuscitate (DNR) order or other advance directive.

An advance directive is an expression of a person's thoughts or wishes for end-of-life care. The Patient Self-determination Act of 1990, revised in 1991, requires hospitals to inform adults of their right to prescribe limits on CPR and lifesaving treatment.[40] Under some circumstances, minors may also express the wish to have life support withheld. This is controversial in children, and laws vary from state-to-state. Only a few states allow prehospital care providers to apply advance directives to children.[41]

Advance directives are always difficult for emergency physicians. They generally do not know the patient or his or her personal wishes about resuscitation. Family members often change their minds when a child approaches death and call EMS because they are ambivalent. Some regions use a bracelet to identify patients who do not want CPR. Several recent court cases have authorized physicians to recognize decisions made by older adolescents regarding the right to withhold resuscitation attempts. Legal uncertainty exists, but if a patient has a living will, it should serve as evidence of the patient's wishes. In the ED, DNR orders should be considered one element of the treatment plan and should not limit other forms of treatment such as admission to an ICU.[37]

In the absence of these findings, and even when the prognosis is dismal, it is still prudent to initiate resuscitation efforts immediately until a more thorough assessment can be made. CPR may be discontinued if no benefit can be expected because the patient's vital function has deteriorated despite maximal therapy for a specific condition such as shock. Prolonged resuscitation for children with pulseless arrests is not likely to be successful.[41] In general, resuscitative efforts may be discontinued if a child has not responded with spontaneous circulation after 20 to 30 minutes.[38,42] It has been noted that failure to respond to 2 doses of epinephrine greatly decreases the chance of survival for a child. After such attempts, and in the absence of ventricular fibrillation, ventricular tachycardia, toxic drug exposure, and primary prearrest hypothermia, resuscitation can be discontinued if there is no return of spontaneous circulation. Hospitals should develop policies on brain death and how this pertains to resuscitated patients in the ED.[37] It should be noted that nonreactive pupils have little predictive value in the outcome of a case and might not be a criterion in itself to halt resuscitation. In one study of pediatric resuscitation, 33% of children with nonreactive pupils survived.[43]

If at all possible, talk with the parents about withholding CPR or avoiding further treatment that might be futile.[37] Parents, if present at the time of resuscitation, have the right to select among medically appropriate options. Parental decisions to withhold CPR or other life-sustaining treatment may be honored if this seems to be in the best interest of the child or if the treatment is futile. In some circumstances, adolescents are granted the authority to decide to withhold resuscitation efforts. Hospital policies should guide practitioners in the ED.[37] When there is doubt about the authority or reasonableness of a guardian's request to withhold CPR, resuscitation should continue until the conflict can be resolved.

## Approach to the Deceased Child and Family

The death of a pediatric patient in the ED places an enormous strain on the medical staff and obviously the child's family (Figure 20.3). Most deaths in the ED are unexpected, and the patients were well children only minutes before a tragic incident. Dealing with such situations

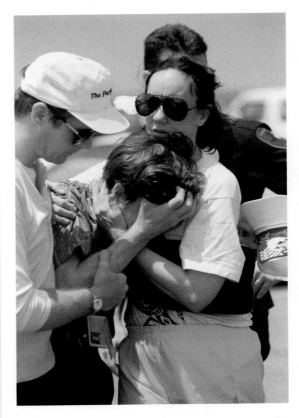

**Figure 20.3** The death of a child creates a highly stressful situation for the family. Dealing with such situations takes great skill and compassion.

takes great skill, compassion, and poise. Knowledge of policies, procedures, and local laws is essential. The American College of Emergency Physicians' Pediatric Committee and the American Academy of Pediatrics Committee on Pediatric Emergency Medicine created a joint policy, "Death of a Child In the Emergency Department."[44,45] This policy outlines the issues to consider when dealing with a death of a child in the ED as well as the grieving family. Clinicians must support family members. They must inform them about the cause of death, whether the death was preventable, whether the child suffered pain, and perhaps whether the child's condition is contagious to others. They must guide them about practical issues such as funeral arrangements. Answers should be provided with truth and compassion.[44,45]

Protocols and written policies for the investigation of a pediatric death in the ED, with accompanying checklists, are important to aid the staff. This will help ensure a thorough examination and notification of proper authorities. It will also contribute to the understanding of SIDS, child abuse and neglect, undiagnosed genetic diseases, and cases of inadequate health care.[44,45] Accurate documentation of the history and physical examination and resuscitation efforts is essential. Investigation at the time of death or at post mortem might include a skeletal survey, drug screen, cultures, photographs of injuries, and forensic evaluation for sexual assault. The ED staff is often responsible for notification of others such as the medical examiner, primary care physician, additional family members, and perhaps a religious leader. The primary care physician can have an important role in supporting the family and reviewing autopsy reports in the future. Child protective services or the police should be notified as appropriate.[44,45]

The hospital should provide a team of physicians, social workers, nursing personnel, and clergy or chaplain who can respond immediately to a sudden death in the ED. They are needed to provide initial and long-term support and assistance. Someone experienced in supportive care should remain with the family for as long as they remain in the ED, even if the nursing and medical staff must depart to take care of other patients. Grief counselors and support groups are available in some communities.

Delivering bad news to a family, especially informing them of the death of their child, is an extremely difficult task. ED staff members generally have no previous relationship with the family and now must give news to them that they will remember forever. The responsible physician should find a private area to meet with the family and review the events and outcome.[46] A designated room in the ED is most helpful. The room should have comfortable seating and only basic accompaniments such as tissues, a telephone, and perhaps water.

The physician who is delegated to deliver news of the child's death should sit at eye level with the family members. He or she should be sympathetic and say he or she is very sorry. An empathetic staff member will be remembered long after the child's death. It is important to use the child's name and not refer to the deceased as a "patient" or even "your child."[47] Use clear words such as "died" or "dead" so there is no misunderstanding of the child's condition. Avoid terms such as "passed on" or "expired." Speak clearly in a soft, sympathetic voice. Allow the family members to absorb the initial information before proceeding on with additional details. Listen and do not falsely reassure them. While saying you are sorry, avoid trite expressions such as, "I know how you feel." There is no way to know how the family feels. Do not offer hope with expressions such as, "You are young and can have other children." Such comments would be inappropriate as the child is not replaceable. Allow the parents time to react or even to sit in silence. Offer help in informing siblings or other family members. Offer information about the next steps, such as contacting a funeral home and the medical examiner. Explain that autopsy is mandatory (usually). Explain in simple terms what this involves and that it will not interfere with funeral plans. Try to reduce the family's feelings of guilt if appropriate.[48]

The ED staff should be prepared for a variety of reactions to the news of a child's death. Some will deny the news, others will be distraught. Some will be violent, or angry with themselves, family members, or the medical staff. Family members should be offered the opportunity to see or sit privately with the deceased child and hold the child, regardless of whether they were present in the ED for the resuscitation. It should be noted that some families have religious or cultural norms that alter their behavior at the time of death. Discuss the merits of seeing their child in a nonjudgmental way.[48] This is a chance to confirm the reality of death, say good-bye, and begin separation.[48,49] Prepare them for the child's appearance beforehand. Many parents would like a memento, such as a lock of hair, a handprint or footprint, and staff should consider offering such to families.[50,51] Make certain the family has transportation and support at home before they leave.[51] Table 20-10 highlights the important features of the approach to the family after the death of a child in the ED.

The medical staff is generally emotionally and physically drained after the death of a child in the ED. Ideally, the staff should be allowed a brief time to recover from such a dramatic event. Even taking a short walk or a moment outside the ED can be helpful. Unfortunately, the pace of the ED does not often allow an immediate recovery time. Critical incident debriefing often helps the medical staff cope with sudden death of a child in the ED. This is best done within 24 hours of the child's death.[44,45] At such sessions, the medical care can be reviewed and feelings can be shared with professionals who can offer guidance. Studies have shown that emergency physicians often feel guilty or inadequate after an unsuccessful pediatric resuscitation, and a significant number admit to feeling impaired during the remainder of their shifts.[49] Many members of the staff have a need to know that they acted properly and what they could do differently in the future. Table 20-11 summarizes the responsibilities of the physician after a pediatric death in the ED.

| TABLE 20-10 Discussion of Death With Family in the ED |
|---|

- Find a private area to deliver news, discuss events.
- Sit with the family at eye level.
- Use a calm, sympathetic voice.
- Show genuine concern; say you are sorry.
- Use clear terms ("died" or "dead").
- Offer explanation—possible cause of death.
- Be a good listener; do not hurry off.
- Relieve guilt if appropriate.
- Avoid giving false hope; avoid reassurance about their future.
- Offer help in contacting others, speaking to siblings.
- Offer opportunity to see or hold the deceased child.
- Offer advice—funeral plans, autopsy, organ donation.

| TABLE 20-11 Physician Responsibilities After Death in the ED |
|---|

- Complete physical examination of child.
- Document carefully.
- Consider forensic investigation (not extensive) for cause of death.
- Assemble support team for family.
- Contact medical examiner, police, and child protective services if indicated.
- Contact primary care physician.
- Complete death certificate.
- Help console, inform other staff members.
- Arrange critical incident debriefing.
- Take time for self.

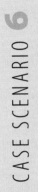

**CASE SCENARIO 6**

A 16-year-old cyclist is brought to the emergency department after being stuck by a motor vehicle. At the scene, EMS personnel arrive to find an apneic and pulseless patient. Resuscitative efforts in the field and in the ED are not successful, and the patient is pronounced dead. The patient's family arrives at the hospital just after resuscitative efforts have ceased. The nursing staff notifies the local organ procurement organization as required by law. The organ procurement service representative arrives at the hospital to discuss organ transplantation possibilities with the family.

1. *Should the organ procurement service be notified before death, immediately after death, or after sufficient time for grieving has passed?*

## Organ Donation

The death of a child in the ED is usually a sudden and unforeseen event. In addition to supporting a grieving family (as previously discussed), the emergency physician has responsibilities related to organ donation. The physician's primary responsibility remains with the patient and the family. The physician must be constantly mindful of this when dealing with all subsequent matters related to the child's death.

Despite an increase in public awareness, organ availability remains limited. Children from birth to 17 years account for approximately 3% of patients on the waiting list for an organ.[52] Existing legislation requires hospitals to refer all potential donors to local organ procurement organizations and to discuss organ donation with families of deceased patients.[52] Although these discussions should occur in conjunction with the physician, the death notification must be uncoupled from the request for organ donation. The rate of consent is substantially increased when this request is made independently and when made by personnel specifically trained in organ procurement.[53] This can include appropriately trained hospital staff or representatives from the local organ procurement organization.

The office of the medical examiner should be notified soon after a child's death. Organ procurement in pediatric patients is often coupled with medical and forensic investigations related to the cause of death.[52] In some cases, the medical examiner will advise against organ donation. However, in many cases, through cooperation of personnel in multiple disciplines, organ donation can still be achieved while preserving important medical and forensic evidence. This cooperation can substantially affect the supply of pediatric organs. For many families, organ donation is very important. Despite their tragic loss, a family might derive significant comfort from the knowledge that their child's organs are being used to benefit others.

## The Medical Examiner

The medical examiner or coroner should be notified of all deaths in the ED.[44,45] Many states require the medical examiner to investigate all deaths that occur as a result of violence, sudden deaths when the patient is in apparent good health (such as SIDS), a suspicious, unusual, or unnatural manner of death,

deaths that occur when the victim is not under the care of a physician for a potentially fatal illness, or any death otherwise unexplained.[44,45,54] A death certificate must be filled out accurately in the ED. This serves to identify high-risk populations and geographic trends. Funding for research and prevention is often allocated based on death certificates.[54]

### KEY POINTS

- A child's death in the ED results in substantial social stress and is associated with legal requirements and additional legal risk.

### THE BOTTOM LINE

- Establish policies for death of a child in the ED.
- Present news of a child's death to parents professionally and clearly, in a quiet environment.
- Physicians must be aware of and comply with legal requirements such as notification of organ procurement services and the medical examiner.

# CHAPTER REVIEW

## Check Your Knowledge

1. In many states the following are characteristics of an emancipated minor, except:
   A. College graduation
   B. High school graduation
   C. Married
   D. Military service
   E. Pregnancy

2. When parents are present during procedures and resuscitations, which of the following is correct?
   A. Children cry more when parents are present because they do not understand why the parents are not helping them
   B. Most parents are at risk of fainting during the procedure
   C. Most parents prefer to be present
   D. Most parents provide technical assistance during the procedure
   E. Studies have demonstrated that procedure success rates are lower when parents are present

3. DNR orders are difficult to carry out in EDs for all of the following reasons except:
   A. Parents frequently change their minds as deterioration approaches
   B. Parents have called 9-1-1 in a panic and resuscitation efforts have already begun
   C. Parents have not previously established a relationship with the emergency physician, who does not know about the child's chronic condition
   D. Primary care physician for the child cannot be reached immediately
   E. There is no written DNR order, but the parents communicate "do not resuscitate" orally

4. Which of the following situations is most likely to result in a successful malpractice lawsuit against a physician?
   A. A child is seen for abdominal pain in the office by a primary care physician, who diagnoses gastroenteritis. Later that night the child is brought to an ED and diagnosed with acute appendicitis. The emergency physician comments that this is a very obvious case of appendicitis. After appendectomy, the child is discharged and recovers well.
   B. A child is seen for worsening abdominal pain of 6 hours' duration. The emergency physician suspects appendicitis. An abdominal CT scan is ordered, which is read as normal. Still, a surgeon is consulted and the patient is hospitalized for observation. The following morning, his pain worsens and the surgeon decides to perform a laparotomy, at which time a perforated appendix is found. He develops peritonitis, requiring a prolonged hospitalization. He sustains multiple future episodes of bowel obstruction due to bowel adhesions, requiring seven hospitalizations and three laparotomies for lysis of bowel adhesions.
   C. An obese boy presents to his primary care physician with limping associated with thigh and knee pain. Radiographs of his knee are ordered and are normal. An ESR and CRP looking for osteomyelitis are normal. He is given a diagnosis of a knee strain and is instructed to rest his knee. One week later, his pain worsens after walking down the stairs. He presents to the ED, radiographs of his hip demonstrate a severely slipped femoral capital epiphysis. An orthopedic surgeon is consulted, and the boy is hospitalized for bedrest, traction, and surgical pinning. He develops avascular necrosis of the femoral head and a prolonged disability.
   D. The parents of a child with a forearm fracture have a long wait time to see a physician then are treated rudely by that physician. The fracture heals well with no permanent disability.

# References

1. Selbst SM, Korin JB. *Preventing Malpractice Lawsuits in Pediatric Emergency Medicine.* Dallas, Tx: American College of Emergency Physicians; 1999:1–196.

2. Ricci JA, Lambert RL, Stefes DG. Pediatrics and professional liability. *Pediatr Emerg Care.* 1986;2:106.

3. Selbst SM, Korin JB. Malpractice and emergency care: doing right by the patient—and yourself. *Contemp Pediatr.* 2000;17:88–106.

4. American Academy of Pediatrics Division of Health Care Finance and Practice. Keep eye on malpractice insurance carrier, not just premium. *AAP News.* August 2001;64–65.

5. Albert T. Malpractice awards pushing insurance premiums higher. *Am Med News.* 2001;44(9):1–2.

6. Hickson GB, Clayton EW, Githers PB et al. Factors that prompted families to file malpractice claims following perinatal injuries. *JAMA.* 1992;267:1359.

7. Laska L (ed). Medical malpractice verdicts, settlements & experts. 1995;11(4):18.

8. Selbst SM. Pediatric emergency medicine legal briefs. *Pediatr Emerg Care.* 1996;12:59–61.

9. Laska L (ed). Medical malpractice verdicts, settlements & experts. 1995;11:16–17.

10. Selbst SM. The febrile child—missed meningitis and bacteremia. *Clin Pediatr Emerg Med.* 2000; 1:164–171.

11. George JE, Quattrone MS. The ED record: legal implications. *Em Phys Leg Bull.* 1984;10:2.

12. Adamson TE, Tschann JM, Guillan DS et al. Physician communication skills and malpractice claims: a complex relationship. *West J Med.* 1989; 150:356–360.

13. Hickson GB, Federspiel CF, Pichert JW et al. Patient complaints and malpractice risk. *JAMA.* 2002;287:2951–2957.

14. Laska L (ed). Medical malpractice: verdicts, settlements and experts. 1995;11(12):11.

15. Selbst SM. Pediatric emergency medicine legal briefs. *Pediatr Emerg Care.* 1995;12(3):236–238.

16. Laska L (ed). Medical malpractice verdicts, settlements & experts. 2002;18(6):15.

17. Selbst SM. Pediatric emergency medicine legal briefs. *Pediatr Emerg Care.* 2002;18(6):456–459.

18. Holliman CJ. The art of dealing with consultants. *J Emerg Med.* 1993;11:633–640.

19. Wilde JA, Pedroni AT. The do's and don'ts of consultations. *Contemp Pediatr.* 1991;8:23–28.

20. O'Riordan WD. Consultations. In: Henry GL, Sullivan DJ, eds. *Emergency Medicine Risk Management: A Comprehensive Review.* 2nd ed. Dallas, Tx: American College of Emergency Physicians; 1997:329–334.

21. Fish RM, Ehrhardt ME. Legal liability for the acts of others; hospitals and emergency physicians. *J Emerg Med.* 1991;9:175–179.

22. Sigman GS, O'Connor C. Exploration for physicians of the mature minor doctrine. *J Pediatr.* 1991;119:520–525.

23. Tsai AK, Schafermeyer RW, Kalifon D et al. Evaluation and treatment of minors: reference on consent. *Ann Emerg Med.* 1993:22:1211–1217.

24. Thewes J, Fitzgerald D, Sulmasy DP. Informed consent in emergency medicine—ethics under fire. *Emerg Med Clin North Am.* 1996;14:245–254.

25. Sheldon M. Ethical issues in the forced transfusion of Jehovah's witness children. *J Emerg Med.* 1996;14:251–257.

26. Health Care Financing Administration. The Emergency Medical Treatment and Active Labor Act, as established under the Consolidated Omnibus Budget Reconciliation Act of 1985. (42 USC 1395 dd) 1985.

27. HCFA Interpretive Guidelines, 1998, V-15. In: Bitterman RA. *Providing Emergency Care under Federal Law: EMTALA.* Dallas, Tx: American College of Emergency Physicians;2000:221.

28. Bresler MJ, Henry GL. In-house coverage of hospitalized patients. *Foresight – American College of Emergency Physicians.* 1995; 35:1–8.

29. Goldman PL. Admitting orders. In: Henry GL, Sullivan DJ, eds. *Emergency Medicine Risk Management: A Comprehensive Review.* Dallas, Tx: American College of Emergency Physicians; 1997:343–345.

30. American College of Emergency Physicians. Writing admission orders [policy statement]. ACEP Web site. Available at http://www.Acep.org/1,687,0.html. Accessed September 23, 2003.

31. Bauchner H, Waring C, Vinci R. Pediatric procedures. Do parents want to watch? *Pediatrics.* 1989;84:907–908.

32. Bauchner H, Waring C, Vinci R. Parental presence during procedures in an emergency room. Results of 50 observations. *Pediatrics.* 1991; 87:544–548.

33. Sacchetti A, Lichenstein R, Carraccio CA et al. Family members presence during pediatric emergency department procedures. *Pediatr Emerg Care.* 1996;12:268–271.

34. Bauchner H, Vinci R, Bak S et al. Parents and procedures: a randomized control trial. *Pediatrics.* 1996;98:861–867.

35. Boie ET, Moore GP, Brummett C, Nelson DR. Do parents want to be present during invasive procedures performed on their children in the emergency department? A survey of 400 parents. *Ann Emerg Med.* 1999;34:70–74.

# CHAPTER REVIEW

36. Sacchetti A, Carraccio C, Leva E, Harris RH. Acceptance of family member presence during pediatric resuscitations in the emergency department: effects of personal experience. *Pediatr Emerg Care.* 2000;16:85–87.

37. Landwirth J. Ethical issues in pediatric and neonatal resuscitation. *Ann Emerg Med.* 1993; 22(pt 2):502–507.

38. Rosenberg N, Klein E, Gittleman MA, Nozicka CA. When to start and when to stop. *Pediatr Emerg Care.* 2001;17:126–129.

39. Holleran RS. When is dead, dead? *Nurs Clin North Am.* 2002;37:11–18.

40. Jefferson LS, White BC, Louis PT et al. Use of the Natural Death Act in pediatric patients. *Crit Care Med.* 1991;19:901.

41. American Academy of Pediatrics, Committee on School Health and Committee on Bioethics. Do not resuscitate orders in schools. *Pediatrics.* 2000;105:878–879.

42. Young KD, Seidel JS. Pediatric cardiopulmonary resuscitation: a collective review. *Ann Emerg Med.* 1999;33:195–205.

43. Nichols DG, Kettrick RG, Swedlow DB et al. Factors influencing outcome of cardiopulmonary resuscitation in children. *Pediatr Emerg Care.* 1986;2:1–5.

44. American Academy of Pediatrics Committee on Pediatric Emergency Medicine and the American College of Emergency Physicians Pediatric Committee. Death of a child in the emergency department. *Pediatrics.* 2002; 110: 839–840.

45. American College of Emergency Physicians Pediatric Committee and American Academy of Pediatrics Committee on Pediatric Emergency Medicine. Death of a child in the emergency department. *Ann Emerg Med.* 2002;40: 409–410.

46. Jukovich GJ, Pierce B, Pananen L, Rivara FP. Giving bad news: the family perspective. *J Trauma.* 2000;48:865–873.

47. Hart RG, Ahrens WR. Coping with pediatric death in the ED by learning from parental experience. *Am J Emerg Med.* 1998;16:67–68.

48. Soulen J, Ludwig S. Chapter 27. Death in the emergency department. In: Selbst SM, Torrey SB, eds. *Pediatric Emergency Medicine for the House Officer.* Baltimore, Md: Williams & Wilkins; 1988:307–314.

49. Ahrens WR, Hart RG. Emergency physicians' experience with pediatric death. *Am J Emerg Med.* 1997;15:642–643.

50. Ahrens B, Hart R. Death in the emergency department (letter). *Ann Emerg Med.* 1999;33:356.

51. Ahrens W, Hart R, Maruyama N. Pediatric death: managing the aftermath in the emergency department. *J Emerg Med.* 1997;15:601–603.

52. American Academy of Pediatrics, Committee on Hospital Care and Section on Surgery. Policy statement: pediatric organ donation and transplantation. *Pediatrics.* 2002;109:982–984.

53. Razek T, Olthoff K, Reilly PM. Issues in potential organ donor management. *Surg Clin North Am.* 2000;81:1021–1032.

54. Bowen KA, Marshall WN. Pediatric death certification. *Arch Pediatr Adolesc Med.* 1998;152: 852–854.

**CASE SUMMARY 1**

A 12-year-old boy is hit by a car while bicycling. He is brought to the emergency department and found to be hypotensive with abdominal distention and a swollen left thigh. The staff begins fluid resuscitation, and blood is ordered for possible transfusion. The child's condition worsens, and perfusion cannot be maintained with saline alone. His parents are told about his serious condition and the need for surgery and blood transfusion. The parents reply that they cannot consent to a blood transfusion because of their religious beliefs.

1. *What should you do now?*

In this case, you should do what is necessary to save the child's life. If a blood transfusion is considered essential for treatment, it should be given. Most courts in the United States will not allow a parent to impose his or her religious beliefs on a minor, especially in a life-threatening situation. A court order will be necessary and should be sought simultaneously as treatment is begun.

**CASE SUMMARY 2**

Paramedics bring in a 4-year-old boy who was rescued from a house fire, along with his uninjured mother. The child is awake and responds to questions but is mildly tachypneic despite receiving supplemental oxygen. Other vital signs are stable. The physical exam is notable for scattered first- and second-degree burns to less than 5% of the body surface area but involving regions on the face and lips. Carbon deposits are noted in the oropharynx. Concern for inhalational injury prompts the decision to perform endotracheal intubation. The child's mother asks to stay with her son as the intubation is performed.

1. *How should you respond to the mother's request?*

This represents an urgent but not emergent clinical situation. The physician should discuss the decision to perform endotracheal intubation and provide the mother with a description of the procedure. Most parents want to remain with their children even during invasive procedures. After receiving the information about her child's care, the mother's request to stay with her child should be granted unless there are strong indications that she would interfere with the procedure.

**CASE SUMMARY 3**

A 4-year-old girl is brought to the emergency department with a history of choking on a peanut. Her past medical history is unremarkable. On examination, she is in mild respiratory distress. Her respiratory rate is 44/minute. She has slight retractions with decreased breath sounds on the right. Chest radiograph is consistent with foreign body aspiration. There is difficulty starting an IV, and the mother has "words" with the nursing staff. When bronchoscopy is suggested, the mother is visibly upset and shouts harshly at the house officer. The mother wants to sign out against medical advice.

1. *How could this situation have been avoided?*
2. *What steps can be taken now to ensure that the child receives the best care possible?*

---

In this case it should be noted that parents have the right to seek a second opinion for their child. However, this situation can be avoided if staff members are counseled on the importance of maintaining a professional attitude at all times. It can be difficult to deal with an irate family, but if the goal is to provide the best care for the child, then maintaining a calm and professional demeanor will help diffuse situations such as that which occurred in this case. The physician must also determine if it is safe for the child to leave the ED if parents wish to sign out against medical advice. If the child is only in mild distress, the physician might allow the parent/patient to leave, only after attempts to keep the child in the ED have failed. Ensure proper documentation of the scenario, as described above. It might be wise to offer assistance to the family and help transport the child to another hospital in such situations.

**CASE SUMMARY 4**

A 3-year-old child presents to a small, rural emergency department with a 24-hour history of abdominal pain. The patient also has fever and vomiting but is clinically stable. The child has a past medical history of developmental delay, cerebral palsy, and epilepsy. The emergency department physician establishes a diagnosis of appendicitis and consults a general surgeon. The surgeon agrees with the diagnosis of appendicitis but recommends transfer to a tertiary care center given the patient's complex medical issues. Citing a lack of bed availability within the hospital, the physician at the tertiary care center refuses to accept the patient. The emergency physician disregards the refusal and sends the patient by ambulance to the tertiary care center.

1. *Should the patient have been transferred under these circumstances?*
2. *Is such a refusal justified?*

---

The emergency physician at the rural hospital established a diagnosis of appendicitis and obtained appropriate surgical consultation. The decision to transfer the patient to a more specialized center is appropriate. However, a physician at the receiving facility must be identified to provide care for the patient. In this case, the receiving facility did not have bed availability for this patient and is justified in its decision to not accept the patient. EMTALA requires more specialized centers to accept transferred patients only if they possess the resources (including bed availability) to provide appropriate care. Transfer to a facility unable to provide necessary care is not beneficial to the patient. The discussion should then have focused on the identification of an alternative center able to provide the necessary care for this patient.

CASE SUMMARY 5

A 3-month-old baby is brought to the emergency department with no pulse and no respirations. The mother had fed the infant at 6:00, and put her back in her crib. She found the infant lifeless at 9:00 and called EMS. The mother attempted CPR before the paramedics arrived, and the paramedics intubated the baby's trachea and continued resuscitation en route to the hospital. In the ED, the baby is noted to have an asystolic rhythm. The temperature is 36°C. Pupils are fixed and dilated.

The ED staff confirm correct placement of the endotracheal tube, place an intraosseous line, and give the infant epinephrine, 3 doses over 15 minutes. The baby has no spontaneous respirations and remains asystolic.

1. *Does the literature support termination of CPR in this case?*
2. *In what clinical situations can prolonged resuscitation be justified?*

Resuscitation may be terminated, as the literature demonstrates very poor to no survival rates in children receiving more than 2 doses of epinephrine without effect.

Clinical situations that can result in meaningful survival after prolonged resuscitations (more than 25 minutes) include ventricular fibrillation, ventricular tachycardia, electrocution, toxic drug exposure, and primary prearrest hypothermia.

CASE SUMMARY 6

A 16-year-old cyclist is brought to the emergency department after being stuck by a motor vehicle. At the scene, EMS personnel arrive to find an apneic and pulseless patient. Resuscitative efforts in the field and in the ED are not successful, and the patient is pronounced dead. The patient's family arrives at the hospital just after resuscitative efforts have ceased. The nursing staff notifies the local organ procurement organization as required by law. The organ procurement service representative arrives at the hospital to discuss organ transplantation possibilities with the family.

1. *Should the organ procurement service be notified before death, immediately after death, or after sufficient time for grieving has passed?*

Legislation requires hospitals to refer all potential donors to local organ procurement organizations. This should take place before death has occurred, if possible. Otherwise, it should occur immediately after death. The medical examiner will help determine if organ donation is feasible in each particular circumstance. However, at least a limited use of organs is possible in many cases, and the emergency physician should facilitate this process with early referrals to both the organ procurement organizations and the medical examiner.

# chapter 21

# Office-Based Emergencies

John P. Santamaria, MD, FAAP, FACEP

## Objectives

1 Explain the importance of preparedness for common pediatric emergencies in the office setting.

2 Describe the need for physician and staff education, including periodic practice sessions, in preparation for office-based emergencies, such as resuscitation.

3 Identify equipment and supplies needed for treatment of office-based emergencies.

4 Assess the stabilization and transport priorities for patients with major trauma presenting in the office setting.

5 Describe minor surgical procedures in the office setting.

## Chapter Outline

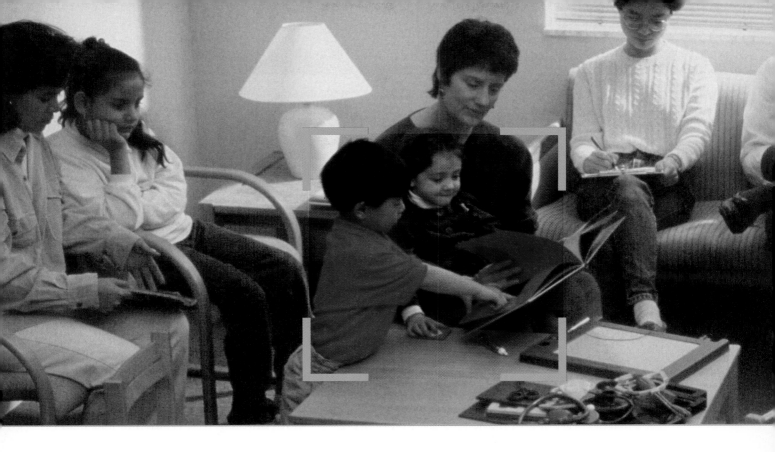

# Introduction

A wide spectrum of pediatric emergencies can be encountered in an office setting. Physicians and their staffs who do not encounter emergencies on a regular basis will feel discomfort when faced with life-threatening situations. Anticipation of the types of emergencies that are likely to be seen, and preparation of the staff and office environment for handling these situations, will alleviate much of this discomfort and greatly facilitate the care of these children. The process of preparedness begins by ensuring that the physicians and office staff are trained in the assessment of an emergency situation and in the methods of resuscitation. Office settings also must be stocked with the correct, appropriately sized equipment to allow maximum effectiveness of trained personnel. Once a patient is stabilized in the office setting, the office staff must be prepared to arrange for expeditious emergency transport to the most appropriate definitive care facility.

It is recommended that an ambulatory site caring for pediatric patients, at a minimum, be prepared to stabilize and refer the emergency conditions cited in Table 21-1.[1,2] Specific evaluation and management of some of these problems are discussed in other sections of this text. This chapter provides a review of issues related to general

| TABLE 21-1 | Pediatric Emergencies Encountered in Physicians' Offices |
|---|---|

- Anaphylaxis
- Respiratory and cardiac arrest
- Respiratory distress (asthma, airway obstruction)
- Seizures/status epilepticus
- Sepsis/shock
- Sickle cell crisis
- Trauma

office preparedness for handling medical and traumatic emergencies and discusses certain office activities, such as telephone triage and education, that have an impact on the prevention, identification, and appropriate handling of potential emergencies. The procedures include step-by-step approaches to minor surgical emergencies that can be treated in the office setting.

In preparing a pediatric or family practice office to care for emergencies, it is important to recognize limitations. Awareness of institutional limitations and the availability of pediatric emergency care in the community can reduce the need for elaborate office preparation. In all cases, coordination of care with local and regional resources best serves the needs of children.

## Section 1 General Office Preparedness

### 1.1 Telephone Triage

Telephone triage proficiency is important for the staff in the physician's office. They must be able to determine which patients are in need of immediate referral to an emergency department, which patients need to be seen immediately but can be evaluated in the office, and which can be scheduled for routine appointments. Parents often are in need of advice and reassurance. Although books with pediatric telephone triage protocols providing guidance are available, it is still essential that staff members receive the proper training.[3] Even with proper training, there are many times when it is difficult or impossible to determine the true severity of an illness or injury by telephone. Office staff should recommend formal medical evaluation whenever there is doubt and participate in periodic training sessions to cover the common and important problems likely to be the basis of calls from parents.

### 1.2 Monitoring the Waiting Area

Early intervention is key to optimal outcome. Educate registration staff about conditions that warrant immediate medical attention or isolation from other children. Instruct the staff to periodically check the waiting area for the possibility of deterioration of patients. Parents can be less vigilant once they have reached the health care facility and might miss signs of deterioration (Tables 21-2 and 21-3).

---

**YOUR FIRST CLUE**

**Worrisome Waiting Room Signs and Symptoms**

- Active seizures
- Altered mental status
- Difficulty breathing
- History of ingestion or overdose
- Pallor or cyanosis

---

### 1.3 Staff Education

Initial training and periodic practice drills require dedication of staff time to the process of developing preparedness. Training in basic life support (BLS) and pediatric advanced life support (PALS) is recommended. BLS training typically requires 1 day, and PALS is a 2-day course. BLS training is a good baseline for all staff; PALS is recommended for all physicians and at least one nurse in the office. *APLS: The Pediatric Emergency Medicine Course* is a 1-day to 2-day comprehensive modular pediatric emergency medicine course desirable for physicians, nurses, and other health care personnel who work in sites in which a substantial amount of emergency care is delivered. This course concentrates on the initial evaluation and management of a broad range of life-threatening pediatric illnesses and injuries. In the majority of cases, early appropriate intervention can prevent deterioration to cardiorespiratory arrest. Once initial training is complete, no more than a few hours per month are required to maintain a reasonable state of preparedness. The American Heart Association (AHA) recommends an annual update for BLS and biannual update for PALS (Table 21-4). The American Academy of Pediatrics (AAP) and the American College of Emergency Physicians (ACEP) recommend continuing study of the APLS materials, attendance at a "live" APLS course, and formal renewal education every 4 years.

Good resuscitation skills are not enough. Emergency stabilization and management require a team effort, a plan, adequate resources, and practice. Once training is completed, periodic practice drills are required to avoid deterioration of newly acquired knowledge and skills. Location of emergency equipment, supplies, and medications must be known at all times. This is especially important in environments in which emergency cases are rare. Such drills also assist the staff in maintaining the ability to locate and assemble emergency equipment quickly. Secretaries and receptionists are key personnel in managing office emergencies

| **TABLE 21-2** **Checklist for Pediatric Office Emergency Preparedness** |
|---|

**Recognition:**

Instruct secretaries and receptionists to recognize indications for immediate medical evaluation:

- Active vomiting or profuse diarrhea
- Actively bleeding wounds
- Altered mental state
- Any patient in pain
- Any patient who needs to lie down
- Difficulty breathing
- History of head injury
- History of ingestion and/or overdose
- Infants younger than 2 months with fever
- Pallor or cyanosis
- Petechiae/purpura (purple rash that resembles bruising)
- Seizures
- Testicular pain or swelling

**Response Plan:**

- Is a staff member assigned to periodically check the waiting area?
- Who will call Emergency Medical Services (EMS)? Is the number clearly posted?
- Is the staff informed about the various prehospital providers in the area and their capabilities?
- Is the staff prepared to quickly provide EMS with the necessary information such as office address, patient age, condition, vital signs, transport destination, need for ALS versus BLS?
- What will be done if the physician is not in the office?
- Are roles preassigned for the resuscitation team?
  - Physician provides medical direction, manages airway.
  - Nurse draws and gives medications and fluids.
  - Aide/tech assists physician, performs chest compressions.
  - Secretary/receptionist activates EMS system, records events, accesses chart.
- Who will call ahead to the receiving facility?

**Equipment:**

Is resuscitation equipment:

- Complete?
- Well organized?
- Easily located by office personnel?
- Periodically restocked and rechecked? By whom?

**Provider Skills:**

- Are all staff members adequately trained to fulfill their roles?
- Are all resuscitation protocols known or readily available?

**Maintaining Readiness:**

Remember what was told to the young man who asked how to get to Carnegie Hall: "Practice, practice, practice!"

- Mock codes
- Scavenger hunts
- Group critique

**Documentation:**

Designate a recorder for:

- Dates and times of all treatments and calls
- Stabilization attempts, medication/fluid doses and responses, child's weight (measured or estimated)
- Conversations with family
- Patient condition upon leaving office

Adapted from: Frush K, Cinoman M. *Office Preparedness for Pediatric Emergencies; Provider Manual*. North Carolina Emergency Medical Services for Children, 1999.

**Section**

**1**

| TABLE 21-3 | Patients Requiring Isolation |
| --- | --- |

- Complaint of possible lice or scabies
- History of exposure to chickenpox, tuberculosis, or measles
- History of immunosuppressive illness
- History of organ transplant surgery

| TABLE 21-4 | Courses | | |
| --- | --- | --- | --- |
| Course | Sponsoring Organization | Duration (days) | Recommended Update |
| BLS | AHA | 1 | Annually |
| PALS | AHA/AAP | 2 | Every 2 years |
| APLS | AAP/ACEP | 1–2 | Every 4 years |

and need to be part of the planning and practice for such events. Assign every staff member a written, assigned role in case of an emergency.[4] Make the emergency response plan comprehensive, including answers to the questions posed in Table 21-2.

Not every drill must be a full mock code. Simply locating and preparing equipment and medications as though they were going to be used for an emergency, and then discussing what would be done in the event of a real emergency can provide a useful experience for the staff with minimal input of resources and time. A physician and a nurse can work together to plan the sessions, and it is a good idea to involve as many of the staff as possible in conducting the sessions. When the mock code format is used, it is best to assign 1 or 2 individuals to observe and to share their observations constructively with the group.[4,5] An important part of the wrapup is ensuring that all participants have had an opportunity to share their observations as well. The involvement of community emergency physicians and EMS personnel can facilitate the implementation of practice sessions and build relationships that further help staff to function effectively under true emergency conditions. Conduct practice sessions regularly, preferably at least monthly, to maintain a reasonable degree of staff readiness, confidence, and comfort.

## 1.4 Equipment and Medications

The equipment and medications listed in Tables 21-5 and 21-6 can be assembled easily without a major investment of time or money and are sufficient for most pediatric or family practice offices. Tables 21-7 and 21-8 provide expanded equipment and medication lists more appropriate for large, busy, or remote sites or for facilities seeing children with complex medical problems. The following considerations are important in deciding on the equipment needs of a specific office:

- Frequency and type of emergencies seen
- Proximity to a hospital emergency department
- Response time for EMS
- Level of training of EMS personnel

Store emergency equipment in a specific location that is easily accessible in an emergency situation. The development of an emergency cart or case is highly recommended. When properly assembled, the contents will enable the resuscitation of patients in a wide range of ages, from the premature newborn to the husky adolescent. Locking tool cabinets on wheels, such as those widely available in hardware stores, are ideal for this use because they have multiple locked drawers and cabinets, allowing for better super-

## TABLE 21-5 Basic Office Equipment and Supplies

**Airway Equipment:**
- Masks for bagging (infant, pediatric, adult)
- Oxygen source with flowmeter
- Self-inflating bag with reservoir (500 cc, 1,000 cc)
- Oxygen masks (simple, Venturi type, and nonrebreather in premature, infant, child, adult sizes)
- Suction, wall or portable/Yankauer suction catheters (8, 10, 14F)
- Cardiac arrest board
- Emergency drug dosing card or Broselow© Pediatric Emergency Tape

**Fluid and Medication Administration:**
- Butterfly needles (23g)
- IV catheters—short over-the-needle (18, 20, 22, 24g), several of each size
- IV boards, tape, alcohol swabs, tourniquet
- Normal saline and tubing
- Syringes
- Sphygmomanometer and blood pressure cuffs (infant, child, adult)

## TABLE 21-6 Basic Emergency Office Medication List

- Albuterol, 0.5% nebulization solution, 20 mL
- Ceftriaxone, 5 g
- Dextrose 25% or 50%, 200 mL
- Epinephrine, 1:1000, 10 amp of 1 mg/mL (also effective when nebulized for croup in place of racemic epinephrine)
- Flumazenil (if stocking a benzodiazepine)
- Lidocaine, 1%, 50-mL vial
- Lorazepam or diazepam
- Naloxone, 1 mg/mL, 2-mL vial
- Tetanus toxoid, (dT) 0.5 mL

## TABLE 21-7 Expanded Equipment and Supplies List

**Airway Equipment:**
- Adhesive tape
- Endotracheal tubes (sizes 3.0 to 8.0)
- Laryngoscope handle with spare batteries
- Magill forceps (pediatric and adult sizes)
- Miller blades (0, 1, 2, 3)
- Nasal airways (infant to adult sizes)
- Nasogastric tubes (8, 10, 14F)
- Oropharyngeal airways (infant to adult sizes)
- Stylets (small and large)

**Fluid and Medication Administration:**
- Intraosseous needles
- Pediatric drip chambers

**Other**
- Cervical collar (several sizes)
- Lumbar puncture kit
- Portable monitor/defibrillator with pediatric paddles and skin electrode contacts (peel and stick)
- Pulse oximeter
- Splints
- Urine dipsticks
- Accucheck blood glucose oxidase reagent strips

## TABLE 21-8 Expanded Office Emergency Medication List

- Activated charcoal, 125 g
- Atropine (0.1 mg/mL), 1-mL vials (at least 5 vials)
- Corticosteroids (methylprednisolone or dexamethasone)
- Diphenhydramine, 50 mg/mL, (at least 1-mL vial)
- Epinephrine, 1:10,000, 10 mL
- Ipratropium for nebulization, 500 micrograms
- Phenytoin, fosphenytoin, or phenobarbital
- Sodium bicarbonate, 4.2%, five 50-mL vials or premeasured syringes

vision and monitoring of resuscitation equipment and medications. Ready-made kits are available. The Broselow/Hinkle Pediatric Emergency System contains seven color-coded nylon packs that correspond to the size ranges on the Broselow tape. This system is relatively expensive but provides a great degree of convenience.

# Section 1

Checking and restocking, although not particularly time-consuming, must be completed on a regular basis. For medications with expiration dates, an arrangement for exchange with a hospital pharmacy or emergency department can assist in keeping costs down. Responsibility for periodically checking and updating equipment and medications is preferably assigned to one person to enhance accountability and reduce oversight of this duty. It is advised that the physician in charge complete an equipment checklist and review it regularly.

## 1.5 Emergency Transport

Staff in a physician's office must be knowledgeable with regard to accessing emergency transportation services. In most of the United States, the emergency response system is contacted by simply dialing 9-1-1. If the office is not located in an area served by a 9-1-1 system, post the specific 7-digit emergency number or numbers prominently in the clinic area. It is also important that the appropriate level of care be requested. A BLS crew can perform oxygen administration, bag-mask ventilation, CPR, splinting, and spinal immobilization. They might also be able to assist patients with certain medication administration (albuterol metered-dose inhaler), but they do not carry any medications in the ambulance. If an intravenous line is initiated in the office, medications are needed, or intubation is performed in the office, an advanced life support (ALS) crew is required.

## 1.6 Patient and Parent Education

Education of parents and patients in regard to preventive measures is a key role of the primary care physician. Effective injury prevention training programs include those that cover installation and use of adequate swimming pool barriers, the use of infant car seats, seat belts, and bicycle helmets, as well as the use of poison centers. Early recognition of age-appropriate signs and symptoms of serious illness is another area of educational need for parents, and this topic leads logically to the discussion of how to proceed when an emergency occurs.[6]

Aftercare instruction is an important part of an office visit. Answer specific questions and give parents guidelines to follow. Instructions might include warning signs and symptoms of complications and when to call the office or go to an emergency department.

# Section 2 Trauma

# Section 2

## 2.1 Major Trauma

The outcome after major trauma is related directly to the interval between the precipitating event and the initiation of therapy. Although the large majority of severely injured pediatric patients are appropriately routed to an emergency department or a trauma center, it is not rare for children with very significant injuries to be brought to the office of their primary care physician. Rapid assessment and management, and contact of EMS for transfer to the emergency department for definitive care, are important to achieve optimal outcome.

## 2.2 Minor Trauma

Minor emergencies account for large numbers of unscheduled urgent care visits not only to the emergency department but also to the physician's office. Emergency physicians as well as office-based pediatricians and family practitioners therefore require a working knowledge of management of such conditions. The management of frequently encountered minor emergencies is summarized in the following sections.

## 2.3 Minor Head Trauma

Head trauma is one of the most common injuries during childhood, accounting for 7,000 deaths, 29,000 permanent disabilities, 95,000 hospital admissions, and more than 500,000 emergency department visits annually.[7–9] No study of children with minor head trauma has been able to identify reliable historical or physical exam criteria that will identify all children with radiographic abnormalities. Also, there has been much written and debated about the clinical significance of radiographically detected intracranial lesions. Adding to the mix, relatively few children with minor head trauma require surgical intervention, even when there is a radiographic abnormality. The initial evaluation of these children has been a topic of much discussion over the years.[7–13]

The American Academy of Pediatrics (AAP) has defined children older than 2 years with minor head injury as "those who have a normal mental status at the initial examination, who have no abnormal or focal findings on neurologic examination, and who have no physical evidence of skull fracture."[9] More severe head injuries and injuries occurring in children with suspected child abuse or a history of preexisting neurologic (e.g., presence of VP shunt) or hematologic illness generally warrant complete evaluation in the emergency department.

### Diagnostic Studies

Computed tomography (CT) imaging is recommended for children with altered mental status, focal neurologic deficits, or evidence of a depressed or basilar skull fracture.[7,9] A history of loss of consciousness, amnesia, seizure, headache, repeated emesis, irritability, and behavioral change is of particular concern when intense and prolonged, and CT should be considered in these cases.[7] The occurrence of an impact seizure is not, by itself, a reason to consider a head injury potentially more severe. Awake, alert, and otherwise asymptomatic children without a history of loss of consciousness do not require imaging.[7,9] Transport to the emergency department (ED) for appropriate imaging and further treatment might be necessary via EMS.

Children younger than 2 years are more likely to sustain an intracranial injury or skull fracture than older children and are more likely to be abused.[10] These children require a lower threshold for imaging than older children. Infants younger than 3 months are especially difficult to assess clinically and require a high index of suspicion for intracranial injury and a more aggressive evaluation. Consider CT imaging for these youngest children if there is a significant mechanism of injury or if there is evidence of a hematoma, even if the history and physical examination are otherwise unremarkable, and arrange for appropriate transport.[7,10]

The need for skull radiographs after minor head trauma has been much debated and studied in recent years.[7,9] Skull radiographs have a limited role in the evaluation of minor head trauma, with CT imaging the diagnostic modality of choice.[9] However, in children younger than 2 years with a significant scalp hematoma who are awake and alert with no associated signs of head injury, skull films can be a useful screen for skull fractures if these children would not otherwise undergo a CT scan.[7] The presence of a skull fracture increases the risk of finding an abnormality on CT scan by 20 times, and therefore would prompt the physician to obtain a head CT.[8]

### Management

For those patients with minor head injury in whom imaging is not necessary, discuss the risk of delayed deterioration, even though it is a rare event. Discharge the child to a competent adult for observation at frequent intervals during the first 24 hours post injury. Instruct the adult to seek immediate medical attention at an ED in the event of any deterioration.[9]

# Section 2

## 2.4 Minor Torso Trauma

In children with blunt trauma to the chest or abdomen, the absence of signs or symptoms of serious injury, and the presence of normal vital signs for age reassure the examining physician that internal injury is unlikely. However, abnormalities in vital signs must be taken seriously. In a recent study of patients admitted to pediatric trauma centers, abnormal vital signs for age were associated with high mortality rates.[14] Accordingly, children who present with abnormal vital signs for age after seemingly trivial trauma warrant immediate evaluation in the hospital by physicians familiar with the initial management of major trauma in the pediatric population.

### Clinical Features

Certain physical findings also warrant immediate evaluation. Children who present with significant chest pain, noisy or rapid breathing, respiratory distress or failure, or bloody sputum might have potentially serious intrathoracic injuries. Children who present with significant abdominal pain, swelling, tenderness, distention, abdominal wall contusions, or vomiting can have potentially serious intra-abdominal injuries. Vomiting is particularly significant when associated with blood or bile. Children who present with mild, localized, superficial chest or abdominal wall tenderness are not likely to have significant injuries, especially if such tenderness is limited to soft tissues located over bony prominences, such as the ribs or pelvis. All children with chest wall injury require careful evaluation for decreased or absent breath sounds and palpation for subcutaneous emphysema, either of which points toward the diagnosis of pneumothorax.

There are, however, certain mechanisms of blunt injury that require a more detailed evaluation. Children who sustain a sharp blow to the epigastrium, particularly from a handlebar during a fall from a bicycle, are at higher than usual risk for hepatic, splenic, and pancreatic injury. Children who sustain a sharp blow to the flank, particularly during contact sports, also are at high risk of renal injury and require ED evaluation.

Hematuria also is an important indicator of intra-abdominal injury. Perform a urine dipstick test for occult blood in children with a history of blunt abdominal trauma. Although significant renal injury is unlikely to have occurred unless there are more than 20 RBCs/hpf on microscopic examination, patients with any degree of hematuria should have a reevaluation within 2 days. If even a few red blood cells persist, a sonogram is indicated because renal abnormalities frequently are heralded by microscopic hematuria after trivial trauma. Evaluation in the ED and CT of the abdomen are indicated if gross or significant microscopic hematuria is found.[14]

---

## YOUR FIRST CLUE

**Serious Signs and Symptoms of Torso Injury**

- Abdominal pain
- Abdominal swelling
- Abdominal tenderness or distention
- Abdominal wall contusions
- Bloody sputum
- Hematuria
- Moderate to severe chest pain
- Noisy or rapid breathing
- Respiratory distress or failure
- Vomiting

---

## 2.5 Soft Tissue Injuries

Soft tissue injuries are treated by pain relief, rest, ice, compression, and elevation of the affected part to the extent possible (Figure 21.1). Ice packs can retard swelling during the first 1 to 2 days but might cause hypothermia and discomfort, especially in small children. After the acute period, warm showers, baths, and soaks or application of a carefully monitored moist heating pad several times daily can promote more rapid reabsorption of blood. Analgesia can be pro-

```
P  ain relief
R  est
I  ce
C  ompression
E  valuation
```

**Figure 21.1** PRICE Mnemonic.

vided by administration of a nonsteroidal anti-inflammatory agent such as ibuprofen. Aspirin-containing analgesics should be avoided in the first couple of days post injury because they might interfere with platelet function and promote hematoma development.

## 2.6 Lacerations

Closure of lacerations can present special technical problems in children, chiefly because the child usually is moving or thrashing about. The use of passive restraints such as the papoose board and involvement of the parent for psychological support of the child during suturing might facilitate the repair. The use of topical anesthetic agents, such as lidocaine-epinephrine-tetracaine (LET), infiltrative anesthetic agents buffered with sodium bicarbonate to reduce pain, and appropriate sedative agents, also can be useful in reducing the anxiety and discomfort traditionally associated with suturing of lacerations in children.[15,16] Suturing techniques are the same for children and adults, but it is wise to remember the following points when suturing children:

- The suture material chosen should be strong enough to withstand reinjury, especially when the laceration is on an extremity.
- Sutures of thin diameter and low reactivity should be used in highly visible areas such as the face.
- Blue or green sutures can be helpful, particularly on the scalp and face, to avoid confusion between suture material and hair at the time of suture removal.

- Use sutures that are large enough, placed far enough apart, and tied loosely enough so they are easy to remove and ensure there is not enough tension to cause unsightly cross-hatching.
- The use of staples on the scalp is another option for laceration closure. It does not require hair removal and has resulted in a more rapid procedure time and a more cosmetically acceptable wound closure.[17]

**Section**

**2**

## 2.7 Suturing

Basic wound management begins with wound assessment (Table 21-9), followed by application of local anesthesia (Table 21-10), wound preparation (Table 21-11), and selection of appropriate suture material (Table 21-12). Most wounds are closed with either a simple interrupted stitch or a horizontal mattress stitch.

### LET Application

LET (lidocaine 4% solution, epinephrine 1:1,000 solution, and tetracaine 0.5% solution) is a topical anesthetic that can be used prior to cleaning, irrigating, or closing lacerations to relieve pain at the wound site. Make sure that the patient has no allergies or sensitivities to any components of the LET solution prior to

| TABLE 21-9 | Wound Assessment |
|---|---|
| • Mechanism of injury | Sharp versus blunt trauma, bite |
| • Time since injury | Suture up to 12 hours; 24 hours on the face. It can be sutured after longer durations, but risk of infection might increase. Consider surgical consultation if closure is delayed. |
| • Foreign body, contamination | Explore for contamination and obtain radiographs for metal, glass, shell, rocks, coral |
| • Functional examination | Nerves, muscles, blood vessels, tendons |

| TABLE 21-10 | Types of Anesthesia | | | |
|---|---|---|---|---|
| Agent | Route of Administration | Dose | Onset | Duration |
| EMLA | Topical to intact skin | Thin layer of cream | 45 min | 1 hr |
| LET† | Topical, avoid mucous membranes | 3 mL (or 1 mL/cm of wound length) | 20 min | 1 hr |
| Lidocaine | Injectable | 4.5 mg/kg, maximum | 10 min | 1 hr |
| Lidocaine plus epinephrine‡ | Injectable | 7 mg/kg, maximum | 10 min | 1 hr |
| Bupivacaine | Injectable | 1.5 mg/kg | 20 min | 4 hr |
| Bupivacaine plus epinephrine‡ | Injectable | 2.5 mg/kg | 20 min | 4 hr |

Note: Use of systemic sedation and analgesia might be necessary to achieve optimal patient compliance.

*Eutectic mixture of local anesthetics.

†Lidocaine/epinephrine/tetracaine.

‡Do not use epinephrine in areas of terminal circulation such as distal parts of digits, ears, nose, or penis. Pain on injection can be lessened with distraction, slow infiltration, warming, and alkalinization (1 in 10 parts sodium bicarbonate).

applying it. Never use LET on fingers, toes, penis, nose, lips, ears, or any other area of terminal circulation. The purpose of LET application is to make the child more comfortable for the wound repair process. If the child does not relax or appears to be significantly distressed, consider the possibility of aborting LET application and using a different technique for anesthesia.

### Technique

1. Explain the procedure to the child and parent.
2. Use clean gloves.
3. Place 3 mL of a premixed solution on a cotton ball and apply it to the wound. For wider wounds, place a single LET-soaked 2×2 sterile gauze pad in the wound after instillation of excess. If a premixed solution is not available, use separate sterile syringes and needles for each medication. Mix equal parts depending on wound size. For wounds less than or equal to 2.5 cm, use 0.2 mL of each drug. For wounds greater than or equal to 2.5 cm, use 0.5 mL of each drug.
4. Place tape over the area and ask the parent to apply single-finger, gentle pressure for 20 minutes. The parent should wear a glove, as medication might be absorbed into skin.

| TABLE 21-11 | Wound Preparation |
|---|---|

- Remove excess dirt/debris by simple washing in sink (if possible).
- Skin can be scrubbed with betadine or other cleansing solution. Do not be timid when scrubbing the skin around a wound; the mechanical effect of scrubbing, independent of the agent used, is an important part of cleaning the skin. Do not instill betadine solution, iodophor, hydrogen peroxide, or hexachlorophene into an open wound.
- Cleanse anesthetized wound by irrigation with sterile normal saline solution using a 20-mL to 60-mL syringe and 18-gauge angiocatheter or splash shield. Another method is to stick an 18-gauge needle in the top of a 1-L bottle to make a hole, then squeeze the bottle. A fenestrated sterile drape will help maintain a sterile field when repairing the laceration.
- Use adequate direct pressure over the wound for at least 5 minutes without interruption to achieve hemostasis. Generally, 5 to 8 minutes with continuous pressure without release is sufficient. Do not send a child home with an open wound until proper hemostasis has been achieved.

| TABLE 21-12 Suture Material | | |
| --- | --- | --- |
| **Suture Type** | **Examples** | **Anatomic Area** |
| **External Skin Sutures** | | |
| Nylon (nonabsorbable) | Ethilon | Body,* face* |
| Nylon coated with polypropylene glycol (Nonabsorbable) | Prolene | Body, face |
| Rapidly degrading absorbable suture material | Vicryl rapide | Body, lips |
| Surgical staples | | Scalp,* noncosmetic areas |
| Wound closure strips | SteriStrips® | Superficial epidermal closure |
| Silk (not recommended unless others are not available) | | |
| **Absorbable "Deep" Sutures** | | |
| Polyglactin | Vicryl | Most commonly used* |
| Catgut (plain or coated) | | Not commonly used |

*Primarily indicated closure type.

5. The application should remain in place for 20 minutes. Effective skin blanching indicates proper absorption.

6. Do not use dry or partially soaked 2×2s as a cover. They act like a wick and draw the medicine into the gauze, thus decreasing the effectiveness of the LET.

## Irrigation of Wounds

Irrigation of a wound will remove particulate matter that can be a nidus of infection.

### Technique

1. In a contaminated wound, scrub the surrounding skin with betadine or equivalent solution. Avoid getting the solution into an open wound; it might inhibit the healing process.

2. For successful irrigation, an adequate volume of solution and adequate pressure are necessary. A 20-mL or larger syringe with an opening equivalent to an 18 to 19 gauge opening is generally effective. Sterile normal saline is an appropriate irrigation solution in most cases.

3. Remove particulate matter.

4. Irrigate wound copiously.

5. If the depth of the wound cannot be clearly visualized, consider the presence of foreign bodies and conduct appropriate investigations to rule out this possibility.

## Suturing Technique

1. The first principle of wound suturing is to match the skin heights up absolutely, which requires eversion of the wound edges. Shadows are cast over a wound closure that is not perfectly flat. Do not allow the wound edge(s) to roll inward.

2. To aid eversion of the wound edges, place sutures so the depth is greater than the width.

3. Ensure adequate exposure and illumination of the wound.

4. Assume a comfortable position; the best position generally is at one end of the long axis of the wound.

5. Preserve and protect all viable tissue. Office suturing is not recommended in certain situations, including any massive injury, an open fracture, an open joint dislocation, a wound in which there is precarious viability or impaired function distal to the wound, and any injury complicated by a compartment syndrome.

6. Immediate wound closure is best accomplished when there is no tension

# Section

## 2

2.7 Suturing

across the suture line. Tension can be reduced by undermining the wound beneath the subcutaneous tissue. The more tension on the wound edge, the closer the stitches should be to the edge. The more tension on the wound, the closer the stitches should be to each other.

7. Tie sutures just tight enough to approximate the wound edges, remembering that the tissues will swell with edema fluid.

8. Whenever possible, avoid the practice of halving an elliptical wound. This often causes bunching and uneven closure of the wound. Instead, work from one end of the wound to the other, sewing the skin the same distance along each side of the wound with each stitch.

### Simple Interrupted Stitch Technique

1. Select appropriate suture material.

2. In a sterile manner, remove the suture material from the packet and arm the tip of the needle holder one third of the way from the swage (needle-suture junction) (**Figure 21.2**). To prevent needlestick, do not use fingers to adjust the needle.

3. Enter the skin 5 mm or less from the laceration with the needle at 90 degrees to the skin surface (**Figure 21.3**).

4. Following the curvature of the needle, complete the stitch by exiting the opposite side of the wound at the same depth and distance from the wound edge as the entrance bite (**Figure 21.4**).

5. Tie a surgical knot with the instrument tie (**Figure 21.5**). Use five knots for nylon, six for coated nylon, and three for polyglactin absorbable or silk. Cut the suture with a 3-mm tail.

6. Arrange all knots symmetrically on the same side of the wound (preferably the side least susceptible to ischemia or cosmetic problems) (**Figure 21.6**).

7. Apply a topical antibiotic and dressing.

### Horizontal Mattress Stitch Technique

The horizontal mattress stitch is useful when a wound is under slight (not extreme) tension.

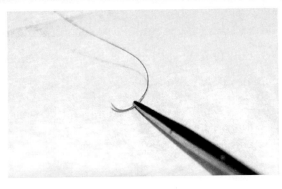

**Figure 21.2** The needle holder grasps the needle one third of the distance from the swage.

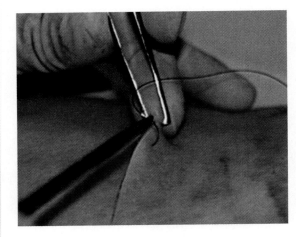

**Figure 21.3** Enter skin approximately 5 mm from the wound edge with the needle at 90 degrees to the skin surface.

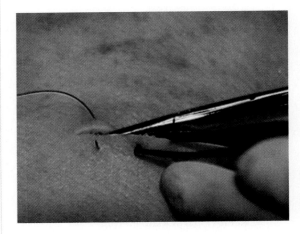

**Figure 21.4** Follow the curvature of the needle and complete the stitch by exiting the opposite side at the same depth and distance from the wound edge as the entrance bite.

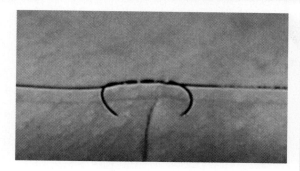

Figure 21.5 A surgical knot should be tied with the instrument tie.

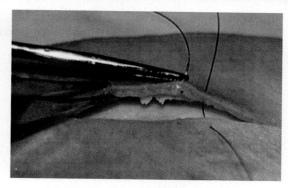

Figure 21.7 Use the horizontal mattress stitch for wounds under slight but not extreme tension.

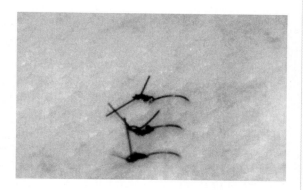

Figure 21.6 All stitches should be symmetrical and the knots should be aligned.

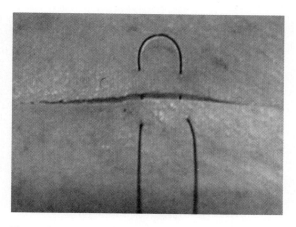

Figure 21.8 The two ends are tied on the same side of the wound.

Do not use in areas of cosmetic importance (e.g., face or hands).

1. Begin with the first stitch as above. Instead of tying this simple stitch, continue to the second half of the horizontal mattress suture by identifying the location you would have placed your next simple stitch (5 mm or less away). Do not cut the suture (Figure 21.7)!

2. Rearm the needle holder and enter the skin in the same manner from the second side to the first side. This is the simple stitch going back to the first side of the wound (Figure 21.8).

3. Tie the stitch on the first side of the wound parallel to the wound. It will look like a little box, with sides parallel to the laceration (Figure 21.9).

4. Instruct the patient to return for suture removal at the appropriate time based on the site of the laceration (Table 21-13).

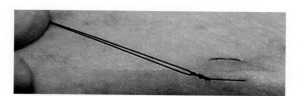

Figure 21.9 Tie as with the simple interrupted stitch to create a horizontal mattress.

## 2.8 Staples[18]

Staples are generally used to close wounds on the scalp only. Large wounds on the extremities could be closed using staples, but staples are never used on cosmetic areas, including the face.

# Section

## 2

2.8 Staples

2.9 Tissue Adhesive Application

| TABLE 21-13 Suture Removal Guidelines | | |
|---|---|---|
| Anatomic Area | Days Until Removal | External Suture Size |
| Face | 3–5 | 6–0* |
| Scalp | 7–10 | Staples, 5–0* |
| Upper body | 7–10 | 4–0 |
| Hand | 7–10 | 5–0 |
| Lower body | 10–14 | 4–0 |
| Over joint (recommend splint) | 14–21 | 4–0 |

*Use a colored suture material (usually green or blue) that will not be confused with the child's facial or scalp hair.

## Technique

1. Carefully select patients for wound closure with staples. Disclose risks and complications of the procedure. Explain advantages and disadvantages of treatment alternatives. Discuss what to expect during the procedure and the importance of keeping the child still during the procedure. Discuss methods of immobilization.

2. Cleanse the skin and irrigate the wound thoroughly, just as for placing sutures.

3. Approximate and slightly evert the skin edges.

4. Hold the stapler at the angle to the skin specified by the manufacturer. Different staplers require the stapler to be held at different angles and placed with varying amounts of downward pressure on the skin.

5. To form the staple, squeeze the handle of the stapler.

6. To release the staple, release pressure on the handle.

7. Check the staple position and replace any poorly placed staples.

## Staple Removal

1. Insert both lower jaw tips of the staple remover completely and symmetrically under the staple.

2. Lift slightly, holding the staple perpendicular to the skin.

3. Gently squeeze the handle while lifting the staple out of the skin.

## 2.9 Tissue Adhesive Application[19,20]

Carefully select patients for wound closure with tissue adhesive. Small children often wet or pick at the wound, weakening or peeling off the tissue adhesive. Avoid tissue adhesive closure in areas of tension (chin, joints, weight-bearing surfaces, wounds that do not easily approximate), areas with hair (scalp, eyebrows), and areas that might be kept moist (fingers that might be sucked). Adequate immobilization is required.

Disclose risks and complications of the procedure. Explain advantages and disadvantages of treatment alternatives. Discuss what to expect during the procedure, including the possibility of heat sensation with application. Discuss the importance of keeping the child from moving during the procedure and methods of immobilization.

## Technique

1. Cleanse the skin and irrigate the wound thoroughly, just as for placing sutures or staples. Because local anesthesia might not be required, there can be temptation to be less aggressive when exploring, scrubbing, and irrigating these wounds.

2. Achieve complete hemostasis. Sutures provide circumferential tension and facilitate hemostasis within the ligature loop; tissue adhesive does not facilitate hemostasis. Optimally, the skin will be dry before application; mixing tissue adhesive with tears is not recommended.

3. Wear tight-fitting vinyl gloves. The tissue adhesive Dermabond adheres to vinyl gloves only weakly compared to its adherence to latex gloves.

4. Position the patient to avoid dripping of tissue adhesive onto sensitive areas (e.g., keep eyes "uphill" from the laceration site). When possible, position the wound surface horizontally to reduce runoff. Tissue adhesive that seeps into the wound and polymerizes can cause the wound to be "glued open" or result in a foreign body reaction and promote infection. Prophylactic application of petroleum jelly or ointment to sensitive areas can reduce adherence of tissue adhesive. Surrounding the laceration with damp gauze can also absorb tissue adhesive and prevent runoff. Moistened gauze is as effective as dry gauze in absorbing tissue adhesive but is much less likely to get glued to the skin.

5. Manually approximate and evert wound edges with a gloved hand or forceps. The wound must be held closed firmly until polymerization is complete, generally 1 minute after the last layer of tissue adhesive is applied. Use metal forceps. Unless specifically made for use with tissue adhesive, plastic forceps are much more likely than metal forceps to get glued to the skin.

6. Remove the applicator from sterile packaging and hold with its tip pointed upward. Crush the inner glass ampule by applying pressure at the midpoint of the outer plastic ampule. Use the tissue adhesive immediately after crushing the inner glass ampule. Polymerization of the tissue adhesive begins even before it is applied to the skin.

7. Apply adequate pressure to the ampule to moisten the fabric applicator tip, evidenced by a color change from white to purple color. Apply gentle pressure to the ampule while using gentle brushing strokes to apply a thin film of liquid over the approximated and everted wound edges. Overzealous pressure on the ampule will increase the likelihood of complications

from tissue adhesive runoff. Apply three or four evenly distributed layers of tissue adhesive at least 0.5 cm on each side of the wound margins. Maintain approximation of the incision edges until a flexible film is formed, usually about 1 minute after applying the last layer.

8. Dab up excessive glue with a moistened cotton-tipped applicator or gauze.

9. There is no need to cover the tissue adhesive, but if desired, the wound can be covered with a dry dressing. Do not apply ointments, medications, or skin strips on top of tissue adhesive.

10. On discharge, provide instructions regarding proper wound care and potential complications, such as infection, allergic reaction, and dehiscence.

11. Instruct parents that the glue should slough off in 5 to 10 days.

12. Parents also should keep the area as clean and dry as possible. Do not expose the wound to prolonged wetness or scrubbing for 7 to 10 days. After this time, the patient should wet the wound so that tissue adhesive breakdown is accelerated and timely sloughing will occur. In some cases, tissue adhesive has been applied excessively; prolonged presence on the skin has been associated with superficial infection.

## Management of Wounds

Given the uncanny ability of children to reinjure the involved areas, do not remove sutures from the extremities until it is clear that complete healing has occurred. This might require up to 2 to 3 weeks after injury over joints. With proper patient selection, certain minor wounds can be closed with tissue adhesive.[21]

Systemic antibiotics are of little use and of potential harm in patients with blunt trauma, even if extensive. Systemic antibiotics also have no proven role in patients with clean lacerations, especially those of the face and scalp, provided they are closed promptly, within 12 to 24 hours of injury. Treat older wounds and tetanus-prone wounds with systemic antibiotics as well as aggressive local care, including debridement of devitalized tissue. Patients with such wounds also require tetanus prophylaxis, including tetanus immune globulin if the immunization series has been deficient.

The importance of timely and appropriate wound care in the prevention of wound infection cannot be overemphasized. Wounds must be thoroughly explored, debrided, and irrigated before closure. Particulate debris in the wound must be picked out, and the wound must be vigorously scrubbed and irrigated. If these measures are inadequate, tissue excision might be necessary. Adequate volume and pressure of irrigation fluid are essential. Surgical consultation might be necessary if the wound is significantly contaminated. For wounds involving penetration of a body cavity, surgical consultation is mandatory.

---

## KEY POINTS

### Management of Wounds

- Provide analgesia.
- Perform wound irrigation and debridement as needed.
- Immobilize child and area to be sutured by nonpharmacologic or pharmacologic means.
- Choose appropriate suture material or tissue adhesive.
- Perform wound closure.
- Explain appropriate wound care to parents.

---

## 2.10 Human and Animal Bites

Bites inflicted by humans and animals can result in grossly contaminated wounds due to the microorganisms that reside in oral cavities. *Staphylococcus* and both aerobic and anaerobic *streptococcus* are found in all species, and *Pasteurella* species are prominent in the oral cavity of cats. Thoroughly clean and meticulously debride all bite wounds, then irrigate liberally. Most can be left open, but if closure is necessary, only loosely approximate the wound edges. With the exception of deep puncture wounds, bite wounds on the head and face can be closed in the usual manner. Tetanus immunization status must be determined and appropriate measures taken if the immunization series is incomplete. Also consider the risk of rabies based on the animal species and circumstances of the attack.

Antibiotics are not necessary for meticulously cleaned, superficial human and dog bite wounds. However, treat puncture wounds and other deep, irregular, or extensive bite wounds with antibiotics, as well as all wounds involving the face, hands, wrists, feet, ankles, and genital area, and all wounds in patients who are immunocompromised or those with asplenism. Treat all cat bites with antibiotics. Amoxicillin-clavulanic acid, in a dose of 40 mg/kg per day of amoxicillin, divided into 2 doses, is a good choice. An alternative is penicillin VK (25 to 50 mg/kg per day) divided into 4 doses, plus cephalexin (25 to 100 mg/kg per day) divided into 2 doses or dicloxacillin (50 mg/kg per day) divided into 4 doses. Erythromycin can be used for penicillin-allergic patients.

After cleansing or closure, the wound should be elevated, immobilized, and observed frequently for signs of cellulitis. At the first sign of infection, immediate hospitalization is required.

---

## Section 3  Foreign Bodies

**Section**

**3**

If clearly visible or palpable, most subcutaneous, subungual, and loose foreign bodies of the eye, ear, or nose can be removed in the ED or physician's office depending on the child's ability to cooperate (**Figure 21.10**). Procedural sedation can facilitate management of such problems but should be undertaken only when the treating physician is experienced in its use and proper monitoring is available. Foreign bodies of the gastrointestinal tract will usually pass sponta-

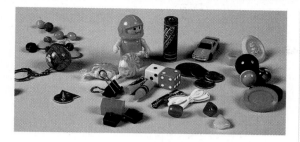

**Figure 21.10** Children sometimes swallow tiny objects or put them in their noses or ears.

neously if allowed to do so. Endoscopic or surgical removal is required for ingested button batteries. Promptly refer all patients with esophageal or tracheobronchial foreign bodies to an ED or qualified specialist. Because esophageal foreign bodies can be asymptomatic, it is appropriate to attempt imaging of any ingested foreign body that might be radioopaque. A hand-held metal detector can also be used to determine passage of metallic foreign bodies into the stomach, thus eliminating the need for routine radiographs.[22]

# 3.1 Subcutaneous Foreign Body Removal

Subcutaneous foreign bodies often can be removed with simple methods appropriately suited to the type of foreign body retained. In general, it is best to attempt office removal of a foreign body only if its exact location can be determined by palpation or visualization. Radiographic localization is often deceptive in that, without fluoroscopy, the foreign body can be much more difficult to localize than anticipated. Surgical consultation, if available, is preferable for removal of foreign bodies that are not easily located.

## Technique

1. Obtain anteroposterior and lateral radiographs of the affected part to localize a radiodense foreign body. Most glass is radiodense.

2. Prepare the site adjacent to the entrance wound with an antiseptic such as betadine.

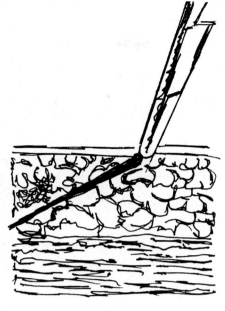

**Figure 21.11** Pass a straight mosquito hemostat into the entrance wound until it makes contact with the foreign body.

3. For a long, sharp, metallic foreign body, such as a needle, pin, or nail:
   - Anesthetize the skin adjacent to the entrance wound and along the shaft of the foreign body with a short-acting local anesthetic such as lidocaine.
   - Slightly enlarge the entrance wound.
   - Press gently over the deep end of the foreign body to elevate the superficial end into the entrance wound.
   - Pass a straight mosquito hemostat into the entrance wound until it makes contact with the foreign body (**Figure 21.11**).
   - Open the jaws of the hemostat, grasp the foreign body, and remove the hemostat and foreign body as a unit.

4. For a horizontally embedded wooden splinter:
   - Anesthetize the skin along the entire length of the splinter with a short-acting local anesthetic such as lidocaine.
   - Incise the skin over the splinter starting over the entrance wound and extend as far as necessary to expose

# Section

# 3

3.1 Subcutaneous Foreign Body Removal

3.2 Nail Bed Splinter Removal

3.3 Ocular Foreign Body Removal

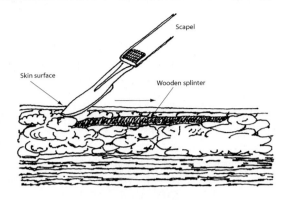

Figure 21.12 Horizontal splinter removal.

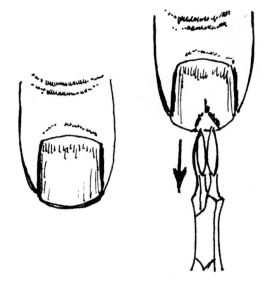

Figure 21.13 Nail bed splinter removal.

the end of the splinter, and then remove the splinter with a straight mosquito hemostat. It is important to visualize the entire foreign body before removal so that the likelihood of retained fragments is reduced (**Figure 21.12**).

- Loosely close the skin if necessary.

5. Because a vertically embedded wooden splinter will not be visualized completely before removal, it is likely that a portion of the splinter will remain in the wound, increasing the risk of subsequent infection and need for surgical consultation later. In general, this type of foreign body is best removed in consultation with a surgeon.

## 3.2 Nail Bed Splinter Removal

1. Use of a digital block can facilitate splinter removal.

2. Pass a straight mosquito hemostat longitudinally along the underside of the nail directly adjacent and parallel to the splinter, just past its tip on each side of the splinter, with the jaws of the hemostat closed.

3. Slightly open the jaws of the hemostat and pass each blade along the underside of the nail, straddling the splinter (**Figure 21.13**).

4. Close the jaws of the hemostat over the splinter and gently extract the hemostat and splinter as a unit.

If the splinter appears likely to fragment during removal or if fragmentation occurs during attempted removal, remove the overlying portion of the nail so that complete splinter removal is ensured under direct visualization:

1. Test effectiveness of digital block.

2. Dissect under the nail with a hemostat, being careful to not injure the nail matrix.

3. Using sharp-pointed scissors, cut out the appropriate nail section to completely expose the splinter.

4. Lift the splinter out carefully and completely.

5. Irrigate the area using normal saline through an 18-gauge needle in a large syringe.

6. Dress the wound with nonadherent gauze, then sterile gauze and tape.

7. Arrange for wound recheck and dressing change the next day.

## 3.3 Ocular Foreign Body Removal

Irrigation of the eye will remove particulate matter that can cause corneal abrasions or ulcerations. Superficial ocular foreign bodies that cannot be dislodged through repetitive blinking or washing the foreign body toward the medial canthus usually can be removed following the procedures described below.

## Eye Irrigation Technique

1. Check visual acuity (OD,OS,OU) before irrigation. The only exception is alkaline exposures to the eye. Immediate removal of particulate matter and irrigation are appropriate in this case.

2. Using a topical anesthetic such as proparacaine (0.5%) can enhance patient tolerance and lead to a better result.

3. Gauze pads are helpful to grasp the periorbital tissue and hold the eye open for irrigation.

4. Whenever possible, pull down the lower eyelid and evert the upper eyelid to irrigate most effectively.

5. In cooperative patients, a Morgan Lens can be helpful for prolonged irrigation (e.g., alkaline exposures).

## Ocular Foreign Body Removal Technique

1. The use of a topical anesthetic such as proparacaine might facilitate foreign body removal.

2. For loose foreign bodies, press the eyelashes against the superior orbital rim. Locate the foreign body and gently brush it downward with a moistened cotton-tipped applicator (**Figure 21.14**).

3. With topical anesthesia and a cooperative patient, a superficially embedded corneal foreign body can be removed with a beveled 18- to 25-gauge needle held tangentially to the corneal surface while scooping out the foreign body. Close ophthalmologic followup is necessary to be sure there are no retained fragments, particularly in the case of a metallic foreign body, which could leave a rust ring with eventual staining of the cornea.

4. If the foreign body cannot be located, evert the eyelid by grasping the eyelashes, pressing downward in the center of the dermal surface of the eyelid with the

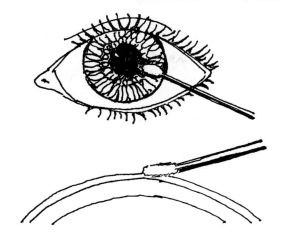

**Figure 21.14** Ocular foreign body removal.

cotton-tipped end of an applicator (**Figure 21.15A**) to rotate the tarsal plate (**Figure 21.15B**), and proceed as above. Vigorous irrigation can aid removal of certain foreign bodies, including those that are difficult to visualize.

5. Refer children with foreign bodies that cannot be removed with these simple measures to an ophthalmologist immediately.

## 3.4 Cerumen/Aural Foreign Body Removal[23]

The only attempts to remove foreign bodies that should be made are those that are likely to end in success. Unsuccessful manipulation can cause bleeding, movement of the foreign body to a less accessible area, and mucosal edema, making the task of removal for an otolaryngology (ENT) consultant even more difficult. Explain the procedure to the parent and child. It is best to accomplish removal without violating the child's trust.

### Technique

Impacted cerumen and loose foreign bodies usually can be removed with the following technique:

1. Assess the need for sedation and administer medications as indicated.

# Section 3

3.4 Cerumen/Aural Foreign Body Removal

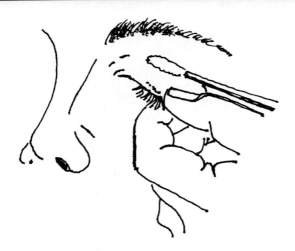

**Figure 21.15A** Evert the eyelid.

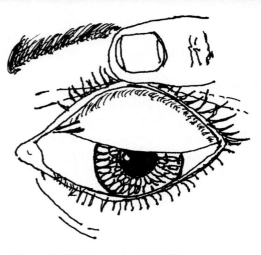

**Figure 21.15B** Rotate the tarsal plate.

2. Ensure adequate immobilization with a sheet or papoose board, along with assistants as needed. Adequate immobilization will reduce the risk of injury to the child and staff

3. Place traction on the pinna, exposing the external auditory canal (**Figure 21.16A**).

4. Insert the operating head of an otoscope into the external auditory canal if necessary to expose the impacted cerumen or foreign body (**Figure 21.16B**).

5. For soft cerumen or foreign bodies such as food matter, pass a long, narrow, cylindric, thin-walled Frazier-type suction device into the external auditory canal until it makes contact with the entrapped matter. Occlude the side port of the suction device and then gently extract the suction device and entrapped matter as a unit.

6. Repeat as necessary.

7. For hard cerumen or hard foreign bodies, pass a cerumen spoon into the external auditory canal along its outer circumference, opposite the impacted cerumen or foreign body, until the tip of the instrument has passed beyond it. Rotate the cerumen spoon until its angulated tip engages the entrapped matter. Then gently extract the instrument, pulling the entrapped matter ahead of it. Avoid scraping the outer circumference of the external auditory canal with the instrument because it is exquisitely sensitive to pain (**Figure 21.17**).

8. In some cases, extraction of a hard foreign body or wax can be facilitated by using a combination of curettage and irrigation. Irrigation can be particularly effective in removal of small foreign bodies close to the tympanic membrane. Do not irrigate in the presence of any foreign body of vegetable origin; swelling and further obstruction can result. Body temperature tap water can be used unless there is perforation of the tympanic membrane. The goal is to deliver an adequate volume of water with a brisk flow rate to a well-defined area. Use a 30- to 60-mL syringe attached to a plastic infusion catheter or butterfly needle tubing cut off 3 inches from the hub. The tubing should be inserted into the lateral portion of the external auditory meatus and directed to flow around a partial obstruction, allowing the foreign body or wax to be washed out along with the effluent irrigation fluid. Refer the patient to an otorhinolaryngologist if entrapped matter cannot be removed using these simple measures.

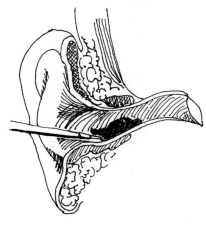

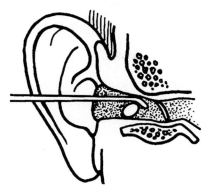

3.5 Nasal Foreign Body Removal

**Figure 21.17** Avoid scraping the outer circumference of the external auditory canal with the instrument.

**Figure 21.16A** Expose the external auditory canal.

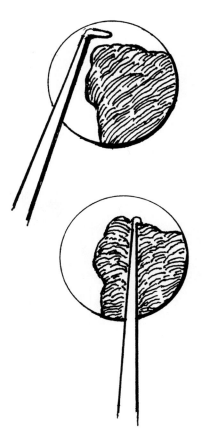

**Figure 21.16B** Insert the operating head of an otoscope into the external auditory canal if necessary to expose the impacted cerumen or foreign body.

## 3.5 Nasal Foreign Body Removal[23]

Again, do not attempt to remove a foreign body unless success is likely. Unsuccessful manipulation can cause bleeding, movement of the foreign body to a less accessible area, and mucosal edema, making the task of removal for an ENT consultant even more difficult. Explain the procedure to the parent and child. It is best to accomplish removal without violating the child's trust.

### Technique

1. Assess the need for sedation and administer medications as indicated.

2. Ensure adequate immobilization with a sheet or papoose board, along with assistants as needed. Adequate immobilization will reduce the risk of injury to the child and staff.

3. Instill a topical vasoconstrictor, such as phenylephrine, cocaine, or epinephrine, to reduce nasal mucosal tissue.

4. With a good headlight or alternative light source for visualization, insert a nasal speculum and open it vertically to avoid injury to the nasal septum.

5. Depending on the shape and size of the foreign body, use one of the following techniques:
   - Using alligator forceps, grasp the foreign body and extract it.
   - Place a wire loop or curette behind the foreign body and extract the foreign body and loop as a unit.
   - Attach a suction apparatus to the foreign body and extract it.
   - Apply an adhesive (e.g., Super Glue) to a cotton-tipped applicator. Once the foreign body has adhered to the applicator, it can be extracted.
   - Pass a Foley or Fogarty catheter (size 8) beyond the object, then inflate the balloon and withdraw it along with the foreign body.

6. Once a foreign body is removed, check for additional objects in the nose and ears.

7. If removal is unsuccessful, immediate ENT consultation should be sought. If immediate removal is not essential, the child can be started on antibiotics and referred to an otorhinolaryngologist for removal.

## Section 4  Minor Burns

### 4.1 Minor Burns

Minor burns can be defined as superficial or partial thickness burns that do not require in-patient or burn center care. Most sunburn, scald, and contact burns that involve less than 10% of total body surface area are considered minor. Children with scald or contact partial thickness burns involving more than 10% of total body surface area or any burns involving the eyes, ears, face, hands, feet, or genitalia, and those crossing a joint space, require consultation with a burn specialist (Figure 21.18). Children with electrical burns and burns associated with inhalation injury or major trauma also are candidates for inpatient care. Burn size can be estimated using the rule of nines modified for use in pediatric patients (Figure 21.19) or the rule of palms, which states that the size of a child's palmar surface of the hand is equal to approximately 1% of body surface area (Figure 21.20).[24,25]

Outpatient management of minor burns begins with gentle cleansing of burned skin with mild soap or detergent (e.g., chlorhexidine scrub), then with sterile water or saline. Once the wound has been cleansed, large and small bullae that have broken are debrided

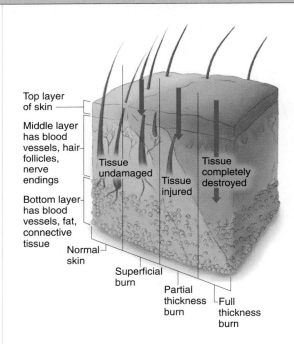

**Figure 21.18** Depth of burn injury.

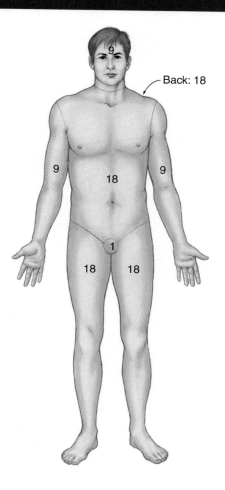

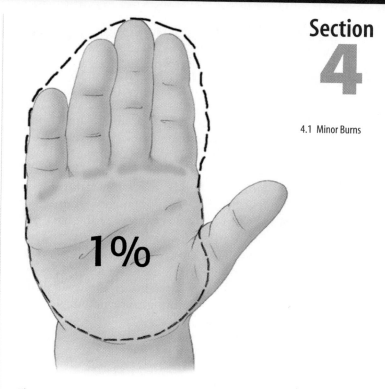

**Figure 21.20** Rule of palms. The palmar surface of the child's hand equals approximately 1% of the body surface area.

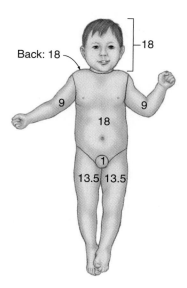

**Figure 21.19** The rule of nines is a quick way to estimate the amount of surface area that has been burned. It divides the body into sections, each approximately 9% of the total body surface area.

carefully with clean instruments. Intact bullae are not opened. Finally, a thin layer of silver sulfadiazine cream (if no sulfa drug allergy exists) is applied to the wound and covered with nonadherent gauze; avoid using silver sulfadiazine on the face. When silver sulfadiazine cannot be used, bacitracin ointment is another option. This process is repeated daily. Followup medical evaluation should be arranged for at least twice weekly. Daily rechecks might be indicated initially for more complex wounds. Prophylactic antibiotics should be avoided because they can promote the emergence of resistant organisms. Tetanus immunization status should be confirmed and toxoid administered as indicated. Oral fluids are encouraged to replace transepidermal water losses that occur when skin is not intact.

# Section 5  Miscellaneous Procedures

## 5.1 Subungual Hematoma Drainage

The decision to drain a subungual hematoma is based on the size of the hematoma, pain experienced by the child, and age of the hematoma. Injuries less than 1 or 2 days old are more likely to be made less painful with drainage. If there is spontaneous drainage of blood from around the edges of the nail, nail trephination is usually not necessary. The relative merits of alternative nonsurgical treatment with elevation and oral analgesics are considered in the decision to drain a subungual hematoma. Subungual hematomas can be decompressed easily.

### Technique

1. Prepare the nail with an antiseptic such as betadine.
2. Consider using a digital block with an anesthetic such as lidocaine. Anesthesia is not necessary if the child is cooperative and the procedure can be done in a controlled manner so the nail bed itself is not penetrated.
3. Unfold a standard paper clip and hold one end in a flame for several seconds until the tip becomes red hot. A battery-operated, hand-held cautery unit or 18-gauge needle can be used instead of a hot paper clip.
4. Immediately apply the hot tip to the nail overlying the center of the hematoma, using gentle pressure until it burns a hole in the nail (**Figure 21.21**). Then remove the paper clip. This permits sufficient decompression of the subungual hematoma to relieve the pain as the remainder of the subungual hematoma spontaneously resorbs. Because small holes in the nail can occlude with clotted blood, making more than one hole in the nail might be a good idea.

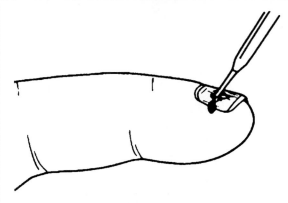

**Figure 21.21** Apply the hot tip to the nail overlying the center of the hematoma.

## 5.2 Paronychia

A paronychia is an infection involving the soft tissue folds of the fingernail or toenail. If there is only erythema and soft tissue swelling, it might be possible to treat with a combination of frequent warm water soaks and oral semi-synthetic penicillin or cephalosporin. If there is fluctuance, definitive treatment must include drainage of the pus. Paronychia can be drained in several ways. It is usually not necessary to remove the nail to drain the paronychium.

### Technique

1. Consider digital block and/or systemic sedation.
2. Soften the epichondrium and nail by soaking them in warm water.
3. At the point of maximal swelling, lift the epichondrium from its attachment to the nail using scissors or hemostats, or pierce the area of maximal swelling with an 18-gauge needle or a scalpel.
4. Hold the instrument parallel to the nail and gently sweep from side to side, breaking up any loculations of pus while minimizing damage to the nail bed (**Figure 21.22**).

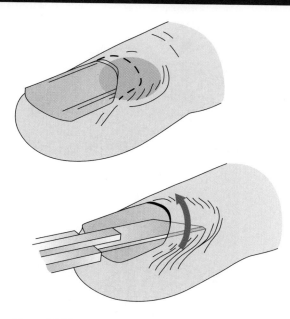

**Figure 21.22** Method for drainage of a simple paronychia.

5. Allow the pus to escape and irrigate the area with normal saline.

6. Place a small piece of gauze between the nail and epichondrium to allow continued drainage.

7. The gauze can be removed at followup 1 to 2 days later.

If subungual pus is present or if the previous methods have been unsuccessful, consider partial nail removal.

1. Place digital block.

2. Lift the epichondrium off the nail using scissors or hemostats.

3. Dissect the portion of the nail to be removed from the nail bed using hemostats, being careful not to damage the nail matrix.

4. Using scissors, make a cut along the longitudinal axis of the fingernail to remove one quarter of the nail.

5. Be sure the portion of the nail to be removed is completely freed from the nail bed all the way back to the nail matrix.

6. Grasp the nail firmly with hemostats and remove.

7. Allow pus to escape and irrigate the area.

8. Obtain hemostasis.

9. Place nonadherent gauze and a sterile dressing over the wound. If nonadherent gauze is not available, an antibiotic ointment can be used.

10. Have the patient follow up in 1 to 2 days.

## 5.3 Skin Abscess Drainage

A skin abscess is a localized infection that has coalesced to form pus. In the early stages of a skin infection, there might be only redness, tenderness, warmth, and swelling. In such cases it is advisable to treat with warm compresses, systemic antibiotics, and frequent reevaluation. However, if there is softening of the area (fluctuance) or if there is any draining of pus from the wound, drainage is necessary.

The drainage procedure used is largely dependent on the size and site of the abscess. Examples of special cases that require surgical consultation include deep tissue abscesses of the face, hand, or foot. Most abscesses encountered in pediatrics do not involve deep tissue structures and can be handled as an outpatient procedure without surgical consultation.

### Technique

1. Scrub the skin with an antibacterial solution such as betadine. Use an expanding spiral pattern, scrub three times, and allow the betadine to dry between applications.

2. Use topical anesthesia (ethyl chloride), or LET and local anesthesia (lidocaine) to provide pain relief. Consider systemic analgesia and sedation.

3. Using a scalpel, incise along the entire length of the abscess cavity (**Figure 21.23A**).

4. Insert and spread hemostats into the abscess cavity to break up any loculations.

5. Irrigate the abscess cavity (**Figure 21.23B**).

6. Look for a shiny, fibrous capsule within the wound, suggesting an infected sebaceous cyst. If not removed at the time of abscess drainage, followup care must be planned to remove the capsule. If not removed, the abscess is likely to recur.

**Section**
**5**

# Section

# 5

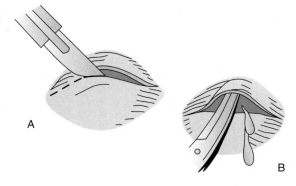

**Figure 21.23A** Make a linear incision through the skin over the full length of the abscess cavity. Pay careful attention to avoid adjacent neurovascular structures.
**Figure 21.23B** Explore and drain the abscess cavity with a hemostat.

7. Loosely pack the abscess cavity with plain Nu-Gauze, leaving a tail outside the wound.

8. Cover the site with a sterile dressing.

9. Send pus to the lab for culture.

10. Arrange followup care for the next day.

## 5.4 Fish Hook Removal

Fish hooks usually can be removed with any of several methods. If the fish hook is not barbed, it will be easily removed by retrograde traction. Do not attempt fish hook removal without subspecialty consultation when removal can lead to tearing through the eyelid margin or other serious complications.

The preferred removal method will depend on patient cooperativeness and physician comfort with each technique. Although simplest to perform, the advance and cut technique requires the use of wire cutters and traumatizes previously undamaged tissue.

### Technique

The needle-over-barb technique can be easily mastered and is generally effective.

1. Prepare the skin adjacent to the entrance wound with an antiseptic such as betadine.

2. Anesthetize the skin overlying the barb with a short-acting local anesthetic such as lidocaine.

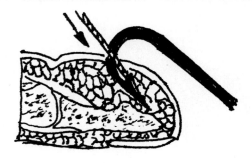

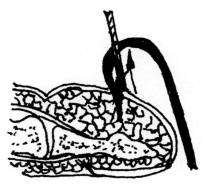

**Figure 21.24A, B** With the beveled tip facing the barb, pass it through the skin so the beveled tip engages the sharp end of the barb; extract the needle and hook as a unit.

3. With the beveled tip facing the barb, pass it through the skin so the beveled tip engages the sharp end of the barb; extract the needle and hook as a unit (**Figure 21.24A, B**).

The string traction method is particularly useful if local anesthesia is not preferred or impossible.

1. Wrap a loop of string around the curve of the fish hook.

2. Depress the shaft of the fish hook using the thumb, then depress the curved portion of the hook with the index finger to disengage the barb from the subcutaneous tissue.

3. Pull sharply and strongly with the string to remove the fish hook.

The advance and cut technique is the most commonly used method to remove barbed fish hooks from the skin.

1. Prepare the skin adjacent to the entrance wound with an antiseptic such as betadine.

2. Anesthetize the skin overlying the barb with a short-acting local anesthetic such as lidocaine.

Figure 21.25 Advance the fish hook, following the curve, until the barb passes outside the skin.

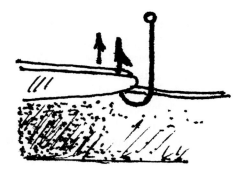

Figure 21.26 Cut the barb from the hook with wire cutters.

3. Advance the fish hook, following the curve of the belly, until the barb passes outside the skin, piercing through from inside the skin (**Figure 21.25**).

4. Cut the barb from the hook with wire cutters and then retract the hook, following the curve until completely removed (**Figure 21.26**).

## 5.5 Ring Removal

Rings entrapped by soft tissue swelling of the digit distal to the ring that cannot be removed with lubricant and circular traction (after elevation of the digit and immersion in cold water) often can be removed using the following technique.

### Technique

1. Use of a digital block can aid cooperation and facilitate ring removal.

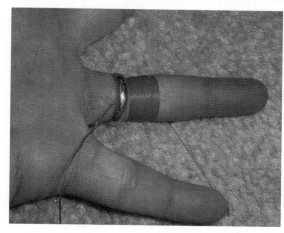

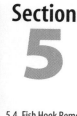

Figure 21.27 Wrap the string so that each turn touches the other.

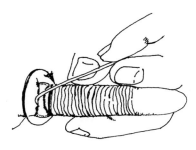

Figure 21.28 The string will lift the ring off the finger as it unravels.

2. Wrap a piece of string, heavy silk suture, or umbilical tape around the finger, starting proximal to the ring and pulling the end under the ring.

3. Continue wrapping tightly around the digit, moving from proximal to a point beyond the distal interphalangeal joint, laying each turn so that it touches the other and in such a way that the outer circumference of each turn is slightly less than the inner circumference of the entrapped ring (**Figure 21.27**).

4. Unwind the proximal end of the string and pull the ring gently but firmly toward the distal end of the digit.

5. The string will lift the ring off the finger as it unravels circumferentially (**Figure 21.28**).

If the ring is not successfully removed by this method, a ring cutter or Dremel tool can be used. If a high-speed cutting tool is used, be sure to protect the skin of the finger from mechanical or thermal injury by irrigating the site with cool water while cutting the ring and by sliding a thin metal barrier between the ring and finger. After cutting through the ring, the cut ends can be spread to facilitate removal.

## 5.6 Contact Lens Removal

Requests for contact lens removal might be due to the inability to "find" the contact lens or actual inability to remove the lens after visualization.

### Technique

1. Perform visual acuity testing. The child can use an ophthalmoscope to reproduce the corrective lens while viewing the eye chart.
2. Examine the eye, looking for a fine, curvilinear shape over the sclera, which represents one edge of the contact lens.
3. Use a topical anesthetic such as proparacaine (0.5%) to facilitate thorough examination and removal.
4. If the lens is not easily visible, evert the eyelid.
5. If the lens still cannot be seen, evert the eyelid and sweep under the eyelid with a moist cotton swab.
6. Do not place fluorescein in the eye without notifying the family that the lens will be permanently discolored.

### Removal

For a hard contact lens, push the edge of the lower eyelid under the edge of the contact lens while pushing the upper lid against the upper edge of the contact lens. Once the contact lens is lifted off the globe, it can easily be lifted out of the eye.

For a soft contact lens, slide the contact lens off the cornea onto the sclera, then pinch the contact lens between the thumb and index finger while lifting it off the globe. Even if the soft contact lens was initially dried out, it should be moistened by the instillation of local anes-

thetic. If the lens is still dry and difficult to bend, additional saline eye drops can be used.

Examine the eye for evidence of conjunctival trauma, retained foreign body, hemorrhage, and corneal ulceration/abrasion. If significant pain or corneal abrasion is present, consider the use of topical mydriatics, oral analgesics, and eye patching for comfort.

## 5.7 Eye Patching

In the past, eye patches in the pediatric emergency setting were used mostly for corneal abrasions. Because the literature suggests that there is no advantage to patching over the use of topical antibiotics and systemic analgesics for patients with small (less than 2 mm) corneal abrasions, eye patches are not frequently indicated for children in the emergency setting. Indications for pressure patching include larger corneal abrasions, chemical injuries, and ultraviolet light injuries. Simple patches can be used to protect a dilated eye from exposure to sunlight. Patches are contraindicated in the presence of an active corneal infection or penetrating injury.

### Placement of a Pressure Patch

The goal of patching is to create adequate pressure under the patch to keep the eyelid closed, thus protecting the cornea from movements of the eyelid.

### Technique

1. Place a topical anesthetic and mydriatic eye drop in the eye to be patched. Always have pilocarpine on hand when instilling a mydriatic agent, especially if there is a family history of narrow-angle glaucoma. If acute eye pain develops after instillation of a mydriatic agent, immediately instill pilocarpine.
2. Have the patient keep both eyes closed during the entire patching procedure.
3. Place a folded, vertically oriented eye patch in the orbital recess.
4. Overlay a horizontally oriented eye patch, holding both in position with one finger.

5. Tape the patch securely in place while maintaining both patches in position using gentle, steady pressure.

6. Pull the tape firmly across the patched eye from cheek to forehead, while the patient or an assistant pulls the lips away from the affected side. This reduces the movement of the tape and patch with lip movements and makes the patch more comfortable for the patient.

7. Repeat the placement of tape 2 or 3 additional times until all areas of the patch are held firmly in place.

8. If age appropriate, have the patient open the unaffected eye and ask if the affected eye remains closed.

9. Have the patient follow up the next day to remove the patch and reexamine the eye.

## 5.8 Tooth Reimplantation and Stabilization

Avulsion of a primary tooth does not require reimplantation. Avulsion of a permanent tooth does require reimplantation as soon as possible; even a 30-minute delay can preclude successful reimplantation. Hold the tooth by the crown, avoiding trauma to the root surface and periodontal ligament. Quickly immerse the tooth in cold milk or place under the tongue of the child (as age appropriate) or parent. Placing the tooth in commercially available Hanks solution, a cell culture medium, might significantly extend the reimplantation window and should be done if possible.

### Technique

1. After proper anesthesia, suction clot from the socket and irrigate the socket with normal saline.

2. Cleanse the tooth gently with irrigation. Avoid scrubbing, which can traumatize the root surface.

3. Place the tooth gently into the socket, then fully seat the tooth with firm pressure.

4. Stabilization can be accomplished with a variety of techniques; two simple, noninvasive methods are described:

   • Commercially available periodontal packs composed of a putty-like substance can be formed around the affected tooth and the teeth on both sides. A resin and catalyst are mixed together to form a paste, which is kneaded to obtain the proper consistency. This is a temporary stabilization technique to be used only with timely dental consultation.

   • Heavy silk suture can be tied in a figure-8 pattern around the reimplanted tooth and adjacent tooth. The teeth are anchored together as the suture is tightened and knotted in place.

5. Advise the patient to avoid further trauma and chewy or hard foods to reduce the risk of loosening the reimplanted tooth.

6. Have the patient follow up with a dentist in 1 or 2 days.

## 5.9 Management of Penile Zipper Injury[26]

Young, uncircumcised boys, usually between the ages of 3 and 6 years, can entrap the foreskin in the zipper mechanism when attempting to zip their pants.

### Technique

1. Splitting the median bar of the zipper mechanism with a bone cutter (or wire cutter) can be accomplished without local or general anesthesia as long as the patient remains cooperative (Figure 21.29). If the clothing can be sacrificed, it is advantageous to cut off the bar at the bottom of the zipper and also cut the zipper away from the clothing.

# Section
# 5

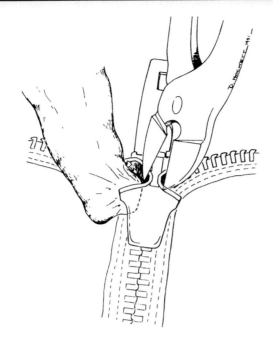

**Figure 21.29** Split median bar of zipper mechanism with wire cutter.

2. If proper cutting equipment is not available, it might be possible to pull the skin free from the zipper. Use a local anesthetic such as lidocaine, then allow liberally applied mineral oil to soak into the foreskin for 10 minutes or more.

3. If the foreskin is caught between the teeth of the zipper only and not in the zipping mechanism, then simply cut the zipper below the entrapment and pull apart the teeth.

4. If none of these strategies is successful, consultation with a urologist and circumcision might be needed, but this is rare.

# 5.10 Reduction of Inguinal Hernia[27]

Inguinal hernias incarcerate in 10% to 12% of cases. The successful reduction of an incar-cerated inguinal hernia allows elective rather than emergency herniorrhaphy. This reduces the complication rate of surgery, lessens the likelihood of bowel strangulation, and relieves the pain associated with incarceration.

**Technique**

1. Place the patient in a slight Trendelenburg position, externally rotating the hip and flexing the knee on the affected side.

2. Place the index and middle fingers of one hand over the hernial bulge in the inguinal canal. Grasp the apex of the hernia with the index and middle fingers of the other hand, providing slow, steady pressure.

If this procedure does not reduce the hernia quickly, consider parenteral sedation and analgesia, but only in the ED or if proper monitoring is available.

1. After sedation and analgesia, observe the patient in a slight Trendelenburg position for at least 20 minutes in a calm environment with a cool compress applied to the hernia sac.

2. If spontaneous reduction does not occur, reattempt manual reduction as described above. Slow, steady pressure is the key to success.

3. Timely elective surgical consultation for repair of an inguinal hernia is indicated after successful reduction. Inguinal hernia incarceration is likely to recur.

4. Avoid forceful repeated attempts to reduce an incarcerated inguinal hernia. Emergency surgery is indicated if manual attempts are unsuccessful.

# 5.11 Reduction of Paraphimosis[27]

A paraphimosis occurs when a phimotic foreskin is retracted proximal to the glans penis and subsequent venous congestion edema prevents repositioning of the foreskin back to its normal position. Paraphimosis is a true urologic emergency that requires rapid reduction to reduce the risk of arterial compromise and necrosis. Immediate reduction also prevents further swelling and pain.

## Technique

Manual Reduction

1. Consider systemic analgesia.

2. Apply topical anesthetic lubricant to the glans penis and inside of the foreskin. Do not apply to the penile shaft: this will make it more difficult to grasp the skin of the penile shaft.

3. If markedly swollen, consider the use of an ice slurry to reduce edema before attempting manual reduction. Fill an examination glove with crushed ice and water to create an ice slurry. Slide the penis into the thumb portion of the glove, holding it in place with gentle compression for 5 to 10 minutes.

4. Identify the location of the phimotic ring.

5. Stabilize the skin of the penile shaft proximal to the phimotic ring by compressing between the index and middle fingers of both hands.

6. Place the thumbs of both hands against the urethral opening using slow, steady, firm pressure to "push" the glans penis through the phimotic ring.

## Phimotic Ring Incision

Consult with a urologist if possible. Use this procedure only when manual reduction is not possible.

1. Using sterile procedure, cleanse the penis and infiltrate locally with 1% lidocaine on and around the dorsal aspect of the phimotic ring.

2. Consider systemic analgesia.

3. Incise perpendicular to the phimotic ring, being careful to avoid injury to the penile shaft.

4. The constricting ring will spring open once it is completely incised.

5. Reduce foreskin back to its normal position.

## 5.12 Reduction of Rectal Prolapse[27]

Partial rectal prolapse is the abnormal protrusion of rectal mucosa and submucosa through the anus. This is most common in the toddler age group and is not usually associated with underlying pathology. Straining with stool and excessive spreading of the gluteal folds (often caused by the use of an adult-sized toilet by a small child) are the most likely culprits. Complete rectal prolapse, or protrusion of the entire rectal wall through the rectum, is more common in older children and is associated with diseases such as cystic fibrosis, rectal polyps, and ascites. There is no contraindication to the procedure, and rectal prolapse should be reduced as soon as possible to avoid rare complications of bleeding, ulceration, and ischemia.

## Technique

1. Adequately relax and/or sedate the child.

2. Place the child in the knee-chest position on the examination table or prone over the parent's lap.

3. Stabilize the position of the buttocks using the nondominant hand.

4. Wrap a gloved index finger of the dominant hand with several layers of toilet tissue.

5. Insert the wrapped index finger into the lumen of the prolapsed rectal tissue, exerting constant, firm pressure while pushing it into the anal orifice.

6. The dry toilet tissue will attach to the rectal mucosa, allowing the index finger pressure to reduce the prolapsed segment. The prolapsed segment can be additionally guided using the fingers of the nondominant hand.

**Section**

**5**

5.12 Reduction of
Rectal Prolapse

7. Once the prolapse has been reduced, remove the gloved index finger and leave the toilet tissue inside the rectum to be passed with the next bowel movement.

8. Refer for followup care to be sure that underlying pathology is sought and the primary causes are addressed. Changes such as using a child-sized toilet seat or stool softeners might be necessary.

## THE BOTTOM LINE

- Preparation of an office for handling pediatric emergencies need not be time-consuming or expensive.

- Proper matching of staff training, supplies, and equipment with the number and type of emergencies anticipated will lead to improved staff confidence and allow the office facility to meet reasonable emergency care needs.

- Attainment of skills to handle minor trauma and the occasional critically ill or injured child will enhance patient care and provide optimal outcome.

# Check Your Knowledge

1. Which of the following statements regarding a paronychia is correct?
   A. Can be treated in the physician's office or ED
   B. Deep space infection of the hands and feet
   C. Usually painless
   D. Usually requires removal of the nail on the affected digit

2. Which of the following statements regarding paraphimosis is correct?
   A. Associated with a phimotic ring of the foreskin
   B. Painless
   C. Can be reduced electively
   D. Should be reduced only by a urologist
   E. Usually seen as part of a febrile illness

3. All of the following are examples of appropriate management of an avulsed permanent tooth except:
   A. Avoiding further trauma after reimplantation
   B. Handling the tooth by the root surface
   C. Reimplanting the tooth as soon as possible
   D. Stabilizing the tooth using a periodontal pack or sutures, if possible

4. Correct application of tissue adhesive includes which of the following?
   A. Complete hemostasis
   B. Debridement of foreign bodies or materials
   C. Immobilization
   D. Thorough wound cleansing and irrigation
   E. All of the above

# References

1. Fuchs S, Jaffe D, Christoffel KK. Pediatric emergencies in office practices: prevalence and office preparedness. *Pediatrics.* 1989;83:931–939.

2. Flores, G, Weinstock DJ. The preparedness of pediatricians for emergencies in the office: what is broken, should we care, and how can we fix it?. *Archives of Pediat Adol Med.* 1996;150;249–256.

3. Schmitt BD. *Pediatric Telephone Protocols, Office Version.* Elk Grove Village, Il: American Academy of Pediatrics; 2002.

4. Frush K, Cinoman M. *Office Preparedness for Pediatric Emergencies;Provider Manual.* North Carolina Emergency Medical Services for Children, 1999. Available at: www.ems-c.org: Products #0797 and #0614.

5. Walsh-Kelly CM, Melzer-Lange M. *Office Preparedness for Pediatric Emergencies.* Poster presentation at: National Congress for Childhood Emergencies: April 17, 2002; Dallas, Tx.

6. Emergency 10 Steps. Available at: www. ems-c.org/downloads/htm/Emerge10.htm. Accessed December 4, 2002.

7. Schutzman SA, Greenes DS. Pediatric minor head trauma. *Ann Emerg Med.* 2001;37(1):65–74.

8. Quayle KS. Minor head injury in the pediatric patient. *Pediatr Clin North Am.* 1999;46: 1189–1199.

9. Committee on Quality Improvement, American Academy of Pediatrics. The management of minor closed head injury in children. *Pediatrics* 1999;104:1407–1415.

10. Dietrich AM, Bowman MJ, Ginn-Pease ME et al. Pediatric head injuries: can clinical factors reliably predict an abnormality on computed tomography? *Ann Emerg Med.* 1993;22:1535–1540.

11. Mitchell KA, Fallat ME, Raque GH et al. Evaluation of minor head injury in children. *J Pediatr Surg.* 1994;29:851–854.

12. Schunk JE, Rodgerson JD, Woodward GA. The utility of head computed tomographic scanning in pediatric patients with normal neurologic examination in the emergency department. *Pediatr Emerg Care.* 1996;12:160–165.

13. Davis RL, Hughes M, Gubler KD et al. The use of cranial CT scans in the triage of pediatric patients with mild head injury. *Pediatrics.* 1995;95:345–349.

14. Gausche M. Genitourinary trauma. In: Barkin RM, ed. *Pediatric Emergency Medicine: Concepts and Clinical Practice.* 2nd ed.. St Louis, Mo: Mosby; 1997:355–370.

15. Schilling CG, Bank DE, Borchert BA et al. Tetracaine, epinephrine (adrenaline), and cocaine (TAC) versus lidocaine, epinephrine, and tetracaine (LET) for anesthesia of lacerations in children. *Ann Emerg Med.* 1995;25:203–208.

# CHAPTER REVIEW

16. Cristoph RA, Buchanan L, Begalia K et al. Pain reduction in local anesthetic administration through pH buffering. *Ann Emerg Med.* 1988;17: 117–120.

17. Khan AN, Dayan PS, Miller S, Rosen M, Rubin D. Cosmetic Outcome of scalp wound closure with staples in the pediatric emergency department: a prospective, randomized trial. *Pediatr Emerg Care.* 2002;18:171–173.

18. Precise™ Disposable Skin Stapler [instructional brochure]. 3M Health Care.

19. Dermabond Topical Skin Adhesive [instructional brochure]. Ethicon: 2001.

20. Yamamoto LG. Preventing adverse events and outcomes encountered using dermabond [letter]. *Am J Emerg Med.* 2000;18(4):511–515.

21. Quinn JV, Drzewiecki A, Li MM et al. A randomized, controlled trial comparing a tissue adhesive with suturing in the repair of pediatric facial lacerations. *Ann Emerg Med.* 1993;22:1130–1135.

22. Ros SP, Cetta F. Successful use of a metal detector in locating coins ingested by children. *J Pediatr.* 1992;120:752–3.

23. Santamaria JP, Abrunzo TJ. Ear, nose, and throat disorders. In: Barkin RM, ed. *Pediatric Emergency Medicine: Concepts and Clinical Practice.* 2nd ed. St. Louis, Mo: Mosby-Year Book Inc; 1997:709–754.

24. O'Neill JA. Burns in children. In: Artz CP, Moncrief JA, Pruitt BA, eds. *Burns: A Team Approach.* Philadelphia, Pa: WB Saunders; 1979:341–350.

25. Coren CV. Burn injuries in children. *Pediatr Ann.* 1987;16:328–332.

26. Gausche M, Seidel J. Releasing penile foreskin trapped in a zipper. *Pediatr Rev.* 1993;14:140.

27. Gausche M. Genitourinary surgical emergencies. *Pediatr Ann.* 1996;25:458–464.

# chapter 22

# Critical Procedures

Brent R. King, MD, FAAP, FACEP, FAAEM
Christopher King, MD, FACEP
Wendy C. Coates, MD, FACEP

## Objectives

1 Demonstrate the maneuvers required for basic management of ill and injured children, including oxygen administration, monitoring, and basic airway maneuvers.

2 Demonstrate orotracheal intubation using a manikin model.

3 Demonstrate placement of an intraosseous needle in a manikin or other model and describe the landmarks for intraosseous needle placement in a child.

4 Describe the indications and technique for needle thoracostomy.

5 Describe indications and technique for pericardiocentesis.

## Chapter Outline

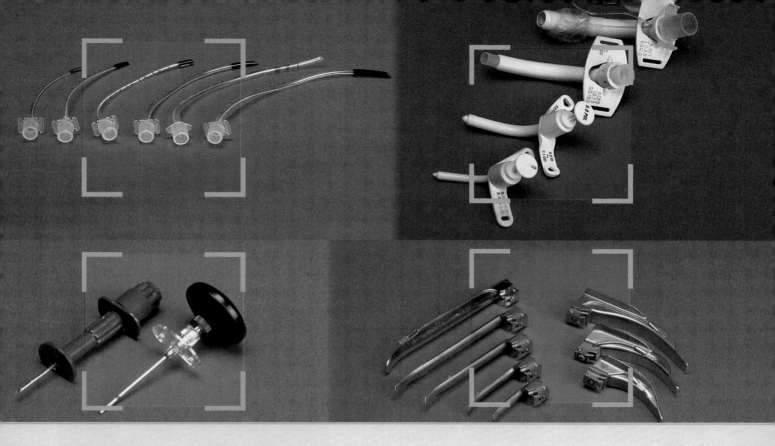

## Introduction

Competence in emergency care is, in part, based on the physician's ability to perform potentially lifesaving procedures. In many cases, performance of the procedure takes precedence over other aspects of treatment. When a child presents in impending respiratory failure or in the early phases of shock, urgent therapy is warranted even in the absence of a specific diagnosis. This chapter addresses the performance of several key emergency procedures. The individual practitioner must determine the extent to which each of these procedures is likely to be required in his or her practice, but all physicians who care for children with serious illnesses and/or injuries must possess, in addition to cognitive skills, the requisite procedural skills. All procedures should be done with universal precautions.

---

# Section 1  Pediatric Length-Based Resuscitation Tape

## Section 1

### 1.1 Pediatric Length-Based Resuscitation Tape

1.1 Pediatric Length-Based Resuscitation Tape

Length-based resuscitation tape permits the rapid determination of size-dependent resuscitation parameters such as drug doses, endotracheal tube (ETT) sizes, mask sizes, vital signs, and so on. This potentially speeds resuscitation efforts and reduces the likelihood of a medical error. The tape is placed at one end of the patient, and the other end of the patient aligns with a color-coded block corresponding to the patient's length-based resuscitation parameters. There might be two sets of blocks, one of which corresponds to tube sizes, vital signs, and so on, while the other indicates drug dosing. Some length-based resuscitation systems will have corresponding color-coded bags or carts that contain the actual resuscitation devices (e.g., tracheal tubes and laryngoscope) and drugs (precalculated unit doses).

### Technique

1. Align the end of the tape to the patient. Alternatively, if the tape is secured to the gurney, adjust the patient's position to

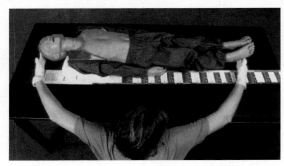

**Figure 22.1** Correct technique for use of the length-based resuscitation tape.

align with the red end of the tape.

2. Identify the inferior end of the patient using the heels, not the toes (**Figure 22.1**).

3. If the child is larger than the tape (>36 kg), proceed as in the case of an adult.

4. Verbalize the color or letter block (on the edge of the tape) and the weight estimate determined by the tape so that this information can be recorded.

5. Use the appropriate color or letter block to identify appropriate drug doses and equipment sizes (**Figure 22.2**).

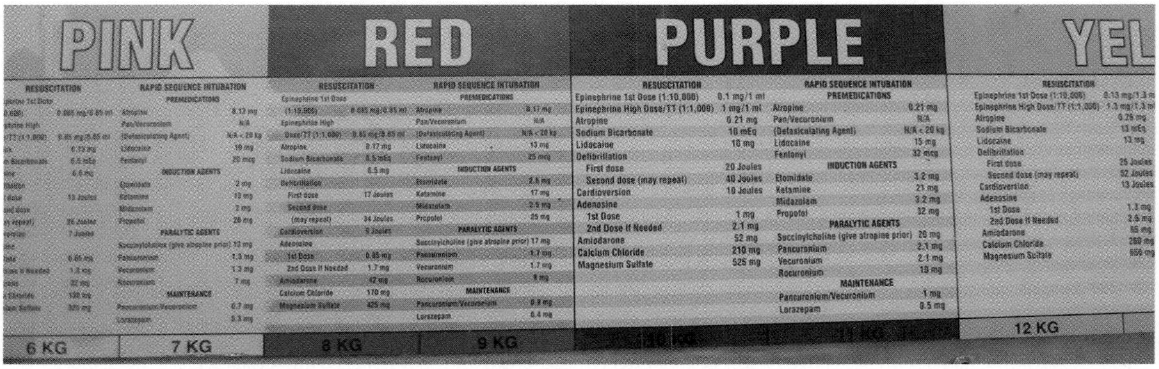

**Figure 22.2** The length-based resuscitation tape.

## Section 2  Cervical Spine Stabilization

### 2.1 Cervical Spine Stabilization

#### Indications

Although cervical spine injuries are relatively rare in children, victims of significant blunt trauma (e.g., falls from heights, auto/pedestrian accidents, moderate to severe motor vehicle crashes, diving injuries) and those who sustain direct injury to the neck (blunt or penetrating) are at risk, and the cervical spine should be protected prior to complete evaluation. Likewise, children and adolescents with symptoms of cervical cord dysfunction after trauma (e.g., numbness and/or tingling or weakness in an extremity) should be appropriately stabilized pending further evaluation, even if the symptoms are transient. Finally, patients who have significant alterations in mental status and who might have been injured should also be stabilized until they can be thoroughly evaluated.

#### Equipment

- Appropriately sized rigid cervical collar (**Figure 22.3**)
- Long spine stabilization board
- Lateral spacing blocks or similar devices*
- Straps or tape*

Required for Infants and Young Children:

- Specially designed long spine stabilization board with cutout or indentation to accommodate the occiput,* or
- Pad placed on the spine board and extending from the child's shoulders to his or her feet*

#### Technique

1. Ensure that adequate personnel are available to assist.
2. Stabilize the patient's head in place by holding the head and keeping the neck in a neutral position (**Figure 22.4A**).
3. Determine the proper size for the cervical

*This equipment can be obtained as part of a kit specially designed for this purpose.

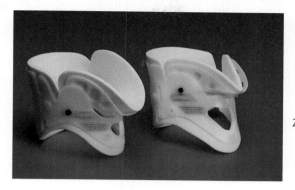

**Figure 22.3**  Rigid cervical collars in pediatric sizes.

collar. The ideally sized collar extends from the top of the shoulders to the bottom of the chin, leaving the neck in neutral position. A collar that is too tall hyperextends the neck, while one that is too short allows for unwanted neck flexion. Both hyperextension and flexion can be disastrous in the face of a cervical spine injury and, therefore, should be avoided.

4. Some cervical collars require assembly prior to use. If necessary, assemble the collar.
5. Open the cervical collar and carefully slide the rear portion behind the neck while an assistant maintains inline stabilization of the patient's head and neck.
6. Bring the front of the collar into position and then attach the front and back portions together using the adhesive straps. The collar should fit snugly but not constrict the airway or restrict blood flow to the skin (**Figure 22.4B**).
7. Ensure that the head remains in neutral position.
8. Secure the patient to a long spine board. If the patient is seated, a short spine board or extrication vest should be secured to the patient to stabilize the head and trunk as a unit. Then place a long spine board beside the patient and, keeping the knees and hips bent, pivot and lower the patient onto the long board. Lower the knees to the board. If

# Section
# 2

2.1 Cervical Spine
Stabilization

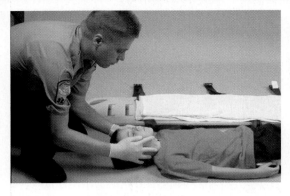

**Figure 22.4A** Align the head and neck in a neutral cervical spine position.

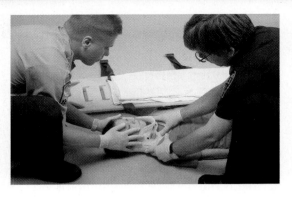

**Figure 22.4B** Apply a size-appropriate rigid cervical collar.

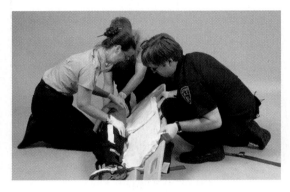

**Figure 22.4C** Transfer the patient as a unit onto a spine board or other stabilization device long enough to support the patient's full length.

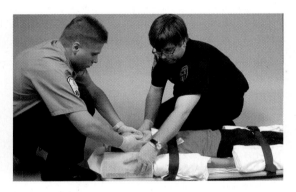

**Figure 22.4D** Stabilize the cervical spine by using blanket rolls or blocks from a cervical stabilization device to block lateral head motion and rotation, and to prevent upward motion of the shoulder.

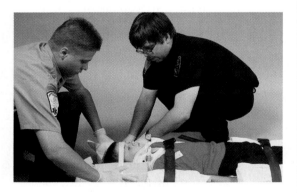

**Figure 22.4E** Secure the head by using tape directly above the patient's eyebrows.

the patient is supine, log-roll the patient onto his or her side, maintaining inline stabilization of the neck. Place the long board on edge behind the patient and roll the patient and the board as a unit back into a supine position (**Figure 22.4C**).

9. Secure the patient to the spine board.

Place soft lateral spacing devices on either side of the patient's head. Heavy objects such as sandbags should be avoided because they can place undue lateral pressure on the spine if the board is inadvertently tilted (**Figure 22.4D**).

10. Using tape or commercial straps, first secure the forehead, then the chin, shoulders, and pelvis to the board (**Figure 22.4E**).

11. Examine the patient to ensure that the stabilization is complete and effective but is not causing neurovascular compromise, and to ensure that neurologic injury has not occurred during stabilization.

For infants and young children, the technique must be modified slightly because children of this age have relatively large occiputs. This can cause the child's neck to be flexed when he or she is placed in a supine position on a flat surface. This problem can be corrected in two ways. Special spine boards designed with indentations or cut-outs to accommodate the head can be used. Alternatively, a pad can be placed over the spine board before the patient is secured to it. The child should then be placed on the board such that his or her shoulders and body are on the pad but the head and neck are not. Elevation of the torso allows the neck to remain in a neutral position. Some recommend that stable, very young infants be stabilized in a car seat (**Figure 22.5**).

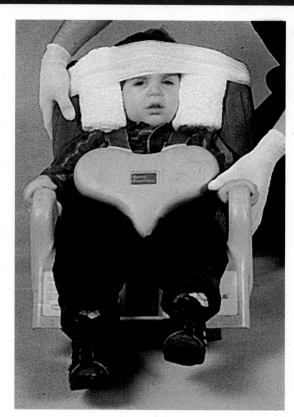

**Figure 22.5** Very young, clinically stable infants can be stabilized in a car seat.

> ### KEY POINTS
>
> **Performing Spinal Stabilization**
> - Clinical cervical spine clearance (without radiographs) in selected patients at low risk.
> - Maintain cervical spine stabilization in nonawake patients.
> - Ensure proper cervical spine stabilization position for children to avoid flexion.
> - Avoid heavy sandbags.

## Complications and Pitfalls

The major risk associated with cervical spine stabilization is accidental injury to the spinal cord. Excessive movement of the patient's neck must be avoided because such movement might convert a stable cervical spine fracture not involving the spinal cord into a cord injury with neurologic deficits. Therefore, stabilization should be performed carefully, avoiding unnecessary movements. Adequate assistance is mandatory to ensure that the uncooperative patient does not harm himself or herself. This technique requires teamwork and should not be undertaken by one person if at all possible. In some cases, attempted stabi-

lization of struggling patients might place them at risk of injury. In such cases, patients can be evaluated without formal stabilization provided that they can remain calm and cooperative during the evaluation. The reasons for the decision not to stabilize should be documented.

Spinal stabilization is an all-or-none procedure. All personnel must understand that a cervical collar alone is not adequate protection, as it allows a significant amount of neck extension and rotation and does not completely eliminate flexion. The straps and lateral supports are an integral part of the system. Effective lateral supports, also called lateral spacing devices, can be made of many materials, including cardboard, foam, or air-filled bladders. Heavy objects, such as sandbags, should not be used because they can put pressure on the lateral side of the neck when the spine board is tilted to one side. Tilting of the

# Section 2

2.1 Cervical Spine Stabilization

board can occur accidentally during movement or deliberately in the transport of a pregnant adolescent or to allow the patient to vomit without aspirating.

Stabilization can compromise circulation or the airway. These must be assessed after the patient is stabilized and at frequent intervals thereafter. The stabilized patient with significant nausea and vomiting can aspirate, and treatment with antiemetics and/or nasogastric suction might be necessary. Personnel should carefully log-roll the patient to one side (preferably the left side) to allow him or her to vomit, if necessary. Adolescent females in the latter stages of pregnancy might require transport with the board tilted to the left side to reduce pressure on the inferior vena cava. Stabilization can also make it more difficult to assess other injuries, particularly head and neck injuries. In these cases it is acceptable to remove the restraint devices in order to examine the patient while assistants maintain inline stabilization.

Finally, it is important that the clinician understand when stabilization can be discontinued. In some cases, cervical restraints can be removed after a clinical examination of the neck. Several studies have demonstrated that patients who do not have neurologic deficits, lack midline cervical spine tenderness, and are able to voluntarily move their necks without experiencing significant pain are unlikely to have sustained a fracture of the cervical spine, provided that the patient has a normal level of consciousness, does not have a second injury causing significant pain (e.g., a long bone fracture), and is not intoxicated.[2,3] Although the mechanism of injury is not a part of these rules, experience suggests that well-restrained patients involved in low-speed motor vehicle crashes are at even lower risk of cervical spine injury. These rules may be cautiously applied to pediatric patients; however, few very young children have been studied, and more conservative evaluation of these patients is recommended.

Unfortunately, the standard 3-view series of radiographs of the cervical spine is only 93%

to 95% sensitive for the presence of a cervical spine fracture. Conscious patients should undergo a thorough examination of the cervical spine after radiographs have demonstrated no fractures. Unconscious patients with normal cervical spine radiographs should remain stabilized unless stabilization is compromising clinical care or causing injury. Likewise, children with neurologic symptoms should remain stabilized even if their radiographs are normal. Initially, it can be difficult or impossible to distinguish patients with occult cervical spine fractures from those who have spinal cord injury without radiographic abnormality (SCIWORA).[4]

Children placed on standard spine boards will likely have their necks in moderate flexion. Lateral cervical spine radiographs taken in this position frequently show C2-3 pseudosubluxation (Figure 22.6A, B). This malalignment can be difficult to distinguish from a true subluxation or fracture injury. Absence of prevertebral soft tissue widening, a history of relatively benign trauma, lack of neck pain in an awake patient without other distracting injuries, and alignment of the anterior cortical margins of the spinous processes of C1, C2, and C3 all suggest (but do not guarantee) that this is a pseudosubluxation and not a true subluxation. It would be preferable to stabilize children properly to avoid cervical spine flexion, which reduces the risk of spinal cord injury and the artifact pseudosubluxation on initial lateral cervical spine radiographs.

## THE BOTTOM LINE

- Optimal cervical spine stabilization requires special positioning for children.
- Children are at lower risk for cervical spine fracture and spinal cord injury compared to adults, but this does not permit clinicians to ignore this risk.

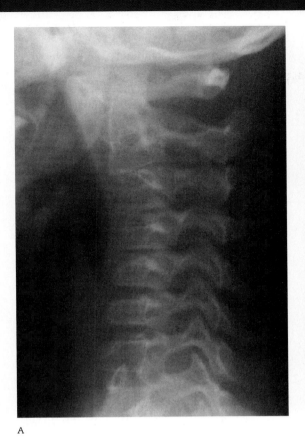

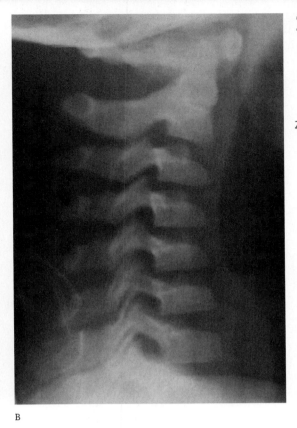

A

B

**Figure 22.6A, B** Two examples of C2-3 pseudosubluxation. Note that the neck is flexed forward.

## Section 3  Monitoring

Monitoring of physiologic parameters is an essential component of modern emergency care. Advances in technology have made it possible to measure several key physiologic indicators in a noninvasive manner. There are seven essential monitoring devices in current use. These are electrocardiographic monitoring (ECG), impedance pneumographic monitoring, blood pressure monitoring, pulse oximetry, exhaled $CO_2$ detection, temperature, and the stethoscope.

Measurement of temperature and auscultation are commonly used by most health care professionals; these techniques will not be described in this chapter.

### 3.1 ECG Monitoring

ECG monitors detect and display the electrical activity produced by the cardiac conducting system. This monitor allows emergency personnel to detect changes in cardiac rhythm. Because these devices measure the difference in electrical potential between two electrodes, several electrodes are required. The standard monitor has three sensing leads. The two upper leads are intended to be placed on the left and right arms, respectively, but in practice are usually placed on the left and right sides of the upper torso. Likewise, the lower left lead is intended for placement on the left leg but might be placed on the lower left side of the abdomen. Some monitors have a fourth lead for the right lower extremity, which is placed on the right leg or on the right side of the lower abdomen. In many cases, the electrodes are labeled so that they can be properly placed. In other cases, they are color-coded. Proper lead placement is important, and each provider should learn the configuration used in his or her institution (**Figure 22.7**).[5,6]

### Equipment

- ECG monitor
- Electrodes
- Alcohol pads

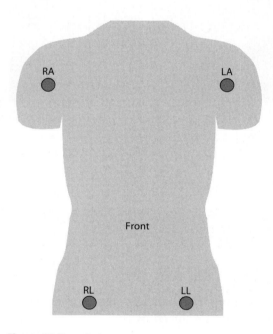

Figure 22.7 Lead placement.

### Technique

1. Ensure that the monitor is functioning properly and that the electrode pads are not damaged. New electrode pads must be used for each patient to prevent the spread of infection and to ensure that the adhesive substance can make adequate contact with the patient's skin.
2. Select the sites for electrode placement and cleanse the patient's skin with alcohol to improve contact.
3. Allow the alcohol to dry and then attach the electrodes.
4. Turn on the monitor.
5. Most monitors have different lead configurations (using different pairs of leads), which will give a different waveform. Select one. Often lead II is selected (**Figure 22.8**).
6. Set the monitor alarms.

### Complications and Pitfalls

ECG monitoring is generally safe. There are, however, a few complications that should be noted. On some monitors, the alarms must be activated before they will function. Failure to activate these alarms can result in a serious dysrhythmia going unrecognized. It is also vital that the staff correctly interpret the data received from the monitor. Apparent dysrhythmias should be checked in a second lead configuration, and the staff must ensure that the electrodes are properly positioned and that the problem is not related to patient movement.

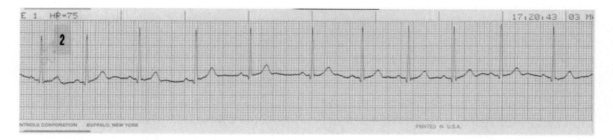

Figure 22.8 Lead II.

## 3.2 Impedance Pneumatography

The impedance pneumatograph uses the ECG electrodes to measure the motion of the chest wall as a surrogate marker for respiratory effort, which is displayed as a waveform (or square waveform) on the monitor.[6]

### Equipment and Technique

Uses the same leads as the ECG monitor.

### Complications and Pitfalls

Like ECG monitoring, impedance pneumatography is subject to artifact caused by patient movement and lead placement problems. However, the most important potential pitfall in the use of impedance pneumatography lies in the understanding that it is measuring chest wall movement, not air flow. Intermittent auscultation is required to ensure that the ventilation is indeed adequate.

## 3.3 Blood Pressure Monitors

Most health care providers were taught to measure blood pressure by auscultation. The modern oscillometric methods used by monitoring devices replace the sound of blood flowing with a measurement of the oscillations in the arterial wall.[6,7]

### Equipment

- Properly sized blood pressure cuff
- The appropriately sized cuff should cover approximately two thirds of the upper arm length and should completely encircle the arm. It should fit snugly but not constrict the arm, as this can affect the result. If in doubt, select a larger cuff rather than a smaller one.
- Blood pressure monitoring device

### Technique

1. Place the cuff on the patient's upper arm (or thigh).
2. Attach the cuff to the monitoring device.

3. Set the frequency of measurement and set the alarms.

### Complications and Pitfalls

Like all monitors, blood pressure monitors are affected by patient movement. Likewise, improperly sized cuffs and air leaks can affect the accuracy of the result. A key issue in the measurement of blood pressure is the understanding that the presence of shock is not determined or ruled out by any specific blood pressure value. This is particularly true in early (compensated) shock. A patient with a normal or near normal blood pressure can exhibit shock physiology.

## 3.4 Pulse Oximetry

The pulse oximeter uses two different wavelengths of light to transcutaneously measure the degree to which the patient's hemoglobin molecules are bound to oxygen. The result is expressed as the percentage of oxygen-saturated hemoglobin. Normally, 97% to 100% of available binding sites are saturated. In hypoxemic states, when the $PaO_2$ is less than 70 mm Hg, the pulse oximeter will display an oxygen saturation value of 90% or less.[8,9]

There are many types of pulse oximeters available. Technological advances have made these devices quite small and portable.

### Equipment

- Pulse oximeter
- Pulse oximeter probe
- Alcohol pads

### Technique

1. Choose a location for the placement of the pulse oximeter probe. The site must allow the light waves to pass through the skin to the receiver probe (Figure 22.9). Fingers, toes, and ear lobes are often used for this purpose. In infants and very young children, the side of the hand or foot can be used.
2. Clean the skin at the site if necessary.

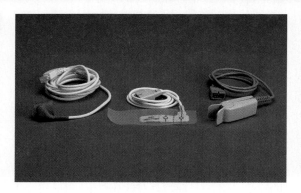
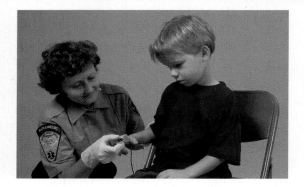

**Figure 22.9** Various pulse oximeter probes wrap around or clip onto a digit or earlobe.

3. Apply the probe, making certain that the transmitting and receiving portions are well aligned.

4. Connect the probe to the monitor and confirm that the heart rate measured by the device correlates with the patient's actual heart rate.

## Complications and Pitfalls

Like all monitoring devices, the pulse oximeter is subject to erroneous readings caused by patient movement. Likewise, the sending and receiving sections of the probe must be relatively well aligned for the device to function effectively. There are rare case reports of falsely elevated pulse oximeter readings caused by ambient light. It is, therefore, important to ensure that the receiving section of the probe is not exposed.

Pulse oximetry is based on the light absorption characteristics of hemoglobin A (i.e., normal adult hemoglobin). It is inaccurate in the presence of carboxyhemoglobin and methemoglobin. It is fairly accurate for fetal hemoglobin and most other hemoglobinopathies.

Pulse oximetry can be falsely elevated by the presence of carboxyhemoglobin (i.e., the pulse oximeter reads 100% when the true oxygen saturation is lower). When carbon monoxide poisoning is suspected, a blood sample for co-oximetry or a carboxyhemoglobin level should be sent. An arterial or venous blood gas measurement will similarly be misleading because it will show a high $PO_2$ and high cal-

culated oxygen saturation, although it might correctly demonstrate a metabolic acidosis. Most blood gas analyzers do not automatically run co-oximetry, which uses four wavelengths (as opposed to only two wavelengths for pulse oximetry) that can accurately detect carboxyhemoglobin presence. A blood gas without the co-oximetry component will have falsely elevated oxygen saturation because it is calculated based on the $PO_2$ and not actually measured. Thus, it is the co-oximetry portion that correctly identifies the presence of carboxyhemoglobin and not the blood gas measurement.

Methemoglobinemia presents a similar but less misleading phenomenon. The accuracy of the pulse oximeter is directly related to the amount of methemoglobin. When more than 30% of the patient's hemoglobin exists as methemoglobin, the oximeter will display an oxygen saturation of approximately 85%. Lesser degrees of methemoglobinemia are associated with higher displayed oxygen saturations. The displayed oxygen saturation might be in the low normal range (e.g., 93% to 95%). The oxygen saturation displayed by the pulse oximeter does not accurately reflect the degree of methemoglobinemia. An arterial blood gas analysis will reveal a high $PO_2$ (especially if the patient is on supplemental oxygen), and the calculated oxygen saturation will be falsely high (usually 100%, despite the lower oxygen saturation measured by pulse oximetry, which is a discrepancy that should lead to this diagnosis). Additionally, the patient's blood will appear to be chocolate brown in color (if

| TABLE 22-1 | Oximetry Measurement Method Differences in Patients With Carbon Monoxide Poisoning and Methemoglobinemia | | | **Section**<br>**3** |
|---|---|---|---|---|
| | Normal Hemoglobin | Carboxyhemoglobin 20% | Methemoglobin 20% | |
| **Room Air (normal lungs)** | | | | |
| pH (ABG) | 7.4 | <7.4 | <7.4 | |
| $PO_2$ (ABG) | 100 mm Hg | 100 mm Hg | 100 mm Hg | |
| Calculated $O_2$sat (ABG) | 99% | 99% | 99% | |
| Color of blood (ABG) | Red | Red | Brown | |
| Pulse oximetry $O_2$sat | 99% | 100% | 90% | |
| Co-oximetry $O_2$sat | 99% | 80% | 80% | |
| Clinical color | Pink | Pink | Dusky/gray | |
| **Supplemental Oxygen 50% $F_{IO_2}$ (normal lungs)** | | | | |
| pH (ABG) | 7.4 | <7.4 | <7.4 | |
| $PO_2$ (ABG) | 350 mm Hg | 350 mm Hg | 350 mm Hg | |
| Calculated $O_2$sat (ABG) | 100% | 100% | 100% | |
| Color of blood (ABG) | Red | Red | Brown | |
| Pulse oximetry $O_2$sat | 100% | 100% | 90% | |
| Co-oximetry $O_2$sat | 100% | 80% | 80% | |
| Clinical color | Pink | Pink/red | Dusky/gray | |

the methemoglobin percentage is high enough), and the patient will appear to be dusky or pale (often described as ashen gray). In other instances where there is doubt as to the accuracy of the pulse oximeter reading, co-oximetry should be obtained.

Note that methemoglobinemia pulse oximetry measurements are low, but they should be lower. This is less misleading than in carbon monoxide poisoning, where the pulse oximetry measurements are usually 99% to 100%. Additionally, while methemoglobinemia patients are dusky, pale, or grayish, carbon monoxide-poisoned patients are pink and can appear to be well oxygenated. Table 22-1 describes the pulse oximetry, arterial blood gas, and co-oximetry differences between normal hemoglobin, carboxyhemoglobin, and methemoglobin.

The pulse oximeter does not measure the patient's hemoglobin concentration, so the patient's oxygen-carrying capacity cannot be fully assessed. A patient with an oxygen saturation of 95% and hemoglobin of 6 mg/dL has a lower oxygen content than a patient with an oxygen saturation of 90% and a hemoglobin of 14 mg/dL.

Finally, the pulse oximeter gives no information regarding the $P_{aCO_2}$ and, therefore, no information about the adequacy of ventilation. It is possible for a child receiving supplemental oxygen to be well oxygenated and yet be hypoventilating.

## 3.5 Exhaled $CO_2$ Monitors

Capnometry devices measure and, in some cases, quantify the exhaled $CO_2$.[10,11]

Following endotracheal intubation, capnography is used to confirm that the tube is located in the trachea; later it is used to ensure the tube remains properly located. $CO_2$ detectors are small plastic devices that are inserted into the ventilation circuit closest to the endotracheal tube (ETT) (Figure 22.10). These devices change color as $CO_2$ flows through the device. The color change visible with each respiration indicates the presence of $CO_2$, confirming endotracheal intubation. End-tidal $CO_2$ ($ETCO_2$) monitors quantify the degree of

# Section 3

3.5 Exhaled CO$_2$ Monitors

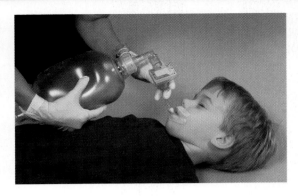

**Figure 22.10** Using the CO$_2$ detector.

exhaled CO$_2$. A sensor is inserted into the ventilation circuit closest to the ETT. The sensor is then connected by wires to an ETCO$_2$ monitor to follow or track ventilation (gas exchange) because the ETCO$_2$ measurement (numeric display on the monitor) usually approximates the arterial P$_{CO_2}$ (except in instances described below). An arterial blood gas analysis should be done to confirm the accuracy of the ETCO$_2$ measurement.

## Complications and Pitfalls

The following conditions can result in capnometry measurements that are lower than the arterial P$_{CO_2}$. This occurs because capnometry requires the CO$_2$ to be exhaled for the device to detect or measure it. In conditions of reduced pulmonary blood flow or poor air exchange, exhaled P$_{CO_2}$ will be lower than the arterial P$_{CO_2}$. For example:

- Low cardiac output, severe hypotension, cardiac arrest (false readings)
- Severe airway obstruction (increases dead space)
- Severe parenchymal lung disease (increases dead space)

## KEY POINTS

**Use of Monitoring Devices in the ED**

- Know limitations of monitoring devices.
- Carbon monoxide poisoning and methemoglobinemia can result in false pulse oximetry readings.
- Presence of end-tidal CO$_2$ indicates endotracheal intubation.
- Lack of end-tidal CO$_2$ suggests esophageal intubation unless pulmonary circulation is poor, in which case it is still possible that the trachea is intubated (requires confirmation by another method such as direct visualization).

## THE BOTTOM LINE

All monitoring devices can provide misleading information under certain conditions.

---

# Section 4   Oxygen Administration

# Section 4

4.1 Nasal Cannula

Supplemental oxygen is indicated for the treatment of documented hypoxemia. Although oxygen is used liberally for other indications, there is scant evidence to support this practice. There are, however, several oxygen delivery devices, and each has its own indications and limitations.

## Equipment

- Oxygen source (e.g., hospital gas system, oxygen cylinder)
- Oxygen delivery device (e.g., nasal cannula, mask, oxygen hood)

## 4.1 Nasal Cannula

This simple device consists of soft rubber tubing fitted with two small prongs, or nipples, intended to direct oxygen into the patient's nares, or at least enrich the oxygen concentration around the nares (Figure 22.11). These devices are available in a variety of sizes and have the advantage of being better tolerated than face masks. They have several disadvantages. Obviously, they are less useful in children with nasal obstruction. Likewise, less oxygen is delivered in the child who is crying excessively

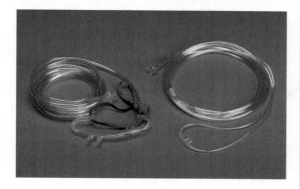

Figure 22.11 Infant and pediatric nasal cannulas.

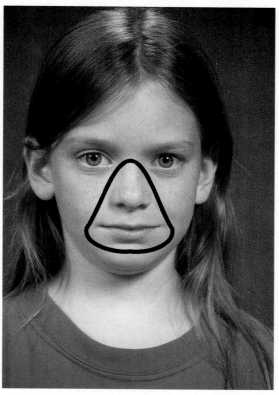

Figure 22.12 A proper size mask extends from the bridge of the nose to the cleft of the chin.

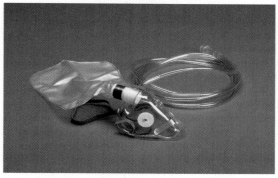

Figure 22.13 Pediatric nonrebreathing mask.

or mouth breathing. Finally, oxygen flow rates higher than 2 to 4 L/min are uncomfortable and might be poorly tolerated. Some children will have oxygen requirements that cannot be met by nasal cannula.

### Technique

1. Choose the correct size for the patient.
2. Insert the nasal prongs into the anterior nares.
3. Drape the tubing behind the ears.
4. Consider securing the tubing to the patient's face with tape.
5. Connect the distal end of the tubing to the oxygen source.
6. Monitor the patient's oxygen saturation.

## 4.2 Oxygen Mask

Oxygen masks are clear plastic masks that fit over the mouth and nose (**Figure 22.12**). They provide more oxygen than a nasal cannula because they create a more closed system. With oxygen flow rates of 6 or more L/min, the patient will receive 30% to 60% $FIO_2$. These masks have exhalation ports and, depending on how well the mask fits, there might be spaces along the sides of the mask. These areas allow the patient to "entrain" room air with each breath and, therefore, dilute the inspired oxygen. Face masks are poorly tolerated by some children.

## 4.3 Nonrebreathing Masks

When a child requires an even higher concentration of oxygen, this can often be provided by a nonrebreathing mask (**Figure 22.13**). These devices are simple face masks with two important modifications. First, the exhalation ports have one-way valves so that the patient cannot inhale room air through them. Second, and most important, the mask is equipped with a reservoir bag for the collection of more oxygen. This reservoir bag provides the patient with a second source of oxygen. The bag must inflate with

# Section 4

oxygen for this to work. With a well-fitting mask and high enough oxygen flow, the patient can receive a $FIO_2$ of well over 90%.

## Technique

1. Choose a mask that fits over the nose and mouth with as few gaps as possible.
2. Secure the mask to the patient's face using the elastic strap.
3. Connect the distal end of the tubing to the oxygen source.
4. The oxygen flow should be at least 6 L/min.
5. The reservoir bag might need to be unfolded and manipulated to inflate.
6. Monitor the patient's oxygen saturation.

## 4.4 Oxygen Hoods

Oxygen hoods can deliver relatively high concentrations of oxygen without the discomfort sometimes associated with a face mask (**Figure 22.14**). They are generally used only in young infants because older children can easily remove them.

## Technique

1. Assemble the hood (if necessary).
2. The patient should be in the supine position.
3. Place the hood over the patient's head.
4. Connect the device to the oxygen source.
5. Monitor the patient's oxygen saturation.

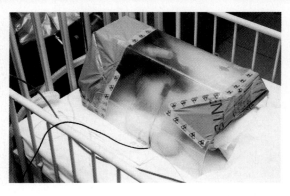

**Figure 22.14** Oxygen hood.

## Complications and Pitfalls

The most significant potential complication of emergency oxygen therapy lies in its misuse. Oxygen therapy is indicated for hypoxemia, not respiratory failure. In order to benefit from oxygen therapy, the patient must have adequate ventilatory effort. The patient with inadequate ventilatory effort might require oxygen therapy but will also require assisted ventilation. Another common error is the use of a self-inflating ventilation bag (discussed later) to deliver blow-by oxygen. This type of ventilation device has a one-way valve that prevents the delivery of oxygen to the mask unless the bag is squeezed (regardless of the oxygen flow rate into the tail of the device). Hospital oxygen delivery systems rarely fail, but oxygen tanks have a limited capacity. This capacity must be taken into consideration when planning treatment.

# Section 5  Suction

# Section 5

The airway can easily become occluded by secretions or foreign material, such as emesis or blood clots. The ability to clear these obstructions using the appropriate suction apparatus is critical to basic and advanced airway management. Appropriately sized equipment should be readily accessible and prepared for use prior to any airway procedures. At least one functioning suction apparatus is required at the head of the patient's bed, and the following functional attachments must be available for use if needed.[12–14]

## 5.1 Suction

### Indications and Equipment

1. Tonsillar tip suction tips—for the removal of solid materials such as vomitus or blood clots from the hypopharynx. Most stiff suction tips have several small holes at the tip that will not permit suctioning of solid debris. To suction solid material, a stiff suction tip with a large end hole must be used.

2. Nasogastric/orogastric tubes—for the removal of gastric secretions and air from the stomach. If not contraindicated, a nasogastric suction device should be placed in every intubated patient.

3. Tracheal suction catheters—these devices are used in combination with a saline wash to remove secretions and mucus from endotracheal tubes or tracheostomy tubes.

### Contraindications

1. Deep tonsillar tip suction in awake or lightly sedated patients should be avoided to prevent gagging, emesis, or laryngospasm.

2. Avoid nasogastric tubes in cases of facial/cranial trauma (use the oral route instead).

3. Use caution when placing orogastric tubes in suspected laryngeal, penetrating neck, or esophageal injury.

4. Avoid vigorous suctioning with tracheal suction catheters in fresh surgical tracheostomies.

### Equipment

- Tonsillar tip (stiff) adult- and pediatric-sized suction catheters. Most of these have several small holes at the tip. Some have a single large hole at the tip (**Figure 22.15**)

- Nasogastric/orogastric tubes of various sizes from 10 Fr to 16 Fr, with connectors to suction tubing (**Figure 22.16**)

- Tracheal suction catheters of various sizes from 5/6 Fr to 14 Fr (**Figure 22.17**)

- Suction source

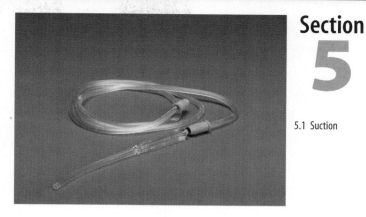

**Figure 22.15** Tonsillar tip.

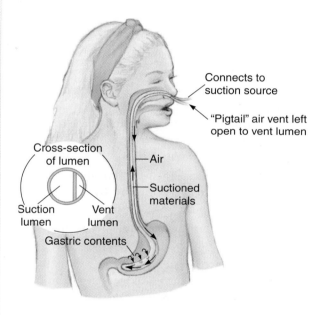

Connects to suction source

"Pigtail" air vent left open to vent lumen

Cross-section of lumen

Air

Suction lumen — Vent lumen

Suctioned materials

Gastric contents

**Figure 22.16** Double lumen sump tube.

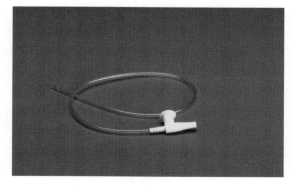

**Figure 22.17** Suction catheter.

# Section

## 5

5.1 Suction

## Technique

Oral suctioning with tonsillar tip:

1. Connect suction apparatus to wall suction or portable suction pump and adjust to medium, continuous pressure (not to exceed 300 mm Hg). If suctioning vomitus, the suction strength will need to be increased to high and a stiff suction tip with a larger hole will be necessary.

2. Preoxygenate patients by increasing oxygen delivery or manually ventilating them.

3. Open the mouth manually and sweep the suction tip across the oropharynx, under direct visualization.

4. Limit suctioning to 10 seconds per attempt, or less depending on the patient's condition.

5. Reoxygenate the patient manually between attempts.

Tracheal suctioning with endotracheal/tracheostomy tube:

1. Connect suction apparatus to wall suction, adjust to low, continuous pressure (not to exceed 100 mm Hg).

2. Preoxygenate the patient by increasing oxygen delivery or manually ventilating the patient.

3. Apply sterile gloves and open sterile suction setup.

4. Advance the sterile catheter beyond the distal tip of the ET tube/tracheostomy tube without applying suction.

5. When the catheter can no longer be easily advanced, withdraw the catheter in a rotating manner while intermittent vacuum pressure is applied.

6. Limit vacuum suction time to 10 to 15 seconds.

7. Reoxygenate the patient manually immediately after suctioning.

8. Suctioning may be repeated as necessary. To loosen mucus plugs, inject 1 to 2 mL of sterile saline into the ET tube between attempts.

9. After airway suctioning, the catheter can be used to suction oropharyngeal secretions.

## Complications and Pitfalls

1. If the suction device becomes completely occluded, then suctioning will fail. Whenever possible, use the adult Yankauer suction tip to avoid clogging the suction apparatus with large particles of debris or blood clots. A second stand by suction apparatus is strongly encouraged. Ideally, this device should be a rigid-tipped suction device for the suctioning of larger debris. Also remember that the suction tubing can be used directly without the Yankauer tip if the tip becomes clogged with debris.

2. In order to function effectively, nasogastric/orogastric tubes must extend into the stomach. These should be measured prior to placement.

3. Nasogastric/orogastric tubes can be accidentally inserted into the trachea. Always check placement with auscultation immediately after placement.

4. Tracheal suctioning can produce significant hypoxemia. The patient should receive supplemental oxygen before the procedure begins, and then be monitored throughout the procedure. The procedure should be limited to 15 seconds.

5. Tracheal suctioning can produce vagally mediated cardiovascular alterations and should be used judiciously with careful monitoring in the unstable patient.

6. All suctioning techniques can produce mucosal irritation. Overly vigorous suctioning, suctioning using very high suction pressure, and excessively frequent suctioning should be avoided.

## Section 6  Opening the Airway

Under the right (or wrong) circumstances, almost any patient can be difficult to intubate, ventilate, or both. Some patients have anatomic features or other limitations that should be recognized as potential impediments to effective airway management prior to the administration of neuromuscular blocking agents. Although some children require immediate airway management, when time permits, it is prudent for the physician to perform a brief evaluation of the airway in an attempt to identify the presence of a "difficult airway." This assessment can afford the physician an opportunity to use an alternative method of airway management and to avoid potential disaster. The assessment of the difficult airway is discussed thoroughly in Chapter 3, The Pediatric Airway in Health and Disease.[15] Potential rescue airway devices are discussed later in this chapter.

The initial step for most children requiring urgent airway intervention will be a basic maneuver designed to relieve the airway obstruction that inevitably accompanies loss of tone in the upper airway. The two techniques that are commonly used are the chin lift maneuver and the jaw thrust maneuver.

## 6.1 Chin-Lift Maneuver

### Indications

The chin-lift maneuver is indicated in children who have a depressed level of consciousness with concomitant upper airway obstruction and who are not victims of trauma.[16,17]

### Contraindications

Because this technique involves movement of the neck, it should not be performed in children who are trauma victims, even if radiographs do not demonstrate a cervical spine fracture.

### Technique

1. Verify unresponsiveness.
2. Place one hand on the forehead and the other on the mandible just lateral to the chin.
3. Gently depress the forehead with one hand to extend the neck while simultaneously lifting the chin anteriorly with the other. Classically, this technique is performed by placing the fingers of the dominant hand beneath the patient's chin and then lifting the chin anteriorly and caudally. In some cases, it might be necessary to firmly grasp the chin and/or skin or to use the lip or teeth to gain the appropriate mechanical advantage. If the latter technique is used, care must be exercised to ensure that the patient is indeed unconscious and unable to bite the rescuer. Hyperextension of the neck should be avoided in infants and young children (**Figure 22.18**).
4. Confirm adequate ventilation by looking for chest wall rise, feeling for exhaled air, and by auscultation.

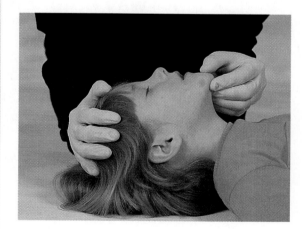

**Figure 22.18** Use the chin-lift maneuver to place the airway in a neutral position.

# Section 6

## Complications and Pitfalls

The chin-lift maneuver can cause or exacerbate cervical spine injury and should not be used in victims of trauma. Hyperextension of the neck in infants and young children can cause, rather than relieve, airway obstruction.

## 6.2 Jaw-Thrust Maneuver

### Indications

The jaw-thrust maneuver is indicated when the movement of the patient's neck is impossible or imprudent (Figure 22.19).[16,17]

### Contraindications

There are no contraindications to this technique; however, it might be ineffective in children with significant mandibular injuries.

### Technique

1. Without moving the neck, place both hands at the mandibular angle and push

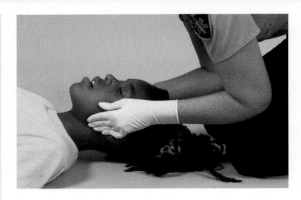

**Figure 22.19** Use the jaw-thrust maneuver in a child with possible spinal injury.

the mandible anteriorly. This is commonly done by using the maxilla/zygoma or forehead region for leverage.

2. Confirm adequate ventilation by looking for chest wall rise, feeling for exhaled air, and by auscultation.

### Complications and Pitfalls

Movement of the neck should be avoided.

# Section 7   Airway Adjuncts

# Section 7

Oropharyngeal airways and nasopharyngeal airways provide a mechanical stent that relieves soft tissue obstruction from the mouth to the glottis (oral airway) or from the nasal opening to the glottis (nasal airway). They can be used in intubated and nonintubated patients. These airways are important in overcoming proximal airway obstruction for effective spontaneous and bag-mask–assisted ventilations.[12]

## 7.1 Oropharyngeal Airways

Oropharyngeal airways are rigid, semicircular tubes (or sometimes H-shaped in cross-section) with a central lumen (Figure 22.20). These devices provide a mechanical stent that relieves soft tissue obstruction of the upper airway.

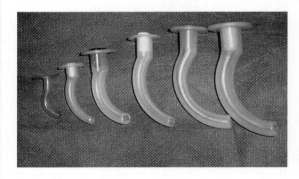

**Figure 22.20** Different sizes of oropharyngeal airways.

They can be used in intubated and nonintubated patients. In the latter case they serve to protect the ETT from being crushed between the patient's upper and lower jaws.

## Indications

Oropharyngeal airways are indicated for:

Relieving upper airway obstruction, serving as a "bite block" to protect the ETT, and facilitating oral and pharyngeal suctioning

## Contraindications

Oropharyngeal airways should not be used in conscious/ semiconscious patients (including lightly sedated or anesthetized patients) who have intact protective airway reflexes. When used in these patients, oropharyngeal airways can cause gagging, vomiting, or catastrophic laryngospasm or bronchospasm. Nasopharyngeal airways are generally better tolerated in awake or semiconscious patients. Do not use either type of airway in cases of suspected foreign body aspiration.

## Equipment

- Properly sized oral airway (available in sizes 55 to 90 mm)—to estimate size, place the airway on the patient's cheek. With the flange at the level of the lips, the distal pharyngeal tip should be at the angle of the mandible (**Figure 22.21**).

## Technique

1. Select the appropriate-sized oropharyngeal airway.
2. Suction the oral cavity if indicated.
3. Open the mouth and place a tongue blade at the base of the tongue.

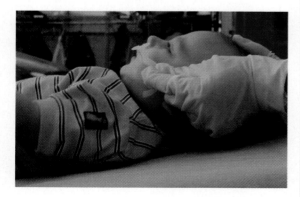

**Figure 22.21** Place an oropharyngeal airway next to the face, with the flange at the level of the central incisors and the bite block segment parallel to the hard palate.

4. Depress and pull the tongue forward with the tongue blade, lifting it off the posterior pharyngeal wall.
5. Insert the airway, leaving 1 to 2 cm protruding beyond the incisors.
6. To complete the insertion, perform a jaw-thrust maneuver with the fingers until the flange is even with the lips.
7. Relax the jaw thrust.
8. Check that the tongue and lips are not caught between the teeth and the airway.

## Alternative Technique

1. Select the appropriately sized oropharyngeal airway.
2. Suction the oral cavity if indicated.
3. Open the mouth and insert the oral airway such that the curved portion of the device depresses the tongue.
4. Rotate the airway 180 degrees into position, leaving 1 to 2 cm protruding beyond the incisors.
5. To complete the insertion, perform a jaw-thrust maneuver with the fingers until the flange is even with the lips.
6. Relax the jaw thrust.
7. Check that the tongue and the lips are not caught between the teeth and the airway.

## Complications and Pitfalls

The oropharyngeal airway must be appropriately sized to function properly. An oral airway that is too large can obstruct the airway and might stimulate potentially lethal laryngospasm and/or bronchospasm. Conversely, an oral airway that is too small will push the tongue base posteriorly into the pharynx, worsening the airway obstruction (**Figure 22.22**).

## 7.2 Nasopharyngeal Airways

A nasopharyngeal airway is a soft rubber or plastic tube that provides a mechanical stent to relieve soft tissue obstruction from the nares to the glottis (**Figure 22.23**).[12]

## Indications

Nasopharyngeal airways can be used in awake or lightly sedated patients when airway obstruction

# Section

## 7

7.2 Nasopharyngeal Airways

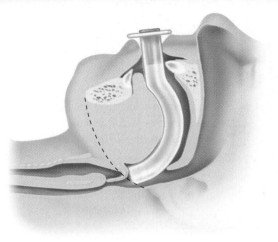

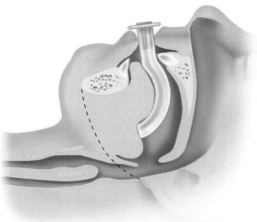

**Figure 22.22** Improperly sized oropharyngeal airways. An airway device that is too large will displace the epiglottis inferiorly over the glottic opening. An airway that is too small will impinge on the tongue, displacing it posteriorly into the hypophyarynx.

Adapted from: Henretig FM, King CC, eds. *Textbook of Pediatric Emergency Procedures*. Baltimore, Md: Williams & Wilkins; 1997:117.

is not relieved with an oropharyngeal airway alone (e.g., large adenoids, swollen tonsillar tissues), and in patients with trismus when placement of an oral airway may be difficult or impossible (e.g., status epilepticus).

## Contraindications

The following may be considered contraindications to NP airway placement:

1. Trauma with suspected nasal or basilar skull trauma or mid-face fractures
2. Coagulopathy (epistaxis)
3. Prior history of nasal facial surgery (e.g., cleft palate repair)

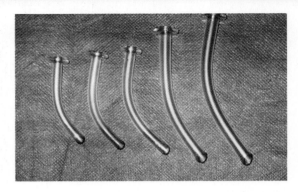

**Figure 22.23** Different sizes of nasopharyngeal airways.

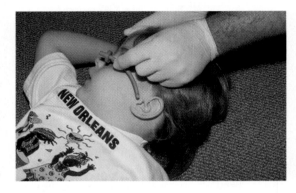

**Figure 22.24** Place the NP airway next to the face and measure from the tip of the nose to the tragus of the ear.

4. Adenoid hypertrophy
5. Suspected foreign body aspiration

## Equipment

- Properly sized nasal airway (available in sizes 16 Fr through 34 Fr)—to estimate size, place the nasopharyngeal airway at the tip of the nose. A properly sized tube will extend to the tragus of the patient's ear (**Figure 22.24**). A shortened ET tube can also be used as a nasal airway.

## Technique

1. Select an appropriately sized nasopharyngeal airway.
2. Suction the nares if indicated.
3. Lubricate the airway with water-soluble lubricant.
4. Hold the tube between the thumb and the first two fingers of the dominant hand

and insert it into the nostril with the bevel facing the patient's nasal septum.

5. On the right:

   a. Pass the tube along the floor of the nasal passage "downward" (i.e., do not aim it upward) toward the posterior pharynx using slow, gentle, steady pressure.

   b. If resistance is felt in the posterior nasopharynx, a gentle anterior-posterior, back-and-forth motion of the nasal airway a few millimeters in each direction, or a gentle rotation in a clockwise or counterclockwise direction while advancing, will help in passing the tube.

   c. If continued resistance is felt, remove the tube and attempt placement attempted in the opposite nostril. Consider the need for a smaller tube.

6. On the left: a. Insert the tube with the bevel toward the septum. The nasopharyngeal airway will be pointed upward and

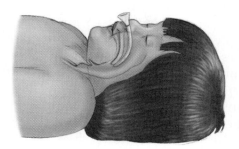

**Section**

**7**

7.2 Nasopharyngeal Airways

**Figure 22.25** If using the left nostril, begin inserting the nasopharyngeal airway with the curvature upward until resistance is felt (about 2 cm), then rotate the device 180 degrees and advance until the flange is against the outside of the nostril.

resistance will be felt at 1 to 2 cm.

b. Rotate the airway 180 degrees into position with the flange resting against the base of the nostril (**Figure 22.25**).

## Complications and Pitfalls

The nasal airway must be appropriately sized to function properly.

# Section 8   Bag-Mask Ventilation

Because resistance to gas flow through a tube increases to the fourth power as the lumen becomes smaller, infants and children have higher baseline airway resistance than adults. They also experience substantially greater increases in resistance with the same amount of airway narrowing (edema, obstruction). Furthermore, the respiratory muscles (intercostals and diaphragm) of infants and children have fewer fatigue-resistant fibers than adults and thus tire (fail) more rapidly.

These characteristics, combined with the rarity of cardiac disease in pediatric patients, account for the fact that most episodes of cardiac arrest in children are secondary events following (primary) respiratory failure and arrest. In adults, cardiac arrest is usually a primary process resulting from ischemia. This is perhaps the most fundamental difference in terms of resuscitation between pediatric and adult patients. For this reason, bag-mask ventilation (BMV) is a crucial skill in managing pediatric arrests. Additionally, while emergent endotracheal intubation will be performed in the ED by physicians, BMV serves as the initial method to maintain ventilation and the method of choice if endotracheal intubation is unsuccessful. Many types of health care professionals (nurses, respiratory therapists, physician assistants) may be called on to perform BMV in a pediatric resuscitation.[18,19]

## 8.1 Bag-Mask Ventilation

### Indications

Indications for BMV include all circumstances in which assisted or controlled ventilation is required. The list of potential etiologies is long and involves a diversity of mechanisms, e.g., neurologic causes (diffuse axonal injury,

**Section**

**8**

8.1 Bag-Mask Ventilation

# Section
# 8

8.1 Bag-Mask
Ventilation

herniation syndromes), infectious causes (sepsis, meningitis), upper airway causes (anaphylaxis, thermal injury), lower airway causes (pneumonia, asthma, pulmonary contusion), among many others. There are few contraindications to this procedure. Relative contraindications include conditions that make performing effective BMV extremely difficult or impossible, such as severe facial/mandibular injuries or complete upper airway obstruction from a foreign body. If the patient has a known pneumothorax, BMV should only be performed for a brief period of time before decompression of the affected hemithorax is performed to avoid precipitating a tension pneumothorax. The two absolute contraindications to BMV are meconium in a depressed newly born infant and known diaphragmatic hernia, which both require immediate endotracheal intubation.

## Equipment

- Manual resuscitator (self-inflating or gas inflated)
- Appropriately sized masks

The most important difference in BMV set-ups is determined by the type of resuscitation bag used, i.e., a self-inflating bag (manual resuscitator) versus a standard anesthesia bag (also known as the Rusch bag). As the name implies, a self-inflating bag is designed to re-inflate automatically after being compressed and released during BMV. While this might make the procedure somewhat easier to perform, rapid re-expansion of the bag with each ventilation allows entrainment of ambient air, even when an oxygen reservoir is used, thereby decreasing the concentration of oxygen delivered to the patient. This disadvantage is also an advantage. Because self-inflating bags are not dependent on an external gas source, they will continue to function even when the oxygen tank is depleted. This allows the patient to be ventilated, albeit with room air, until the oxygen tank can be replaced (Figure 22.26).

By contrast, an anesthesia bag will inflate only if there is sufficient oxygen inflow, a closed system is maintained (good mask seal),

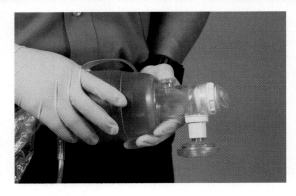

Figure 22.26 A self-inflating bag.

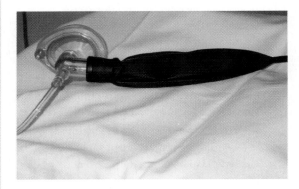

Figure 22.27 An anesthesia bag.

and the adjustable pressure leak valve is set appropriately (Figure 22.27). Although these requirements make BMV more complicated, failure of the bag to re-expand provides a valuable indication that a significant problem exists and must be corrected. Such problems

## KEY POINTS

**Basic Airway Management**

- Position the head.
- Open the airway using jaw-thrust or chin-lift, or by placing an oropharyngeal or nasopharyngeal airway.
- Select the appropriate oxygen delivery device.
- Provide assisted ventilation (BMV).

(e.g., depletion of an oxygen tank or a poor mask seal) do not prevent re-expansion of a self-inflating resuscitation bag and might therefore go undetected.

This is especially relevant in the ED, because BMV circuits with self-inflating bags are used by prehospital and emergency personnel far more commonly than anesthesia bag circuits. For this reason, only the use of self-inflating bag circuits is described here.

## Technique

As with most aspects of pediatric advanced life support, performing BMV in an infant or child begins with the ABCs (airway, breathing, circulation). First, determine whether the child requires BMV using the "look, listen, and feel" method if necessary. Look at the chest wall for any respiratory effort and/or signs of respiratory distress (belly breathing, retractions). Listen, with one ear close to the child's nose and mouth, for any air movement. Feel, with one cheek close to the child's nose and mouth, for any air movement. These steps might not be necessary, as with a child in cardiac arrest, but they can be useful in many circumstances. This aspect of the assessment should take at most only a few seconds.

If the child is not moving adequate air, position the head and neck so that the upper airway is most likely to be patent. This is generally best accomplished by flexing the neck slightly and rotating the head upward in a "sniffing position" (**Figure 22.28**). For patients with no risk of neck trauma, use the chin-lift maneuver to open the airway. For trauma patients, use the jaw-thrust maneuver to reduce neck movement. If necessary, place a small pad under the patient's head to produce neck flexion. This will not usually be required with young infants because they have a relatively large occiput, which causes neck flexion whenever they are supine on a firm, flat surface. In infants it might be necessary to place a small towel under the shoulders to level the plane of the airway.

If the patient continues to have inadequate respirations after appropriate airway maneuvers, begin performing BMV.

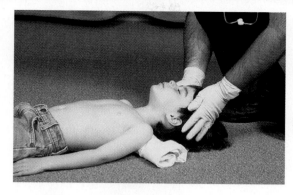

**Figure 22.28** The airway should be placed in a neutral sniffing position to keep the trachea from kinking when the neck is flexed or hyperextended.

First, select the smallest mask that completely covers the nose and mouth. A mask that is too large will compress the eyes, causing injury and/or bradycardia. A mask that is too small will make it impossible to establish and maintain an adequate mask seal on the face. Measure the mask from the bridge of the nose to the cleft of the chin.

Next, select a bag that is appropriately sized for the patient. Remember that it is always possible to ventilate with a bag that is too large—and never possible with one that is too small.

Do not hesitate to change to a better size of bag or mask, even during the procedure, if this seems necessary. A process of trial and error is often required in selecting the best equipment for this procedure. Do not make the mistake of trying to manage with improperly sized equipment.

Apply the mask to the face with the nondominant hand while positioning the head and neck optimally to maintain airway patency. The index finger and thumb gently compress the mask onto the face (C-grip), and the long, ring, and small fingers are placed on the angle of the jaw, forming an "E." The entire hand placement for BMV is called the EC clamp. The fingers on the jaw should pull the patient's chin into the mask, creating a good mask seal.

Compress the resuscitation bag with the dominant hand at an age-appropriate rate (**Figure 22.29**). It is helpful to control rate and

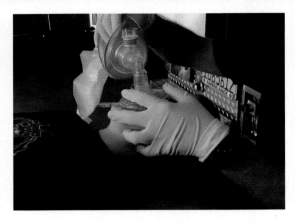

**Figure 22.29** Compress the resuscitation bag with the dominant hand.

volume by saying, "Squeeze, release, release." Squeeze the bag just until chest rise is initiated and then release.

It might be preferable to use a two-person technique in which one person uses both hands to apply the mask using the EC clamp and the other person compresses the bag. If two individuals perform BMV, the more experienced person should generally apply the mask and maintain the airway while the other person compresses the resuscitation bag. An assistant (if available) should apply cricoid pressure (Sellick maneuver).

Carefully monitor the patient at all times while performing BMV. Compress the bag so that the patient's chest excursions approximate a normal deep inspiration. Once chest rise is visible, enough volume has been delivered to the patient, so begin releasing the bag. Less than this will not provide an adequate tidal volume; more will cause air entry into the stomach, increasing the risk of vomiting and aspiration. Monitor the heart rate and, if available, pulse oximetry and/or capnometry to ensure that the procedure is being properly performed. Bradycardia, hypoxia, and hypercapnia are all possible indications of poor technique.

## Complications and Pitfalls

The most common serious complication that occurs with BMV is aspiration pneumonitis. Patients who require BMV often have diminished or absent protective airway reflexes and, in the prehospital and ED settings, a full stomach. Unlike endotracheal intubation, BMV does not provide protection against aspiration of gastric contents into the lungs. The risk of this complication can be reduced by applying cricoid pressure and by ventilating the patient with an appropriate tidal volume (i.e., monitoring chest excursions). The other serious complication associated with BMV (or any other method of positive pressure ventilation) is barotrauma resulting in a pneumothorax and, potentially, a tension pneumothorax. The likelihood of this complication can be reduced by carefully monitoring chest wall excursions to avoid administering excessive tidal volumes. Finally, minor and generally self-limited complications include eye injury due to compression with the mask, facial nerve neurapraxia caused by excessive pressure on the mask, and allergic reactions resulting from contact with the materials used to manufacture the mask.

# Section 9  Management of Upper Airway Foreign Bodies With Magill Forceps

Management of the patient with a foreign object occluding, or partially obstructing, the upper airway is dependent on several factors. If the child is awake and has evidence of partial airway obstruction (e.g., stridor), then the best course of action will almost certainly be to administer high-flow oxygen or a helium-oxygen mixture, allow the patient to find the most comfortable position, and transport the child to a location where the object can be removed by those with the most expertise under controlled circumstances. On the other hand, the child with impending respiratory failure or complete airway obstruction must be treated immediately.

Depending on age, such children should be treated with back blows and chest thrusts for infants (<12 months) or the Heimlich maneuver or abdominal thrusts for children (>1 year). When these techniques have failed and the patient has lost consciousness, the next step in the treatment algorithm is attempted removal of the object using direct laryngoscopy and Magill (or other) forceps.

## 9.1 Management of Upper Airway Foreign Bodies With Magill Forceps

### Equipment

- Laryngoscope
- Magill forceps (Figure 22.30). If Magill forceps are not available, other forceps or clamps may be substituted. In fact, it is wise to have a variety of tools available, including suction devices and gynecologic tenacula so that oddly shaped or slippery objects can be grasped.

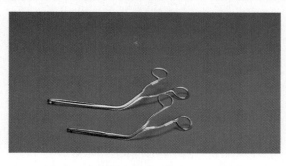

Figure 22.30  Magill forceps, adult and pediatric sizes.

- Equipment for airway management, including endotracheal tubes
- Equipment for surgical airway

### Technique

1. Open the mouth and insert the laryngoscope as described for endotracheal intubation.

2. Using the light from the laryngoscope, attempt to visualize the foreign object.

3. If the object cannot be seen, have an assistant administer abdominal thrusts in an attempt to bring the object into view.

4. Once the object is visualized, grasp it with the forceps and remove it from the upper airway. Some objects can be difficult to grasp. In such cases, consider a different tool or a suction device (Figure 22.31).

5. If the patient does not begin breathing spontaneously, proceed with appropriate airway management.

6. If the object cannot be visualized or removed, the clinician has further options:

    a. Attempt to pass an ETT and, in so doing, force the object further into the airway so that it enters one mainstem bronchus, leaving the other open,

    b. Perform a surgical airway, bypassing the occlusion, or

# Section 9

**c.** Perform repeated basic maneuvers to dislodge a foreign body in the esophagus or one below the level of the vocal cords.

9.1 Management of Upper Airway Foreign Bodies With Magill Forceps

### Complications and Pitfalls

This technique should generally be reserved for unconscious patients with complete airway obstruction. Attempted removal of objects in awake patients with partial airway obstruction can dislodge the object and cause complete occlusion of the airway. Blind attempts to grasp objects can damage the vocal cords and cause bleeding, which makes further efforts to visualize objects more difficult.[20]

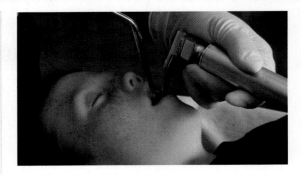

**Figure 22.31** Insert Magill forceps into the mouth.

## Section 10  Emergent Intubation

# Section 10

10.1 Endotracheal Intubation

There is perhaps no procedure more important in pediatric resuscitation than endotracheal intubation. For the child who is not adequately breathing, the most immediate priority is always establishing a stable airway, and the definitive method of accomplishing this is endotracheal intubation. The methods involved with performing this procedure can be broadly divided into two categories depending on the clinical circumstances: emergent and nonemergent (elective). While the goal in both situations is the same (successful insertion of a tube into the trachea), the challenges that the clinician will confront differ substantially. Elective intubations, such as those for scheduled procedures in the operating room, are performed in patients who are hemodynamically stable, have an empty stomach, and have previously been evaluated for any potential airway problems.

With emergent intubations, which are most commonly performed in the ED and prehospital settings, patients are usually acutely ill and often rapidly deteriorating. They must always be presumed to have a full stomach, putting them at much greater risk for vomiting and aspiration of stomach contents. The clinician is rarely afforded a prior opportunity to carefully assess the patient's airway anatomy to identify possible impediments to intubation. Many clinicians who perform emergent intubations in adult patients with great confidence and expertise become extremely anxious when the same procedure must be performed in a child.

Although there are important differences between adults and children that must be understood when performing this procedure, the similarities far outnumber the differences. Some of the most problematic characteristics of adults are rarely if ever present in children (morbid obesity, beards, arthritic cervical vertebrae, false teeth). With proper training and experience, emergency personnel can develop a high level of skill and proficiency in performing this procedure, using the same careful, systematic approach used for other complex emergency procedures.

## 10.1 Endotracheal Intubation

### Indications

Indications for this procedure are similar to those for BMV. As such, the list of potential indications for emergent endotracheal intubation in children is a long one, encompassing virtually all causes of acute respiratory compromise that affect the pediatric population. However, it is useful to consider how the indications and contraindications for these two procedures differ to better understand the unique aspects of endotracheal intubation.

For example, unlike BMV, which delivers positive pressure ventilation to the entire upper airway, endotracheal intubation also protects the airway so that entry of secretions and stomach contents into the lungs is minimized. This is one reason why tracheal suctioning is indicated, and BMV is contraindicated, for the management of the depressed newly born infant after meconium delivery—the presence of a properly positioned ETT prevents further soilage of the lungs.

Another major difference between BMV and endotracheal intubation is that an ETT delivers air only to the lungs, while BMV almost always causes air entry into the lungs and the stomach. This is why patients with respiratory distress resulting from a diaphragmatic hernia should undergo immediate endotracheal intubation and should not receive BMV. If the diaphragm herniates into the stomach, a "ball valve" effect can occur, allowing air to enter but not escape. As the stomach progressively expands and displaces the lung, respiratory distress worsens, and the patient can develop tension physiology (similar to a tension pneumothorax). BMV, which forces more air down the esophagus and into the stomach, exacerbates this effect. In children requiring ventilatory support for other reasons, excessive air entry into the stomach increases the likelihood of vomiting and aspiration and can impede expansion of the chest wall.

Thus, while BMV can be effectively used as a temporizing measure, emergent endotracheal intubation is indicated for any child requiring assisted or controlled ventilation for a more prolonged period of time. In addition, emergent intubation is indicated for airway protection (e.g., depressed mental status) and to provide direct access to the trachea to facilitate pulmonary toilet.

## Equipment

In children younger than 8 years, the narrowest point along the trachea is not at the vocal cords (as with adults) but at the cricoid ring. With adults, the largest ETT that can pass through the cords is still small relative to the subglottic diameter of the trachea. For this reason, a balloon (cuff) is needed to fill the surrounding space. This prevents a large air leak (air flowing out into the hypopharynx instead of into the lungs), which would significantly limit effective administration of positive pressure ventilation. By contrast, a properly sized tube for a younger child will pass through the cords and then wedge in position at the cricoid ring, preventing any significant air leak without the use of a cuff. For this reason, uncuffed ETTs are generally used in emergency settings for younger patients (usually age 8 years and younger) (Figure 22.32). It should be noted, however, that cuffed tubes might be appropriate even for children younger than 8 years of age if high inspiratory pressures are required, as with a patient who has greatly diminished lung compliance (e.g., a near-drowning). With higher pressures, a large air leak will often occur despite having an uncuffed tube that fits properly. Use of a cuffed tube in such situations should only be a temporizing measure, because excessive pressure on the wall of the trachea for prolonged periods can lead to the development of subglottic stenosis.

Another important decision regarding equipment when performing an emergent endotracheal intubation involves choosing a laryngoscope blade (Figure 22.33). For both

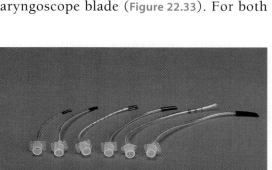

**Figure 22.32** Uncuffed endotracheal tubes in pediatric sizes 2.5, 3.0, 3.5, 4.0, 4.5, and 5.0.

# Section

# 10

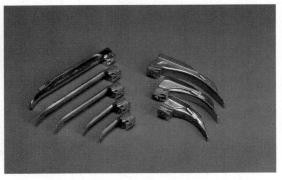

**Figure 22.33** Pediatric laryngoscope blades: straight blades (0, 1, 2, 3, 4), and curved blades (2, 3, 4).

children and adults, selecting the correct laryngoscope blade involves asking two questions: Should a straight or curved blade be used? Which size is right for the patient? With adults, curved (Macintosh) laryngoscope blades are preferred by most clinicians because they are comparatively easy to use. Except in rare cases, visualization of the vocal cords is readily accomplished by simply inserting the blade tip into the vallecula and pulling upward on the laryngoscope handle. This causes tension in the hyoepiglottic ligament, which in turn retracts the epiglottis and thereby reveals the cords. Use of a straight blade for an adult is generally reserved for the patient who is anticipated to have an especially difficult airway or when laryngoscopy with a curved blade has failed.

Conversely, a curved laryngoscope blade is not recommended for use in children younger than 8 years because of two important characteristics of the immature airway: greatly increased laxity of the hyoepiglottic ligament, and a relatively large, floppy epiglottis. In these younger patients, inserting the tip of a curved laryngoscope blade into the vallecula and pulling up might not adequately retract the epiglottis. In fact, the epiglottis might not move at all. Consequently, straight (Miller) blades should be used for such patients because they allow the clinician to directly lift the epiglottis using the blade tip so that the vocal cords can then be visualized. Guidelines

for selecting the proper laryngoscope blade are shown in Table 22-6. Although the airway of a child is considered to become more "adult-like" at about 8 years of age, significant variability can be seen in this regard among individual patients. For this reason, many sources recommend the use of a straight laryngoscope blade for emergent intubation of any pediatric patient who is not yet adult-sized.[21]

The difference between straight and curved blades is traditionally described in this manner, but it should be noted that: Some clinicians (and some studies) use curved blades for young children, and that use of a straight blade is sometimes directed initially into the vallecula, and subsequently used to directly lift the epiglottis only if the epiglottis fails to retract.

## 10.2 Rapid Sequence Intubation

Rapid sequence intubation (RSI, also known as rapid sequence induction) is the process of administering a sedative and muscle relaxant (inducing pharmacologic flaccid paralysis) to facilitate the process of endotracheal intubation. There are three major advantages of RSI as follows:

- RSI creates a controlled clinical environment to facilitate endotracheal intubation in pediatric patients who are frightened, anxious, and uncooperative. RSI provides rapid onset of unconsciousness and muscle relaxation.

- The combination of anesthetic agents and neuromuscular blockade used in RSI decreases the stimulation of potentially harmful autonomic reflexes associated with endotracheal intubation and their associated side effects (e.g., elevated intracranial pressure, hypertension, bradycardia).

- RSI with cricoid pressure minimizes risks for pulmonary aspiration during intubation. The effectiveness of RSI depends on the rapid intravenous administration of two drugs—an anesthetic and a neuromuscular blocking agent administered sequentially.[22,23]

## Indications

RSI is indicated for most patients who will undergo emergent endotracheal intubation.

## Contraindications

RSI should be attempted with caution, if at all, in patients who might have difficult airways. Once the neuromuscular blocking agent has been administered, the patient will be irreversibly paralyzed for at least a few minutes. RSI should also be used with caution in children who have a history or a family history of untoward reactions to anesthetic agents. Although not contraindicated, RSI might be unnecessary in patients who are unconscious.

## Equipment

Making sure you have all essential equipment in place can best be aided by the mnemonic SOAP-ME (suction, oxygen, airway equipment, pharmacology, and monitoring equipment). The essential airway equipment is listed in Table 22.2. This equipment must be immediately available and known to be functioning properly before the RSI agents are administered. All equipment must be available in the appropriate size(s) for the patient.

### Pharmacologic Agents

Many pharmacologic agents are useful in the performance of RSI. Tables 22-3 through 22-5 provide information about the advantages and disadvantages of each agent. The actual agents used by an individual physician will likely be dictated by availability, institutional policy, familiarity, and clinical advantages/disadvantages of each agent with respect to the clinical requirements of the patient.

## Management

The discussion regarding selection of sedatives, neuromuscular blocking agents, and adjunctive agents can be rather involved, but it can be broken down into three basic categories: head injury without hemodynamic compromise, status asthmaticus, and any condition with hemodynamic compromise. By examining the benefits and cautions of

---

**Section**

# 10

10.2 Rapid Sequence Intubation

---

### TABLE 22-2. Airway Equipment for RSI

**Essential Airway Equipment**
- Ventilation face masks
- Ventilation bags
- Oropharyngeal airways (with tongue blades)
- Nasopharyngeal airways (with lubrication gel)
- Endotracheal tubes (with syringes for the cuff)
- Stylets
- Laryngoscope handles
- Laryngoscope blades
- Magill forceps

**Difficult Airway Equipment**
- Laryngeal mask airway
- Combitube (16 years old or older)
- Gum elastic bougie (or other airway guide 14 years old or older)
- Specialized laryngoscopes
- Lighted stylet

**Surgical Airway Equipment**
- Transtracheal ventilation equipment

---

## KEY POINTS

**Performing RSI**
- Select patient who will benefit from the procedure.
- Prepare equipment (SOAP-ME).
- Monitor the patient.
- Administer appropriate sedation based on the patient's clinical status:
  - hypotension—etomidate
  - status asthmaticus—ketamine
  - head injury—thiopental or etomidate
- Administer appropriate neuromuscular blocking agent—succinylcholine versus rocuronium.
- Perform endotracheal intubation.
- Perform clinical assessment and use $ETCO_2$ monitor/detector to confirm endotracheal intubation.

---

| TABLE 22-3 | Sedative Agents | | | | |
|---|---|---|---|---|---|
| Agent | Dose | Onset | Duration | Benefits | Caution |
| Thiopental | 3–5 mg/kg | 30–40 sec | 10–30 min | Lowers ICP | Hypotension, Laryngospasm |
| Midazolam | 0.1 mg/kg | 1–2 min | 20–30 min | Reversible Amnestic Anticonvulsant | Apnea<br><br>Variable dose |
| Ketamine | 1–2 mg/kg | 1 min | 30–60 min | Bronchodilator Dissociative amnesia | Increases secretions Increases ICP Possible emergence reactions |
| Etomidate | 0.3 mg/kg | < 1 min | 10–20 min | Lowers ICP Lowers IOP Supports BP | Myoclonic excitation Vomiting Low cortisol states (sepsis) |

| TABLE 22-4 | Neuromuscular Blocking Agents—Succinylcholine | | | | |
|---|---|---|---|---|---|
| Adult Dose | Infant/Child Dose | Onset | | Duration | Benefits |
| 1–1.5 mg/kg | 1–2 mg/kg | 30–60 sec | | 3–8 min | Rapid onset Short duration |

<u>Complications of succinylcholine</u>
Bradyarrhythmias
Increased intragastric, intraocular, and intracranial pressure
Hyperkalemia
Fasciculation induced musculoskeletal trauma
Masseter spasm
Malignant hyperthermia
Prolonged apnea with pseudocholinesterase deficiency
Histamine release
Cardiac arrest

each sedative, the following can be determined: thiopental and etomidate are useful agents for head injury without hemodynamic compromise; ketamine is useful for status asthmaticus; and etomidate, ketamine, and midazolam are the least likely to compromise blood pressure (BP) in the hemodynamically compromised patient. (However, consider that no sedative might be preferable if the degree of hemodynamic compromise is severe.)

The choice of neuromuscular blocking agent comes down to physician preferences for onset time, duration, and adverse effects when comparing succinylcholine with one of the nondepolarizing neuromuscular blocking agents, of which rocuronium is the most useful is rocuronium for most patients.

## Technique

1. While personnel, equipment, and pharmacologic agents are being assembled and intravenous access is being obtained, the patient should receive high-flow oxygen through a nonrebreather mask. The objective is to completely saturate all available

## TABLE 22-5 Neuromuscular Blocking Agents—Nondepolarizing Agents

| Agent | Dose | Onset | Duration | Complications |
|---|---|---|---|---|
| Rocuronium | 0.6–1 mg/kg | 1–3 min | Intermediate 30–45 min | Tachycardia |
| Vecuronium | 0.08–0.15 mg/kg 0.15–0.28 mg/kg (high dose) | 2–4 min | Intermediate/long 25–40 min 60–120 m (high dose) | Prolonged recovery in obese patients and those with hepatorenal dysfunction |
| Atracurium | 0.4–0.6 mg/kg | 2–3 min | Intermediate 25–45 min | Histamine release Hypotension Bronchospasm |
| Mivacurium | 0.15–0.2 mg/kg | 2–3 min | Short 10–20 min | Histamine release |

Adjunctive Medications

Atropine 0.4–0.6 mg (adolescent) to reduce secretions.

Atropine 0.01–0.02 mg/kg (min 0.1-max 0.4 mg) (Child)—Use with Succinylcholine if ≤5 years old to prevent bradycardia.

Lidocaine 1.5 mg/kg IV—May be beneficial in head trauma patients to reduce ICP.

hemoglobin binding sites so that the patient can tolerate a protracted period of apnea if necessary.

2. Briefly assess the patient for a potentially difficult airway (See Chapter 3, The Pediatric Airway in Health and Disease).

3. Prepare all equipment.

4. Secure vascular access and monitor the patient.

5. Administer atropine if indicated.

6. Administer the sedative agent.

7. Administer any adjunctive agents (e.g., lidocaine) if indicated.

8. Administer the neuromuscular blocking agent while an assistant holds cricoid pressure (Sellick maneuver).

9. Proceed with endotracheal intubation.

The first aspect of preparing the patient is usually preoxygenation. When time and circumstances permit, always preoxygenate the patient using 100% oxygen, either by having the patient breathe spontaneously through a nonrebreather face mask, or if necessary, by administering assisted or controlled BMV. Effective preoxygenation allows the longest period of "safe" apnea (i.e., the patient does not develop hypoxemia), which provides the greatest amount of time for the clinician to perform laryngoscopy and tube insertion. Confirm that the patient has a reliable means of intravenous access so that RSI medications can be administered if needed. Position the patient close to the head of the bed and raise/lower the bed to a comfortable height for performing the procedure.

Next ensure that all the necessary equipment is easily accessible and functioning properly. Select the ETT most likely to be the correct size for the patient, and since this is only an estimate, have two additional tubes (1 size smaller and 1 size larger) readily available. Refer to Table 22-6, use the formula (Age/4) + 4, or use a length-based system such as the Broselow tape to determine the appropriate ETT size.[21,24,25]

Attach the laryngoscope blade to the handle and snap it into position to verify that the light on the blade is working and bright. If a cuffed tube is to be used, check to see that the balloon inflates easily and has no air leak. Ask for any drugs that might be needed to be drawn up in syringes and confirm the appropriate dosages. Insert a stylet (if used) into the ETT.

## Section 10

10.2 Rapid Sequence Intubation

Administer atropine if indicated. This is considered optional in adolescents but recommended in younger children who are more susceptible to bradycardia with laryngoscopy. Atropine is also beneficial if succinylcholine (reduces the risk of bradycardia) or ketamine (reduces the risk of excessive secretions) is to be used.

Next, administer any other adjunctive agents, then the selected sedative and neuromuscular blocking agent. Which of these should go first or second is controversial, but the sedative and neuromuscular blocking agent should be given in rapid sequence regardless of order. It might be preferable to give some sedatives (such as thiopental) slowly, which argues in favor of giving the neuromuscular blocking agent first so that its time of onset coincides with the completion of sedative administration. However, others recommend that the sedative be given first to ensure unconsciousness before paralyzing the patient.

Once the sedative or neuromuscular blocking agent is administered, a staff member should be dedicated to the single task of providing cricoid pressure sufficient to gently occlude the esophageal lumen (Sellick maneuver), which reduces the risk of passive regurgitation (Figure 22.34). This should be maintained until endotracheal intubation is confirmed.

While achieving a successful emergent endotracheal intubation involves several coordinated actions, the procedure itself essentially consists of two steps—direct laryngoscopy and tube insertion. Once the patient is fully paralyzed (usually 60 to 90 seconds after the administration of the neuromuscular blocking

### TABLE 22-6  RSI Drugs, Doses (mg/kg), Sizes, Distances

| Age | 2 mo | 6 mo | 1 yr | 3 yr | 5 yr | 7 yr | 9 yr | 11 yr | 12 yr | 14 yr | 16 yr | Adult |
|---|---|---|---|---|---|---|---|---|---|---|---|---|
| **Average weight (kg)** | 5 | 8 | 10 | 15 | 19 | 23 | 29 | 36 | 44 | 50 | 58 | 65 |
| Preoxygenation | | | | | | | | | | | | |
| Adjunctive agents (optional): | | | | | | | | | | | | |
| Atropine (0.01–0.02 mg/kg): Use in all children or with ketamine. | | | | | | | | | | | | |
| | 0.1 | 0.15 | 0.2 | 0.3 | 0.3 | 0.4 | 0.5 | 0.5 | 0.5 | 0.5 | 0.5 | 0.5 |
| Lidocaine (1.5 mg/kg): Lowers ICP | | | | | | | | | | | | |
| | 8 | 12 | 15 | 22 | 28 | 35 | 44 | 54 | 66 | 75 | 90 | 100 |
| Sellick maneuver | | | | | | | | | | | | |
| Sedative | | | | | | | | | | | | |
| Hypotension | | | | | | | | | | | | |
| Etomidate (0.3 mg/kg): | 1.5 | 2.4 | 3 | 4.5 | 6 | 7 | 9 | 11 | 13 | 15 | 17 | 20 |
| Head trauma without hypotension | | | | | | | | | | | | |
| Etomidate (see above) or | | | | | | | | | | | | |
| Thiopental (3–5 mg/kg): | 15–25 | 24–40 | 30–50 | 45–75 | 57–95 | 70–115 | 90–145 | 110–180 | 130–220 | 150–250 | 170–290 | 195–325 |
| Status asthmaticus: | | | | | | | | | | | | |
| Ketamine (1–2mg/kg): | 5–7 | 8–16 | 10–20 | 15–30 | 19–38 | 23–46 | 29–58 | 36–72 | 44–88 | 50–100 | 58–100 | 65–100 |
| Paralyzing agent: | | | | | | | | | | | | |
| Succinylcholine (1–2 mg/kg): | 8 | 12 | 15 | 25 | 30 | 40 | 50 | 55 | 60 | 65 | 70 | 80 |
| Rocuronium (0.6–1 mg/kg): | 4 | 6 | 9 | 12 | 15 | 20 | 25 | 30 | 40 | 45 | 50 | 60 |
| Intubate (tube size): | 3.5 | 3.5 | 4.0 | 4.5 | 5.0 | 5.5 | 6.0 | 6.5 | 7.0 | 7.0 female, 8.0 male | | |
| Tube depth at lip (cm): | 11 | 12 | 13 | 14 | 15 | 16 | 18 | 19 | 20 | 22 | 22 | 22 |
| Laryngoscope blade size: | 1 | 1 | 1 | 2 | 2 | 2 | 2 | 2 | 3 | 3 | 3 | 3–4 |

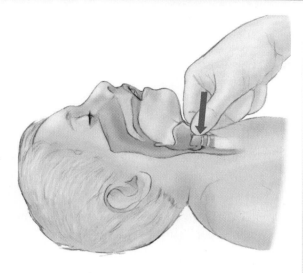

Figure 22.34 Cricoid pressure occludes the esophagus to prevent gastric reflux.

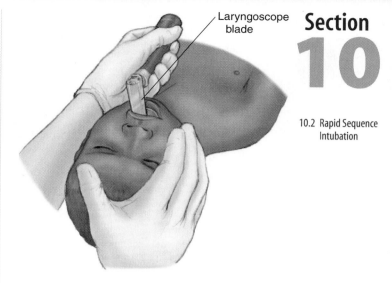

Laryngoscope blade

Figure 22.35 Insert the pediatric straight laryngoscope blade into the patient's mouth.

agent), open the patient's mouth and insert the laryngoscope blade, taking care not to injure the lips, teeth, or tongue (Figure 22.35). Most sources recommend inserting the blade on the right side of the patient's mouth and "sweeping" the tongue to the left, especially when using a curved blade. However, in most cases it is also acceptable to insert the blade along the midline and slide it over the tongue into the proper position.

If a curved blade is used, insert it into the hypopharynx until the tip of the blade meets resistance at the vallecula, and then pull the handle upward at a 45-degree angle to retract the epiglottis and reveal the vocal cords (Figure 22.36). If a straight blade is used, advance it under direct visualization (by retracting the tongue) until the epiglottis is seen. If desired, make one attempt to retract the epiglottis with the technique used with a curved blade, (i.e., by inserting the blade tip into the vallecula and lifting upward). If this reveals the cords, then proceed with tube insertion. However, if the epiglottis continues to obscure the glottic opening (as will happen in most instances), withdraw the blade slightly and use a scooping motion to directly lift the epiglottis from view with the blade tip. This might take more than one attempt, as the epiglottis will sometimes

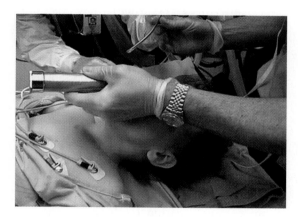

Figure 22.36 Place gentle traction upward along the axis of the laryngoscope handle at 45 degrees.

slip off the tip of the blade with even the slightest movement of the laryngoscope handle.

Next, insert the ETT without losing sight of the glottic opening and vocal cords (Figure 22.37). This is greatly facilitated by having an assistant retract the right cheek slightly by pulling it laterally and holding the tube close by and providing it when needed. Retracting the cheek allows the tube to be inserted from the right side of the hypopharynx so that it does not obscure the cords (Figure 22.38). This also makes it possible to watch the tip of the tube as it enters

# Section

# 10

10.2 Rapid Sequence
Intubation

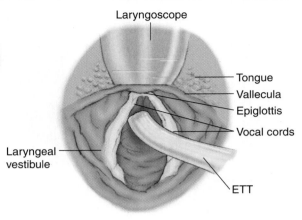

Figure 22.37 View of normal anatomic landmarks for advancing the ETT using a straight blade.

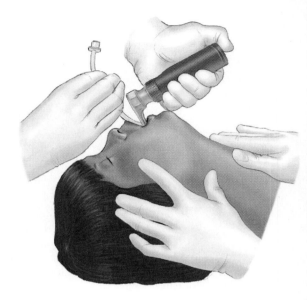

Figure 22.38 Advance the ETT from the right corner of the mouth past the vocal cords and into the trachea.

the glottis, which is the best way to ensure a successful intubation. Remember to always keep both eyes open during this step of the procedure to preserve depth perception. As with threading a needle, maintaining depth perception makes inserting the tube between the vocal cords and into the trachea much easier. Confirm intratracheal placement of the tube (and exclude any possibility of an esophageal intubation) by listening for breath sounds in both lungs, listening over the stomach, and most importantly, by seeing good color change on a colorimetric $CO_2$ detector and/or good waveforms on a capnograph ($ETCO_2$ monitor).

Once the ETT has been properly inserted, position it so that the tip lies at an appropriate distance from the carina to achieve midtracheal placement (1 to 2 cm in younger children; 2 to 3 cm in older children). The depth of tube placement can be estimated by multiplying 3 times the ETT size; this value will be the appropriate depth in centimeters. For example, a child who is intubated with a 4-mm ETT should have the depth of placement measuring about 12 cm at the lip. Correct depth can also be found on the Broselow tape. Table 22-6 provides the expected tube length that should be at the patient's lips for each age group. Although these methods are highly reliable, a chest radiograph should be performed after the tube is secured to verify correct placement.

Finally, secure the tube using adhesive tape and/or cloth tape, or if preferred, a commer-

cially produced device designed for this purpose. There is a variety of methods advocated for taping an ETT, but in general, the tube should be anchored well enough that even an inadvertent yank will not dislodge it. Unexpected tube dislodgement often results in a frantic scramble for equipment to provide ventilatory support pending reintubation. Unrecognized tube dislodgement can be fatal, thus, carefully securing the ETT will usually prevent undoing the good work of a successful intubation.

## Complications and Pitfalls

Whenever possible, equipment and devices should be tested to ensure that they will function properly during the procedure (e.g., the light in the laryngoscope blade, the balloon of a cuffed ETT, wall suction, oxygen source).

Several potentially serious complications can be associated with performing an emergent endotracheal intubation. The most common of these include adverse physiologic effects of the procedure, inadequate oxygenation, barotrauma, mechanical trauma, and aspiration pneumonitis. Adverse physiologic effects are normally only a significant problem with patients who have severe cardiovascular compromise. For example, direct laryngoscopy is a potent inducer of vagal stimulation, especially in infants and younger children. In a healthy child, this is unlikely to produce any deleterious effects; in a child with unstable hemodynamics, however, profound bradycardia (even asystole) can occur, resulting in an abrupt cardiovascular collapse. Additionally, direct laryngoscopy is suspected to increase ICP in children.

The most serious complication of RSI is failure of the intubation attempted in a patient who cannot be ventilated (the so-called cannot intubate/cannot ventilate situation). In such patients, a rescue airway technique must be used immediately to avoid significant hypoxemic injury. Additionally, each of the pharmacologic agents is associated with one or more potential complications. Agents must be chosen with the clinical situation and patient factors (e.g., allergies) in mind.

Inadequate oxygenation, typically caused by an esophageal intubation, is generally the most disastrous complication of this procedure. Two ways that esophageal intubation most commonly occurs are by inserting the tube into the esophagus during intubation, and by dislodging the tube from the trachea into the esophagus after intubation. It is important to remember that everyone who performs this procedure enough times encounters an esophogeal intubation. It is the failure to recognize an esophageal intubation that must be avoided at all costs. Consequently, whenever a child who has recently been intubated has sudden and unexpected hemodynamic decompensation, the prudent clinician will take immediate measures to exclude any possibility of an unrecognized esophageal intubation or dislodgement of the ETT from the trachea.

Barotrauma, as the name implies, occurs as a complication of endotracheal intubation when excessive pressure causes injury to the patient. The most common type of pressure-related complication is a pneumothorax resulting from the administration of excessive tidal volume during positive pressure ventilation. The high level of intrapulmonary pressure induced overcomes the normal elastic properties of the tissues and produces a rup-

ture in the lung. This problem can normally be avoided by carefully observing the patient while performing positive pressure ventilation to ensure that only tidal volumes sufficient to cause chest rise are administered.

Although a significant injury, a simple pneumothorax rarely causes the patient major harm as long as it is recognized and treated appropriately. However, if the problem is not recognized and the patient continues to receive positive pressure ventilation, a much more serious (and potentially fatal) tension pneumothorax can develop. This complication occurs when the "ball valve" effect is created, in which air can enter the thoracic cavity (through the rupture in the lung) but cannot escape. With each positive pressure ventilation, more air is forced into the thoracic cavity, increasing the pressure in the affected hemithorax and eventually causing the mediastinum to shift away from the affected side. As this shift increases, deformation of the vena cava prevents adequate venous return to the heart, producing a rapid drop in blood pressure. This dramatic and rapid decompensation takes place within, at most, a few minutes and must be treated immediately with needle decompression of the chest. Because of this potential cascade of events, any pneumothorax identified in a patient who will continue to receive positive pressure ventilation must be treated early with tube thoracostomy.

Mechanical trauma during an emergent intubation occurs when injury to the tissues is caused by improper manipulation of the laryngoscope and/or ETT. Great care must be taken during direct laryngoscopy to avoid using the upper teeth (or in babies, the upper gingival ridges) as a leveraging fulcrum, which can avulse a tooth or lacerate the gingiva. The lips and tongue can also be contused or lacerated during laryngoscopy. Aside from the obvious detriment of harming the patient, excessive bleeding from such an injury can make intubation much more difficult. Improper insertion of the tube can cause permanent damage to the vocal cords, resulting in lifelong abnormalities of the voice. Therefore, the tube must never be forced.

# Section 10

10.2 Rapid Sequence Intubation

Aspiration pneumonitis is another serious potential complication of emergent intubation. Any patient with a full stomach and diminished or absent upper airway reflexes (either from a depressed mental status or administration of a paralytic agent) is at risk for aspiration of stomach contents into the lungs. This is precisely the type of situation encountered (or induced) with many patients requiring emergent endotracheal intubation. Measures must be taken to prevent aspiration whenever possible. This is best accomplished by having an assistant apply cricoid pressure (Sellick maneuver) from the time that a patient first receives assisted or controlled ventilation with a BMV setup until the time that the ETT is inserted into the trachea. When performed properly, cricoid pressure minimizes air entry into the stomach during BMV, greatly reducing the likelihood of vomiting, and limits reflux of stomach contents into the hypopharynx during direct laryngoscopy and tube insertion.

## THE BOTTOM LINE

- Although the task of performing an emergent endotracheal intubation in a pediatric patient is one of the more challenging undertakings a clinician can face, there are few accomplishments in medicine more rewarding than saving the life of a child in severe respiratory distress.

- Because it will be a relatively rare occurrence in the lifetime of most clinicians, the value of preparation (reading, conducting inservice meetings, assembling a pediatric airway tray) and practice (airway workshops, animal labs, mock codes) cannot be overstated.

- In the end, it is our duty as emergency care professionals to do whatever we can to ensure that any young patient who requires an emergent endotracheal intubation will undergo this procedure in the safest and most effective manner possible.[21,22,26]

---

## Section 11   Rescue Airway Techniques

# Section 11

11.1 Supraglottic Devices

Most children who require urgent or emergent airway management will respond to standard techniques such as BMV and endotracheal intubation. However, if an experienced intubator has made three unsuccessful attempts despite changing the laryngoscope blade length and type, then the intubation has failed.[26]

When standard techniques fail and a patient can neither be intubated nor mask ventilated, an alternative approach is indicated. These alternative approaches can be categorized as follows: supraglottic devices, special laryngoscopes, airway guides, and surgical techniques. A complete discussion of these techniques is beyond the scope of this chapter. However, several of the more commonly used approaches are addressed.

## 11.1 Supraglottic Devices

### Indication

These devices may be used to manage the airway in a child who cannot be intubated or effectively ventilated and who does not have upper airway obstruction.

### Contraindications

These devices are generally ineffective in patients with upper (extrathoracic) airway obstruction because they do not form a tight seal against the airway. Other contraindications include grossly distorted upper airway anatomy and significant oropharyngeal trauma. Most supraglottic airway devices do not provide ad-

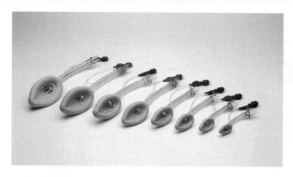

Figure 22.39 Different sizes of LMAs. Courtesy of LMA North America.

equate protection against aspiration of stomach contents. However, when intubation has failed, the benefit of effective ventilation generally outweighs the risk of aspiration.

## 11.1A Laryngeal Mask Airway

The laryngeal mask airway (LMA) was originally designed for elective surgery. However, it is an easy-to-use rescue airway device available in a variety of sizes (Figure 22.39).

### Technique

1. Choose the correct size LMA based on the child's weight in kilograms. The size for weight and the mL needed to inflate the LMA cuff are printed on the side of the device (Figure 22.40).

2. Remove the LMA from its package and inspect the cuff for damage.

3. Completely deflate the cuff. The manufacturer has developed a special deflator for this purpose. Alternatively, the LMA can be placed with the ventilating port against a flat surface (e.g., a countertop). The index and middle fingers of one hand are placed on either side of the device and over the cuff to deflate the cuff. Lubricate the cuff with water-soluble lubricant.

4. Insert the LMA into the mouth with the ventilating port facing down (onto the tongue). Guide the cuff against the palate with one or two fingers.

5. When the device cannot be advanced any further, inflate the cuff. The LMA should seat itself over the glottis.

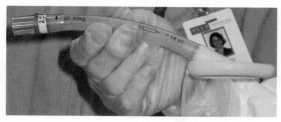

Figure 22.40 Choose the correct size LMA based on the child's weight in kilograms.

**Section**

# 11

11.1 Supraglottic Devices

11.1A Laryngeal Mask Airway

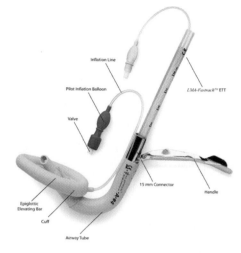

Figure 22.41 LMA-Fastrach. Courtesy of LMA North America.

6. Connect the manual resuscitator and begin ventilation.

### Alternative Technique: The Reverse Rotation Technique

Steps 1 and 2 are identical to those described for LMA use.

3. Insert the LMA into the mouth with the ventilating port facing the hard palate instead of the tongue; the black line of the LMA will be facing the patient's feet.

4. Advance the LMA and rotate the ventilating port 180 degrees into position simultaneously.

5. Inflate the cuff and begin ventilation.

The LMA comes in two styles. The standard LMA is designed to serve as a supraglottic ventilation tool, although some have described ways to use this device as a "bridge" to intubation. A newer device is the intubating LMA (LMA-Fastrach, The Laryngeal Mask

## LMA–Fastrach Insertion

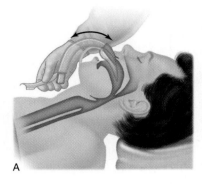

A

Figure 22.42A Deflate the cuff of the mask and apply a water-soluble lubricant to the posterior surface. Rub the lubricant over the anterior hard palate.

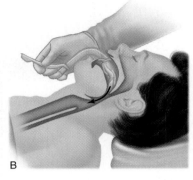

B

Figure 22.42B Ensure the curved metal tube is in contact with the chin and the mask tip is flat against the palate prior to rotation.

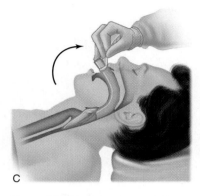

C

Figure 22.42C Swing the mask into place with a circular motion, maintaining pressure against the palate and posterior pharynx.

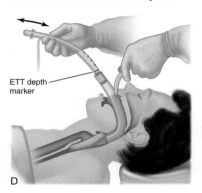

ETT depth marker

D

Figure 22.42D Visually inspect and inflate ETT to verify cuff integrity and symmetry. Deflate cuff, lubricate ETT, and pass through LMA-Fastrach tube (rotate with up/down movement) to distribute lubricant. Pass the ETT to the 15-cm depth marker or the transverse line on the LMA-Fastrach ETT, which corresponds to passage of tube tip through the epiglottic elevating bar.

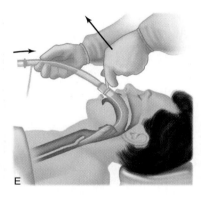

E

Figure 22.42E Use the handle to gently lift the device 2 to 5 cm as the ETT is advanced. Carefully advance until intubation is complete. Do not force. Inflate ETT cuff and confirm intubation.

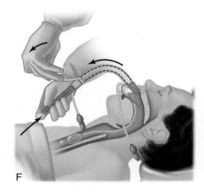

F

Figure 22.42F Remove connector and gently ease the LMA-Fastrach out over the ETT into the oral cavity. Use a stabilizer rod to hold the ETT in position as LMA-Fastrach is withdrawn over tube.

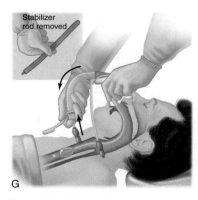

Stabilizer rod removed

G

Figure 22.42G Remove the stabilizer rod and hold onto the ETT at the level of the incisors.

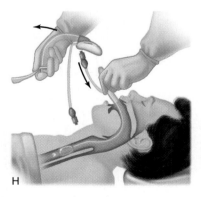

H

Figure 22.42H Remove the LMA-Fastrach completely, gently unthreading the inflation line and pilot balloon of the ETT.

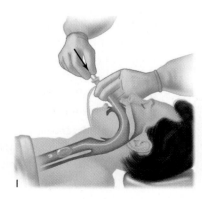

I

Figure 22.42I Replace the ETT connector.

Company Limited, Henley on Thames Oxon, UK). This device can be used like a standard LMA but is also designed to serve as a conduit for the insertion of a special flexible ETT (**Figure 22.41**). Although the Fastrach is somewhat different in appearance, it is inserted in the same manner as the standard LMA and can be used to ventilate the patient in the same way. Then, the flexible ETT can be passed into the device.

When the tip of the ETT reaches the laryngeal mask, it lifts a special lever designed to lift the epiglottis and allow the tube unrestricted access to the airway. An indicator mark can be found on the side of the ETT. When this mark reaches the proximal portion of the ventilation port, the tip of the tube will be about to pass into the airway. A rubber stabilizing rod is then attached to the proximal end of the tube and the ETT is advanced into the airway. The LMA is removed over the trachea tube and stabilizing rod, the stabilizing rod is removed, and the adapter is placed on the proximal end of the ETT. An $ETCO_2$ detector should be used to demonstrate that the ETT is in the airway. Then ventilation can begin in the standard manner (**Figure 22.42A-I**).

## 11.1B Combitube

The Combitube is a true rescue airway (**Figure 22.43**) designed specifically as an airway management tool for office-based practitioners. It is available in two sizes and is appropriate for adolescents who are at least 4 feet tall. It is not available for smaller children. The larger balloon is made of latex so this device should not be used in latex-sensitive individuals.

### Technique

1. Remove the Combitube from its package and inspect the balloons for damage.
2. Ensure that both balloons are deflated.
3. Insert the Combitube blindly into the oropharynx and advance it until the central incisors lie between the black marks on the proximal portion of the tube.
4. Inflate the smaller balloon (5 to 15 mL of air) and then inflate the larger balloon (85 to 100 mL of air).

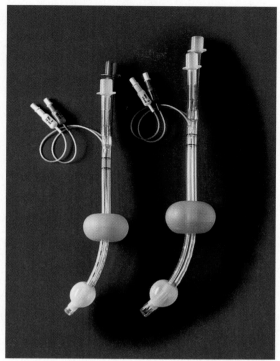

**Figure 22.43** Combitube.

5. Attempt to ventilate via the esophageal port (blue, labeled number 1). In well over 90% of cases, the Combitube is located in the esophagus. The small balloon occludes the esophagus and the larger balloon occludes the oral cavity. When this is the case, oxygen/air from the esophageal port can only enter the trachea. The chest should rise, and breath sounds should be heard over the lung fields. The arterial oxygen saturation will be maintained in the normal range. $ETCO_2$ detection can be used to confirm endotracheal ventilation.

6. If ventilation via the esophageal port is ineffective, the tube might have been inserted into the trachea. Disconnect the bag-mask device from the esophageal port and attempt to ventilate via the tracheal port (clear, shorter tube, labeled number 2). If ventilation through this port is effective, the large balloon can be deflated and the combitube can function as a standard ETT. $ETCO_2$ detection can be used to confirm tracheal ventilation.[27,28]

# Section 11

## 11.2 Specialized Laryngoscopes

### Indications

These devices may be used on children who cannot be successfully intubated using a standard laryngoscope.

### Contraindications

There are no absolute contraindications. Those devices that rely on fiberoptic technology can be difficult to use in cases of significant oral or oropharyngeal trauma. The presence of secretions and blood can obscure the viewing port. An extremely small mouth opening can also be a contraindication. When a surgical airway is urgently required, these devices cannot serve as a substitute.

## 11.2A Fiberoptic Scopes

A variety of fiberoptic scopes is available. Familiarize yourself with the device to ensure proper usage. The key issue is the relationship between the viewing port and the ETT. If the viewing port is at the tip of the stylet onto which the tube is placed, the vocal cords should be seen in the center of the field of vision. If the tube is mounted to the right of the viewing port, the cords should be placed in the right side of the visual field so that they are aligned with the position of the tube.

### Technique

1. Prepare the patient for intubation in the standard manner.
2. Assemble the laryngoscope and connect the fiberoptic light source.
3. Place the tube in the proper location on the scope.
4. Clean the distal fiberoptic port with defogging solution.
5. Suction the oropharynx.
6. Insert the laryngoscope and align the vocal cords as described.
7. Pass the tube into the cords under direct vision.
8. Remove the fiberoptic scope from the ETT (similar to removing a stylet).
9. Confirm proper ETT location using ETCO$_2$ and secure the tube.

## 11.3 Laryngoscopes With Special Blades

A complete discussion of even a few of these devices would be beyond the scope of this chapter. Most commonly, these blades allow extra manipulation (e.g., a flexible tip) for better visualization. In general, they are used exactly like standard laryngoscopes except that, if an adequate laryngoscopic view is not obtained, the tip or blade of the laryngoscope can be moved, (by depressing a lever or by some other means) to improve the view.

## 11.3A Lighted Stylet

The lighted stylet is a device that does not depend on an adequate laryngoscopic view of the airway (**Figure 22.44**).[21,28,29]

### Indications

The lighted stylet works very well in circumstances in which the laryngoscopic view might be obscured by blood or secretions. It also requires little or no movement of the neck.

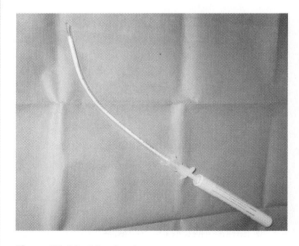

**Figure 22.44** Lighted stylet.

## Contraindications

The lighted stylet should not be used in circumstances in which the normal airway anatomy is likely to be significantly distorted or in cases of partial or complete tracheal transection.

## Technique

1. Choose a properly sized stylet for the patient.

2. Connect the stylet to the light handle and check to make sure that the light is functioning properly.

3. Lubricate the stylet and place the ETT over the stylet so that the light source is near the distal end of the ETT. Many ETTs have a small hole in the side wall of the tube. This hole is sometimes referred to as the Murphy eye. When using these tubes, the light source should be aligned with the Murphy eye of the tube.

4. Bend the distal portion of the stylet (many of these devices have a label indicating where to bend the stylet) at about a 90 to 110 degree angle with respect to the proximal portion of the stylet.

5. Prepare the patient for intubation.

6. Open the patient's mouth and lift the mandible using the nondominant hand.

7. Have an assistant dim the lights.

8. With the dominant hand, place the tube/stylet into the patient's mouth so that it is aligned with the midline of the tongue.

9. Following the tongue in the midline, advance the tube/stylet toward the airway. Initially, the handle of the lighted stylet will be nearly parallel to the patient's body, and the distal portion of the ETT/stylet will be parallel and adjacent to the middle of the tongue. As the tube is advanced, the handle of the lighted stylet is gently pulled upward to between 45 and 90 degrees with respect to the patient's body. This motion, coupled with

the proper bend in the tube, pushes the tube anteriorly into the trachea.

10. Tracheal location of the tube is indicated by a concentrated uniform glow seen in the patient's anterior neck in the region of the thyroid cartilage. A more diffuse glow or a glow that is seen laterally suggests that the tube is not located in the trachea.

11. When the location of the light suggests that the tube is within the trachea, advance the tube and stylet approximately 2 to 5 cm. Some types of lighted stylet are designed to allow the rigid portion to be withdrawn while the light source remains in the ETT. If this is the case, withdraw the rigid stylet slightly as the tube is advanced. Correct location is indicated by a glow at the sternal notch.

12. Remove the stylet and advance the tube into the trachea.

13. Confirm proper ETT location using $ETCO_2$ and secure the tube.

## 11.4 Tracheal Guides

Tracheal guides are devices designed to facilitate placement of the ETT in the same way that a guidewire is used in the Seldinger technique.[30,31] A variety of these devices may be used. Some are semirigid tubes that allow oxygenation/ventilation and $ETCO_2$ detection, while others are solid flexible guides.

Airway guides can be used in a variety of ways, as follows:

- A guide can be passed through a properly located ETT that is damaged or is too small, and then used as a guide for tube replacement.

- A guide can be passed through an LMA and into the trachea. Tracheal position is suggested by the feel as the guide crosses the tracheal rings. If the guide is hollow, tracheal location can be confirmed by $ETCO_2$ detection. Once the guide is in place, the LMA can be removed and an ETT passed below the cords and into the trachea.

**Section**

# 11

**Section**
**11**

11.4 Tracheal Guides

- If laryngoscopy affords only a partial view of the airway, the guide can be passed below the epiglottis and tracheal position and confirmed as described earlier.

### Contraindications

Airway guides are contraindicated in cases of tracheal injury.

## Section 12 Surgical Airway Techniques

**Section**
**12**

12.1 Needle Cricothyrotomy

Surgical airway techniques are the final option for management of the difficult airway. These techniques are the most invasive form of airway management and are associated with the most complications.

### 12.1 Needle Cricothyrotomy

Needle cricothyrotomy is the simplest form of surgical airway management. This technique involves the passage of a needle through the cricothyroid membrane. The needle is then used as a conduit for ventilation.[32–34]

#### Indications

Needle cricothyrotomy is indicated in the patient who cannot be intubated and who cannot be ventilated by less invasive means. It is often considered in cases of significant facial trauma and life-threatening upper airway obstruction (e.g., epiglottitis, foreign body at the level of the vocal cords).

#### Contraindications

Given that this technique is intended for use in children who might otherwise die, there are no true contraindications. Significant injury to the neck might make the procedure difficult or impossible to perform. If the needle is placed for transtracheal jet ventilation (beyond the scope of this chapter), it should be understood that the role of transtracheal ventilation in cases of complete upper airway obstruction remains controversial.[32]

#### Equipment

- Sterile gloves and mask
- Sterile prep solution
- 18- to 14-gauge (depending on the size of the child) plastic over-the-needle intravenous catheter
- 10-mL syringe
- Adapter from a 3.0 ETT
- Ventilation bag

#### Technique

1. Attach the syringe to the needle.
2. Identify the cricothyroid membrane (**Figure 22.45**).

In older children (and adults), the membrane is identified by locating the laryngeal prominence. This is the thyroid cartilage. The inferior border of the thyroid cartilage is the superior border of the cricothyroid membrane. In younger children, identification of the membrane is difficult. It might be possible to follow the trachea superiorly until the cricoid cartilage is palpated. The membrane lies just superior to the cartilage. It is also wise to palpate the area above the thyroid cartilage and attempt to identify the hyoid bone. The thyroid membrane is between these two structures. This membrane lies above the vocal cords and is not an appropriate site for insertion. Knowing the location of the thyroid membrane might prevent this complication. In the dying child, inadvertent puncture of the trachea is preferable to the alternative; the clinician should proceed with the procedure even if he

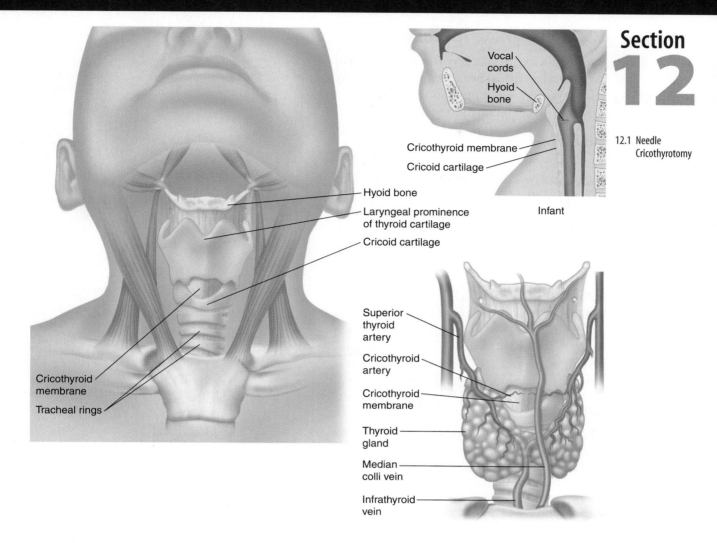

**Figure 22.45** Cricothyroid membrane.
Adapted from: Henretig FM, King CC, eds. *Textbook of Pediatric Emergency Procedures.* Baltimore, Md: Williams & Wilkins; 1997: 240.

or she is not completely confident that the cricothyroid membrane has been identified.

3. Prep the neck in standard fashion.

4. Insert the catheter with the needle directed inferiorly and aspirate while advancing. Tracheal location is indicated by aspiration of air.

5. Remove the needle, advance the catheter, and attach the adapter from the 3.0-mm ETT into the hub of the catheter.

6. Attach the ventilation bag to the adapter and begin ventilation, taking care not to kink the catheter. Ideally, a designated team member should hold the catheter hub securely to prevent it from kinking. There will be significant resistance to bag ventilation, but adequate ventilation can usually be provided (i.e., the bag must be squeezed very hard to deliver a sufficient tidal volume to make the chest rise).

## Complications and Pitfalls

Tracheal puncture can lead to subcutaneous emphysema. Likewise, vascular structures can be injured, with resultant bleeding. If the puncture site is infected or if sterile technique is not used, the patient can develop an airway infection.

## Section 12

## 12.2 Retrograde Intubation

Retrograde intubation involves the passage of a guidewire into the airway through the cricothyroid membrane and then using this guide to direct an ETT into the trachea.[21,33,34]

### Indications

Retrograde intubation is most useful in an awake, sedated patient with a predicted difficult airway. It can be used to secure the airway in the "cannot intubate/can ventilate" situation; however, it is fairly time-consuming, so it would be difficult to use this procedure in such a situation.

### Contraindications

This technique should not be used when the anatomy of the neck is severely distorted, when there is a known obstruction that will prevent passage of the ETT, or when the skin overlying the cricothyroid membrane is infected.

### Equipment

All or most of the necessary equipment can be found in a commercial retrograde intubation kit. If such a kit is unavailable, the following equipment is required:

- Sterile gloves and drapes
- Sterile prep solution
- 18- to 14-gauge over-the-needle catheter
- Syringe
- Guidewire—must have a flexible tip and be of sufficient length
- Kelly clamp or needle drivers (at least two)
- Magill forceps
- ETT
- Introducer (optional)

### Technique

1. Prepare for and perform the procedure as described for needle cricothyrotomy.
2. Once the catheter is located within the trachea, it should be directed superiorly (Figure 22.46A).
3. Insert the flexible tip of the guidewire into the hub of the catheter and advance

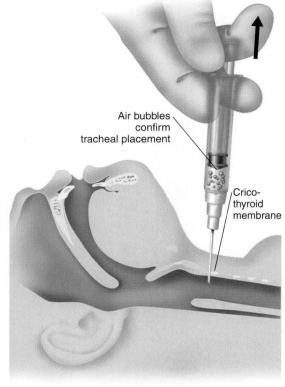

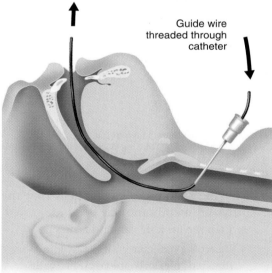

Air bubbles confirm tracheal placement

Cricothyroid membrane

Guide wire threaded through catheter

**Figure 22.46A** Guidewire threaded through catheter. Adapted from: Henretig FM, King CC, eds. *Textbook of Pediatric Emergency Procedures*. Baltimore, Md: Williams & Wilkins; 1997: 218.

it superiorly until the wire can be visualized in the hypopharynx or mouth.

4. Grasp the wire with clamps or Magill forceps and bring it out of the oral cavity,

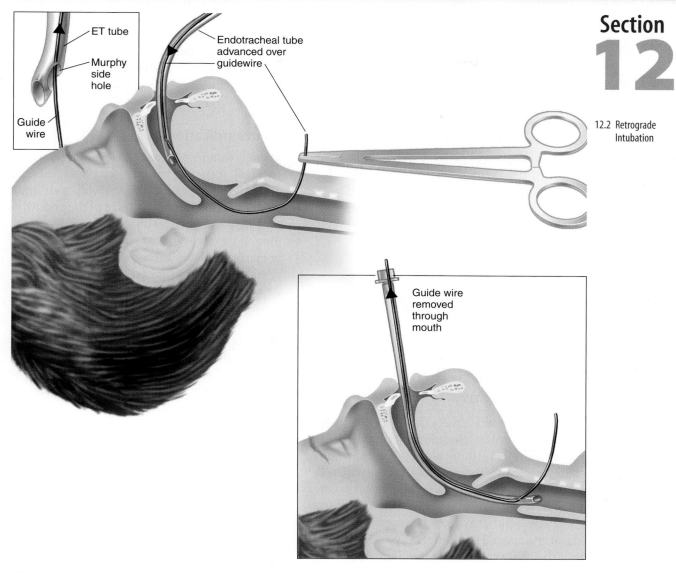

**Figure 22.46B** Advance guidewire.
Adapted from: Henretig FM, King CC, eds. *Textbook of Pediatric Emergency Procedures.* Baltimore, Md: Williams & Wilkins; 1997: 219.

then continue to advance the guidewire until sufficient wire extends from the oral cavity to allow for ETT placement (**Figure 22.46B**).

5. Optional step—pass an introducer over the wire and down the airway until it will not advance further. "Tenting" of the skin overlying the cricothyroid membrane might be noted as the tip of the tube pushes up against the small hole in the cricothyroid membrane.

6. Pass the ETT over the wire or introducer and down the airway. Some experts recommend passing the wire through the Murphy eye of the ETT (in an outside-to-inside manner) rather than through the lumen of the tube.

7. The tube might encounter resistance at the level of the arytenoids or epiglottis. In this circumstance, it can be manipulated into position by repositioning or with Magill forceps.

8. Once the ETT has reached the level of the cricothyroid membrane, the wire can be removed. Some authorities recommend cutting the wire and then removing it from the oral cavity. Others recommend simply pulling the wire out from either end. There are arguments in favor of either of these approaches. However, all agree that gentle downward pressure should be maintained on the ETT to avoid inadvertent dislodgement of the ETT during wire removal.

9. Advance the ETT into the airway and secure it in the usual manner.

## Complications and Pitfalls

Injury to the trachea or vocal cords, airway infection, and injury to nearby structures are possible.

## 12.3 Wire-Guided Cricothyrotomy

This technique is identical to retrograde intubation except that the (much shorter) wire is passed distally into the airway. An incision is then made into the membrane immediately adjacent to the guidewire (to enlarge the cricothyroid membrane opening around the guidewire), and a small tracheostomy tube resting over a special introducer is passed distally into the airway over the guidewire. Once the tube is in position, the introducer and guidewire are removed and the patient is ventilated through the ventilating port of the tracheostomy tube.[33,34]

## 12.4 Surgical Cricothyrotomy

In the older child or adolescent who can be neither intubated nor ventilated, the procedure of choice is cricothyrotomy.[33–35]

### Indications

Surgical cricothyrotomy is indicated under two circumstances. Most commonly it will be used in patients who can be neither intubated nor ventilated and in whom less invasive alterna-tive techniques cannot be used. It might also be chosen as the primary means of airway management when the anatomy of the face and oral cavity have been very distorted such that other airway management techniques are likely to fail.

### Contraindications

There is some debate regarding the age at which surgical cricothyrotomy replaces needle cricothyrotomy as the management technique of choice. Given the small size of the cricothyroid membrane in young children, most authorities agree that this technique should not be performed in patients younger than 5 or 6 years. Some recommend that this technique be used only in those older than 8 years and those younger children with the body habitus of an older child. This technique can be very difficult to perform when the anatomy of the neck is distorted. In a life-or-death situation, however, this should not be considered a contraindication.

### Equipment

- Sterile gloves and drapes
- Local anesthetic and syringe (for awake patients)
- Sterile prep solution
- Scalpel (#11 blade recommended, #15 blade optional)
- Trousseau dilator (not for use in the smaller child)
- Tracheal hook
- Curved hemostats (two sets)
- Small Mayo scissors
- Appropriately sized tracheostomy tube (Shiley 0 to 4)
- Appropriately sized ETT (4 mm to 6 mm, cuffed if available)
- Tape or sutures to secure the tracheostomy tube or ETT

### Technique

Note that several variations on this technique are described. A complete description of each of these is beyond the scope of this chapter.

The method presented below is a standard approach to the procedure.

1. Prep the skin in the usual manner.

2. Apply sterile drapes.

3. Identify the cricothyroid membrane as described above.

4. In the awake patient, if time permits, lidocaine should be infiltrated into the incision site.

5. Using the thumb and middle finger of the nondominant hand, stabilize the larynx.

6. Taking care to incise only the skin and subcutaneous tissue, make a vertical incision approximately 2 cm in length in the midline over the cricothyroid membrane (**Figure 22.47A**).

7. An assistant should be assigned to provide retraction of the skin and subcutaneous tissue using standard retractors (e.g., Army/Navy retractor or Weitlaner).

8. Palpate the cricothyroid membrane with the index finger of the nondominant hand to confirm that the incision has been made in the appropriate location (**Figure 22.47B**).

9. Bluntly dissect through the sternohyoid muscle to visualize the cricothyroid membrane (**Figure 22.47C**).

10. Using the scalpel, make a 1-cm horizontal incision into the membrane. Incision in the lower half of the membrane helps to avoid inadvertent ligation of the superior cricothyroid artery (**Figure 22.47D**).

11. Insert the tracheal hook into the superior portion of the incision and gently lift the thyroid cartilage. Once placed, the hook should be passed to an assistant.

12. Place the Trousseau dilator a short distance into the anterior portion of the wound with the blades oriented so that the incision is dilated in a cephalad to caudad manner. Alternatively, curved hemostats can be used for this purpose. These should be inserted "upside down" in a caudal direction with the tip of the jaws directed anteriorly (**Figure 22.47E**). The jaws should be placed so as to dilate the lateral wound margins.

13. Insert the tracheostomy tube or tracheal tube into the incision, confirm proper position, and secure the tube in place (**Figure 22.47F**).

### Complications and Pitfalls

There are many potential complications of this procedure. The reported incidence of these complications is approximately 20%, with most being minor. However, major hemorrhage and serious injury to the airway or esophagus can occur. Nonetheless, this technique is intended to be used in situations in which the alternative is death or severe hypoxemic injury. In such cases, the benefits of the procedure far outweigh its potential complications. Electrocautery should be avoided because high-flow oxygen is generally in use during such an emergency procedure, which might result in explosive combustion.

## 12.5 Tracheostomy Management[1]

Tracheostomy care is described in more detail in Chapter 19, Children With Special Health Care Needs. The most common complication of tracheostomy placement in a child is obstruction of the tube by hardened secretions. The following technique describes steps to assess and manage the tracheostomy for obstruction.

### Technique

1. Ensure that the ventilation bag device is connected to an oxygen source.

2. Ensure that the suction device is functioning.

3. Draw 2 mL of normal saline into a 3-mL syringe. Remove the needle (if present) from the syringe and discard the needle.

4. Open glove and catheter package(s). Apply a glove to the hand that will hold the suction catheter. With the gloved hand holding the suction catheter, connect the catheter to the suction device (connecting tubing). Maintain aseptic technique throughout the procedure.

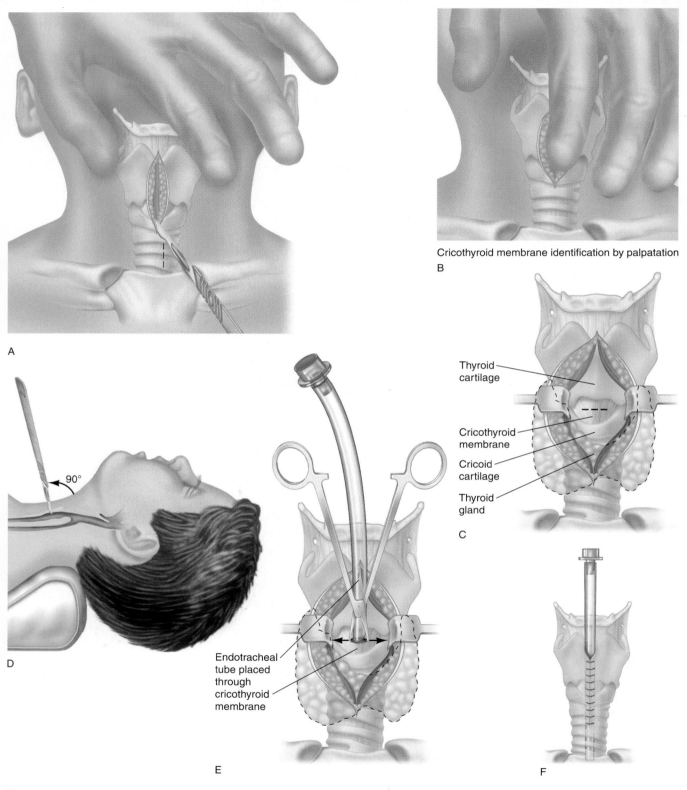

A

Cricothyroid membrane identification by palpatation
B

Thyroid cartilage
Cricothyroid membrane
Cricoid cartilage
Thyroid gland
C

90°
D

Endotracheal tube placed through cricothyroid membrane
E

F

**Figure 22.47A** Make a vertical incision approximately 2 cm in length in the midline over the cricothyroid membrane.
**Figure 22.47B** With the index finger of the nondominant hand, palpate the cricothyroid membrane to confirm the appropriate location.
**Figure 22.47C** Dissect through the sternohyoid muscle to visualize the cricothyroid membrane.
**Figure 22.47D** Make a 1-cm horizontal incision into the membrane.
**Figure 22.47E** Place Trousseau dilator or curved hemostats into wound to dilate opening to receive tracheostomy or endotracheal tube.
**Figure 22.47F** Insert the tracheostomy or endotracheal tube into the incision and secure in place.
Adapted from: Henretig FM, King CC, eds. *Textbook of Pediatric Emergency Procedures.* Baltimore, Md: Williams & Wilkins; 1997: 354.

5. Place a ventilation bag on the end of the tracheostomy tube and attempt to ventilate. If a mechanical ventilator is used, disconnect the ventilator and assist ventilation with a ventilation bag device.

6. If there is no chest rise, remove the ventilation bag device from the tracheostomy tube. Instill 2 mL of normal saline into the tracheostomy tube. Insert a sterile suction catheter through the tracheostomy tube until resistance is met. Suction up to a maximum of 10 seconds while withdrawing the catheter proximally.

7. Attempt to ventilate.

8. Repeat the procedure.

9. If assisted ventilation with a ventilation bag does not result in chest rise after suctioning, remove the entire tracheostomy device.

10. Begin BMV over the mouth with an assistant holding a gauze sponge over the tracheostomy stoma to prevent air leakage.

11. If no chest rise is achieved with BMV, insert the appropriately sized replacement tracheostomy tube or ETT (if available) into the tracheostomy stoma.

   a. ETT size is determined by using a length-based resuscitation tape, width of child's little fingernail, or the formula (Age/4) +4.

   b. If using an ETT, advance it approximately half the distance of that used for orotracheal insertion.

12. Attach the BMV device and begin to ventilate.

13. Assess for chest rise and fall. Repeat assessment and management as needed.

## THE BOTTOM LINE

- Preparation (equipment availability and practice) is crucial.
- Determine a set of rescue methods before they are actually needed.
- The skills to perform a rescue airway cannot be learned in an emergency.

# Section 13  Cardioversion and Defibrillation

## 13.1 Cardioversion and Defibrillation

### Indications

The indications for defibrillation are the presence of ventricular fibrillation or pulseless ventricular tachycardia. The indications for cardioversion include the presence of a dysrhythmia that might respond to cardioversion (e.g., supraventricular tachycardia, perfusing ventricular tachycardia) accompanied by circulatory compromise, or when chemical cardioversion has failed. Overall, life-threatening dysrhythmias are unusual in children, and ventricular tachycardia and ventricular fibrillation are especially rare. These facts, while reassuring, are a mixed blessing.

## Section 13

13.1 Cardioversion and Defibrillation

On one hand, normal children are unlikely to require cardioversion or defibrillation. On the other hand, physicians, nurses, and other health care providers who primarily treat children are less familiar with these procedures than are their counterparts who care for adults. Furthermore, health care providers should become familiar with the operation of the automated external defibrillator (AED), although it is less likely to be of benefit. The staff must also learn to recognize and treat the most common pediatric rhythm disturbances, especially supraventricular tachycardia. While this holds true for most pediatric practitioners, a growing population of children have had cardiac surgery. These children are at greater risk for significant dysrhythmias than their normal peers.

### Equipment

- Standard defibrillator/monitor or AED
- Appropriately sized paddles or appropriately sized contact pads —for children weighing less than 10 kg, the American Heart Association (AHA) recommends paddles 4.5 cm in diameter; for those weighing more than 10 kg, the AHA recommends paddles 8 cm in diameter.
- Conductive gel for use with the paddles

### Technique

Synchronized Cardioversion:

1. If the patient is conscious, administer sedation.
2. Attach monitor leads to the patient.
3. Turn on the defibrillator and select the lead displaying the tallest R waves.
4. Set the defibrillator to synchronized mode. The R waves shown on the monitor should appear to be tagged with an extra thick stripe in the center of the wave.
5. If paddles are being used, apply conductive gel to them. If contact pads are used, there is no need to apply gel because the pads have a conductive material within them.

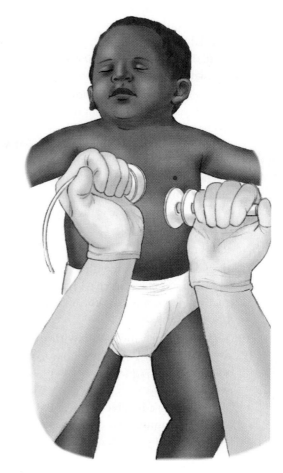

**Figure 22.48** Site for paddles on anterior chest wall.

6. Place the paddles or pads into contact with the patient's chest. Two positions are acceptable.
   a. One paddle/pad can be placed on the sternum and the other at the cardiac apex (located in the anterior axillary line just below the nipple) (**Figure 22.48**).
   b. One paddle is placed on the anterior chest over the heart and the other on the posterior chest and aligned with the first (**Figure 22.49**).
7. Ensure that the pads are not touching each other and are not connected by conductive material.
8. Charge the unit. For cardioversion, the initial charge selected is 0.5 J/kg. The

energy is doubled and then remains constant at this level for each subsequent attempt.

9. Ensure that the patient is not touching any metal parts of the bed.

10. Initiate a "clearing chant." Say, "I am going to shock on three."

    a. "One. I am clear." The operator should make certain that he or she is not touching the patient or the bed.

    b. "Two. You are clear." The operator should ensure that all other personnel are not in contact with the bed or patient.

    c. "Three. Everyone clear." The operator should check to make sure that everyone is indeed clear.

11. If paddles are used, press them firmly against the chest.

12. Press the discharge buttons and hold them until the shock is delivered. In synchronized cardioversion, there can be a delay of a few seconds before the dose of electricity is delivered.

13. After the cardioversion attempt, check the patient's rhythm to determine the need, if any, for further treatment.

14. If necessary, double the energy level, recharge the unit, and make another attempt.

## 13.2 Automated External Defibrillator[36,37]

The automated external defibrillator represents a significant advance in the care of patients with ventricular fibrillation and pulseless ventricular tachycardia. The 2005 resuscitation guidelines published in *Circulation* (December 13, 2005, Volume 112, Issue 24 supplement) recommend that AEDs be used for children 1 to 8 years of age who have no signs of circulation. Ideally, the device should deliver a pediatric dose. In addition, the arrhythmia detection algorithm used in the device should demonstrate high specificity for pediatric shockable rhythms (i.e., it will not recommend delivery of a shock for nonshockable rhythms).

---

> ## KEY POINTS
>
> ### Performing Defibrillation or Cardioversion
>
> - Defibrillation is indicated for ventricular fibrillation and pulseless ventricular tachycardia.
> - The most common indication for cardioversion in children is for unstable paroxysmal supraventricular tachycardia (PSVT) or for PSVT refractory to drug conversion.
> - AEDs are more likely to be available in a nonhospital setting.
> - Practice the "clearing chant."

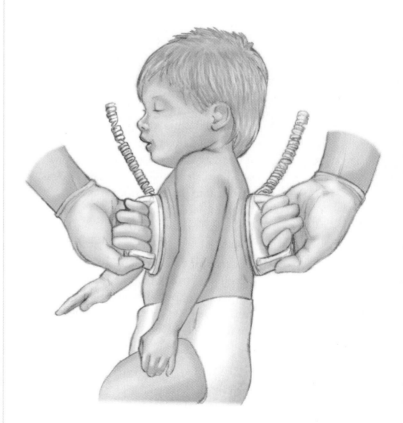

**Figure 22.49** Site for paddles with child on side and paddles placed anterior-posterior.

# Cardioversion and Defibrillation

## Section
## 13

13.2 Automated External Defibrillator

## Technique

1. Remove the AED from its storage container.
2. If not already done by the manufacturer, attach the pads to the cables and the cables to the unit.
3. Attach the pads to the patient as described for cardioversion.
4. Power on the AED.
5. Many newer units will "talk" the operator through the rest of the process.
6. If the unit is fully automated, it should begin analyzing the rhythm right away. If the unit is not fully automated, press the "Analyze" button. The AED will analyze the rhythm. This can take up to 15 seconds. During the time the unit is analyzing the rhythm, there is a small theoretical possibility that other devices producing an electromagnetic field might interfere with the unit. Therefore, cell phones and radios should not be used while the unit is analyzing. If such devices must be used, they should be kept well away from the patient.
7. If ventricular fibrillation or pulseless ventricular tachycardia is present, the unit will recommend a shock. Fully automated units may perform the clearing chant and deliver the shock without human assistance. Otherwise the process of administering the electrical shock is identical to that described for synchronized cardioversion. The discharge button on the AED is clearly labeled.
8. The machine will reanalyze the rhythm. In the presence of persistent ventricular fibrillation or pulseless ventricular tachycardia, the AED will call for another shock. Up to 3 successive shocks can be delivered

as quickly as is allowed by analysis and charging. For children 1 to 8 years old, the AHA recommends that a pediatric dose-attenuator system be used. (Source: ECC Committee, Subcommittees, and Task Forces of the American Heart Association. 2005 American Heart Association guidelines for cardiopulmonary resuscitation and emergency cardiovascular care: part 5: electrical therapies. *Circulation*. 2005; 112(Suppl I):IV-39.)

## Standard Defibrillator

1. Turn on the defibrillator.
2. Select appropriately sized paddles/pads as described for cardioversion.
3. If the patient is not on a monitor, the paddles/pads can be used for a "quick look" rhythm interpretation by placing them as described for synchronized cardioversion and turning the selector switch to the setting that allows the paddles to be used as sensing leads. As described in cardioversion, if paddles are used, they should be prepared with conductive gel prior to use.
4. If the rhythm is either ventricular fibrillation or pulseless ventricular tachycardia, then charge the machine. For defibrillation, the correct energy dose is 2 J/kg for the first attempt and 4 J/kg for subsequent attempts. The maximum dose of energy for the initial shock is 200 J; for the second, 300 J; and for the third and subsequent shocks, 360 J.
5. As with cardioversion, ensure that the patient is not touching metal parts of the bed and perform the clearing chant as described previously.
6. If paddles are used, press them firmly against the chest and discharge the device to deliver the shock.

**7.** After the shock is delivered, reevaluate the rhythm. If the patient remains in ventricular fibrillation or pulseless ventricular tachycardia, deliver up to 3 stacked shocks before beginning CPR, performing endotracheal intubation, or administering medications.

---

**THE BOTTOM LINE**

Children are not likely to need defibrillation or cardioversion, but when it is necessary, practice and familiarization with defibrillation/cardioversion equipment are essential.

**Section**
**13**

13.2 Automated External Defibrillator

---

## Section 14  Vascular Access

Intravenous fluids and medications are often required in the treatment of ill and injured children. In most cases, catheters placed into peripheral veins are sufficient. However, sometimes central venous access is required. Central venous catheters can be used to monitor central venous pressure, pulmonary artery wedge pressure, and central venous oxygen saturation. On occasion, a central venous catheter will be placed after several attempts to place a peripheral venous catheter have failed.

## 14.1 Peripheral Venous Catheter Placement

### Equipment

- Catheters—the catheter size chosen should be appropriate for the vein selected. If a standard over the needle intravenous catheter is unavailable, a butterfly or similar needle can be used as a temporary alternative.
- Rubber or elastic tourniquet
- Antiseptic soap or wipes
- Syringes
- Flush solution
- Tape
- Dressing material
- Clear dressing material (optional)
- Local anesthetic cream (optional)

- Local anesthetic injection (optional)
- 18- to 20-gauge needle (optional)

### Technique

Easily accessible peripheral veins are located in several anatomic areas. The most commonly cannulated veins are located on the dorsum of the hand (branches of the cephalic and basilic veins) (**Figure 22.50**), the antecubital fossa (cephalic vein, basilic vein, medial cubital vein) (**Figure 22.51**), the forearm (cephalic vein), the dorsum of the foot (dorsal arch veins), the medial side of the foot (saphenous vein, medial marginal vein), and the lateral side of the foot (small saphenous vein, lateral marginal vein) (**Figure 22.52A–B**). Less commonly, the external jugular veins (**Figure 22.53**) or the scalp veins are used.

**Section**
**14**

14.1 Peripheral Venous Catheter Placement

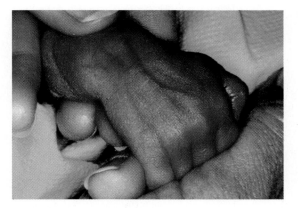

Figure 22.50 Dorsum of the hand.

14.1 Peripheral Venous
Catheter
Placement

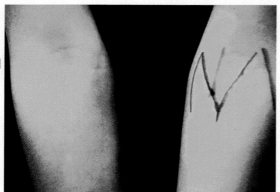

**Figure 22.51** Antecubital sites.

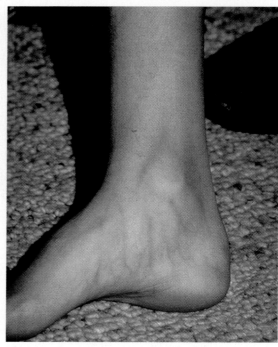

A

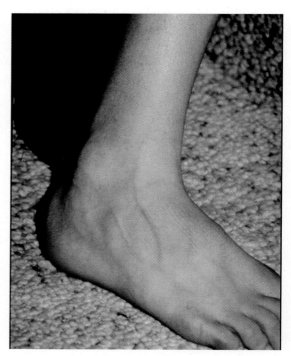

B

**Figure 22.52A–B** IV sites on the foot.

1. Select the vein into which the catheter will be placed. When time permits, local anesthetic cream can be applied to the site. This can reduce the discomfort associated with intravenous catheter placement, but takes approximately 30 minutes to 1 hour for the medication to have a significant anesthetic effect. Alternatively, a small amount of local anesthetic can be injected at the insertion site immediately before the needlestick. This method of anesthesia is, unfortunately, associated with a second needlestick.

2. Apply a tourniquet (exception: external jugular vein—see below) proximal to the site. A rubber band around the head makes a good tourniquet for scalp vein access.

3. Clean the site with alcohol or sterile preparation liquid.

4. Visualize and/or palpate the vein to be cannulated, if possible. Some veins (e.g., the saphenous vein) are reliably located near anatomic landmarks, and these veins can be accessed blindly, if need be.

5. Some physicians choose to make a hole in the dermis with a larger gauge needle prior to catheter insertion. They argue that this technique avoids damage to the plastic catheter as it passes through the skin. This step is optional.

6. Insert the catheter through the skin at a shallow angle parallel to the vein. Some

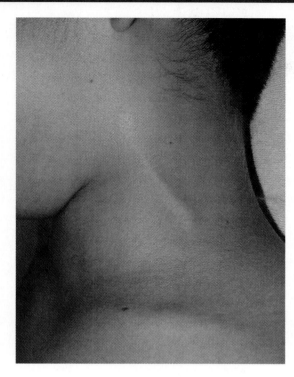

**Figure 22.53** The external jugular veins can also be used.

10. The catheter should be flushed with normal saline. During this process, it is important to observe the surrounding tissues for evidence of infiltration of fluid into the surrounding tissues. This is particularly critical for intravenous lines that will be used to administer certain medications that might cause significant tissue injury if they are extravasated.

11. Secure the line with tape or a clear plastic dressing. In younger children, it might be necessary to wrap the site in gauze or to restrain the child's upper extremities so that he or she cannot remove the intravenous catheter.[35]

authorities recommend inserting the catheter with the bevel facing down in very small or collapsed veins. This technique is intended to prevent accidental penetration of the posterior wall of the vein.

7. Advance the catheter until blood return is seen in the hub and then advance 1 to 3 mm further to ensure that both the needle and the catheter are located within the vein.

8. Using the index finger of the dominant hand or the thumb and index finger of the nondominant hand, gently advance the catheter into the vein. Blood should flow freely from the catheter, but lack of blood flow does not necessarily mean that the catheter has not been properly placed. This is especially true in the case of external jugular veins.

9. If blood is needed for laboratory studies, it might be possible to obtain it from the catheter prior to infusion of flush or intravenous fluid.

## 14.2 External Jugular Vein Cannulation

The technique for placing a catheter in the external jugular vein varies slightly from that used in cannulating other veins. The external jugular veins are located in the lateral neck (**Figure 22.54**). They are most prominent when the patient is supine (in the Trendelenburg position) or when intrathoracic pressure is high (e.g., vigorous crying). It might be necessary to place a small towel roll under the child's neck and turn his or her head away from the insertion site in order to access the vein. Additionally, the position of the mandible can interfere with placement, and the insertion needle might need to be bent slightly in order for the catheter to pass below it. In order to stabilize the vein, the skin should be taut at the insertion site. Furthermore, it might be useful to make a small hole in the skin prior to insertion of the catheter. It is not unusual to have little or no spontaneous blood return from the catheter even when it is in the correct location. However, on aspiration with a syringe, blood should return relatively easily.[39]

### Complications and Pitfalls

Peripheral intravenous cannulation is safely accomplished hundreds of times each day by medical professionals of all types. It is rela-

# Section
# 14

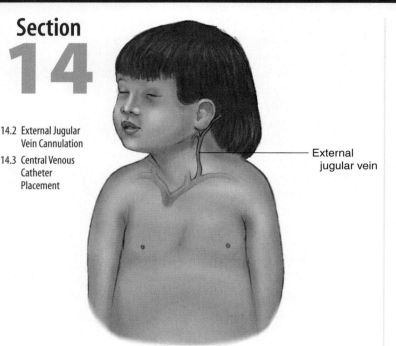

External jugular vein

**Figure 22.54** The external jugular veins are good IV sites in toddlers and older children.

tively free of serious complications. The most common and important complications are:

- Injury to a contiguous structure (e.g., an artery or a nerve)
- Extravasation of fluid into the tissues leading to compartment syndrome or, in the case of certain toxic medications, leading to damage to the tissues
- Infection
- Phlebitis/thrombophlebitis

Almost all of these complications can be avoided with attention to proper technique. However, the most serious problem with peripheral intravenous catheterization is failure to recognize when the technique has failed. Repeated attempts to obtain peripheral access in a critically ill child are not warranted. Once three or four skilled nurses and/or physicians have failed to place a peripheral catheter, an alternative method of vascular access should be chosen. When a child is in shock, it is not appropriate to delay vascular access via intraosseous access, central venous catheter placement, or venous cutdown.

## 14.3 Central Venous Catheter Placement

### Indications

Central venous access is required for central venous and pulmonary artery wedge pressure monitoring and for the placement of a transvenous cardiac pacing device. It might also be necessary for fluid infusion or blood transfusion if a peripheral IV cannot be established.[40,41]

### Equipment

- Sterile gloves
- Sterile gown and mask (optional)
- Sterile prep solution
- Local anesthetic
- Central venous catheter kit—a number of different types of kits are available. All have the use of the Seldinger over the wire technique for placement. Likewise, the type of catheter inserted varies with its intended purpose. A multiple lumen catheter might be needed to infuse several different types of vasoactive medications, while a large-bore catheter is better for infusing a large volume of fluid or as a port for inserting a Swan-Ganz catheter.
- Syringes
- Sterile flush solution
- Suture material (might be included in the kit)
- Dressing material

### Technique

The three central veins most commonly used for catheter insertion are the femoral vein, the internal jugular vein, and the subclavian vein. The insertion technique is as follows:

1. Determine the vein into which the catheter will be inserted and identify the external landmarks.

   a. Femoral vein: The femoral vein lies in the medial portion of the anterior thigh (groin). The portion of the vein distal to the inguinal ligament is most commonly used as a site for catheter insertion (**Figure 22.55**). This section of

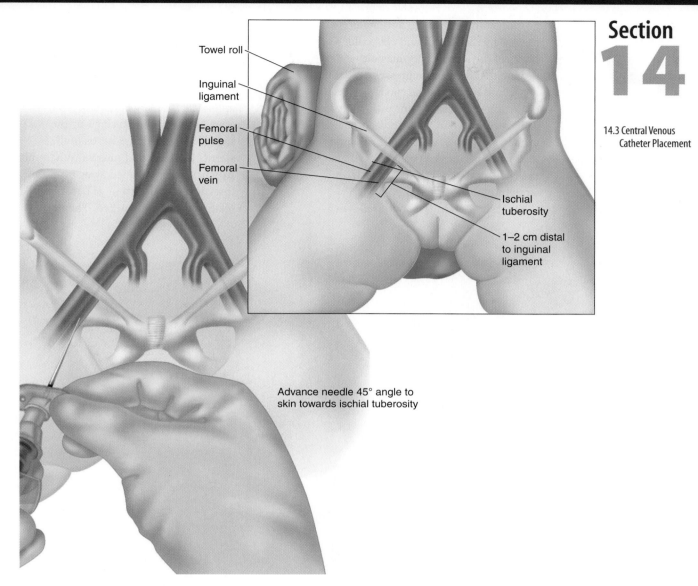

Towel roll

Inguinal
ligament

Femoral
pulse

Femoral
vein

Ischial
tuberosity

1–2 cm distal
to inguinal
ligament

Advance needle 45° angle to
skin towards ischial tuberosity

**Figure 22.55** Femoral vein.
Adapted from: Henretig FM, King CC, eds. *Textbook of Pediatric Emergency Procedures.* Baltimore, Md: Williams & Wilkins; 1997:269.

the vein is medial to and slightly posterior to the femoral artery, and both the vein and the artery are somewhat superficial. To identify the correct site for insertion, identify the arterial pulse 1 to 2 cm distal to the inguinal ligament. A towel roll placed beneath the ipsilateral buttock can improve exposure. The correct site for insertion is 1 to 2 cm medial to the femoral arterial pulse. The needle is directed along the course of the vein and at a 45-degree angle to the skin.[40]

**b.** Internal jugular vein: The internal jugular (IJ) vein is located in the anterior neck. The more cephalad portions of the vein are located somewhat deep within the neck, but the caudal portions are more superficial. The location of the vein is best understood in relation to the sternocleidomastoid muscle. For much of its course, the vein runs directly beneath the muscle. However, its more cephalad section lies just medial to the sternal head of the muscle. Its medial

# Section

# 14

14.3 Central Venous
     Catheter
     Placement

portion courses through a triangle formed by the sternal and clavicular heads of the sternocleidomastoid muscle. As the vein progresses caudally, it is found medial to the clavicular head of the muscle. The IJ veins ultimately join the subclavian veins to become the innominate veins, which in turn empty into the superior vena cava (SVC). On the right side, the IJ forms a nearly straight pathway into the SVC; therefore, the right IJ is preferred when

possible. The carotid artery lies medial to and slightly posterior to the vein. Several approaches to cannulation of the IJ have been described. Of these, the most popular is the "median" approach. The key landmark is the apex of the triangle formed by the sternal and clavicular heads of the sternocleidomastoid muscle. When the patient's head is turned away from the insertion site, this triangle becomes relatively easily identified. The needle

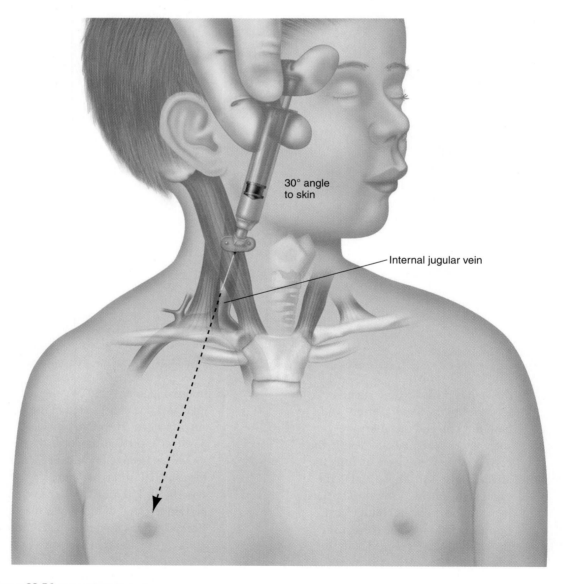

**Figure 22.56** Internal jugular vein.
Adapted from: Henretig FM, King CC, eds. *Textbook of Pediatric Emergency Procedures*. Baltimore, Md: Williams & Wilkins; 1997:271.

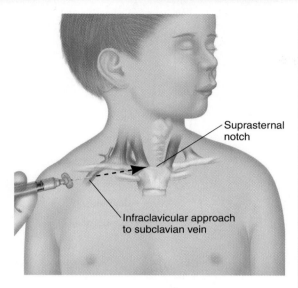

Suprasternal
notch

Infraclavicular approach
to subclavian vein

**Figure 22.57** Subclavian vein.
Adapted from: Henretig FM, King CC, eds. *Textbook of
Pediatric Emergency Procedures.* Baltimore, Md: Williams &
Wilkins; 1997:273.

is inserted at the apex at an
approximately 30-degree angle with
the skin and is directed toward the
ipsilateral nipple (**Figure 22.56**).[40]

c. Subclavian vein: The subclavian veins
lie just beneath the clavicles. They are
less often chosen as an insertion site
because attempted cannulation of the
subclavian veins is associated with
many potentially serious complications.
The most commonly used approach to
the subclavian is the so-called
infraclavicular approach. The insertion
site is the junction of the distal and
middle thirds of the clavicle. This site
should be approximately 1 cm lateral to
the lateral border of the clavicular head
of the sternocleidomastoid. The needle
is inserted into the skin, and the tip is
directed toward the sternal notch. The
needle is then guided beneath the
clavicle but is continually directed
toward the notch (**Figure 22.57**).[40]

2. Prepare the area with sterile prep solution
and apply sterile drapes.

3. Recheck landmarks and administer a small
amount of local anesthetic medication into
the skin and subcutaneous tissue without
puncturing the vein.

4. Attach a 5 to 10-mL syringe to the needle.
Insert the needle using the landmarks
above and advance the needle while
aspirating continuously.

5. The easy aspiration of dark-colored venous
blood indicates that the needle is in the
correct location. If the blood is bright red,
the syringe should be removed from the
needle. Pulsatile blood return suggests that
the needle has entered the arterial lumen.
If this occurs, the needle should be
removed and pressure held on the site.

6. Once the clinician is reasonably certain
that the needle is within the lumen of
the vein, the syringe is removed and the
guidewire inserted into the needle. The
flexible, or "soft," end of the guidewire
should be inserted into the vein first.
The guidewire should then be advanced
well into the vein. If the needle and
wire are in the proper location, there
should be almost no resistance to wire
advancement. Significant resistance
indicates that the needle and wire are
improperly located. In such cases, the
wire should be removed and the needle
repositioned or removed and reinserted.

7. When the wire is positioned, withdraw
the needle. Keep one hand firmly holding
the wire at all times.

8. Using a #11 scalpel blade (often supplied
in the kit), make a small nick in the skin
over the guidewire. Take care not to
injure the underlying vessel.

9. Pass the dilating device down the wire
and insert it fully into the vessel lumen.
As previously described, one hand must
be firmly holding the wire.

10. Remove the dilating device and insert the
central venous catheter by passing it down
the guidewire and into the vessel. A slight
twisting motion can facilitate placement.

11. Remove the guidewire and confirm
proper location by aspirating blood from
the catheter.

12. Infuse fluids into the catheter to keep the
lumen patent and secure the catheter in
place with sutures. Apply a sterile
dressing to the site.

# Section 14

## 14.4 Umbilical Vein Catheterization[1]

Umbilical vein catheterization should be considered as a potential intravenous access site in infants up to 2 weeks old. The procedure is indicated for neonates with shock or cardiopulmonary failure.

### Equipment

- 5 or 8 French catheter, or a 5 French feeding tube
- 10-mL syringe
- Umbilical cord tape or suture to tie the base of the cord
- Flush solution

### Technique

1. Place the infant beneath a radiant warmer and restrain the extremities.
2. Prepare the abdomen and umbilicus with antiseptic solution (surgical prep).
3. Drape the umbilical area in a sterile manner. The infant's head is exposed for observation.
4. To anchor the line after placement, place a constricting loop of umbilical tape at the base of the cord. Using a scalpel blade, trim the umbilical cord to 1 to 2 cm above skin surface.
5. Identify the umbilical vessels. The umbilical vein is a single, thin-walled, large-diameter lumen, usually located at 12 o'clock. The arteries are paired and have thicker walls with a small-diameter lumen (**Figure 22.58**).
6. Obtain an umbilical vascular catheter (5 Fr). Flush the catheter with heparinized saline (1 unit per mL) and attach it to a 3-way stopcock.
7. Measure and mark 5 cm from the tip of the catheter.
8. Close the ends of a pair of smooth forceps, then insert the end into the lumen of the umbilical vein. Dilate the opening by allowing the ends of the forceps to separate, then insert the

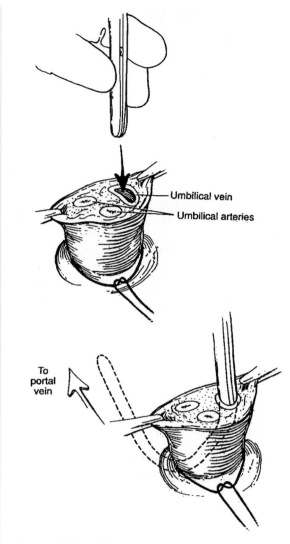

**Figure 22.58** Umbilical vein catheterization.

catheter into the lumen of the umbilical vein and advance it gently toward the liver for 4 to 5 cm or until blood return is noted.

9. If resistance to advancement of the catheter is encountered, the tip might be in the portal vein or the ductus venosus. The catheter should be pulled back until blood can be withdrawn smoothly.
10. Remove the catheter when resuscitation is complete and peripheral vascular access has been obtained.

## Complications and Pitfalls

Central venous catheterization is an invasive form of vascular access, and many potential complications are associated with this technique. Some of these potential complications are common to all sites of insertion, while others are site specific. The complications common to all insertion sites are as follows:

- Arterial injury: The most common complication of this technique is accidental puncture and/or cannulation of the adjacent artery. In most cases, this results in a minor injury to the artery that can be easily managed with direct pressure at the insertion site or by application of a pressure dressing. Obviously, it is much harder to control significant bleeding of one of the carotid arteries, but fingertip pressure applied directly to the site might be sufficient. Use of the vein dilator or a mishap with the scalpel can result in more serious injury to the artery, necessitating the involvement of a vascular surgeon. If possible, it is best to avoid injuring the artery.

- Infection: Central venous catheters are foreign bodies and can, like any such object, become colonized by bacteria. Central venous catheter infections can have devastating consequences, particularly in critically ill children. Furthermore, the emergence of multiple-resistant bacteria in many hospitals increases the risks substantially. Attention to sterile technique is critical. When time permits, those involved in the placement should don sterile gowns and wear masks and hats. Large sterile drapes can prevent inadvertent contamination of the guidewire and catheter prior to insertion.

- Thrombosis: Just as any foreign object can become infected, almost any foreign object can become a nidus for thrombus formation. The risk is highest with polyvinylchloride catheters and when the rate of infusion through the catheter is less than 3 mL/hr. Flushing the catheter with

heparin when it is not in use and using heparinized fluid when the rate of infusion is less than 3 mL/hr might prevent thrombus formation. Catheters made of Teflon have surface characteristics that are not conducive to the thrombus formation. Unfortunately, these catheters are also quite stiff and can injure vascular structures. Likewise, catheters that are impregnated with heparin are less often associated with thrombus formation.

- Guidewire misplacement: In rare instances, the guidewire enters the central venous circulation and must be retrieved by an angiographer or a surgeon. This complication can be avoided by ensuring that one hand remains in firm contact with the wire at all times.

- Air embolus: Allowing a bolus of air to enter the catheter can result in an air embolus when the end of the needle or catheter is open to the air and the venous pressure is low. This complication is most likely to occur when the catheter is placed into the IJ vein or the subclavian vein. An air embolus can be avoided by covering the open end of the catheter with the thumb after the guidewire has been removed, before connecting the intravenous fluids, and by positioning the patient with the insertion site slightly dependent. Such positioning has the added benefit of aiding catheter placement because it dilates the veins. Aspirating the catheter before flushing will remove air within the catheter. Older patients can be asked to perform a Valsalva maneuver during IJ and subclavian cannulation to avoid negative pressure within the vein.

## Site-Specific Complications[40,41]

- Femoral Vein: Few significant complications are associated with femoral vein cannulation. The most potentially serious complication is inadvertent penetration of the peritoneal cavity or rectum. This complication can be avoided by ensuring the site of insertion is below

# Section 14

the inguinal ligament and the needle is not directed too posteriorly or inserted too deeply.

- IJ Vein: Cannulation of the IJ vein is also relatively safe but less so than femoral vein cannulation. As previously described, inadvertent puncture of the carotid artery can be problematic. Accidental injury to the brachial plexus has also been described. The most important potential complication is accidental pneumothorax.

- Subclavian Vein: The location of the subclavian vein is such that it is possible for the needle to inadvertently penetrate the pleural space and create a pneumothorax. This complication occurs in up to 5% of attempted subclavian line placements. More skilled operators have a lower incidence of this complication, so subclavian cannulation is recommended only for those who have experience with this technique.

- Umbilical Vein Catheterization: This should be used for temporary vascular access only, and the catheter should be removed once the patient is stable and vascular access has been secured via other sites. Umbilical vein catheterization can cause hepatic thrombosis, infection, and hemorrhage due to vessel perforation.

## 14.5 Intraosseous Needle Placement

### Indications

Intraosseous (IO) access is indicated under two circumstances. In the moribund child, it might be wise to first insert an IO needle for the immediate infusion of fluids and medications and then attempt to insert an intravenous or central venous catheter. Alternatively, IO access might be required in the treatment of a child who requires urgent vascular access and when attempts to place standard intravenous catheters have failed.

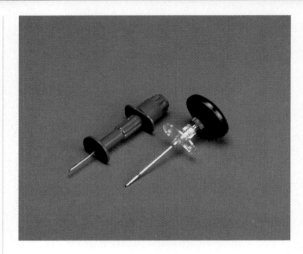

**Figure 22.59** IO needles.

### Equipment

- Antiseptic prep solution
- Local anesthetic (optional in the moribund patient)
- IO needles (**Figure 22.59**) —IO needles and bone marrow aspiration needles are made by several different manufacturers, an 18- to 20-gauge spinal needle can be used as an alternative.
- Syringe
- Flush solution (saline or sterile water)
- Gauze pads and tape (optional)

### Technique

Several bones contain active marrow. In theory, any of these can be used as a site for IO infusion. In practice, three locations are most commonly used. The three sites are the distal femur, proximal tibia, and distal tibia (medial malleolus). Of the three sites, the proximal tibia is most commonly used. The technique is as follows:

1. Select the location for insertion and identify the landmarks:

   a. Proximal tibia (**Figure 22.60**)—the landmark is on the medial side of the tibia, 1 to 2 cm below and avoiding the tibial tuberosity, approximately half the distance between the prominent

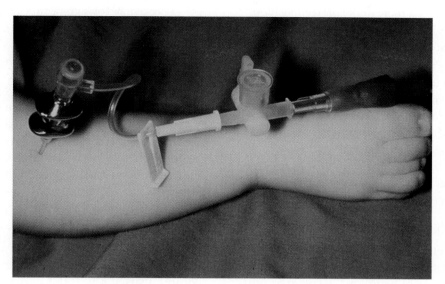

**Figure 22.60**  An IO needle in the proximal tibia, distal to the tibial tuberosity.

anterior ridge of the tibia and its medial edge.

**b.** Distal femur—the femur is a triangular bone with the point of the triangle on its anterior aspect. Its shape makes needle insertion somewhat challenging. The site of needle insertion should be 1 to 2 cm proximal to the superior border of the patella and slightly medial or lateral to the anterior ridge. The bone is flatter in these locations, and access is easier.

**c.** Distal tibia—the insertion site is located approximately 1 to 2 cm proximal to the medial malleolus in the center of the bone.

**2.** Prep the area. In the alert child, 1 to 3 mL of lidocaine may be infiltrated into the skin and down to the periosteum before proceeding. When time is of the essence, however, this step may be omitted.

**3.** Grasp the needle in the dominant hand and place it on the insertion site with the point angled slightly away from the joint space. When possible, pinch the needle itself with the thumb and forefinger of the dominant hand and allow the hub of the

needle to rest against the palm or the hypothenar area. Do not allow the patient's limb to rest in your nondominant hand, because accidental slip or penetration of both cortices of the bone can result in a needlestick injury with its attendant risk of acquiring a blood-borne disease.

**4.** Use firm downward pressure and rotate the needle back and forth. It will gradually penetrate the cortex of the bone. A sudden decrease in resistance can often be felt as the needle penetrates the cortex. This decrease in resistance might be immediately preceded by or accompanied by a popping sound. At this point, the needle may be advanced a few millimeters more to ensure placement into the marrow cavity.

**5.** Remove the trochar (or stylet) and, if possible, attempt to confirm that the needle is in the marrow space. This can be done by aspirating marrow or by infusing a sufficient volume of fluid to determine that fluid flows easily into the space and there is no extravasation of fluid into the soft tissues around the insertion site. When the device is determined to be in the correct position, it may be used to infuse medications or fluids.

6. There is some debate about the best way to secure an IO line. The needle is in a bone and, when placed in a child who is not moving, it is unlikely to become dislodged. One option for securing the IO needle that allows visualization of the site is taping the needle in a "goal-post" manner (similar to an umbilical vessel catheter).[42,43]

## Complications and Pitfalls

IO line placement is often successful and is relatively free of complications. The most significant potential problems associated with this procedure are:

- Failure to place the needle into the marrow space. This technique does occasionally fail. When this occurs, it is generally best to move to another bone rather than attempt to place the needle into the same bone.

- Fracture—there is some risk of fracture. This is especially true in infants and young children. In theory, the most significant potential complication of fracture is damage to the growth plate. In practice, this has not been reported.

- Infection—improper attention to sterile technique can result in a variety of infectious complications ranging from cellulitis to osteomyelitis. Additionally, the risk of osteomyelitis increases when the needle is left in place for more than 24 hours. This complication can be minimized by establishing an intravenous line once the child is adequately resuscitated and then removing the IO needle.

- Compartment syndrome—compartment syndrome can result from extravasation of fluid into the soft tissues or possibly from a fracture at the insertion site. The area of greatest potential risk is the proximal tibia. Insertion sites, even sites of failed insertions, should be examined periodically in the hours after the

procedure for significant edema or tension.[42,44,45]

## 14.6 Venous Cutdown

When it is impossible to secure venous access by standard methods, can be considered a surgical cutdown. The most common sites are the greater saphenous vein (at the ankle or groin), cephalic vein, or basilic vein. Of these, the two saphenous vein techniques are the most commonly used and are described here.[44–47]

### Indications

Venous cutdown is indicated when the patient requires resuscitative fluids or drugs and other methods of venous access are impossible or contraindicated. Situations in which venous cutdown might be considered include hypovolemic shock, trauma, thermal burns, and cardiac arrest.

### Contraindications

Potential contraindications to venous cutdown include:

- Known vascular or orthopedic injury proximal to cutdown site
- Major blunt or penetrating trauma to groin or abdomen
- Infection at the proposed site of cutdown
- Standard venous access is available

### Equipment

- Sterile prep solution, local anesthetic, syringes, needles
- Scalpels (#10 and #11 blades)
- Curved Kelly hemostats, straight mosquito hemostats, Iris scissors, needle holder, fine tooth forceps
- Suture material: 3-0 and 4-0 silk, 4-0 nylon; for infants, 5-0 silk and 6-0 nylon
- IV needle/catheters (22 to 14 gauge), IV extension tubing, saline flush
- Resuscitative fluids or medications
- Sterile 4×4 gauze, antibiotic ointment

## Technique: Distal Saphenous Vein Cutdown

1. Stabilize the extremity with an armboard if the patient is awake.

2. Prep the medial ankle with sterile prep solution.

3. Identify landmarks: The saphenous vein lies 1 to 2 cm superior and anterior to the medial malleolus (**Figure 22.61**).

4. Anesthetize the skin in an awake patient. (Omit in cardiac or traumatic arrest.)

5. With a #10 blade, make a 2-cm (infant) to 4-cm (adolescent) transverse superficial incision superior and anterior to the medial malleolus.

6. With the curved hemostat (tip pointing downward), bluntly dissect subcutaneous tissue down to the tibia.

7. Locate the saphenous vein against the periosteum and bluntly dissect surrounding adventitious tissue to isolate it.

8. Elevate the vein with the hemostat, grasp the silk suture in the middle with the hemostat, and pull it under the vein. Cut the suture material in half, leaving two strands perpendicularly under the vein. Bluntly dissect a space under the vein so that the two sutures are separated by at least 1 cm.

9. Tie off the distal suture (ligating the vein), leaving long ends to use as a handle to elevate the vein.

10. Leave the proximal suture untied, and use it as handle to elevate and isolate the vein.

11. Using a #11 blade, perform a venotomy (small nick) on the superficial surface of the vein. Hold both ends of the vein by the suture material and nick the vein transversely with an upward motion of the scalpel. Do not transect the vein. The venotomy must include the lumen of the vein for successful venous access. Once the lumen is entered, bleeding can be controlled by upward tension on the proximal suture, which will pinch the vein and prevent further bleeding.

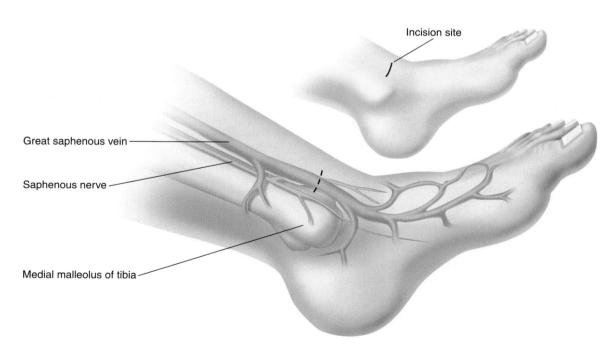

Incision site

Great saphenous vein

Saphenous nerve

Medial malleolus of tibia

**Figure 22.61** Distal saphenous vein cutdown site.
Adapted from: Henretig FM, King CC, eds. *Textbook of Pediatric Emergency Procedures*. Baltimore, Md: Williams & Wilkins; 1997:280.

## Section

# 14

14.6 Venous Cutdown

12. Insert a catheter (angiocatheter or IV tubing) into the venotomy site. Advance the catheter by reducing tension on the proximal suture. Aspirate the catheter to confirm blood return, and then flush the catheter with intravenous fluid.

13. Tie the proximal suture around the vein with the catheter in place to secure it.

14. Attach IV tubing and fluids. Medications can also be administered via this route.

15. Close the incision with fine sutures.

16. Apply antibiotic ointment and a dressing.

17. Perform routine wound care and remove sutures in 7 to 10 days. Bleeding from catheter removal can be controlled with sustained direct pressure.

## Technique: Saphenofemoral Venous Cutdown

The saphenous vein remains superficial until it joins the femoral vein in the groin. A cutdown in this region enables more aggressive fluid resuscitation. Once access is secured, the procedure is identical to the distal saphenous procedure described earlier.

1. Thoroughly cleanse the groin area with a sterile prep solution.

2. Identify the landmarks. The saphenous vein at the groin is located medial to the femoral artery and vein, 2 to 4 cm inferior to the inguinal ligament and near the junction of the thigh crease and the scrotal or labial folds (Figure 22.62).

3. Anesthetize the area if indicated.

4. Make a 4-cm to 6-cm superficial transverse incision.

5. Using a curved hemostat, bluntly dissect through the adventitious tissue and isolate the saphenous vein. The vein is located just below the Scarpa fascia.

6. Secure vascular access in a manner identical to that for the distal saphenous vein (steps 8 to 17, above). Larger diameter catheters can be used in the proximal location.

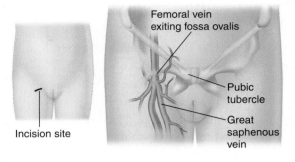

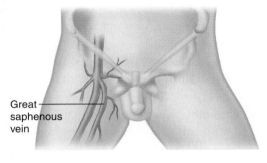

**Figure 22.62** Proximal saphenous vein cutdown site. Adapted from: Henretig FM, King CC, eds. *Textbook of Pediatric Emergency Procedures.* Baltimore, Md: Williams & Wilkins; 1997:281.

## Complications and Pitfalls

Complications of venous cutdown procedures include hematoma formation, infection, thrombophlebitis, hemorrhage, injury to adjacent structures, failure to identify the vein, and failure to cannulate the true lumen. Therefore, venous cutdown procedures should be reserved for critical patients in whom it is impossible to secure access by more conventional means. The distal end of the vein is ligated, so its future functionality is doubtful.[44–47]

## THE BOTTOM LINE

### Vascular Access in Infants and Children

- Immediate vascular access is best obtained via peripheral IV or IO.

- Central venous and peripheral vein cutdown requires more time but has other advantages.

## Section 15  Thoracic Procedures

### 15.1 Needle Thoracostomy (Thoracentesis)

When intrapleural pressure exceeds atmospheric pressure, an existing pneumothorax can progress to a tension pneumothorax. The patient is unable to ventilate due to the increased intrathoracic pressure. Cardiac function can be compromised. Absence of breath sounds, tracheal deviation, and jugular venous distention are often noted. Following the insertion of a needle to relieve pressure, a chest tube is usually inserted to maintain stability.

#### Indications

There are several indications for the performance of a needle thoracostomy. In some circumstances, this technique can be used to definitively or temporarily treat a pneumothorax. However, the emergency practitioner is most likely to use this technique when he or she suspects a tension pneumothorax based on the patient's clinical findings.[48–50]

#### Equipment

- Sterile prep solution
- 14-gauge angiocatheter (a smaller catheter or a butterfly needle may be used in infants)
- Syringe (use a large syringe for a tension pneumothorax)
- Optional stopcock

#### Technique

1. Elevate the head of the bed to 30 degrees if possible.
2. Identify the second intercostal space in the midclavicular line (alternative location—fourth intercostal space in the anterior axillary line) (**Figure 22.63**).
3. Cleanse the site with sterile prep solution in the usual manner.
4. Attach the syringe to the angiocatheter or needle and insert it perpendicular to the chest wall. In order to avoid injury to

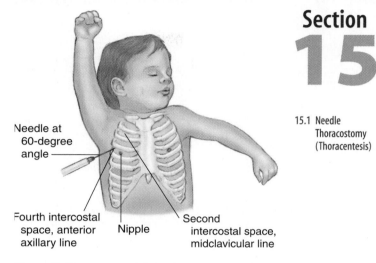

**Section**
# 15

15.1 Needle Thoracostomy (Thoracentesis)

Needle at 60-degree angle

Fourth intercostal space, anterior axillary line    Nipple    Second intercostal space, midclavicular line

**Figure 22.63**  Position the child and identify entry sites.

vascular structures (which lie under the rib), insert the needle at the superior margin of the third rib (**Figure 22.64**).

5. Apply negative pressure (aspirate) the syringe as the needle is advanced. A rush of air denotes entrance into the pleural space and partial or nearly total relief of the pneumothorax. However, for a tension pneumothorax, continued repeated aspiration might be required to improve heart rate, blood pressure, and oxygenation. Stopcock closure between syringe aspiration cycles is generally not necessary when evacuating a tension pneumothorax.
6. Listen for the return of breath sounds.
7. Perform the tube thoracostomy procedure once the patient has stabilized.

#### Complications and Pitfalls

The major complication associated with this procedure is the failure to recognize the presence of a tension pneumothorax. This diagnosis should be made clinically and not with radiographs. If the needle is inserted near the lower margin of the second rib, vascular structures can be damaged. It can be difficult or impossible to perform this procedure in large, muscular adolescents.[48]

## Section

# 15

15.2 Tube
Thoracostomy

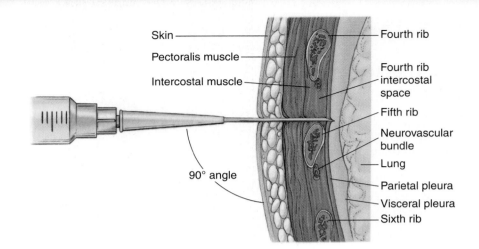

Skin
Pectoralis muscle
Intercostal muscle

Fourth rib
Fourth rib intercostal space
Fifth rib
Neurovascular bundle
Lung
Parietal pleura
Visceral pleura
Sixth rib

90° angle

**Figure 22.64** Insert the needle over the top of the rib margin in the fourth intercostal space (pictured) at the anterior axillary line, or in the second intercostal space at the midclavicular line.

## 15.2 Tube Thoracostomy

The purpose of a chest tube is to drain an abnormal collection of air, blood, or other fluid from the pleural space and permit full re-expansion of the affected lung tissue.[48,49]

### Indications

The following are indications for placement of a chest tube:

1. The presence of a pneumothorax (air collection in the pleural space) resulting from chest trauma or occurring spontaneously. If a tension pneumothorax is suspected clinically and if the patient is symptomatic, a needle thoracostomy should be performed first, followed by the insertion of the chest tube.

2. The presence of a hemothorax (blood collection in the pleural space), usually resulting from trauma.

3. Tube thoracostomy is sometimes used in the treatment of pleural effusion, empyema, or chylothorax.

### Contraindications

The following are potential contraindications to this procedure:

1. The presence of a coagulopathy

2. The presence of massive hemothorax, prior to fluid resuscitation

3. The patient with a recognized need for open thoracotomy

4. The presence of pulmonary adhesions, or blebs

### Equipment

Many centers have a prepared tray for chest tube placement.

- Sterile prep solution, sterile gloves, drapes, face shields
- Local anesthetic, syringes, needles
- Scalpel, curved Kelly hemostats (two or more), suture scissors
- Chest tube of appropriate size
- Water-sealed drainage apparatus
- Needle holder, forceps
- Suture material, 3-0 and 4-0 silk, 4-0 nylon
- Sterile petroleum jelly gauze, sterile 4×4 gauze, antibiotic ointment, adhesive tape

### Technique

1. Place the patient in the supine position. Elevate the head of bed 30 degrees, if possible.

2. Have the patient place his or her ipsilateral arm behind his or her head.

3. Provide adequate analgesia and/or sedation.

4. Prep the area in the usual manner.

5. Anesthetize the skin at the site of the planned incision (usually the fourth intercostal space) (**Figure 22.65**).

6. Anesthetize the subcutaneous tissues (i.e., muscle, periosteum of rib, pleura) with a longer needle. Direct the needle along the top surface of the rib to prevent injury to the neurovascular bundle. Aspirate while advancing the needle.

7. Make an incision 1 cm (infant) to 4 cm (adolescent) over the fifth rib at the anterior axillary line, through the skin to the muscle layer.

8. Using firm pressure, advance and dissect over the fifth rib with a curved hemostat. The tips should be pointed toward the thoracic cavity, using small opening and closing motions.

9. When the Kelly hemostat reaches the pleura, guide it over the rib until it passes through the pleura. This is heralded by loss of resistance and a rush of air or fluid.

10. Enlarge the opening by spreading the tips of the hemostat.

11. In a large child, place a gloved finger into the hole that was just created and attempt to palpate lung tissue and/or the inner chest wall. Assure yourself that this is the proper location. (Avoid placement into solid organ.)

12. Discard the trochar from the chest tube and place a closed curved hemostat into a distal side hole of the chest tube.

13. With the tip pointing toward the thoracic cavity, advance the chest tube through the incision, over the rib, and into the thoracic cavity.

14. Guide the chest tube posteriorly and superiorly until all drainage holes are within the pleural space. Posterior placement can be facilitated by rotating the hemostat, holding the chest tube 90 degrees so that the points are directed posteriorly and then opening the clamp and advancing the tube. Posterior placement is not always required. For example, if the lung is severely collapsed,

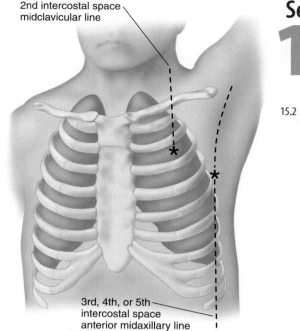

2nd intercostal space midclavicular line

3rd, 4th, or 5th intercostal space anterior midaxillary line

**Figure 22.65** Possible sites for chest tube placement. Adapted from: Henretig FM, King CC, eds. *Textbook of Pediatric Emergency Procedures*. Baltimore, Md: Williams & Wilkins; 1997:281.

the lung will re-expand when negative pressure is applied to the chest tube. Only then can it be determined whether the chest tube is posterior or anterior to the lung.

15. Connect the proximal end of the tube to the water seal.

16. Confirm proper placement by observing bubbles in the pleural drainage system when the patient coughs (if possible).

17. Consider using an autotransfusion device for patients with brisk bleeding.

18. Secure the chest tube to the skin using a purse string suture.

19. Wrap the tube with petroleum jelly gauze to prevent leakage of air.

20. Cover with a dressing.

## Complications and Pitfalls

The following are potential complications of tube thoracostomy:

1. Damage to the thoracic neurovascular bundle that lies beneath the superior rib.

2. The hemothorax might have been tamponading a bleeding vessel and its removal can result in severe hemorrhage. Clamp the chest tube to reinstate the tamponade, pending definitive surgical care.

3. Infection at the site or resultant empyema.

4. Penetration of solid organs, stomach, diaphragm, or mediastinal structures.

5. Subcutaneous emphysema resulting from incorrect placement of the tube dissecting subcutaneously instead of in the pleural space.

## 15.3 Emergency Thoracotomy

This lifesaving procedure requires technical expertise and proper judgment as to when it should be performed. Although survival rates for patients undergoing emergency thoracotomy are low, those whose underlying conditions are detected and repaired early have a chance of survival to hospital discharge.[51–53] Patients with penetrating trauma who arrest in transit or in the ED have the greatest likelihood of survival and are the best candidates for this procedure. Patients who suffer blunt trauma have little, if any, chance of benefiting from this procedure. The physician should have a clear understanding of the sequence of events that will be performed after the chest is opened. Necessary equipment should be readily available, and a surgeon should be available to provide definitive care if the patient is resuscitated. Opening the chest of a pediatric patient is a dramatic procedure that is rarely successful. In the victim of penetrating chest trauma who sustains circulatory arrest in the ED, thoracotomy can provide one last opportunity to save his or her life. Preparation and teamwork are the keys to successful performance of this procedure.

### Indications

An emergency department thoracotomy should be considered in the following types of patients:

1. The child or adolescent who is a victim of penetrating chest trauma and who sustains a circulatory arrest a few minutes before arrival or while present in the emergency department

2. The patient with penetrating chest trauma who is in shock and who fails to respond to aggressive fluid resuscitation

3. The victim of blunt trauma who sustains a circulatory arrest in the ED during the resuscitation

### Contraindications

This procedure is contraindicated in victims of blunt trauma who sustain a circulatory arrest in the field, in patients who have clearly lethal injuries (e.g., decapitation), and in those who have less severe injuries and can be managed by more conservative means or can be safely transferred to the operating room. Lack of a surgeon who can provide definitive management after the emergency thoracotomy should be considered a relative contraindication. Likewise, this procedure should not be performed in mass casualty situations because the providers should devote their efforts to the care of patients who are likely to survive.

### Equipment

A prepared tray with all necessary equipment should be available.

- Sterile prep solution, sterile gloves, drapes, face shields/masks
- Scalpel (#10 blade)
- Chest wall retractor (child and adult sizes available)
- Mayo and Metzenbaum scissors, forceps, curved hemostats, right-angle clamps, Liebsche knife or sternal saw
- Foley catheters (various sizes), sutures, pledgets, needle holder
- Chest tubes
- Vascular clamps, aortic cross clamp instrument

### Technique

1. With the patient supine, rapidly sterilize the entire thorax with a sterile prep solution.

2. Locate the left fifth intercostal space (under nipple).

3. Make an incision extending from the sternum to the posterior axillary line, following the natural curve of the rib. Incise through the skin and chest wall muscles.

4. Using Mayo scissors, cut the intercostal tissues and pleura.

5. Insert rib spreaders with the ratchet side down and the handle pointing toward the head.

6. Spread the chest open.

7. Use suction to remove any blood that might obstruct the view of the heart (consider autotransfusion).

8. Identify and repair sources of bleeding, if possible, then proceed.

9. Identify and carefully open the pericardium widely with Metzenbaum scissors to relieve tamponade, and remove clots and/or identify cardiac injury. Remember to keep the heart warm by bathing it in warm saline.

10. Repair ventricular injury by inserting a Foley catheter into the opening and inflating the balloon. The lumen can be used to infuse fluids, if necessary.

11. Other methods for cardiac repair include horizontal mattress sutures or application of sutures with Teflon pledgets.

12. Injuries to coronary arteries should be managed by applying direct pressure until definitive repair can be performed.

13. Open cardiac massage and/or internal defibrillation may be performed.

14. If abdominal injury is suspected, cross-clamp the aorta with a vascular clamp by rotating the left lung anteriorly and dissecting the aorta from the fascia of the spine posteriorly and esophagus anteriorly. Cross-clamping the aorta is done to preferentially perfuse the heart and brain with available blood. The aorta may also be occluded using direct pressure or an aortic occlusion device.

15. If no obvious injury exists, prepare to extend the incision to the right hemithorax, using sternal saw/Liebsche knife (to transect the sternum), scalpel,

and Mayo scissors. Follow the curve of the fifth rib, opening the chest in a "clam shell" manner.

16. Identify and ligate the internal mammary artery.

17. Identify and repair the source of bleeding.

18. If resuscitation is successful, consult with a surgeon regarding definitive care.

## Complications and Pitfalls

Many serious complications are associated with this procedure. However, if the procedure succeeds, a child who would otherwise have died might survive. Therefore, in properly selected patients, the potential benefits outweigh the risks. The most significant complications of thoracotomy are as follows:

1. Inadvertent cutting of breast tissue or breast bud on initial incision

2. Injury to vascular tissues: intercostal, coronary, or intrathoracic vessels

3. Infection, postoperative pericarditis, dysrhythmias

4. Injuries to the heart, lungs, and/or aorta

### THE BOTTOM LINE

**Emergency Thoracic Procedures**
- Immediate thoracentesis followed by tube thoracostomy for a tension pneumothorax
- Emergency thoracotomy for penetrating trauma–related cardiac arrest

## 15.4 Pericardiocentesis

The normal pericardial sac contains 20 to 30 cc of fluid. Larger volumes of fluid are often well tolerated, especially when the fluid accumulates slowly. In some cases, however, the volume of fluid is great enough to significantly affect cardiac function. In such cases, the patient experiences cardiac tamponade. Many patients with cardiac tamponade will eventually require surgery, but, as a temporizing measure, some of the

# Section

# 15

15.4 Pericardiocentesis

fluid can be drained percutaneously, thus restoring normal or near-normal cardiac function.[54]

## Indications

Pericardiocentesis is indicated for the emergent correction of immediately life-threatening cardiac tamponade. The mere presence of excessive pericardial fluid is generally not an indication for this procedure. Pericardiocentesis is not without risks and should only be performed when there is evidence of circulatory compromise.[54]

## Equipment

- Sedative agents (optional)
- Local anesthetic
- Sterile prep solution
- Sterile drapes
- Sterile gloves
- Mask
- 3-mL syringe and needle (for local anesthetic)
- 20 to 60-mL syringes
- Needle for procedure:
  – Infant: 1 inch (2.5 cm), 20-gauge needle
  – Older child: 1.5 to 2 inch (3 to 5 cm), 20-gauge needle
  – Adolescent: 3 inch (7.5 cm), 18- to 20-gauge needle
- ECG monitor
- Alligator clip attached to one precordial lead

## Technique

1. If time and the patient's clinical condition permit, administer sedation and monitor the patient. The patient should be in the supine position.
2. Apply sterile prep solution to the precordial area.
3. Apply sterile drapes.
4. Administer local anesthetic (as appropriate) at a point approximately 1 cm to the left of and immediately inferior to the xiphoid process.
5. Place the patient slightly into the reverse Trendelenburg position, if possible.
6. Attach the needle to the syringe and attach the alligator clip to the proximal portion of the needle. If the alligator clip is not available or if time is short, the procedure can be performed using anatomic landmarks alone.
7. Insert the needle into the skin (on the left side and just below the xyphoid) at a 45-degree angle to the skin surface and direct it toward the tip of the left scapula. In older children and adolescents, some authorities prefer to insert the needle in the left fifth intercostal space, immediately adjacent to the sternum. The needle is inserted perpendicular to the skin and advanced as described below.
8. Advance the needle slowly, aspirating continuously.
9. If fluid is obtained, the pericardial space should be drained as completely as possible.
10. If an ECG lead has been attached to the needle, contact with the ventricular wall is indicated by ECG changes. The most common manifestations are ST segment changes, QRS complex widening, or PVCs. If any of these are seen, the needle should be withdrawn slightly until the ECG change disappears. If the ECG tracing does not normalize, remove the needle. If no ECG lead is used, then assign an assistant to watch the cardiac monitor for changes.
11. Accurate needle placement can be aided by ultrasonography/echocardiography, if available.

## Complications and Pitfalls

Pericardiocentesis is associated with several potentially severe complications. However, in the setting of cardiac tamponade, the risks of the procedure are outweighed by its potential benefits. The most significant complications associated with the procedure are:

1. Pneumothorax
2. Injury to coronary arteries with subsequent ischemic injury to the heart
3. Infection
4. Injury to the heart
5. Creation of a pericardial effusion/tamponade when none was initially present[54]

# Section 16 Miscellaneous Procedures

## 16.1 Nasogastric/Orogastric Intubation

### Indications

A nasogastric (NG) or orogastric (OG) tube may be used to decompress the stomach in cases of bowel obstruction or to improve the effectiveness of mechanical ventilation by reducing intra-abdominal pressure. Likewise, NG and OG tubes may be used in gastric decontamination for accidental poisoning and for administration of activated charcoal. Finally, many children will not voluntarily drink oral contrast material for CT and will require an NG or OG tube for administration of this material. Sometimes enteral rehydration and enteral nutrition using an NG tube can be more efficient than administering fluids and nutrition parenterally.[55,56]

The choice between OG and NG intubation will be dictated by the clinical situation. For simple gastric decompression or enteral rehydration, a small NG tube is often well tolerated. NG tubes also offer the advantage of being easy to secure, and they cannot be bitten. On the other hand, gastric lavage after ingestion of particulate matter might require a large-bore tube, and such tubes often cannot be passed via the NG route. Likewise, in the patient with facial trauma, NG intubation is contraindicated. Trauma to the face can disrupt the cribriform plate, and attempted passage of an NG tube under such circumstances can result in passage of the tube into the cranium. Other relative contraindications to NG intubation include bleeding disorders, severe epistaxis, and nasal obstruction.

Neither NG nor OG intubation should be attempted blindly in the patient with a depressed gag reflex before the airway is secure. The absence of an intact gag reflex places the patient at risk for inadvertent endotracheal intubation.

### Equipment

- Phenylephrine (optional—NG)
- Viscous lidocaine or lidocaine jelly (optional—NG)
- Nebulized lidocaine (optional—NG/OG)
- 20% benzocaine spray (optional—NG/OG)
- Water-soluble lubricant
- An appropriately sized NG or OG tube
- Tape

### Technique

1. Determine the correct length of tube to be inserted. The time-honored way to accomplish this is to measure along the external surface of the body from the tip of the nose along the side of the face and down to the left side of the epigastric area. For OG insertion, the measurement is made from the corner of the mouth to the left epigastric area. An alternative method to determine depth of insertion has recently been described. This method involves the use of a height-based graph (**Figure 22.66**).[55]

2. When time permits, insertion can be made more comfortable and less traumatic by the following:

   a. If not contraindicated, a small amount of phenylephrine or similar substance sprayed into the nostril will minimize the risk of bleeding.

## KEY POINTS

**Use of OG and NG Tubes in Children**

- Advantages:
  - NG—smaller, easier to tolerate
  - OG—larger lumen for lavage and/or charcoal
- Disadvantages:
  - NG—epistaxis, can enter the cranium if the cribriform is fractured
  - OG—more noxious, patient might bite it

# Section

# 16

16.1 Nasogastric/
Orogastric
Intubation

b. Swabs coated with viscous lidocaine or lidocaine jelly may be inserted into the nostril. This process, while effective, takes several minutes.

c. For OG administration, local anesthetic spray can be used to anesthetize the mouth and throat.

d. Alternatively, a cooperative patient can inhale nebulized lidocaine in a standard nebulizer for 5 to 10 minutes.

3. Lubricate the tube well with water-soluble lubricant.

4. Using the dominant hand, insert the tube into the nose. The tube should be parallel to the floor of the nostril (i.e., directed posteriorly and not superiorly) and not directed up toward the cribriform plate. For OG insertion, the tube is placed into the mouth and directed posteriorly. In older children, a bite block might be required to prevent biting of the tube.

5. Having the patient flex his or her neck will facilitate gastric intubation.

6. Older children can be directed to swallow and, in the case of NG insertion, babies can be allowed to suck a pacifier.

7. Once the tube has been inserted to the desired length, its position should be confirmed. Traditionally, this determination is made by having one member of the team inject 60 cc of air into the tube while another auscultates the epigastric area. Aspiration of the tube with the return of gastric contents also indicates that the end of the tube is in the stomach. Cooperative patients should be asked to speak. The ability to speak in a normal voice confirms that the tube is not between the vocal cords. Similarly, infants who are crying loudly are not likely to have the tube between the vocal cords, but a muffled or hoarse cry suggests endotracheal placement.

8. NG tubes can be easily secured to the nose with standard tape. OG tubes are more difficult to secure but can often be taped to the side of the face with standard tape.

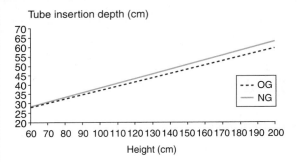

Tube insertion depth (cm)

**Figure 22.66** Estimated esophageal length for gastric tube insertion. Graph of formulas, determined on the basis of height, to determine depth of gastric tube insertion by the graphic method.

## Complications and Pitfalls

Most complications associated with NG and OG intubation are minor. The most common of these is epistaxis, although there are several more significant complications. The tube can injure the tonsil or adenoid and cause bleeding. As previously described, injury to the cribriform plate can permit the very unusual but devastating complication of intracranial tube placement. Finally, the tube can be improperly placed, either coiled in the esophagus or, worse, placed in the trachea. This latter complication can be devastating if unrecognized, especially if substances such as activated charcoal are administered through the tube.[56]

THE BOTTOM LINE

**Placement of NG and OG Tubes**

- Tubes might go where they are not wanted.
- Avoid the cribriform plate: Direct NG tube back (posteriorly), not up (superiorly).
- Use OG route in facial trauma.
- Avoid endotracheal placement. If the tube is correctly placed, the patient must be able to talk or cry loudly.

## 16.2 Catheterization of the Bladder

### Indications

Bladder catheterization is a common procedure in most emergency departments. It is the most reliable method for obtaining a sterile urine specimen in infants and children too young for a "clean catch" specimen. Bladder catheters are also used to monitor urine output in children with dehydration, hemorrhage, and other critical illnesses. In some cases, contrast material must be infused into the lower genitourinary tract for imaging studies. In fact, a urethrogram demonstrating an intact urethra is mandatory before proceeding with bladder catheterization in children with lower abdominal and pelvic trauma. Urinary bladder catheters are used for this purpose. Lastly, urinary catheters are occasionally required to drain the bladder in cases of urethral obstruction (e.g., posterior urethral valves) or neurogenic bladder or when medications have caused urinary retention.

### Equipment

- Sterile gloves, prep solution, and drapes
- Syringes
- Water-soluble lubricant
- An appropriately sized catheter

### Technique

1. Determine the size of the catheter to be placed. When a Foley catheter will be used, the size can be determined by using the standard formula for ETT size selection (Age/4) + 4 and then doubling the result. For example, a 4-year-old requires a 5.0-mm ETT and a 10 French Foley. Alternatively, one can use an 8 French catheter can be used for an infant, a 10 French catheter for a young child, and a 12 French catheter for an older child.

2. Apply sterile prep solution to the genital area. If necessary, the nondominant hand can be used to manipulate the labia or penis. In uncircumcised boys, the nondominant hand can be used to gently retract the foreskin. The dominant hand should remain sterile, and only this hand should touch the catheter. Apply sterile drapes.

3. Procedure for female patients (**Figure 22.67**):

   a. Separate the labia. (The presence of labial adhesions can make catheterization impossible. If adhesions are present, the labia should not be forced apart.)

   b. The urethra is located just anterior to the vaginal introitus. It is best visualized by lateral and anterior traction. An assistant can perform this maneuver or the clinician can use his or her nondominant hand.

   c. Insert the lubricated catheter into the urethra until urine is obtained, and then advance the catheter further to ensure that the balloon is within the bladder.

   d. Inflate the balloon and withdraw the catheter until the balloon abuts the internal wall of the bladder.

4. Procedure for male patients (**Figure 22.68**):

   a. Grasp the penis in the nondominant hand and apply gentle traction such that the shaft is straight and approximately 90 degrees from the body.

   b. Insert the lubricated catheter until urine is obtained. Resistance at the external bladder sphincter can be overcome by application of gentle constant pressure and by having the patient relax his or her abdominal musculature.

   c. Advance the catheter until the balloon is well within the bladder, inflate it, and withdraw the catheter until the balloon rests against the internal wall of the bladder.

5. If the catheter is not to remain in place, a simple bladder catheter can be used instead of a Foley, and the catheter can be removed once its purpose has been served.

## Section

# 16

16.2 Catheterization
of the Bladder

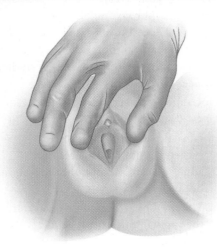

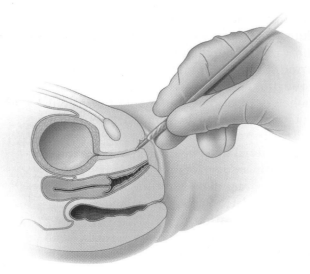

**Figure 22.67** With girls, the urethra is short and generally easily catheterized with adequate visualization of the urethral meatus.
  Adapted from: Henretig FM, King CC, eds. *Textbook of Pediatric Emergency Procedures*. Baltimore, Md: Williams & Wilkins; 1997:993.

## Complications and Pitfalls

Bladder catheterization is generally quite safe. The most common potential complication is the introduction of bacteria into the bladder and subsequent development of a urinary tract infection. Attention to sterile technique is, therefore, very important. Male patients can sustain damage to the penile urethra if an overly large catheter is inserted or excessive force is applied during insertion. Likewise, it is important to ensure that the balloon is deflated before removing a Foley catheter. Failure to return the foreskin to its normal position in an uncircumcised patient can cause a paraphimosis.[57]

## THE BOTTOM LINE

### Bladder Catheterization

- Female patients: Labial/vulvar adhesions are a contraindication.
- Uncircumcised male patients: Do not forcibly retract the foreskin.
- All patients: Determine correct catheter size and do not use excessive force in catheter placement.

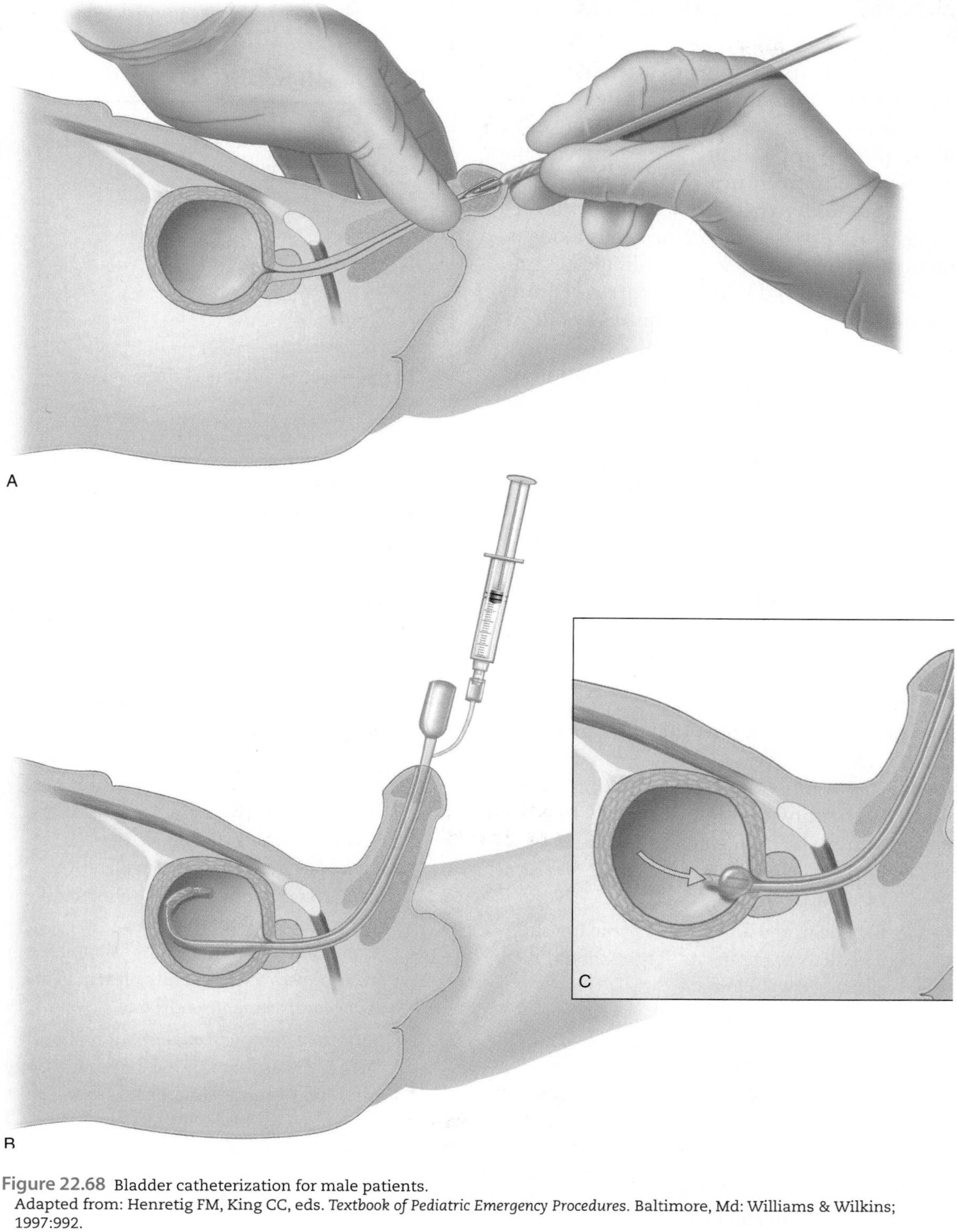

A

B

C

**Figure 22.68** Bladder catheterization for male patients.
Adapted from: Henretig FM, King CC, eds. *Textbook of Pediatric Emergency Procedures.* Baltimore, Md: Williams & Wilkins;
1997:992.

## Section 17  Orthopedic Procedures

**Section**

# 17

17.1 Compartment
Syndrome

Bone and soft tissue injuries are among the most common reasons children and adolescents are brought in for emergency treatment. Most of these injuries are minor and can be managed definitively in an ED or a physician's office. Some, however, will require the involvement of an orthopedic surgeon. If one is immediately available, he or she should be consulted and involved in the patient's care from the outset. However, some injuries result in restricted blood flow to distal extremities. Because a significant delay in restoration of circulation can leave the patient permanently disabled, the emergency physician might need to take the necessary steps to ensure adequate blood flow before the patient is transferred to the care of an orthopedic surgeon. The procedures described in this section are those required to adequately assess and, if necessary, treat extremity injuries with vascular compromise.

### Clinical Features

The presence of ischemia distal to an injury can be subtle. The prudent physician will perform a rapid but complete evaluation of the injured extremity prior to treatment. The evaluation should be performed as follows:

1. Ensure adequate exposure of the extremity.
2. Pain, fear, and anxiety will make the child less likely to cooperate. These should be addressed as follows:
   a. If possible, apply a splint that encompasses the injury and the points above and below the injury. This step alone can significantly reduce the child's discomfort.
   b. If necessary, narcotic analgesics can be administered. The goal is to reduce the child's pain and anxiety without creating sedation. Morphine sulfate (0.05 to 0.2 mg/kg) or fentanyl (1 to 3 mcg/kg) can be titrated to achieve the desired effect.

> ## YOUR FIRST CLUE
>
> **The Six P's of Circulatory Compromise to an Extremity**
> - Pain
> - Pallor
> - Paresis
> - Pulselessness
> - Paresthesias
> - Poikilothermia
>
> The presence of any one of these suggests circulatory insufficiency.

3. Briefly examine the extremity, looking for signs of circulatory compromise. Comparing the injured extremity to the contralateral, uninjured extremity is a good idea. Remember the "six P's" that suggest circulatory compromise. These are: 1) Pain out of proportion to the injury or distal to the injury, 2) pallor distal to the injury, 3) paresthesias distal to the injury, 4) paresis, 5) pulselessness (or diminished pulses) distal to the injury, and 6) poikilothermia (coolness) of the extremity distal to the injury. Presence of any one of these suggests circulatory insufficiency. Conversely, the absence of these signs does not rule out a compartment syndrome. For example, strong pulses are frequently present in an acute compartment syndrome.
4. Perform a complete examination of both the injured and uninjured extremities. Pay attention to subtle differences between the extremities and look for less obvious changes such as diminished capillary refilling time and mild sensory changes.

## 17.1 Compartment Syndrome

In some cases, injuries to the forearm or lower extremity (below the knee) will result in damage to muscle tissue. Because the muscles are encased within fascial sheaths, there is little room for the tissue to expand to compensate for edema or hematoma formation, and the pressures within the muscle compartment rise. Over time, this elevated pressure can decrease perfusion of the extremity distal to the injury. Most commonly, a compartment syndrome occurs as a result of either blunt or penetrating trauma to the extremity. Rarely, however, recurrent injury to the extremity can result in compartment syndrome as well. When the intracompartmental pressure has become high enough to cause vascular compromise, the patient might be expected to have some of the signs of impaired circulation described above. However, these are late findings (often too late); thus, the diagnosis must be made earlier than this, before irreversible injury occurs. A common misconception is to believe that ischemia occurs when the compartment pressure exceeds arterial pressure, but ischemia and potential infarction occur at intracompartmental pressures well below the arterial pressure.

## Clinical Features

Of the six P's, only pain and paresthesia are usually present during the initial presentation of a compartment syndrome. It is typical yet paradoxical that the patient will often complain of pain together with diminished sensation. Muscle tenderness not associated with a fracture or another injury is considered to be a sensitive early sign. Likewise, pain with passive or active stretching of the muscle group also suggests the possibility of a compartment syndrome. Paresis (weakness or paralysis), together with pain and paresthesia, is highly suggestive of acute compartment syndrome. Pulselessness and pallor will occur with an arterial transection or occlusion (e.g., embolization), but a compartment syndrome is actually a venous infarction, so pulselessness and pallor will be absent until infarction has already occurred (i.e., too late). Excessive swelling of the extremity should lead the clinician to consider compartment syndrome, but this sign is not always present. Splints and casts can also cause a compartment syndrome.

---

**YOUR FIRST CLUE**

**Signs and Symptoms of Compartment Syndrome**

- Extremity injury or infection or presence of cast
- Excessive swelling of the extremity
- Pain and paresthesia
- Pain on passive or active motion of the extremity
- Paresis or weakness

## Diagnostic Studies

Once a compartment syndrome is suspected, the diagnosis is made by measuring the intracompartmental pressure. Portable, battery powered devices are made exclusively for this purpose and should be used if available. However, three other methods have been described.[58–61] Intracompartmental pressures between 30 and 45 mmHg are high risk and can represent a compartment syndrome. The actual numbers are controversial, but intracompartmental pressures in this range or higher require a stat surgical consultation or surgical intervention. Failure to diagnose a compartment syndrome or intervene in a timely manner will result in irreversible extremity damage (contracture, paralysis, paresis, gangrene, chronic pain). Identification of a compartment syndrome requires immediate orthopedic consultation and surgical intervention to restore perfusion.

## Method 1—The Manometer Method

This method is the most complex of the three (and it might not work), but it has the advantage of requiring equipment available in most physician's offices and EDs.

### Equipment

- A standard mercury manometer
- Two lengths of clear intravenous line tubing at least 10 to 20 cm long
- A 3-way stopcock

- Sterile saline or sterile water
- Several sterile 18-gauge needles
- Local anesthetic
- A sterile 20-mL syringe
- 5- to 10-mL syringe
- Sterile prep material

### Technique

1. Attach one length of tubing to the manometer and then to the rear port of the 3-way stopcock (**Figure 22.69**).
2. Attach the other length of tubing to the front port of the 3-way stopcock.
3. Draw about 15 mL of air into the 20-mL syringe and attach this to the top port of the stopcock.
4. Attach an 18-gauge needle to the tubing attached to the front port of the stopcock.
5. Open the stopcock to the top and front ports and insert the 18-gauge needle into the bag or bottle of saline or sterile water.
6. Use the syringe to draw saline or sterile water into the system so that liquid fills about one half of the length of the front tubing.
7. Close the front port of the stopcock and exchange the needle for a new one.

8. Sterilize the skin over the site of needle insertion.
9. Anesthetize the site, taking care not to inject a significant amount of anesthetic into the muscle compartment, thereby increasing the intracompartmental pressure.
10. Insert the 18-gauge needle into the muscle compartment.
11. Open the stopcock to all three ports.
12. Apply steady pressure to the plunger of the 20-mL syringe. The pressure in the mercury manometer will rise.
13. The manometer reading when the saline in the front tubing just begins to move toward the needle represents the intracompartmental pressure (**Figure 22.70**).

## Method 2—The IV Infusion Pump Method

This method is the easiest but it requires an IV infusion pump that has a manometer feature to measure pressure within the IV line.

### Equipment

- An intravenous infusion pump with an internal manometer with a digital readout

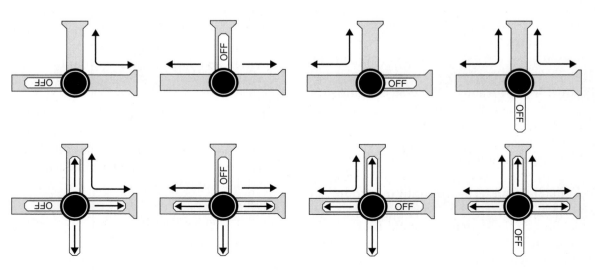

**Figure 22.69** Diagram of the stopcock.

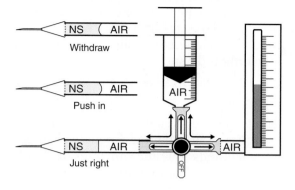

**Figure 22.70** Diagram of the manometer method.

### KEY POINTS

**Diagnosis of Compartment Syndrome**

- The classic 6 P's of compartment syndrome are a pitfall. Only the pain, paresthesia, and paresis are early signs.
- Pallor, pulselessness, poikilothermia are NOT signs of an early compartment syndrome. By the time the above occur, it is too late.
- Once a compartment syndrome is suspected, the intracompartmental pressure must be measured and immediate orthopedic consultation must be obtained.

- A length of IV tubing
- Normal saline or sterile water
- 18-gauge needles
- Sterile prep material
- Local anesthetic

### Technique

1. Attach a bag of IV fluid to the infusion pump in the standard manner.
2. Attach a sterile 18-gauge needle to the distal end of the IV tubing.
3. If the pump can move up and down, it should be moved to the level of the injured extremity. Alternatively, the bed can be raised or lowered.
4. Set the pump to infuse a small amount of fluid (e.g., 2 mL/hr).
5. Obtain a baseline reading by pressing and holding the pressure button before the needle is inserted. Ideally, this baseline number will be zero, but it might not be. If the baseline number is negative, it is important to know that some pumps place a limit on the amount of negative pressure that can be accurately reported. Lower pressures are simply reported as the lowest number that the pump can report.
6. Record the baseline pressure.
7. Prep and drape the area in the standard manner.
8. Anesthetize the skin with local anesthetic as previously described.

9. Insert the needle into the compartment and press the start or pressure button again.
10. Record the pressure obtained and then add or subtract the baseline number as appropriate to obtain the intracompartmental pressure.

## Method 3—The Arterial Line Monitor Method

### Equipment

- A standard multichannel monitor with a module for monitoring the blood pressure using an arterial line manometer
- Sterile saline or sterile water
- 18-gauge needles
- Sterile prep solution
- Local anesthetic

### Technique

1. Prep and drape the area in the standard manner.
2. Anesthetize the skin with local anesthetic as previously described.
3. Set up and zero the monitor/manometer as would be done for an arterial line.
4. Insert the needle into the compartment.
5. The intracompartmental pressure will appear where one would expect to find the arterial line blood pressure.

# Section 17

## THE BOTTOM LINE

### Compartment Syndrome

- Compartment syndrome must be recognized early when pain and paresthesia are present.
- Several methods are available to measure compartment pressure.
- Immediate orthopedic consultation and surgical intervention are required to restore perfusion.

## 17.2 Dislocations

Many dislocations are minor and are easily treated in an office or ED setting. However, some dislocations compromise the distal circulation by compressing, stretching, or tearing major arteries. These dislocations often require urgent reduction to avoid permanent disability.

### Equipment and Personnel

- Sedative medications and equipment for monitoring and resuscitation
- Splinting materials
- Assistant

## 17.3 Shoulder Dislocation

The shoulder joint is hypermobile and prone to dislocation with traction when the upper extremity is raised over the head. Common motions associated with a shoulder dislocation include forceful throwing, spiking a volleyball, and serving a tennis ball. Falling onto the shoulder area when the upper extremity is outstretched can also cause a dislocation. Most shoulder dislocations are "anterior" dislocations (the humerus is anterior to the glenoid). A bulge will be visible and/or palpable anterior to the shoulder. This might not be obvious if the patient is obese or very muscular. A fracture can mimic a dislocation or occur in conjunction with a dislocation. Thus, x-rays should be obtained to rule out a fracture prior to a reduction attempt. Posterior dislocations are uncommon and sometimes associated with severe direct trauma or a seizure. Posterior dislocations usually require reduction by an orthopedic surgeon.

### Technique

Parenteral analgesia and/or sedation is optional and is based on patient preference. There are many methods to reduce an anterior shoulder dislocation. The external rotation method is described as follows:

1. Have the patient remain supine or sitting up. The affected upper arm should be adducted against the torso. Flex the elbow to 90 degrees.
2. Grasp the patient's hand and slowly externally rotate the humerus by using the forearm as a lever (**Figure 22.71**). If the patient complains of pain, administer IV analgesia and/or encourage the patient to relax. Once the pain subsides and muscle relaxation is achieved, continue external rotation.
3. As the forearm approaches the coronal plane, reduction occurs spontaneously. This method has the advantage of not requiring strength, traction, or weights.
4. Once reduction has occurred, check for light touch sensation over the lateral portion of the deltoid, then place the patient in a shoulder immobilizer.

### Complications and Pitfalls

A branch of the axillary nerve can be injured during a shoulder dislocation. This can be assessed by checking the axillary nerve dermatome over the lateral aspect of the deltoid. Fractures can mimic a dislocation. Even minor trauma can cause a fracture if the bone is weak in this area. The proximal humerus is a common area for bone cysts that can predispose the patient to a pathologic fracture (**Figure 22.72**). Shoulder dislocations are fairly common in older teens, but they are uncommon in younger children. Young children are more likely to have a fracture. Obtaining x-rays prior to a reduction attempt is recommended (exception might be those patients who experience recurrent dislocations).

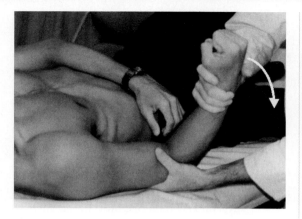

Figure 22.71 External rotation technique for reduction of an anterior shoulder dislocation.

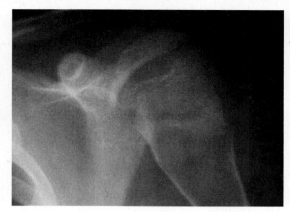

Figure 22.72 Bone cyst of the proximal humerus and an associated pathologic fracture sustained during minor trauma.

## 17.4 Elbow Dislocation

Posterior elbow dislocations can occur when a child falls onto the hand of a hyperextended arm. Adolescent males are the most common victims. In more than half of reported cases, the dislocation is accompanied by a fracture of the distal humerus, the radial head, or the coronoid process.

### Technique

1. Administer sedation/analgesia and monitor the patient.

2. Place the patient prone on an examination table. Allow the affected arm to hang over the side of the table.

3. Slightly flex the elbow and apply gentle traction to the proximal forearm. If necessary, an assistant can provide gentle countertraction.

4. Place the thumb of the hand not providing traction onto the patient's olecranon process and apply gentle forward and downward force while simultaneously gently flexing the elbow.

5. Once the dislocation has been reduced, maintain the elbow in 90 degrees of flexion with a posterior splint (**Figure 22.73**).

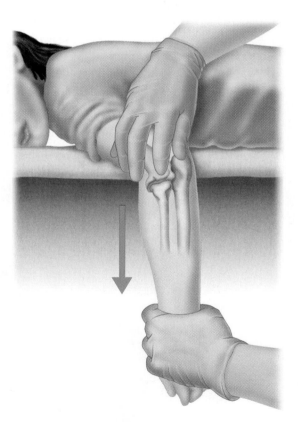

Figure 22.73 Technique for reduction of elbow joint dislocation.
Adapted from: Henretig FM, King CC, eds. *Textbook of Pediatric Emergency Procedures*. Baltimore, Md: Williams & Wilkins; 1997:1097.

## Section

# 17

### Complications and Pitfalls

The brachial artery or the median or ulnar nerve can become entrapped during reduction. Entrapment is more likely if the elbow is hyperextended or pronated during the reduction. Since associated fractures are common, these should be identified.

## 17.5 Knee Dislocation

Dislocation of the knee is a truly serious injury. The popliteal artery is relatively fixed within the popliteal fossa, and in approximately 30% to 40% of knee dislocations the artery is torn. Failure to restore adequate circulation to the knee within 6 hours is associated with an 85% incidence of limb loss. The type of dislocation depends on the relative position of the tibia and the femur. When the tibia is positioned forward relative to the femur, the patient has sustained an anterior dislocation. When the tibia is posterior to the femur, the patient has sustained a posterior dislocation.

### Technique

1. Administer sedation/analgesia and monitor the patient.

2. Have an assistant apply longitudinal traction to the extremity (Figure 22.74).

3. To reduce an anterior dislocation, lift the femur anteriorly or push the tibia posteriorly.

4. To reduce a posterior dislocation, ensure that the knee is extended but not hyperextended and then lift the tibia anteriorly.

5. After reduction, an evaluation by an orthopedic surgeon and/or a vascular surgeon is mandatory. Most authorities recommend that the patient undergo angiography as soon as possible after the reduction so that injuries to the popliteal artery can be identified and repaired.

6. The knee should be maintained in a knee immobilizer or a posterior splint after reduction.

7. If transfer to another facility is required, it should occur promptly.

### Complications and Pitfalls

As previously discussed, the most common complication is injury to the popliteal artery. Injury to the peroneal nerve is also possible. Tibial spine

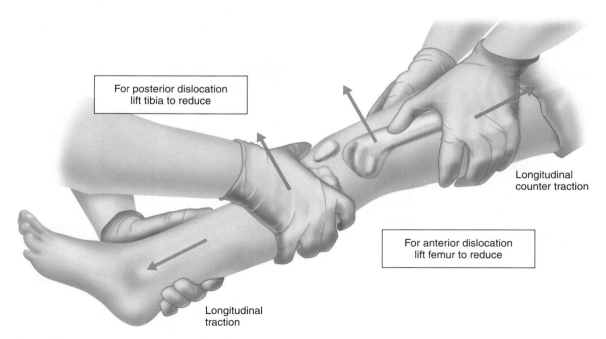

For posterior dislocation lift tibia to reduce

Longitudinal counter traction

For anterior dislocation lift femur to reduce

Longitudinal traction

**Figure 22.74** Technique for reduction of knee joint dislocation.
Adapted from: Henretig FM, King CC, eds. *Textbook of Pediatric Emergency Procedures*. Baltimore, Md: Williams & Wilkins; 1997:1098.

fractures and other fractures of the femur and tibia can occur in association with this injury. In some cases, the dislocation is not reducible. This can occur when soft tissues or bone fragments are interposed between the bones. This is a true medical emergency and warrants an urgent evaluation by an orthopedic surgeon.

## 17.6 Hip Dislocation

Like a knee dislocation, a hip dislocation represents a true medical emergency. Fortunately, this injury is rare in children. In older children and adolescents, hip dislocation often results from significant trauma, and the patient can have other serious injuries. On the other hand, younger children, presumably because they have more ligamentous laxity, can sustain a hip dislocation with less serious trauma.

Hip dislocations are potentially serious because they place the sciatic nerve and the vascular structures at risk. Posterior dislocations are less often associated with neurovascular injury than are anterior dislocations, though posterior dislocations can injure the sciatic nerve. Anterior dislocations are generally reduced in the operating room under general anesthesia. This reduction should occur within 6 hours, if possible, in order to minimize the risk of neurovascular compromise. Posterior dislocations can, however, be reduced in the ED. The technique for reduction of posterior dislocations is discussed below.

### Technique

1. Administer sedation/analgesia and monitor the patient.

2. Position the patient on the stretcher in either a prone or a supine position with the knee in 90 degrees of flexion. The hip should be slightly internally rotated and adducted.

3. Apply anterior traction to the leg in order to fatigue the muscle and overcome muscle spasm. If the patient is in the supine position, the person providing traction can either stand or kneel on the stretcher itself in order to gain mechanical advantage.

4. Using a gentle external rotary motion of the femur, guide the femoral head laterally and anteriorly over the posterior rim of the acetabulum and into proper position.

5. Once the dislocation is reduced, as evidenced by easy extension of the hip and knee, apply longitudinal traction to maintain the reduction.

6. The patient should be admitted or transferred.

### Complications and Pitfalls

Failure of the reduction is the most frequent complication of this procedure. Most failed reductions require reduction in the operating room under general anesthesia. Avascular necrosis of the femoral head complicates approximately 10% of hip dislocations.

## 17.7 Splinting

### Indications

Splints serve to immobilize and protect injured extremities. They can be used to stabilize fractures pending definitive management, immobilize injured joints, and protect sensitive wounds.[62,63]

### Equipment

- Cotton stocking/sleeve (cotton stocking material)—optional
- Soft cotton cast padding roll
- Splint materials—one of the following:
  - Commercial fiberglass or plaster splint material
  - Plaster or fiberglass casting material
  - Preformed metal or plastic splint
- Elastic bandage roll
- Sling (optional)
- Crutches (optional)

### Technique

1. Determine the length of splint material required. Measuring of the uninjured extremity is usually more comfortable for

the patient. Once the correct length of splint has been determined, the splint material can be prepared as follows:

   **a.** Commercial splint material can be cut to the desired length.

   **b.** Plaster or fiberglass casting material often comes in strips or rolls. Several layers (usually 5 to 15) are usually required to make a strong splint. Roll out the first layer to the desired length, then fold the material and roll out a second layer in the opposite direction. Continue the process until the desired number of layers has been added. If one roll is inadequate, additional rolls can be used. If the correct number of layers is reached using a part of a roll, then tear or cut the plaster at that point.

   **c.** Plastic or metal splints for arms and legs are generally preformed and sized; simply select the correct size for the patient. However, some metal finger splints are long strips of padded metal that can be cut to the correct length.

**2.** If cotton stocking material is to be used, it should be cut to the appropriate length and then applied like a sleeve. If the hand is to be incorporated into the splint, cut a thumb hole in the cotton stocking material. Cotton stocking material has the advantage of protecting the skin but the disadvantage of requiring manipulation of the injured extremity. The cotton stocking material must be loose enough to accommodate swelling of the extremity.

**3.** Roll 1 or 2 layers of cast padding over the cotton stocking material or, if no cotton stocking material has been used, directly onto the skin. As is the case with cotton stocking material, the cast padding should not be so tight as to constrict the extremity.

**4.** Wet the splint or cast material. In general, fiberglass material requires less water than plaster. Cool or cold water should be used for two reasons. First, the chemical reaction that causes the plaster to harden releases heat, and if the splint is already warm it can seem uncomfortable to the patient as it hardens. Second, hot water can accelerate the process of hardening, which might not allow enough time for the splint to be applied and shaped.

**5.** Apply the splint material and shape it into the general shape needed.

**6.** Roll the elastic wrap over the splint material. The elastic wrap should be only tight enough to hold the splint in place.

**7.** Finish shaping the splint.

**8.** Keep the extremity and splint in the correct position until the splint has hardened (30 to 60 seconds, in most cases).[63]

## 17.7A Volar Arm Splint

### Indications

Forearm fractures, Colles fractures, wrist fractures, metacarpal fractures, dislocations, lacerations.

### Technique

To place a splint on the volar surface of the palm and forearm (**Figure 22.75**), proceed as follows:

**1.** Measure from the proximal interphalangeal joint (PIP) or metacarpal-phalangeal joint (MCP) joint to:

   **a.** the mid-forearm for hand injuries

   **b.** 6 to 10 cm distal to the elbow for wrist injuries

   **c.** the midhumerus for forearm injuries.

**2.** Shape the splint with the elbow at 90 degrees flexion, wrist neutral, and the MCP joint at 45 to 90 degrees flexion.

## 17.7B Sugar-Tong Splint (Forearm)

### Indications

Forearm injuries. Can be combined with upper arm sugar-tong splint to immobilize the elbow.

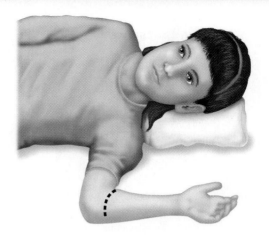

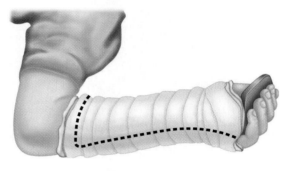

**Figure 22.75** Volar arm splint.
Adapted from: Henretig FM, King CC, eds. *Textbook of Pediatric Emergency Procedures.* Baltimore, Md: Williams & Wilkins; 1997:1033.

## Technique

To place the splint on the dorsal and volar sides of the forearm, looping around the elbow, proceed as follows:

1. Measure from the palmar PIP joint to the dorsal PIP joint, looping around the elbow.
2. Shape the splint with the elbow in 90 degrees flexion, wrist neutral, and the MCP joint in 45 to 90 degrees flexion.

## 17.7C Ulnar Gutter Splint

### Indications

Injuries to the middle, ring, and/or small finger, ulnar styloid fractures.

## Technique

To place a splint on the ulnar side of forearm, proceed as follows:

1. Measure from the tip of the longest finger included (often the ring finger), to 7 to 10 cm distal to the antecubital fossa (**Figure 22.76**).
2. Shape the splint with the wrist neutral and the MCP joint in 50 to 80 degrees of flexion.

## 17.7D Thumb Spica Splint

### Indications

Injuries to the thumb, scaphoid fracture, de Quervain tenosynovitis.

### Technique

To place a splint on the radial side of the forearm and hand, incorporating the thumb but no other digits (**Figure 22.77**), proceed as follows:

1. Measure from the tip of the thumb to 7 to 10 cm distal to the antecubital fossa.
2. Shape the splint with the wrist neutral, thumb slightly abducted and flexed. The thumb end of the splint should partially encircle the thumb to immobilize it.

## 17.7E Sugar-Tong Splint (Upper Extremity)

### Indications

Most often combined with forearm sugar-tong splint for stable elbow injuries.

### Technique

To place a splint on the medial and lateral sides of the humerus, looping around the elbow, proceed as follows:

1. Measure from 5 to 10 cm distal to the axilla, around elbow, to mid-deltoid.
2. Shape the splint with the elbow at 90 degrees.

# Section

# 17

17.7E Sugar-Tong Splint (Upper Extremity)

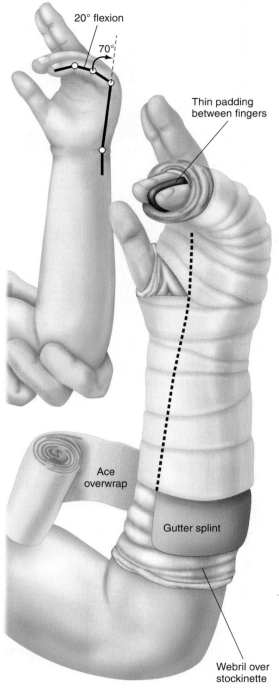

**Figure 22.76** Ulnar gutter splint.
Adapted from: Henretig FM, King CC, eds. *Textbook of Pediatric Emergency Procedures.* Baltimore, Md: Williams & Wilkins; 1997:1031.

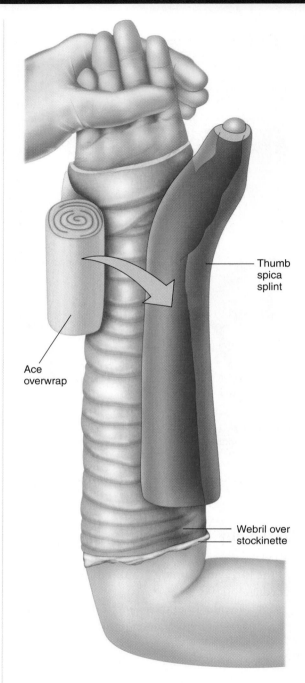

**Figure 22.77** Thumb spica splint.
Adapted from: Henretig FM, King CC, eds. *Textbook of Pediatric Emergency Procedures.* Baltimore, Md: Williams & Wilkins; 1997:1032.

## 17.7F Finger Splints

### Indications

Finger injuries.

### Technique

To place a splint on the palmar and/or dorsal sides of the finger:

1. Measuring depends on the injury. If the MCP joint is involved, the splint should extend from the finger tip to 2 to 5 cm proximal to the wrist.

2. Shape the splint with the wrist neutral, MCP joint neutral, PIP and distal interphalangeal joint (DIP) joints in slight flexion. Small finger fractures can usually be splinted with padded malleable aluminum or metal splints by curving the splint to a position of comfort and applying an elastic bandage starting at the wrist, encompassing the hand, then the injured finger with a neighboring finger, then back to the hand and wrist to finish.

## 17.7G Posterior Splint (Lower Extremity)

### Indications

Lower limb injuries. If the splint is extended above the knee, it can make a "poor man's" knee immobilizer.

### Technique

To place a splint on the plantar surface of the foot and posterior leg: (**Figure 22.78**).

1. Measuring depends on the injury. For ankle, foot, and distal tibia/fibula, the splint should extend from the great toe to 7 to 10 cm distal to the popliteal fossa. For distal femur, knee, and proximal tibia/fibula, it should extend above the knee to a point approximately half the distance from the popliteal fossa and the lower gluteal fold.

2. Shape the splint with the ankle neutral. If the knee is incorporated into the splint, it should be slightly flexed to allow for crutch walking.

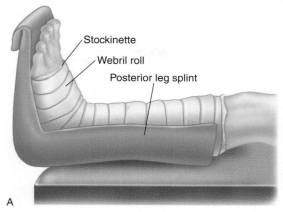

Stockinette
Webril roll
Posterior leg splint

A

**Figure 22.78** Posterior splint, lower extremity. Adapted from: Henretig FM, King CC, eds. *Textbook of Pediatric Emergency Procedures*. Baltimore, Md: Williams & Wilkins; 1997:1036.

## 17.7H Sugar-Tong Splint (Lower Extremity)

### Indications

Ankle injuries (including sprains). When combined with a posterior splint, the sugar-tong splint (also called stirrup splint) can be used for more serious injuries (**Figure 22.79**).

### Technique

To place a splint on the lateral and medial aspects of the lower leg, looping under the foot:

1. Measure about 6 to 9 cm distal to the popliteal fossa on either side of the leg.

2. Shape the splint with the ankle neutral.

### Complications and Pitfalls

The most serious complication associated with splinting is ischemic injury to the extremity secondary to constriction by the splint. This can occur because either the cotton stocking material, cast padding, or elastic wrap is put on too tightly or because it is too tight to allow for limb edema. Other complications include mechanical injury to the underlying skin associated with an improperly padded splint and (usually minor) thermal injury when the splint is hardening.

# Section 17

17.7H Sugar-Tong Splint (Lower Extremity)

17.8 Crutch Walking

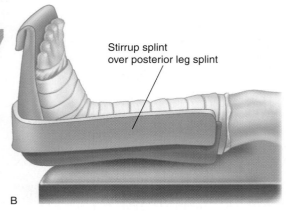

Stirrup splint over posterior leg splint

B

**Figure 22.79** Sugar-tong splint, lower extremity. Adapted from: Henretig FM, King CC, eds. *Textbook of Pediatric Emergency Procedures.* Baltimore, Md: Williams & Wilkins; 1997:1036.

## KEY POINTS

### Splinting

- Perform emergent reduction procedures before splinting.
- Knee dislocation is a true emergency to restoring blood flow.
- Obtain orthopedic consultation on dislocations and fractures that might result in neurovascular compromise.
- Review and practice splinting methods.

## THE BOTTOM LINE

### Splinting

- Splinting an injured extremity reduces pain, swelling, and complications of the injury.
- Splinting is a temporizing measure prior to definitive orthopedic care.

## 17.8 Crutch Walking

When a fracture of an extremity is suspected, put the extremity to rest and splint it in the anatomic position of function to include the joints above and below the area of injury. Immobilization will reduce pain and reduce the likelihood of further injury to soft tissues as a result of fracture fragment movement. The use of crutches can help rest lower extremity injuries.

### Fitting

- Determine the height of the patient.
- Choose child, youth, or adult size—each has the range of appropriate patient height written on it.
- Adjust the top of the crutch to a height 2 fingerbreadths below the axilla.

### Teaching Use to the Patient

- Grasp handles with both hands simultaneously and place crutches a comfortable distance in front (approximately 6 to 12 inches) and to the sides of the planted foot.
- Shift weight to the arms, swinging lower body forward while stepping ahead with uninjured leg. Keep injured leg or foot off the ground by flexing the knee.
- Do not allow the top of the crutch to come in contact with the axilla.

### Points to Emphasize to the Patient

- The purpose of crutches is to protect and rest the injured limb.
- Climb stairs only with assistance.
- Avoid slippery surfaces.
- Wear nonslip footwear. Do not wear flip-flops or sandals.
- Support body weight with the handgrips. Do not press the crutches into the armpits. Hold the elbows straight, with the tops of the crutches pressed against the sides of the upper chest.

# CHAPTER REVIEW

## Check Your Knowledge

1. All of the following statements regarding impedance pneumanography are true except:
   A. Display can be affected by patient movement
   B. Measures chest wall movement
   C. Measures respiratory effort
   D. Measures ventilation
   E. Uses the ECG monitor leads

2. Which of the following statements regarding basic airway management is correct?
   A. Chin-lift maneuver is acceptable for most trauma victims
   B. Chin-lift maneuver is acceptable for unconscious trauma victims as long as cervical spine films are normal
   C. Jaw-thrust maneuver is preferred for trauma victims
   D. Nasal airways can only be used in conscious patients
   E. Oral airways work best in conscious patients

3. Which of the following statements regarding pericardiocentesis is correct?
   A. Any pericardial effusion requires emergency drainage
   B. ECG changes, including ST segment changes and PVCs, suggest that the needle is in contact with the heart muscle
   C. Injury to the coronary arteries during pericardiocentesis has never been described
   D. Normal pericardial space contains less than 5 mL of fluid
   E. Not possible for a pneumothorax to be created during pericardiocentesis

4. Which of the following statements regarding compartment syndrome is correct?
   A. Most patients with compartment syndrome experience pain out of proportion to their clinical findings
   B. Muscle tenderness not associated with an underlying fracture or other severe injury is an important sign of compartment syndrome
   C. Pulselessness is a late finding (too late)
   D. Untreated compartment syndrome can result in permanent damage to the extremity
   E. All of the above

## References

1. Gausche M et al (eds). *APLS: The Pediatric Emergency Medicine Course Instructor Manual.* Dallas, Tx: American College of Emergency Physicians and Elk Grove Village, Il: American Academy of Pediatrics; 1998.
2. Viccellio P, Simon H, Pressman BD et al. A prospective multicenter study of cervical spine injury in children. *Pediatrics.* 2001;108:e20.
3. Hoffman JR, Mower WR, Wolfson AB et al, for the National Emergency X-Radiography Utilization Study Group. Validity of a set of clinical criteria to rule out injury to the cervical spine in patients with blunt trauma. *N Engl J Med.* 2000;343:94–99.
4. Woodward GA, Kunkel NC. Cervical spine immobilization and imaging. In: Henretig FM, King CC, eds. *Textbook of Pediatric Emergency Procedures.* Baltimore, Md: Williams & Wilkins: 1997:329–341.
5. Nobel JJ. ECG monitors. *Pediatr Emerg Care* 1993;9:52.
6. Maller JS, Gorelick MH. Use of monitoring devices. In: Henretig FM, King CC, eds. *Textbook of Pediatric Emergency Procedures.* Baltimore, Md: Williams & Wilkins; 1997: 33–37.
7. Ramsey M. Knowing your monitoring equipment. Blood pressure monitoring: automated oscillometric devices. *J Clin Monit* 1991;7:56.
8. Fuerst RS. Use of pulse oximetry. In: Henretig FM, King CC, eds. *Textbook of Pediatric Emergency Procedures.* Baltimore, Md: Williams & Wilkins; 1997:823–828.
9. Sinex JE. Pulse oximetery: principles and limitations. *Am J Emerg Med.* 1999;17:59.
10. Jones BR, Dorsey MJ. Disposable end tidal $CO_2$ detector: Minimal $CO_2$ requirements. *Anesthesiology.* 1989;71:A358.
11. Gonzalez del Rey JA. End tidal $CO_2$. In: Henretig FM, King CC, eds. *Textbook of Pediatric Emergency Procedures.* Baltimore, Md: Williams & Wilkins; 1997:829–837.
12. Scarfone RJ. Airway adjuncts, oxygen delivery, and suctioning the upper airway. In: Henretig

# CHAPTER REVIEW

FM, King CC, eds. *Textbook of Pediatric Emergency Procedures*. Baltimore, Md: Williams & Wilkins; 1997:101–118.

13. Lacher ME. Suctioning the trachea. In: Henretig FM, King CC, eds. *Textbook of Pediatric Emergency Procedures*. Baltimore, Md: Williams & Wilkins; 1997:863–870.

14. Barnes CA, Kirchhoff KT. Minimizing hypoxemia due to endotracheal suctioning: A review of the literature. *Heart Lung*. 1986;15:164.

15. American Society of Anesthesiologists Task Force on Management of the Difficult Airway. Practice guideline for management of the difficult airway. *Anesthesiology* 1993;78:597–602.

16. The American Heart Association in Collaboration with the International Liason Committee on Resuscitation. Pediatric basic life support. *Circulation* 2000;102 (suppl I): I 253.

17. Bausher JC, McAneny CM. Basic life support. In: Henretig FM, King CC, eds. *Textbook of Pediatric Emergency Procedures*. Baltimore, Md: Williams & Wilkins; 1997: 85–99.

18. Finer NN, Barrington KJ, Al-Fadley F, Peters KL. Limitations of self-inflating resuscitators. *Pediatrics*. 1986;77:1.

19. King C, Dorsey AT. Bag-valve-mask ventilation. In: Henretig FM, King CC, eds. *Textbook of Pediatric Emergency Procedures*. Baltimore, Md: Williams & Wilkins; 1997:119–140.

20. Poirier MP, Ruddy RM. Acute upper airway foreign body removal-the choking child. In: Henretig FM, King CC, eds. *Textbook of Pediatric Emergency Procedures*. Baltimore, Md: Williams & Wilkins; 1997:621–629.

21. King C, Stayer SA. Emergent endotracheal intubation. In: Henretig FM, King CC, eds. *Textbook of Pediatric Emergency Procedures*. Baltimore, Md: Williams & Wilkins; 1997:161–237.

22. Decker JM, Lowe DA. Rapid sequence induction. In: Henretig FM, King CC, eds. *Textbook of Pediatric Emergency Procedures*. Baltimore, Md: Williams & Wilkins; 1997:141–159.

23. Gerardi MJ, Sacchetti AD, Cantor RM et al. Pediatric Emergency Medicine Committee of the American College of Emergency Physicians. Rapid sequence induction of the pediatric patient. *Ann Emerg Med*. 1996;28:55.

24. King BR, Baker MD, Braitman LE et al. Endotracheal tube size selection in children: a comparison of four methods. *Ann Emerg Med*. 1993;22:530.

25. Luten RC, Wears RL, Broselow J et al. Length-based endotracheal tube and emergency equipment in pediatrics. *Ann Emerg Med*. 1992;21:900.

26. The American Heart Association in Collaboration with the International Liaison Committee on Resuscitation. Pediatric advanced life support. *Circulation*. 2000;102 (suppl I):I291.

27. Minkowitz HS. Laryngeal mask airway and esophageal tracheal combitube. In: Hagberg C, ed. *Handbook of Difficult Airway Management*. Philadelphia, Pa: Churchill Livingstone: 2000;171–183.

28. Pollack CV. The laryngeal mask airway: a comprehensive review for the emergency physician. *J Emerg Med*. 2001;20:53–66.

29. Davis L et al. Lighted stylet tracheal intubation: a review. *Anesth Analg*. 2000;90:745–756.

30. Minkowitz HS. Airway gadgets. In: Hagberg C, ed. *Handbook of Difficult Airway Management*. Philadelphia, Pa: Churchill Livingstone; 2000:171–183.

31. Nitahara K et al. Intubation of a child with a difficult airway using a laryngeal mask airway and a guidewire and jet stylet. *Anesthesiology*. 1999;91:330–331.

32. Greenfield RH. Percutaneous transtracheal ventilation. In: Henretig FM, King CC, eds. *Textbook of Pediatric Emergency Procedures*. Baltimore, Md: Williams & Wilkins; 1997:239–249.

33. Wong MEK, Bradrick JP. Surgical approaches to airway management for anesthesia practitioners. In: Hagberg C, ed. *Handbook of Difficult Airway Management*. Philadelphia, Pa: Churchill Livingstone; 2000: 185–218.

34. Walls RM, Vissers RJ. Surgical airway techniques. In: Walls RM, ed. *Manual of Emergency Airway Management*. Baltimore, Md: Lippincott, Williams & Wilkins; 2000:89–104.

35. Strange GR, Niederman LG. Surgical cricothyrotomy. In: Henretig FM, King CC, eds. *Textbook of Pediatric Emergency Procedures*. Baltimore, Md: Williams & Wilkins; 1997:351–356.

36. Tang W, Weil MH, Jorgenson D et al. Fixed energy biphasic waveform defibrillation in a pediatric model of cardiac arrest and resuscitation. *Crit Care Med*. 2002;30:2736.

37. VF treated with CPR and automated external defibrillation. In: Cummins RO, ed. *ACLS Provider Manual*, 2001. Dallas, Tx: The American Heart Association; 2001:63–73.

38. Cecchin F, Jorgenson DB, Berul CI et al. Is arrhythmia detection by automatic external defibrillator accurate for children? *Circulation*. 2001; 103:2483.

39. Bhende MS. Venipuncture and peripheral venous acccess. In: Henretig FM, King CC, eds. *Textbook of Pediatric Emergency Procedures*. Baltimore, Md: Williams & Wilkins; 1997:797–810.

40. Lavelle J, Costarino AT. Central venous access and central venous pressure monitoring. In: Henretig FM, King CC, eds. *Textbook of Pediatric*

*Emergency Procedures*. Baltimore, Md: Williams & Wilkins; 1997:251–278.

41. Goutail-Flaud MF, Sfez M, Berg A et al. Central venous catheter-related complications in newborns and infants: a 587-case survey. *J Pediatr Surg.* 1991;26:645.

42. Hodge D. Intraosseous infusion. In: Henretig FM, King CC, eds. *Textbook of Pediatric Emergency Procedures*. Baltimore, Md: Williams & Wilkins; 1997:289–298.

43. Miner WF, Corneli HM, Bolte RG et al. Prehospital use of intraosseous infusion by paramedics. *Pediatr Emerg Care.* 1989;5:5.

44. Kirkham JH. Infusion into the internal saphenous vein at the ankle. *Lancet.* 1945;2:815.

45. Gauderer MWL. Vascular access techniques and devices in the pediatric patient. *Surg Clin North Am.* 1992;72:1267.

46. McIntosh BB, Dulchavsky SA. Peripheral vascular cutdown. *Crit Care Clin.* 1992;8:807.

47. Vinci RJ. Venous Cutdown Catheterization. In: Henretig FM, King CC, eds. *Textbook of Pediatric Emergency Procedures*. Baltimore, Md: Williams & Wilkins; 1997:279–287.

48. Connors KM, Terndrup TE. Tube thoracostomy and needle decompression of the chest. In: Henretig FM, King CC, eds. *Textbook of Pediatric Emergency Procedures*. Baltimore, Md: Williams & Wilkins; 1997:389–407.

49. Miller KS, Sahn SA. Chest tubes: indications, technique, management, and complications. *Chest.* 1987;91:258.

50. Hamilton AD, Archer GJ. Treatment of pneumothorax by simple aspiration. *Thorax.* 1983;38:934.

51. Rothenberg SS, Moore EE, Moore FA et al. Emergency department thoracotomy in children: a critical analysis. *J Trauma.* 1989;29:1322.

52. Sheika AA, Culbertson CB. Emergency department thoracotomy in children: rationale for selective application. *J Trauma.* 1993;34:323.

53. King BR, Wagner DK. Emergency thoracotomy. In: Henretig FM, King CC, eds. *Textbook of*

*Pediatric Emergency Procedures*. Baltimore, Md: Williams & Wilkins; 1997:415–427.

54. Reeves SD. Pericardiocentesis. In: Henretig FM, King CC, eds. *Textbook of Pediatric Emergency Procedures*. Baltimore, Md: Williams & Wilkins; 1997:777–782.

55. Klasner AE, Luke DA, Scalzo AJ. Pediatric orogastric and nasogastric tubes: a new formula evaluated. *Ann Emerg Med.* 2002;39:268.

56. Simon HK, Lewander W. Gastric intubation. In: Henretig FM, King CC, eds. *Textbook of Pediatric Emergency Procedures*. Baltimore, Md: Williams & Wilkins; 1997:909–914.

57. Boenning DA, Henretig FM. Bladder Catheterization. In: Henretig FM, King CC, eds. *Textbook of Pediatric Emergency Procedures*. Baltimore, Md: Williams & Wilkins; 1997: 991–998.

58. Allen MJ, Stirling AJ, Crawshaw CV, Barnes MR. Intracompartmental pressure monitoring of leg injuries. *J Bone Joint Surg.* 1985;67-B:53.

59. Mubarak SJ, Hargens AR, Owen CA et al. The wick catheter technique for measurement of intramuscular pressure. *J Bone Joint Surg.* 1976; 58-A:1016.

60. Freedman SH, King BR. Approach to fractures with neurovascular compromise. In: Henretig FM, King CC, eds. *Textbook of Pediatric Emergency Procedures*. Baltimore, Md: Williams & Wilkins; 1997:1105–1121.

61. Uliasz A, Ishida JT, Fleming JK, Yamamoto LG. Comparing the methods of measuring compartment pressures in acute compartment syndrome. *Am J Emerg Med.* 2003 Mar;21(2):143–145.

62. Young GM. Reduction of common joint dislocations and subluxations. In: Henretig FM, King CC, eds. *Textbook of Pediatric Emergency Procedures*. Baltimore, Md: Williams & Wilkins; 1997:1075–1100.

63. Klig JE. Splinting procedures. In: Henretig FM, King CC, eds. *Textbook of Pediatric Emergency Procedures*. Baltimore, Md: Williams & Wilkins; 1997:1025–1038.

# Check Your Knowledge Answers

## Chapter 1: Preparedness for Pediatric Emergencies

1. **D**, A Level II triage, and requires immediate medical attention. Based on the Canadian Triage and Acuity Scale, young children who present with high fevers are at risk for a serious infection. They require immediate attention.

2. **A**, Involves both décor and safety- proofing the room. The décor is important to children. Use soft colors and appropriate decorations. In addition, the room must be safe; include safety plugs, and all equipment or supplies should be out of reach of a child.

3. **D**, None of the above. Surveys have shown gaps in all areas of pediatric preparedness in US hospitals.

4. **D**, Most children are transported by caregivers to the ED.

## Chapter 2: Pediatric Assessment

1. **C**, Heart rate. Although heart rate is important, it is not a part of the Pediatric Assessment Triangle. The components of the Pediatric Assessment Triangle include appearance, work of breathing, and circulation to the skin.

2. **A**, Appearance and circulation. Abnormalities in appearance and work of breathing would indicate respiratory distress. Abnormalities in circulation alone could indicate compensated shock, as would occur with diarrhea. However, the combination of abnormalities in appearance and circulation to skin could indicate decompensated shock, as could occur with severe gastroenteritis or a multisystem blunt injury.

3. **D**, Work of breathing. Work of breathing is not an indicator of compensated or decompensated shock. A child in shock might not interact normally with his environment due to poor brain perfusion. Quality of pulses is a good measure of peripheral circulation and shock. Effortless tachypnea and hyperpnea occur in shock as a way of compensating for metabolic acidosis.

4. **C**, Offer distractions. A 6 to 12-month-old infant is socially interactive, yet has stranger and separation anxiety. Keeping the infant with his parent, getting down to his level, and offering a distraction such as a penlight, will make the assessment easier. In addition, working from toe to head will not be as threatening to the child.

## Chapter 3: The Pediatric Airway in Health and Disease

1. **A**, High-risk groups for severe bronchiolitis include infants with congenital heart disease and bronchopulmonary dysplasia. Respiratory syncytial virus (RSV) is the most common pathogen causing bronchiolitis. Initial RSV infections are usually more symptomatic. Most children have been infected with RSV by their second birthday. Infants with congenital heart disease and chronic lung disease are at increased risk for severe disease. Corticosteroids can reduce duration of symptoms but have not been shown to reduce admission rates.

2. **B**, Humidified oxygen. In a child with moderate to severe croup, racemic epinephrine or L-epinephrine and dexamethasone have shown benefit in outcomes and should be administered early in the treatment course. Humidified oxygen has a theoretical benefit, but

randomized trials have not shown improvement in patient outcomes.

**3.A**, Bronchoscopy is the gold standard for diagnosis and treatment of FB aspiration. Bronchoscopy is nearly 100% successful in the diagnosis and treatment of airway FB. The most commonly aspirated items are food items, with peanuts being the most common. Physical examination is often normal in these patients and should not lower the index of suspicion for FB aspiration. The most common sites of obstruction are in the lower airways. Plain radiographs are normal in approximately one quarter of children with airway FB. Most FBs are not radio–opaque.

**4.C**, Infants and children are more likely to experience oxygen desaturation. Infants and young children are more susceptible to air swallowing and emesis due to crying, diaphragmatic breathing, and a short esophagus. Infants are more likely to develop bradycardia and oxygen desaturation and have increased rates of oxygen consumption, lower lung compliance, and diminished functional residual capacity. Rapid sequence intubation for critically ill infants is a common procedure that is well tolerated.

## Chapter 4: Cardiovascular System

**1.B**, Ductus arteriosus. The ductus arteriosus closes in response to the decrease in pulmonary artery pressure and the reversal of flow through the ductus that begins the closure process. Because the newborn no longer requires flow through the ductus, it is a perinatal developmental change that results in increased flow through an infant's lungs ("right side").

**2.B**, Tetralogy of Fallot. The cyanotic congenital heart lesions are the five T's

(transposition of the great vessels, tetralogy of Fallot, truncus arteriosus, tricuspid atresia, and total anomalous pulmonary venous return) as well as severe aortic stenosis and hypoplastic left heart. Ventricular septal defect is the most common structural congenital heart condition (noncyanotic unless associated with other cardiac malformations).

**3.D**, Prostaglandin $E_1$. Prostaglandin $E_1$ will help reverse closure of the ductus arteriosus when the CHF is secondary to the need for the shunt. It can be a lifesaving maneuver until the definitive surgical correction or extracorporeal membrane oxygenation (ECMO) is performed.

**4.C**, Erythema marginatum. The major criteria for ARF include: arthritis, carditis, chorea, and erythema marginatum (rash) and subcutaneous nodules.

## Chapter 5: Central Nervous System

**1.C**, Serum glucose. Many perfumes contain significant quantities of alcohol and can therefore cause hypoglycemia. A bedside glucose is indicated. The other laboratory studies will not provide any additional information. The only other test that might be useful is a blood alcohol level.

**2.D**, Mild hyperventilation. Mild hyperventilation causes immediate vasoconstriction of blood vessels and thus can lower intracranial pressure (ICP). While steroids are helpful with mass lesions, they do not act quickly. Midline positioning of the neck facilitates venous drainage and is simply a preventive measure. Hyperoxygenation has not been shown to lower ICP.

**3.A**, Acute renal failure. Bacterial meningitis has been associated with syndrome of inappropriate secretion of antidiuretic hormone (SIADH), seizures, and subdural effusions. Clinicians must be wary of these potential complications. No association between bacterial meningitis and acute renal failure has been described.

4. **C**, Fever greater than 40°C. Criteria needed to classify a seizure as a simple febrile one include age between 6 months and 5 years, generalized seizure lasting less than 15 minutes, and no neurologic deficit on evaluation. The seizure must be associated with a fever, but no specific fever threshold is defined.

## Chapter 6: Metabolic Disease

1. **B**, High serum glucose concentration at presentation. Recent studies have demonstrated that the risk of cerebral edema in diabetic ketoacidosis (DKA) is increased in children with higher initial blood urea nitrogen (BUN) concentrations, lower initial $PCO_2$ levels, smaller increases in measured serum sodium concentration during treatment of DKA, and treatment with bicarbonate. The initial glucose concentration was not associated with risk for cerebral edema, after adjusting for other variables.

2. **A**, Acanthosis nigricans. Ambiguous genitalia and hyperpigmentation are findings seen in congenital adrenal hyperplasia and primary adrenal insufficiency. Midline facial defects and microphallus might be seen in patients with hypopituitarism and secondary adrenal insufficiency. Acanthosis nigricans is a dermatologic finding associated with increased risk for type 2 diabetes.

3. **D**, Fluid restriction unless the patient is seizing or severely lethargic/comatose. Fluid restriction alone is the treatment of choice for syndrome of inappropriate secretion of antidiuretic hormone (SIADH) unless the patient has seizures or is extremely lethargic or comatose. Oral sodium or normal saline infusion will not be effective. Rapid correction of hyponatremia in the absence of neurologic signs should be avoided because of the risk of central pontine myelinolysis. Hydrocortisone is used to treat adrenal insufficiency.

4. **C**, Rare in older children with diabetes insipidus (DI) and normal thirst mechanisms. Older children with DI and a normal thirst mechanism generally will maintain the serum sodium concentration in the normal range by consuming large quantities of fluids. Hypernatremia is more commonly a feature of DI in infants. Symptomatic children with hyponatremia (not hypernatremia) might require treatment with 3% saline solution.

## Chapter 7: Environmental Emergencies

1. **B**, Heat exhaustion. This child's symptoms are consistent with heat exhaustion. Heat cramps are manifested by severe cramps of heavily exercised muscles occurring after exercise. Usually, patients with heat cramps have been drinking large amounts of hypotonic fluids. Heat syncope is exhibited by syncopal episodes, which this child did not have. Patients with heat stroke usually have core temperature greater than 41°C and altered mental status. Often these children have an absence of sweating, though sweating might be present.

2. **C**, Start an IV of normal saline at 20 mL/Kg and obtain a CBC, electrolytes, BUN, and creatinine. The management of heat exhaustion includes placing the patient in a cool environment, starting fluids with normal saline to treat dehydration, and obtaining a panel of laboratory studies. Antipyretics are ineffective in patients

with heat stroke and heat exhaustion. The use of ice water enemas or placing the patient in a tub of ice water can be appropriate therapies for management of heat stroke but are not needed in this case.

**3.D**, Warmed oxygen by tracheal tube plus IV fluids heated to 40°C. The protection of the child's airway is warranted in this case, requiring intubation. However, warmed humidified $O_2$ alone is not the most effective way of increasing this child's core temperature. Warm blankets plus heat lamps are useful only for the mildest cases of hypothermia. Forced air rewarming devices have been effective in similar cases; however, they are not widely available and would not provide airway protection.

**4.C**, Signs of neurologic involvement. Paresthesia, weakness, diplopia, and bulbar signs are seen with coral snake envenomation. Pain and edema are minimal with coral snake envenomations but might not be present in "dry bites" of pit vipers. Unlike pit vipers, antivenin is recommended for any patient with documented coral snake bite because it is more difficult to monitor the progression of signs and symptoms.

## Chapter 8: Toxicological Emergencies

**1.A**, Ferrous sulfate. Iron ions are too small to be absorbed by activated charcoal. All other options are well absorbed and bound by charcoal and might benefit from multidose regimens.

**2.C**, Isopropanol. Although isopropanol can cause an elevated osmolar gap, it typically causes a state of respiratory alkalosis rather than an elevated anion gap metabolic acidosis. All of the other ingestions cause metabolic acidosis and an elevated anion gap.

**3.B**, Flumazenil. The benzodiazepine antagonist flumazenil should not be administered in poisoned, comatose patients with an unclear etiology because its administration can induce seizure activity in mixed drug ingestions (e.g., TCAs) or induce life-threatening benzodiazepine withdrawal in chronic users. However, in the comatose child with a documented acute benzodiazepine overdose, this is an effective antidote and might prevent the child from requiring emergent intubation and subsequent ventilatory support.

**4.B**, 60 to 90 minutes. In room air, the half-life of carbon monoxide is approximately 4 hours (240 minutes). On 100% oxygen, it is 60 to 90 minutes. Only in hyperbaric conditions with oxygen does it decrease to 15 to 30 minutes.

## Chapter 9: Trauma

**1.C**, Most commonly due to respiratory failure and shock. Secondary brain injury refers to a further insult to the traumatically injured brain as a result of an ongoing physiologic abnormality. The most common causes of secondary brain injury are failure to recognize and treat respiratory failure and shock. The consequences of secondary brain injury are similar to primary brain injury, and the degree of secondary brain injury is temporally related to the time when appropriate resuscitation is instituted rather than a specific time frame such as 6 hours. Because children have an exaggerated cerebrovascular response to injury compared with adults, secondary brain injury is a preeminent cause of morbidity and mortality.

**2.D**, Rapid sequence intubation using sedation and paralysis after preoxygenation. This child has obvious evidence of traumatic brain injury and requires effective airway control with rapid sequence intubation (RSI). RSI with appropriate sedation and use of lidocaine will facilitate intubation, reduce adrenergic response to intubation, and reduce intracranial pressure caused by intubation. Direct oral intubation would be too traumatic and would probably raise intracerebral pressure. Nasotracheal intubation is not appropriate for children because of the acute angle of the posterior nasopharynx. The other options are not adequate therapy.

**3. C**, 35 torr. The ideal level of ventilation is about 35 torr. This provides effective ventilation and allows rescue hyperventilation if such is required. $PaCO_2$ levels below 25 torr induce ischemia from inappropriate vasospasm in the face of attenuated autoregulation. Levels above 40 torr will result in vasodilatation and increase in intracranial pressure. Recent reports suggest that hyperventilation effectively treats increased intracranial hypertension; however, it can induce ischemia in areas of injured neurons, the so-called penumbra of injury.

**4. E**, All of the above. Only the surgeon can make the decision to operate or observe. Any child with a suspicion of intra-abdominal injury must be evaluated by an appropriately trained and credentialed surgeon.

## Chapter 10: Child Maltreatment

**1. D**, All of the above. All of the scenarios presented should raise concern that the injury was intentionally inflicted. Often a child with a major injury presents with a history of some minor mishap, or the child's injuries are attributed to a young sibling who is incapable of inducing the trauma. Alternatively, the child is alleged to have sustained the injury doing some activity that the child is developmentally incapable of doing. In each of these cases, the health care provider must be concerned that the child is the victim of inflicted trauma.

**2. A**, Abusive head injury. Head injuries remain the major cause of death from inflicted trauma. Hemorrhage, cerebral edema, and diffuse axonal injury are the physiologic changes responsible for the fatal outcome.

**3. C**, Skeletal dysplasia. Infants with environmental failure to thrive have growth impairment related to impaired nurturing (impaired mother-infant relationship and interactions), and disturbed social skills manifested by findings such as a watchful, wary gaze and poor eye contact. The presence of skeletal dysplasia suggests a potential medical etiology for growth impairment.

**4. B**, Mother who administers ipecac to her healthy child and complains about intractable vomiting. Munchausen syndrome by proxy (MSBP) occurs when a parent lies about, fabricates, or induces illness in a child. Administration of ipecac to induce vomiting represents MSBP. Parental refusal to provide lifesaving health care can represent a form of medical neglect. The use of complementary and/or alternative medicines is widely practiced and, in some cases, provides some benefits.

## Chapter 11: Nontraumatic Surgical Emergencies

**1. C**, Necrotizing enterocolitis. The only listed condition typically associated with both rectal bleeding and abdominal distention is necrotizing enterocolitis.

**2. C**, Nuclear medicine scan. Pneumatosis intestinalis and intrahepatic air can be seen on plain film radiographs. Sonographic visualization of portal circulation air bubbles is typical of necrotizing enterocolitis (NEC). MRI and CT are also capable of visualizing pneumatosis intestinalis and intrahepatic air.

3.**D**, Midgut volvulus. Midgut volvulus is the most serious acute complication. If the midgut volvulus is not surgically relieved soon, an extensive bowel infarction results.

4.**D**, Roughly half or more than half of the cases of appendicitis present in a nontypical manner. Younger children such as infants are even more likely to present with nonspecific symptoms and signs of appendicitis. Ultrasonography is dependent on the skill of the individual performing the procedure but can be highly accurate in experienced hands. Discharge sheets for any patient with abdominal pain should outline signs and symptoms that are of concern and require further evaluation.

## Chapter 12: Nontraumatic Orthopedic Emergencies

1.**A**, Can be bilateral. Legg-Calvé-Perthes disease is bilateral in up to 10% of children. It affects children between 4 and 9 years old and tends to affect smaller children. There are multiple radiographic findings, depending on the stage of disease.

2.**C**, Often presents as knee pain. Slipped capital femoral epiphysis can present as hip, thigh, groin, or knee pain. The physician must examine the hips of any child presenting with knee pain, as hip pain can be referred to the knee. The femoral head slips posterior and inferior relative to the femoral neck. Slipped capital femoral epiphysis presents in the early teen years and is treated surgically.

3.**D**, Treated with joint drainage and intravenous antibiotics. It most commonly presents in children younger than 4 years. Pathogens vary by age, but *N meningitidis* is not a common cause. Synovial cultures are positive in approximately 50% of cases.

4.**B**, Have increased pain when they squat with the knee in full flexion. Children with Osgood-Schlatter disease can reproduce the pain while squatting with knees in full flexion. They tend to be physically active in sports that require repeated contraction of the quadriceps. There is swelling over the tibial tubercle but no knee effusion.

## Chapter 13: Medical Emergencies

1.**C**, Parvovirus B19. Parvovirus B19 has been associated with aplastic crises in patients with sickle cell disease. Encapsulated organisms are a common source of infection due to the relative asplenia seen in sickle cell patients. *Salmonella* can lead to osteomyelitis.

2.**D**, Relief of pain with scrotal elevation (Prehn sign) is reliable in differentiating between testicular torsion and epididymitis. Prehn sign is unreliable in differentiating between testicular torsion and epididymitis and should not be the deciding factor for obtaining an urologic consultation or testicular scan. Significant scrotal swelling can be present in both acute testicular torsion and epididymitis, and up to 50% of patients can have a normal urinalysis with epididymitis. A urethral discharge should raise the suspicion for a sexually transmitted disease, and the patient should be treated for both gonorrhea and chlamydia infections.

3.**D**, Obtain a blood culture, give an intravenous normal saline bolus and intravenous antibiotics. Lethargy, tachycardia, tachypnea, and poor peripheral perfusion are classic signs of shock. The etiology of shock in this child is most likely hypovolemic (history of vomiting) or septic (febrile). After evaluation of the ABCs, the next priority is to treat for suspected hypovolemia (with an intravenous normal saline bolus) and sepsis (with intravenous antibiotics). If possible, it is helpful to obtain a blood culture prior to antibiotic therapy. The lumbar puncture should be deferred until the child is clinically stable.

4. **D**, Vasovagal. This child most likely had vasovagal syncope as a result of prolonged standing on a hot summer day. There were no associated symptoms, and the physical examination was unremarkable. A seizure is usually associated with tonic-clonic movements and incontinence and might have a postictal state. Although dysrhythmia is a possibility, the lack of warning signs (palpitations, tachycardia, chest pain), quick recovery, and normal exam make it an unlikely etiology. Breath-holding spells are usually seen in children younger than 4 years and have a clear history.

## Chapter 14: Neonatal Emergencies

1. **C**, Dry the infant while suctioning the airway. Although moving quickly to bag-mask ventilation is appropriate, in the newly born a brief time should be taken to ensure the airway is patent by suctioning any mucus present from the delivery.

2. **A**, A full sepsis evaluation and admit. Fever in the first few weeks of life in an infant with any abnormal physical examination findings should be considered caused by sepsis until proved otherwise. The differential diagnosis also includes metabolic disease, child maltreatment, hypoxia, and hypoglycemia.

3. **A**, Do you abuse alcohol? The other questions are important to evaluate potential need for newborn resuscitation and to prepare ED resources for delivery. Although maternal alcohol use can have teratogenic effects on the fetus, it is not directly associated with depression of the newborn at the time of delivery. Twins often are delivered prematurely, and the ED must prepare to receive two infants. The due date is important to determine if a premature newborn will be delivered. Prematurity increases the risk of delivering a newborn requiring resuscitation. Finally, color of amniotic fluid helps to determine if meconium has passed into the fluid, which if present, will increase the likelihood for resuscitation.

4. **A**, Begin bag-mask ventilation. If the newborn does not respond to drying and warming, rapidly begin assisted ventilation with bag-mask ventilation and then assess heart rate and the need for chest compressions.

## Chapter 15: Procedural Sedation and Analgesia

1. **B**, Class II. Patients with mild systemic disease are categorized as Class II.

2. **E**, All of the above. The child described in this case would present a challenge for intravenous access. A nonintravenous method of delivery would be preferred, and all of the agents listed would be considered possible options. Because each of these choices has its own advantages and disadvantages, the correct choice in this case would depend more on individual physician preference and ED capabilities. Rectal methohexital is effective and safe and would be easy to administer in this patient, although the degree of sedation produced by this route might be more than would be warranted

for this study in this child and the child would need to be monitored more closely for respiratory depression. Oral midazolam is an option, but its variability in dosing and response might make it difficult to titrate if the initial dose is ineffective. Ketamine (IM) would be a good sedative, but the risk of its effects on intracranial pressure (ICP) is not well delineated. In this case, the infant is awake and alert with a normal neurologic exam, so it is unlikely that ketamine will have any deleterious effect on ICP. Chloral hydrate is effective and simple to administer, although its onset time and duration of action would be longer than the other drugs.

3. **D**, Return to baseline respiratory status. At the very least, a child must demonstrate baseline respiratory activity before discharge can be considered. Some children will have some residual sleepiness or lack of coordination after procedural sedation, but this is not a contraindication to discharge. No set time frame can be used for any child for procedural sedation discharge. Some agents have durations of action of under 10 minutes, while others are longer than 2 hours.

4. **A**, 14 mL. 7 mg/kg of lidocaine with epinephrine is the recommended maximum for safely infiltrating wounds. Since 1% lidocaine with epinephrine contains 10 mg/mL, the 140 mg maximum is contained in 14 mL of solution.

## Chapter 16: Interface With EMS

1. **C**, Respiratory distress. While seizures are a common reason for EMS response, this is more common in the younger age group. Respiratory distress can include obstructed airway, bronchiolitis, and asthma. These conditions can be seen in a variety of age groups and frequently result in an EMS response. While submersion, poisonings, and even rashes can result in an EMS call, they are less common than respiratory problems.

2. **D**, They require frequent refreshing of pediatric knowledge and skills. Children make up 10% of ambulance transports. Critically ill or injured children are a small fraction of this 10%. Therefore, frequent refreshing of pediatric knowledge and skills is needed to improve prehospital provider comfort with caring for these patients.

3. **D**, Manual defibrillation. An EMT-B can provide assisted ventilation, cardiac compressions, immobilization, and transport. Only those with a special certification (EMT-D) can provide defibrillation with an automated external defibrillator (AED) only (not with a manual defibrillator).

4. **D**, Providing funding for issues pertaining to EMSC. Most funding for EMSC issues comes from the federal or state governments, not individuals. Physician involvement in EMSC could include all of the other answers.

## Chapter 17: Disaster Management

1. **D**, 72 hours. Disaster relief agencies such as the Red Cross and the Federal Emergency Management Agency recommend that families and critical businesses such as hospitals be prepared to be self-sufficient for the first 72 hours following a disaster. Federal relief resources (such as the military and NDMS teams) take time to activate and mobilize. Travel into the affected area can also be difficult due to transportation system disruption. Relief resources might be available more quickly in anticipated disasters such as hurricanes, as response

teams are mobilized and staged outside of the projected impact zone before the disaster strikes.

2. **E**, All of the above. All of the factors listed can adversely influence the health and behavior of children with traditional and nontraditional special health care needs such as ventilator dependency, diabetes, dialysis, asthma, and behavioral and psychiatric disorders. Lack of power and refrigeration can affect life-support systems and monitors as well as compromise medication efficacy. Environmental allergens might be unavoidable by asthmatics and atopic children in disrupted housing. Stress and the disruption of daily routines can cause children with behavioral or psychiatric disorders to decompensate.

3. **A**, An objective triage system helps to optimize patient classification and resource allocation. An objective triage system that guides decision-making based on the physiologic state of each victim helps to eliminate emotional influences and ensure that resources are allocated to work toward the survival of the greatest number of victims, regardless of age. Triage personnel should process victims as they encounter them, rather than inefficiently skipping around looking for a particular type of patient. Children should be triaged as objectively as adults and not automatically given a higher subjective value by overtriaging them. In the mass casualty incident setting, patients of any age in full cardiopulmonary arrest have little chance of salvage; resuscitation should be attempted only if it is certain that critical resources are not being withheld from more salvageable victims.

4. **E**, All of the above. Hospital disaster plans should be risk-specific and consider incidents that occur inside the hospital as well as those that occur in the community. An explicit command structure helps to control and coordinate a hospital's response to a disaster and maintains consistency from incident to incident, despite staff turnover. Critical incident stress management, both proactive and reactive, will assist staff members in dealing with the disaster and help to sustain the efficient functioning of the hospital after a disaster.

## Chapter 18: Preparedness for Acts of Nuclear, Biological, and Chemical Terrorism

1. **D**, A severe influenza epidemic. The incubation period of infectious agents would signify a delay in presentation from point and time of exposure. However, this intentional epidemic would likely be more compressed in time, with higher morbidity and mortality, and involve an exotic disease for a given region.

2. **C**, Febrile prodrome. A nonspecific febrile prodrome with fatigue, malaise, and headache of 1 to 3 days of duration is characteristic of anthrax, plague, smallpox, and viral hemorrhagic fevers.

3. **C**, Intact sensation. Intact sensation and sensorium are distinctive features of botulism, along with the descending nature of the paralysis and prominent early bulbar dysfunction.

4. **C**, Children exposed to high doses of ionizing radiation. Children with even high-dose radiation exposure are not "radioactive" and pose no risk to health care staff unless they are additionally contaminated with radioactive residue, as from a "dirty bomb" explosion. Smallpox is extremely contagious, and even persons who were vaccinated many years before can be susceptible to infection. Pneumonic plague is highly infectious and requires droplet precautions for caregivers. Both mustard and nerve

agents are very hazardous to caregivers via secondary spread from contaminated skin and clothing, and personal protective gear must be worn until careful decontamination is accomplished.

## Chapter 19: Children With Special Health Care Needs: The Technologically Dependent Child

1. **D**, Suction tracheostomy. Assessment and management of the ABCs (airway, breathing and circulation) include first attention to the equipment such as the tracheostomy tube (e.g., suctioning to remove a mucus plug) and the ventilator (ensuring that all connections are intact and settings are correct). Then assess breathing (auscultate chest), then circulation (assess color).

2. **A**, Coca-Cola. Obstructed gastrostomy tubes can be cleared with either a proteolytic enzyme solution or Coca-Cola. Forcing fluid under higher pressure through the tube does not work. If the tube cannot be cleared by these means, it should be replaced. Pancrease, hydrogen peroxide, and ginger ale do not work.

3. **D**, A regular needle can be used to access an implanted port. Tunneled central venous catheters are placed surgically. They are inserted directly into a central vein, most commonly the subclavian, cephalic, or jugular. There are three common types: Broviac, Hickman, and Groshong. The first two are most common in children. The distal ends rest outside the chest and can have one to three ports. Implanted vascular access ports (Port-A-Cath, PAS Port, and Med-A-Ports) are also common in children. The insertion sites and method are the same as for the tunneled central venous catheters. The distal end of the catheter

consists of a reservoir covered with a self-healing rubber septum. This reservoir rests subcutaneously, and a special (Huber) needle is needed to access this line.

4. **B**, Cushing's triad. While signs and symptoms of a shunt obstruction include headache, nausea, vomiting, irritability, altered mental status, ataxia, change in vital signs, and a bulging fontanel in an infant. Late and very worrisome signs include those of the Cushing triad: bradycardia, irregular respirations, and hypertension.

## Chapter 20: Medical-Legal Considerations

1. **A**, College graduation. Nearly all college graduates are 18 years old or older, so this is not a criterion for being an emancipated minor. All the others can qualify a minor as being emancipated depending on statute (which varies between states).

2. **C**, Most parents prefer to be present. Studies have failed to demonstrate lower procedural success rates; however, these results might be confounded by other factors. Children might cry more when parents are present for the reason listed in A, but this has not been proved in any studies to date. It is clear that most parents prefer to be present, and whether this hinders or helps care for the child is not clear.

3. **E**, There is no written DNR order, but the parents communicate "do not resuscitate" orally. The circumstances in choice E clearly indicate that the parents do not want their child to be resuscitated. This should be just as valid as a paper document. All the other items are issues that make a DNR order difficult to carry out in an emergency. Resuscitation care must be started immediately to improve

the probability of success; therefore, the decision to initiate resuscitation is not afforded the luxury of time and discussion.

**4. C**, An obese boy presents to his primary care physician with limping associated with thigh and knee pain. Radiographs of his knee are ordered and are normal. An ESR and CRP looking for osteomyelitis are normal. He is given a diagnosis of a knee strain and is instructed to rest his knee. One week later, his pain worsens after walking down the stairs. He presents to the ED, radiographs of his hip demonstrate a severely slipped femoral capital epiphysis. An orthopedic surgeon is consulted, and the boy is hospitalized for bedrest, traction, and surgical pinning. He develops avascular necrosis of the femoral head and a prolonged disability. Choices A and D have good outcomes so there is not basis to sue. Choice B has a bad outcome with long-term complications, but the standard of medical care was met in which an advanced imaging study was used and a surgical consultant's clinical evaluation and judgment did not initially justify surgical intervention. Choice C has a bad outcome and an error of omission in the patient's care in that radiographs of the child's hip were not obtained during the initial evaluation.

## Chapter 21: Office-Based Emergencies

**1. A**, Can be treated in the physician's office or ED. A paronychia is an infection involving the soft tissue folds of the fingernail or toenail, not the deep tissue spaces. It is typically quite painful and can usually be treated by lifting the lateral nail fold off the nail, allowing the pus to drain, or by piercing the area of maximal swelling with an 18-gauge needle or a scalpel. Nail removal is usually not necessary. This procedure is well suited to the physician's office or ED, usually requiring only a digital block to achieve adequate anesthesia.

**2. A**, Associated with a phimotic ring of the foreskin. Paraphimosis is a urologic emergency and must be reduced to avoid prolonged pain and ischemia to the glans penis. Paraphimosis is very painful, and the need for immediate reduction precludes the luxury of always waiting for a urologist to perform the procedure. Paraphimosis begins as a mechanical problem; the glans penis is not able to fit through the phimotic section of the retracted foreskin. There is no association with febrile illness.

**3. B,** Handling the tooth by the root surface. Avulsion of a permanent tooth requires reimplantation as soon as possible; even a 30-minute delay might preclude successful reimplantation. Hold the tooth by the crown, avoiding trauma to the root surface and periodontal ligament. After reimplantation, it is important to prevent further trauma that could avulse the tooth or change its position. The use of a periodontal pack or sutures can help stabilize the tooth.

**4. E,** All of the above. Wound preparation for closure with tissue adhesive must be as meticulous as that for closure with sutures. Inadequate wound cleansing can lead to wound infection. Inadequate hemostasis can lead to hemorrhage within the wound. Sutures provide circumferential tension and facilitate hemostasis within the ligature loop. Tissue adhesive does not facilitate hemostasis. Inadequate immobilization can lead to dripping of tissue adhesive onto unintended areas, causing gluing of body parts (like eyelids) or seeping of tissue adhesive into the wound (e.g., when a wound is "glued open").

## Chapter 22: Critical Procedures

**1. D**, The impedance pneumograph measures ventilation. The impedance pneumograph measures chest wall movement and can be used as a surrogate marker for respiratory effort. It uses the external ECG leads and can be affected by patient movement. However, it does not directly measure air flow. In a patient with upper airway obstruction, the chest wall can be moving while ventilation is poor. Therefore, intermittent auscultation is important.

**2. C**, The jaw-thrust maneuver is preferred for trauma victims. Because the chin-lift maneuver involves movement of the neck, it should not be used in trauma victims. This caveat extends to those who have normal cervical spine films but cannot be assessed clinically (e.g., unconscious patients). A small number of such patients have fractures or cord injury even though their films are normal. Nasal airways can be used in patients who are either conscious or unconscious. On the other hand, only those who are unconscious can tolerate oral airways.

**3. B**, ECG changes, including ST segment changes and PVCs, suggest that the needle is in contact with the heart muscle. If performed using ECG guidance, contact with the cardiac muscle is indicated by ECG changes such as PVCs and ST segment abnormalities. The normal pericardial space contains up to 30 mL of fluid. Larger volumes of fluid may be well tolerated and do not mandate immediate pericardiocentesis. However, the presence of cardiac tamponade is an indication for immediate pericardiocentesis. Pericardiocentesis is a very invasive procedure. It has been associated with several complications, including injury to the coronary arteries and pneumothorax.

**4. E**, All of the above. Because the muscles of the forearm and lower leg are enclosed within fascial sheaths and are surrounded by bones and other muscles, significant injury to these areas can result in localized edema significant enough to compromise circulation. Unless the situation is corrected promptly, permanent ischemic injury can occur. Although the "six P's" (pain, poikilothermia, paresthesia, paresis, pulselessness, and pallor) are described as the classic signs of compartment syndrome, only pain and paresthesia occur early. Pulselessness and pallor are signs of arterial embolization. By the time pulselessness and/or pallor occurs in a compartment syndrome, irreversible infarction is likely. Significant muscle tenderness in the absence of an underlying fracture or serious contusion is another worrisome sign.

Note to reader: Page references with the letter "t" refer to tables. Page references with the letter "f" refer to figures.

# Symbols

# A